DNA REPAIR

Edited by **Inna Kruman**

DNA Repair
Edited by Inna Kruman

Published by InTech

Janeza Trdine 9, 51000 Rijeka, Croatia

Publishing Process Manager Alenka Urbancic

Technical Editor Teodora Smiljanic

Cover Designer InTech Design Team

Additional hard copies can be obtained from orders@intechopen.com

DNA Repair, Edited by Inna Kruman
p. cm.
ISBN 978-953-307-697-3

For EU product safety concerns:
IN TECH d.o.o., Prolaz Marije Krucifikse Kozulić 3, 51000 Rijeka, Croatia,
info@intechopen.com or visit our website at intechopen.com.

Meet the editor

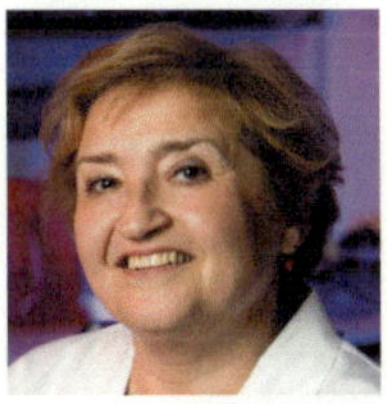

Dr. Kruman received her PhD in Cellular Biology from Moscow State University (Russia). She is an Associate Professor in the department of Pharmacology and Neuroscience, Texas Tech University Health Sciences Center, USA. Her research interests focus on mechanisms of apoptosis and DNA damage response in postmitotic neurons. She has authored over 50 scientific publications, including articles in major peer reviewed journals such as Neuron and Journal Neuroscience, book chapters and invited reviews.

Contents

Preface

The stability of the genome is of crucial importance. Every day, mammalian cells accumulate an estimated 100,000 lesions in their DNA as a result of exposure to reactive oxygen species, chemical deterioration of their bases, and exposure to exogenous agents such as ultraviolet and ionizing radiation. The cells have evolved complex response mechanisms to recognize and repair such injury in order to maintain genomic integrity. With the development of sophisticated molecular techniques, the spectrum of diseases benefitting from the research effort to understand the mechanisms of DNA damage response has grown to include virtually all fields where genotoxic stress plays a role in disease initiation, evolution, and treatment. One of the most important is cancer biology. It is becoming increasingly clear that DNA damage plays an essential role in neurodegeneration. However, the molecular mechanisms of cellular responses to DNA injury and how they influence mutagenesis and cell death remain unclear. This book reviews a number of important DNA repair-related topics.

The book consists of 31 chapters, divided into six parts. Each chapter is written by one or several experts in the corresponding area. The scope of the book ranges from the DNA damage response and DNA repair mechanisms, to evolutionary aspects of DNA repair, providing a snapshot of current understanding of DNA repair processes. A collection of articles presented by active and laboratory-based investigators gives a clear understanding of the recent advances in the field of DNA repair in various cell types, including bacteria (Davydov et al.; Wang and Maier), germ (Leduc et al.), and neurons (Kruman; Coppedè).

The first part is devoted to various aspects of DNA damage response, focusing on BRCA1 (Boutou et al.; Ratanaphan), BRCA2 (Brown), TopBP1 (Forma et al.), Rad51 (Popova et al.; Boutou et al.), DDB2 (Jones et al.; Chao) and E2F1 (Zhang and Chen; Dagnino et al.) factors, the role of cell cycle machinery in DNA damage response of postmitotic cells (Kruman), the involvement of DNA-repair proteins in centrosome maintenance (Mikio), transcriptional regulatory networks controlling DNA repair pathways (Welch et al.) and on the function of microRNA in DNA damage response (Chen and Chen).

The second part of the book deals with an evolutionary view of DNA repair, focusing on meiosis as an evolutionary adaptation for DNA Repair (Bernstein et al.) and evolution of DNA repair in plants (Vuosku et al.).

The third part discusses the mechanisms of DNA repair, particularly non-homologous end-joining (Kamdar and Matsumoto), homologous recombination (Korolev), global genome nucleotide excision repair (Sugasawa) and the gratuitous repair on undamaged DNA formed by unusual DNA structures generating genomic instability (Pan et al.).

The fourth and fifth parts cover roles of DNA repair gene mutations in carcinogenesis and neurodegeneration (Long et al.; Ankathil; Hansen and Vogel; Coppede), and the role of DNA repair machinery in telomere maintenance (Uchiumi et al., Ueno). In the last part, Dr. Azqueta and colleagues review various applications of the comet assay for quantification of DNA repair capacity, including DNA repair analysis at the level of specific genome regions.

Together, the chapters are a collection of contemporary works on DNA injury and the associated cellular response. While not every topic in the DNA damage response domain could be reviewed in the book, I do believe the authors have done an outstanding job in providing timely and relevant discussions on their respective subjects, allowing the reader to become more familiar with the field. I assume the information contained in this book underscores the significance of DNA repair in the fields of cancer research and neurodegeneration, and the need for continued investigation in this area.

The editor wishis to acknowledge Ms. Alenka Urbancic for her tireless efforts in collecting and organizing all of the manuscripts from our illustrious contributors.

Inna Kruman
Associate Professor
Department of Pharmacology and Neuroscience
Texas Tech University Health Sciences Center (TTUHSC)
Texas
USA

Part 1

DNA Damage Response

1

A Recombination Puzzle Solved: Role for New DNA Repair Systems in *Helicobacter pylori* Diversity/Persistence

Ge Wang and Robert J. Maier
Department of Microbiology, University of Georgia, Athens Georgia

1. Introduction

1.1 Helicobacter pylori pathogenesis

Helicobacter pylori is a gram-negative, slow-growing, microaerophilic, spiral bacterium. It is one of the most common human gastrointestinal pathogens, infecting almost 50% of the world's population [1]. Peptic ulcer disease is now approached as an infectious disease, and *H. pylori* is responsible for the majority of duodenal and gastric ulcers [2]. There is strong evidence that *H. pylori* infection increases the risk of gastric cancer [3], the second most frequent cause of cancer-related death. *H. pylori* infections are acquired by oral ingestion and is mainly transmitted within families in early childhood [2]. Once colonized, the host can be chronically infected for life, unless *H. pylori* is eradicated by treatment with antibiotics.

H. pylori is highly adapted to its ecologic niche, the human gastric mucosa. The pathogenesis of *H. pylori* relies on its persistence in surviving a harsh environment, including acidity, peristalsis, and attack by phagocyte cells and their released reactive oxygen species [4]. *H. pylori* has a unique array of features that permit entry into the mucus, attachment to epithelial cells, evasion of the immune response, and as a result, persistent colonization and transmission. Numerous virulence factors in *H. pylori* have been extensively studied, including urease, flagella, BabA adhesin, the vacuolating cytotoxin (VacA), and the cag pathogenicity island (cag-PAI) [5]. In addition to its clinical importance, *H. pylori* has become a model system for persistent host-associated microorganisms [6]. How *H. pylori* can adapt to, and persist in, the human stomach has become a problem of general interest in both microbial physiology and in pathogenesis areas.

1.2 Genetic diversity of *H. pylori*

H. pylori displays exceptional genetic variability and intra-species diversity [7]. Allelic diversity is obvious as almost every unrelated isolate of *H. pylori* has a unique sequence when a sequenced fragment of only several hundred base pairs is compared among strains for either housekeeping or virulence genes [8-10]. Approximately 5% nucleotide divergence is commonly observed at the majority of gene loci between pairs of unrelated *H. pylori* strains [11]. *H. pylori* strains also differ considerably in their gene contents, the genetic macro-diversity. The two sequenced strains 26695 and J99 share only 94% of their genes, whereas approximately 7% of the genes are unique for each strain [12, 13]. Supporting studies using whole-genome microarray detected numerous genomic changes in the paired sequential isolates of *H. pylori* from the same patient [14, 15].

Mechanisms proposed to account for the observed genetic variability include mainly the high inherent mutation rate and high frequency of recombination [16]. The spontaneous mutation rate of the majority of *H. pylori* strains lies between 10^{-5} and 10^{-7} [17]. This is several orders of magnitude higher than the average mutation rate of *Escherichia coli*, and similar to that of *E. coli* strains defective in mismatch repair functions (mutator strains) [18]. While mutation is essential for introducing sequence diversity into the species, a key role in generating diversity is played by recombination.

H. pylori is naturally competent for DNA transformation, and has a highly efficient system for recombination of short-fragment involving multiple recombination events within a single locus [19, 20]. A special apparatus homologous to type IV secretion system (T4SS, encoded by *comB* locus) is dedicated to a DNA uptake role [21, 22] and a composite system involving proteins at the *comB* locus and ComEC mediates two-step DNA uptake in *H. pylori* [23]. T4SS systems are known to transport DNA and proteins in other bacteria, but *H. pylori* is the only species known to use a T4SS for natural competence [24]. Unlike several other bacterial species, *H. pylori* does not require specific DNA sequences for uptake of related DNA [25]. Instead, numerous and efficient restriction modification systems take over the function as a barrier to horizontal gene transfer from foreign sources [26, 27].

Population genetic analyses of unrelated isolates of *H. pylori* indicated that recombination was extremely frequent in *H. pylori* [9, 28]. There is evidence that humans are occasionally infected with multiple genetically distinct isolates and that recombination between *H. pylori* strains can occur in humans [29, 30]. Using mathematical modeling approaches on sequence data from 24 pairs of sequential *H. pylori* isolates, Falush et al. [31] estimated that the mean size of imported fragments was only 417 bp, much shorter than that observed for other bacteria. The recombination rate per nucleotide was estimated as 6.9×10^{-5}, indicating that every pair of strains differed on average by 114 recombination events. Compared to other bacteria studied in this way [32-34], the recombination frequency within *H. pylori* is extraordinarily high. The *H. pylori* genome also has extensive repetitive DNA sequences that are targets for intragenomic recombination [35].

2. Overview of DNA repair in *H. pylori*

Oxidative DNA damage represents a major form of DNA damage. Among the many oxidized bases in DNA, 8-oxo-guanine is a ubiquitous biomarker of DNA oxidation [36]. In addition, acid (low pH) conditions may result in DNA damage via depurination [37]. *H. pylori* survives on the surface of the stomach lining for the lifetime of its host and causes a chronic inflammatory response. Several lines of evidence suggest that *H. pylori* is exposed to oxidative damage soon after infection [38, 39]. Under physiological conditions, *H. pylori* is thought to frequently suffer oxidative and acid stress [40, 41]. In addition to diverse oxidant detoxification enzymes (e.g. superoxide dismutase, catalse, and peroxiredoxins) [42] and potent acid avoidance mechanisms (mainly urease) [43], efficient DNA repair systems are required for *H. pylori* to survive in the host.

2.1 DNA repair systems in *H. pylori*

The whole genome sequences of *H. pylori* revealed it contains several DNA repair pathways that are common to many bacterial species, while it lacks other repair pathways or contains only portions of them. *H. pylori* encodes the homologues of all four members of the nucleotide excision repair (NER) pathway; these are UvrA, UvrB, UvrC, and UvrD, all of which are well conserved in bacteria. NER deals with DNA-distorting lesions, in which an excinuclease removes a 12- to 13- nucleotide segment from a single strand centered around the lesion; the resulting gap is then filled in by repair synthesis [44]. Loss of *uvrB* in *H. pylori* was shown to confer sensitivity to UV light, alkylating agents and low pH, suggesting that the *H. pylori* NER pathway is functional in repairing a diverse array of DNA lesions [45]. *H. pylori* UvrD was shown to play a role in repairing DNA damage and limiting DNA recombination, indicating it functions to ultimately maintain genome integrity [46].

The methyl-directed mismatch repair system (MMR), consisting of MutS1, MutH, and MutL, is conserved in many bacteria and eukaryotes, and it plays a major role in maintaining genetic stability. MMR can liberate up to 1000 nucleotides from one strand during its function to correct a single mismatch arising during DNA replication [47]. Notably, MMR does not exist in *H. pylori*, contributing to the high mutation rates observed in *H. pylori* [17]. *H. pylori* has a MutS homologue that belongs to the MutS2 family. *H. pylori* MutS2 was shown to bind to DNA structures mimicking recombination intermediates and to inhibit DNA strand exchange, thus it may play a role in maintaining genome integrity by suppressing homologous and homeologous DNA recombination [48]. In addition, *H. pylori* MutS2 appears to play a role in repairing oxidative DNA damage, specifically 8-oxo-guanine [49].

Damaged bases can be repaired by a variety of glycosylases that belong to the base excision repair (BER) pathway. All glycosylases can excise a damaged base resulting in an apurinic/apyrimidinic (AP) site, while some of them additionally nick the DNA deoxyribose-phosphate backbone (via an AP lyase activity). *H. pylori* harbors the glycosylase genes *ung, mutY, nth,* and *magIII,* whereas several other genes appear to be absent from the *H. pylori* genome, e.g. *tag, alkA,* and *mutM*. The *H. pylori* endonuclease III (*nth* gene product), which removes oxidized pyrimidine bases, was shown to be important in establishing long-term colonization in the host [50]. The *H. pylori* MutY glycosylase is functional in removing adenine from 8-oxoG:A mispair, and the loss of MutY leads to attenuation of the colonization ability [51-53].

To repair DNA double strand breaks and blocked replication forks, *H. pylori* is equipped with an efficient system of DNA recombinational repair, which is the main focus of this review (See section 4).

2.2 *H. pylori* response to DNA damage

Many bacteria encode a genetic program for a coordinated response to DNA damage called the SOS response. The best known *E. coli* SOS response is triggered when RecA binds ssDNA, activating its co-protease activity towards LexA, a transcriptional repressor [54]. Cleavage of LexA results in transcriptional induction of genes involved in DNA repair, low-fidelity polymerases, and cell cycle control. However, the *H. pylori* genome contains neither a gene for LexA homolog nor the genes for low-fidelity polymerases, and an SOS response pathway seems to be absent in *H. pylori* [12, 13].

To define pathways for an *H. pylori* DNA damage response, Dorer et al. [55] used cDNA based microarrays to measure transcriptional changes in cells undergoing DNA damage. In both ciprofloxacin treated cells and the Δ*addA* (a major DNA recombination gene, see section 4.4 below) mutant cells, the same set of genes were induced which include genes required for energy metabolism, membrane proteins, fatty acid biosynthesis, cell division, and some translation factors, although the contribution of these genes to survival in the face of DNA damage is not understood. No DNA repair genes, a hallmark of the SOS response, were induced in either the antibiotic-treated cells or the recombination gene deleted strain. Surprisingly, several genes involved in natural competence for DNA transformation (*com* T4SS components *comB3*, *comB4* and *comB9*) were induced significantly. Indeed, natural transformation frequency was shown to be increased under DNA damage conditions. Another DNA damage-induced gene was a lysozyme-encoding gene. Experimental evidence was provided that a DNA damage-induced lysozyme may target susceptible cells in culture and provide a source of DNA for uptake [55]. Taken together, DNA damage (mainly DSBs in their experiments) induces the capacity for taking up DNA segments from the neighboring cells of the same strain (homologous) or co-colonizing strain (homeologous) that may be used for recombinational DNA repair.

3. Mechanisms of DNA recombinational repair known in model bacteria

Although the bulk of DNA damage affects one strand of a duplex DNA segment, occasionally both DNA strands opposite each other are damaged; the latter situation necessitates recombinational repair using an intact homologous DNA sequence [56, 57]. DNA double-strand breaks (DSB) occur as a result of a variety of physical or chemical insults that modify the DNA (e.g. DNA strands cross-links). In addition, if a replication fork meets damaged bases that cannot be replicated, the fork can collapse leading to a DSB. In *E. coli*, 20-50% of replication forks require recombinational repair to overcome damage [58].

Homologous recombinational repair requires a large number of proteins that act at various stages of the process [56]. The first stage, **pre-synapsis**, is the generation of 3' single-stranded (ss) DNA ends that can then be used for annealing with the homologous sequence on the sister chromosome. In *E. coli*, the two types of two-strand lesions (double strand end and daughter strand gap) are repaired by two separate pathways, RecBCD and RecFOR, respectively [57]. The second and most crucial step in DNA recombination is the introduction of the 3' DNA overhang into the homologous duplex of the sister chromosome, termed **synapsis**. This is performed by RecA in bacteria. RecA binds to ssDNA in an ATP-dependent manner, and RecA-bound ssDNA (in a right-handed helix structure) can invade homologous duplex DNA and mediate strand annealing, accompanied by extrusion of the other strand that can pair with the remaining 5' overhang of the DSB (called D-loop formation).

During DNA recombination, the single stranded DNA (ssDNA) is always coated (protected) by ssDNA-binding protein (SSB), which has a higher affinity to ssDNA than RecA. RecA needs to be loaded (during pre-synapsis stage), either by RecBCD or RecFOR, onto the generated ssDNA that is coated with SSB. During the third step in recombination, **post-synapsis**, RecA-promoted strand transfer produces a four-stranded exchange, or Holliday junctions (HJ) [59]. The RecG and RuvAB helicases are two pathways that process the branch migration of HJ. Finally, RuvC resolves HJ in an orientation determined by RuvB, and the remaining nicks are sealed by DNA ligase.

Several other genes (recJ, recQ, recN) are also required for recombination, although their functions are unclear [60, 61]. Single stranded exonuclease RecJ and RecQ helicase are sometimes needed to enlarge the gap for RecFOR to act [62]. RecN, RecO, and RecF were found to be localized to distinct foci on the DNA in *Bacillus subtilis* cells after induction of DSBs [63]. These proteins form active repair centers at DSBs and recruit RecA, initiating homologous recombination. RecN was shown to play an important role in repairing DSBs, probably coordinating alignment of the broken segments with intact duplexes to facilitate recombination [64].

4. DNA recombinational repair factors in *H. pylori*

While some genes that are predicted to be involved in DNA recombinational repair, including *recA, recG, recJ, recR, recN, and ruvABC,* were annotated from the published *H. pylori* genome sequences, many genes coding for the components that are involved in the pre-synapsis stage, such as RecBCD, RecF, RecO, and RecQ, were missing. Considering that *H. pylori* is highly genetic diverse with a high recombination frequency, this has been a big puzzle over the past decade. Recent studies revealed the existence of both pathways, AddAB (RecBCD-like) and RecRO, for initiation of DNA recombinational repair in *H. pylori.* In the following sections we will summarize the current understanding of DNA recombinational repair in *H. pylori* by reviewing the literature accumulated in recent years.

4.1 The central recombination protein RecA

The RecA protein is a central component of the homologous recombination machinery and of the SOS system in most bacteria. The relatively small RecA protein contains many functional domains including different DNA-binding sites and an ATP-binding site. *E. coli* RecA has also coprotease activities for the LexA repressor and other factors involved in SOS response. However, *H. pylori* genome does not contain a LexA homolog and an SOS response pathway is likewise absent in *H. pylori.* Thus, a coprotease activity may be dispensable for the *H. pylori* RecA protein. Nevertheless, RecA is required for DNA damage response observed in *H. pylori,* although the underlying mechanism is unclear [55].

Before the genome era, the roles of *H. pylori* RecA in DNA recombination and repair have been studied genetically [65, 66]. *H. pylori* RecA (37.6 kDa protein) is highly similar to known bacterial RecA proteins. The *H. pylori* recA mutants were severely impaired in their ability to survive treatment with DNA damaging agents such as UV light, methyl methanesulfonate, ciprofloxacin, and metronidazole. *H. pylori* RecA also played a role in survival at low pH in a mechanism distinct from that mediated by urease [66]. Disruption of *recA* in *H. pylori* abolished general homologous recombination [65]. Interestingly, *H. pylori* RecA protein is subject to posttranslational modifications that result in a slight shift in its electrophoretic mobility [67]. One putative mechanism for RecA modification is protein glycosylation. *H. pylori* RecA protein was shown to be membrane associated, but this association is not dependent on the posttranslational modification. The RecA modification is required for full activity of DNA repair [67].

In recent years, the phenotypes of *H. pylori recA* mutants have been further characterized in comparison with other mutants. Among the mutants of DNA recombination and repair genes, *recA* mutants displayed the most severe phenotypes. For example, *recA* mutants were much more sensitive to UV or Gamma radiation than the *recB* or *recO* single mutants, and were similar to the *recBO* double mutant [68-70]. The *recA* mutants completely lost the ability to undergo natural transformation [68-70]. The intra-genomic recombination frequency of the *recA* mutant was also much lower than that of the *recR* or *recB* single mutants [68, 71]. Finally, the *recA* mutants completely lost the ability to colonize mouse stomachs [69]. In competition experiments (mixed infection with wild type and mutant strains), *recA* mutant bacteria were never recovered, while some *addA* or *addB* mutant bacteria were recovered from mouse stomachs.

4.2 Post-synapsis proteins RuvABC and RecG

In addition to the synapsis protein RecA, the genes for post-synapsis proteins (RuvABC and RecG) are also well conserved among bacteria [72]. Genes for RuvABC proteins are present in *H. pylori*, thus *H. pylori* seems to be able to restore Holliday Junctions in a similar way to *E. coli*. RuvC is a Holliday junction endonuclease that resolves recombinant joints into nicked duplex products. A *ruvC* mutant of *H. pylori* was more sensitive (compared to the wild type) to oxidative stress and other DNA damaging agents including UV light, mitomycin C, levofloxacin and metronidazole [73]. As Macrophage cells are known to produce an oxidative burst to kill bacterial pathogens, the survival of *H. pylori ruvC* mutant within macrophages was shown to be 100-fold lower than that of the wild type strain [73]. Furthermore, mouse model experiments revealed that the 50% infective dose of the *ruvC* mutant was approximately 100-fold higher than that of the wild-type strain. Although the *ruvC* mutant was able to establish colonization at early time points, infection was spontaneously cleared from the murine gastric mucosa over long periods (36 to 67 days) [73]. This was the first experimental evidence that DNA recombination processes are important for establishing and maintaining long-term *H. pylori* infection. Further studies suggested that RuvC function and, by inference, recombination facilitate bacterial immune evasion by altering the adaptive immune response [74], although the underlying mechanisms remain obscure.

RuvAB proteins are involved in the branch migration of Holliday junctions. The annotated *H. pylori* RuvB (HP1059) showed extensive homology (52% sequence identity) to *E. coli* RuvB, particularly within the helicase domains. However, unlike in *E. coli*, *ruvA*, *ruvB*, and *ruvC* are located in separate regions of the *H. pylori* chromosome, which may predict possible functional differences. In contrast to *E. coli ruvB* mutants, which have moderate susceptibility to DNA damage, the *H. pylori ruvB* mutant has intense susceptibility to UV, similar to that of a *recA* mutant [75]. Similarly, the *H. pylori ruvB* mutant has a significantly diminished MIC (minimal inhibitory concentration) for ciprofloxacin, an agent that blocks DNA replication fork progression, to the same extent as the *recA* mutant. In agreement with these repair phenotypes, the *ruvB* mutant has almost completely lost the ability of natural transformation of exogenous DNA (frequency of $<10^{-8}$), similar to the *recA* mutant. In an assay measuring the intra-genomic recombination (deletion frequency between direct repeats), the *ruvB* mutants displayed significantly (four- to sevenfold) lower deletion frequencies than the background level. All four phenotypes of the *ruvB* mutant suggested that *H. pylori* RuvAB is the predominant pathway for branch migration in DNA recombinational repair [75].

In *E. coli*, an alternative pathway processing branch migration of Holliday junctions is the RecG helicase. In marked contrast to *E. coli*, *H. pylori recG* mutants do not have defective DNA repair, as measured by UV-light sensitivity and ciprofloxacin susceptibility [76]. Furthermore, *H. pylori recG* mutants have increased frequencies of intergenomic recombination and deletion, suggesting that branch migration and Holliday junction resolution are more efficient in the absence of RecG function [75, 76]. Thus, the effect of *H. pylori* RecG seems to be opposite to that of the RuvAB helicase. In the RuvABC pathway, the RuvC endonuclease nicks DNA, catalyzing Holliday junction resolution into double-stranded DNA. Although the resolvase in the RecG pathway has not been completely elucidated, it has been hypothesized that RusA may serve this function in *E. coli* [77]. By introducing *E. coli rusA* into *H. pylori ruvB* mutants, the wild-type phenotypes for DNA repair and recombination were restored [75]. A hypothesis was proposed that RecG competes with RuvABC for DNA substrates but initiates an incomplete repair pathway (due to the absence of the RecG resolvase RusA) in *H. pylori*, interfering with the RuvABC repair pathway [75].

4.3 *H. pylori* RecN

Bacterial RecN is related to the SMC (structure maintenance of chromosome) family of proteins in eukaryotes, which are key players in a variety of chromosome dynamics, from chromosome condensation and cohesion to transcriptional repression and DNA repair [78]. SMC family proteins have a structural characteristic of an extensive coiled-coil domain located between globular domains at the N- and C-termini that bring together Walker A and B motifs associated with ATP-binding [79]. *E. coli* RecN is strongly induced during the SOS response and was shown to be involved in RecA-mediated recombinational repair of DSBs [64]. In *Bacillus subtilis*, RecN was shown to be recruited to DSBs at an early time point during repair [63, 80, 81]. In vitro, RecN was shown to bind and protect 3' ssDNA ends in the presence of ATP [82].

In the published *H. pylori* genome sequence [12], HP1393 was annotated as a *recN* gene homolog. The *H. pylori recN* mutant is much more sensitive to mitomycin C, an agent that predominantly causes DNA DSBs, indicating RecN plays an important role in DSB repair in *H. pylori* [83]. In normal laboratory growth conditions, an *H. pylori recN* mutant does not show a growth defect, but its survival is greatly reduced under oxidative stress which resembles the *in vivo* stress condition. While very little fragmented DNA was observed in either wild type or *recN* mutant strain when cells were cultured under normal microaerobic conditions; after oxidative stress treatment the *recN* mutant cells had a significantly higher proportion of the DNA as fragmented DNA than did the wild type [83]. Similar roles of RecN in protection against oxidative damage have been demonstrated in *Neisseria gonorrhoeae* [84, 85]. In addition, the *H. pylori recN* mutant is much more sensitive to low pH than the wild type strain, suggesting that RecN is also involved in repair of acid-induced DNA damage [83]. This could be relevant to its physiological condition, as *H. pylori* appears to colonize an acidic niche on the gastric surface [41].

As mentioned in the sections above, loss of *H. pylori* RecA, RuvB or RuvC functions results in a great decrease of DNA recombination frequency. Similarly, the *H. pylori recN* mutant has a significant decrease of DNA recombination frequency, suggesting that RecN is a critical factor in DNA recombinational repair [83]. In contrast, loss of UvrD or MutS2 in *H. pylori* resulted in an increase of DNA recombination frequency [46, 48]. Suppression of DNA recombination by UvrD or MutS2, and facilitation of DNA recombination by RecN, may play a role in coordinating DNA repair pathways. Recombinational repair could be mutagenic due to homeologous recombination or cause rearrangement due to recombination with direct repeat sequences. In addition, recombinational repair systems are much more complex and require more energy to operate, compared to nucleotide excision repair (NER) and base excision repair (BER) systems. Thus UvrD, as a component of NER, and MutS2 as a likely component of a BER (8-oxoG glycosylase) system [49], both suppress DNA recombination. Both NER and BER systems would be expected to continuously function in low stress conditions. Under a severe stress condition when large amounts of

DSBs are formed, RecN perhaps recognizes DSBs and recruits proteins required for initiation of DNA recombination.

The role of *H. pylori* RecN *in vivo* has been demonstrated, as the *recN*-disrupted *H. pylori* cells are less able to colonize hosts than wild type cells [83]. However, the mouse colonization phenotype of the *recN* strain seems to be less severe than those observed for the *recA* or *ruvC* mutants. In contrast to RecA or RuvC which are major components of DNA recombination machinery, RecN is a protein specific for repairing DSBs by linking DSB recognition and DNA recombination initiation. It was proposed that the attenuated ability to colonize mouse stomachs by *recN* cells was mainly due to the strain's failure to repair DSBs through a DNA recombinational repair pathway.

4.4 AddAB helicase-nuclease

DNA helicases play key roles in many cellular processes by promoting unwinding of the DNA double helix [86]. Bacterial genomes encode a set of helicases of the DExx family that fulfill several, sometimes overlapping functions. Based on the sequence homology, bacterial RecB, UvrD, Rep, and PcrA were classified as superfamily I (SF1) helicases [86-88]. In the well-studied *E. coli*, RecBCD form a multi-functional enzyme complex that processes DNA ends resulting from a double-strand break. RecBCD is a bipolar helicase that splits the duplex into its component strands and digests them until encountering a recombinational hotspot (Chi site). The nuclease activity is then attenuated and RecBCD loads RecA onto the 3' tail of the DNA [89]. Another bacterial enzyme complex AddAB, extensively studied in *Bacillus subtilis*, has both nuclease and helicase activities similar to those of RecBCD enzyme [90, 91].

The genes for RecBCD or AddAB were missing in the published *H. pylori* genome [12, 13]. However, HP1553 from strain 26695 was annotated as a gene encoding a putative helicase [12], and the corresponding gene from strain J99 was annotated as *pcrA* [13]. Amino acid sequence alignment of HP1553 to *E. coli* RecB (or to *B. subtilis* AddA) revealed 24% identity (to both heterologous systems) at the N-terminal half (helicase domain), and no significant homology at the C-terminal half (including nuclease domain). Thus, HP1553 could be a RecB (or AddA)-like helicase [69, 92]. Furthermore, by using the highly conserved AddB nuclease motif "GRIDRID" in BLAST search, HP1089 was identified as the putative AddB homolog [69]. Now it is accepted that HP1553 and HP1089 are termed *addA* and *addB* respectively in *H. pylori* with a reminder that previous *recB* [20, 68, 70, 92] was the equivalent of *addA* [69, 71, 93]. Both genes *addA* and *addB* are present in 56 *H. pylori* clinical isolates from around the world [94]; thus they are considered core genes that are not strain variable.

The biochemical activities of *H. pylori* AddAB helicase-nuclease have been demonstrated [69]. Cytosolic extracts from wild-type *H. pylori* showed detectable ATP-dependent nuclease activity with ds DNA substrate, while the *addA* and *addB* mutants lack this activity. Cloned *H. pylori addA* and *addB* genes express ATP-dependent exonuclease in *E. coli* cells. These genes also conferred ATP-dependent DNA unwinding (helicase) activity to an *E. coli recBCD* deletion mutant, indicating that they are the structural genes for this enzyme [69]. The roles of individual (helicase, exonuclease) activity of the AddA and AddB in DNA repair, recombination, and mouse infection have been further studied by site-directed mutagenesis approach [93].

H. pylori addA and *addB* mutant strains showed heightened sensitivity to mitomycin C and the DNA gyrase inhibitor ciprofloxacin, both of which lead to DNA ds breaks [69, 92]. The level of sensitivity was similar to that seen for a *recA* mutant, but more severe than for the *recN* mutant. It is thus concluded that AddAB plays a major role in the repair of DNA ds breaks [69, 92]. On the other hand, the *addA* and *addB* mutants were markedly less sensitive to UV irradiation than a *recA* mutant, suggesting that AddAB does not play a major role in repair of UV damage in *H. pylori* [69]. AddA was shown to be important for *H. pylori* protection against oxidative stress-induced damage, as the *addA* mutant cells were significantly more sensitive to oxidative stress and contained a large amount of fragmented DNA [92]. Furthermore, loss of AddA resulted in reduced frequencies of apparent gene conversion between homologous genes encoding outer membrane proteins (*babA* to *babB*) [69]. Finally, it was shown that the *addA* and *addB* mutant strains display a significantly attenuated ability to colonize mouse stomachs, in both competition experiments and during single-strain infections [69, 92].

While *addA* and *addB* are adjacent in the chromosome in most bacteria, including other epsilon Proteobacteria, this is not the case in *H. pylori*. However, the phenotypes of *H. pylori addA* and *addB* mutants are indistinguishable. Thus, it was proposed [69] that the AddA and AddB act together in a complex, as do the RecBCD polypeptides and AddAB polypeptides of other bacteria. If so, the control of the unlinked *H. pylori addA* and *addB* genes to maintain the proper stoichiometry of the two polypeptides remains an interesting question.

Regarding the role of *H. pylori* AddA in DNA recombination during natural transformation, conflicting results were reported from different studies. The *addA* (note: it was named *recB* in certain references) mutant showed enhanced [68, 70], decreased [20, 71, 92], or no change [27, 69] in transformation frequency. Indeed, a high degree of variability (>100-fold) in transformation frequency in *H. pylori* was observed between different strains and different experiments. The use of different assay systems may partly explain the discrepancy in transformation results. For example, the total genomic DNA from antibiotic-resistant strain was used for the transformation assay in certain studies, while in others the defined linear DNA fragments of small size [92]. Use of the transformation frequency as an indicator of DNA recombination frequency is based on the assumption that the wild type *H. pylori* and its isogenic *rec* strains are equally competent for DNA uptake. However, it is now known that this assumption is not valid because DNA damage triggers genetic exchange in *H. pylori* [55]. *H. pylori addA* mutant cells suffered more DNA damage [92], and have an enhanced competence for DNA uptake [55]. Thus, the accumulation of unrepaired DNA damage and subsequent poor growth, as well as unknown strain differences, could be the main cause of the high degree of variability in *H. pylori* transformation frequency [27].

4.5 *H. pylori* RecRO pathway

RecFOR is a highly conserved DNA recombination pathway in bacteria, and is mainly used for ssDNA gap repair [72]. In the published *H. pylori* genome sequences, only the *recR* gene was annotated [12, 13]. Although RecF historically served as a reference for RecFOR pathway, it is absent from genomes of many bacteria including *H. pylori* [72]. By bioinformatics analysis, Marsin et al [68] identified HP0951 as a novel RecO orthologue, although its sequence identity with the *E. coli* protein is lower than 15%. Recent studies in *E. coli* indicated that RecOR in the absence of RecF can perform recombination by loading RecA [95, 96]. Whereas the RecO protein can displace ssDNA-binding protein (SSB) and bind to ssDNA, RecR is the key component for loading RecA onto ssDNA [95, 97]. Likely, the RecRO pathway (with no RecF) is present in *H. pylori*.

The *recR* and *recO* mutants showed marked sensitivity to DNA damaging agents metronidazole and UV light, indicating roles of RecR and RecO in DNA repair. Unlike the *addA* (*recB*) mutant, the *recR* and *recO* mutants did not show significant sensitivity to ionizing radiation (IR) and to mitomycin C [68, 71], suggesting that RecRO pathway is not responsible for repairing DNA damage induced by these agents, most likely double strand breaks. This is in contrast to *E. coli* where the RecFOR pathway sometimes substitutes for the RecBCD pathway and in *Deinococcus radiodurance* where the RecFOR pathway plays a major role in double strand break repair [98, 99]. On the other hand, *H. pylori recR* and *recO* mutants were shown to be much more sensitive to oxidative stress and to acid stress than the wild type strain [71], indicating that *H. pylori* RecRO pathway is involved in repairing DNA damage induced by these stress conditions. The *addA recO* double mutant (deficient in both AddAB and RecRO pathways) was significantly more sensitive to atmospheric oxygen than the *recO* single mutant, indicating that both RecRO and AddAB pathways are important for survival of oxidative damage. Similar roles of the RecBCD and the RecFOR pathways for survival of oxidative damage were also observed in *E. coli* [57, 100] and in *Neisseria gonorrhoeae* [84]. In those bacteria, however, the RecBCD appeared to be the predominant (over the RecFOR) repair pathway for oxidative damage. Our results suggest that the two pathways in *H. pylori* play similarly important roles in repairing oxidative stress-derived DNA damage [71]. In accordance with the sensitivity to oxidative and acid stress in vitro, *H. pylori recR* and *recO* mutants were shown to be less able to colonize mouse stomachs [71]. Furthermore, the mouse colonization ability of the *addA recO* double mutant was significantly lower than that of the *addA* or *recO* single mutant. Therefore, both AddAB- and RecRO-mediated DNA recombinational repair in *H. pylori* play an important role in bacterial survival and persistent colonization in the host.

Although differing results regarding the effect of *addA* gene on transformation frequency were reported by different research groups, it was agreed that the RecRO-pathway is not involved in recombination of exogenous DNA into the *H. pylori* genome in the process of transformation [68, 71]. The RecRO pathway is known to have a major role in intragenomic recombination at repeat sequences [101]. Using an assay to assess the deletion frequency resulting from recombination on direct repeat sequences (358 bp long), Marsin et al [68] showed that the *recR* and *recO* mutants exhibited a statistically significantly lower deletion frequency than the wild type strain, suggesting a role of RecRO in intragenomic recombination. Recently we adopted a similar assay using DNA constructs (deletion cassettes) that contain identical repeat sequences of different length (IDS100 and IDS350) [71]. The results indicated that the intra-genomic recombination of 100 bp-long direct repeat sequences in *H. pylori* is partially dependent on RecR and RecA, yet a large portion of the recombination event is RecA-independent. This is basically in agreement (with small variance) with the results of Aras et al [35] who reported that the repeat sequences of 100 bp or shorter recombined through a RecA-independent pathway. For the deletion cassette containing repeat sequences of 350 bp in length, inactivation of *recR* or *recA* resulted in a significant 4-fold or 35-fold decrease respectively in deletion frequency, indicating that RecR plays a significant role in recombination of IDS350, while this recombination was highly dependent on RecA.

5. Concluding remarks and perspectives

Severe *Helicobacter pylori*-mediated gastric diseases are associated with the bacterium's persistence in the host and its adaptability to host differences, which in turn is associated with its remarkable genetic variability. DNA recombination is an extraordinarily frequent event in *H. pylori*, and this manifests itself into a bacterium with unusual flexibility in stress-combating enzymes, repair mechanisms, and other adaptability characteristics. Nearly every *H. pylori* recombination-related gene studied thus far by a gene directed mutant analysis approach has documented they are individually important in stomach colonization ability; this underscores the importance of these recombination repair processes in bacterial survival in the host. It is well recognized that homologous DNA recombination is a special system in bacteria for repairing stalled replication forks and double strand breaks, while generating genetic diversity as an advantageous byproduct [102]. *H. pylori* may be an especially fruitful organism in which to learn the ultimate boundaries in roles of recombination repair enzymes, as *H. pylori* is subject to intense and prolonged host mediated stress and it displays an enormous genetic diversity.

Substantial progress has been made recently in unraveling the complex systems of DNA recombinational repair in *H. pylori*. As expected, whole genome sequencing has been a powerful tool to aid in identifying recombination-related proteins in *H. pylori*. For example, *recA, recR, recN,* and *ruvABC* were identified and confirmed to play important roles in *H. pylori* as could be expected from results for other bacteria. Some recombination-related proteins (e.g. MutS2, RecG), however, play unique roles in *H. pylori*. Most of the genes for the major components of the two pre-synapsis pathways (RecBCD and RecFOR) were not annotated from *H. pylori* genome sequences, which drove researchers' interest to search for additional novel systems required for *H. pylori* DNA recombinational repair. Recent studies revealed the existence of both pathways, AddAB and RecRO, in *H. pylori*. Although they display a limited level of sequence homology to the known recombination enzymes, both AddAB and RecRO were shown to play important roles in *H. pylori* DNA recombinational repair, conferring resistance to oxidative and acid stress.

The major components of DNA recombinational repair machinery in *H. pylori* are listed in Table 1. *H. pylori* RecN protein may recognize DNA double strand breaks and recruits AddAB helicase-nuclease complex for further processing. While not being involved in repair of DNA double strand breaks, *H. pylori* RecRO proteins play a major role in intra-genomic recombination at repeat sequences. Both pre-synapsis pathways (AddAB and RecRO) require RecA for catalyzing DNA strand exchange (synapsis) and *H. pylori* RuvABC is the predominant pathway for DNA branch migration and Holliday Junction resolution (post-synapsis). Although the major functions of these components are similar to those observed in model bacteria, some novel attributes of these components have been discovered, which may be related to the highly-specific lifestyle of *H. pylori*. Additional new components that work synergistically with these pathways could be found in this unique bacterium via future biochemical and genetic approaches.

6. Acknowledgements

The work on *H. pylori* DNA repair in our laboratory was supported by NIH grant R21AI076569 and by the University of Georgia Foundation.

Gene	HP # (a)	Activity / function	Main phenotypes of mutant (b)	reference
recN	1393	Initiates DSB-induced recombination.	Sensitive to DSB damage; Sensitive to oxidative stress; Attenuated mouse colonization.	[83]
recJ	0348	5'-3' ssDNA exonuclease.	Not studied experimently.	
addA	1553	AddAB Helicase-nuclease; Initiates DSB-induced recombination.	Sensitive to DSB damage; Sensitive to oxidative stress; Attenuated mouse colonization.	[69, 92]
addB	1089			
recR	0925	RecRO recombination pathway; Initiates ssDNA gap repair.	Not sensitive to DSB damage; Sensitive to oxidative stress; Attenuated mouse colonization.	[68, 71]
recO	0951			
recA	0153	DNA recombinase; Catalyzes DNA pairing and strand exchange.	Sensitive to DNA damaging agents; Decreased recombination frequency; Defective mouse colonization.	[65, 66, 69]
recG	1523	Holiday junction helicase.	Not sensitive to DNA damaging agents; Increased recombination frequency.	[76]
ruvA	0883	Holliday junction recognition.	Not studied experimently.	
ruvB	1059	Holiday junction helicase.	Sensitive to DNA damaging agents; Decreased recombination frequency.	[75]
ruvC	0877	Holliday junction resolvase.	Sensitive to DNA damaging agents; Decreased recombination frequency; Attenuated mouse colonization.	[73]

(a) HP# refers to the gene number in the genome sequence of strain 26695 [12].
(b) DSB (double strand breaks) damage refers to those damages caused e.g. by ionizing radiation, mitomycin C, or ciprofloxacin.

Table 1. *H. pylori* genes involved in DNA recombinational repair

7. References

[1] Dunn BE, Cohen H, Blaser MJ. Helicobacter pylori. Clin Microbiol Rev 1997;10(4):720-41.

[2] Suerbaum S, Michetti P. Helicobacter pylori infection. N Engl J Med 2002;347(15):1175-86.

[3] Uemura N, Okamoto S, Yamamoto S, *et al.* Helicobacter pylori infection and the development of gastric cancer. N Engl J Med 2001;345(11):784-9.

[4] McGee DJ, Mobley HL. Mechanisms of Helicobacter pylori infection: bacterial factors. Curr Top Microbiol Immunol 1999;241:155-80.

[5] Kusters JG, van Vliet AH, Kuipers EJ. Pathogenesis of Helicobacter pylori infection. Clin Microbiol Rev 2006;19(3):449-90.

[6] Kang J, Blaser MJ. Bacterial populations as perfect gases: genomic integrity and diversification tensions in Helicobacter pylori. Nat Rev Microbiol 2006;4(11):826-36.

[7] Suerbaum S. Genetic variability within Helicobacter pylori. Int J Med Microbiol 2000;290(2):175-81.

[8] Falush D, Wirth T, Linz B, *et al.* Traces of human migrations in Helicobacter pylori populations. Science 2003;299(5612):1582-5.

[9] Suerbaum S, Smith JM, Bapumia K, Morelli G, Smith NH, Kunstmann E, Dyrek I, Achtman M. Free recombination within Helicobacter pylori. Proc Natl Acad Sci U S A 1998;95(21):12619-24.

[10] Kansau I, Raymond J, Bingen E, *et al.* Genotyping of Helicobacter pylori isolates by sequencing of PCR products and comparison with the RAPD technique. Res Microbiol 1996;147(8):661-9.

[11] Wang G, Humayun MZ, Taylor DE. Mutation as an origin of genetic variability in Helicobacter pylori. Trends Microbiol 1999;7(12):488-93.

[12] Tomb JF, White O, Kerlavage AR, *et al.* The complete genome sequence of the gastric pathogen Helicobacter pylori. Nature 1997;388(6642):539-47.

[13] Alm RA, Ling LS, Moir DT, *et al.* Genomic-sequence comparison of two unrelated isolates of the human gastric pathogen Helicobacter pylori. Nature 1999;397(6715):176-80.

[14] Salama N, Guillemin K, McDaniel TK, Sherlock G, Tompkins L, Falkow S. A whole-genome microarray reveals genetic diversity among Helicobacter pylori strains. Proc Natl Acad Sci U S A 2000;97(26):14668-73.

[15] Israel DA, Salama N, Krishna U, Rieger UM, Atherton JC, Falkow S, Peek RM, Jr. Helicobacter pylori genetic diversity within the gastric niche of a single human host. Proc Natl Acad Sci U S A 2001;98(25):14625-30.

[16] Kraft C, Suerbaum S. Mutation and recombination in Helicobacter pylori: mechanisms and role in generating strain diversity. Int J Med Microbiol 2005;295(5):299-305.

[17] Bjorkholm B, Sjolund M, Falk PG, Berg OG, Engstrand L, Andersson DI. Mutation frequency and biological cost of antibiotic resistance in Helicobacter pylori. Proc Natl Acad Sci U S A 2001;98(25):14607-12.

[18] Horst JP, Wu TH, Marinus MG. Escherichia coli mutator genes. Trends Microbiol 1999;7(1):29-36.

[19] Lin EA, Zhang XS, Levine SM, Gill SR, Falush D, Blaser MJ. Natural transformation of helicobacter pylori involves the integration of short DNA fragments interrupted by gaps of variable size. PLoS Pathog 2009;5(3):e1000337.

[20] Kulick S, Moccia C, Didelot X, Falush D, Kraft C, Suerbaum S. Mosaic DNA imports with interspersions of recipient sequence after natural transformation of Helicobacter pylori. PLoS One 2008;3(11):e3797.

[21] Hofreuter D, Odenbreit S, Haas R. Natural transformation competence in Helicobacter pylori is mediated by the basic components of a type IV secretion system. Mol Microbiol 2001;41(2):379-91.

[22] Karnholz A, Hoefler C, Odenbreit S, Fischer W, Hofreuter D, Haas R. Functional and topological characterization of novel components of the comB DNA transformation competence system in Helicobacter pylori. J Bacteriol 2006;188(3):882-93.

[23] Stingl K, Muller S, Scheidgen-Kleyboldt G, Clausen M, Maier B. Composite system mediates two-step DNA uptake into Helicobacter pylori. Proc Natl Acad Sci U S A 2010;107(3):1184-9.

[24] Alvarez-Martinez CE, Christie PJ. Biological diversity of prokaryotic type IV secretion systems. Microbiol Mol Biol Rev 2009;73(4):775-808.

[25] Saunders NJ, Peden JF, Moxon ER. Absence in Helicobacter pylori of an uptake sequence for enhancing uptake of homospecific DNA during transformation. Microbiology 1999;145 (Pt 12):3523-8.

[26] Aras RA, Small AJ, Ando T, Blaser MJ. Helicobacter pylori interstrain restriction-modification diversity prevents genome subversion by chromosomal DNA from competing strains. Nucleic Acids Res 2002;30(24):5391-7.

[27] Humbert O, Dorer MS, Salama NR. Characterization of Helicobacter pylori factors that control transformation frequency and integration length during inter-strain DNA recombination. Mol Microbiol 2011;79(2):387-401.
[28] Go MF, Kapur V, Graham DY, Musser JM. Population genetic analysis of Helicobacter pylori by multilocus enzyme electrophoresis: extensive allelic diversity and recombinational population structure. J Bacteriol 1996;178(13):3934-8.
[29] Kersulyte D, Chalkauskas H, Berg DE. Emergence of recombinant strains of Helicobacter pylori during human infection. Mol Microbiol 1999;31(1):31-43.
[30] Salama NR, Gonzalez-Valencia G, Deatherage B, Aviles-Jimenez F, Atherton JC, Graham DY, Torres J. Genetic analysis of Helicobacter pylori strain populations colonizing the stomach at different times postinfection. J Bacteriol 2007;189(10):3834-45.
[31] Falush D, Kraft C, Taylor NS, Correa P, Fox JG, Achtman M, Suerbaum S. Recombination and mutation during long-term gastric colonization by Helicobacter pylori: estimates of clock rates, recombination size, and minimal age. Proc Natl Acad Sci U S A 2001;98(26):15056-61.
[32] Achtman M, Zurth K, Morelli G, Torrea G, Guiyoule A, Carniel E. Yersinia pestis, the cause of plague, is a recently emerged clone of Yersinia pseudotuberculosis. Proc Natl Acad Sci U S A 1999;96(24):14043-8.
[33] Guttman DS, Dykhuizen DE. Clonal divergence in Escherichia coli as a result of recombination, not mutation. Science 1994;266(5189):1380-3.
[34] Linz B, Schenker M, Zhu P, Achtman M. Frequent interspecific genetic exchange between commensal Neisseriae and Neisseria meningitidis. Mol Microbiol 2000;36(5):1049-58.
[35] Aras RA, Kang J, Tschumi AI, Harasaki Y, Blaser MJ. Extensive repetitive DNA facilitates prokaryotic genome plasticity. Proc Natl Acad Sci U S A 2003;100(23):13579-84.
[36] Martinez GR, Loureiro AP, Marques SA, *et al.* Oxidative and alkylating damage in DNA. Mutat Res 2003;544(2-3):115-27.
[37] Foster JW, Bearson B. Acid-sensitive mutants of Salmonella typhimurium identified through a dinitrophenol lethal screening strategy. J Bacteriol 1994;176(9):2596-602.
[38] Algood HM, Cover TL. Helicobacter pylori persistence: an overview of interactions between H. pylori and host immune defenses. Clin Microbiol Rev 2006;19(4):597-613.
[39] Chaturvedi R, Cheng Y, Asim M, *et al.* Induction of polyamine oxidase 1 by Helicobacter pylori causes macrophage apoptosis by hydrogen peroxide release and mitochondrial membrane depolarization. J Biol Chem 2004;279(38):40161-73.
[40] Ding SZ, Minohara Y, Fan XJ, *et al.* Helicobacter pylori infection induces oxidative stress and programmed cell death in human gastric epithelial cells. Infect Immun 2007;75(8):4030-9.
[41] Scott DR, Marcus EA, Wen Y, Oh J, Sachs G. Gene expression in vivo shows that Helicobacter pylori colonizes an acidic niche on the gastric surface. Proc Natl Acad Sci U S A 2007;104(17):7235-40.
[42] Wang G, Alamuri P, Maier RJ. The diverse antioxidant systems of Helicobacter pylori. Mol Microbiol 2006;61(4):847-60.

[43] Pflock M, Kennard S, Finsterer N, Beier D. Acid-responsive gene regulation in the human pathogen Helicobacter pylori. J Biotechnol 2006;126(1):52-60.
[44] Sancar A. Mechanisms of DNA excision repair. Science 1994;266(5193):1954-6.
[45] Thompson SA, Latch RL, Blaser JM. Molecular characterization of the Helicobacter pylori uvr B gene. Gene 1998;209(1-2):113-22.
[46] Kang J, Blaser MJ. UvrD helicase suppresses recombination and DNA damage-induced deletions. J Bacteriol 2006;188(15):5450-9.
[47] Modrich P. Mismatch repair, genetic stability, and cancer. Science 1994;266(5193):1959-60.
[48] Pinto AV, Mathieu A, Marsin S, Veaute X, Ielpi L, Labigne A, Radicella JP. Suppression of homologous and homeologous recombination by the bacterial MutS2 protein. Mol Cell 2005;17(1):113-20.
[49] Wang G, Alamuri P, Humayun MZ, Taylor DE, Maier RJ. The Helicobacter pylori MutS protein confers protection from oxidative DNA damage. Mol Microbiol 2005;58(1):166-76.
[50] O'Rourke EJ, Chevalier C, Pinto AV, Thiberge JM, Ielpi L, Labigne A, Radicella JP. Pathogen DNA as target for host-generated oxidative stress: role for repair of bacterial DNA damage in Helicobacter pylori colonization. Proc Natl Acad Sci U S A 2003;100(5):2789-94.
[51] Eutsey R, Wang G, Maier RJ. Role of a MutY DNA glycosylase in combating oxidative DNA damage in Helicobacter pylori. DNA Repair (Amst) 2007;6(1):19-26.
[52] Mathieu A, O'Rourke EJ, Radicella JP. Helicobacter pylori genes involved in avoidance of mutations induced by 8-oxoguanine. J Bacteriol 2006;188(21):7464-9.
[53] Huang S, Kang J, Blaser MJ. Antimutator role of the DNA glycosylase mutY gene in Helicobacter pylori. J Bacteriol 2006;188(17):6224-34.
[54] Butala M, Zgur-Bertok D, Busby SJ. The bacterial LexA transcriptional repressor. Cell Mol Life Sci 2009;66(1):82-93.
[55] Dorer MS, Fero J, Salama NR. DNA damage triggers genetic exchange in Helicobacter pylori. PLoS Pathog 2010;6(7):e1001026.
[56] Cromie GA, Connelly JC, Leach DR. Recombination at double-strand breaks and DNA ends: conserved mechanisms from phage to humans. Mol Cell 2001;8(6):1163-74.
[57] Kuzminov A. Recombinational repair of DNA damage in Escherichia coli and bacteriophage lambda. Microbiol Mol Biol Rev 1999;63(4):751-813, table of contents.
[58] Cox MM, Goodman MF, Kreuzer KN, Sherratt DJ, Sandler SJ, Marians KJ. The importance of repairing stalled replication forks. Nature 2000;404(6773):37-41.
[59] Liu Y, West SC. Happy Hollidays: 40th anniversary of the Holliday junction. Nat Rev Mol Cell Biol 2004;5(11):937-44.
[60] Fernandez S, Ayora S, Alonso JC. Bacillus subtilis homologous recombination: genes and products. Res Microbiol 2000;151(6):481-6.
[61] Skaar EP, Lazio MP, Seifert HS. Roles of the recJ and recN genes in homologous recombination and DNA repair pathways of Neisseria gonorrhoeae. J Bacteriol 2002;184(4):919-27.
[62] Courcelle J, Donaldson JR, Chow KH, Courcelle CT. DNA damage-induced replication fork regression and processing in Escherichia coli. Science 2003;299(5609):1064-7.
[63] Kidane D, Sanchez H, Alonso JC, Graumann PL. Visualization of DNA double-strand break repair in live bacteria reveals dynamic recruitment of Bacillus subtilis RecF,

RecO and RecN proteins to distinct sites on the nucleoids. Mol Microbiol 2004;52(6):1627-39.
[64] Meddows TR, Savory AP, Grove JI, Moore T, Lloyd RG. RecN protein and transcription factor DksA combine to promote faithful recombinational repair of DNA double-strand breaks. Mol Microbiol 2005;57(1):97-110.
[65] Schmitt W, Odenbreit S, Heuermann D, Haas R. Cloning of the Helicobacter pylori recA gene and functional characterization of its product. Mol Gen Genet 1995;248(5):563-72.
[66] Thompson SA, Blaser MJ. Isolation of the Helicobacter pylori recA gene and involvement of the recA region in resistance to low pH. Infect Immun 1995;63(6):2185-93.
[67] Fischer W, Haas R. The RecA protein of Helicobacter pylori requires a posttranslational modification for full activity. J Bacteriol 2004;186(3):777-84.
[68] Marsin S, Mathieu A, Kortulewski T, Guerois R, Radicella JP. Unveiling novel RecO distant orthologues involved in homologous recombination. PLoS Genet 2008;4(8):e1000146.
[69] Amundsen SK, Fero J, Hansen LM, Cromie GA, Solnick JV, Smith GR, Salama NR. Helicobacter pylori AddAB helicase-nuclease and RecA promote recombination-related DNA repair and survival during stomach colonization. Mol Microbiol 2008;69(4):994-1007.
[70] Marsin S, Lopes A, Mathieu A, Dizet E, Orillard E, Guerois R, Radicella JP. Genetic dissection of Helicobacter pylori AddAB role in homologous recombination. FEMS Microbiol Lett 2010;311(1):44-50.
[71] Wang G, Lo LF, Maier RJ. The RecRO pathway of DNA recombinational repair in Helicobacter pylori and its role in bacterial survival in the host. DNA Repair (Amst) 2011; 10: 373-379.
[72] Rocha EP, Cornet E, Michel B. Comparative and evolutionary analysis of the bacterial homologous recombination systems. PLoS Genet 2005;1(2):e15.
[73] Loughlin MF, Barnard FM, Jenkins D, Sharples GJ, Jenks PJ. Helicobacter pylori mutants defective in RuvC Holliday junction resolvase display reduced macrophage survival and spontaneous clearance from the murine gastric mucosa. Infect Immun 2003;71(4):2022-31.
[74] Robinson K, Loughlin MF, Potter R, Jenks PJ. Host adaptation and immune modulation are mediated by homologous recombination in Helicobacter pylori. J Infect Dis 2005;191(4):579-87.
[75] Kang J, Blaser MJ. Repair and antirepair DNA helicases in Helicobacter pylori. J Bacteriol 2008;190(12):4218-24.
[76] Kang J, Tavakoli D, Tschumi A, Aras RA, Blaser MJ. Effect of host species on recG phenotypes in Helicobacter pylori and Escherichia coli. J Bacteriol 2004;186(22):7704-13.
[77] Sharples GJ, Ingleston SM, Lloyd RG. Holliday junction processing in bacteria: insights from the evolutionary conservation of RuvABC, RecG, and RusA. J Bacteriol 1999;181(18):5543-50.
[78] Hirano T. At the heart of the chromosome: SMC proteins in action. Nat Rev Mol Cell Biol 2006;7(5):311-22.

[79] Haering CH, Lowe J, Hochwagen A, Nasmyth K. Molecular architecture of SMC proteins and the yeast cohesin complex. Mol Cell 2002;9(4):773-88.
[80] Kidane D, Graumann PL. Dynamic formation of RecA filaments at DNA double strand break repair centers in live cells. J Cell Biol 2005;170(3):357-66.
[81] Sanchez H, Kidane D, Castillo Cozar M, Graumann PL, Alonso JC. Recruitment of Bacillus subtilis RecN to DNA double-strand breaks in the absence of DNA end processing. J Bacteriol 2006;188(2):353-60.
[82] Sanchez H, Alonso JC. Bacillus subtilis RecN binds and protects 3'-single-stranded DNA extensions in the presence of ATP. Nucleic Acids Res 2005;33(7):2343-50.
[83] Wang G, Maier RJ. Critical role of RecN in recombinational DNA repair and survival of Helicobacter pylori. Infect Immun 2008;76(1):153-60.
[84] Stohl EA, Seifert HS. Neisseria gonorrhoeae DNA recombination and repair enzymes protect against oxidative damage caused by hydrogen peroxide. J Bacteriol 2006;188(21):7645-51.
[85] Stohl EA, Criss AK, Seifert HS. The transcriptome response of Neisseria gonorrhoeae to hydrogen peroxide reveals genes with previously uncharacterized roles in oxidative damage protection. Mol Microbiol 2005;58(2):520-32.
[86] Singleton MR, Wigley DB. Modularity and specialization in superfamily 1 and 2 helicases. J Bacteriol 2002;184(7):1819-26.
[87] Petit MA, Ehrlich D. Essential bacterial helicases that counteract the toxicity of recombination proteins. Embo J 2002;21(12):3137-47.
[88] Lestini R, Michel B. UvrD controls the access of recombination proteins to blocked replication forks. Embo J 2007;26(16):3804-14.
[89] Singleton MR, Dillingham MS, Gaudier M, Kowalczykowski SC, Wigley DB. Crystal structure of RecBCD enzyme reveals a machine for processing DNA breaks. Nature 2004;432(7014):187-93.
[90] Kooistra J, Haijema BJ, Hesseling-Meinders A, Venema G. A conserved helicase motif of the AddA subunit of the Bacillus subtilis ATP-dependent nuclease (AddAB) is essential for DNA repair and recombination. Mol Microbiol 1997;23(1):137-49.
[91] Yeeles JT, Dillingham MS. A dual-nuclease mechanism for DNA break processing by AddAB-type helicase-nucleases. J Mol Biol 2007;371(1):66-78.
[92] Wang G, Maier RJ. A RecB-like helicase in Helicobacter pylori is important for DNA repair and host colonization. Infect Immun 2009;77(1):286-91.
[93] Amundsen SK, Fero J, Salama NR, Smith GR. Dual nuclease and helicase activities of Helicobacter pylori AddAB are required for DNA repair, recombination, and mouse infectivity. J Biol Chem 2009;284(25):16759-66.
[94] Gressmann H, Linz B, Ghai R, *et al.* Gain and loss of multiple genes during the evolution of Helicobacter pylori. PLoS Genet 2005;1(4):e43.
[95] Sakai A, Cox MM. RecFOR and RecOR as distinct RecA loading pathways. J Biol Chem 2009;284(5):3264-72.
[96] Handa N, Morimatsu K, Lovett ST, Kowalczykowski SC. Reconstitution of initial steps of dsDNA break repair by the RecF pathway of E. coli. Genes Dev 2009;23(10):1234-45.
[97] Inoue J, Honda M, Ikawa S, Shibata T, Mikawa T. The process of displacing the single-stranded DNA-binding protein from single-stranded DNA by RecO and RecR proteins. Nucleic Acids Res 2008;36(1):94-109.

[98] Ivancic-Bace I, Peharec P, Moslavac S, Skrobot N, Salaj-Smic E, Brcic-Kostic K. RecFOR function is required for DNA repair and recombination in a RecA loading-deficient recB mutant of Escherichia coli. Genetics 2003;163(2):485-94.

[99] Bentchikou E, Servant P, Coste G, Sommer S. A major role of the RecFOR pathway in DNA double-strand-break repair through ESDSA in Deinococcus radiodurans. PLoS Genet;6(1):e1000774.

[100] Imlay JA, Linn S. Mutagenesis and stress responses induced in Escherichia coli by hydrogen peroxide. J Bacteriol 1987;169(7):2967-76.

[101] Galitski T, Roth JR. Pathways for homologous recombination between chromosomal direct repeats in Salmonella typhimurium. Genetics 1997;146(3):751-67.

[102] Cox MM. Historical overview: searching for replication help in all of the rec places. Proc Natl Acad Sci U S A 2001;98(15):8173-80.

2

RloC: A Translation-Disabling tRNase Implicated in Phage Exclusion During Recovery from DNA Damage

Gabriel Kaufmann et al.*
Tel Aviv University
Israel

1. Introduction

Bacteria respond to DNA damage by inducing the expression of numerous proteins involved in DNA repair and the reversible arrests of DNA replication and the cell division cycle (Fernandez De Henestrosa *et al*, 2000). This general rule may be violated by a conserved bacterial protein termed RloC (Davidov & Kaufmann, 2008). RloC combines structural-functional properties of two unrelated proteins (i) the universal DNA-damage-responsive/DNA-repair protein Rad50/SbcC (Williams *et al*, 2007) and (ii) the translation-disabling, phage-excluding anticodon nuclease (ACNase) PrrC (Blanga-Kanfi *et al*, 2006). These seemingly conflicting features may be reconciled in a model where RloC is mobilized as an antiviral back-up function during recovery from DNA damage (Davidov & Kaufmann, 2008), when DNA restriction, the cell's primary immune system is temporarily shut-off (Thoms & Wackernagel, 1984). Another intriguing feature of RloC is its ability to excise its substrate's wobble nucleotide (Davidov & Kaufmann, 2008). This harsh lesion is expected to encumber reversal by phage enzymes that repair the tRNA nicked by PrrC (Amitsur *et al*, 1987). Evaluating RloC's salient features and purported role requires prior description of its more familiar distant homolog PrrC and a DNA-damage-sensing device RloC shares with Rad50/SbcC. We conclude with an account of cellular RNA and DNA repair tools related to the phage tRNA repair mechanism that counteracts PrrC and may be frustrated by RloC.

2. PrrC – A potential phage-excluding tool counteracted by tRNA repair enzymes

2.1 A host-phage survival cascade yields an RNA repair pathway

RNA repair may seem unnecessary because damaged RNA molecules can be readily replenished by re-synthesis. Yet, there exist situations where RNA repair could be the preferred or only possible option. A case in point is presented by an RNA repair pathway triggered by the ACNase PrrC. This conserved bacterial protein was detected in quest of roles of two phage T4-encoded enzymes: 3'-phosphatase/5'-polynucleotide kinase (PseT/Pnk,

---

* Elena Davidov, Emmanuelle Steinfels-Kohn, Ekaterina Krutkina, Daniel Klaiman, Tamar Margalit, Michal Chai-Danino and Alexander Kotlyar
Tel Aviv University, Israel

henceforth Pnk) (Richardson, 1965;Becker & Hurwitz, 1967;Cameron & Uhlenbeck, 1977) and RNA ligase 1 (Rnl1, Silber *et al*, 1972;Ho & Shuman, 2002). The combined activities of Pnk and Rnl1 seemed tailored to fix RNA nicks, converting 3'-phosphoryl or 2',3'-cyclic phosphate and 5'-OH cleavage ends into 3'→5' phosphodiester linkages (Kaufmann & Kallenbach, 1975;Amitsur *et al*, 1987). Suggested alternative roles in DNA metabolism (Novogrodsky *et al*, 1966;Depew & Cozzarelli, 1974) were assigned in later years to a related eukaryal DNA kinase-phosphatase essential for genome stability and a possible therapeutic target in cancer cells rendered resistant to genotoxic drugs (Weinfeld *et al*, 2011).

Pnk and Rnl1 are dispensable for T4 growth on common *E. coli* laboratory strains but required on a rare host encoding the optional locus *prr* (*pnk* and *rnl1* restriction) (Depew & Cozzarelli, 1974; Sirotkin *et al*, 1978; Runnels *et al*, 1982; Jabbar & Snyder, 1984). Mutating a minuscule T4 orf termed *stp* (*s*uppressor of *t*hree-prime *p*hosphatase) abrogates *prr* restriction (Depew & Cozzarelli, 1974;Depew *et al*, 1975;Chapman *et al*, 1988;Penner *et al*, 1995). These facts reinforced the notion that Pnk and Rnl1 cooperate in RNA nick repair. They also led to the detection of the *prr*-encoded latent ACNase comprising the core ACNase PrrC and PrrC's silencing partner, the associated type Ic DNA restriction-modification (R-M) system EcoprrI (Levitz *et al*, 1990;Linder *et al*, 1990;Amitsur *et al*, 1992;Tyndall *et al*, 1994). EcoprrI and PrrC are also genetically linked, the ACNase core gene *prrC* is flanked by the genes encoding the three R-M subunit types *hsdMSR/prrABD* (Fig. 1A).

Type I R-M systems to which EcoprrI belongs recognize with their HsdS subunit a bipartite target containing a variable 6-8nt long spacer such as EcoprrI's CCAN$_7$RTGC (Tyndall *et al*, 1994). HsdS associates with two HsdM protomers to form a site-specific DNA methylase (HsdM$_2$S). Further attachment of two HsdR protomers yields a full-fledged R-M protein (HsdR$_2$M$_2$S). The R-M protein ignores a fully methylated target and readily methylates a hemi-methylated one. A fully unmodified target, usually of foreign DNA, induces the helicase domains of the HsdR protomers to pump-in DNA flanking the target sequence at the expense of ATP hydrolysis. This translocation and consequent DNA looping go on until an obstacle is encountered and cleavage occurs, usually far away from the specific recognition site. The type I R-M proteins are divided into families by antigenic cross-reactivity, subunit interchangeability and sequence similarity. PrrC is invariably linked to type Ic family members while RloC may interact with type Ia or the distantly related type III R-M proteins. For detailed coverage of DNA restriction and anti-restriction the readers are encouraged to consult relevant reviews (Murray, 2000;Dryden *et al*, 2001;Youell & Firman, 2008;Janscak *et al*, 2001).

EcoprrI normally silences PrrC's ACNase activity in the uninfected cell (Fig. 1B). The significance of this masking interaction is indicated by the "double-edged" nature of the T4 encoded peptide Stp, mutations in which suppress *prr* restriction. Thus, Stp inhibits EcoprrI's DNA restriction, probably its intended function; and activates the latent ACNase, its host co-opted task (Penner *et al*, 1995). Once activated PrrC nicks cellular tRNA^{Lys} 5' to the wobble base, yielding 2', 3'-cyclic phosphate and 5'-OH termini. Since T4 shuts-off host transcription (Mathews, 1994) and does not encode tRNA^{Lys} (Schmidt & Apirion, 1983) the lesion inflicted by PrrC could disable T4 late translation and contain the infection (Sirotkin *et al*, 1978). However, T4 overcomes also this hurdle by using Pnk and Rnl1 to resuscitate the damaged tRNA^{Lys}. Pnk heals the cleavage termini, converting them into a 3'-OH and 5'-P pair that Rnl1 seals (Amitsur *et al*, 1987)(Fig. 1B). In other words, this host-phage survival cascade gave rise to an RNA repair pathway. The ability of the *prr*-encoded latent ACNase to restrict only tRNA repair-deficient phage invokes the possible existence of a "smarter" ACNase able to encumber phage reversal. Later we ask if RloC could be one.

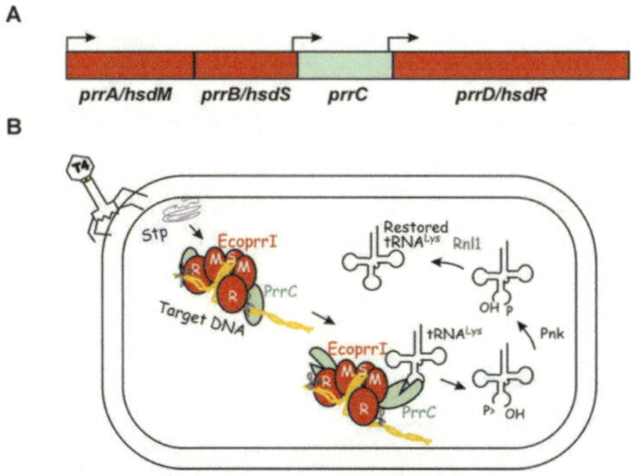

Fig. 1. A host-phage survival cascade gives rise to an RNA repair pathway. A. The optional host locus *prr* comprises the core ACNase gene *prrC* and flanking genes encoding the type Ic DNA R-M protein EcoprrI that silences PrrC's ACNase activity. Arrows mark transcription start sites. B. Cleavage-ligation of $tRNA^{Lys}$ in phage T4 infected *E. coli* prr^{+}. T4's anti-DNA restriction factor Stp inhibits EcoprrI and activates the latent ACNase. The resultant disruption of $tRNA^{Lys}$ is reversed by the T4's tRNA repair enzymes Pnk and Rnl1.

Nested *prr* loci where *prrC* intervenes a type Ic *hsd* locus (Fig 1A) appear sporadically in distantly related bacteria. They are present in some strains of a given species but not in others, as would a niche-function (Blanga-Kanfi *et al*, 2006). They abound among *Proteobacteria*, are less frequent in *Bacteroidetes* and *Firmicutes*, rare in *Actinobacteria* and apparently absent from *Cyanobacteria*. PrrC's phylogenic tree does not match the bacterial, unlike the associated type Ic R-M protein, which only rarely teams with PrrC. In contrast, a stand-alone *prrC* gene has not been detected so far. These facts hint that PrrC can be readily transmitted by horizontal gene transfer (HGT), possibly from a *prr* donor to an *hsd* acceptor. The dependence of PrrC's function on its detoxifying partner, the linked R-M system is indicated also by their coincident inactivation in a *Neisseria meningitidis* strain (Meineke and Shuman, pers. comm.). This addiction and the similar ACNase activities of various PrrC orthologs examined (Davidov & Kaufmann, 2008;Meineke *et al*, 2010) further suggest that PrrC acts in general as a translation-disabling, antiviral contingency mobilized when the linked R-M system is compromised.

The host-phage survival cascade depicted in Fig. 1B entails some caveats. Namely, the DNA of T4 and related phages incorporates 5-hydromethylcytosine (5-HmC) instead of cytosine and 5-HmC is further glucosylated at the DNA level (Morera *et al*, 1999). Due to this hyper-modification the phage DNA is refractory to many DNA restriction nucleases (Miller *et al*, 2003b) including EcoprrI and, hence, need not be protected from them by Stp. Moreover, a T4 mutant with unmodified cytosine in its DNA succumbs to EcoprrI's restriction, notwithstanding Stp's presence. The failure of Stp to protect this EcoprrI-sensitive mutant can be accounted for by the delayed-early schedule of its expression, a few minutes after the onset of the infection (Jabbar & Snyder, 1984;David *et al*, 1982). Due to these reasons EcoprrI's DNA restriction and Stp's anti-restriction activities were investigated using surrogate lambdoid phages (Jabbar & Snyder, 1984;Penner *et al*, 1995). Yet, the conservation of Stp's sequence among T4-like phages (Penner *et al*, 1995) http://phage.ggc.edu/,

indicates that this anti-DNA restriction factor provides selective advantage, e.g., preventing nucleases related to EcoprrI from cleaving nascent, not yet glucosylated progeny DNA.
The importance of Pnk and Rnl1 as PrrC's countermeasures is suggested by the following observations. First, docking tRNA on the crystal structure of T4 Pnk or Rnl1 places the anticodon loop at their respective active sites. These outcomes have been taken to indicate that both Pnk and Rnl1 evolved to repair a disrupted anticodon loop (Galburt *et al*, 2002;El Omari K. *et al*, 2006). Second, T4-related phages expected to infect *prr*-encoding bacteria feature both Pnk and Rnl1 (Miller *et al*, 2003a;Blondal *et al*, 2005;Blondal *et al*, 2003) whereas T4-related cyanophages, which are less likely to encounter *prr*, lack these tRNA repair proteins (http://phage.ggc.edu/).

2.2 PrrC's functional organization

PrrC comprises a regulatory motor domain occupying the N-proximal two thirds of its 396aa polypeptide (*Eco*PrrC). The remaining part constitutes the ACNase domain (Fig. 2A). The N-domain resembles ATP Binding Cassette (ABC) ATPases. These are universal motor components found in membrane-spanning transporters and in soluble proteins engaged in DNA repair, translation and related functions (Hopfner & Tainer, 2003). PrrC's N-domain differs from typical ABC ATPases in certain sequence attributes and in its unusual nucleotide specificity. The ABC ATPase motifs found in it partake in binding and hydrolysis of the nucleotide triphosphate moiety (Chen *et al*, 2003). However, the nucleobase recognizing motif of many transporter ABC ATPases termed A- or Y-loop (Ambudkar *et al*, 2006) is missing from PrrC. On the other hand, PrrC contains between its Walker A and Q-loop motifs a unique 16-residue motif rich in aromatic, acidic and other hydrophilic residues (Fig. 2A). This PrrC Box motif is highly degenerate (or rudimental) in RloC and is missing from other ABC ATPases and any other protein in the public database (Amitsur *et al*, 2003;Blanga-Kanfi *et al*, 2006). The PrrC Box candidates as a Y-loop substitute, responsible perhaps for PrrC's unusual specificity, the ability to simultaneously interact with its two different effector nucleotides GTP and dTTP (Blanga-Kanfi *et al*, 2006; unpublished data).
PrrC's ACNase domain harbors a catalytic ACNase triad (Arg^{320}-Glu^{324}-His^{356} in *Eco*PrrC) shared also by most RloC's orthologs except for a few cases where Glu is replaced by Asp. By analogy with the catalytic triad of RNase T1 (Gerlt, 1993;Steyaert, 1997), in the PrrC/RloC triad Glu and His could function as respective general base and acid catalysts while Arg could stabilize the pentameric transition state phosphate. The ACNase domain contains also residues implicated in recognition of the substrate's anticodon. Mutating one of them, *Eco*PrrC's Asp^{287} impairs the reactivity of the natural substrate and enhances that of analogs with a hypomodified or heterologous wobble base. These compensations hint that Asp^{287} interacts with the wobble base modifying side chain (Meidler *et al*, 1999;Jiang *et al*, 2001;Jiang *et al*, 2002).
When PrrC is expressed by itself it exhibits overt (core) ACNase activity. This core activity purifies with an oligomeric PrrC form, possibly a dimer of dimers. The N-domains of each dimer are expected to create two nucleotide binding sites (NBS) at their anti-parallel dimerization interfaces, as do typical ABC ATPases (Hopfner *et al*, 2000;Chen *et al*, 2003). In contrast, the ACNase C-domains are thought to dimerize in parallel, judged from the (i) behavior of a peptide mimic of a PrrC region implicated in the recognition of the tRNA substrate and (ii) ability of single to-Cys replacements in an overlapping PrrC region to induce disulphide-bond-dependent subunit dimerization (Klaiman *et al*, 2007).

Accordingly, the PrrC dimer of dimers assumes a phosphofructokinase-like topology (Schirmer & Evans, 1990) (Fig. 2B).

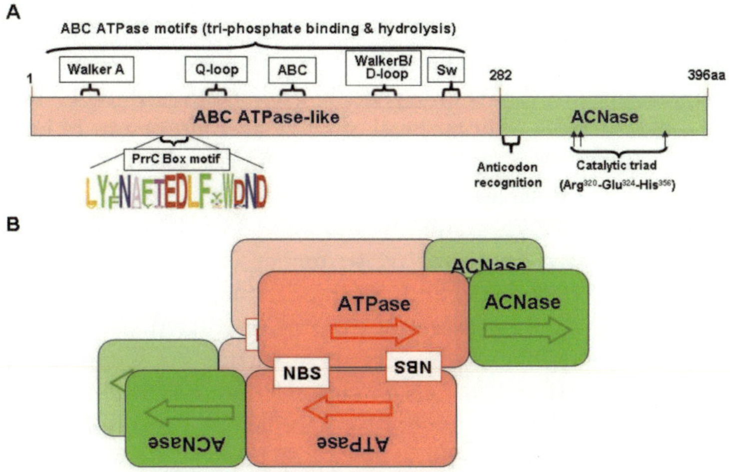

Fig. 2. Functional structure and possible quaternary organization of PrrC. **A.** PrrC's N-proximal ABC-ATPase domain features motifs involved in binding and hydrolysis of the nucleotide's triphosphate moiety (Walker A, Q-loop, ABC signature (ABC), Walker B, D-loop and linchpin Switch region (SW) but not the nucleobase recognizing Y-loop motif. The unique PrrC Box motif shown in WebLogo format, a putative functional substitute of the Y-loop, could confer the unusual GTP/dTTP specificity of PrrC. **B.** Antiparallel dimerization of the N-domains (Moody & Thomas, 2005) and anticipated parallel dimerization of the C-domains (Klaiman *et al*, 2007) suggest that PrrC assumes a phosphofructokinase-like quaternary topology (Schirmer & Evans, 1990). NBS - nucleotide binding site.

2.3 Players in PrrC's silencing and activation

As mentioned, PrrC's toxic activity is normally silenced, being unleashed only during phage infection. The requisite switches are provided in the case of *Eco*PrrC by its silencing partner EcoprrI, the phage T4-encoded anti-DNA restriction factor Stp and the motor domains of the ACNase protein itself. Insights into the underlying mechanisms were provided by the discrepant behaviors of the latent ACNase holoenzyme and the core ACNase activity of the unassociated PrrC. Thus, *in vitro* activation of the latent ACNase requires besides the Stp peptide, the DNA tethered to EcoprrI, GTP hydrolysis and the presence of dTTP. In contrast, the overt activity of the core ACNase is refractory to Stp, DNA and GTP but rapidly decays without dTTP (Amitsur *et al*, 2003;Blanga-Kanfi *et al*, 2006). These differences have been taken to indicate that Stp triggers the activation of the latent ACNase, GTP hydrolysis drives conformational changes needed to turn it on while the binding of dTTP stabilizes the ACNase once activated. The possible role of EcoprrI's DNA ligand is discussed later in this section.

GTP and dTTP probably exert their respective ACNase activating and stabilizing functions by interacting with PrrC's N-domains. This is suggested by their binding to full-sized PrrC protein or PrrC's isolated N-domains with vastly differing affinities (mM- and μM-range, respectively) and without displacing each other (Amitsur *et al*, 2003;Blanga-Kanfi *et al*, 2006; and unpublished data). This unusual specificity distinguishes PrrC from its distant homolog RloC and other ABC ATPase-containing proteins, which bind and hydrolyze ATP or GTP (Guo *et al*, 2006) and are not expected to avidly bind dTTP (our unpublished data).

The biological significance of PrrC's idiosyncratic interaction with dTTP has been hinted at by the dramatic increase in the cellular level of dTTP early in phage T4 infection, when the ACNase is induced (Amitsur *et al*, 2003;Blanga-Kanfi *et al*, 2006). The increased level of dTTP benefits the phage by safeguarding effective and faithful replication of its AT-rich DNA. In fact, delaying dTTP's accretion by mutating T4's dCMP deaminase (Cd) elicits a mutator phenotype indicated by increased frequency of AT→GC transitions (Sargent & Mathews, 1987). The Cd deficiency, and, by implication, the consequent delay in dTTP's accretion, also reduce 2-3 fold the extent of the PrrC-mediated cleavage of $tRNA^{Lys}$. This partial inhibition does not suffice to suppress *prr* restriction but is synthetically suppressive with a leaky *stp* mutation that also fails to suppress *prr* restriction by itself (Klaiman & Kaufmann, 2011). Thus, dTTP's accretion is another T4 contraption expatiated by the bacterial host, in that case to stabilize the activated ACNase.

PrrC's ability to "gauge" changes in dTTP's level could benefit its host also by precluding the toxicity of any free PrrC molecules that could arise in the uninfected cell due to their translation in excess over EcoprrI or dissociation from the latent holoenzyme. Their excessive translation may be stochastic or programmed to saturate the silencing partner. PrrC's dissociation from the latent holoenzyme may be accidental or due to EcoprrI's disruption in response to DNA damage (Restriction Alleviation, RA) (Makovets *et al*, 2004) (see also section 3.6). Free PrrC's cytotoxicity has been indicated by the coincident inactivation of *prrC* and linked *hsd* genes, by the self-limiting expression of free PrrC (Meidler *et al*, 1999;Blanga-Kanfi *et al*, 2006) and the rapid *in vivo* inactivation of the core ACNase (Amitsur *et al*, 2003). The ACNase enhancing effects of dTTP's accretion during phage T4 infection (Klaiman & Kaufmann, 2011) and *in vitro* stabilization of the core ACNase by dTTP (Amitsur *et al*, 2003) suggest that the *in vivo* instability of the core ACNase owes to the relatively low dTTP level in the uninfected cell. Although this level far exceeds that needed to stabilize the core ACNase *in vitro*, the actual level availed to PrrC in the cell could be prohibitively low due to localization of the nucleotide pools (Wheeler *et al*, 1996). In sum, we propose that PrrC's ability to gauge dTTP's level not only stabilizes its activated form but also confines the toxicity of this ACNase to the viral target.

Yet another player in PrrC's regulation is the DNA tethered to EcoprrI (Amitsur *et al*, 2003). Its possible role is suggested by three observations. First, short nonspecific ssDNA oligonucleotides avidly bind PrrC and competitively inhibit its ACNase activity (Fig. 3A and unpublished results), hinting that ssDNA encountered by PrrC in the uninfected cell helps silence the ACNase. Second, the type Ic DNA R-M protein EcoR124I unwinds short DNA stretches flanking its target sequence (van Noort *et al*, 2004;Stanley *et al*, 2006), suggesting a possible source for the putative ACNase-inhibiting ssDNA. Third, within a latent ACNase complex tethered to an EcoprrI DNA ligand PrrC was UV-crosslinked to DNA regions flanking EcoprrI's recognition site (Fig. 3B). These facts underlie a model where DNA unwound by EcoprrI helps silence PrrC and its rewinding due to Stp's interaction with EcoprrI unleashes the ACNase (Fig. 3C).

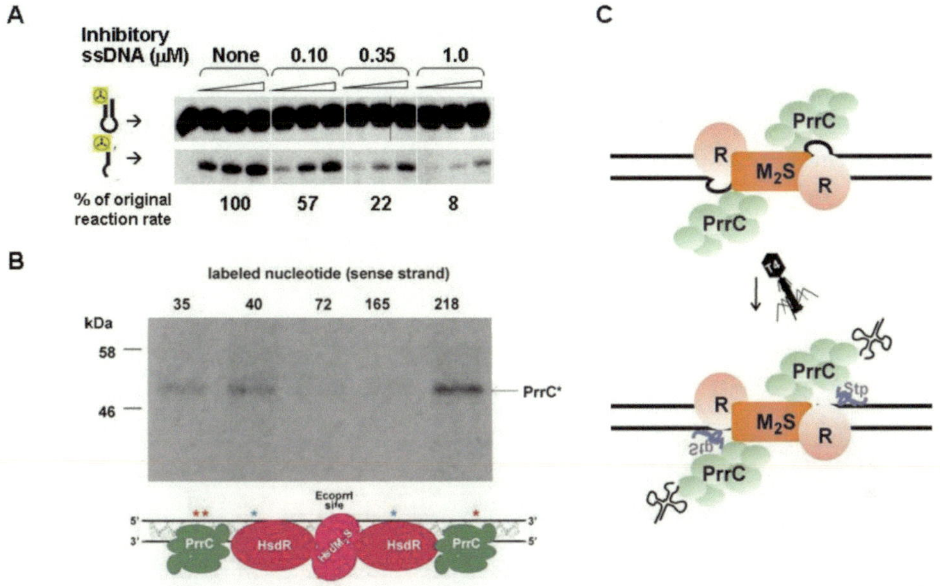

Fig. 3. DNA tethered to EcoprrI could figure in PrrC's regulation. A. ssDNA inhibits PrrC ACNase. PrrC ACNase was assayed using a 5'-^{32}P labeled anticodon stem loop substrate and increasing levels of a nonspecific 17nt PCR primer. B. PrrC contacts DNA regions flanking EcoprrI's target. A 249bp DNA fragment with a near-central EcoprrI site was singly ^{32}P-labeled at specific sites and tethered to the EcoprrI-PrrC complex. Following UV-irradiation, DNase I digestion, the photo-labeled PrrC was immunoprecipitated, separated by SDS-PAGE and monitored by autoradiography. Brown and blue asterisks indicate sites PrrC did or did not crosslink to, respectively. C. In this model DNA unwound by EcoprrI silences PrrC and its rewinding due to Stp's interaction with EcoprrI unleashes the ACNase.

3. RloC - A translation-disabling and potential DNA-damage-sensing protein

3.1 Functional organization

RloC is a conserved bacterial protein that shares PrrC's overall organization into a motor N-domain and ACNase C-domain (Fig. 4) (Davidov & Kaufmann, 2008). However, RloC is about twice as large, its orthologs ranging in size between 650 to 900 residues compared to 350-420 with PrrC. This increase is mainly due to a long coiled-coil forming sequence inserted between RloC's Walker A and ABC signature motifs. This coiled-coil sequence contains near its center a loop featuring the conserved zinc-hook motif CXXC. A similar coiled-coil insert in an ABC ATPase head-domain characterizes the universal DNA-damage-checkpoint/DNA-repair protein Rad50/SbcC (Hopfner *et al*, 2002;Connelly *et al*, 1998). Rad50's insert protrudes from the ATPase head-domain as an antiparallel coiled-coil presenting the zinc-hook motif at its apex. The apical ends of two such protrusions dimerize by coordinating Zn^{++} to their four cysteines. This zinc-hook linkage can arise intra-molecularly, connecting the two coiled-coil protrusions of the same Rad50 dimer. Alternatively, when Rad50's ATPase head-domains are bound to DNA the two protrusions straighten. In this form they can dimerize only inter-molecularly, bridging in this manner distant DNA molecules (Moreno-Herrero *et al*, 2005). Other proteins belonging to the SMC (Structure Maintenance of Chromosomes) super-family exhibit similar DNA bridging activity but link their coiled-coil protrusions via apical hydrophobic domains (Hirano, 2005). RloC is the only known protein other than Rad50/SbcC with a coiled-coil/zinc-hook containing ABC-ATPase domain. Therefore, cellular functions imparted by Rad50/SbcC may provide clues to RloC's.

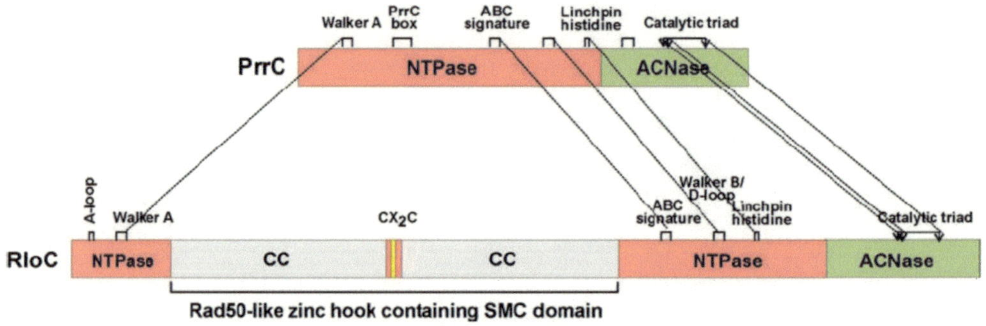

Fig. 4. RloC and PrrC share the same functional organization. The alignment of *Gka*RloC and *Eco*PrrC sequences reveals shared ABC ATPase and ACNase motifs and presence in RloC's N-domain of a large coiled-coil (CC) stretch interrupted by a loop containing the zinc hook motif CXXC (adapted from ref. 4).

3.2 RloC's occurrence and genomic attributes

RloC genes appear in major bacterial phyla except for *Cyanobacteria*. They are often encased within a cryptic mobile element as a single cargo gene. This pattern and a phylogenic tree not matching the bacterial suggest that RloC is readily transmitted by HGT, like PrrC. RloC's genes are also sporadically distributed but they occur ~3-fold more frequently than PrrC's. These facts suggest that the niche function RloC provides is more beneficial to its bacterial host.

RloC was originally identified as one of various open reading frames that intervene type Ia *hsd* loci in different *Campylobacter jejuni* strains (Restriction Linked Orf, Miller *et al*, 2005). This fact and the overall resemblance to PrrC could be taken to indicate that RloC is a related ACNase also silenced by an associated Hsd protein (Davidov & Kaufmann, 2008). Yet, only ~10% of the identified RloC orthologs turned out to be linked to type Ia or the distantly related type III DNA R-M system. Nonetheless, other genomic attributes suggested that the majority of the non-linked RloC orthologs team with an R-M system *in trans*. First, most bacteria encoding them encode also a suitable R-M system while in those lacking it RloC often features poor ATPase or ACNase motifs, as if inactivated. Second, some *rloC* genes are flanked by a cryptic *hsd* locus, a full-fledged homologue of which exists elsewhere in the genome, hinting that a past Hsd-RloC interaction *in cis* was superseded by one *in trans*. Third, RloC is occasionally linked to an ArdC-like anti-DNA restriction factor (Belogurov *et al*, 2000) with or without an adjacent R-M system, suggesting its possible regulation by an R-M system in either case. Fourth, non-linked *rloC* and *hsd* genes of one species, but not their respective flanking genes can be missing both from related, syntenic species [e.g., *Acinetobacter* sp. ADP1 *rloC* and *hsd* (ACIAD0152, ACIAD3430-2) but not flanking genes are missing from various *A. baumannii* strains] (http://www.cns.fr/agc/microscope/mage/viewer.php?S_id=36&wwwpkgdb =aa12fda27bb61b62ac34913acfd35916.)

The role ascribed to the R-M proteins in RloC's ACNase regulation need not contradict the existence of additional or alternative switches provided by the coiled-coil/zinc-hook insert. For example, silencing of the ACNase function by the latter device could be advantageous when RloC is introduced by HGT into a new host. Namely, silencing by a pre-existing R-M system could require a highly promiscuous interaction between the two partners. The possibility that RloC is endowed with an internal ACNase silencing mechanism agrees with properties of the ortholog encoded by the thermophile *Geobacillus kaustophilus* (*Gka*RloC) to be described in the following sections.

3.3 RloC wobble-nucleotide-excising activity

Due to its potential toxicity, RloC's ACNase activity was expected to be as unstable as PrrC's (Blanga-Kanfi *et al*, 2006). Indeed, among several RloC orthologs investigated, only *Gka*RloC proved sufficiently stable to warrant its *in vitro* characterization (Davidov & Kaufmann, 2008). Yet, even *Gka*RloC's ACNase is intrinsically unstable. Its *in vitro* activity is highest at 25°C and undetectable at 45°C (our unpublished results) although *G. kaustophilus* grows optimally at 65°C (Takami *et al*, 2004). When expressed in *E. coli* *Gka*RloC preferentially cleaved $tRNA^{Glu}$. However, identifying RloC's natural substrate must await physiological studies. This reservation is based on the experience gained with PrrC, the over-expression of which results in cleavages of secondary substrates that overwhelm the natural (Meidler *et al*, 1999).
A more striking difference between RloC and PrrC is the ability of the former to cleave its tRNA substrates successively, first 3' and then 5' to the wobble position (Davidov & Kaufmann, 2008). Such an excision reaction using as a substrate yeast $tRNA^{Glu}$ radiolabeled 3' to the wobble base is shown in Fig. 5. The incision of this substrate 3' to the wobble base yields a labeled 5' fragment containing residues 1-34. This intermediate is further cleaved immediately upstream, yielding the labeled wobble-nucleotide. Under these *in* vitro conditions *Gka*RloC inadvertently incises the substrate also 5' to the wobble base but this reaction yields a dead-end product that is not further cleaved. This is indicated by the accumulation of this product when the overall reaction declines; and of RloC to cleave it when generated by PrrC, which normally cleaves its substrates 5' to the wobble position. Such a 5' incision product of GkaRloC is not detected *in vivo* and, therefore, is considered an *in vitro* artifact. The excision of the wobble nucleotide has been observed with different tRNA and anticodon-stem-loop substrates and was catalyzed also by a mesophilic RloC species of *E. coli* APECO1 (Davidov & Kaufmann, 2008; unpublished data).

3.4 RloC may frustrate phage reversal

The harsh lesion inflicted by *Gka*RloC could render this ACNase a more potent antiviral device than PrrC. Namely, RloC could perform the successive cleavages of its substrate in a processive manner, i.e., without releasing the incision intermediate. The phage tRNA repair enzymes would in that case process and ligate back the fragments lacking the wobble nucleotide and yield a defective product. Conversely, if *Gka*RloC's incision intermediate were accessible, the repair enzymes would faithfully restore the original tRNA substrate. Simulated *in vitro* encounters between *Gka*RloC and T4 Pnk or both tRNA repair enzymes indicated that a sizable fraction of its incision intermediate was occluded from the repair enzymes (Davidov & Kaufmann, 2008; and unpublished data). It is possible that under physiological conditions RloC's would more effectively occlude its incision intermediate.

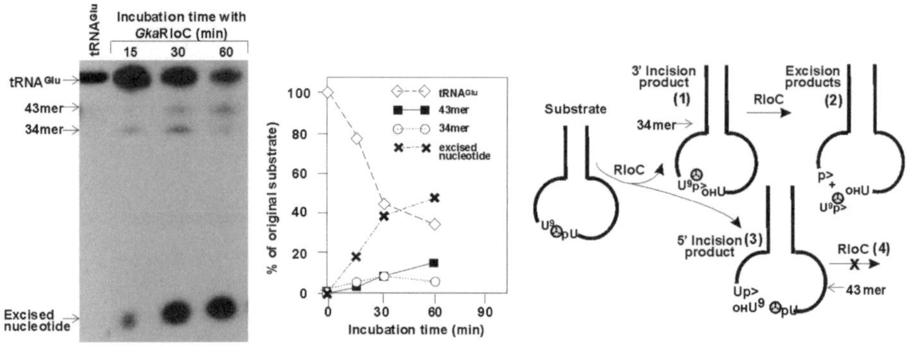

Fig. 5. RloC excises the wobble nucleotide. Yeast $tRNA^{Glu}$ ^{32}P-labeled 3' to the wobble base was incubated with *Gka*RloC. The 34mer resulting from incision 3' to the wobble base is further cleaved, yielding the wobble nucleotide. The 43mer resulting from incision 5' to the wobble base is a dead-end product that is not further cleaved. It is considered an *in vitro* artifact, as explained in the text. In the cartoon depicting these reactions the substrate is schematically represented by the anticodon stem loop outline. ⊛ marks the labeled phosphate. U^9 is the modified wobble base 5-methoxycarbonylmethyl-2-thiouridine. (mcm^5s^2U).

Moreover, repeated cleavage-ligation cycles would diminish the proportion of any incision intermediate ligated back by phage enzymes. On the other hand, the existence of tRNA repair enzymes that more efficiently extract RloC's incision intermediate and generate perhaps repair products immune to re-cleavage (Chan *et al*, 2009b) cannot be excluded. Clearly, whether RloC does frustrate phage reversal remains to be examined in situations closer to the natural.

3.5 RloC's DNA bridging domain regulates its ACNase

RloC's second striking feature is the coiled-coil/zinc-hook insert in its ABC ATPase head-domain. The presence of this structure raised the possibility that RloC is endowed with Rad50-like DNA bridging activity and uses such a faculty to respond to DNA damage cues by turning on its ACNase. That RloC is in fact endowed with DNA bridging activity is indicated by an electrophoresis mobility shift experiment and by scanning force microscopy (AFM) imaging. In the first experiment we compared *Gka*RloC constructs with an intact or mutated zinc-hook. The first protein aggregated a dsDNA probe that the second only bound (Fig. 6). Their discrepant behavior suggests that the aggregation was due to the formation of zinc-hook-dependent DNA bridges. Preliminary AFM imaging data reinforce this assumption (Fig. 7).

That RloC's ACNase is regulated by the protein's coiled-coil/zinc-hook and ATPase head-domain is indicated by several observations. First, mutating RloC's zinc-hook dramatically enhances its ACNase activity *in vivo* and *in vitro* (Davidov & Kaufmann, 2008). Second, *Gka*RloC's ACNase activity is modestly enhanced by ATP and further stimulated when the protein is also tethered to DNA (Fig. 8). In contrast, DNA alone has no effect on the ACNase and the residual ACNase activity seen without added ATP is abolished by the non-hydrolyzable analog AMP-PNP. Presumably, RloC's interaction with DNA turns on its ATPase to drive conformational changes that activate the ACNase. Interestingly, mutating the zinc-hook renders the ACNase refractory to these various agents, uncoupling the ACNase from the protein's internal controls (not shown). Together, these facts suggest that RloC's mode of interaction with DNA, which is sensed by its coiled-coil/zinc-hook monitoring device and relayed by the ATPase (Fig. 9), determines if the protein's ACNase will be silenced or turned on.

The ability to activate *Gka*RloC's ACNase by ATP hydrolysis in the presence of tethered DNA is in stark contrast with the behavior of PrrC's ACNase. As mentioned, PrrC's ACNase is activated by nucleotide hydrolysis only when associated with its silencing partner EcoprrI. However, its unassociated form exhibits overt ACNase activity refractory to nucleotide hydrolysis. This discrepancy raises the possibility that RloC's ACNase can be regulated by the internal device of the protein, the coiled-coil/zinc-hook and the ATPase domain that harbors this structure.

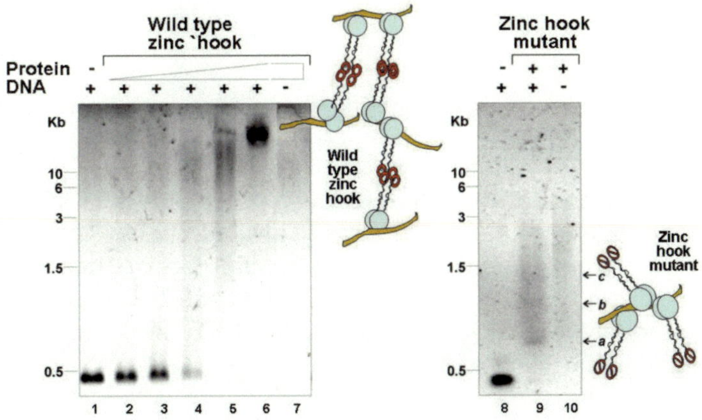

Fig. 6. *Gka*RloC aggregates DNA in a zinc-hook-dependent manner. A 485bp DNA fragment was incubated with increasing levels of GkaRloC's ACNase-null mutant E696A (lanes 2-6) or with its ZH mutant derivative E696A-C291G (lane 9). Lanes 1 and 8 contain only DNA, 7,10 only the indicated protein. The cartoons depict the assumed bridged DNA aggregate formed by E696A (right) and the simpler complex formed by E696A-C291G (left). The ACNase-null mutation allows high level expression and facilitates the isolation of the RloC proteins.

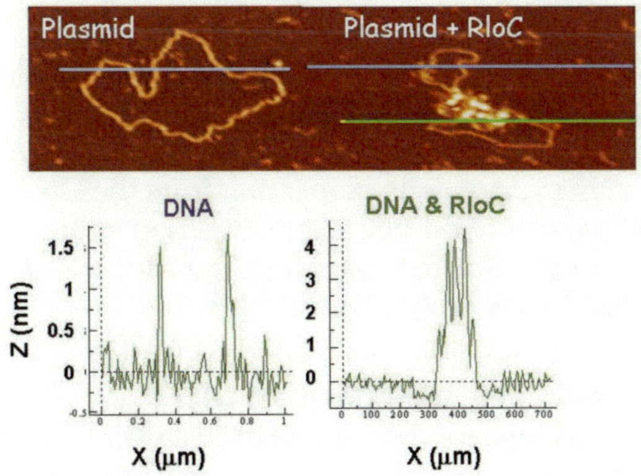

Fig. 7. AFM images of plasmid pUC19 (DNA) and its complex with RloC-E696A (DNA and RloC). Blue lines stretch over pure DNA regions, green lines also over regions containing the bound protein. Regions transected by the green line feature virtual heights both of the DNA alone (~1.5nm) and of the presumptive RloC-DNA complexes (~4.5nm).

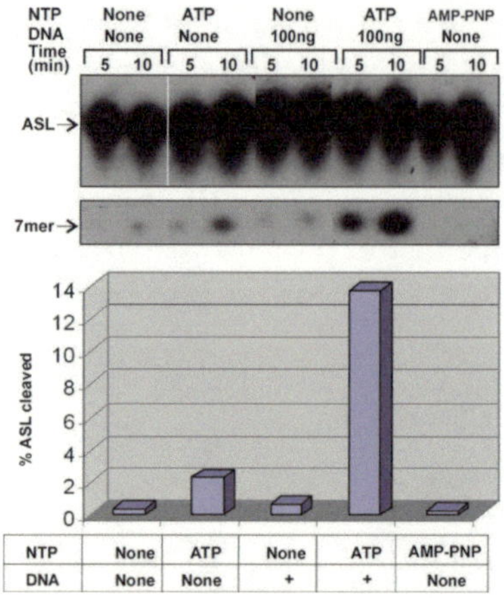

Fig. 8. *Gka*RloC's ATPase and tethered DNA cooperatively regulate its ACNase function. *Gka*RloC's ACNase activity was assayed using as a substrate a 5'-^{32}P labeled anticodon-stem-loop analog corresponding to mammalian tRNA^{Lys3} (ASL). The reaction was performed in the absence or presence of 2mM of ATP and/or 10ng/µl of BstE II digested λ DNA, or in the presence of the non-hydrolyzable ATP analog AMP-PNP. The 7mer is a radiolabeled fragment resulting from the final excision reaction

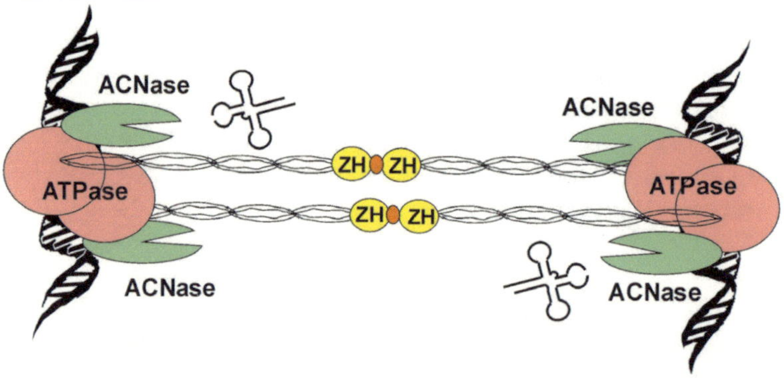

Fig. 9. RloC's anticipated DNA bridging activity. By analogy with Rad50, RloC bridges DNA through Zn^{++} (orange circles) coordinated at zinc-hook (ZH) dimerization interfaces (yellow circles) at the apical tips of the coiled-coils protruding from the DNA-borne ATPase head domains (pink circles). The status of the bound DNA sensed by RloC determines if its ATPase will be activated and drive structural changes needed to switch on the ACNase domains (split green ovals) toward tRNA cleavage.

3.6 Is RloC a suicidal DNA-damage-responsive device?

If RloC can be regulated by its internal devices, what role plays the anticipated interaction of RloC with a DNA R-M protein? Do these external and internal devices cooperate or act separately, responding to the same or different environmental cues? The present state of RloC's research does not permit us to distinguish between these possibilities, let alone assign to this protein specific biological functions. However, cues provided by Rad50/SbsC, the only other known coiled-coil/zinc-hook containing entity, may facilitate the formulation of useful guiding hypotheses. Here it will suffice to briefly summarize pertinent features of this universal DNA-damage-responsive, DNA-repair protein. For comprehensive coverage several recent reviews are suggested (Hirano, 2006;Stracker & Petrini, 2011;Williams *et al*, 2010;Paull, 2010) as well as relevant chapters in this book.

Archaeal Rad50 and the bacterial SbcC counterparts associate with the respective dimeric DNases Mre11 or SbcD. The eukaryal Rad50-Mre11 complex (MR) further associates with an adapter protein termed Nbs1 (Xrs2 in yeast), which links the ternary complex to key DNA damage checkpoints. The ternary MRN complex controls key sensing, signaling, regulating, and effecter responses triggered by DNA double-strand breaks (DSB). These responses include the activation of master regulators such as ATM as well as roles in homologous recombinational repair (HRR), microhomology-mediated end joining (MMEJ) and, occasionally, non-homologous end-joining (NHEJ). Rad50 figures in these transactions as a DNA-bridging SMC protein, using its coiled-coil/zinc-hook and ATPase to properly orient the DNA molecules it bridges and its associated protein partners (Hirano, 2005;Stracker & Petrini, 2011;Williams *et al*, 2010;Paull, 2010;Stracker & Petrini, 2011). As mentioned, Rad50's coiled-coils bend when the ATPase domains are free and stretches when tethered to DNA (van *et al*, 2003;Moreno-Herrero *et al*, 2005). This flexibility also allows the linked ATPase domain to communicate nucleotide binding and DNA ligand signals across distances and between components of the complex. These transmissions depend, among others, on the binding of Mre11 to the coiled-coil portion closest to the ATPase domain, which positions the DNase to resect DSB ends (Williams *et al*, 2011).

Rad50's bacterial homologue SbcC may likewise exert its function as a DNA bridging protein, directing SbcD to cleave hairpin structures that impede DNA replication and initiate DSB that drive HRR (Darmon *et al*, 2010;Storvik & Foster, 2011;White *et al*, 2008). Interestingly, over-expressed in *E. coli*, *SbcC* co-localizes with the replication factory whereas SbcD is dispersed throughout the cytoplasm. Their discrepant behaviors underlie the proposal that at its low, natural level SbcC constantly checks the replication fork for misfolded DNA, recruiting SbcD only when repair is required. A different distribution in *B. subtilis* suggests that in this organism SbcCD partakes also in NHEJ (Mascarenhas *et al*, 2006; Darmon *et al*, 2007).

*Gka*RloC could use its DNA bridging activity (Figs. 5, 6) to monitor the status of cellular DNA molecules like Rad50 and SbcC. However, there is no evidence that RloC associates with a DNase corresponding to Mre11 or SbcD. On the other hand, RloC's regulatory domain, Rad50/SbcC's counterpart is uniquely appended to the translation-disabling ACNase domain. It is tempting to speculate therefore that the ACNase C-domain interacts with the regulatory N-domain in a manner analogous to Mre11's, i.e., tethers to the proximal portion of the coiled-coil fiber emerging from the ATPase head-domain. Such a contact could help transduce DNA damage signals sensed by RloC's DNA monitoring device and relayed by the ATPase to the ACNase effecter domain. The existence of such a signal transduction pathway agrees with the effects of RloC's zinc-hook mutations, ATPase and tethered DNA on its ACNase function (Davidov & Kaufmann, 2008) (Fig 8).

The suggestions that RloC's ACNase is activated in response to DNA damage and, consequently, arrests translation may seem self-contradictory. After all, bacteria normally respond to DNA insults by enhancing the synthesis of DNA repair and other stress responsive proteins (Fernandez De Henestrosa *et al*, 2000). This apparent contradiction may be reconciled by considering the phenomenon of DNA restriction alleviation (RA) (Thoms & Wackernagel, 1984). RA is enacted in response to genotoxic stress as a protective measure intended to prevent degradation of self DNA. In the best documented RA case, the restriction subunit HsdR of the type Ia R-M protein EcoKI is degraded by the protease ClpXP (Makovets *et al*, 2004). In the case of the type Ic protein EcoR124I, RA may entail dissociation or functional occlusion of the HsdR subunit (Youell & Firman, 2008). RA prevents the degradation of fully unmodified portions of the cellular DNA synthesized during the recovery from DNA damage, mainly by HRR. In fact, exposure of an RA-deficient mutant to DNA damage causes DSB and eventual cell death (Cromie *et al*, 2001;Makovets *et al*, 2004;Blakely & Murray, 2006).

RA exacts also a price. Namely, inactivation of the cell's primary immune system renders it highly vulnerable to phage infection (Yamagami & Endo, 1969;Blakely & Murray, 2006). In theory, RloC could benefit its host in this situation by acting as an antiviral back-up device, mobilized when the cell is infected by a phage during recovery from DNA damage. The activation of RloC under these circumstances would prevent the spread of the phage to other members of the vulnerable bacterial population. In this regard RloC could resemble PrrC, which fails to rescue the cell in which it is turned on but can contain the infection. However, the proposed mode of RloC's activation calls for combined inputs of DNA damage and phage infection. Namely, phage infection alone would be offset by the functional DNA restriction nuclease while DNA damage alone would be effectively dealt with by the SOS response (Friedberg *et al*, 2006). It is noteworthy that exposure of an RloC encoding species to mytomycin C did not induce detectable ACNase activity (unpublished results).

Clearly, the above model raises more questions than it attempts to answer. For example, how does the anticipated RloC-Hsd interaction fit in this scheme? Do the genotoxic and viral stress signals cooperate or act separately? Can RloC frustrate phage encoded tRNA repair? To address these issues it will be necessary to employ experimental systems based on natural RloC-encoding hosts and cognate T4-like phages that activate RloC and encode a tRNA repair system.

4. RNA damage repair

4.1 Why repair damaged RNA?

The emergence of an RNA cleavage-ligation pathway in the wake of a host-parasite encounter (Fig. 1) brought to the fore the rather overlooked subject of RNA damage repair. RNA is susceptible to the same agents that threaten DNA. Radiation and chemicals that break the DNA backbone and modify its bases have similar effects on RNA and its precursors. RNA is also attacked by stress responsive RNases (Thompson & Parker, 2009) and various secreted ribotoxins (Wool *et al*, 1992;Masaki & Ogawa, 2002;Lu *et al*, 2005). What is more, its backbone is more sensitive to spontaneous hydrolysis than DNA's. Yet, the repair of damaged RNA seems necessary only in cases where its replenishment by re-synthesis is not possible, e.g., when a DNA template to transcribe from is missing.

Thus, it is conceivable that RNA repair tools played a critical role in sustaining the genomes of the hypothetical RNA and RNA/Protein Worlds (Cech, 2009). One may further speculate that some of these tools could have evolved into extant devices with similar RNA repair tasks or expatiated roles in other RNA transactions (Abelson *et al*, 1998;Sidrauski *et al*, 1996) or even in DNA repair (Aas *et al*, 2003;Tell *et al*, 2010).

RNA repair can be the only option also in extant situations, especially when a DNA template to transcribe from is missing. A relevant example already given here is the reliance of phage T4 on its tRNA repair proteins as a means to overcome the disruption of $tRNA^{Lys}$ by the host's ACNase PrrC (section 2.1). Another relevant example is the AlkB RNA demethylase of certain single stranded plant RNA viruses. The intended role of this demethylase is probably the removal of toxic methyl groups from the viral genomic RNA (van den *et al*, 2008). Homologous bacterial and human RNA-specific AlkB methylases could save the resources and/or time needed to re-synthesize damaged RNAs. In fact, these enzymes have been found able to resuscitate damaged RNA models while distinguishing between natural base modifications and toxic ones. However, the biological relevance of these findings remains uncertain (Aas *et al*, 2003;Ougland *et al*, 2004). Another DNA repair protein with possible roots in RNA metabolism is the abasic DNA endonuclease APE1 (Tell *et al*, 2010). Below we focus on recently discovered cellular tools able to repair nicked RNA, as do the phage T4-encoded proteins Pnk and Rnl1 that counteract PrrC and are frustrated perhaps by RloC.

4.2 Cellular RNA nick repair systems

The RNA phosphodiester linkage is vulnerable to nucleophilic attack. Deprotonation of its adjacent 2' oxygen, subsequent formation of a pentameric phosphate intermediate and 5'-O protonation disrupt it, yielding 2', 3' cyclic phosphate and 5'-OH cleavage ends. This reaction occurs spontaneously and nonspecifically under physiological conditions but is also catalyzed at critical target sites by stress-responsive tRNases (Thompson & Parker, 2009) and secreted ribotoxins (Wool *et al*, 1992;Masaki & Ogawa, 2002;Lu *et al*, 2005;Jablonowski *et al*, 2006;Klassen *et al*, 2008). Some of the small self-cleaving ribozymes that catalyze it also catalyze the reverse reaction, converting 2',3'-cyclic-P and 5'-OH ends into a 3'-5' phosphodiester linkage (Ferre-D'Amare & Scott, 2010). A similar RNA ligase activity involved in tRNA splicing was detected early on in HeLa cell extracts (Filipowicz & Shatkin, 1983) and later in an archaeon (Gomes & Gupta, 1997). The protein catalyzing it termed RtcB has been recently identified in an archaeon, human cells and bacteria (Englert *et al*, 2011;Popow *et al*, 2011;Tanaka & Shuman, 2011). The archaeal and human proteins join 5' and 3' exons of tRNAs and the human possibly also those of the mRNA of an unfolded-protein-response factor (Englert *et al*, 2011;Popow *et al*, 2011). A role for the bacterial RtcB has not been assigned yet. However, its possible participation in an RNA-nick-repair pathway is suggested by the operon RtcB shares with the RNA 3'-P cyclase RtcA. RtcA turns the 3'-P end into 2', 3'-P> through an adenylated intermediate, analogous to the manner in which RNA and DNA ligases activate 5'-P termini (Genschik *et al*, 1998). Thus, combined, RtcAB could convert a 3'-P and 5'-OH pair into a 3'-5' phosphodiester linkage. Unlike RtcA, the RtcB mediated transesterification reaction does not require an energy source although it may be allosterically directed by bound GTP (Tanaka & Shuman, 2011). Given their ability to repair such RNA nicks, RtcAB or RtcB alone could mend accidentally broken RNAs, restore RNAs temporarily inactivated by stress-responsive RNases (Neubauer *et al*, 2009;Zhang *et al*, 2005) or counteract ribotoxins secreted by rival cells (Masaki & Ogawa, 2002). Moreover, the existence of both RtcA and RtcB in all three domains of life (Tanaka & Shuman, 2011;Englert *et al*, 2011;Popow *et al*, 2011) suggests that their cooperation could be rather widespread.

A more intricate RNA-nick-repair pathway is catalyzed by the bacterial proteins PnkP and Hen1. PnkP and Hen1 share the same operon and form a tetrameric P_2H_2 complex (Martins & Shuman, 2005;Chan *et al*, 2009b). The reactions catalyzed by the PnkP component of the complex resemble those mediated by phage T4 Pnk and Rnl1 (section 1) and the yeast and plant tRNA splicing ligase (Abelson *et al*, 1998). What makes this repair system unique is its ability to render the restored phosphodiester linkage immune to re-cleavage by virtue of the 2'-O methylase activity of Hen1 (Chan *et al*, 2009b). PnkP comprises an N-terminal kinase domain, a central metallophosphoesterase domain and a C-terminal ligase domain. Thus, it comprises functions similar to those of the yeast tRNA splicing ligase but differs in domain order and different origin of the phosphoesterase domain (Apostol *et al*, 1991;Martins & Shuman, 2005). Interestingly, by itself the bacterial PnkP heals 2', 3'-cyclic P and 5'-OH termini pairs and undergoes the first step in the RNA ligase reaction, its auto-adenylation, but does not proceed to activate the 5'-P end and generate the phosphodiester linkage (Martins & Shuman, 2005). This deficiency is corrected by expressing PnkP with the 2'-O methylase Hen1. Within the resultant PnkP/Hen1 complex PnkP heals and seals the cleavage termini while Hen1 2'-O methylates the dephosphorylated 3'-end prior to the ligation step. This modification renders the restored ligation junction immune to re-cleavage (Chan *et al*, 2009b). The bacterial Hen1 is so named because it resembles in sequence and structure the methylase domain of eukaryal miRNA methyltransferase Hen1 (Chan *et al*, 2009a). The eukaryal Hen1 protects the 3'-terminal ribose of miRNA from exonucleolytic degradation or utilization as replication primer (Chen, 2005).

As with bacterial RtcAB, the biological role of the PnkP/Hen1 is not known. Noteworthy in this regard is that PnkP/Hen1 is most abundant among *Actinobacteria.* In contrast, RtcAB is more prevalent among *Proteobacteria* and has not been detected yet in *Actinobacteria.* This coincidence raises the possibility that the two systems provide similar benefits to their respective hosts. In theory, PnkP/Hen1 complexes could defend their host cells from secreted ribotoxins more efficiently than RtcAB due to the ability to prevent re-cleavage of the susceptible RNA. It is noteworthy though that colicin-like ribotoxins that target rRNA (Bowman *et al*, 1971;Senior & Holland, 1971) or tRNA anticodon loops (Masaki & Ogawa, 2002) have not been identified yet in bacteria likely to accommodate PnkP/Hen1.

If PnkP/Hen1 were to counteract an ACNase that cleaves its substrate 3' to the wobble base like colicin E5 (Ogawa *et al*, 1999), then the repaired tRNA would contain a 2'-O methylated wobble nucleotide. Such a protective modification need not impair the tRNA's function since it exists in some natural bacterial tRNAs (Juhling *et al*, 2009). However, it cannot be excluded that PnkP/Hen1 plays additional or other roles and may be exploited differently in different bacterial hosts. One example of such a different role is hinted at by the juxtaposition of the PnkP/Hen1 and CRISPR-Cas loci of *Microscilla marina*. The CRISPR-Cas system confers adaptive immunity against foreign nucleic acids. During its antiviral interference activity specific RNA portions of the CRISPR transcript are used to target a Cas protein to cleave the invasive nucleic acid (Deveau *et al*, 2010). Hence, it may be asked if *M. marina* PnkP/Hen1 catalyze some RNA processing and/or modification steps during CRISPR RNA maturation. Finally, in a reversal of roles, one could envisage PnkP/Hen1 encoding phage able to prevent re-cleavage of a tRNA by the ACNase they counteract.

4.3 An essential eukaryal DNA repair protein is related to T4 Pnk

There are a number of examples of DNA repair devices that could have originated from RNA-specific progenitors, some of them already alluded to above. Here it will suffice to describe just one of them, related to the phage T4-encoded end healing protein Pnk. This conserved eukaryal protein termed interchangeably PNKP and Pnk1 contains 5'-kinase and 3'-phosphatase domains resembling those of T4 Pnk but arranged in the reverse order, the phosphoesterase domain preceding the kinase domain. The mammalian PNKP is also endowed with an N-terminal FHA (Fork Head Associated) phosphopeptide binding domain that links PNKP to the scaffold proteins XRCC1 and XRCC4 (Bernstein *et al*, 2009). The latter recruit PNKP to exercise its functions in base excision repair (Hegde *et al*, 2008) or NHEJ (Lieber, 2008). PNKP's essential role in these ssDNA and DSB repair pathways is to convert 3'-P and 5'-OH DNA termini into 3'-OH and 5'-P pairs that are ligatable or fit for gap-filling by a DNA polymerase. A wide DNA binding cleft accounts for the ability of this protein to prefer nicked duplexes and recessed 5'-termini over ssDNA substrates and distinguishes it from the RNA end healing phage counterpart. The 3'-P and 5'-OH DNA termini are caused by ionizing radiation, genotoxic chemicals and enzymatic reactions. Specific examples include excision of abasic sites (Hazra *et al*, 2002), DSB generated by DNase II (Evans & Aguilera, 2003) and release of camptothecin- trapped topoisomerase I-DNA adducts by a tyrosine-DNA specific phosphodiesterase (Pouliot *et al*, 1999). Failure to repair such lesions underlies several inborn neural disorders. Conversely, PNKP can render cancer cells resistant to certain genotoxic drugs and, therefore, is considered itself a potential therapeutic target (Weinfeld *et al*, 2011).

5. Conclusions

In this chapter we addressed the possible biological role of the conserved bacterial anticodon nuclease RloC that combines two seemingly conflicting properties. One, predicted by resemblance of its regulatory region to the universal DNA-damage-checkpoint/DNA repair protein Rad50/SbcC is monitoring DNA insults. The second, predicted by its tRNase activity is disabling the translation apparatus. The co-existence of such functions in the same molecule and the regulation of one by the other suggests that RloC is designed to block translation in response to DNA damage. Such a response is suicidal since it prevents recovery from DNA damage. Hence, it must be executed only under special circumstances where cell death is advantageous. One possibility considered here is that RloC benefits its host cell by acting as an antiviral contingency during recovery from DNA damage. Under these conditions bacterial cells may shut off their primary antiviral defense, i.e., their DNA restriction activity. RloC's suicidal activity would not rescue the infected cell but would prevent the spread of the infection to other vulnerable members of the population recovering from DNA damage.

Another unique property, which could make RloC particularly suited to thwart phage infection, is the ability of this ACNase to excise its substrate's wobble nucleotide. In this regard RloC differs from its distant homologue the ACNase PrrC, which only incises its tRNA substrate and is counteracted by phage tRNA repair enzymes. Therefore, it seems conceivable that the harsher lesion inflicted by RloC will encumber such phage reversal. The possibility that RloC is a more efficient antiviral device than PrrC is also hinted at by its ~3-fold more frequent occurrence among bacteria.

While these notions are supported by some demonstrated properties of RloC, testing them and identifying RloC's true call requires studying this protein under physiological conditions; ideally, using a natural host encoding it and cognate phages endowed with tRNA repair enzymes.

The RNA repair pathway instigated by PrrC and possibly avoided by RloC brings to the fore the rather overlooked issue of RNA damage repair. Such repair would seem necessary only under circumstances such as the absence of a DNA template to transcribe from. Nonetheless, recent discoveries of various cellular RNA repair devices distributed in the three domains of life suggest that RNA damage repair is more prevalent, exercised perhaps also during responses to nutritional, pathogenic and other forms of stress. RNA repair is also of interest because many of its devices seem to have evolved to serve in other RNA transactions and even in DNA repair. Conversely, the vast repertoire of DNA repair, RNA splicing and RNA editing reactions may be exploited by investigators to discover novel RNA repair phenomena.

Work in G.K's laboratory was supported by grants from the Israeli Science Foundation, Jerusalem, the United States-Israel Bi-national Science Foundation and the Israeli Ministry of Science. G.K. is an incumbent of the Louise and Nahum Barag Chair in Cancer Molecular Genetics.

6. References

Aas,P.A., Otterlei,M., Falnes,P.O., Vagbo,C.B., Skorpen,F., Akbari,M., Sundheim,O., Bjoras,M., Slupphaug,G., Seeberg,E., & Krokan,H.E. (2003) Human and bacterial oxidative demethylases repair alkylation damage in both RNA and DNA. *Nature*, 421, 859-863.

Abelson,J., Trotta,C.R., & Li,H. (1998) tRNA splicing. *Journal of Biological Chemistry*, 273, 12685-12688.

Ambudkar,S.V., Kim,I.W., Xia,D., & Sauna,Z.E. (2006) The A-loop, a novel conserved aromatic acid subdomain upstream of the Walker A motif in ABC transporters, is critical for ATP binding. *FEBS Lett.*, 580, 1049-1055.

Amitsur,M., Benjamin,S., Rosner,R., Chapman-Shimshoni,D., Meidler,R., Blanga,S., & Kaufmann,G. (2003) Bacteriophage T4-encoded Stp can be replaced as activator of anticodon nuclease by a normal host cell metabolite. *Mol.Microbiol.*, 50, 129-143.

Amitsur,M., Levitz,R., & Kaufmann,G. (1987) Bacteriophage T4 anticodon nuclease, polynucleotide kinase and RNA ligase reprocess the host lysine tRNA. *The EMBO Journal*, 6, 2499-2503.

Amitsur,M., Morad,I., Chapman-Shimshoni,D., & Kaufmann,G. (1992) HSD restriction-modification proteins partake in latent anticodon nuclease. *The EMBO Journal*, 11, 3129-3134.

Apostol,B.L., Westaway,S.K., Abelson,J., & Greer,C.L. (1991) Deletion analysis of a multifunctional yeast tRNA ligase polypeptide. Identification of essential and dispensable functional domains. *Journal of Biological Chemistry*, 266, 7445-7455.

Becker,A. & Hurwitz,J. (1967) The enzymatic cleavage of phosphate termini from polynucleotides. *Journal of Biological Chemistry*, 242, 936-950.

Belogurov,A.A., Delver,E.P., Agafonova,O.V., Belogurova,N.G., Lee,L.Y., & Kado,C.I. (2000) Antirestriction protein Ard (Type C) encoded by IncW plasmid pSa has a high similarity to the "protein transport" domain of TraC1 primase of promiscuous plasmid RP4. *Journal of Molecular Biology*, 296, 969-977.

Bernstein,N.K., Hammel,M., Mani,R.S., Weinfeld,M., Pelikan,M., Tainer,J.A., & Glover,J.N. (2009) Mechanism of DNA substrate recognition by the mammalian DNA repair enzyme, Polynucleotide Kinase. *Nucleic Acids Res.*, 37, 6161-6173.

Blakely,G.W. & Murray,N.E. (2006) Control of the endonuclease activity of type I restriction-modification systems is required to maintain chromosome integrity following homologous recombination. *Mol.Microbiol.*, 60, 883-893.

Blanga-Kanfi,S., Amitsur,M., Azem,A., & Kaufmann,G. (2006) PrrC-anticodon nuclease: functional organization of a prototypical bacterial restriction RNase. *Nucleic Acids Res.*, 34, 3209-3219.

Blondal,T., Hjorleifsdottir,S., Aevarsson,A., Fridjonsson,O.H., Skirnisdottir,S., Wheat,J.O., Hermannsdottir,A.G., Hreggvidsson,G.O., Smith,A.V., & Kristjansson,J.K. (2005) Characterization of a 5'-polynucleotide kinase/3'-phosphatase from bacteriophage RM378. *J Biol.Chem.*, 280, 5188-5194.

Blondal,T., Hjorleifsdottir,S.H., Fridjonsson,O.F., Aevarsson,A., Skirnisdottir,S., Hermannsdottir,A.G., Hreggvidsson,G.O., Smith,A.V., & Kristjansson,J.K. (2003) Discovery and characterization of a thermostable bacteriophage RNA ligase homologous to T4 RNA ligase 1. *Nucleic Acids Res.*, 31, 7247-7254.

Bowman,C.M., Dahlberg,J.E., Ikemura,T., Konisky,J., & Nomura,M. (1971) Specific inactivation of 16S ribosomal RNA induced by colicin E3 in vivo. *Proc.Natl.Acad.Sci.U.S.A*, 68, 964-968.

Cameron,V. & Uhlenbeck,O.C. (1977) 3' Phosphatase activity in T4-polynucleotide kinase. *Biochemistry*, 16, 5120-5126.

Cech,T.R. (2009) Evolution of biological catalysis: ribozyme to RNP enzyme. *Cold Spring Harb.Symp.Quant.Biol.*, 74, 11-16.

Chan,C.M., Zhou,C., Brunzelle,J.S., & Huang,R.H. (2009a) Structural and biochemical insights into 2'-O-methylation at the 3'-terminal nucleotide of RNA by Hen1. *Proc.Natl.Acad.Sci.U.S.A.*

Chan,C.M., Zhou,C., & Huang,R.H. (2009b) Reconstituting Bacterial RNA Repair and Modification in Vitro. *Science*, 326, 247.

Chapman,D., Morad,I., Kaufmann,G., Gait,M.J., Jorissen,L., & Snyder,L. (1988) Nucleotide and deduced amino acid sequence of *stp*: the bacteriophage T4 anticodon nuclease gene. *Journal of Molecular Biology*, 199, 373-377.

Chen,J., Lu,G., Lin,J., Davidson,A.L., & Quiocho,F.A. (2003) A tweezers-like motion of the ATP-binding cassette dimer in an ABC transport cycle. *Mol.Cell*, 12, 651-661.

Chen,X. (2005) MicroRNA biogenesis and function in plants. *FEBS Lett.*, 579, 5923-5931.

Connelly,J.C., Kirkham,L.A., & Leach,D.R. (1998) The SbcCD nuclease of Escherichia coli is a structural maintenance of chromosomes (SMC) family protein that cleaves hairpin DNA. *Proc.Natl.Acad.Sci.U.S.A*, 95, 7969-7974.

Cromie,G.A., Connelly,J.C., & Leach,D.R. (2001) Recombination at double-strand breaks and DNA ends: conserved mechanisms from phage to humans. *Mol.Cell*, 8, 1163-1174.

Darmon,E., Eykelenboom,J.K., Lincker,F., Jones,L.H., White,M., Okely,E., Blackwood,J.K., & Leach,D.R. (2010) E. coli SbcCD and RecA control chromosomal rearrangement induced by an interrupted palindrome. *Mol.Cell*, 39, 59-70.

Darmon,E., Lopez-Vernaza,M.A., Helness,A.C., Borking,A., Wilson,E., Thacker,Z., Wardrope,L., & Leach,D.R. (2007) SbcCD regulation and localization in Escherichia coli. *Journal of Bacteriology*, 189, 6686-6694.

David,M., Borasio,G.D., & Kaufmann,G. (1982) Bacteriophage T4-induced anticodon-loop nuclease detected in a host strain restrictive to RNA ligase mutants. *Proceedings of the National Academy of Sciences U.S.A.*, 79, 7097-7101.

Davidov,E. & Kaufmann,G. (2008) RloC: a wobble nucleotide-excising and zinc-responsive bacterial tRNase. *Mol.Microbiol.*, 69, 1560-1574.

Depew,R.E. & Cozzarelli,N.R. (1974) Genetics and physiology of bacteriophage T4 3'-phosphatase: evidence for the involvement of the enzyme in T4 DNA metabolism. *Journal of Virology*, 13, 888-897.

Depew,R.E., Snopek,T.J., & Cozzarelli,N.R. (1975) Characterization of a new class of deletions of the D region of the bacteriophage T4 genome. *Virology*, 64, 144-145.

Deveau,H., Garneau,J.E., & Moineau,S. (2010) CRISPR/Cas system and its role in phage-bacteria interactions. *Annu.Rev.Microbiol.*, 64, 475-493.

Dryden,D.T., Murray,N.E., & Rao,D.N. (2001) Nucleoside triphosphate-dependent restriction enzymes. *Nucleic Acids Res.*, 29, 3728-3741.

El Omari K., Ren,J., Bird,L.E., Bona,M.K., Klarmann,G., LeGrice,S.F., & Stammers,D.K. (2006) Molecular architecture and ligand recognition determinants for T4 RNA ligase. *Journal of Biological Chemistry*, 281, 1573-1579.

Englert,M., Sheppard,K., Aslanian,A., Yates,J.R., III, & Soll,D. (2011) Archaeal 3'-phosphate RNA splicing ligase characterization identifies the missing component in tRNA maturation. *Proc.Natl.Acad.Sci.U.S.A*, 108, 1290-1295.

Evans,C.J. & Aguilera,R.J. (2003) DNase II: genes, enzymes and function. *Gene*, 322, 1-15.

Fernandez De Henestrosa,A.R., Ogi,T., Aoyagi,S., Chafin,D., Hayes,J.J., Ohmori,H., & Woodgate,R. (2000) Identification of additional genes belonging to the LexA regulon in Escherichia coli. *Mol.Microbiol.*, 35, 1560-1572.

Ferre-D'Amare,A.R. & Scott,W.G. (2010) Small self-cleaving ribozymes. *Cold Spring Harb.Perspect.Biol.*, 2, a003574.

Filipowicz,W. & Shatkin,A.J. (1983) Origin of splice junction phosphate in tRNAs processed by HeLa cell extract. *Cell*, 32, 547-557.

Friedberg,E.C., Walker,G.C., Siede,W., Wood,R.D., & Ellenberger,T. (2006) *DNA Repair And Mutagenesis,* Second edn, p. 1. ASM Press, Washington, DC.

Galburt,E.A., Pelletier,J., Wilson,G., & Stoddard,B.L. (2002) Structure of a tRNA Repair Enzyme and Molecular Biology Workhorse: T4 Polynucleotide Kinase. *Structure*, 10, 1249-1260.

Genschik,P., Drabikowski,K., & Filipowicz,W. (1998) Characterization of the Escherichia coli RNA 3'-terminal phosphate cyclase and its sigma54-regulated operon. *Journal of Biological Chemistry*, 273, 25516-25526.

Gerlt,J.A. (1993) Mechanistic principles of enzyme-catalyzed cleavage of phosphodiester bonds. Nucleases (ed. by S. M. Linn, R. S. Lloyd, & R. J. Roberts), pp. 1-34. Cold Spring Harbor Laboratory Press, Plainview NY.

Gomes,I. & Gupta,R. (1997) RNA splicing ligase activity in the archaeon Haloferax volcanii. *Biochem.Biophys.Res.Commun.*, 237, 588-594.

Guo,X., Chen,X., Weber,I.T., Harrison,R.W., & Tai,P.C. (2006) Molecular basis for differential nucleotide binding of the nucleotide-binding domain of ABC-transporter CvaB. *Biochemistry*, 45, 14473-14480.

Hazra,T.K., Izumi,T., Boldogh,I., Imhoff,B., Kow,Y.W., Jaruga,P., Dizdaroglu,M., & Mitra,S. (2002) Identification and characterization of a human DNA glycosylase for repair of modified bases in oxidatively damaged DNA. *Proc.Natl.Acad.Sci.U.S.A*, 99, 3523-3528.

Hegde,M.L., Hazra,T.K., & Mitra,S. (2008) Early steps in the DNA base excision/single-strand interruption repair pathway in mammalian cells. *Cell Res.*, 18, 27-47.

Hirano,T. (2006) At the heart of the chromosome: SMC proteins in action. *Nat.Rev.Mol.Cell Biol.*, 7, 311-322.

Hirano,T. (2005) SMC proteins and chromosome mechanics: from bacteria to humans. *Philos.Trans.R.Soc.Lond B Biol.Sci.*, 360, 507-514.

Ho,C.K. & Shuman,S. (2002) Bacteriophage T4 RNA ligase 2 (gp24.1) exemplifies a family of RNA ligases found in all phylogenetic domains. *Proceedings National Academy of Sciences USA*, 99, 12709-12714.

Hopfner,K.P., Craig,L., Moncalian,G., Zinkel,R.A., Usui,T., Owen,B.A., Karcher,A., Henderson,B., Bodmer,J.L., McMurray,C.T., Carney,J.P., Petrini,J.H., & Tainer,J.A. (2002) The Rad50 zinc-hook is a structure joining Mre11 complexes in DNA recombination and repair. *Nature*, 418, 562-566.

Hopfner,K.P., Karcher,A., Shin,D.S., Craig,L., Arthur,L.M., Carney,J.P., & Tainer,J.A. (2000) Structural biology of Rad50 ATPase: ATP-driven conformational control in DNA double-strand break repair and the ABC-ATPase superfamily. *Cell*, 101, 789-800.

Hopfner,K.P. & Tainer,J.A. (2003) Rad50/SMC proteins and ABC transporters: unifying concepts from high-resolution structures. *Curr.Opin.Struct.Biol.*, 13, 249-255.

Jabbar,M.A. & Snyder,L. (1984) Genetic and physiological studies of an Escherichia coli locus that restricts polynucleotide kinase- and RNA ligase-deficient mutants of bacteriophage T4. *Journal of Virology*, 51, 522-529.

Jablonowski,D., Zink,S., Mehlgarten,C., Daum,G., & Schaffrath,R. (2006) tRNAGlu wobble uridine methylation by Trm9 identifies Elongator's key role for zymocin-induced cell death in yeast. *Mol.Microbiol.*, 59, 677-688.

Janscak,P., Sandmeier,U., Szczelkun,M.D., & Bickle,T.A. (2001) Subunit assembly and mode of DNA cleavage of the type III restriction endonucleases EcoP1I and EcoP15I. *Journal of Molecular Biology*, 306, 417-431.

Jiang,Y., Blanga,S., Amitsur,M., Meidler,R., Krivosheyev,E., Sundaram,M., Bajji,A.C., Davis,D.R., & Kaufmann,G. (2002) Structural features of tRNALys favored by anticodon nuclease as inferred from reactivities of anticodon stem and loop substrate analogs. *Journal of Biological Chemistry*, 277, 3836-3841.

Jiang,Y., Meidler,R., Amitsur,M., & Kaufmann,G. (2001) Specific Interaction between Anticodon Nuclease and the tRNA(Lys) Wobble Base. *Journal of Molecular Biology*, 305, 377-388.

Juhling,F., Morl,M., Hartmann,R.K., Sprinzl,M., Stadler,P.F., & Putz,J. (2009) tRNAdb 2009: compilation of tRNA sequences and tRNA genes. *Nucleic Acids Res.*, 37, D159-D162.

Kaufmann,G. & Kallenbach,N.R. (1975) Determination of recognition sites of T4 RNA ligase on the 3'-OH and 5' -P termini of polyribonucleotide chains. *Nature*, 254, 452-454.

Klaiman,D., Amitsur,M., Blanga-Kanfi,S., Chai,M., Davis,D.R., & Kaufmann,G. (2007) Parallel dimerization of a PrrC-anticodon nuclease region implicated in tRNALys recognition. *Nucleic Acids Res.*, 35, 4704-4714.

Klaiman,D. & Kaufmann,G. (2011) Phage T4-induced dTTP accretion bolsters a tRNase-based host defense. *Virology*, 414, 97-101.

Klassen,R., Paluszynski,J.P., Wemhoff,S., Pfeiffer,A., Fricke,J., & Meinhardt,F. (2008) The primary target of the killer toxin from Pichia acaciae is tRNA(Gln). *Mol.Microbiol.*

Levitz,R., Chapman,D., Amitsur,M., Green,R., Snyder,L., & Kaufmann,G. (1990) The optional *E. coli prr* locus encodes a latent form of phage T4-induced anticodon nuclease. *The EMBO Journal*, 9, 1383-1389.

Lieber,M.R. (2008) The mechanism of human nonhomologous DNA end joining. *Journal of Biological Chemistry*, 283, 1-5.

Linder,P., Doelz,R., Gubler,M., & Bickle,T.A. (1990) An anticodon nuclease gene inserted into a *hsd* region encoding a type I DNA restriction system. *Nucleic Acids Res.*, 18, 7170.

Lu,J., Huang,B., Esberg,A., Johansson,M.J., & Bystrom,A.S. (2005) The Kluyveromyces lactis gamma-toxin targets tRNA anticodons. *RNA.*, 11, 1648-1654.

Makovets,S., Powell,L.M., Titheradge,A.J., Blakely,G.W., & Murray,N.E. (2004) Is modification sufficient to protect a bacterial chromosome from a resident restriction endonuclease? *Mol.Microbiol.*, 51, 135-147.

Martins,A. & Shuman,S. (2005) An end-healing enzyme from Clostridium thermocellum with 5' kinase, 2',3' phosphatase, and adenylyltransferase activities. *RNA.*, 11, 1271-1280.

Masaki,H. & Ogawa,T. (2002) The modes of action of colicins E5 and D, and related cytotoxic tRNases. *Biochimie*, 84, 433-438.

Mascarenhas,J., Sanchez,H., Tadesse,S., Kidane,D., Krisnamurthy,M., Alonso,J.C., & Graumann,P.L. (2006) Bacillus subtilis SbcC protein plays an important role in DNA inter-strand cross-link repair. *BMC.Mol.Biol.*, 7, 20.

Mathews,C.K. (1994) An overview of the T4 develpmental program. Molecular Biology of bacteriophage T4 (ed. by J. D. Karam, J. W. Drake, K. N. Kreuzer, G. Mosig, D. W. Hall, F. A. Eiserling, L. W. Black, E. K. Spicer, E. Kutter, K. Carlson, & E. S. Miller), pp. 1-8. American Society for Microbiology, Washigton, DC.

Meidler,R., Morad,I., Amitsur,M., Inokuchi,H., & Kaufmann,G. (1999) Detection of Anticodon Nuclease Residues Involved in tRNALys Cleavage Specificity. *Journal of Molecular Biology*, 287, 499-510.

Meineke,B., Schwer,B., Schaffrath,R., & Shuman,S. (2010) Determinants of eukaryal cell killing by the bacterial ribotoxin PrrC. *Nucleic Acids Res.*

Miller,E.S., Heidelberg,J.F., Eisen,J.A., Nelson,W.C., Durkin,A.S., Ciecko,A., Feldblyum,T.V., White,O., Paulsen,I.T., Nierman,W.C., Lee,J., Szczypinski,B., & Fraser,C.M. (2003a) Complete genome sequence of the broad-host-range vibriophage KVP40: comparative genomics of a T4-related bacteriophage. *J Bacteriol.*, 185, 5220-5233.

Miller,E.S., Kutter,E., Mosig,G., Arisaka,F., Kunisawa,T., & Ruger,W. (2003b) Bacteriophage T4 Genome. *Microbiology and Molecular Biology Reviews*, 67, 86-156.

Miller,W.G., Pearson,B.M., Wells,J.M., Parker,C.T., Kapitonov,V.V., & Mandrell,R.E. (2005) Diversity within the Campylobacter jejuni type I restriction-modification loci. *Microbiology*, 151, 337-351.

Moody,J.E. & Thomas,P.J. (2005) Nucleotide binding domain interactions during the mechanochemical reaction cycle of ATP-binding cassette transporters. *J.Bioenerg.Biomembr.*, 37, 475-479.

Moreno-Herrero,F., de,J.M., Dekker,N.H., Kanaar,R., Wyman,C., & Dekker,C. (2005) Mesoscale conformational changes in the DNA-repair complex Rad50/Mre11/Nbs1 upon binding DNA. *Nature*, 437, 440-443.

Morera,S., Imberty,A., schke-Sonnenborn,U., Ruger,W., & Freemont,P.S. (1999) T4 phage beta-glucosyltransferase: substrate binding and proposed catalytic mechanism. *Journal of Molecular Biology*, 292, 717-730.

Murray,N.E. (2000) Type I restriction systems: sophisticated molecular machines (a legacy of Bertani and Weigle). *Microbiology and Molecular Biology Reviews*, 64, 412-434.

Neubauer,C., Gao,Y.G., Andersen,K.R., Dunham,C.M., Kelley,A.C., Hentschel,J., Gerdes,K., Ramakrishnan,V., & Brodersen,D.E. (2009) The structural basis for mRNA recognition and cleavage by the ribosome-dependent endonuclease RelE. *Cell*, 139, 1084-1095.

Novogrodsky,A., Tal,M., Traub,A., & Hurwitz,J. (1966) The enzymatic phosphorylation of ribonucleic acid and deoxyribonucleic acid. II. Further properties of the 5'-hydroxyl polynucleotide kinase. *Journal of Biological Chemistry*, 241, 2933-2943.

Ogawa,T., Tomita,K., Ueda,T., Watanabe,K., Uozumi,T., & Masaki,H. (1999) A Cytotoxic Ribonuclease Targeting Specific Transfer RNA Anticodons. *Science*, 283, 2097-2100.

Ougland,R., Zhang,C.M., Liiv,A., Johansen,R.F., Seeberg,E., Hou,Y.M., Remme,J., & Falnes,P.O. (2004) AlkB restores the biological function of mRNA and tRNA inactivated by chemical methylation. *Mol.Cell*, 16, 107-116.

Paull,T.T. (2010) Making the best of the loose ends: Mre11/Rad50 complexes and Sae2 promote DNA double-strand break resection. *DNA Repair (Amst)*, 9, 1283-1291.

Penner,M., Morad,I., Snyder,L., & Kaufmann,G. (1995) Phage T4-coded Stp: double-edged effector of coupled DNA and tRNA-restriction systems. *Journal of Molecular Biology*, 249, 857-868.

Popow,J., Englert,M., Weitzer,S., Schleiffer,A., Mierzwa,B., Mechtler,K., Trowitzsch,S., Will,C.L., Luhrmann,R., Soll,D., & Martinez,J. (2011) HSPC117 is the essential subunit of a human tRNA splicing ligase complex. *Science*, 331, 760-764.

Pouliot,J.J., Yao,K.C., Robertson,C.A., & Nash,H.A. (1999) Yeast gene for a Tyr-DNA phosphodiesterase that repairs topoisomerase I complexes. *Science*, 286, 552-555.

Richardson,C.C. (1965) Phosphorylation of nucleic acid by an enzyme from T4 bacteriophage infected E. coli. *Proceedings National Academy of Sciences USA*, 54, 158-165.

Runnels,J., Soltis,D., Hey,T., & Snyder,L. (1982) Genetic and physiological studies of the role of RNA ligase of bacteriophage T4. *Journal of Molecular Biology*, 154, 273-286.

Sargent,R.G. & Mathews,C.K. (1987) Imbalanced deoxyribonucleoside triphosphate pools and spontaneous mutation rates determined during dCMP deaminase-defective bacteriophage T4 infections. *Journal of Biological Chemistry*, 262, 5546-5553.

Schirmer,T. & Evans,P.R. (1990) Structural basis of the allosteric behaviour of phosphofructokinase. *Nature*, 343, 140-145.

Schmidt,F.J. & Apirion,D. (1983) T4 transfer RNAs: Pardigmatic System for the Study of RNA Processing. Bacteriophage T4 (ed. by C. K. Mathews, E. M. Kutter, G. Mosig, & P. B. Berget), pp. 193-217. American Society for Microbiology, Washington.

Senior,B.W. & Holland,I.B. (1971) Effect of colicin E3 upon the 30S ribosomal subunit of Escherichia coli. *Proc.Natl.Acad.Sci.U.S.A*, 68, 959-963.

Sidrauski,C., Cox,J.S., & Walter,P. (1996) tRNA ligase is required for regulated mRNA splicing in the unfolded protein response. *Cell*, 87, 405-413.

Silber,R., Malathi,V.G., & Hurwitz,J. (1972) Purification and properties of bacteriophage T4-induced RNA ligase. *Proceedings National Academy of Sciences USA*, 69, 3009-3013.

Sirotkin,K., Cooley,W., Runnels,J., & Snyder,L. (1978) A role in true-late gene expression for the T4 bacteriophage 5'-polynucleotide kinase 3'-phosphatase. *Journal of Molecular Biology*, 123, 221-233.

Stanley,L.K., Seidel,R., van der,S.C., Dekker,N.H., Szczelkun,M.D., & Dekker,C. (2006) When a helicase is not a helicase: dsDNA tracking by the motor protein EcoR124I. *The EMBO Journal*, 25, 2230-2239.

Steyaert,J. (1997) A decade of protein engineering on ribonuclease T1--atomic dissection of the enzyme-substrate interactions. *Eur.J Biochem.*, 247, 1-11.

Storvik,K.A. & Foster,P.L. (2011) The SMC-like protein complex SbcCD enhances DNA polymerase IV-dependent spontaneous mutation in Escherichia coli. *Journal of Bacteriology*, 193, 660-669.

Stracker,T.H. & Petrini,J.H. (2011) The MRE11 complex: starting from the ends. *Nat.Rev.Mol.Cell Biol.*, 12, 90-103.

Takami,H., Nishi,S., Lu,J., Shimamura,S., & Takaki,Y. (2004) Genomic characterization of thermophilic Geobacillus species isolated from the deepest sea mud of the Mariana Trench. *Extremophiles.*, 8, 351-356.

Tanaka,N. & Shuman,S. (2011) RtcB is the RNA ligase component of an Escherichia coli RNA repair operon. *Journal of Biological Chemistry*.

Tell,G., Wilson,D.M., III, & Lee,C.H. (2010) Intrusion of a DNA repair protein in the RNome world: is this the beginning of a new era? *Mol.Cell Biol.*, 30, 366-371.

Thompson,D.M. & Parker,R. (2009) Stressing out over tRNA cleavage. *Cell*, 138, 215-219.

Thoms,B. & Wackernagel,W. (1984) Genetic control of damage-inducible restriction alleviation in Escherichia coli K12: an SOS function not repressed by lexA. *Mol.Gen.Genet.*, 197, 297-303.

Tyndall,C., Meister,J., & Bickle,T.A. (1994) The Escherichia coli prr region encodes a functional type IC DNA restriction system closely integrated with an anticodon nuclease gene. *Journal of Molecular Biology*, 237, 266-274.

van den,B.E., Omelchenko,M.V., Bekkelund,A., Leihne,V., Koonin,E.V., Dolja,V.V., & Falnes,P.O. (2008) Viral AlkB proteins repair RNA damage by oxidative demethylation. *Nucleic Acids Res.*, 36, 5451-5461.

van Noort,J., van der Heijden,T., Dutta,C.F., Firman,K., & Dekker,C. (2004) Initiation of translocation by Type I restriction-modification enzymes is associated with a short DNA extrusion. *Nucleic Acids Res.*, 32, 6540-6547.

van,N.J., van Der,H.T., de,J.M., Wyman,C., Kanaar,R., & Dekker,C. (2003) The coiled-coil of the human Rad50 DNA repair protein contains specific segments of increased flexibility. *Proc.Natl.Acad.Sci.U.S.A*, 100, 7581-7586.

Weinfeld,M., Mani,R.S., Abdou,I., Aceytuno,R.D., & Glover,J.N. (2011) Tidying up loose ends: the role of polynucleotide kinase/phosphatase in DNA strand break repair. *Trends Biochem.Sci.*

Wheeler,L.J., Ray,N.B., Ungermann,C., Hendricks,S.P., Bernard,M.A., Hanson,E.S., & Mathews,C.K. (1996) T4 phage gene 32 protein as a candidate organizing factor for the deoxyribonucleoside triphosphate synthetase complex. *Journal of Biological Chemistry*, 271, 11156-11162.

White,M.A., Eykelenboom,J.K., Lopez-Vernaza,M.A., Wilson,E., & Leach,D.R. (2008) Non-random segregation of sister chromosomes in Escherichia coli. *Nature*, 455, 1248-1250.

Williams,G.J., Lees-Miller,S.P., & Tainer,J.A. (2010) Mre11-Rad50-Nbs1 conformations and the control of sensing, signaling, and effector responses at DNA double-strand breaks. *DNA Repair (Amst)*, 9, 1299-1306.

Williams,G.J., Williams,R.S., Williams,J.S., Moncalian,G., Arvai,A.S., Limbo,O., Guenther,G., Sildas,S., Hammel,M., Russell,P., & Tainer,J.A. (2011) ABC ATPase signature helices in Rad50 link nucleotide state to Mre11 interface for DNA repair. *Nat.Struct.Mol.Biol.*, 18, 423-431.

Williams,R.S., Williams,J.S., & Tainer,J.A. (2007) Mre11-Rad50-Nbs1 is a keystone complex connecting DNA repair machinery, double-strand break signaling, and the chromatin template. *Biochem.Cell Biol.*, 85, 509-520.

Wool,I.G., Gluck,A., & Endo,Y. (1992) Ribotoxin recognition of ribosomal RNA and a proposal for the mechanism of translocation. *Trends Biochem.Sci.*, 17, 266-269.

Yamagami,H. & Endo,H. (1969) Loss of lysis inhibition in filamentous Escherichia coli infected with wild-type bacteriophage T4. *Journal of Virology*, 3, 343-349.

Youell,J. & Firman,K. (2008) EcoR124I: from plasmid-encoded restriction-modification system to nanodevice. *Microbiology and Molecular Biology Reviews*, 72, 365-77, table.

Zhang,Y., Zhang,J., Hara,H., Kato,I., & Inouye,M. (2005) Insights into the mRNA cleavage mechanism by MazF, an mRNA interferase. *J Biol.Chem.*, 280, 3143-3150.

3

The Role of DDB2 in Regulating Cell Survival and Apoptosis Following DNA Damage - A Mini-Review

Chuck C.-K. Chao
Department of Biochemistry and Molecular Biology
Graduate Institute of Biomedical Sciences, Chang Gung University, Taiwan
Republic of China

1. Introduction

Nucleotide excision repair (NER) represents a central cellular process for the removal of structurally and chemically diverse DNA lesions [Friedberg et al., 2006]. Mutations in genes involved in NER are associated with rare autosomal recessive syndromes such as xeroderma pigmentosum (XP), a condition characterized by sensitivity to UV light, neurological abnormalities, and a propensity to develop skin cancer (Cleaver, 2005). The observation that cells from XP subgroup E (XP-E cells XP2RO and XP3RO) are defective in recognizing damaged DNA and performing NER highlighted the physiological importance of the protein termed DNA damage-binding protein, or DDB [Chu & Chang, 1988]. The DDB protein, sometimes also referred to as UV-DDB due to its high affinity and specificity for UV-damaged DNA, contains two principal subunits, DDB1 and DDB2 [Grossman, 1976; Keeney et al., 1993; Takao et al., 1993]. The DDB protein complex also binds to non-UV-damaged DNA, like cisplatin-modified DNA, although with much lower affinity. Although the history of DDB spans more than two decades, the complete understanding of its physiological functions remains to be clarified. The activity of DDB has been repeatedly described in crude mammalian cell extracts by electrophoretic mobility shift assays or filter-binding assays performed by different laboratories since the first report of its discovery [Feldberg & Grossman, 1976]. Notably, micro-injections of DDB complexes into the nucleus of XP-E cells restored NER activity [Keeney et al., 1994], supporting the notion that DDB participates in chromatin NER. The *DDB1* gene from simian cells was the first *DDB* gene to be identified [Takao et al., 1993]. The human *DDB1* and *DDB2* genes were subsequently sequenced [Dualan et al., 1995; Lee et al., 1995]. Soon after, DNA sequencing from Linn's laboratory revealed that *DDB2* is mutated in XP-E cells which lack DDB activity [Nichols et al., 1996; Tang & Chu, 2002]. The predicted DDB2 protein sequence was shown to contain several functional domains, including WD40 repeats, post-translation modification sites (e.g. acetylation, phosphorylation, and ubiquitination), DDB1- and DNA-binding sites, as well as a DWD box. Notably, in a majority of XP-E cell lines, DDB2 was found to be altered at domains other than the one required for binding DNA. Thus, DDB appears to be regulated at several levels in UV-irradiated cells, including by transcriptional activation of DDB2 mRNA, post-translational modification, translocation to the nucleus, complex formation, and proteolytic degradation of DDB2 protein through ubiquitination [for a recent review, see Sugasawa, 2010]. Notably, 60% of chromatin-bound DDB2 is degraded within 4 hrs of UV irradiation. After 48 hrs, DDB2 mRNA levels increase several fold above the level seen in non-irradiated cells [Nichols et al., 2000; Rapic-Otrin et al., 2002]. Interestingly, the majority of UV-induced DNA photoproducts in human cells are repaired by this time [Mitchell et al., 1985].

2. DDB2 recognizes DNA damage during global genome NER

NER removes diverse DNA lesions, ranging from UV-induced cyclobutane pyrimidine dimers (CPD) and 6-4 pyrimidine-pyrimidone photoproducts (6-4PP) to a variety of bulky adducts formed by environmental carcinogens. Mammalian NER comprises global genome NER (GG-NER) and transcription-coupled NER (TC-NER). These two processes involve similar but distinct repair proteins that process DNA damage and chromatin proteins like histones may significantly regulate the activity of repair proteins (reviewed by Friedberg et al., 2006). One such multiprotein complex involved in GG-NER and containing both DDB1 and DDB2 is closely related to a complex containing DDB1 and the Cockayne syndrome group A (CSA) protein in TC-NER. In GG-NER, DNA is initially surveyed for lesions by XP group C (XPC) protein-RAD23B (Sugasawa et al., 1998) and the UV-DDB complex (Fitch et al., 2003; Moser et al., 2005; Sugasawa et al., 2005). DDB2 binds to DDB1 to form the DDB complex which may recognize UV-induced DNA damage and recruit proteins of the NER pathway to initiate GG-NER (Hwang et al., 1999; Tang et al., 2000). The DDB complex preferentially binds to UV-induced CPD, 6-4PP, apurinic sites, and short mismatches (Fujiwara et al., 1999; Kulaksiz et al., 2005; Sugasawa et al., 2005; Wittschieben et al., 2005). While XPC functions as a versatile factor that senses abnormal DNA structures, DDB appears to recognize more specific types of lesions, particularly UV-induced 6-4PP, whereas binding to CPD is much weaker but nonetheless detectable [Payne & Chu, 1994]. Strikingly, structural analysis of DDB bound to DNA duplex containing 6-4PP has revealed that the DDB2 subunit is responsible for the interaction, and this subunit induces the movement of the two affected bases into a binding pocket, therefore indicating that DDB has evolved to specifically recognize dinucleotide lesions, like UV photolesions [Figure 1; Scrima et al., 2008]. Furthermore, accumulating evidence has confirmed the existence of multiple forms of DDB2 mRNA splicing variants, including isoforms D1 and D2, which do not interact with DDB1, but inhibit UV-damaged DNA repair (Inoki et al., 2004). DDB2 is ubiquitously expressed in human tissues, with the highest level being found in corneal endothelium and the lowest level in the brain. Isoform D1 is highly expressed in brain and heart tissues, whereas isoforms D2, D3, and D4 are weakly expressed in these tissues (Inoki et al., 2004). Interestingly, repair of DNA damage induced by UV light appears to be less active in brain and heart tissues which are naturally protected against UV irradiation and express high levels of isoform D1.

3. DDB2 links DNA repair to protein ubiquitination

Another breakthrough that links protein ubiquitination with GG-NER is the finding that DDB is part of an ubiquitin ligase (E3) complex. Epitope-tagged DDB2 purified from cells was found in complex with CUL4A, ROC1, DDB1, and the COP9 signalosome [Groisman et al., 2003]. Besides its function as part of the DDB-protein complex, DDB2 may function as a substrate-recognition module within the CUL4A ubiquitination complex. CUL4 is one of

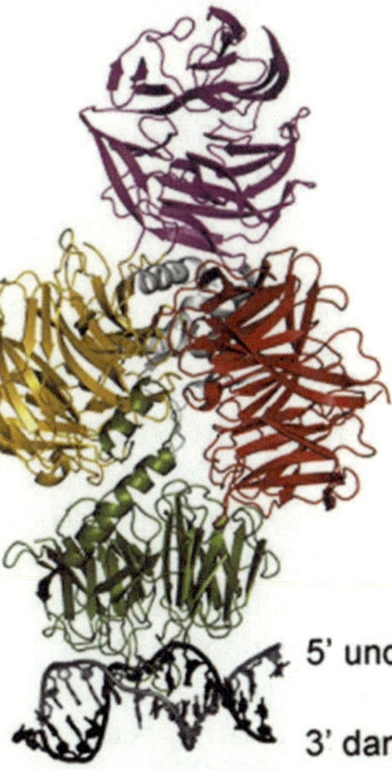

Fig. 1. Overall structure of the DDB1-DDB2-DNA complex. Ribbon representation of the DDB-DNA$^{6\text{-}4PP}$ complex: DDB2; DDB1-BPA; DDB1-BPB; DDB1-BPC; DDB1-CTD. The DNA$^{6\text{-}4PP}$ damaged and undamaged DNA strands are depicted in black and gray, respectively. DNA binding is carried out exclusively by the DDB2 subunit via its WD40 domain. The DDB1 structure consists of three WD40 β-propeller domains (BPA, BPB, and BPC) and a C-terminal helical domain (CTD, shown at the center). DDB2 binds to an interface between the DDB1 propellers BPA and BPC, where its helix-loop-helix motif inserts into a cavity formed by the two propellers. The structures reveal the molecular mechanism underlying high-affinity recognition of UV lesions (damaged DNA strand) that are refractory to detection by XPC. The structures also suggest a mechanism for the assembly of the DDB-CUL4 ubiquitin ligase in chromatin and provide a framework for understanding the ubiquitination of proteins proximal to damage sites. [For detail, see Scrima et al., 2008].

three founding cullins that are conserved from yeast to humans. A large number of E3 ubiquitin-protein ligase complexes are part of the DCX proteins (short for DDB1-CUL4-X-box). Components of the CUL4-DDB-ROC1 (also known as CUL4-DDB-RBX1) include CUL4A or CUL4B, DDB1, DDB2, and RBX1 (Chen et al., 2001; Groisman et al., 2003). Other CUL4-DDB-ROC1 complexes may also exist in which DDB2 is replaced by a subunit that targets an alternative substrate. These targeting subunits are generally known as DCAF proteins (short for DDB1- and CUL4-associated factor) or CDW (short for CUL4-DDB1-associated WD40-repeat; for reviews, see Lee & Zhou, 2007; Jackson & Xiong, 2009; Sugasawa, 2009). Many CUL4 complexes are involved in chromatin regulation and are frequently hijacked by viruses (reviewed by Jackson & Xiong, 2009). The DDB1-CUL4-ROC1 complex may ubiquitinate histones H2A, H3, and H4 at sites of UV-induced DNA damage (Wang et al., 2006; Kapetanaki et al., 2006; Guerrero-Santoro et al., 2008). The ubiquitination of histones may facilitate their removal from the nucleosome and promote assembly of NER components for subsequent DNA repair. Furthermore, the DDB1-CUL4-ROC1 complex ubiquitinates XPC and DDB2, which may enhance DNA binding by XPC and promote NER (El-Mahdy et al., 2006; Sugasawa et al., 2005). Structural analysis support the notion that CUL4 uses DDB1 as a large β-propeller protein and as a linker to interact with a subset of WD40 proteins like DDB2, which serves as substrate receptors, forming as many as 90 E3 complexes in mammals [Jackson & Xiong, 2009]. Taken together, these results indicate that DDB complex is a component of the CUL4A-based ubiquitin ligase DDB1-CUL4A^{DDB2}, and that DDB2 may coordinate the ubiquitination of various proteins at DNA damage sites during GG-NER.

In addition, CUL4B also binds to UV-damaged chromatin as a part of the DDB1-CUL4B^{DDB2} E3 ligase in the presence of functional DDB2. Nevertheless, CUL4B is localized in the nucleus and facilitates the transfer of DDB1 into the nucleus independently of DDB2 [Guerrero-Santoro et al., 2008]. Notably, DDB1-CUL4B^{DDB2} is more efficient than DDB1-CUL4A^{DDB2} in mono-ubiquitinating histone H2A in vitro, suggesting that the DDB1-CUL4B^{DDB2} E3 ligase may have a distinctive function in modifying the chromatin structure at sites of UV lesions and promoting efficient GG-NER. Intriguingly, the CSA protein, a WD40 motif protein defective in a complementation group of Cockayne's syndrome, forms a similar E3 complex in place of DDB2 at damage sites during TC-NER. Although not detected in the DDB2 and CSA complex, CUL4B is highly expressed in mammalian cells, and the two CUL4 isoforms CUL4A and CUL4B appear to be redundant, at least for some cellular functions [Higa et al., 2003; Hu et al., 2004].

4. DDB2 inhibits apoptosis in cultured cell lines and *Drosophila*

Although the regulation of the DDB2 gene is complex, evidence on the biological function of DDB2 in response to apoptotic stimuli has accumulated. Evidence from biochemical experiments has shown how DDB2 interacts with proteins, DNAs, and RNAs. Most strikingly, structural studies using X-ray crystallography support the evidence of biochemical studies, as seen for example with GG-NER. Nevertheless, a complete understanding of the biological roles of DDB2 remains to be fully elucidated. To assess this question, we explored the role of DDB2 in regulating UV sensitivity in both human cells and *Drosophila* [Sun et al., 2010]. As such, a full-length DDB2 open reading frame sequence was overexpressed in cells that express low or no DDB2. Conversely, DDB2 expression was suppressed in cells that endogenously express high levels of DDB2 by stable expression of full-length anti-sense cDNA. Using this strategy, we found that DDB2 displays a protective role against UV irradiation and cell surface death receptor signaling in both cisplatin-selected human HeLa cells and hamster V79 cells [Sun et al., 2002a; Sun et al., 2002b; Sun & Chao, 2005a]. Furthermore, cFLIP expression was upregulated by DDB2 in a dose- and time-dependent manner in HeLa cells, a process associated with inhibition of apoptosis [Sun & Chao, 2005a]. Inhibition of cFLIP by anti-sense oligonucleotides substantially inhibited apoptosis induced by UV irradiation and death receptor signaling in HeLa and other cell lines. Importantly, the protective effect of DDB2 was only detected in cells in which cFLIP is elicited during apoptotic stimuli. In contrast, DDB2 did not show a protective effect against apoptotic stimuli in human cell lines in which cFLIP expression was not induced [Sun et al., 2010]. A transcription reporter assay also showed that DDB2 induces the transcription of cFLIP in a p38/MAPK-dependent manner [Sun & Chao, 2005b], suggesting that the DDB2/cFLIP pathway may be active in specific cell conditions [Figure 2]. Surprisingly, overexpression of a DDB2 mutant (82TO) that does not significantly enhance DDB activity (Nichols et al., 1996), also protected HeLa cells from both UV- and Fas-induced cell death (Sun et al., 2002a; Sun & Chao, 2005a), suggesting that the protection effect of DDB2 may be independent of its DNA repair activity. Furthermore, ectopic expression of human DDB2 in *Drosophila* dramatically reduced UV-induced animal death compared to control GFP expression. On the other hand, expression of DDB2 in *Drosophila* failed to rescue a different type of apoptosis induced by the genes *reaper* or *eiger* [Sun et al., 2010]. Depletion of DDB2 in HeLa cells did not affect apoptosis induced by cisplatin or mitomycin C (Sun et al., 2002a). In addition, overexpression or inhibition of DDB2 in HeLa cells only slightly affected cisplatin-induced caspase-8 signaling and apoptosis (Sun & Chao, 2005a), probably due to the observation that cisplatin primarily induces mitochondrial apoptotic signaling (Gonzalez et al., 2001). These observations suggest that the modulation of apoptosis by DDB2 may be unique.

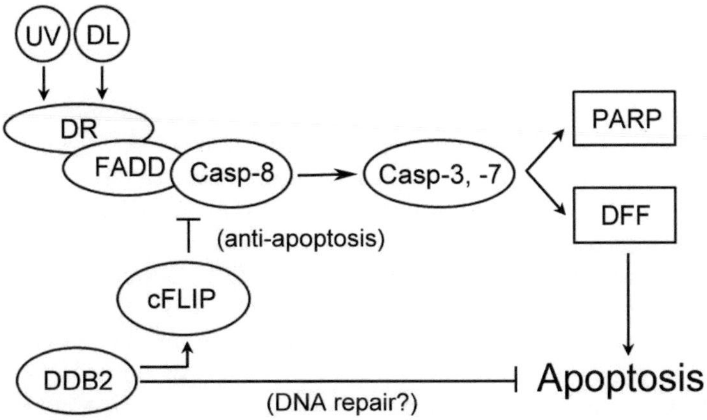

Fig. 2. Model illustrating the role of DDB2 in regulating non-DNA damage-induced apoptosis. An anti-apoptotic effect is proposed for DDB2 against death ligand- or UV-induced stress through cFLIP up-regulation. DDB2 transactivation of cFLIP is required to enhance their apoptosis-inhibitory function. UV- or death receptor-induced apoptosis is attenuated by the up-regulated cFLIP; consequently, activation of initiator caspases (3 and 7), cleavage of protein substrates (PARP and DFF), and apoptosis are inhibited. DDB2 may also attenuate UV-induced apoptosis through repair of DNA damage. However, evidence from protective DDB2 mutants suggests possible alternative pathways. DL, death ligands; DR, death receptors. [Modified from Sun and Chao, 2005a]

Cross-resistance to UV was found in cisplatin-selected cells, which overexpress DDB2 [Chu & Chang, 1990; Chao et al., 1991]. DDB2 is a transcriptional partner of E2F1; however, the target of DDBs/E2F1 has not been identified (Hayes et al., 1998; Shiyanov et al., 1999). We found that the overexpression of DDB2 increases the expression of cFLIP at both the mRNA and protein levels in resistant cells in which DDB2 has been genetically suppressed [Sun and Chao, 2005a]. E2F1 was also shown to regulate the expression of cFLIP (Stanelle et al., 2002). Therefore, cFLIP may represent the first potential target of DDB2/E2F1. E2F1 promotes TNF-induced apoptosis by stabilizing the TRAF2 protein (Phillips et al., 1999). However, the possibility that DDB2/E2F1 may co-activate cFLIP expression suggests a possible dual role for E2F1 in regulating cell survival and death. Additional overexpression of E2F1 does not increase endogenous cFLIP expression more than overexpression of DDB2 alone (Peng, 2008). Thus, the increased level of E2F1 observed in resistant cells is not enough to support the apoptotic resistance mediated by DDB2-cFLIP. Although induction of cFLIP by DDB2 is required to protect cells against UV-induced apoptosis, at least in HeLa cells, we could not exclude the possibility that other genes are also involved in mediating the anti-apoptotic effect of DDB2.

5. Ectopic expression of DDB2 induces apoptosis in DDB2-deficient cells

An extensive review of XP-E and DDB has been presented by Itoh who focused on XP-E and DDB2 as well as the classification of photosensitive diseases [Itoh, 2006]. Surprisingly, XP-E cell strains proved to be abnormally resistant to UV irradiation and possessed reduced caspase-3 activity. Since the apoptotic defect in XP-E strains could be rescued by exogenous p53 expression, DDB2 was also proposed to regulate p53-mediated apoptotic pathway after UV irradiation in human primary cell strains [Itoh et al, 2000; 2003]. Cells from DDB2-knockout mice also showed abnormal resistance and impaired p53 response to UV irradiation similar to human XP-E cell strains [Itoh et al., 2004]. Furthermore, a recent study has demonstrated that mouse embryonic fibroblasts and human HeLa that express DDB2 shRNA are resistant to apoptosis induced by a variety of DNA-damaging agents despite the activation of p53 and other pro-apoptotic genes [Stoyanova et al., 2009]. Also, these DDB2-deficient cells are resistant to E2F1-induced apoptosis, probably due to the observation that these cells undergo p21Waf1/Cip1-associated cell cycle arrest following DNA damage. Notably, DDB2 targets p21Waf1/Cip1 for proteolysis and this process involves Mdm2 in a manner that is distinct from the p53-regulatory activity of Mdm2 [Stoyanova et al., 2009]. These results suggest a new regulatory loop involving DDB2, Mdm2, and p21Waf1/Cip1 that is critical in determining the cellular fate between apoptosis and cell cycle arrest (for DNA repair) in response to DNA damage. The existence of this regulatory loop may be strengthened by showing that forced expression of DDB2 renders XP-E or DDB2-deficient cells sensitive to apoptotic stimuli.

6. Cancer-prone DDB2-deficient mice

DDB2-knockout mice have been shown to be prone to cancer formation [Itoh et al., 2004]. Importantly, mice with single DDB2 allele knockout showed enhanced skin cancer following UV-B exposure, suggesting that DDB2 heterozygotes may be predisposed to skin cancer [Itoh et al., 2004]. In addition, XP mouse models were reported to be prone to the formation of papillomas induced by 7,12-dimethylbenz[a]anthracene (DMBA) [de Bohr et al., 1999; Nakane et al., 1995; de Vries et al., 1995], a carcinogen that produces bulky DNA adducts usually repaired by the NER system. On the other hand, p53-knockout mice are prone to spontaneous tumors [Donehower et al., 1992; Jacks et al., 1994], but not to tumors induced by DMBA or 12-O-tetradecanoyl-phorbol-13-acetate (TPA) [Kemp et al.,1993]. Taken together, these observations suggest that DDB2 may be involved in cancer formation through p53-mediated pathways. However, it is unclear whether re-introducing DDB2 in DDB2-knockout mice may prevent cancer formation.

7. Concluding remarks and future perspectives

The various results cited above suggest that the genetic integrity or gene expression status of the cells may be critical in determining the regulatory effects of DDB2 in response to apoptotic stimuli. The level of DDB2, p53, E2F1, and other proteins such as anti-apoptotic cFLIP and cell-cycle arrest p21, for instance, should be considered. The pro-apoptotic activity of p53 could vary between primary and cultured cell lines. For example, p53 activity in HeLa cells is hijacked by the human papillomavirus (HPV) E6 protein, a process that weakens apoptotic signaling in these cells. High levels of DDB2 may up-regulate and potentiate p53 activity by up-regulating apoptotic proteins in p53-normal cells. As such, HeLa cells, which harbor nearly null-p53 activity and additional anti-apoptotic cFLIP activity elicited by DDB2, may become resistant to apoptosis in response to cytotoxic DNA damage. These cellular responses are not surprising if the cultured cell lines were transformed by viruses or chemical means. Unfortunately, the cell lines used for the studies mentioned above are often treated this way. Furthermore, the expression of DDB2 isoforms, including the inhibitory D1 isoform, is often overlooked and the differential expression of such isoforms may dictate the cellular responses observed. Accordingly, alternative splicing of DDB2 transcripts and alteration of these genetic factors by other means in cell lines must be considered while evaluating the role of DDB2 in regulating apoptosis. In fact, there is no evidence so far that the apoptotic resistance of DDB2-defective XP-E, DDB2-knockout mouse cells, or DDB2-deficient human cells could be rescued by re-introducing DDB2 expression. In this sense, DDB2 is required to suppress apoptosis, but it does not suffice to be apoptotic. Furthermore, DDB2 as a proteasome component can target various proteins, such as p21 which is involved in cell cycle arrest, subsequently dysregulating cell cycle arrest during stress repair and leading to apoptosis. The cisplatin-selected HeLa cells used in our study do not display G1 arrest following mild, repairable DNA damage [Lin-Chao & Chao, 1994], which may explain the negligible, pro-apoptotic influence of DDB2 found by others [Stoyanova et al., 2009]. Therefore, an updated model is proposed in Figure 3, in

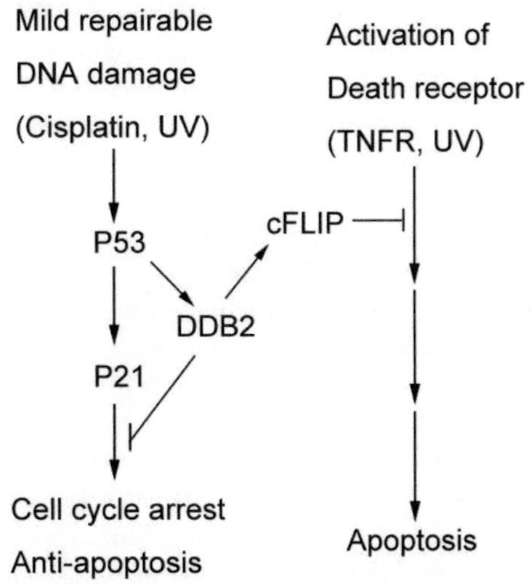

Fig. 3. Updated model for the regulation of DNA damage-induced apoptosis by DDB2. In this model, DNA damage applied to cells was mild and reached repairable level, leading to inhibition of apoptosis and cell cycle arrest for stress repair. The regulatory effect of DDB2 can be pro-apoptotic in cells experiencing mild DNA damage through p21 degradation which is targeted by DDB2. On the other hand, DDB2 can also be anti-apoptotic in cells harboring non-DNA damage apoptotic stimuli (e.g., death receptor) with up-regulation of anti-apoptotic cFLIP. Accordingly, the final outcome may be influenced by intrinsic mutations or extrinsic viral hijacking that can impair checkpoint for G1 arrest via p53 and p21.

which the regulatory effect of DDB2 can be either pro-apoptotic in cells that respond to mild DNA damage or anti-apoptotic in cells that respond to non-DNA damage apoptotic stimuli and that show up-regulation of the anti-apototic cFLIP. Notably, we found that human DDB2 may play a protective role against UV irradiation in the fruit fly *Drosophila* which does not express DDB2 as seen in the DDB2-defective cultured cell models. Therefore, the seemingly contrasting results mentioned above may be explained by our models, and primary cell cultures which are more representative of in vivo situations may represent a better choice for future studies of the biological functions of DDB2.

8. Acknowledgements

The author would like to thank the members of his research group for helpful discussions. The author also appreciates the help of Jan Martel during preparation of the manuscript. This review is partly supported by the National Science Council (Taiwan), Chang Gung University, and the Foundation for the Advancement of Outstanding Scholarship.

9. References

de Bohr, J., van Steeg, H., Berg, R.J.W., Garssen, J., de Wit, J., van Oostrum, C.T.M., Beems, R.B., van der Horst, G.T., van Kreijl, C.F., de Gruijl, F.R., Bootsma, D., Hoeijmakers, J.H., Weeda, G. (1999). Mouse model for the DNA repair/basal transcription disorder trichothiodystrophy reveals cancer predisposition. *Cancer Res.,* 59, 3489-3494

Chao, C.C., Huang, S.L., Huang, H.M., and Lin-Chao, S. (1991). Cross-resistance to UV radiation of a cisplatin-resistant human cell line: overexpression of cellular factors that recognize UV-modified DNA. *Mol. Cell. Biol.,* 11, 2075-2080

Chen, X., Zhang, Y., Douglas, L., Zhou, P. (2001). UV-damaged DNA-binding proteins are targets of CUL-4A-mediated ubiquitination and degradation. *J. Biol. Chem.,* 276, 48175-48182

Chu, G., Chang, E. (1988). Xeroderma pigmentosum group E cells lack a nuclear factor that binds to damaged DNA. *Science,* 242, 564-567

Chu, G., Chang, E. (1990). Cisplatin-resistant cells express increased levels of a factor that recognizes damaged DNA. *Proc. Natl. Acad. Sci. USA,* 87, 3324-3327

Cleaver, J.E. (2005) Cancer in xeroderma pigmentosum and related disorders of DNA repair. *Nat Rev Cancer* 5, 564-573

Donehower, L.A., Harvey, M., Slagle, B.L., McArthur, M.J., Montogomery, Jr. C.A., Butel, J.S., Bradley A. (1992). Mice deficient for p53 are developmentally normal but susceptible to spontaneous tumours. *Nature,* 356, 215-221

Dualan, R., Brody, T., Keeney, S., Nichols, A.F., Admon, A., Linn, S. (1995). Chromosomal localization and cDNA cloning of the genes (DDB1 and DDB2) for the p127 and p48 subunits of a human damage specific DNA-binding protein. *Genomics,* 29, 62-69

El-Mahdy, M.A., Zhu, Q., Wang, Q.E., Wani, G., Praetorius-Ibba, M., Wani, A.A. (2006). Cullin 4A-mediated proteolysis of DDB2 protein at DNA damage sites regulates in vivo lesion recognition by XPC. *J. Biol. Chem.,* 281: 13404–13411

Feldberg, R.S., Grossman, L. (1976). A DNA binding protein from human placenta specific for ultraviolet damaged DNA. *Biochemistry,* 15, 2402-2408

Fitch, M.E., Nakajima, S., Yasui, A., Ford, J.M. (2003). In vivo recruitment of XPC to UV-induced cyclobutane pyrimidine dimers by the DDB2 gene product. *J. Biol. Chem.*, 278, 46906-46910

Friedberg, E.C., Walker, G.C., Siede, W., Wood, R.D., Schultz, R.A., Ellenberger, T. (2006). *DNA repair and mutagenesis*. Second Edition, ASM Press, Washington, DC

Fujiwara, Y., Masutani, C., Mizukoshi, T., Kondo, J., Hanaoka, F., Iwai, S. (1999). Characterization of DNA recognition by the human UV-damaged DNA-binding protein. *J. Biol. Chem.*, 274, 20027-20033

Gonzalez, V.M., Fuertes, M.A., Alonso, C., Perez, J.M. (2001). Is cisplatin-induced cell death always produced by apoptosis? *Mol. Pharmacol.*, 59, 657–663

Groisman, R., Polanowska, J., Kuraoka, I., Sawada, J., Saijo, M., Drapkin, R., Kisselev, A.F., Tanaka, K., Nakatani, Y. (2003). CSA complexes is differentially regulated by the COP9 signalosome in response to DNA damage. *Cell*, 113, 357-367

Guerrero-Santoro, J., Kapetanaki, M.G., Hsieh, C.L., Gorbachinsky, I., Levine, A.S., Rapic-Otrin, V. (2008). The cullin 4B-based UV-damaged DNA-binding protein ligase binds to UV-damaged chromatin and ubiquitinates histone H2A. *Cancer Res.*, 68, 5014-5022

Hayes, S., Shiyanov, P., Chen, X., Raychaudhuri, P. (1998). DDB, a putative DNA repair protein, can function as a transcriptional partner of E2F1. Mol. Cell Biol.,18, 240–249

Higa, L.A., Mihaylov, I.S., Banks, D.P., Zheng, J., Zhang, H. (2003). Radiation-mediated proteolysis of CDT1 by CUL4-ROC1 and CSN complexes constitutes a new checkpoint. *Nat. Cell Biol.*, 5, 1008-1015

Hu, J., McCall, C.M., Ohta, T., Xiong, Y. (2004). Targeted ubiquitination of CDT1 by the DDB1-CUL4A-ROC1 ligase in response to DNA damage. *Nat. Cell Biol.*, 6, 1003–1009

Hwang, B.J., Ford, J.M., Hanawalt, P.C., Chu, G. (1999). Expression of the p48 xeroderma pigmentosum gene is p53-dependent and is involved in global genomic repair. *Proc. Natl. Acad. Sci. U.S.A.*, 96, 424-428

Inoki, T., Yamagami, S., Inoki, Y., Tsuru, T., Hamamoto, T., Kagawa, Y., Mori, T., Endo, H. (2004). Human DDB2 splicing variants are dominant negative inhibitors of UV-damaged DNA repair. *Biochem. Biophys. Res. Commun.*, 314, 1036-1043

Itoh, T., Linn, S., Ono, T., Yamaizumi, M. (2000). Reinvestigation of the classification of five cell strains of xeroderma pigmentosum group E with reclassification of three of them. *J. Invest. Dermatol.*, 114,1022-1029

Itoh, T., O'Shea, C., Linn, S. (2003). Impaired regulation of tumor suppressor p53 caused by mutations in the xeroderma pigmentosum DDB2 gene: mutual regulatory interactions between p48 DDB2 and p53. *Mol. Cell. Biol.*, 23, 7540-7553

Itoh, T., Cado, D., Kamide, Y., Linn, S. (2004). DDB2 disruption leads to skin tumors and resistance to apoptosis after exposure to ultraviolet light but not a chemical carcinogen. *Proc. Natl. Acad. Sci. USA*, 101, 2052-2057

Itoh, T. (2006). Xeroderma pigmentosum group E and DDB2, a smaller subunit of damage-specific DNA binding protein: Proposed classification of xeroderma pigmentosum, Cockayne syndrome, and ultraviolet-sensitive syndrome. *.J Dermatol. Sc.i*, 41, 87-96

Jacks, T., Remington, L., Williams, B.O., Schmitt, E.M., Halachmi, S., Bronson, R.T., Weinberg, R.A. (1994).Tumor spectrum analysis in p53-mutant mice. *Curr Biol*, 4,1-7

Jackson, S., Xiong, Y. (2009). CRL4s: the CUL4-RING E3 ubiquitin ligases. *Trends Bochem. Sci.*, 34, 562-570

Kamarajan, P., Sun, N.-K., Chao, C.C.-K. (2003). Upregulation of FLIP in cisplatin-selected HeLa cells causes cross-resistance to Fas death signaling. *Biochem. J.*, 376, 253-260

Kapetanaki, M.G., Guerrero-Santoro, J., Bisi, D.C., Hsieh, C.L., Rapic-Otrin, V., Levine, A.S. (2006). The DDB1-CUL4ADDB2 ubiquitin ligase is deficient in xeroderma pigmentosum group E and targets histone H2A at UV-damaged DNA sites. *Proc. Natl. Acad. Sci. U.S.A.*, 103, 2588-2593

Keeney, S., Chang, G.J., Linn, S. (1993). Characterization of a human DNA damage binding protein implicated in xeroderma pigmentosum E. *J. Biol. Chem.*, 268, 21293-21300.

Keeney, S., Eker, A.P.M., Brody, T., Vermeulen, W., Bootsma, D., Hoeijmakers, J.H.J., Linn, S. (1994). Correction of the DNA repair defect in xeroderma pigmentosum group E by injection of a DNA damage binding protein. *Proc. Natl. Acad. Sci. U.S.A.*, 91, 4053-4056

Kemp, C.J., Donehower, L.A., Bradley, A., Balmain, A. (1993). Reduction of p53 gene dosage does not increase initiation or promotion but enhances malignant progression of chemically induced skin tumors. *Cell*, 74, 813-822

Kulaksiz, G., Reardon, J.T., Sancar, A. (2005). Xeroderma pigmentosum complementation group E protein (XPE/DDB2): purification of various complexes of XPE and analyses of their damaged DNA binding and putative DNA repair properties. *Mol. Cell. Biol.*, 25, 9784-9792

Lee, J., Zhou, P. (2007). DCAFs, the missing link of the CUL4-DDB1 ubiquitin ligase. *Molecular Cell*, 26, 775-780

Lee, T.H., Elledge, S.J., Butel, J.S. (1995). Hepatitis B virus X protein interacts with a probable cellular DNA repair protein., *J. Virol.*, 69, 1107–1114

Lin-Chao, S., Chao, C.C.-K. (1994). Reduced inhibition of DNA synthesis and G_2 arrest in the cell cycle progression of resistant HeLa cells in response to *cis*-diamminedichloroplatinum(II). *J. Biomed. Sci.*, 1, 131-138

Mitchell, D.L., Haipek, C.A., Clarkson, J.M. (1985). (6-4) Photoproducts are removed from the DNA of UV-irradiated mammalian cells more efficiently than cyclobutane pyrimidine dimers. *Mutat. Res.*, 143, 109–112

Moser, J., Volker, M., Kool, H., Alekseev, S., Vrieling, H., Yasui, A., van Zeeland, A.A., Mullenders, L.H. (2005). The UV-damaged DNA binding protein mediates efficient targeting of the nucleotide excision repair complex to UV-induced photo lesions. *DNA Repair*, 4, 571–582

Nakane, H., Takeuchi, S., Yuba, S., Siajo, M., Nakatsu, Y., Murai, H., Nakatsuru, Y., Ishikawa, T., Hirota, S., Kitamura, Y., Kato, Y., Tsunoda, Y., Miyauchi, H., Horio, T., Tokunaga, T., Matsunaga, T., Nikaido, O., Nishimune, Y., Okada a, Y., Tanaka, K. (1995). High incidence of ultraviolet-B- or chemical-carcinogen induced skin tumours in mice lacking the xeroderma pigmentosum group A gene. *Nature*, 377,165-168

Nichols, A.F., Ong, P., Linn, S., (1996). Mutations specific to the xeroderma pigmentosum group-E DDB(−) phenotype. *J. Biol. Chem.*, 271, 24317-24320

Nichols, A.F., Itoh, T., Graham, J.A., Liu, W., Yamaizumi, M., Linn, S. (2000). Human damage-specific DNA-binding protein p48: characterization of XPE mutations and regulation following UV irradiation. *J. Biol. Chem.*, 275, 21422–21428

Payne, A., Chu, G., (1994). Xeroderma pigmentosum group E binding factor recognizes a broad spectrum of DNA damage. *Mutat. Res.,* 310, 89–102

Peng, K.-Y. (2008). *Effects of DDB2 overexpression on UV toxicity and cell growth.* Master thesis, Chang Gung University, Taiwan

Phillips, A.C., Ernst, M.K., Bates, S., Rice, N.R., Vousden, K.H. (1999). E2F-1 potentiates cell death by blocking antiapoptotic signaling pathways. *Mol. Cell* 4, 771–781

Rapic-Otrin, V., McLenigan, M.P., Bisi, D.C., Gonzalez, M., Levine, A.S. (2002). Sequential binding of UV DNA damage binding factor and degradation of the p48 subunit as early events after UV irradiation. *Nucleic Acids Res.,* 30, 2588–2598

Scrima, A., Konickova, R., Czyzewski, B.K., Kawasaki, Y., Jeffrey, P.D., Nakatani, R.Y., Iwai, S., Pavletich, N.P., Thoma, N.H. (2008). Structural basis of UV DNA damage recognition by the DDB1-DDB2 complex. *Cell,* 135, 1213–1223

Shiyanov, P., Hayes, S.A., Donepudi, M., Nichols, A.F., Linn, S., Slagle, B.L., Raychaudhuri, P. (1999).The naturally occurring mutants of DDB are impaired in stimulating nuclear import of the p125 subunit and E2F1-activated transcription. *Mol. Cell Biol.,* 19, 4935–4943

Stanelle, J., Stiewe, T., Theseling, C.C., Peter, M., Putzer, B.M. (2002). Gene expression changes in response to E2F1 activation. *Nucleic Acids Res.,* 30,1859–1867

Stoyanova, T., Roy, N., Kopanja, D., Bagchi, S., Raychaudhuri, P. (2009). DDB2 decides cell fate following DNA damage. *Proc Natl Acad Sci USA,* 106, 10690–10695

Sugasawa, K., Ng, J.M., Masutani, C., Iwai, S., van der Spek, P.J., Eker, A.P., Hanaoka, F., Bootsma, D., and Hoeijmakers, J.H. (1998). Xeroderma pigmentosum group C protein complex is the initiator of global genome nucleotide excision repair. *Mol. Cell,* 2, 223–232

Sugasawa, K., Okuda, Y., Saijo, M., Nishi, R., Matsuda, N., Chu, G., Mori, T., Iwai, S., Tanaka, K., Tanaka, K., Hanaoka, F. (2005). UV-induced ubiquitylation of XPC protein mediated by UV-DDB-ubiquitin ligase complex. *Cell,* 121, 387–400

Sugasawa, K. (2009). UV-DDB: A molecular machine linking DNA repair with ubiquitination. *DNA Repair,* 8, 969-972

Sugasawa, K. (2010). Regulation of damage recognition in mammalian global genomic nucleotide excision repair. *Mutat. Res.,* 685, 29–37

Sun, C.-L., Chao, C.C.-K. (2005a). Cross-resistance to death ligand-induced apoptosis, in cisplatin-selected HeLa cells, associated with overexpression of DDB2 and subsequent induction of cFLIP. *Mol. Pharmacol.,* 67, 1307-1314

Sun, C.-L., Chao, C.C.-K. (2005b). Potential attenuation of p38 signaling by DDB2 as a factor in acquired TNF resistance. *Int. J. Cancer,* 115, 383-389

Sun, N.-K., Kamarajan, P., Huang, H., Chao, C.C.-K. (2002a). Restoration of UV sensitivity in UV-resistant HeLa cells by antisense-mediated depletion of damaged DNA-binding protein 2 (DDB2). *FEBS Lett.,* 512, 168-172

Sun, N.-K., Lu, H.-P., Chao, C.C.-K. (2002b). Overexpression of damaged DNA-binding protein 2 (DDB2) potentiates UV resistance in hamster V79 cells. *Chang Gung Med. J.,* 25, 686-695

Sun, N.-K., Sun, C.-L., Lin, C.-H., Pai, L.-M., Chao, C.C.-K. (2010). Damaged DNA-binding protein 2 (DDB2) protects against UV irradiation in human cells and *Drosophila. J. Biomed. Sci.,* 17, 27

Takao, M., Abramic, M., Moos, M., Otrin, V.R., Wootton, J.C., McLenigan, M., Levine, A.S., Protic', M. (1993). A 127 kDa component of a UV-damaged DNA-binding complex, which is defective in some xeroderma pigmentosum group E patients, is homologous to a slime-mold protein, *Nucleic Acids Res.* 21 (1993) 4111–4118.

Tang, J.Y., Hwang, B.J., Ford, J.M., Hanawalt, P.C., Chu, G. (2000). Xeroderma pigmentosum p48 gene enhances global genomic repair and suppresses UV-induced mutagenesis. *Mol. Cell*, 5, 737-744

Tang, J., Chu, G. (2002). Xeroderma pigmentosum complementation group E and UV-damaged DNA-binding protein. *DNA Repair*, 1, 601–616

de Vries, A., van Oostrom, C.T.M., Hofhuis, F.M.A., Dortant, P.M., Berg, R.J.W., de Gruiji, F.R., Wester, P.W., van Kreijl, C.F., Capel, P.J., van Steeg, H., Verbeek, S.J. (1995). Increased susceptibility to ultraviolet-B and carcinogens of mice lacking the DNA excision repair gene XPA. *Nature* 377, 169-173

Wang, H., Zhai, L., Xu, J., Joo, H.-Y., Jackson, S., Erdjument-Bromage, H., Tempst, P., Xiong, Y., Zhang, Y. (2006). Histone H3 and H4 ubiquitylation by the CUL4-DDB-ROC1 ubiquitin ligase facilitates cellular response to DNA damage. *Mol. Cell*, 22, 383-394

Wittschieben, B.O., Iwai, S., Wood, R.D. (2005). DDB1-DDB2 (xeroderma pigmentosum group E) protein complex recognizes a cyclobutane pyrimidine dimer, mismatches, apurinic/apyrimidinic sites, and compound lesions in DNA. *J. Biol. Chem.*, 280, 39982-39989

4

The Potential Roles of DNA-Repair Proteins in Centrosome Maintenance

Mikio Shimada, Akihiro Kato and Junya Kobayashi
Radiation Biology Center, Kyoto University
Japan

1. Introduction

The centrosome, an organelle that regulates microtubules, is necessary for proper cell division in mammalian cells (Doxsey, 2001; Nigg, 2002, 2007). The existence of centrosomes was first reported 100 years ago by Theodor Boveri (Boveri, 2008). A centrosome is composed of two centrioles and is surrounded by pericentriolar material (PCM), which provides a binding site for the γ-tubulin ring complex (γ-TuRC). The γ-TuRC acts as a microtubule nucleation template, and it attaches to the PCM to form microtubules (Fig. 1). The number of centrosomes is precisely regulated, and the duplication cycle is synchronized to the cell cycle. Centrosomes duplicate once in the S phase and mature in the G2 phase, and in the M phase, centrosomes are divided into daughter cells (Fig. 2). The number of centrosomes and their functions are regulated by many proteins including centrosome proteins, cell-cycle proteins, and DNA-repair proteins, and recently, the role of DNA-repair proteins in centrosome maintenance has been clarified. In this chapter, we introduce recent findings about the roles of DNA-repair proteins in centrosome maintenance.

2. Centrosomes and aneuploidy

Many cancer cells possess extra centrosomes, which is called centrosome amplification and means overduplication of centrosomes. Extra centrosomes can lead to multipolar cell divisions, subsequent aneuploidy, and cell death (Kwon et al., 2008). Although almost all multipolar cell division results in cell death via mitotic catastrophe (Ganem et al., 2009), some multipolar cells divide into daughter cells to maintain aneuploidy. Aneuploidic cells are believed to potentially cause tumorigenesis. Recent studies suggest that aneuploidic cells are produced by a clustering of extra centrosomes, which accumulate at the two poles, and microtubules from each of the extra centrosomes attach to the chromosomes prior to mitosis (Kwon et al., 2008) (Fig. 2). The tension created by the extra centrosomes leads to improper chromosome segregation (Godinho et al., 2009).

Several environmental factors and chemicals, or carcinogens, including ionizing radiation and benzopyrene, can induce extra centrosomes (Sato et al., 2000). Thus, failure of the centrosome duplication cycle could cause tumorigenesis via chromosome aneuploidy.

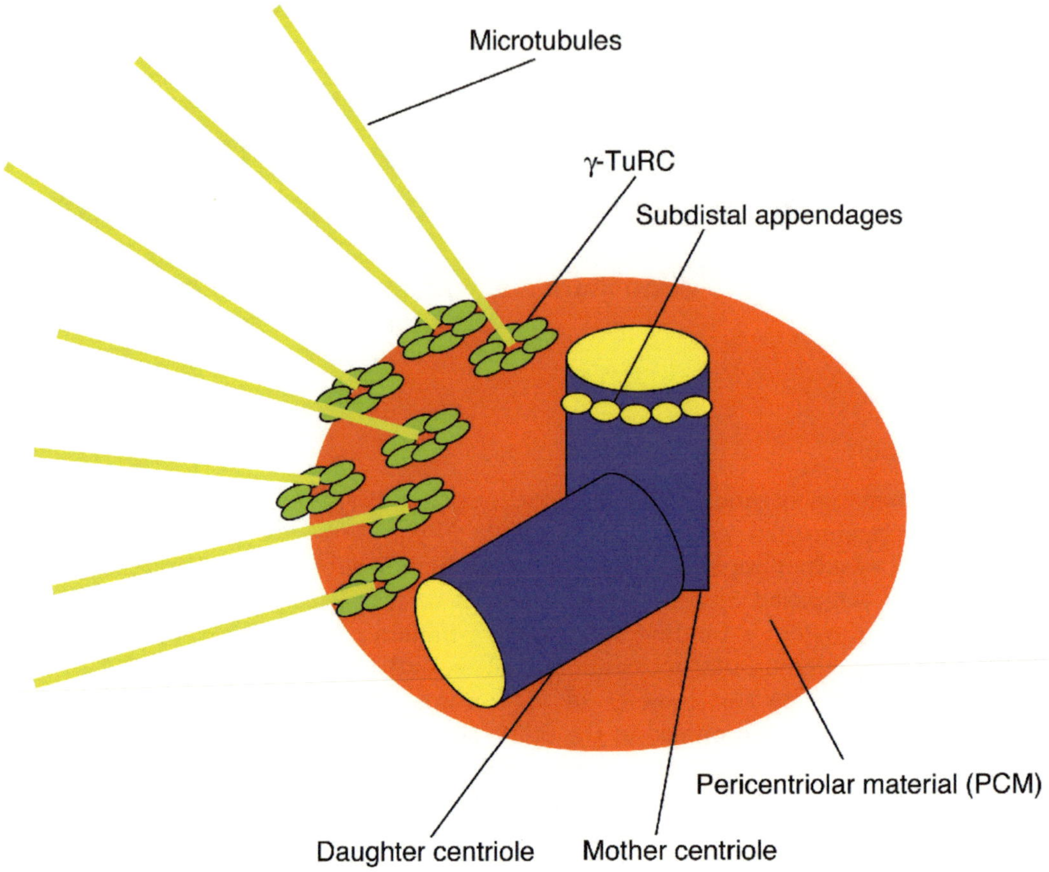

Centrosomes are located at the periphery of the nucleus and consist of a mother centriole and a daughter centriole, surrounded by the pericentriolar material (PCM). The γ-tubulin ring complex (γ-TuRC) binds to the PCM to form microtubules.

Fig. 1. Centrosome structure.

3. Centrosomes and the cell cycle

Centrosome duplication is controlled by several cell-cycle regulators (Fukasawa, 2007). The cyclin E/CDK2 complex is responsible for initiating DNA synthesis and regulates cell-cycle progression (Matsumoto et al., 1999). This complex also contributes to centrosome duplication (Fig. 3). Cyclin E contains the centrosome localization signal (CLS), and overexpression of mutated cyclin E through a CLS deletion results in failed centrosome duplication (Matsumoto and Maller, 2002). The *CDKN1A* product, p21, is a negative regulator of CDK2. As the expression of p21 is regulated by p53-dependent transcription, the absence of p53 abrogates p21-dependent repression of CDK2 and subsequently leads to centrosome duplication. The DNA synthesis inhibitor, hydroxyurea (HU), induces cell-cycle arrest at the G1/S phase. Cells possessing wild-type p53 prevent HU-induced overduplication of centrosomes by inhibiting CDK2 through p53/p21. In contrast, the absence of functional p53 abolishes the p21-dependent repression of CDK2, leading to centrosome amplification. p53

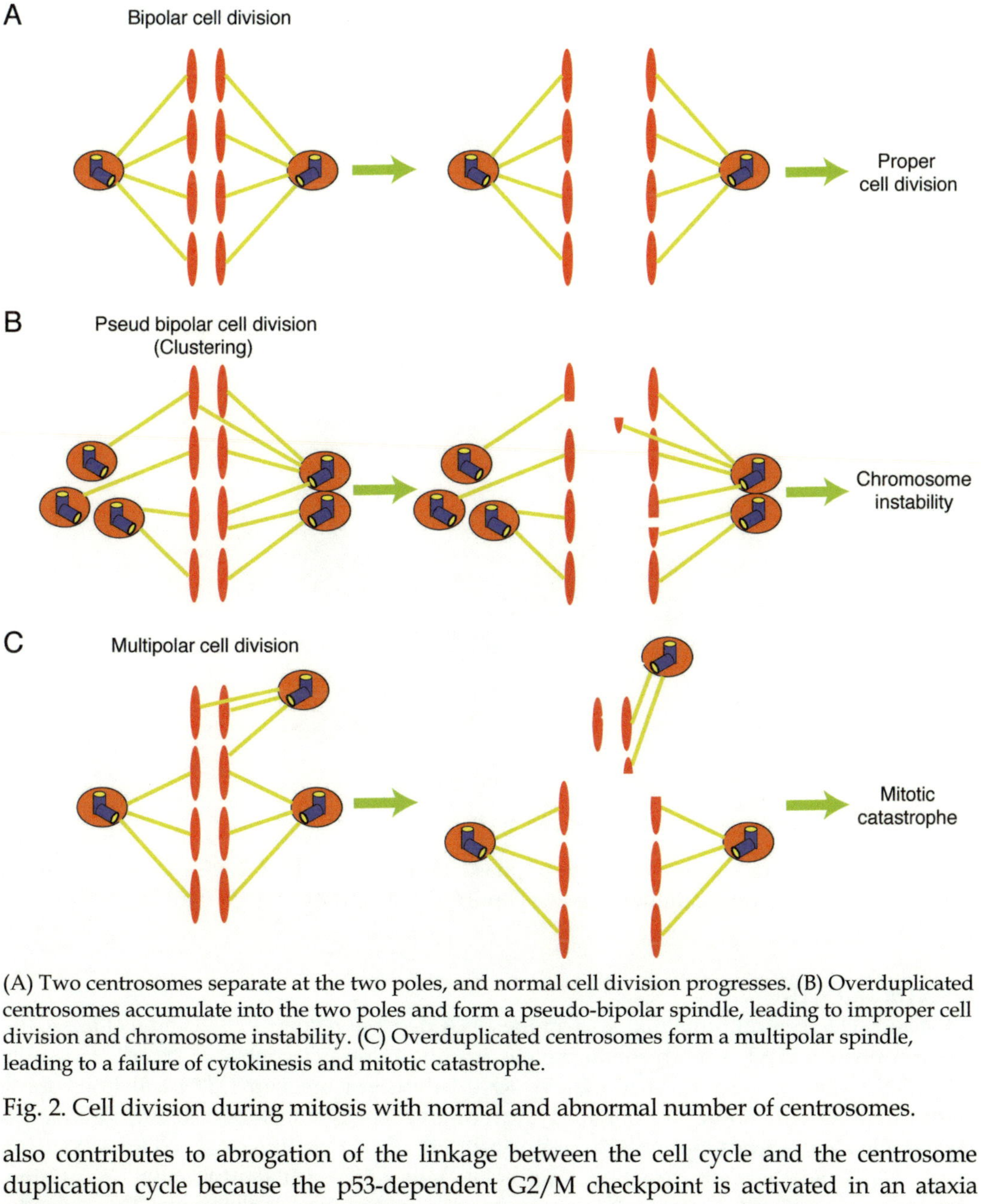

(A) Two centrosomes separate at the two poles, and normal cell division progresses. (B) Overduplicated centrosomes accumulate into the two poles and form a pseudo-bipolar spindle, leading to improper cell division and chromosome instability. (C) Overduplicated centrosomes form a multipolar spindle, leading to a failure of cytokinesis and mitotic catastrophe.

Fig. 2. Cell division during mitosis with normal and abnormal number of centrosomes.

also contributes to abrogation of the linkage between the cell cycle and the centrosome duplication cycle because the p53-dependent G2/M checkpoint is activated in an ataxia telangiectasia mutated (ATM)/ATM- and Rad3-related (ATR)-dependent manner after DNA damage such as from irradiation.

4. Centrosomes and DNA-repair proteins

DNA-repair-related proteins, including ATM, ATR, checkpoint kinase 1 (CHK1), CHK2, PARP1, Nijmegen breakage syndrome (NBS1), BRCA1, BRCA2, RAD51, RAD51 paralogs, and TOPBP1 localize at centrosomes, and defects in these proteins cause several functional aberrations in centrosomes (Fig. 4).

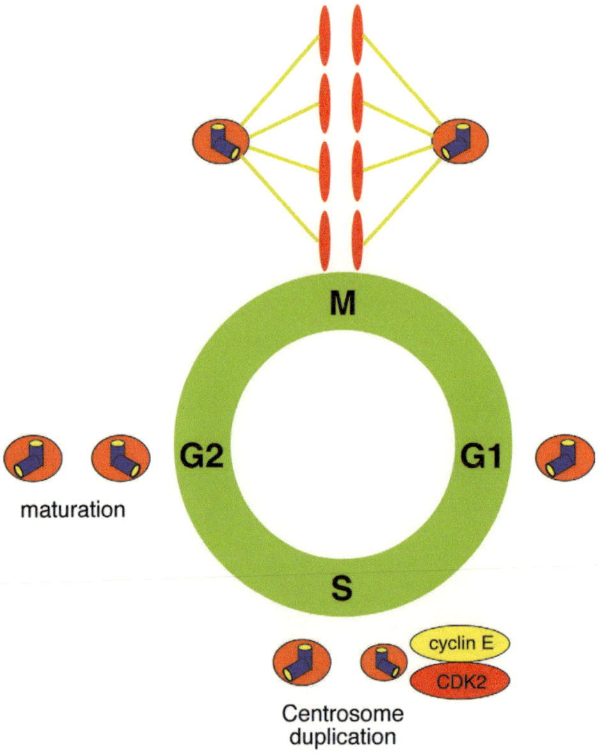

Fig. 3. Centrosome duplication and the cell cycle.

Centrosomes are duplicated once in S phase and mature in G2 phase. In M phase, centrosomes divide into daughter cells. Cyclin E/CDK2 activity is important for centrosome duplication.

4.1 ATM and ATR

ATM and ATR, central protein kinases in the DNA damage response (Bensimon et al., 2010), phosphorylate CEP63, a centrosomal protein, leading to proper control of spindle assembly after DNA damage (Smith et al., 2009). Rad51-deficient chicken DT40 cell lines show centrosome amplification, but a Rad51/Atm-double knockout DT40 cell line revealed a decrease in centrosome amplification compared to Rad51-single knockout cell lines (Dodson et al., 2004). Furthermore, treating Rad51-deficient cells with wortmannin or caffeine, inhibitors of ATM and ATR, results in a decrease in centrosome amplification. These results suggest that ATM could contribute to centrosome amplification in Rad51-deficient cells by regulating the G2/M checkpoint or an unknown function in the centrosome duplication pathway. ATR is mutated in some individuals with Seckel Syndrome (ATR Seckel), which is an autosomal recessive disorder that includes intrauterine growth retardation and microcephaly. Seckel syndrome patient cells have aberrant centrosome and checkpoint regulation (Alderton et al., 2004). *Pericentrin* is a mutated gene in PCNT Seckel syndrome

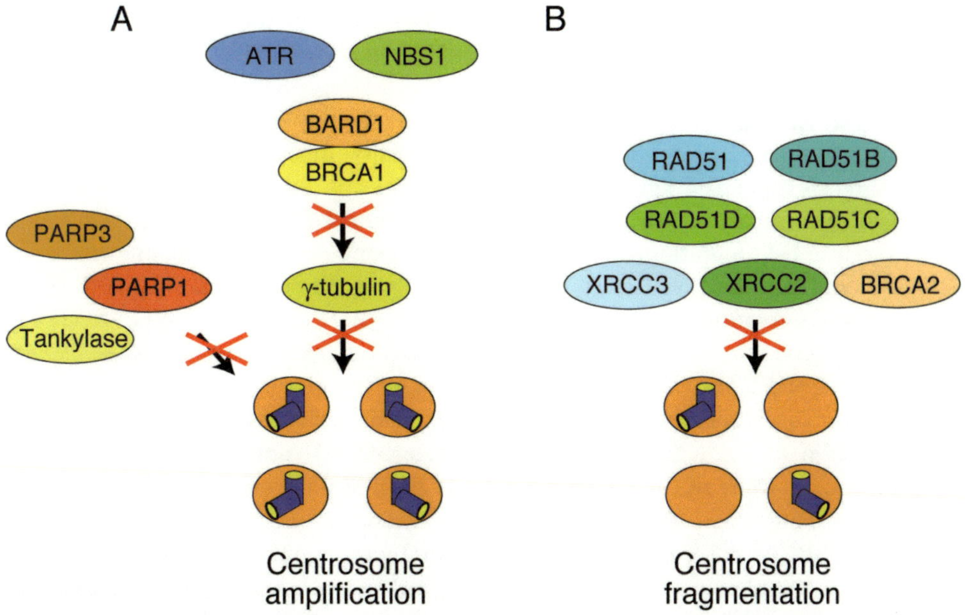

(A) Ataxia telangiectasia mutated (ATM) and Rad3-related (ATR), Nijmegen breakage syndrome (NBS)1, and BRCA1-BARD1 complex-dependent γ-tubulin monoubiquitination is important for centrosome duplication. Defects in these proteins result in centrosome amplification. A defect in PARP-1, PARP-3, or tankylase also leads to centrosome amplification. (B) In contrast, a defect in RAD51, RAD51 paralogs, or BRCA2 results in centrosome fragmentation.

Fig. 4. DNA-repair proteins and centrosome maintenance.

(Griffith et al., 2008; Rauch et al., 2008) that is involved in the ATR-dependent DNA damage signaling pathway. Exposure to UV light or HU induces the activation of ATR, and activated ATR phosphorylates CHK1. Phosphorylated CHK1 accumulates at the centrosome and its localization causes inhibition of Cdc25 activity, which prevents activation of cyclin B/CDK1. Hence, the ATR-dependent G2/M checkpoint may contribute to centrosome amplification.

4.2 CHK1, CHK2

CHK1 is an essential gene for mammalian cells and functions in the cell-cycle checkpoint (Shimada et al., 2008). Loss of functional Chk1 in human or chicken cell lines causes a G2/M checkpoint deficiency and increased sensitivity to DNA damage treatment (Bourke et al., 2007). CHK1 localizes at the centrosome. Chk1-deficient chicken cell lines abolish irradiation-induced centrosome amplification. CHK1 interacts with MCPH1 and pericentrin in the centrosome, and MCPH1 knockdown decreases the accumulation of Chk1 and pericentrin in centrosomes (Tibelius et al., 2009). These results suggest that CHK1 accumulation in the centrosome is dependent on MCPH1. Thus, Chk1 participates in the regulation of centrosome number through checkpoint control or phosphorylation of unknown substrates by Chk1.

Chk2 is another important cell-cycle checkpoint kinase that is activated in response to DNA damage (Tsvetkov et al., 2003; Golan et al., 2010). Chk2 and Plk1, which are mitotic kinases, co-localize at the centrosome. This interaction may be important for the DNA mitotic damage-dependent checkpoint, although the details remain unknown.

4.3 BRCA1 and BRCA2

About 10% of women diagnosed with breast cancer have inherited mutations in *BRCA1* or *BRCA2* (Irminger-Finger and Jefford, 2006). Both *BRCA1* and *BRCA2*, products of the familial breast cancer susceptibility gene, are involved in several cellular functions, such as DNA repair, transcriptional regulation, cell-cycle checkpoints, and centrosome maintenance. BRCA1 forms a heterodimer complex with BRCA1-associated RING domain (BARD1), which functions as an E3 ubiquitin ligase. Both BRCA1 and BARD1 contain a RING domain, which mediates DNA–protein and protein–protein interactions, a nuclear export signal sequence at their N-terminus, and tandem BRCT (BRCA1 carboxy-terminal) domains. The BRCA1–BARD1 complex monoubiquitylates γ-tubulin at Lysine 48 and Lysine 344, and overexpression of mutated γ-tubulin at the K48 ubiquitination site results in centrosome amplification and aberration of microtubule nucleation (Starita et al., 2005; Simons et al., 2006). Overexpression of mutated γ-tubulin (K344R) results in an aberration of microtubule nucleation only, suggesting that BRCA1 controls centrosome function by monoubiquitination of γ-tubulin. The BRCA1–BARD1 complex also ubiquitylates the nucleolar phosphoprotein nucleophosmin (NPM also known as B23), which functions in nucleolar organization, cell-cycle regulation, and centrosome duplication. The BRCA1–BARD1 complex polyubiquitinates NPM, leading to its degradation. Aurora A, which localizes at the centrosome and is an important factor for mitotic progression, phosphorylates BRCA1, which contributes to regulation of centrosome duplication. Furthermore, the BRCA1–BARD1 complex regulates microtubule organization through a Ran-dependent import pathway.

A BRCA2 mutation is involved in approximately 50% of hereditary breast cancers (Yoshida and Miki, 2004). BRCA2 has no sequential or structural similarity with either BRCA1 or BARD1 and localizes at the centrosome. Interaction of BRCA2 with plectin, a cytoskeletal cross-linker protein, is necessary for centrosome anchoring to the nucleus (Niwa et al., 2009). BRCA2 also forms a complex at the centrosome with NPM and ROCK2, an effector of Rho small GTPase. A definite BRCA2 deletion can abrogate the association of BRCA2 with NPM, and cells expressing this deletion mutant show centrosome amplification (Wang et al., 2011), suggesting that the BRCA2–NPM complex maintains centrosome duplication and controls cell division.

4.4 NBS1

NBS, which is caused by an *NBS1* gene mutation, is characterized by growth retardation, a birdlike face, immunodeficiency, predisposition to malignancy, and microcephaly (Matsuura et al., 1998). NBS patient cells have a defect in the cell-cycle checkpoint and hyper-radiosensitivity. NBS1 is a multifunctional protein that participates in homologous recombination repair, DNA replication, the cell-cycle checkpoint, and apoptosis (Tauchi et al., 2002). NBS1 forms a complex with MRE11 and RAD50 (MRN complex), and this complex is required for recruitment of ATM to DNA damage sites and for efficient phosphorylation of ATM substrates (Iijima et al., 2008). NBS1 contains a forkhead-associated (FHA) domain and a BRCT domain at the N-terminus, the binding motif for MRE11, ATM, and RNF20, which is a E3 ubiquitin ligase for H2B, at the C-terminus (Nakamura et al., 2011). The NBS1 FHA domain is required for ATR interaction (Shimada et al., 2009). NBS1 knockdown by siRNA in human or mouse cells causes centrosome amplification and decreases BRCA1-dependent monoubiquitination of γ-tubulin. Furthermore, the NBS1 N-terminus, which interacts with ATR, is indispensable for the monoubiquitination of γ-tubulin. NBS1 potentially plays a role in genome integrity via centrosome and nucleus volume control (Shimada and Komatsu, 2009; Shimada et al., 2010).

4.5 PARP family

PARP1 catalyzes the formation of long branched polyADP-ribosylation covalently attached to target proteins using NAD^+ as a substrate. Many proteins are poly(ADP-ribosyl)ated by PARP1, and this modification may be involved in transcriptional regulation and DNA repair (Miwa and Masutani, 2007). PARP1$^{-/-}$ mouse cell lines show centrosome amplification (Kanai et al., 2003). Other PARP family proteins, such as PARP3 and tankylase (also known as PARP5a), localize at the centrosome (Smith and de Lange, 1999; Augustin et al., 2003). These reports suggest that PARP family proteins are involved in the control of centrosome duplication.

4.6 RAD51 paralogs

RAD51 and five paralogs, RAD51B (RAD51L1), RAD51C (RAD51L2), RAD51D (RAD51L3), XRCC2, and XRCC3, play important roles in homologous recombination (HR) repair (Date et al., 2006; Renglin Lindh et al., 2007; Cappelli et al., 2011). These proteins have a consensus domain including Walker A and B ATPase domains and are necessary for chromosome stability and the control of chromosome segregation. In mammalian cells, XRCC2 forms a complex with RAD51B and RAD51C, and XRCC3 forms a complex with RAD51C. The XRCC2 complex is involved in the RAD51 loading step to ssDNA in HR repair. The XRCC3 complex is involved in Holliday junction resolution. Loss of RAD51, RAD51B, RAD51C, RAD51D, XRCC2, or XRCC3 leads to centrosome amplification and chromosome instability. RAD51C, XRCC2, or XRCC3-deficient cell lines show centrosome amplification in the M phase, but only XRCC2-deficient cell lines show centrosome amplification at interphase (Renglin Lindh et al., 2007), suggesting that RAD51C and XRCC3, but not XRCC2, may be involved in the same centrosome duplication pathway.

4.7 Nonhomologous end-joining repair proteins

Nonhomologous end-joining (NHEJ) repair proteins such as DNA-PKcs also localize at centrosomes (Zhang et al., 2007). Our previous reports showed that DNA-PKcs-deficient cell lines (SCID) have a slightly increased centrosome number compared to wild-type cell lines. Moreover, another NHEJ factor, Ku70, found in a Ku70-deficient cell line also has a slight increase in centrosome number compared to complementary cell lines (Shimada et al., 2010), indicating that NHEJ factors may be involved in centrosome functions different from HR factors.

4.8 Other DNA-repair-related proteins

TopBP1, a sensor protein involved in the DNA damage response, localizes at the centrosome during mitosis but not at interphase (Bang et al., 2011). TopBP1 interacts with the centrosome through its C-terminus and eliminates TopBP1 localization, resulting in a delay in mitotic progression. SMC1, a condensin protein important during chromosome condensation, also localizes at the centrosome but its role in centrosome maintenance is unclear.

5. Conclusion

DNA-repair proteins are necessary for genome integrity. Their main functions are to control DNA repair and control the cell-cycle checkpoint. Recent studies have not clarified the role of DNA damage repair proteins in centrosome maintenance, although interactions between DNA-repair proteins and centrosomal proteins may have an important role in centrosome maintenance and microtubule regulation such as ATM/ATR-dependent CEP63 phosphorylation. How these interactions contribute to centrosome maintenance and microtubule regulation is unclear, so investigating the relationship between DNA-repair proteins and centrosomal proteins is important. Furthermore, the linkage between centrosome amplification and tumorigenesis is key to developing clinical targets. Inhibitors of the DNA-repair protein PARP-1 and the centrosomal protein Aurora A could be a focus for anticancer drugs. Investigations into the molecular signaling pathway of DNA-repair proteins during centrosome maintenance may contribute to advanced options for clinical therapeutics.

6. Acknowledgments

This work was supported by grants from the Ministry of Education, Culture, Sports, Science, and Technology, Japan. We thank M. Takado for critical reading of the manuscript.

7. References

Alderton, G.K., H. Joenje, R. Varon, A.D. Borglum, P.A. Jeggo, and M. O'Driscoll. 2004. Seckel syndrome exhibits cellular features demonstrating defects in the ATR-signalling pathway. *Hum Mol Genet*. 13:3127–3138.

Augustin, A., C. Spenlehauer, H. Dumond, J. Menissier-De Murcia, M. Piel, A.C. Schmit, F. Apiou, J.L. Vonesch, M. Kock, M. Bornens, and G. De Murcia. 2003. PARP-3 localizes preferentially to the daughter centriole and interferes with the G1/S cell cycle progression. *J Cell Sci*. 116:1551–1562.

Bang, S.W., M.J. Ko, S. Kang, G.S. Kim, D. Kang, J. Lee, and D.S. Hwang. 2011. Human TopBP1 localization to the mitotic centrosome mediates mitotic progression. *Exp Cell Res*. 317:994–1004.

Bensimon, A., A. Schmidt, Y. Ziv, R. Elkon, S.Y. Wang, D.J. Chen, R. Aebersold, and Y. Shiloh. 2010. ATM-dependent and -independent dynamics of the nuclear phosphoproteome after DNA damage. *Sci Signal*. 3:rs3.

Bourke, E., H. Dodson, A. Merdes, L. Cuffe, G. Zachos, M. Walker, D. Gillespie, and C.G. Morrison. 2007. DNA damage induces Chk1-dependent centrosome amplification. *EMBO Rep*. 8:603–609.

Boveri, T. 2008. Concerning the origin of malignant tumours by Theodor Boveri. Translated and annotated by Henry Harris. *J Cell Sci*. 121 Suppl 1:1–84.

Cappelli, E., S. Townsend, C. Griffin, and J. Thacker. 2011. Homologous recombination proteins are associated with centrosomes and are required for mitotic stability. *Exp Cell Res*. 317:1203–1213.

Date, O., M. Katsura, M. Ishida, T. Yoshihara, A. Kinomura, T. Sueda, and K. Miyagawa. 2006. Haploinsufficiency of RA-51B causes centrosome fragmentation and aneuploidy in human cells. *Cancer Res*. 66:6018–6024.

Dodson, H., E. Bourke, L.J. Jeffers, P. Vagnarelli, E. Sonoda, S. Takeda, W.C. Earnshaw, A. Merdes, and C. Morrison. 2004. Centrosome amplification induced by DNA damage occurs during a prolonged G2 phase and involves ATM. *EMBO J*. 23:3864–3873.

Doxsey, S. 2001. Re-evaluating centrosome function. *Nat Rev Mol Cell Biol*. 2:688–698.

Fukasawa, K. 2007. Oncogenes and tumour suppressors take on centrosomes. *Nat Rev Cancer*. 7:911–924.

Ganem, N.J., S.A. Godinho, and D. Pellman. 2009. A mechanism linking extra centrosomes to chromosomal instability. *Nature*. 460:278–282.

Godinho, S.A., M. Kwon, and D. Pellman. 2009. Centrosomes and cancer: how cancer cells divide with too many centrosomes. *Cancer Metastasis Rev*. 28:85–98.

Golan, A., E. Pick, L. Tsvetkov, Y. Nadler, H. Kluger, and D.F. Stern. 2010. Centrosomal Chk2 in DNA damage responses and cell cycle progession. *Cell Cycle*. 9:2645–2654.

Griffith, E., S. Walker, C.A. Martin, P. Vagnarelli, T. Stiff, B. Vernay, N. Al Sanna, A. Saggar, B. Hamel, W.C. Earnshaw, P.A. Jeggo, A.P. Jackson, and M. O'Driscoll. 2008. Mutations in pericentrin cause Seckel syndrome with defective ATR-dependent DNA damage signaling. *Nat Genet*. 40:232–236.

Iijima, K., M. Ohara, R. Seki, and H. Tauchi. 2008. Dancing on damaged chromatin: functions of ATM and the RAD50/MRE11/NBS1 complex in cellular responses to DNA damage. *J Radiat Res (Tokyo)*. 49:451–464.

Irminger-Finger, I., and C.E. Jefford. 2006. Is there more to BARD1 than BRCA1? *Nat Rev Cancer*. 6:382–391.

Kanai, M., W.M. Tong, E. Sugihara, Z.Q. Wang, K. Fukasawa, and M. Miwa. 2003. Involvement of poly(ADP-Ribose) polymerase 1 and poly(ADP-Ribosyl)ation in regulation of centrosome function. *Mol Cell Biol*. 23:2451–2462.

Kwon, M., S.A. Godinho, N.S. Chandhok, N.J. Ganem, A. Azioune, M. Thery, and D. Pellman. 2008. Mechanisms to suppress multipolar divisions in cancer cells with extra centrosomes. *Genes Dev*. 22:2189–2203.

Matsumoto, Y., and J.L. Maller. 2002. Calcium, calmodulin, and CaMKII requirement for initiation of centrosome duplication in *Xenopus* egg extracts. *Science*. 295:499–502.

Matsumoto, Y., K. Hayashi, and E. Nishida. 1999. Cyclin-dependent kinase 2 (Cdk2) is required for centrosome duplication in mammalian cells. *Curr Biol*. 9:429–432.

Matsuura, S., H. Tauchi, A. Nakamura, N. Kondo, S. Sakamoto, S. Endo, D. Smeets, B. Solder, B.H. Belohradsky, V.M. Der Kaloustian, M. Oshimura, M. Isomura, Y. Nakamura, and K. Komatsu. 1998. Positional cloning of the gene for Nijmegen breakage syndrome. *Nat Genet*. 19:179–181.

Miwa, M., and M. Masutani. 2007. PolyADP-ribosylation and cancer. *Cancer Sci*. 98:1528–1535.

Nakamura, K., A. Kato, J. Kobayashi, H. Yanagihara, S. Sakamoto, D.V. Oliveira, M. Shimada, H. Tauchi, H. Suzuki, S. Tashiro, L. Zou, and K. Komatsu. 2011. Regulation of homologous recombination by RNF20-dependent H2B ubiquitination. *Mol Cell*. 41:515–528.

Nigg, E.A. 2002. Centrosome aberrations: cause or consequence of cancer progression? *Nat Rev Cancer*. 2:815–825.

Nigg, E.A. 2007. Centrosome duplication: of rules and licenses. *Trends Cell Biol*. 17:215–221.

Niwa, T., H. Saito, S. Imajoh-ohmi, M. Kaminishi, Y. Seto, Y. Miki, and A. Nakanishi. 2009. BRCA2 interacts with the cytoskeletal linker protein plectin to form a complex controlling centrosome localization. *Cancer Sci*. 100:2115–2125.

Rauch, A., C.T. Thiel, D. Schindler, U. Wick, Y.J. Crow, A.B. Ekici, A.J. van Essen, T.O. Goecke, L. Al-Gazali, K.H. Chrzanowska, C. Zweier, H.G. Brunner, K. Becker, C.J. Curry, B. Dallapiccola, K. Devriendt, A. Dorfler, E. Kinning, A. Megarbane, P. Meinecke, R.K. Semple, S. Spranger, A. Toutain, R.C. Trembath, E. Voss, L. Wilson,

R. Hennekam, F. de Zegher, H.G. Dorr, and A. Reis. 2008. Mutations in the pericentrin (*PCNT*) gene cause primordial dwarfism. *Science*. 319:816–819.

Renglin Lindh, A., N. Schultz, N. Saleh-Gohari, and T. Helleday. 2007. RAD51C (RAD51L2) is involved in maintaining centrosome number in mitosis. *Cytogenet Genome Res*. 116:38–45.

Sato, N., K. Mizumoto, M. Nakamura, H. Ueno, Y.A. Minamishima, J.L. Farber, and M. Tanaka. 2000. A possible role for centrosome overduplication in radiation-induced cell death. *Oncogene*. 19:5281–5290.

Shimada, M., and K. Komatsu. 2009. Emerging connection between centrosome and DNA repair machinery. *J Radiat Res (Tokyo)*. 50:295–301.

Shimada, M., H. Niida, D.H. Zineldeen, H. Tagami, M. Tanaka, H. Saito, and M. Nakanishi. 2008. Chk1 is a histone H3 threonine 11 kinase that regulates DNA damage-induced transcriptional repression. *Cell*. 132:221–232.

Shimada, M., R. Sagae, J. Kobayashi, T. Habu, and K. Komatsu. 2009. Inactivation of the Nijmegen breakage syndrome gene leads to excess centrosome duplication via the ATR/BRCA1 pathway. *Cancer Res*. 69:1768–1775.

Shimada, M., J. Kobayashi, R. Hirayama, and K. Komatsu. 2010. Differential role of repair proteins, BRCA1/NBS1 and Ku70/DNA-PKcs, in radiation-induced centrosome overduplication. *Cancer Sci*. 101:2531–2537.

Simons, A.M., A.A. Horwitz, L.M. Starita, K. Griffin, R.S. Williams, J.N. Glover, and J.D. Parvin. 2006. BRCA1 DNA-binding activity is stimulated by BARD1. *Cancer Res*. 66:2012–2018.

Smith, E., D. Dejsuphong, A. Balestrini, M. Hampel, C. Lenz, S. Takeda, A. Vindigni, and V. Costanzo. 2009. An ATM- and ATR-dependent checkpoint inactivates spindle assembly by targeting CEP63. *Nat Cell Biol*. 11:278–285.

Smith, S., and T. de Lange. 1999. Cell cycle dependent localization of the telomeric PARP, tankyrase, to nuclear pore complexes and centrosomes. *J Cell Sci*. 112 (Pt 21):3649–3656.

Starita, L.M., A.A. Horwitz, M.C. Keogh, C. Ishioka, J.D. Parvin, and N. Chiba. 2005. BRCA1/BARD1 ubiquitinate phosphorylated RNA polymerase II. *J Biol Chem*. 280:24498–24505.

Tauchi, H., J. Kobayashi, K. Morishima, D.C. van Gent, T. Shiraishi, N.S. Verkaik, D. vanHeems, E. Ito, A. Nakamura, E. Sonoda, M. Takata, S. Takeda, S. Matsuura, and K. Komatsu. 2002. Nbs1 is essential for DNA repair by homologous recombination in higher vertebrate cells. *Nature*. 420:93–98.

Tibelius, A., J. Marhold, H. Zentgraf, C.E. Heilig, H. Neitzel, B. Ducommun, A. Rauch, A.D. Ho, J. Bartek, and A. Kramer. 2009. Microcephalin and pericentrin regulate mitotic entry via centrosome-associated Chk1. *J Cell Biol*. 185:1149–1157.

Tsvetkov, L., X. Xu, J. Li, and D.F. Stern. 2003. Polo-like kinase 1 and Chk2 interact and co-localize to centrosomes and the midbody. *J Biol Chem*. 278:8468–8475.

Wang, H.F., K. Takenaka, A. Nakanishi, and Y. Miki. 2011. BRCA2 and nucleophosmin coregulate centrosome amplification and form a complex with the Rho effector kinase ROCK2. *Cancer Res*. 71:68–77.

Yoshida, K., and Y. Miki. 2004. Role of BRCA1 and BRCA2 as regulators of DNA repair, transcription, and cell cycle in response to DNA damage. *Cancer Sci*. 95:866–871.

Zhang, S., P. Hemmerich, and F. Grosse. 2007. Werner syndrome helicase (WRN), nuclear DNA helicase II (NDH II) and histone gammaH2AX are localized to the centrosome. *Cell Biol Int*. 31:1109–1121.

5

Shared Regulatory Motifs in Promoters of Human DNA Repair Genes

Lonnie R. Welch[1], Laura M. Koehly[2] and Laura Elnitski[3]
[1]*School of Electrical Engineering and Computer Science, Ohio University, Athens, Ohio*
[2]*Social and Behavioral Research Branch, National Human Genome Research Institute, NIH, Bethesda, Maryland*
[3]*Genome Technology Branch National Human Genome Research Institute, NIH, Bethesda, Maryland*
USA

1. Introduction

This manuscript presents methods used to test, and resulting evidence to support the hypothesis that specialized transcription factor binding sites coordinate the expression of DNA repair genes. Building on the seminal work of the Elnitski laboratory (Yang et al. 2007), which identified the most complete set of human transcripts under the control of bidirectional promoters and identified the first putative regulatory networks that make use of the bidirectional promoter structure, the authors present additional details of these regulatory networks.

Much of the work regarding the regulation of DNA repair proteins is aimed at the level of protein-protein interactions and post-translational processing events (Hurley et al. 2007, Jensen et al. 2011, Shibata et al. 2010). However, transcriptional activation of DNA repair genes is likely to utilize shared factors, especially in cases of induced activation, which have not been thoroughly evaluated. Yang, Koehly and Elnitski reported the discovery and characterization of 5,653 bidirectional promoters in the human genome (Yang et al. 2007). Prior to that date, bidirectional promoters were annotated only for protein-coding genes, and only 1,352 examples had been reported in the human genome. The work of Yang et al. included evidence from all noncoding-RNA genes, as well. Each bidirectional promoter regulates the expression of two genes, oriented in opposite directions with transcription start sites within 1000 bp of one another. The authors developed a novel approach to map all bidirectional promoters by analyzing the public expressed-sequence-tag (EST) data. The prevalence of this promoter structure led the authors to explore the hypothesis that it plays a role in regulation of certain classes of genes. They discovered that many more DNA repair genes have bidirectional promoters than previously reported and that many genes with somatic mutations in cancer have bidirectional promoters. The relevance of DNA repair genes to cancers (Kinsella et al. 2009, Liang et al. 2009, Smith et al. 2010, Kelley et al. 2008, Li et al. 2009, Bellizii et al. 2009, Naccarati et al. 2007, Berwick et al. 2000)) and the association of bidirectional promoters with DNA repair genes suggested that bidirectional promoters might indicate a higher-order type of regulatory structure that could be detected through common features at the DNA sequence level. If true, these features should discriminate bidirectional promoters and unidirectional promoters of genes with DNA repair functions.

Thus, this chapter presents additional evidence of these regulatory networks. Specifically, this chapter provides evidence that there are distinct regulatory signatures for (1) genes involved in certain types of cancers, (2) bidirectional versus unidirectional promoters and (3) specific DNA repair pathways. The authors have identified transcription factor binding sites in bidirectional promoters of genes implicated in breast and ovarian (B/O) cancers. Additionally, they have discovered novel transcription factor binding sites that may serve as regulatory elements to distinguish DNA repair genes with bidirectional promoters from DNA repair genes with unidirectional promoters. Applications of this work extend to a collection of novel transcription factor binding sites shared among genes acting as checkpoint factors of DNA repair pathways. These findings have important implications - as evidence of novel regulatory mechanisms, and new insights into cancer biology (i.e., genomic elements relevant to transcriptional regulation) are gained.

2. Regulatory features of genes implicated in breast and ovarian cancers

This section provides evidence to support the hypothesis that there are distinct regulatory control systems among bidirectional and unidirectional promoters. Additionally, this section presents transcription factor binding sites discovered in bidirectional promoters of genes implicated in breast and ovarian cancers.

As reported in Yang et al. 2007, we identified transcription factor binding sites for known factors in genes implicated in B/O cancers. The enrichment of bidirectional promoters in several cancer genes, and in additional genes having functions in DNA repair, suggests common mechanisms of regulation. We used expression clustering and enrichment of genes with bidirectional promoters to group the cancer genes into expression groups from the full genome to address features common among the clusters that might indicate the presence of regulatory networks. The cancer-related genes that were identified and studied are listed below, along with their descriptions from GeneCards (Safran et al. 2010). The Elnitski group was the first to report that this set of genes has bidirectional promoters.

All genes were assessed for the top most related gene expression profiles in the genome using the gene sorter tool at the UCSC Genome Browser and expression data from the Novartis GNF Atlas2 (containing expression profiles for 96 tissues). Each cluster was then compared to all the others to identify intersection points (by gene names) among the lists of co-expressed genes. Using a process of multidimensional scaling, the gene lists were compared and a putative regulatory network was generated (Figure 1). The *MLH1* gene appeared in several co-expression clusters and therefore occupied a central location with connections to 7 other genes (*BARD1, FANCA, BRCA1, CHK2, BRCA2, TP53* and *FANCF*). Two additional genes co-occupied the central position with *MLH1*. *COMMD3* (an uncharacterized protein) and *ITGB3BP*, a regulator of apoptosis in breast cancer cells.

2.1 Network visualization

The bidirectional promoters that are associated with the breast and ovarian cancer genes were considered an affiliation network or a bipartite graph. In this example nodes represent the genes in the co-expression clusters and edges connect the genes appearing in more than one list. The higher the number of appearances of any gene from the ten co-expression lists, the more central its position in the network. Geodesic distances between genes were computed (e.g. length of the shortest path between genes through promoters, and the geodesic distance matrix was scaled using a metric multidimensional scaling (MDS)

Gene	Description from GeneCards (Safran 2010)
BARD1	This gene encodes a protein which interacts with the N-terminal region of *BRCA1*.
BRCA1	This gene encodes a nuclear phosphoprotein that plays a role in maintaining genomic stability, and it also acts as a tumor suppressor.
BRCA2	Inherited mutations in *BRCA1* and this gene, *BRCA2*, confer increased lifetime risk of developing breast or ovarian cancer.
CHK2	In response to DNA damage and replication blocks, cell cycle progression is halted through the control of critical cell cycle regulators. The protein encoded by this gene is a cell cycle checkpoint regulator and putative tumor suppressor.
ERBB2	This gene encodes a member of the epidermal growth factor (EGF) receptor family of receptor tyrosine kinases.
TP53	This gene encodes tumor protein *p53*, which responds to diverse cellular stresses to regulate target genes that induce cell cycle arrest, apoptosis, senescence, DNA repair, or changes in metabolism.
FANCA	DNA repair protein that may operate in a post-replication repair or a cell cycle checkpoint function. May be involved in inter-strand DNA cross-link repair and in the maintenance of normal chromosome stability.
FANCB	DNA repair protein required for *FANCD2* ubiquitination.
FANCD2	Required for maintenance of chromosomal stability. Promotes accurate and efficient pairing of homologs during meiosis. Involved in the repair of DNA double-strand breaks, both by homologous recombination and single-strand annealing. May participate in S phase and G2 phase checkpoint activation upon DNA damage. Promotes *BRCA2/FANCD1* loading onto damaged chromatin.
FANCF	DNA repair protein that may operate in a postreplication repair or a cell cycle checkpoint function. May be implicated in interstrand DNA cross-link repair and in the maintenance of normal chromosome stability.

Table 1. The B/O cancer-related genes that were studied.

algorithm (in UCINET 6; Borgatti et al., 2002). The distance between the 10 B/O cancer genes represents their similarity based on the number of shared genes found in the co-expression clusters. Genes in the center of the network were present in the largest number of gene clusters, seven out of 10, indicating that co-expression clusters intersect through common regulatory nodes.

2.2 Transcription factor binding site analysis

A systematic search of transcription factor binding sites in the list of bidirectional promoters was used to assess regulatory connections at the DNA level, and revealed several in common (using a motif finding algorithm we searched for the motifs reported in (Xie et al. 2005)). Notably, identical *ELK1* binding sites were located at the same distance from *ERBB2*, *FANCD2*, and *BRCA2* transcription start sites (Yang et al. 2007). *ETS* factor binding sites were present as a trio with SP1 and *PAX4/RXR* binding sites in the majority of the promoters. The transcription factors for which binding motifs were found in all of the promoters along with their descriptions from GeneCards (Safran et al. 2010) are reported in Table 2.

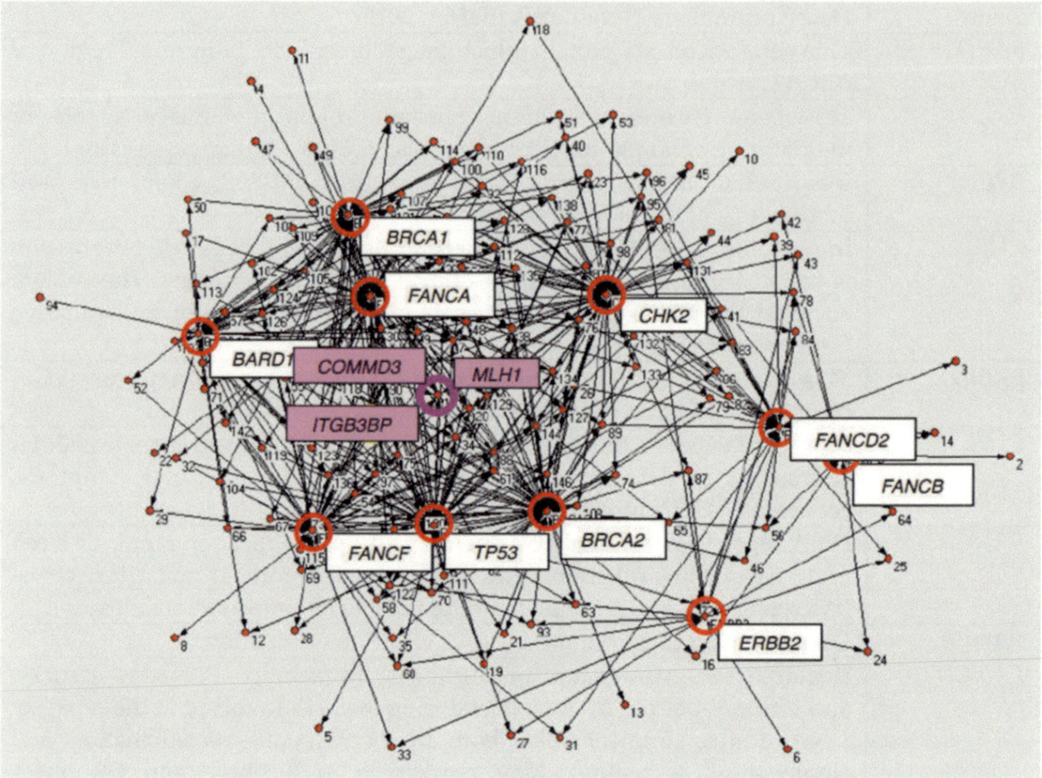

Fig. 1. Co-expression clustering analysis of 10 DNA repair genes finds intersecting nodes.

Transcription Factor	**Description from GeneCards**
Sp1	Transcription factor that can activate or repress transcription in response to physiological and pathological stimuli. Regulates the expression of a large number of genes involved in a variety of processes such as cell growth, apoptosis, differentiation and immune responses. May have a role in modulating the cellular response to DNA damage.
NFAT	The nuclear factor of activated T-cells family of transcription factors.
EGR-1	The protein encoded by this gene belongs to the EGR family of *C2H2*-type zinc-finger proteins. It is a nuclear protein and functions as a transcriptional regulator. Studies suggest this is a cancer suppressor gene.
PAX4	This gene is a member of the paired box (*PAX*) family of transcription factors. These genes play critical roles during fetal development and cancer growth.
ELK1	*ELK1* is a member of *ETS* oncogene family. The protein encoded by this gene is a nuclear target for the ras-raf-MAPK signaling cascade.

Table 2. Transcription factor binding sites in the promoters of the B/O cancer genes.

3. Unbiased assessment of transcription factor binding sites in two subgroups of genes from DNA repair pathways

The research reported in (Yang et al. 2007) provides strong evidence that a unique set of regulatory proteins control genes that contain bidirectional promoters by comparing co-expression clusters of genes enriched for bidirectional promoters versus those depleted for bidirectional promoters. This section reports on a study that identified transcription factor binding sites that are specific to genes in DNA repair pathways (Lichtenberg et al. 2009). The promoters of genes from the DNA repair pathways were partitioned into two groups, those that are bidirectional (32 promoters) and those that are unidirectional (42 promoters).

3.1 Assessment of individual sites

Each group of promoters was analyzed to discover putative transcription factor binding sites. The analysis was performed with WordSeeker motif discovery software (Lichtenberg et al. 2010), which employs high performance supercomputer-based algorithms to perform motif enumeration and to construct Markov models. Our analysis revealed that the average nucleotide G+C content of the bidirectional promoters was slightly higher than the unidirectional promoters, 59.87% versus 50.84%, respectively. These differences were rigorously controlled by the use of the Markov model, which examines background frequencies of each nucleotide in the collection of sequences. Unique sets of binding sites were identified for each group, some of which represent novel binding sites.

A statistical analysis of the promoters of the DNA repair genes revealed a number of significant DNA binding site motifs. Some of the discovered motifs correspond to recognition sequences of known proteins. These are listed in Table 3, along with their *p*-values and the corresponding transcription factors known to bind to the motifs (as determined by the TRANSFAC database (Wingender et al. 2000) and the JASPAR database (Bryne et al. 2008)). In addition, novel motifs, representing uncharacterized transcription factor binding sites, were discovered in the bidirectional and unidirectional promoters from DNA repair pathway genes (see Table 4 for the motifs and their *p*-values).

Motif (bidirectional promoters)	*p*-Value	Transcription Factor	Motif (unidirectional promoters)	*p*-Value	Transcription Factor
AGGGCCGT	0.04142	*MYB*	ACCCGCCT	0.00656	*SP1*
CAGGGGCC	0.02841	*V$WT1_Q6*	AGGAAACA	0.03295	*NFAT*
CGTGGGGG	0.04701	*E2F*	ATTAAAAT	0.05372	*OCT1*
GGCCCGCC	0.06682	*SP1*	CGGAAACC	0.04210	*AREB6*
TCCCGGCT	0.05408	*ELK1*	GCAGGGCG	0.07134	*PF0096*
TCCCGGGA	0.06861	*STAT5A*	GGGGAGTA	0.03321	*FOXC1*
TCGCGCCA	0.01539	*PF0112*	GGGGCTGC	0.06212	*LRF*
TCTGAGGA	0.01350	*TFIIA*	TGGGCGGA	0.06334	*GC*

Table 3. Enriched motifs matching characterized transcription factor binding sites discovered in the bidirectional promoters (columns 1 and 2) and in the unidirectional promoters (columns 3 and 4).

Motif (bidirectional promoters)	P-Value	Motif (unidirectional promoters)	P-Value
ACTCCAGC	0.06212	AGCCGGCT	0.05007
AGAAAAGA	0.02756	ATTCCCAG	0.05599
AGGGAGGG	0.07159	CCTCTTTA	0.03381
CAGCAGCC	0.10540	CGCCCCTT	0.11386
CGACTCCG	0.02756	CGGCGGCG	0.04742
CGCGGCCG	0.03377	CTCCCGCT	0.05998
CGGGCCGA	0.06548	CTTCTTTC	0.03773
GCCCCTCC	0.07021	GCGCCGCG	0.09760
GCCGGCGA	0.03662	GGGCGCCC	0.08390
GGCAGGGA	0.10334	GTGCGTTT	0.06286
GGGCCAGG	0.09632	TCCGCCGG	0.05794
GGGGCCGG	0.05265	TCTCCCCT	0.07881
TCTGGGAT	0.01466	TCTTCTTC	0.04649
TGAAGCCA	0.05699	TGCGCCGA	0.04148
TGCCCGCG	0.08277	TTGGTCTC	0.08543
TGCGGAAT	0.02132	TTTCTCCA	0.06840
TGCTGAGA	0.03377	TTTTTTGA	0.04742

Table 4. Uncharacterized motifs discovered in the promoters of DNA repair genes. Words are ordered alphabetically.

3.2 Assessment of paired binding sites

To identify putative regulatory modules (co-acting regulatory elements), we identified statistically overrepresented pairs of DNA motifs in each set of promoters. Motif pairs are shown in Table 5. The motif pair scores are computed as the product of (1) the number sequences, S, in which the pair occurs and (2) the natural log of the ratio of S and the expected value of S, E_s; i.e., the score is $S \cdot \ln(S/E_s)$. The genomic signatures (significant DNA motifs and motif pairs) of the bidirectional promoters were virtually non-overlapping with the signatures of unidirectional promoters. This provides strong support for the hypothesis that the regulatory mechanisms of bidirectional promoters are unique. Additionally, this work contributes a significant enhancement to the available knowledge about transcriptional regulation of genes involved in DNA repair pathways, and implicates the presence of a regulatory network.

4. Unbiased assessment of transcription factor binding sites of checkpoint factor genes from DNA repair pathways

We have performed a focused, detailed characterization of the checkpoint factors in DNA repair pathways (Elnitski et al. 2010). The checkpoint factors (Kanehisa et al. 2008, Wood 2005, Helleday et al. 2008) are activated upon detection of DNA damage, resulting in halting the cell cycle so that subsequent DNA repair pathways can mend the damage. In addition to examining the most recognized promoter in each gene (the 5′ end of the full-length transcription unit), we assessed alternative start sites for each checkpoint factor gene as independent regulatory units, to discover putative transcription factor binding sites. In this

Co-Occurring Motif Pair (Bidirectional Promoters)		Score	Co-Occurring Motif Pair (Unidirectional Promoters)		Score
TCTGAGGA	TCGCGCCA	12.1158	GTTCATTC	TCCGCCGG	11.2184
ACTCCAGC	TCGCGCCA	11.8387	CTGTGTGC	TGCGCCGA	11.1966
GCCCAGCC	TCCGCCGC	11.1827	TGACGCGA	CTCCCGCT	10.9997
GCCCAGCC	CGGAGCGC	10.8711	AGCCGGCT	GGGGAGTA	10.0590
TGCCCGCG	TCCCGGGA	10.7404	ATTGCAGG	ATTCTCTC	9.5459
GGCAGGGA	GGGCCAGG	9.8609	GGGGAGTA	AGGAAACA	9.3177
TCCCGGGA	TCGCGCCA	9.8112	CTGGGAGC	GTTCATTC	9.0337
AGCCTGTC	TCCCGGGA	9.7646	CCTTCCGA	CTGGGAGC	8.8439
GGAGGCTG	TCGCGCCA	9.7250	TGGGCGGA	ACCCGCCT	8.7895
TCCGCCGC	GCCCCTCC	9.6830	TTTCTCCA	CGGAAACC	8.6446
AGAAAAGA	TCGCGCCA	9.4042	CCCCCGCG	ACCCGCCT	8.5339
GCCCAGCC	GCCCCTCC	9.2808	TCCGCCGG	GGGGCTGC	7.7522
TGCCAAAA	GCCGGCGA	9.2604	AGCTGGCT	CCAGGCTG	7.7192
CAGCAGCC	TGCGGAAT	9.1297	TTGGTCTC	AGGAAACA	7.6068
AGGGCCGT	TCCCGGCT	9.1249	CTGGGAGC	TCCGCCGG	7.3021

Table 5. Putative transcription factor binding modules discovered in promoters of DNA repair genes.

section we report the DNA motifs that were discovered, along with several clusters of related genes and promoters. We hypothesize that these similar components implicate regulatory networks responsible for co-regulation of the checkpoint factor genes.

We studied fourteen checkpoint factor genes, which are listed in Table 6. The number of alternative promoters per gene, shown in parentheses, varied for each gene. Because most of the genes have alternative promoters, we analyzed a total of thirty promoters. The complete set of alternative promotes is shown in Table 7. Alternative promoters were identified using annotations of genes in the UCSC Human Genome Browser. Transcription start sites of transcript isoforms served as the coordinates around which 900 bp upstream and 100 bp downstream were defined as the putative promoter region. Alternative promoters with significant overlap were truncated or removed from the analysis. DNA sequences were obtained for the forward and reverse strands of the genome to ensure coverage of words that might have biased nucleotide content and be subject to omission during the Markov model analysis stage.

Gene	Description from GeneCards (Safran 2010)
ATM (5)	The protein encoded by this gene (ataxia telangiectasia mutated) belongs to the PI3/PI4-kinase family. This protein functions as a regulator of a wide variety of downstream proteins, including *p53, BRCA1, CHK2, RAD17, RAD9,* and *NBS1*. This protein and the closely related kinase ATR are thought to be master controllers of cell cycle checkpoint signaling pathways, required for cell response to DNA damage and for genome stability.
ATR (2)	The protein encoded by this gene (ataxia telangiectasia and Rad3 related) belongs the PI3/PI4-kinase family, and is most closely related to ATM. Both proteins share similarity with

	Schizosaccharomyces pombe rad3, a cell cycle checkpoint gene required for cell cycle arrest and DNA damage repair in response to DNA damage. This kinase has been shown to phosphorylate *CHK1, RAD17,* and *RAD9* and *BRCA1*. Transcript variants utilizing alternative polyA sites exist.
ATRIP (1)	The product of this gene (ATR interacting protein) is an essential component of the DNA damage checkpoint, and binds to single-stranded DNA coated with replication protein A that accumulates at sites of DNA damage. The encoded protein interacts with the ataxia telangiectasia and Rad3 related protein, a checkpoint kinase, resulting in accumulation of the kinase at intranuclear foci induced by DNA damage. Multiple transcript variants encoding different isoforms have been found for this gene.
CHEK1 (3)	Required for checkpoint mediated cell cycle arrest in response to DNA damage or the presence of unreplicated DNA. May also negatively regulate cell cycle progression during unperturbed cell cycles. Binds to and phosphorylates *CDC25A, CDC25B* and *CDC25C*. Binds to and phosphorylates *RAD51*. Binds to and phosphorylates *TLK1*. May also phosphorylate multiple sites within the C-terminus of *TP53*, which promotes activation of *TP53* by acetylation and enhances suppression of cellular proliferation.
CHEK2 (2)	The protein encoded by this gene is a cell cycle checkpoint regulator and putative tumor suppressor. It contains a forkhead-associated protein interaction domain essential for activation in response to DNA damage and is rapidly phosphorylated in response to replication blocks and DNA damage. This protein interacts with and phosphorylates *BRCA1*, allowing *BRCA1* to restore survival after DNA damage. Three transcript variants encoding different isoforms have been found for this gene.
CLK2 (2)	This gene encodes a member of the *CLK* family of dual specificity protein kinases. *CLK* family members have been shown to interact with, and phosphorylate, serine- and arginine-rich (SR) proteins of the spliceosomal complex, which is a part of the regulatory mechanism that enables the SR proteins to control RNA splicing.
HUS1 (1)	The protein encoded by this gene is a component of an evolutionarily conserved, genotoxin-activated checkpoint complex that is involved in the cell cycle arrest in response to DNA damage. This protein forms a heterotrimeric complex with checkpoint proteins *RAD9* and *RAD1*. DNA damage induced chromatin binding has been shown to depend on the activation of the checkpoint kinase ATM, and is thought to be an early checkpoint signaling event.
MDC1 (2)	The protein encoded by this gene (mediator of DNA-damage checkpoint) is required to activate the intra-S phase and G2/M phase cell cycle checkpoints in response to DNA damage. This nuclear protein interacts with phosphorylated histone H2AX near sites of DNA double-strand breaks through its *BRCT* motifs, and facilitates

	recruitment of the ATM kinase and meiotic recombination 11 protein complex to DNA damage foci.
NBS1 (1)	The encoded protein is a member of the *MRE11/RAD50* double-strand break repair complex which consists of 5 proteins. This gene product is thought to be involved in DNA double-strand break repair and DNA damage-induced checkpoint activation.
P53/TP53 (3)	This gene encodes tumor protein *p53*, which responds to diverse cellular stresses to regulate target genes that induce cell cycle arrest, apoptosis, senescence, DNA repair, or changes in metabolism.
PER1 (1)	This gene is a member of the Period family of genes and is expressed in a circadian pattern in the suprachiasmatic nucleus, the primary circadian pacemaker in the mammalian brain. Genes in this family encode components of the circadian rhythms of locomotor activity, metabolism, and behavior. The specific function of this gene is not yet known. Alternative splicing has been observed in this gene; however, these variants have not been fully described.
RAD1 (2)	This gene encodes a component of a heterotrimeric cell cycle checkpoint complex, known as the 9-1-1 complex, that is activated to stop cell cycle progression in response to DNA damage or incomplete DNA replication. The 9-1-1 complex is recruited by *RAD17* to affected sites where it may attract specialized DNA polymerases and other DNA repair effectors. Alternatively spliced transcript variants of this gene have been described.
RAD17 (3)	The protein encoded by this gene is highly similar to the gene product of Schizosaccharomyces pombe rad17, a cell cycle checkpoint gene required for cell cycle arrest and DNA damage repair in response to DNA damage. This protein recruits the *RAD1-RAD9-HUS1* checkpoint protein complex onto chromatin after DNA damage,. The phosphorylation of this protein is required for the DNA-damage-induced cell cycle G2 arrest, and is thought to be a critical early event during checkpoint signaling in DNA-damaged cells. Eight alternatively spliced transcript variants of this gene, which encode four distinct proteins, have been reported.
RAD9A (2)	This gene product is highly similar to Schizosaccharomyces pombe rad9, a cell cycle checkpoint protein required for cell cycle arrest and DNA damage repair in response to DNA damage. This protein is found to possess 3' to 5' exonuclease activity, which may contribute to its role in sensing and repairing DNA damage. It forms a checkpoint protein complex with *RAD1* and *HUS1*. This complex is recruited by checkpoint protein *RAD17* to the sites of DNA damage, which is thought to be important for triggering the checkpoint-signaling cascade. Use of alternative polyA sites has been noted for this gene.

Table 6. The checkpoint factors genes that were studied. The number of alternative promoters is shown in parentheses next to each gene name.

Checkpoint Factors	Alternative promoters (hg18 coordinates)
ATM	*(ATM5)* chr11:107662328-107663378_+ *(ATM5)* chr11:107662328-107663378_- *(ATM2)* chr11:107643346-107644396_+ *(ATM2)* chr11:107643346-107644396_- *(ATM3)* chr11:107597768-107598818_+ *(ATM3)* chr11:107597768-107598818_- *(ATM4)* chr11:107671910-107672960_+ *(ATM4)* chr11:107671910-107672960_- *(ATM5)* chr11:107679611-107680661_+ *(ATM5)* chr11:107679611-107680661_-
ATR	*(ATR1)* chr3:143780308-143781358_+ *(ATR1)* chr3:143780308-143781358_- *(ATR2)* chr3:143671051-143672101_+ *(ATR2)* chr3:143671051-143672101_-
ATRIP	chr3:48462221-48463271_+ chr3:48462221-48463271_-
CHEK1	*(CHEK13)* chr11:125000333-125001383_+ *(CHEK13)* chr11:125000333-125001383_- *(CHEK12)* chr11:125018185-125019235_+ *(CHEK12)* chr11:125018185-125019235_- *(CHEK13)* chr11:124999245-125000295_+ *(CHEK13)* chr11:124999245-125000295_-
CHEK2	*(CHEK22)* chr22:27467772-27468822_+ *(CHEK22)* chr22:27467772-27468822_- *(CHEK22)* chr22:27460665-27461715_+ *(CHEK22)* chr22:27460665-27461715_-
CLK2	*(CLK22)* chr1:153509855-153510905_+ *(CLK22)* chr1:153509855-153510905_- *(CLK22)* chr1:153514075-153515125_+ *(CLK22)* chr1:153514075-153515125_-
HUS1	chr7:47985721-47986771_+ chr7:47985721-47986771_-

MDC1	*($MDC1_2$)* chr6:30792781-30793831_+ *($MDC1_2$)* chr6:30792781-30793831_- *($MDC1_2$)* chr6:30789060-30790110_+ *($MDC1_2$)* chr6:30789060-30790110_-
NBS1	chr8:91066025-91067075_+ chr8:91066025-91067075_-
P53 (TP53)	*($TP53_3$)* chr17:7519486-7520536_+ *($TP53_3$)* chr17:7519486-7520536_- *($TP53_2$)* chr17:7531538-7532588_+ *($TP53_2$)* chr17:7531538-7532588_- *($TP53_3$)* chr17:7520612-7521662_+ *($TP53_3$)* chr17:7520612-7521662_-
PER1	chr17:7996377-7997427_+ chr17:7996377-7997427_-
RAD1	*($RAD1_2$)* chr5:34954089-34955139_+ *($RAD1_2$)* chr5:34954089-34955139_- *($RAD1_2$)* chr5:34951438-34952488_+ *($RAD1_2$)* chr5:34951438-34952488_-
RAD17	*($RAD17_3$)* chr5:68699879-68700929_+ *($RAD17_3$)* chr5:68699879-68700929_- *($RAD17_2$)* chr5:68723716-68724766_+ *($RAD17_2$)* chr5:68723716-68724766_- *($RAD17_3$)* chr5:68701287-68702337_+ *($RAD17_3$)* chr5:68701287-68702337_-
RAD9A	*($RAD9A_2$)* chr11:66918716-66919766_+ *($RAD9A_2$)* chr11:66918716-66919766_- *($RAD9A_2$)* chr11:66914998-66916048_+ *($RAD9A_2$)* chr11:66914998-66916048_-

Table 7. Alternative promoters, indicated by their genomic coordinates, of genes involved in cell-cycle checkpoint factor pathways.

Statistical analysis of thirty promoters found several interesting DNA words, which predict DNA elements that participate in the regulation of the DNA repair checkpoint factors. The most significant words discovered are listed in Table 8. Words that are shared among the gene sets identify regulatory relationships. Reverse complement words are reported separately, as internal verification on the process. Words without a reverse complement example indicate a particular bias in the nucleotide content.

Word	Promoters	Sln(S/Es)
ACAGCCAT	ATM_2	5.41
	$CHEK2_2$	
	$CLK2_1$	
ATGGCTGT	ATM_2	5.41
	$CHECK2_2$	
	$CLK2_1$	
GCCTGGGA	ATR_1	5.40
	$CHEK2_1$	
	$CLK2_2$	
	$MDC1_1$	
	$MDC1_2$	
	$RAD1_2$	
TCCCAGGC	ATR_1	5.40
	$CHEK2_1$	
	$CLK2_2$	
	$MDC1_1$	
	$MDC1_2$	
	$RAD1_2$	
ACTCCCTA	ATM_3	5.29
	$CHEK2_1$	
	$RAD17_2$	
TAGGGAGT	ATM_3	5.29
	$CHEK2_1$	
	$RAD17_2$	
AGCGGCCA	ATR_1	5.24
	ATR_2	
	$CHEK1_1$	
TGGCCGCT	ATR_1	5.24
	ATR_2	
	$CHEK1_1$	
GAAATGAA	ATM_2	5.24
	ATM_3	
	ATR_2	
	$CLK2_2$	
	HUS1	
	$MDC1_1$	
TTCATTTC	ATM_2	5.24
	ATM_3	
	ATR_2	
	$CLK2_2$	
	HUS1	
	$MDC1_1$	
AATGCAGG	$RAD1_1$	4.97
	$TP53_1$	
	$TP53_2$	
	$TP53_3$	

CCTGCATT	$RAD1_1$	4.97
	$TP53_1$	
	$TP53_2$	
	$TP53_3$	
ATCCCTGA	ATRIP	4.73
	$CHEK1_3$	
	$RAD1_2$	
	$RAD17_1$	
TCAGGGAT	ATRIP	4.73
	$CHEK1_3$	
	$RAD1_2$	
	$RAD17_1$	
GTATTTTA	ATM_4	4.58
	$CHEK1_2$	
	NBS1	
	$RAD17_1$	
	ATR_2	
	$TP53_1$	
	HUS1	
	$RAD17_1$	

Table 8. Top 15 enumerated DNA words, based on the $S \cdot \ln(S/E_S)$ overrepresentation score, and the alternative promoters, identified by subscript.

5. Visualization and interpretation of data

Shared words among the checkpoint factor genes suggested the presence of regulatory networks. We assessed the relationships by generating network depictions in the form of interaction networks (Figure 2) and a circos diagram (Figure 3) constructed from the summary data in Table 9. To derive Figure 2, a metric MDS was conducted on the affiliation network defined in Table 9. The resulting graph was then spring-embedded, with node repulsion, to facilitate visualization (Borgatti, 2002). The interaction network depicts the distribution of the DNA words among the genes (note that each gene appears once, representing all alternative promoters as a single node). Genes are denoted by blue squares and words are represented with red circles. Bold lines indicate multiple occurrences of a word. Reverse complement words are shown independently.

The circos diagram represents the information in a closed circular space, wherein connections between words on one side of the diagram extend to genes on the other side. The putative nodes of the regulatory networks are defined by multiple edges, representing a characterized transcription factor or a novel DNA binding site, or a checkpoint factor gene.

Some of the discovered words correspond to known binding sites for transcription factors, reported in the JASPAR and TRANSFAC databases of transcription factors (see Table 10). The relationships between the top fifteen words and the transcription factors are depicted in the circos diagram in Figure 4. Note that multiple binding site motifs were discovered for many of the transcription factors, and that several of the sites match the binding patterns of more than one transcription factor.

Row segments

Column segments

	ATM	ATR	ATRIP	CHEK1	CHEK2	CLK2	HUS1	MDC1	NBS1	P53	PER1	RAD1	RAD17	RAD9A
ACAGCCAT	1	0	0	0	1	1	0	0	0	0	0	0	0	0
ATGGCTGT	1	0	0	0	1	1	0	0	0	0	0	0	0	0
GCCTGGGA	0	1	0	0	1	1	0	2	0	0	0	1	0	0
TCCCAGGC	0	1	0	0	1	1	0	2	0	0	0	1	0	0
ACTCCCTA	1	0	0	0	1	0	0	0	0	0	0	0	1	0
TAGGGAGT	1	0	0	0	1	0	0	0	0	0	0	0	1	0
AGCGGCCA	0	2	0	1	0	0	0	0	0	0	0	0	0	0
TGGCCGCT	0	2	0	1	0	0	0	0	0	0	0	0	0	0
GAAATGAA	2	1	0	0	0	1	1	1	0	0	0	0	0	0
TTCATTTC	2	1	0	0	0	1	1	1	0	0	0	0	0	0
AATGCAGG	0	0	0	0	0	0	0	0	0	3	0	1	0	0
CCTGCATT	0	0	0	0	0	0	0	0	0	3	0	1	0	0
ATCCCTGA	0	0	1	1	0	[illegible]	0	0	0	0	0	1	1	0
TCAGGGAT	0	0	1	1	0	0	0	0	0	0	0	1	1	0
GTATTTTA	1	0	0	1	0	0	0	0	1	0	0	0	1	0

Cell value

Table 9. The top ranked words (rows of the table), based on statistical significance ($S \cdot \ln(S/E_s)$), and the number of occurrences of each word in the promoter regions of genes (columns).

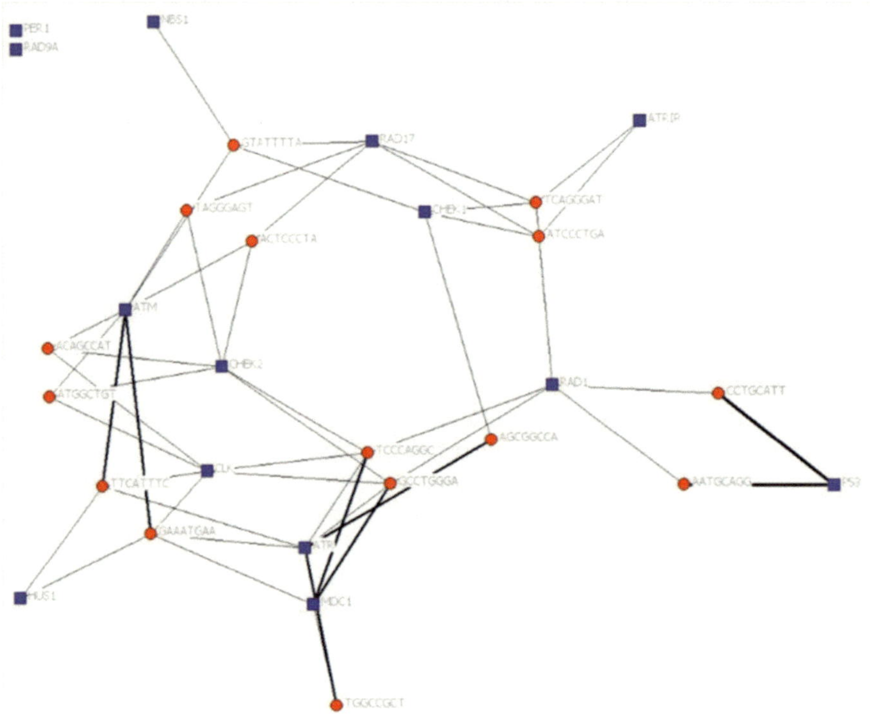

Fig. 2. Model of the checkpoint regulatory network using multidimensional scaling.

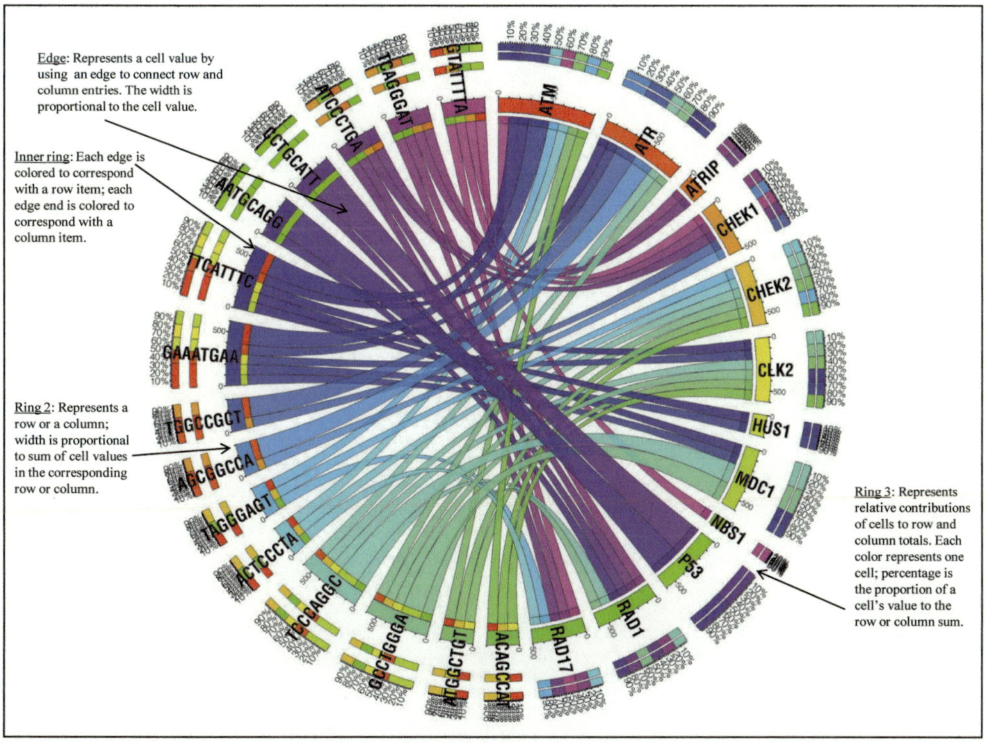

Fig. 3. Circos 2diagram of the top 15 words, based on statistical significance, and their occurrences in gene promoter regions.

TFBS	$S\ \ln(S/E_s)$	TF
ACCCCCAC	3.76	*PF0091, Pax-4*
ACTCCCTA	4.67	*Helios A, p300*
ATGGCTGT	5.42	*Cap*
ATTAAAGA	3.72	*Pax-2*
CGGAGCCC	3.95	*LF-A1*
CTGAAATT	3.80	*STAT1, STAT6*
CTTTTGAA	3.83	*TCF-4*
GAAAAATT	3.76	*CIZ*
GCACCTGC	3.68	*PF0035, AP-4, cap, Lmo2 complex*
GTGGCTGC	3.64	*cap*
TACTTTTT	3.82	*FOXC, CIZ, RUSH-1alpha1*
TATATTTA	3.82	*FOXL1, PF0028, PF0054*
TCCTTTCT	3.70	*Pax-2*
TTTTTATA	3.64	*FOXL1*

Table 10. Known transcription factor binding sites (with significance scores and corresponding transcription factor) discovered in the promoters of the checkpoint factors genes.

Additional insight into the regulatory network for the checkpoint factors can be seen in Figure 5, which replaces the DNA binding site motifs with the names of implicated transcription factors for each DNA repair gene. The diagram indicates the discovery of specific transcription factors involved in the control of each gene and shared among multiple genes. Up to seven transcription factors were discovered for each gene.

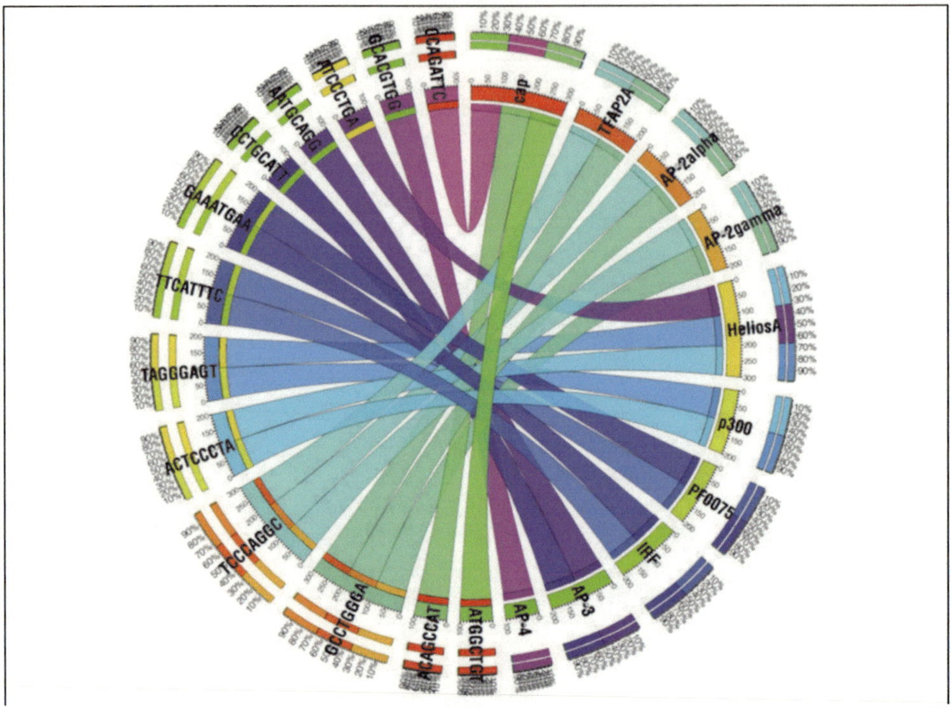

Fig. 4. Circos diagram showing the top 15 DNA motifs found in promoters of checkpoint factor genes and their related transcription factors (number of occurrences are multiplied by 100).

6. Conclusions

This chapter provides a summary of research into transcriptional regulatory networks controlling DNA repair pathways, bidirectional versus unidirectional promoters of DNA repair genes, and bidirectional promoters of breast and ovarian cancer genes. DNA words are shared among these promoters, and these words represent both known and unknown binding sites for transcription factors. When possible, we report the highest scoring assignment of transcription factor to DNA word. Our research represents a novel approach to identifying factors involved in transcriptional regulation of DNA repair genes. Many of these proteins have dual roles in transcription and DNA repair. Although many of the regulatory relationships are characterized at the level of protein-protein interactions, little research is available on the transcriptional regulatory networks that control DNA repair gene expression. We present evidence that regulatory networks exist among these genes, and support the claim that bidirectional promoters (implicated in B/O cancers) have a distinct network from unidirectional promoters. The identification of putative binding sites provides the first step in the elucidation of higher-order interdependencies among DNA repair genes in the cell. We also report preliminary findings on pairs of binding sites that represent regulatory modules. Furthermore, we show that there is much overlap among promoters of DNA repair genes, and that shared DNA binding motifs can be distributed among a collection of alternative promoters, each having distinct combinations of regulatory elements. The complex nature of the data can be simplified for visual interpretation using visualization techniques such as network modeling and circos diagrams.

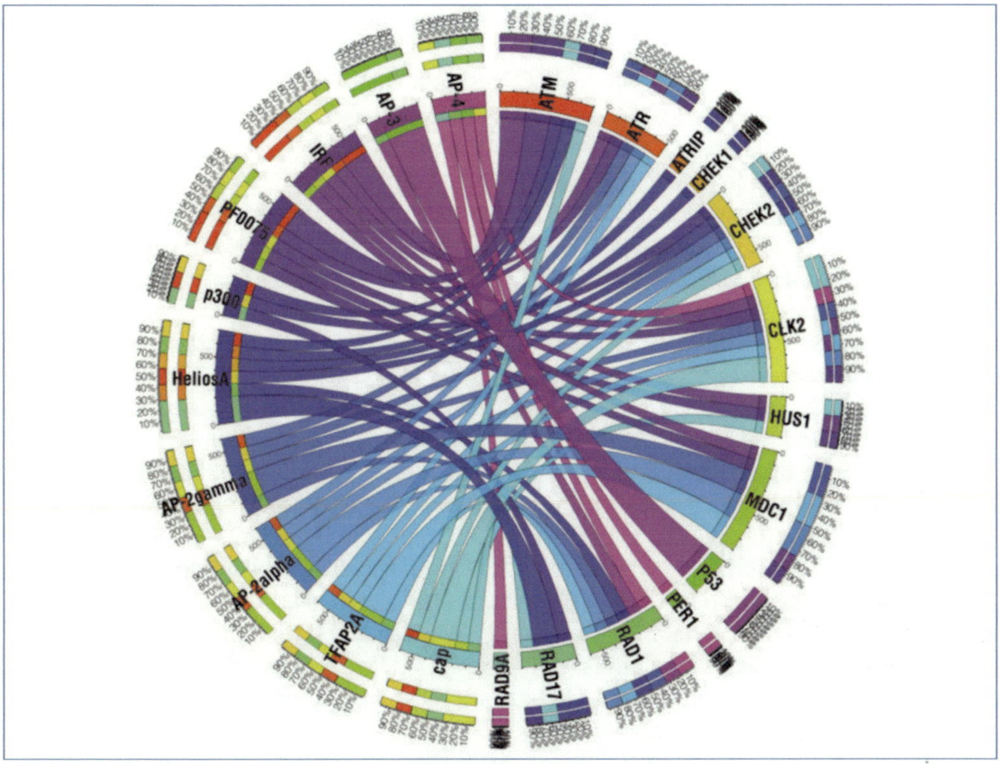

Fig. 5. Relationships between genes and transcription factors.

7. Acknowledgments

This work was supported by the Intramural Research Program of NHGRI (LE and LK) and by the Ohio Plant Biotechnology Consortium, the Choose Ohio First Program of the University System of Ohio, and the Ohio University Graduate Research and Education Board (LW).

8. References

Bellizzi, A.M., & Frankel, W.L. Colorectal cancer due to deficiency in DNA mismatch repair function: a review. *Adv Anat Pathol.* 2009 Nov;16(6):405-17.

Berwick, M. & Vineis, P. Markers of DNA repair and susceptibility to cancer in humans: an epidemiologic review. *J Natl Cancer Inst.* 2000 Jun 7;92(11):874-97.

Borgatti, S.P., Everet, M.G., and Freeman, L.C. 2002. Ucinet 6 for Windows: Software for Social Network Analysis. Harvard: Analytic Technologies.

Bryne, J.C., & Valen, E., Tang, M.H., Marstrand, T., & Winther, O. JASPAR, the open access database of transcription factor-binding profiles: new content and tools in the 2008 update. *Nucleic Acids Res* 2008, 36:D102-106.

Elnitski, L., Lichtenberg, J., & Welch, L.R.Regulatory network nodes of checkpoint factors in DNA repair pathways. *BCB '10: Proceedings of the First ACM International Conference on Bioinformatics and Computational Biology*, 529-536. 2010.

Helleday, T., Petermann, E., Lundin, C., Hodgson B., & Sharma, R.A. DNA repair pathways as targets for cancer therapy, *Nature Reviews Cancer* (2008) 8 (3): 193-204.

Hurley, P.J. & Bunz, F. ATM and ATR: components of an integrated circuit. *Cell Cycle*. 2007 Feb 15;6(4):414-7.

Jensen, N.M., Dalsgaard, T., Jakobsen, M., Nielsen, R.R., Sørensen, C.B., Bolund, L., & Jensen, T.G. An update on targeted gene repair in mammalian cells: methods and mechanisms. *J Biomed Sci*. 2011 Feb 2;18:10.

Kanehisa, M., Araki, M., Goto, S., Hattori, M., Hirakawa, M., Itoh, M., Katayama, T., Kawashima, S., Okuda, S., Tokimatsu, T., & Yamanishi, Y. KEGG for linking genomes to life and the environment. *Nucleic Acids Research* (2008) 36:D480-D484.

Kelley, M.R. & Fishel, M.L. DNA repair proteins as molecular targets for cancer therapeutics. *Anticancer Agents Med Chem*. 2008 May;8(4):417-25.

Kinsella, T.J. Understanding DNA damage response and DNA repair pathways: applications to more targeted cancer therapeutics. *Semin Oncol*. 2009 Apr;36(2 Suppl 1):S42-51.

Li, C., Wang, L.E., & Wei, Q. DNA repair phenotype and cancer susceptibility--a mini review. *Int J Cancer*. 2009 Mar 1;124(5):999-1007.

Liang, Y., Lin, S.Y., Brunicardi, F.C., Goss, J., & Li, K. DNA damage response pathways in tumor suppression and cancer treatment. *World J Surg*. 2009 Apr;33(4):661-6.

Lichtenberg, J., Jacox, E., Welch, J.D., Kurz, K., Liang, X., Yang, M.Q., Drews, F., Ecker, K., Lee, S.S., Elnitski, L., & Welch, L.R. Word-based characterization of promoters involved in human DNA repair pathways. *BMC Genomics* 10(Suppl 1):S18. 2009.

Lichtenberg, J., Kurz, K., Liang, X., Al-ouran, R., Neiman, L. Nau, L.J., Welch, J.D., Jacox, E., Bitterman, T., Ecker, K., Elnitski, L., Drews, F., Lee, S.S., & Welch, L.R. WordSeeker: Concurrent bioinformatics software for discovering genome-wide patterns and word-based genomic signatures. *BMC Bioinformatics*, 2010, 11(Suppl 12):S6.

Naccarati, A., Pardini, B., Hemminki, K., &Vodicka, P. Sporadic colorectal cancer and individual susceptibility: a review of the association studies investigating the role of DNA repair genetic polymorphisms. *Mutat Res*. 2007 May-Jun;635(2-3):118-45.

Safran, M., Dalah, I., Alexander, J., Rosen, N., Iny Stein, T., Shmoish, M., Nativ, N., Bahir, I., Doniger, T., Krug, H., Sirota-Madi, A., Olender, T., Golan, Y., Stelzer, G., Harel, A., & Lancet, D. GeneCards Version 3: the human gene integrator. *Database* (Oxford). 2010 Aug 5;2010:baq020.

Shibata, A., Barton, O., Noon, A. T., Dahm, K., Deckbar D., Goodarzi, A.A., Löbrich, M., & Jeggo, P.A. Role of ATM and the damage response mediator proteins 53BP1 and MDC1 in the maintenance of G(2)/M checkpoint arrest. *Mol Cell Biol*. 2010 Jul;30(13):3371-83.

Smith, J., Tho, L.M., Xu, N., & Gillespie, D.A. The ATM-Chk2 and ATR-Chk1 pathways in DNA damage signaling and cancer. *Adv Cancer Res*. 2010;108:73-112.

Wingender, E., Chen, X., Hehl, R., Karas, H., & Liebich, I. TRANSFAC: an integrated system for gene expression regulation. *Nucleic Acids Res* 2000, 28:316-319.

Wood R.D., Mitchell, M., & T. Lindahl, Human DNA repair genes, 2005, *Mutation Res* (2005) 577 (1-2): 275-83.

Xie, X., Lu J., Kulbokas, E.J., Golub, T.R., Mootha, V., Lindblad-Toh, K., Lander, E.S., & Kellis, M. Systematic discovery of regulatory motifs in human promoters and 3' UTRs by comparison of several mammals. *Nature*. 2005 Mar 17;434(7031):338-45.

Yang, M.Q., Koehly, L.M., & Elnitski, L.L. Comprehensive annotation of bidirectional promoters identifies co-regulation among breast and ovarian cancer genes. *PLoS Comput Biol*. 2007 Apr 20;3(4):e72.

6

Mitochondrial DNA Damage: Role of Ogg1 and Aconitase

Gang Liu[1] and David W. Kamp[2]
[1]Clinical Medicine Research Center, Affiliated Hospital of Guangdong Medical College
[2]Department of Medicine, Northwestern University Feinberg School of Medicine and Jesse Brown VA Medical Center
[1]PR China
[2]USA

1. Introduction

Mitochondria have a vital role in respiration-coupled energy production, amino acid and fatty acid metabolism, Fe^{2+}/Ca^{2+} homeostasis and the integration of apoptotic signals that regulate cellular life and death (Babcock et al., 1997; Loeb et al., 2005; Taylor & Turnbull, 2005; Kroemer et al., 2007). Given the importance of these cellular functions regulated by the mitochondria with implications for aging, degenerative diseases and carcinogenesis, it is not surprising that this organelle has been the subject of intensive investigation for decades and continues to challenge investigators. Mitochondria produce nearly 90% of all the energy made in the body by oxidative phosphorylation that occurs via the electron transport chain (ETC). Mitochondria are the major cellular site of reactive oxygen species (ROS) production. It is estimated that 1–5% of the oxygen consumed in the mitochondrial ETC is converted to ROS (Kroemer et al., 2007). Mammalian mitochondria have a covalently closed round mitochondrial DNA (mtDNA) that is replicated and expressed within the mitochondria in close proximity to the ETC and potentially damaging ROS (Clayton 1982; Clayton 1984; Kroemer et al., 2007). Mammalian mtDNA contains 37 genes that encode 13 proteins (all of which are involved in the ETC), 22 tRNAs, and 2 rRNAs (Anderson et al., 1981). The remaining mitochondrial ETC proteins, the metabolic enzymes, the DNA and RNA polymerases and the ribosomal proteins are all encoded by nuclear genome.

Oxidative stress-induced mtDNA damage is implicated in a wide range of pathologic processes including carcinogenesis, aging and degenerative diseases of various organs and tissues (Bohr et al., 2002; Van Houten et al., 2006; Kroemer et al., 2007; Gredilla et al., 2010). In this review, we summarize the evidence that mtDNA damage augments mitochondria-regulated (intrinsic) apoptosis; an event that underlies the pathophysiologic mechanisms of diverse diseases. We focus our attention on one form of oxidative stress, exposure to asbestos fibers, which are well known to cause pulmonary fibrosis (asbestosis) and malignancies (e.g. mesothelioma and lung cancer). Specifically, we examine the role of a mitochondrial oxidative DNA repair enzyme (8-oxoguanine DNA glycosylase; Ogg1) and a recently described novel mechanism whereby mitochondrial Ogg1 acts as a mitochondrial aconitase chaperone protein to prevent oxidant-induced alveolar epithelial cell (AEC) mitochondrial dysfunction and intrinsic apoptosis. We discuss studies showing that mitochondrial aconitase, a crucial Kreb cycle enzyme, also functions in mtDNA maintenance and are a mitochondrial redox-sensor that is susceptible to oxidative degradation. Finally, we review accumulating evidence for important crosstalk between p53, which is a crucial DNA damage response protein, Ogg1, mtDNA damage and apoptosis.

2. MtDNA damage: Role of mitochondrial ROS

Individual cells contain several thousand copies of mtDNA, and in normal individuals, almost all of the mtDNA is similar. However, in some cases, especially in mitochondrial diseases, wild-type and variant mtDNAs coexist. The mutation rate of mtDNA is several folds higher in mtDNA than nuclear DNA (Bohr et al 2002; Van Houten et al 2006; Gredilla et al., 2010). There are three reasons for the high mutation rate in mtDNA. The first is that mtDNA, which is located along the mitochondrial inner membrane, is vulnerable to ROS-induced damage due to its close proximity to high levels of ROS produced from the ETC (Nass 1969; Albring et al., 1977; Chance et al., 1979; Shigenaga et al., 1994; Gredilla et al., 2010). The second reason is that mtDNA has no histone-containing protein shield as does the nuclear genome, so that mtDNA is uniquely susceptible to ROS-induced stress. Finally, mitochondria have a limited DNA repair systems as compared to what is present in the nucleus (see for review: Gredilla at al 2010). Collectively, these conditions cause mtDNA to accumulate various somatic mtDNA mutations in mitotic (Michikawa et al., 1999) and post-mitotic tissues (Soong et al., 1992; Corral-Debrinski et al., 1992; Liu et al., 1998). Mitochondrial DNA mutations and insertions/deletions have been observed in many types of human cancer (Bohr et al 2002). Mitochondrial functional defects have also been observed due to abnormal expression of mtDNA encoded proteins and defective oxidative phosphorylation (Kroemer et al 2007). Mitochondrial dysfunction and mtDNA mutations are also implicated in the development and complications of diabetic cardiomyopathy as well as directly associated with different types of neurodegenerative diseases (Medikayala et al., 2011). An emerging regulatory role for mitochondrial topoisomerases appears important for mtDNA integrity in the myocardium (Medikayala et al., 2011).

The most frequently formed mitochondrial ROS are hydrogen peroxide (H_2O_2), superoxide anion ($O_2{\bullet}^-$), singlet oxygen, and hydroxyl radicals ($OH{\bullet}$). Nearly 1-5% of the total molecular oxygen utilized by mammalian mitochondria is converted into ROS (Boveris & Chance 1977). Not surprisingly, mitochondria are one of the main cellular targets of oxidative damage resulting in relatively high levels of oxidized proteins, lipids and nucleic acids in mammalian mitochondria under normal metabolic conditions (see for reviews Raha & Robinson, 2000; Kroemer et al 2007). Generation of ROS produce a variety of lesions in cellular DNA, such as single or double strand breaks, intra- and inter-strand cross-linking and base damage (see for reviews Upadhyay & Kamp, 2003; Gredilla et al., 2010). Persistent DNA damage can cause cell cycle arrest, induction of transcription, induction of signal transduction pathways, replication errors, and genomic instability. Mitochondrial ROS can induce oxidative mitochondrial as well as nuclear DNA damage that results in apoptosis, if cells survive, promotes DNA mutations. For example, DNA damage is an early event in asbestos-exposed cells that can trigger apoptosis by inducing mitochondrial ROS production that may in part account for its malignant potential (see for reviews Kamp et al., 1992; Hardy & Aust, 1995; Jaurand 1997; Shukla et al., 2003; Liu et al., 2010).

Mitochondrial-associated gene expression, which is significantly different in cancer cells as compared to normal cells, identifies the changes in mitochondrial function emerging in developing cancer cells (see for review Ralph et al., 2010). Cancer cell development is dependent on the interactions of key oncogenes and tumor suppressor genes and their encoded products (see for review Janicke et al., 2008; Ralph et al., 2010). Studies in yeast show that mtDNA mutations can either reduce or extend life span depending upon the severity, context, and developmental stage of mtDNA damage (Powell et al., 2000). Unexpectedly, complete absence of mtDNA in yeast is associated with increased life span (Powell et al., 2000). Mice with a homozygous mutation in the exonuclease domain of mtDNA polymerase gamma (POLG) have been used as a model of mitochondrial dysfunction and aging. These mice possess an mtDNA mutator phenotype, accumulating lot of deletions and point mutations in mtDNA. These mice do not display signs of elevated ROS generation, but instead exhibit increased apoptosis, a number of age-related phenotypes, and a shortened life span (Kujoth et al., 2005; Trifunovic et al., 2004). As recently reviewed elsewhere (Kamp et al., 2011), chronic inflammation can promote all stages of tumorigenesis including mtDNA damage important in regulating mitochondrial function that coordinates life and death signaling pathways. Lung mesothelial cell mtDNA damage is evident following exposure to a four-fold lower concentration of crocidolite asbestos than required for causing nuclear DNA damage (Shukla et al., 2003). Several lines of evidence implicate mtDNA oxidative injury as a key trigger of apoptosis that can result in inflammation-associated cancer including: (1) cell death is often associated with mtDNA oxidative lesions, (2) mtDNA damage result in ATP depletion and mitochondrial dysfunction, (3) enhancing mtDNA repair can prevent cell death, and (4) defective mtDNA repair enhances cell death (see for review Kamp et al., 2011).

Apoptosis, or programmed cell death, is an important mechanism by which cells with extensive DNA damage, including mtDNA damage, are eliminated without inciting an inflammatory response. Notably, cell-sorting experiments established that persistent mtDNA damage is necessary for triggering mitochondrial dysfunction and apoptosis (Santos et al., 2003). Although much is known about the complex molecular pathways regulating apoptosis, the precise mechanisms involved remain incompletely understood (see for reviews: Kroemer et al., 2007; Kim et al., 2008; Youle & Strasser, 2008; Franco et al., 2009). The two major pathways regulating apoptosis include the mitochondria (intrinsic) death pathway and the death receptor (extrinsic) pathway. The intrinsic death pathway is activated by various stimuli, such as ROS, DNA damage, and calcium, that result in permeabilization of the outer mitochondrial membrane (OMM), a reduction in mitochondrial membrane potential change ($\triangle\psi m$) and the release of apoptogenic proteins, including cytochrome c that activate caspase-9 and, ultimately caspase-3. Notably, mtDNA damage that occurs following oxidative stress or mutations in mitochondrial DNA polymerase are implicated in premature aging as well as tumor metastasis (Trifunovic et al., 2004; Ishikawa et al., 2008)

ROS and DNA damage, including that caused by asbestos, trigger intrinsic apoptosis that can be blocked by antioxidants and iron chelators (Kroemer et al., 2007; Youle & Strasser, 2008; Franco et al., 2009; Kamp et al., 1995; Aljandali 2001; Panduri 2003; Panduri 2004). Herein we focus on asbestos-induced apoptosis to lung cells. Accumulating evidence over the past decade convincingly demonstrate that all forms of asbestos fibers, as opposed to inert particulates (e.g. titanium dioxide [TiO_2]), cause apoptosis in AEC as well as mesothelial cells via the mitochondria-regulated death pathway (reviewed in Kamp et al., 2011). Our group used human A549 cell and rat primary cells isolated alveolar type II to show that asbestos causes both a dose- and time-dependent reduction in $\Delta\psi m$ that was associated with release of cytochrome c from the mitochondria to the cytoplasm as well as activation of caspase-9 (Panduri et al., 2003). In this study, both an iron chelator (phytic acid) and a free radical scavenger (sodium benzoate) blocked asbestos-induced reductions in $\Delta\psi m$ and caspase-9, implying the importance of both iron-derived ROS and the mitochondrial death pathway. Furthermore, asbestos-induced apoptosis in A549 cells that stably overexpress Bcl-xl, an anti-apoptotic Bcl-2 family member, was significantly attenuated as compared to wild-type cells as evidenced by preservation of the OMM integrity and reduced DNA fragmentation (Panduri et al., 2003). Using confocal microscopy and Western blotting of mitochondrial proteins, we showed that asbestos stimulates mitochondrial translocation of pro-apoptotic Bax and that these effects are blocked by phytic acid (Panduri et al., 2006). Notably, using A549-ρ0 cells that lack mtDNA and a functional electron transport chain necessary for mitochondrial ROS generation, asbestos-induced ROS production, caspase-9 activation, and intrinsic apoptosis were all completely blocked (Panduri et al., 2006). These findings establish an important role for mitochondrial ROS in mediating asbestos-induced AEC apoptosis.

3. Ogg1 and mitochondrial base excision repair

Oxidative stress can induce many types of DNA base damage including two of the most abundant lesions, 8-hydroxyguanine (8-oxoG) and thymine glycol (TG) (Demple & Harrison, 1994; Dizdaroglu 1992; Bohr et al., 2002; Gredilla et al., 2010). Further, 8-oxoG is more susceptible to oxidative attack than guanine itself, resulting in the formation of oxidation products such as guanidinohydantoin and spiroiminodihydantoin (Bjelland & Seeberg, 2003; Hailer et al., 2005). The 8-oxoG residue exists predominantly in its keto form at physiological pH, resulting in the normal anti conformation around the *N*-glycosylic bond, and forming a common Watson-Crick base pair with cytosine. 8-oxoG adopts a *syn* conformation and base pairs with adenine leading to transversion mutations in replicating cells (Shibutani 1991), which may play a role in the development of cancer and the process of aging (Ames 1989; Lindahl 1993). In contrast, TG strongly blocks DNA replication (Ide et al., 1985; Clark & Beardsley, 1987) and transcription (Hatahet et al., 1994; Htun & Johnston, 1992) and must be efficiently removed and repaired to maintain genetic stability. Therefore, inefficient repair of oxidative mtDNA damage augments the accumulation of mtDNA damage and mutations that can lead to mitochondrial dysfunction and apoptosis. In this section we focus attention on repair of 8-oxoG by mitochondrial 8-oxoguanine DNA glycosylase 1 (mt-Ogg1) since it is among the best characterized mitochondrial base excision repair (BER) proteins.

The BER pathway accounts for the repair of the majority of spontaneously formed oxidized bases in mtDNA important for preserving the genome stability required for long-term cell survival (Barnes & Lindahl, 2004; Gredilla et al. 2010). All mitochondrial DNA repair enzymes, including those involved in BER, are encoded in the nucleus and imported into the mitochondria (Gredilla et al. 2010). The BER pathway removes small covalent modifications, which do not distort the DNA helix, such as the base modifications generated by ROS and single-strand breaks. The BER pathway in mitochondria and nucleus is highly conserved in all cellular organisms, from bacteria to man. BER is carried out in four sequential enzymatic steps catalyzed by the enzymes DNA glycosylase, AP-endonuclease, DNA polymerase and DNA ligase (Dianova et al., 2001; Gredilla et al., 2010). The initial steps in the BER pathway are recognition and removal of the aberrant base by a DNA glycosylase. Most DNA glycosylases remove several structurally different damaged bases, and some of them have overlapping substrate specificities, which may indicate that they serve as back-up systems for each other (Dianovet al., 2001). The mammalian DNA glycosylase, Ogg1, recognizes and removes 8-oxoG that is base-paired with cytosine in DNA (Aburatani et al., 1997; Radicella et al., 1997). Ogg1 is a bifunctional DNA glycosylase, with an associated AP-lyase activity, cleaving DNA at abasic sites through a β-elimination mechanism (Bjoras et al., 1997). The human OGG1 gene is located on chromosome 3p26.2. Studies of mice that are deficient in Ogg1 demonstrate that this enzyme is responsible for most of the BER activity that is initiated at 8-oxoG in mammalian cells (Klungland et al., 1999). Interestingly, using fluorometric techniques to identify the site of Ogg1 DNA repair activity following exposure to oxidative stress, the mitochondria, rather than the nucleus, was primary site of Ogg1 DNA repair activity (Mirbahai et al., 2010). In Ogg1 knockout mice, the mitochondrial genome contains almost nine times more 8-oxoguanine than control animals, whereas in the nuclear DNA the level of 8-oxoguanine is increased only twofold (Souza-Pinto et al., 2001). OGG1 gene mutations or polymorphisms increase the risk of various malignancies including lung, kidney, gastric, and colorectal cancer, as well as leukemia (Chevillard et al., 1998; Shinmura et al., 1998; Audebert et al., 2000; Bohr et al., 2002; Elahi et al., 2002; Fortini et al., 2003; Russo et al., 2004; Mambo et al., 2005). Furthermore, reduced Ogg1 activity is a risk factor in lung and head and neck cancer (Paz-Elizur et al., 2008).

Several groups have demonstrated that overexpression of mitochondria-targeted Ogg1 prevents mtDNA damage and intrinsic apoptosis caused by ROS-exposed vascular endothelial and asbestos-exposed cells (Dobson et al., 2002; Ruchko et al., 2005; Rachek et al., 2006; Harrison et al., 2007; Panduri et al., 2009; Ruchko et al., 2010). This suggests a prominent role of mt-Ogg1 in regulating intrinsic apoptosis in diverse settings of oxidative stress. Alternative splicing of the OGG1 transcript results in two isoforms: α-Ogg1 and β-Ogg1 (Gredilla et al., 2010). β-Ogg1 levels in the mitochondria are 20-fold greater than α-Ogg1 levels yet, curiously, β-Ogg1 lacks 8-oxoG DNA glycosylase activity (Hashiguchi et al., 2004). This finding suggests a role for Ogg1 that is independent of DNA repair. Our group recently reported that overexpression of mitochondrial α-Ogg1 mutants lacking 8-oxoG DNA repair activity were as effective as wild type mt-Ogg1 in preventing oxidant-induced caspase-9 activation and intrinsic apoptosis. Mitochondria-targeted Ogg1 did not alter the levels of mitochondrial ROS produced but, interestingly, preserved mitochondrial aconitase suggesting a novel role for Ogg1 as discussed further below (Panduri et al., 2009).

4. Aconitase and mitochondrial DNA

Aconitase, an enzyme that is vital for carbohydrate and energy metabolism, is responsible for the interconversion of citrate and isocitrate in the tricarboxcylic acid (TCA) cycle (Emptage et al., 1983). The importance of mitochondrial aconitase is suggested by the observation that citrate levels in the human prostate appear important for promoting oncogenic conditions. Normal citrate-producing prostate epithelial cells can develop into citrate-oxidizing malignant cells that result in a net increase of 22 ATP/mol glucose that affords energy for malignant-associated activities (Costello & Franklin, 1994). It has been suggested that mitochondrial aconitase is a key enzyme associated with this bioenergy transformation since loss of its activity reduces cellular survival (Singh et al., 2006).

Mitochondrial aconitase is an iron-sulfur protein that is vulnerable to oxidative inactivation and is implicated as a mitochondrial redox-sensor (Gardner et al., 1994; Bulteau et al., 2003). Aconitase inactivation can further promote oxidant generation by releasing redox-active Fe from the $(4Fe–4S)^{2+}$ center following exposure to oxidants such as $O_2{\bullet}^-$ (Gardner et al., 2000) or deficiency of mitochondrial manganese superoxide dismutase (MnSOD) (Williams et al., 1998). Oxidative-inactivation of aconitase is associated with decreased Drosophila lifespan (Yan et al., 1997). Reduced aconitase activity has also been described in a number of neurodegenerative diseases, including progressive supranuclear palsy (Park 2001), Friedreich's ataxia (Bradley 2000), and Huntington's disease (Tabrizi 1999).

Collectively, the above findings suggested a key role for mitochondrial aconitase beyond the TCA cycle. In this regard, a provocative finding in yeast showed that mitochondrial aconitase preserves mtDNA independent of aconitase's catalytic activity (Chen et al., 2005). This was the first suggestion of a dual role for aconitase as a mitochondrial TCA enzyme as well as in mtDNA maintenance, mitochondrial aconitase co-precipitates with frataxin, which is an iron chaperone protein that prevents aconitase oxidative inactivation and/or augments aconitase reactivation (Bulteau et al., 2004). This study suggested that prevention of oxidative inactivation of mitochondrial aconitase may be important for the pathogenesis of a degenerative disease (e.g. Friedrich's ataxia). Further evidence for this possibility was our recent finding that mt-Ogg1 overexpression completely blocks oxidant induced decreases in AEC mitochondrial aconitase activity and protein expression (Panduri et al., 2009). Moreover, using immunoprecipitation to explore the possible interactive effects between mitochondrial Ogg1 and aconitase, mitochondrial aconitase coprecipitated with both wild-type and mutant mt-Ogg1. Notably, overexpression of mitochondrial aconitase eliminated oxidant induced AEC apoptosis whereas Ogg1 underexpression using shRNA techniques reduced basal mitochondrial aconitase levels and augmented oxidant-induced AEC apoptosis (Panduri et al., 2009). These latter findings are in accord with several recent studies showing that Ogg1 deficiency increases oxidant-induced apoptosis (Youn et al., 2007; Bacsi et al., 2007; Xie et al., 2008). Collectively, these results suggest a novel interaction between an mtDNA repair enzyme (mt-Ogg1) and aconitase in preventing intrinsic AEC apoptosis following exposure to oxidative stress (e.g. asbestos or H_2O_2).

The underlying mechanisms that account for the interactive protective effect of mt-Ogg1 and aconitase require further study but there are at least two possibilities, which are not mutually exclusive. First, mt-Ogg1 may block key oxidative modification sites on mitochondrial aconitase responsible for triggering degradation by mitochondrial Lon protease (Bota & Davies, 2002; Bota et al., 2005). Lon protease selectively degrades oxidatively modified aconitase at a much higher rate than unexposed aconitase; a finding that may be important in defending the mitochondria against the accumulation of oxidized proteins as well as ensuring that such cells will undergo intrinsic apoptosis (Wallace, 1999; Bota et al., 2005; Bota & Davies, 2002; Panduri et al. 2009). Support for this possibility is our finding that MG132, a protease inhibitor that blocks mitochondrial Lon protease (Granot et al., 2007), attenuates asbestos-induced reductions in mitochondrial aconitase activity (Panduri et al., 2009). Second, overexpression of mt-Ogg1 or aconitase may preserve mtDNA levels necessary to prevent activation of intrinsic apoptosis. Future studies are required to clarify these possibilities as well as to determine precisely how mt-hOgg1 interacts with aconitase and whether other mtDNA repair proteins act similarly.

5. p53 and mitochondrial DNA repair

p53 functions as the "gatekeeper" of the genome by integrating various signals and initiating appropriate biological responses including cell cycle arrest, differentiation, apoptosis, senescence, and anti-angiogenesis (see for reviews Levine 1997; Vogelstein et al., 2000; Vousden et al., 2009). Previous studies have shown that the functions of p53 are mediated by transcriptional activation that regulates expression of downstream target genes (El-Deiry 1998). Expression of some cellular genes, including WAF1, CIP1, p21, IGF-BP3, mdm2, cyclin G, PCNA, and GADD45, are directly regulated by p53-mediated transactivation (Ko & Prives, 1996). p53 is also a redox-sensitive transcription factor whose function is integrally connected to ROS production as well as mediating the down-stream cellular effects following oxidative stress including the induction of apoptotic cell death (reviewed in Sablina et al., 2005; Janicke et al., 2008; Vaseva et al., 2009; Liu et al., 2010). ROS can induce p53 expression whereas p53 stabilization can augment further ROS production, often via effects on the mitochondria (Janicke et al., 2008; Liu et al., 2010). The mitochondria are an important target of transcription-dependent and -independent actions of p53 required to trigger apoptosis. By regulating thousands of genes, either directly or indirectly, p53 is implicated in numerous key cellular roles, including a recently described role for mtDNA maintenance (El-Deiry et al., 1992; Janicke et al., 2008, Bakhanashvili et al., 2008; Lebedeva et al., 2009).

The mechanism by which p53 regulates cellular responses following exposure to oxidative stress generally depends on the levels of ROS. A biphasic response is seen in which low basal p53 expression promotes ROS homeostasis and cell survival by augmenting anti-oxidant defenses as one of its tumor-suppressing mechanisms while higher levels of ROS induce persistent p53 expression that blocks the cell cycle enabling time for DNA repair and, if repair is insufficient, triggers apoptosis (Bensaad et al., 2005; Janicke et al., 2008; Vousden et al., 2009). Notably, p53 also enhances Ogg1 activity for 8-oxoG removal suggesting a link between Ogg1, p53 and mtDNA (Achanta & Huang , 2004). A recently described role for p53 in mtDNA maintenance following exposure to mitochondrial ROS is evidenced by its involvement in maintaining mtDNA copy number and mtDNA synthesis (Bakhanashvili et al., 2008; Lebedeva et al., 2009). Cells that are p53-depleted exhibit significant disruption of cellular ROS homeostasis that are characterized by reduced mitochondrial biogenesis and increased H_2O_2 production (Lebedeva et al., 2009). In contrast, thymic lymphomas derived from the $p53^{-/-}$ mouse (a common model of carcinogenesis) have highly significant upregulation of mitochondrial biogenesis, mitochondrial protein translation, mtDNA copy number, ROS levels, anti-oxidant defenses, proton transport, ATP synthesis, hypoxia response, and glycolysis, indicating important mitochondrial bioenergetic profile changes of cells occurs during the process of malignant transformation (Samper et al., 2009). Hypoxia stimulates mitochondrial ROS production, which activates p53 stabilization and localization to the mitochondria where p53 has many effects including inhibiting MnSOD thereby promoting $O_2{\bullet}^-$ formation and greater oxidative damage (Ralph et al., 2010) as well as regulating mtDNA repair and replication as noted above. Taken together, the emerging evidence strongly implicate that p53 is a key regulator of mitochondrial function, including ROS production and associated mtDNA repair following oxidative damage, as well as mtDNA replication and mitochondrial biogenesis (Ralph et al., 2010).

It is known well that most human tumors contain mutations in one or more p53 gene family members (see for reviews Janicke et al., 2008; Vousden & Prives, 2009). In this section we focus on the role of p53 in the lungs exposed to asbestos fibers. Altered p53 expression has been implicated in the pathophysiology of pulmonary fibrosis, including that due to asbestos, as well as asbestos-associated malignancies, especially bronchogenic lung cancer (Nelson et al., 2001; Mishra et al., 1997; Burmeister et al., 2004; Plataki et al., 2005). Asbestos activates p53 and p21 expression in lung epithelial and mesothelial cells that result in cell cycle arrest (Levresse et al., 1997; Matsuoka et al., 2003; Kopnin et al., 2004). Furthermore, increased p53 levels are detected in lung cancers of patients with asbestosis (Nuorva et al., 1994) and p53 point mutations are present in the lung epithelium of smokers and asbestos-exposed individuals (Husgafvel-Pursiainen et al., 1997). Crocidolite asbestos promotes p53 gene mutations predominantly in axons 9 through 11 in BALB/c-3 T3 cells (Lin et al., 2000). Finally, studies in lung epithelial and mesothelial cells using gene expression microarray techniques have established that induction of p53 gene expression following asbestos fiber exposure is an important event (Nymark et al., 2007; Hevel et al., 2008). Thus, p53 has a crucial role regulating lung cellular DNA damage response following exposure to oxidative stress as occurs with asbestos and tobacco smoke.

The mechanisms by which p53 regulate apoptosis are complex and incompletely understood. One established pathway involves intrinsic apoptosis via p53 crosstalk with the mitochondria by increasing transcription of pro-apoptotic stimuli (e.g. Bax and BH3-only proteins) while inhibiting gene expression of anti-apoptotic Bcl-2 family members (Miyashita et al., 1995; Oda et al., 2000; Nakano et al., 2001; Janicke et al., 2008; Vousden & Prives, 2009). There is considerable evidence that p53 phosphorylation at the Ser15 position following exposure to DNA damaging agents, including asbestos, is in part responsible for p53 stabilization and its subsequent mitochondrial translocation. Several different proteins have been implicated in the phosphorylation of p53 at Ser15, including members of the phosphatidylinostitol 3-kinase-related kinase (PI3K) family such as DNA-activated protein kinase (DNA-PK) and ataxia-telangiectasia mutated (ATM) kinase, as well as members of the mitogen-activated protein kinase (MAPK). In one study, suppression of DNA-PK coupled with a mutated form of ATM inhibited asbestos-induced Ser15 phosphorylation and accumulation of p53 (Matsuoka et al., 2003). Considerable evidence has established that p53 is a crucial regulator of mitochondrial function, including ROS generation and mtDNA repair following oxidative damage as well as mitochondrial biogenesis and mtDNA replication (see for review Liu et al., 2010). For example, p53 mediates asbestos-induced mitochondria-regulated apoptosis in lung epithelial cells and this is blocked in cells incapable of producing mitochondrial ROS (Panduri et al., 2006). Notably, loss of p53 results in mtDNA depletion, altered mitochondrial function and increased H_2O_2 production (Lebedeva et al., 2009).

The above data are providing insights into the molecular mechanisms by which p53 regulates the cellular response to DNA damage caused by exposure to oxidative stress that is likely important in the pathogenesis of inflammation-associated cancer (see for review: Kamp et al., 2011). An important link between p53 and Ogg1 is suggested by the finding that Ogg1 is under transcriptional regulation by p53 in colon and renal epithelial cells (Youn et al., 2007). In this study, the expression and activity of Ogg1 were decreased in HCT116p53$^{-/-}$ cells. Further, gel-shift assays showed that p53 binds to the putative cis-elements within the OGG1 promoter while supplementing p53 in HCT116p53$^{-/-}$ cells enhanced OGG1 transcription. In renal epithelial cells, tuberin also regulates OGG1 expression since transcriptional activity of the OGG1 promoter is decreased in tuberin-null cells; an effect that in part is mediated by the transcription factor NF-YA (Habib et al., 2008).

p53 modulates cellular metabolism by enhancing aerobic respiration and blocking glycolysis in most cell types; findings that are likely important in cellular malignant transformation (Bensaad et al., 2006; Bensaad et al., 2007). Interestingly, there is some evidence that p53 impacts mitochondrial aconitase levels since thymoquinone, a p53-dependent antineoplastic drug, reduces aconitase enzyme activity in isolated rat liver mitochondria (Roepke et al., 2007). Also, mitochondrial aconitase gene expression in prostate carcinoma cells is inhibited by both endogenous p53 induction by camptothecin treatment and exogenous p53 induction by transient overexpression of p53 (Tsui et al., 2011). Further, these investigators showed that mitochondrial aconitase is a p53-downregulated gene. Camptothecin did not affect mitochondrial aconitase reporter activity in p53-null PC-3 cells suggesting that the decrease in mitochondrial aconitase gene expression by camptothecin occurs via p53 activation. The relevance of these findings to other cell types as well as the *in vivo* significance requires further study.

6. Conclusion

In this review we have summarized emerging evidence demonstrating an important interactive effect between mitochondrial Ogg1, mitochondrial aconitase, and p53 in mtDNA repair and oxidant-induced intrinsic apoptosis. Although we focused on the role of oxidative stress caused by exposure to asbestos fibers, it is likely that many of the described interactive effects between mt-Ogg1, aconitase, p53 and intrinsic apoptosis will have broader implications but this awaits future investigations. Additional studies are necessary to further characterize the role of mitochondrial Ogg1 and aconitase in preventing mtDNA damaging (including following asbestos exposure), p53 activation and intrinsic apoptosis. It will also be of considerable interest to better understand the molecular mechanisms by which mitochondrial Ogg1 binds aconitase. Finally, and perhaps most importantly, we reason that the asbestos paradigm will continue to provide insights into the molecular mechanisms underlying the interactive effects between mt-Ogg1, aconitase, p53 and intrinsic apoptosis that should shed light into the pathogenesis of other more common diseases, such as lung cancer and idiopathic pulmonary fibrosis, for which more effective management regimens are urgently required. Strategies aimed at augmenting mtDNA integrity by increasing mt-Ogg1 and/or aconitase levels to mitigate the deleterious effects of oxidative stress may prove useful for developing novel therapeutic treatments for tumors and degenerative diseases as well as modulating the effects of aging.

7. Abbreviations

Electron transport chain (ETC)
outer mitochondrial membrane (OMM)
alveolar epithelial cell (AEC)
reactive oxygen species (ROS)
mitochondrial human 8-oxoguanine-DNA glycosylase 1 (mt-hOgg1)
alveolar type II (AT2) cells
hydrogen peroxide (H_2O_2),
superoxide anion (O_2-)
hydroxyl radical (HO•)
8-hydroxydeoxyguanosine (8OHdG)

mitochondrial DNA (mtDNA)
tricarboxcylic acid (TCA)
mitochondrial membrane potential ($\triangle\psi m$)
titanium dioxide (TiO_2)
thymine glycol (TG)
base excision repair (BER)
8-hydroxyguanine (8-oxoG)
manganese superoxide dismutase (MnSOD)

8. References

Aburatani, H.; Hippo, Y.; Ishida, T.; Takashima, R., Matsuba, C.; Kodama, T. et al. (1997). Cancer Res 57: 2151–2156.

Achanta, G.; Huang, P.;(2004). "Role of p53 in sensing oxidative DNA damage in response to reactive oxygen species-generating agents." Cancer Res 64(17):6233-9.

Albring, M.; Griffith, J.; Attardi, G. (1977). "Association of a protein structure of probable membrane derivation with HeLa cell mitochondrial DNA near its origin of replication." Proc Natl Acad Sci U S A 74: 1348–1352.

Aljandali, A.; Pollack, H.; Yeldandi, A.; Li, Y.; Weitzman, S. A.; Kamp, D. W. (2001). "Asbestos causes apoptosis in alveolar epithelial cells: role of iron-induced free radicals." J Lab Clin Med 137 (5): 330–339.

Ames, B. N. (1989). "Endogenous oxidative DNA damage aging and cancer." Free Radic. Res. Commun. 7: 121–128.

Anderson, S.; Bankier, A. T.; Barrell, B. G.; de Bruijn, M. H.; Coulson, A. R.; Drouin, J.; Eperon, I. C.; Nierlich, D. P.; Roe, B. A.; Sanger, F.; Schreier, P. H.; Smith, A. J.; Staden, R.; Young, I. G. (1981). "Sequence and organization of the human mitochondrial genome." Nature 290: 457–465.

Audebert, M.; Chevillard, S.; Levalois, C.; Gyapay, G.; Vieillefond,A.; Klijanienko J et al. (2000). Cancer Res 60: 4740–4744.

Babcock, D. F.; Herrington, J.; Goodwin, P. C.; Park, Y. B. and Hille, B. (1997). "Mitochondrial participation in the intracellular Ca2. Network." J Cell Biol 136: 833–844.

Bacsi, A.; Chodaczek, G.; Hazra, T. K.; Konkel, D.; Boldogh, I. (2007). "Increased ROS generation in subsets of OGG1 knockout fibroblast cells." Mech. Ageing Dev. 128(11–12): 637–649.

Bakhanashvili,M.; Grinberg, S.; Bonda, E.; Simon, A.J.; Moshitch-Moshkovitz, S.; Rahav, G.(2008). "p53 in mitochondria enhances the accuracy of DNA synthesis." Cell Death Differ 15(12):1865-74.

Barnes, D. E.; Lindahl, T. (2004). "Repair and genetic consequences of endogenous DNA base damage in mammalian cells." Annu. Rev. Genet. 38: 445–476.

Bensaad, K.; Tsuruta, A.; Selak, M. A.; Vidal, M. N. C.; Nakano, K.; Bartrons, R.; Gottlieb, E.; Vousden, K. H. (2006). "TIGAR, a p53-inducible regulator of glycolysis and apoptosis." Cell 126: 107–120.

Bensaad, K.; Vousden, K. H. (2005). "Savior and slayer: the two faces of p53." Nat. Med. 11: 1278–1279.

Bensaad, K.; Vousden, K. H. (2007). "p53:New roles in metabolism." Trends Cell Biol 17: 286–291.

Bjelland, S.; Seeberg, E. (2003). "Mutagenicity, toxicity and repair of DNA base damage induced by oxidation." Mutat. Res. 531: 37–80.

Bjoras, M.; Luna, L.; Johnsen, B.; Hoff, E.; Haug, T.; Rognes, T.; Seeberg, E. (1997). "Opposite base-dependent reactions of a human base excision repair enzyme on DNA containing 7,8-dihydro-8-oxoguanine and abasic sites." EMBO J. 16: 6314–6322.

Bohr, V. A.; Stevnsner, T.; de Souza-Pinto, N. C. (2002). "Mitochondrial DNA repair of oxidative damage in mammalian cells." Gene 286: 127–134.

Bota, D. A.; and Davies, K. J. A. (2002). "Lon protease preferentially degrades oxidized mitochondrial aconitase by an ATP-stimulated mechanism." Nat. Cell Biol. 4 (9): 674–680

Bota, D.A.; Ngo, J.K.; Davies, K.J. (2005). "Downregulation of the human Lon protease impairs mitochondrial structure and function and causes cell death." Free Radic Biol Med 38(5):665-77.

Bota, D. A.; Van Remmen, H.; Davies, K. J. (2002). "Modulation of Lon protease activity and aconitase turnover during aging and oxidative stress." FEBS Lett. 532 (1–2): 103–106.

Boveris, A.; Chance, B. (1977). "The mitochondrial generation of hydrogen peroxide." General properties and effect of hyperbaric oxygen. Biochem. J. 134: 707–716.

Bradley, J.L.; Blake, J.C.; Chamberlain, S.; Thomas, P.K.; Cooper, J.M.; Schapira,A.H.(2000). "Clinical, biochemical and molecular genetic correlations in Friedreich's ataxia." Hum Mol Genet 9(2):275-82.

Bulteau, A. L.; Ikeda-Saito, M.; Szweda, L. I. (2003). "Redox-dependent modulation of aconitase activity in intact mitochondria." Biochemistry 42 (50): 14846–14855.

Bulteau, A. L.; O'Neill, H. A.; Kennedy, M. C.; Ikeda-Saito, M.; Isaya, G.; Szweda, L. I. (2004). "Frataxin acts as an iron chaperone protein to modulate mitochondrial aconitase activity." Science 305 (5681): 242–245.

Burmeister, B.; Schwerdtle, T.; Poser, I.; Hoffmann, E.; Hartwig, A.; Muller, W. U.; Rettenmeier, A. W.; Seemayer, N. H.; Dopp, E. (2004). "Effects of asbestos on initiation of DNA damage, induction of DNA-strand breaks, P53-expression and apoptosis in primary, SV40-transformed and malignanthumanmesothelial cells." Mutat. Res. 558 (1–2): 81–92.

Chance, B.; Sies, H.; Boveris, A. (1979). "Hydroperoxide metabolism in mammalian organs." Physiol Rev 59: 527–605.

Chen, X. J.; Wang, X.; Kaufman, B. A.; Butow, R. A. (2005). "Aconitase couples metabolic regulation to mitochondrial DNA maintenance." Science 307 (5710):714–717.

Chevillard, S.; Radicella, J. P.; Levalois, C.; Lebeau, J.; Poupon, M. F.; Oudard, S.; Dutrillaux, B.; Boiteux, S. (1998). "Mutations in OGG1, a gene involved in the repair of oxidative DNA damage, are found in human lung and kidney tumors." Oncogene 16:3083–3086.

Clark, J. M.; Beardsley, G. P. (1987). "Functional effects of cis-thymine glycol lesions on DNA synthesis in vitro." Biochemistry 26: 5398–5403.

Corral-Debrinski, M.; Horton, T.; Lott, M. T.; Shoffner, J. M.; Beal, M. F.; Wallace, D. C. (1992). "Mitochondrial DNA deletions in human brain: regional variability and increase with advanced age." Nat Genet 2: 324–329.

Costello, L. C.; Franklin, R. B. (1994). "The bioenergetic theory of prostate malignancy." Prostate 25:162–166.

Clayton, D. A. (1982). "Replication of animal mitochondrial DNA." Cell 28: 693–705.

Clayton, D. A. (1984). "Transcription of the mammalian mitochondrial genome." Annu Rev Biochem 53:573–594.

Demple, B.; Harrison, L. (1994). "Repair of oxidative damage to DNA: enzymology and biology."Annu. Rev. Biochem. 63: 915–948.

De Souza-Pinto, N. C.; Eide, L.; Hogue, B. A.; Thybo, T.; Stevnsner, T.; Seeberg, E.; Klungland, A.; Bohr, V. A. (2001). "Repair of 8-oxodeoxyguanosine lesions inmitochondrial 498 DNA depends on the oxoguanine DNA glycosylase (OGG1) gene and 8-499 oxoguanine accumulates in the mitochondrial DNA of OGG1-defective mice." Cancer Res. 61: 5378–5381.

Dianov, G.L.;Souza-Pinto,N.; Nyaga,S.G.; Thybo,T.; Stevnsner,T.;Bohr,V.A.(2001)."Base excision repair in nuclear and mitochondrial DNA." Prog Nucleic Acid Res Mol Biol 68:285-97.

Dianova I.I.; Bohr, V. A.; and Dianov, G. L. (2001). "Interaction of human AP endonuclease 1 with flap endonuclease 1 and proliferating cell nuclear antigen involved in long-patch base excision repair." Biochem 40: 12639-12644.

Dizdaroglu, M. (1992). "Oxidative damage to DNA in mammalian chromatin." Mutat. Res. 275: 331–342.

Dobson, A. W.; Grishko, V. S.; LeDoux, P.; Kelley, M. R.; Wilson, G. L.; Gillespie, M. N. (2002) "Enhanced mtDNA repair capacity protects pulmonary artery endothelial cells from oxidant-mediated death." Am. J. Physiol. Lung Cell Mol. Physiol. 283 (1): 205–210.

Dobson, A. W.; Xu, Y.; Kelley, M. R.; LeDoux, S. P.; Wilson, G. L. (2000). "Enhanced mitochondrial DNA repair and cellular survival after oxidative stress by targeting the human 8-oxoguanine glycosylase repair enzyme to mitochondria." J Biol Chem 275: 37518–37523.

Elahi,A.; Zheng, Z.;Park, J.;Eyring, K.; McCaffrey,T.;Lazarus,P.(2002). "The human OGG1 DNA repair enzyme and its association with orolaryngeal cancer risk." Carcinogenesis 23(7):1229-34.

El-Deiry, W. S.; Kern, S. E.; Pietenpol, J. A.; Kinzler, K. W.; Vogelstein, B. (1992). "Definition of a consensus binding site for p53, Nat." Genet. 1: 45–49.

El-Deiry, W. S. (1998). "Regulation of p53 downstream genes, Semin." Cancer Biol. 8:345–357.

Emptage, M. H.; Kent, T. A.; Kennedy, M. C.; Beinert, H.; Munck, E. (1983). "Mossbauer and EPR studies of activated aconitases: Development of a localized valence state at a subsite of the [4Fe-4S] cluster on binding of citrate." Proc Natl Acad Sci U S A 80: 4674–4678.

Fortini, P.; Pascucci, B.; Parlanti, E.; D'Errico, M.; Simonelli, V.; Dogliotti, E. (2003). "8-Oxoguanine DNA damage: at the crossroad of alternative repair pathways." Mutat Res 531:127–139.

Franco, R.; Sanchez-Olea, R.; Reyes-Reyes, E. M.; Panayiotidis, M. I. (2009). "Environmental toxicity, oxidative stress and apoptosis: menage a trois." Mutat. Res. 674 (1–2): 3–22.

Gardner, P. R. (1997). "Superoxide-driven aconitase Fe–S center cycling." Biosci Rep 17: 33–42.

Gardner, P. R.; Nguyen, D. D.; White, C. W. (1994). "Aconitase is a sensitive and critical target of oxygen poisoning in cultured mammalian cells and in rat lungs." Proc Natl Acad Sci U S A 91(25): 12248-12252.

Granot,Z.;Kobiler,O.;Melamed-Book,N.;Eimerl,S.;Bahat,A.;Lu,B.;Braun,S.;Maurizi,M.R.;Suzuki, C.K.;Oppenheim,A.B.;Orly,J.(2007). "Turnover of mitochondrial steroidogenic acute regulatory (StAR) protein by Lon protease: the unexpected effect of proteasome inhibitors." Mol Endocrinol 21(9):2164-77.

Gredilla, R.; Bohr, V.A.; Stevnsner, T.(2010)" Mitochondrial DNA repair and association with aging--an update." Exp Gerontol. 45(7-8):478-88.

Habib, S. L.; Riley, D. J.; Mahimainathan, L.; Bhandari, B.; Choudhury, G. G.; Abboud, H. E. (2008). "Tuberin regulates the DNA repair enzyme OGG1." Am. J. Physiol. Renal Physiol. 294 (1): F281–290.

Hailer, M. K.; Slade, P. G.; Martin, B. D.; Rosenquist, T. A.; Sugden, K. D. (2005). "Recognition of the oxidized lesions spiroiminodihydantoin and guanidinohydantoin in DNA by the mammalian base excision repair glycosylases NEIL1 and NEIL2." DNA Repair 4: 41–50.

Hardy, J. A.; Aust, A. E. (1995). "The effect of iron binding on the ability of crocidolite asbestos to catalyze DNA single-strand breaks." Carcinogenesis 16 (2): 319–325.

Harrison, J. F.; Rinne, M. L.; Kelley, M. R.; Druzhyna, N. M.; Wilson, G. L.; Ledoux, S.P. (2007). "Altering DNA base excision repair: use of nuclear and mitochondrial-targeted N-methylpurine DNA glycosylase to sensitize astroglia to chemotherapeutic agents." Glia. 55: 1416–1425.

Hashiguchi, K.; Stuart, J. A.; de Souza-Pinto, N. C.; Bohr, V. A. (2004). "The C-terminal α-O helix of human Ogg1 is essential for 8-oxoguanine DNA glycosylase activity: the mitochondrial β-Ogg1 lacks this domain and does not have glycosylase activity." Nucleic Acids Res. 32: 5596–5608.

Hatahet, Z.; Purmal, A. A.; Wallace, S. S. (1994). "Oxidative DNA lesions as blocks to in vitro transcription by phage T7 RNA polymerase." Ann. NY Acad. Sci. 726: 346–348.

Hevel, J.M.; Olson-Buelow, L.C.; Ganesan, B.; Stevens, J.R.; Hardman, J.P.; Aust, A.E.(2008). "Novel functional view of the crocidolite asbestos-treated A549 human lung epithelial transcriptome reveals an intricate network of pathways with opposing functions." BMC Genomics 9:376.

Htun, H.; Johnston, B. H. (1992). "Mapping adducts of DNA structural probes using transcription and primer extension approaches." Methods Enzymol. 212: 272–294.

Husgafvel-Pursiainen, K.; Kannio, A.; Oksa, P.; Suitiala, T.; Koskinen, H.; Partanen, R.; Hemminki, K.; Smith, S.; Rosenstock-Leibu, R.; Brandt-Rauf, P. W. (1997). "Mutations, tissue accumulations, and serum levels of p53 in patients with occupational cancers from asbestos and silica exposure." Environ. Mol. Mutagen. 30 (2): 224–230.

Ide, H.; Kow, Y. W.; Wallace, S. S. (1985). "Thymine glycols and urea residues in M13 DNA constitute replicative blocks in vitro." Nucleic Acids Res. 13: 8035–8052.

Ishikawa,K.; Takenaga,K.; Akimoto,M.; Koshikawa,N.; Yamaguchi,A.; Imanishi,H.; Nakada,K.; Honma,Y.; Hayashi,J.(2008). "ROS-generating mitochondrial DNA mutations can regulate tumor cell metastasis." Science. 320(5876):661-4.

Janicke, R. U.; Sohn, D.; Schulze-Osthoff, K. (2008). "The dark side of a tumor suppressor: anti-apoptotic p53." Cell Death Differ. 15 (6): 959–976.
Jaurand, M. C. (1997). "Mechanisms of fiber-induced genotoxicity." Environ Health Perspect 105 (Suppl. 5): 1073–1084.
Kamp, D. W.; Graceffa, P.; Pryor, W. A.; Weitzman, S. A. (1992). "The role of free radicals in asbestos-induced diseases". Free Radic. Biol. Med. 12 (4): 293–315.
Kamp, D. W.; Israbian, V. A.; Preusen, S. E.; Zhang, C. X.; Weitzman, S. A. (1995). "Asbestos causes DNA strand breaks in cultured pulmonary epithelial cells: role of iron-catalyzed free radicals." Am. J. Physiol. 268 (3 Pt 1): L471–480.
Kamp, D.W., Shacter E, Weitzman SA. Chronic inflammation and cancer: The role of the mitochondria. Oncology 2011; 25:400-13.
Ke-Hung Tsui, Tsui-Hsia Feng, Yu-Fen Lin, Phei-Lang Chang, Horng-Heng Juang. (2011). "p53 Downregulates the Gene Expression of Mitochondrial Aconitase in Human Prostate Carcinoma Cells." The Prostate 71: 62-70.
Kim, I.; Xu, W.; Reed, J. C. (2008). "Cell death and endoplasmic reticulum stress: disease relevance and therapeutic opportunities." Nat. Rev. Drug Discov. 7 (12): 1013–1030.
Klungland, A.; Rosewell, I.; Hollenbach, S.; Larsen, E.; Daly, G.; Epe, B. et al. (1999). Proc Natl Acad Sci USA 96: 13300–13305.
Ko, L. J.; Prives, C. (1996). " p53: puzzle and paradigm." Genes Dev. 10: 1054-1072.
Kopnin, P. B.; Kravchenko, I. V.; Furalyov, V. A.; Pylev, L. N.; Kopnin, B. P. (2004). "Cell typespecific effects of asbestos on intracellular ROS levels, DNA oxidation and G1 cell cycle checkpoint." Oncogene 23 (54): 8834–8840.
Kroemer, G.; Galluzzi, L.; Brenner, C. (2007). "Mitochondrial membrane permeabilization in cell death." Physiol. Rev 87 (1): 99–163.
Kujoth, G. C.; Hiona, A.; Pugh, T. D.; Someya, S.; Panzer, K.; Wohlgemuth, S. E.; Hofer, T.; Seo, A. Y.; Sullivan, R.; Jobling, W. A. et al. (2005). "Mitochondrial DNA mutations, oxidative stress, and apoptosis in mammalian aging." Science 309: 481–484.
Lebedeva, M. A.; Eaton, J. S.; Shadel, G. S. (2009). "Loss of p53 causes mitochondrial DNA depletion and altered mitochondrial reactive oxygen species homeostasis." Biochim. Biophys. Acta. May 1787 (5): 328-34.
Levine, A. J. (1997). "p53, the cellular gatekeeper for growth and division." Cell 88: 323–331.
Levresse, V.; Renier, A.; Fleury-Feith, J.; Levy, F.; Moritz, S.; Vivo, C.; Pilatte, Y.; Aurand, M. C. (1997). "Analysis of cell cycle disruptions in cultures of rat pleural mesothelial cells exposed to asbestos fibers." Am. J. Respir. Cell Mol. Biol. 17 (6): 660–671.
Lindahl, T. (1993). "Instability and decay of the primary structure of DNA." Nature 362: 709–715.
Lin, F.; Liu, Y.; Keshava, N.; Li, S. (2000). "Crocidolite induces cell transformation and p53 gene mutation in BALB/c-3T3 cells." Teratog. Carcinog. Mutagen. 20 (5): 273–281.
Liu, V. W.; Zhang, C.; Nagley, P. (1998). "Mutations in mitochondrial DNA accumulate differentially in three different human tissues during ageing." Nucleic. Acids Res. 26: 1268–1275.
Liu, G.; Beri, R.; Mueller, A.; Kamp, D.W. "Molecular mechanisms of asbestos-induced lung epithelial cell apoptosis." Chemico-Biol Interactions 2010; 188:309-18.
Loeb, L. A.; Wallace, D. C. and Martin, G. M. (2005). "The mitochondrial theory of aging and its relationship to reactive oxygen species damage and somatic mtDNA mutations." Proc. Natl. Acad. Sci. U S A 102: 18769–18770.

Mambo, E.; Chatterjee, A.; de Souza-Pinto, N. C.; Mayard, S.; Hogue, B. A.; Hoque, M. O.; Dizdaroglu, M.; Bohr, V. A.; Sidransky, D. (2005). "Oxidized guanine lesions and hOgg1 activity in lung cancer." Oncogene 24: 4496–4508.

Lebedeva, M. A.; Eaton, J. S.; Shadel, G. S.(2009). "Loss of p53 causes mitochondrial DNA depletion and altered mitochondrial reactive oxygen species homeostasis." Biochimica et Biophysica Acta 1787:328–334.

Matsuoka, M.; Igisu, H.; Morimoto, Y. (2003). "Phosphorylation of p53 protein in A549 human pulmonary epithelial cells exposed to asbestos fibers." Environ. Health Perspect. 111 (4): 509–512.

Medikayala, S.; Piteo, B.; Zhao, X. and Edwards, J. G. (2011). "Chronically elevated glucose compromises myocardial mitochondrial DNA integrity by alteration of mitochondrial topoisomerase function." Am. J. Physiol. Cell Physiol. 300: C338–C348.

Michikawa, Y.; Mazzucchelli, F.; Bresolin, N.; Scarlato, G.; Attardi, G. (1999). "Aging-dependent large accumulation of point mutations in the human mtDNA control region for replication." Science 286: 774–779.

Mirbahai,L.; Kershaw,R.M.; Green,R.M.; Hayden,R.E.; Meldrum,R.A.; Hodges,N.J.(2010). "Use of a molecular beacon to track the activity of base excision repair protein OGG1 in live cells." DNA Repair (Amst) 9(2):144-52.

Mishra, A.; Liu, J. Y.; Brody, A. R.; Morris, G. F. (1997). "Inhaled asbestos fibers induce p53 expression in the rat lung." Am. J. Respir. Cell Mol. Biol. 16 (4): 479–485.

Miyashita, T.; Reed, J. C. (1995). "Tumor suppressor p53 is a direct transcriptional activator of the human bax gene." Cell, 80 (2): 293–299.

Nakano, K.; Vousden, K. H. (2001). "PUMA, a novel proapoptotic gene, is induced by p53." Mol. Cell 7 (3):683–694.

Nass, M. M. (1969). "Mitochondrial DNA. I. Intramitochondrial distribution and structural relations of single- and double-length circular DNA." J. Mol. Biol. 42: 521–528.

Nelson, A.; Mendoza, T.; Hoyle, G. W.; Brody, A. R.; Fermin, C.; Morris, G. F. (2001). "Enhancement of fibrogenesis by the p53 tumor suppressor protein in asbestos-exposed rodents." Chest 120 (1 Suppl): 33S–34S.

Nuorva, K.; Makitaro, R.; Huhti, E.; Kamel, D.; Vahakangas, K.; Bloigu, R.; Soini, Y.; Paakko, P. (1994). "p53 protein accumulation in lung carcinomas of patients exposed to asbestos and tobacco smoke." Am. J. Respir. Crit. Care Med. 150 (2): 528–533.

Nymark, P.; Lindholm, P.M.; Korpela, M.V.; Lahti, L.; Ruosaari, S.; Kaski, S.; Hollmen, J.; Anttila,S.; Kinnula,V.L.; Knuutila,S. (2007). "Gene expression profiles in asbestos-exposed epithelial and mesothelial lung cell lines." BMC Genomics 8:62.

Oda, E.; Ohki, R.; Murasawa, H.; Nemoto, J.; Shibue, T.; Yamashita, T.; Tokino, T.; Taniguchi, T.; Tanaka, N. (2000). "Noxa, a BH3-only member of the Bcl-2 family and candidate mediator of p53-induced apoptosis." Science 288 (5468): 1053–1058.

Panduri, V.; Liu, G.; Surapureddi, S.; Kondapalli, J.; Soberanes, S.; de Souza-Pinto, N. C.; Bohr, V. A.; Budinger, G. R.; Schumacker, P. T.; Weitzman, S. A.; Kamp, D. W. (2009). "Role of mitochondrial hOGG1 and aconitase in oxidant-induced lung epithelial cell apoptosis." Free Radic. Biol. Med. 47 (6): 750–759.

Panduri, V.; Weitzman, S. A.; Chandel, N.; Kamp, D. W. (2003). "The mitochondria regulated death pathway mediates asbestos-induced alveolar epithelial cell apoptosis." Am. J. Respir. Cell Mol. Biol. 28 (2): 241–248.

Panduri, V.; Weitzman, S. A.; Chandel, N. S.; Kamp, D. W. (2004). "Mitochondrial-derived free radicals mediate asbestos-induced alveolar epithelial cell apoptosis." Am. J. Physiol. Lung Cell Mol. Physiol. 286 (6): L1220–L1227.

Panduri, V. S.; Surapureddi, S.; Soberanes, S. A.; Weitzman, N.; Chandel, D.; Kamp, W. (2006). "P53 mediates amosite asbestos-induced alveolar epithelial cell mitochondria-regulated apoptosis." Am. J. Respir. Cell Mol. Biol. 34 (4) : 443–452.

Paradies, G.; Petrosillo, G.; Paradies, V.; Ruggiero, F. M. (2010). "Oxidative stress, mitochondrial bioenergetics, and cardiolipin in aging." Free Radic. Biol. Med. 48: 1286–1295.

Park, L. C. (2001). J. Neurosci. Res. 66 : 1028-1034.

Plataki, M.; Koutsopoulos, A. V.; Darivianaki, K.; Delides, G.; Siafakas, N. M.; Bouros, D. (2005). "Expression of apoptotic and antiapoptotic markers in epithelial cells in idiopathic pulmonary fibrosis." Chest. 127 (1): 266–274.

Powell, C. D.; Quain, D. E. and Smart, K. A. (2000). "he impact of media composition and petite mutation on the longevity of a polyploid brewing yeast strain." Lett. Appl. Microbiol. 31: 46–51.

Rachek, L. I.; Grishko, V. I.; Ledoux, S. P.; Wilson, G. L. (2006). "Role of nitric oxide-induced mtDNA damage in mitochondrial dysfunction and apoptosis." Free Radic. Biol. Med. 40 (5): 754–762.

Rachek, L. I.; Thornley, N. P.; Grishko, V. I.; LeDoux, S. P.; Wilson, G. L. (2006). "Protection of INS-1 cells from free fatty acid-induced apoptosis by targeting hOGG1 to mitochondria." Diabetes 55: 1022–1028.

Radicella, J. P.; Dherin, C.; Desmaze, C.; Fox, M. S.; Boiteux, S. (1997). Proc. Natl. Acad. Sci. U S A 94: 8010–8015.

Raha, S. ; Robinson, B. H. (2000). "Mitochondria, oxygen free radicals, diseases and ageing." Trends Biochem. Sci. 25: 502–508.

Ralph, S. J.; Rodríguez-Enríquez, S.; Neuzil, J.; Saavedra, E.; Moreno-Sánchez, R. (2010). "The causes of cancer revisited: "Mitochondrial malignancy" and ROS-induced oncogenic transformation - Why mitochondria are targets for cancer therapy." Molecular Aspects of Medicine 31: 145–170.

Roepke, M.; Diestel, A.; Bajbouj, K.; Walluscheck, D.; Schonfeld, P.; Roessner, A.; Schneider-Stock, R.; Gali-Muhtasib, H. (2007). "Lack of p53 augments thymoquinone-induced apoptosis and caspase activation in human osteosarcoma cells." Cancer Biol. Ther. 6: 160–169.

Ruchko, M.; Gorodnya, O.; LeDoux, S. P.; Alexeyev, M. F.; Al-Mehdi, A. B.; Gillespie, M. N. (2005). "Mitochondrial DNA damage triggers mitochondrial dysfunction and apoptosis in oxidant-challenged lung endothelial cells." Am. J. Physiol. Lung Cell. Mol. Physiol. 288: L530–L535.

Ruchko, M. V.; Gorodnya, O. M.; Zuleta, A.; Pastukh, V. M.; Gillespie, M. N. (2010). "The DNA glycosylase Ogg1 defends against oxidant-induced mtDNA damage and apoptosis in pulmonary artery endothelial cells." Free Radic Biol Med 50(9):1107-13.

Russo, M. T.; De Luca, G.; Degan, P.; Parlanti, E.; Dogliotti, E.; Barnes, D. E.; Lindahl, T.; Yang, H.; Miller, J. H.; Bignami, M. (2004). "Accumulation of the oxidative base lesion 8-hydroxyguanine in DNA of tumor-prone mice defective in both the Myh and Ogg1 DNA glycosylases." Cancer Res. 64: 4411–4414.

Sablina, A. A.; Budanov, A.V.; Ilyinskaya, G. V.; Agapova, L. S.; Kravchenko, J. E.; Chumakov, P. M. (2005). "The antioxidant function of the p53 tumor suppressor." Nat. Med. 11:1306–1313.

Samper, E.; Morgado, L.; Estrada, J. C.; Bernad, A.; Hubbard, A.; Cadenas, S.; Melov, S. (2009). "Increase in mitochondrial biogenesis, oxidative stress, and glycolysis in murine lymphomas." Free Radic. Biol. Med. 46: 387–396.

Santos, J. H.; Hunakova, L.; Chen,Y.; Bortner,Carl.; Van Houten, B. (2003). "Cell sorting experiments link persistent mitochondrial DNA damage with loss of mitochondrial membrane potential and apoptotic cell death." J. Biol. Chem 278(3):1728-1734.

Shibutani, S.; Takeshita, M.; Grollman, A. P. (1991). "Insertion of specific bases during DNA synthesis past the oxidation-damaged base 8-oxodG." Nature 349: 431–434.

Shigenaga, M. K.; Hagen, T. M.; Ames, B. N. (1994). "Oxidative damages and mitochondrial decay in aging." Proc. Natl. Acad. Sci. U S A 91: 10771–10778.

Shinmura,K.;Kohno,T.;Kasai,H.;Koda,K.;Sugimura,H.;Yokota,J.(1998). "Infrequent mutations of the hOGG1 gene, that is involved in the excision of 8-hydroxyguanine in damaged DNA, in human gastric cancer." Jpn J Cancer Res 89(8):825-8.

Shukla, A.; Gulumian, M.; Hei, T.; Kamp, D. W.; Rahman, Q.; Aust, A. E. (2003). Mossman, B.T. "Multiple roles of oxidants in the pathogenesis of asbestos-induced diseases." Free Radic Biol Med 34 (9): 1117–1129.

Soong, N. W.; Hinton, D. R.; Cortopassi, G.; Arnheim, N. (1992). "Mosaicism for a specific somatic mitochondrial DNA mutation in adult human brain." Nature Genet. 2: 318–323.

Shukla, A.; Jung, M.; Stern, M.; Fukagawa, N. K.; Taatjes, D. J.; Sawyer, D. (2003). "Asbestos induces mitochondrial DNA damage and dysfunction linked to the development of apoptosis." Am. J. Physiol. Lung Cell Mol. Physiol. 285(5): L1018-1025.

Singh, K. K.; Desouki, M. M.; Franklin, R. B.; Costello, L. C. (2006). "Mitochondrial aconitase and citrate metabolism in malignant and nonmalignant human prostate tissues." Mol. Cancer 5:14.

Tabrizi,S.J.;Cleeter,M.W.;Xuereb,J.;Taanman,J.W.;Cooper,J.M.;Schapira,A.H.(1999). "Biochemical abnormalities and excitotoxicity in Huntington's disease brain." Ann Neurol 45(1):25-32.

Tamar, P. E.; Ziv, S.; Yael, L. D.; Dalia, E.; Laila, C. (2008). "Roisman, Zvi Livneh DNA repair of oxidative DNA damage in human carcinogenesis: Potential application for cancer risk assessment and prevention." Cancer Letters 266: 60–72.

Taylor, R. W. and Turnbull, D. M. (2005). "Mitochondrial DNA mutations in human disease. " Nat. Rev. Genet. 6: 389 –402.

Trifunovic, A.; Wredenberg, A.; Falkenberg, M.; Spelbrink, J. N.; Rovio, A. T.; Bruder, C. E.; Bohlooly-Y, M.; Oldfors, A.; Wibom, R. (2004). "Premature ageing in mice expressing defective mitochondrial DNA polymerase." Nature 429: 417–423.

Trifunovic, A.; Hansson, A.; Wredenberg, A.; Rovio,A.T.; Dufour, E.; Khvorostov, I.; Spelbrink, J.N.; Wibom, R.; Jacobs, H.T.; Larsson, N.G.(2005). "Somatic mtDNA mutations cause aging phenotypes without affecting reactive oxygen species production." Proc Natl Acad Sci U S A 102(50):17993-8.

Upadhyay, D.; Kamp, D. W. (2003). "Asbestos-induced pulmonary toxicity: role of DNA damage and apoptosis." Exp Biol Med 228 (6): 650–659.

Van, H. B.; Woshner, V.; Santos,J.H.(2006). "Role of mitochondrial DNA in toxic responses to oxidative stress." DNA Repair (Amst). 5(2):145-52.

Vaseva, A. V.; Moll, U. M. (2009). "The mitochondrial p53 pathway." Biochim. Biophys. Acta 1787: 414–420.

Vásquez-Vivar, J.; Kalyanaraman, B.; Kennedy, M. C. (2000). "Mitochondrial aconitase is a source of hydroxyl radical: an electron spin resonance investigation." J. Biol. Chem. 275: 14064–14069.

Vogelstein, B.; Lane, D. ; Levine, A. J. (2000). "Surfing the p53 network." Nature 408: 307–310.

Vousden, K. H.; Prives, C. (2009). "Blinded by the light: the growing complexity of p53." Cell 137 (3):413–431.

Wallace DC.(1999). "Mitochondrial diseases in man and mouse." Science 283(5407):1482-8.

Williams, M. D.; Van Remmen, H.; Conrad, C. C.; Huang, T. T.; Epstein, C. J. and Richardson, A. (1998) J. Biol. Chem. 273: 28510-28515.

Xie, Y.; Yang, H.; Miller, J. H.; Shih, D. M.; Hicks, G. G.; Xie, J.; Shiu, R. P. (2008). "Cells deficient in oxidative DNA damage repair genes My hand Ogg1 are sensitive to oxidants with increased G2/Marrest and multinucleation." Carcinogenesis 29 (4): 722–728.

Yan,L. J.; Levine, R. L.; Sohal, R. S. (1997). "Oxidative damage during aging targets mitochondrial aconitase." Proc Natl Acad Sci U S A 94(21):11168-72.

Youn, C. K.; Song, P. I.; Kim, M. H.; Kim, J. S.; Hyun, J. W.; Choi, S. J.; Yoon, S. P.; Chung, M. H.; Chang, I. Y.; You, H. J. (2007) "Human 8-oxoguanine DNA glycosylase suppresses the oxidative stress induced apoptosis through a p53-mediated signaling pathway in human fibroblasts." Mol. Cancer Res. 5(10): 1083-1098.

Youle, R. J. ; Strasser, A. (2008). "The BCL-2 protein family: opposing activities that mediate cell death." Nat. Rev. Mol. Cell Biol. 9 (1): 47–59.

7

Structure-Function Relationship of DNA Repair Proteins: Lessons from BRCA1 and RAD51 Studies

Effrossyni Boutou[1,2], Vassiliki Pappa[3],
Horst-Werner Stuerzbecher[4] and Constantinos E. Vorgias[1]
[1]*Department of Biochemistry & Molecular Biology*
Faculty of Biology, School of Sciences Athens University, Athens
[2]*Prenatal Diagnosis Lab, Laiko Hospital, Athens*
[3]*2nd Propaedeutic Pathology Clinic, Medical School, Athens University, Athens*
[4]*Molecular Cancer Biology Group, Institute of Pathology, UK-SH, Luebeck*
[1,2,3]*Greece*
[4]*Germany*

1. Introduction

Accurate transfer of genetic information is vital for all living organisms in order to guarantee species survival. DNA damage occurs spontaneously during a cell's life due to either endogenous causes such as Reactive Oxygen Species (ROS) produced during metabolism or due to exogenous insults such as Ionizing Radiation (IR) or genotoxic agents in food / water and environment, to which an organism is exposed. Endogenous damage, due to intrinsic instability of chemical bonds in DNA structure, occurs spontaneously under normal physiologic conditions and is calculated to be approximately 10^4 events per cell, per day (Lindahl, 1993). Moreover, during DNA replication base adducts can cause collapse of replication forks and DNA double strand breaks (DSBs) are introduced in order to reinitiate genome duplication process.

As the genome carries all necessary information for life and evidently preservation of genome integrity is critical for cell survival, a number of mechanisms have evolved over time to ensure the most effective performance of the genome repair procedure. DNA repair mechanisms are capable of repairing practically all different types of chromosomal lesions (single and double strand breaks, base modifications, etc.) ensuring that genetic information is accurately transferred to the next generation. The cell's response to DNA damage (DNA Damage Response, DDR) encompasses a complex network of proteins, consisting of DNA damage recognition, signal transduction, transcriptional regulation, cell cycle control, DNA repair and verification of the repair efficiency, depending on the type of lesion, the replication status of the genome as well as the cell cycle stage. (scheme 1). Many excellent recent reviews as well as other chapters in the current volume extensively cover this topic (Rogakou, 1999; Lisby & Rothstein 2005; Murphy & Moynahan, 2010).

Defects in repair efficiency are the consequence of dysfunction of either upstream damage signalling or the central repair process. The current chapter covers topics referring to

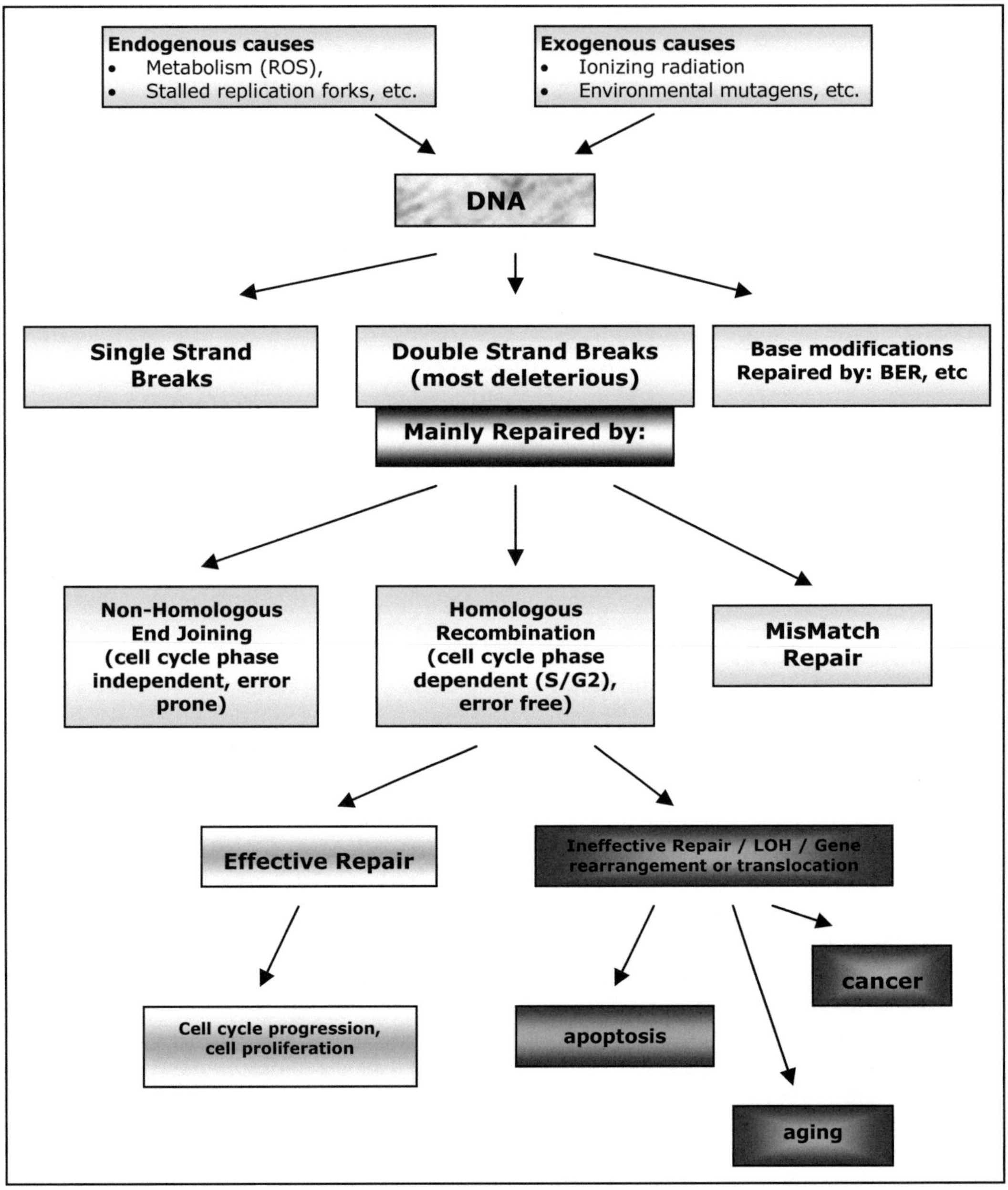

Scheme 1. Simplified diagram of DNA damage response network

factors/events influencing the structure - function relation of key molecules involved in each of the two processes, namely the BRCA1 and RAD51/Rad51 proteins, respectively. The breast cancer susceptibility gene 1 (brca1), isolated by reverse genetics in 1994, encodes for a large multifunctional protein (BRCA1) whose function is regulated by multiple post-translational modification events, driving the multi tasks performed, by which BRCA1 conducts almost all steps of DDR. The important anti-tumorigenic role of BRCA1 is strongly supported by its correlation with increased breast & ovarian familial cancer susceptibility in individuals carrying BRCA1 mutations. On the other hand, RAD51 is a relatively small and rigid protein playing a basic role (homology search strand and strand exchange) in the high fidelity DNA repair mechanism of Homologous Recombination (HR). RAD51 appears absolutely vital for cell survival, as its depletion results in embryonic lethality, it is highly conserved throughout evolution and up to now there is not a single mutation in the amino acid sequence detected in any type of cancer, although there is a strong correlation between its expression levels and both cancer development and cancer progression.

2. Consequences of genomic instability

Loss or insufficiency of DDR and genome repair can lead to an increased susceptibility to cancer due to the consequential genomic instability. Ineffective repair may result in subsequent mutations of genes required for cellular replication and division. The genome repair pathways also communicate with processes involved in induction of senescence and apoptosis when the damage cannot be repaired. Carefully balanced signalling cascades and regulatory systems are implicated in the maintenance of healthy cell survival in order to unfavour tumorigenesis and maintain stem and progenitor cells for renewal (anti-ageing) (Seviour & Lin 2010). Therefore, an effectively repaired genome is crucial not only for cancer prevention but also for lifespan extension. This notion is even more enhanced by the emerging benefit of the response of HR defective tumors to double strand break (DSB) producing therapies a promising and continuously evolving field. A clearer understanding of the biochemical, structural and genetic processes in conjuction with clinical data will lead to the development of more effective treatment strategies for both cancer and ageing processes.

2.1 Genomic instability and cancer

It is generally accepted that tumors are derived from a single genetically unstable cell, and that the unstable cell population as a whole continues to acquire further chromosomal abnormalities over time, although the precise mechanisms of acquisition of these abnormalities still remain unclear. Hereditary cancers are often characterized by the presence of a specific type of genomic instability, termed chromosomal instability. In these cancers, chromosomal instability can often be attributed to mutations in DNA repair genes, suggesting that the driving force behind tumor development is an increase in spontaneous genetic mutations resulting from lack of appropriate management of DNA damage. A second form of genomic instability, termed microsatellite instability, is also associated with defects in DNA repair, namely the mismatch repair system. However, in non-hereditary sporadic tumors, the picture is less clear. It should be emphasized that cancer is an extremely complex set of diseases, and that cancer cells develop many different mechanisms to achieve a similar phenotype of independent and uncontrolled growth (Hanahan & Weinberg, 2000; Luo et al., 2009 as reviewed by Schild & Wiese 2010).

Many of the DDR components including BRCA1 are known to be lost or mutated in human tumors. While loss of BRCA1 has been shown to lead to the development of mammary tumors in mouse models, the genetic diversity within those tumors suggests that the loss of BRCA1 may not directly be responsible for tumorigenesis. It is more likely, therefore, that the role of BRCA1 in the initiation of cancer is a result of its effects on DNA repair and the maintenance of genomic integrity. BRCA1 -/- tumors are shown to display numerous chromosomal aberrations. Analysis of BRCA1 -/- mouse models, coupled with the study of human BRCA1 -/- tumors, has revealed prevalence for p53 mutations in these tumors, which is likely to be caused by the decrease in genomic stability associated with the defects in DNA repair. Overall, these and many other data suggest that the loss of cell cycle checkpoints confers a selection advantage to cells with DNA repair defects, thereby triggering tumorigenesis in genetically unstable cells. Moreover, an increase in genomic instability is significantly correlated with the metastatic potential of the tumor. Further studies are required to determine whether this involvement in metastasis is a result of acquired genetic mutations resulting from DNA repair defects, or whether other mechanisms are required for this process (Murphy & Moynahan, 2010).

DNA repair by the high fidelity mechanism of homologous recombination, termed as Homologous Recombinational Repair (HRR) is practically the only 'error free' repair mechanism of the cell and as it requires a sister chromatid, normally is active in late S and G2 phases of the cell cycle. HRR involves a compex network of recombination mediators and co-mediators. Defects in recombination mediators and co-mediators, leading to impaired HRR, are indicated as major contributors in carcinogenesis and particularly in breast cancer (reviewed by Pierce et al., 2001; Henning & Stuerzbecher, 2003; Murphy & Moynahan, 2010). Nevertheless, up to now not a single mutation in the coding region of RAD51, the central recombinase in the HRR pathway, has been found in many tumor types examined. However, many primary tumor cells and cancer cell lines express significantly modified levels of RAD51 (Maacke et al., 2000; Henning & Stuerzbecher 2003; Klein 2008) and at least partly, this misregulation in protein expression levels is correlated with the polymorphism G->C in the 5'untranslated region of rad51 mRNA, as shown in some cases of hereditary breast tumors with BRCA2 mutation. As extensively discussed in the excellent and comprehensive review of Schild & Wiese 2010, RAD51 overexpression presumably complements initial HRR defects, thereby limiting genomic instability during carcinogenic progression and may explain the high frequency of *TP53* mutations in human cancers, as wild-type p53 represses RAD51 expression. Notably, both positive and negative regulations of HRR are required to maintain genomic stability by precise repair and suppression of deleterious rearrangements.

2.2 Genomic instability and ageing

DNA damage is a prominent cause of cancer in frequently dividing cells since cell proliferation is a prerequisite for the manifestation of genetic changes as permanent mutations. In contrast, DNA damage in infrequently dividing cells is likely a prominent cause of ageing (Best, 2009). Therefore, in addition to its role in the maintenance of genomic integrity, the DDR has been hypothesized to play a critical role in organismal ageing. Supporting to this hypothesis is the observation that DNA repair disorders such as Werner's syndrome, Bloom's syndrome and Ataxia telangiectasia, syndromes also characterised by premature ageing and / or retarded growth, are often called "segmental progerias" ("accelerated ageing diseases"). Individuals suffering from such diseases appear elderly and suffer from ageing-related diseases at an abnormally young age, while not manifesting all the symptoms of old age.

Ageing, resulting from the accumulation of damage to molecules, cells, organs and tissues over time, is believed to be caused by two cellular processes: senescence and apoptosis.

2.2.1 Senescence and DNA damage

Senescence, a phenomenon describing the irreversible cease of cell division, was initially described by Hayflick and Moorhead in 1961 and includes replicative senescence and oncogene-induced senescence, both of which involve aspects of the DDR.

Replicative senescence results from progressive shortening of telomeres with repeated rounds of cell replication. p53–dependent senescence serves as a tumor suppressor mechanism and is activated by the uncapping of critically shortened telomeres which are recognised as damaged DNA (Feldser and Greider, 2007). Recent studies argue that p53 can either activate or suppress senescence in cells, depending on their specific transcriptional activities and its interaction with partner molecules. As described by Vigneron & Vousden, 2010, the role of p53 in cell fate determination is even more complex as it involves epigenetic modifications of chromosomal DNA and relates chronic DDR signalling with increased levels of p53 acetylation. In addition to p53 other DNA damage response proteins like ATM have been associated with replicative senescence. ATM depletion in mice results in an increase in both chromosomal end-to-end fusion events and cell cycle-dependent telomere loss. These mice exhibit a premature ageing phenotype as defined by increased hair graying, alopecia and marked weight loss. Expression of mutant BRCA1 in mice also results in premature ageing, accompanied by an increase in cellular senescence and an increased susceptibility to certain cancers. The enhanced senescence observed in these mice may interfere with the fact that senescent cells have been noted to modify their tissue microenvironment. This phenomenon is thought to synergize with the accumulation of DNA damage over time to encourage cancer growth.

Oncogene-induced senescence can be induced by the overexpression of oncogenes by among others the induction of DNA damage resulting from both the generation of reactive oxygen species (ROS) and the hyper-replication of DNA. Both of these mechanisms activate the DNA damage response, which result in senescence by similar processes that induce replicative senescence.

2.2.2 Apoptosis and DNA damage

The accumulation of DNA damage can also lead to apoptosis. Activation of p53 by DNA damage and its role in the regulation of expression of pro-apoptotic proteins has been well documented. This is further supported by the fact that functional p53 is not detected to the majority of tumors. In cases of decline of the immune system an increase in p53 mediated apoptosis has been observed, linking ageing with apoptotic function. Moreover, constitutively activated p53 in mice also showed that, while high levels of p53 protect against cancer, it also accelerates the ageing process by reducing the mass of various tissues. The human condition Ataxia telangiectasia, which results from mutations in ATM, is associated with substantial neuro-degeneration. This has been shown in a mouse model to result from an accumulation of neurons harboring genomic damage, due to the inability of the mutant ATM protein to stimulate the p53 apoptotic cascade. Chk2 has also been shown to regulate apoptosis in a p53-dependent manner *in vitro* and *in vivo* in response to DNA damage (Seviour & Lin, 2010). Notably, the major recombinase of HR, Rad51, seems also to interact with p53, possibly serving as a tool for monitoring the extension as well the effectiveness of DNA repair processes (Henning & Sturzbecher Toxicology, 2003; Morita et al., 2010).

Consequently, impaired DDR appears to have dramatic effects on both tumorigenesis and premature ageing. At the molecular level, DDR impairment could be attributed to irregular interactions between the complexes involved in each process due to structural changes of DDR components resulting from either mutagenesis, modified post-translational modifications of altered protein levels, guiding equilibrium in favour of abnormal decisions.

3. Structural & functional integrity is essential for protein interactions with partner molecules

The efficient performance of DNA repair processes requires the coordinated actions of many players and mainly depends on proper interactions between the protein components of each pathway involved which in turn mainly relies on their functional structure (structure – function relationship). At least three major mechanisms influence protein function due to or independently of its tertiary structure:

a. Missense mutations in the coding region can modify the primary structure of a protein resulting in dys-functional folding of the protein, and / or instability in the cellular environment.
b. Post-translational modifications (phosphorylation, ubiquitination, ribosylation and acetylation) regulating distinct interactions with partner molecules driving the various pathways in which the protein in question is implicated.
c. Regulation of the protein levels, availability through regulation of the quantity of the protein, which can drive cell decisions in improper pathways, leading to abnormal cell cycle progression, cell division and possibly malignant transformation or aggressive tumor progression.

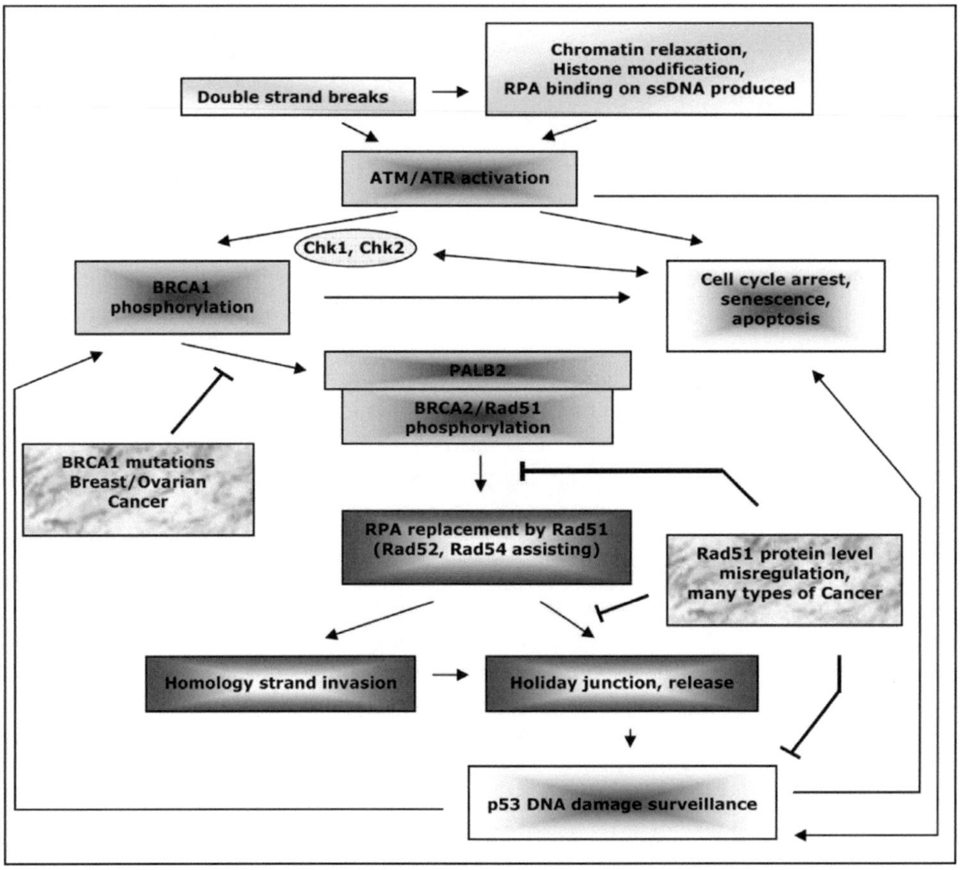

Scheme 2. Simplified Scheme of major steps of DNA Double strand break repair by Homologous Recombination.

The fundamental proteins involved in the HRR pathways are highly conserved in almost all organisms ranging from bacteria to human. The significance of this repair system is also indicated by the fact that defects in HRR cause human hereditary cancers as well as sporadic tumors. In many cases the dysfunction of proteins observed in many tumors helps to elucidate all three categories of the mechanisms mentioned above and to clarify different aspects of DDR pathways (Murphy & Moynahan, 2010).

Herein we will focus on current information regarding the structure - function relationship of two key players in regulation and performance of DSB repair - the most deleterious reported lesion of the genome - BRCA1 and RAD51. BRCA1 is a core component of many multi-molecular complexes involved in DNA damage detection, HR regulation, cell cycle regulation and genome transcription. RAD51, a key factor of HRR, replaces RPA on the produced single strands of damaged DNA and performs the search for homologous DNA strand and exchange in order to restore the damaged DNA sequence according to its sister chromatid. Moreover, RAD51 is implicated in telomere maintenance via ALT pathway and is also involved in mitochondrial DNA repair. Via at least its indirect interaction with BRCA1 as well as with direct p53 complex formation, RAD51 seems to be an interplayer responsible for communication between DNA repair effectiveness, cell replication, apoptosis or senescence decisions.

3.1 The BRCA1 structure – function relation paradigm

The Breast Cancer Susceptibility Gene 1 protein (BRCA1) is a multifunctional nuclear phosphoprotein of 1863 residues (220-240 kDa). BRCA1 was attributed the role of a tumor suppressor involved in multiple cellular functions (Starita & Parvin, 2003). Most of BRCA1 is located in the cell nucleus and is phosphorylated in a cell cycle-dependent manner by a number of kinases (reviewed by Ouchi, 2006). Depending on the position and the number of phosphorylated residues, BRCA1 participates in different multiprotein complexes performing diverse tasks. Therefore, BRCA1 has been implicated in a variety of functions required for the maintenance of genomic stability (Rowling et al., 2010).

Regarding DDR, BRCA1 has been attributed many roles in regulation of genome integrity including DNA replication, cell cycle checkpoint control, apoptosis, regulation of transcription, chromatin unfolding and protein ubiquitination. The ascribed functions are exerted through an extensive number of protein interactions reported (Jasin M. 2002 as cited in Murphy & Moynahan 2010). In brief, upon detection of chromatid relaxation due to breakage of both strands of the double helix of DNA, BRCA1 - being activated by ATR kinase - is recruited to the damage breakpoint assisting assembly of the BRCA2 - RAD51 complex in order to replace RPA and restore damage by the high fidelity process of HRR. In parallel, BRCA1 interaction with Fanconi Anemia (FA) and other complexes regulates G1/S and G2/M checkpoints. BRCA1 implication in cell cycle regulation is assisted by complex formation with BRCA1 interacting protein C-terminal helicase (BRIP1) and CtIP which are activated in S-phase by post-translational modifications. A graphical representation of the BRCA1 protein, including sites of both post-translational modifications and regions involved in protein-protein interactions, is depicted in Fig 1.

The amino-terminal region of BRCA1 contains a distinct ~100aa RING finger motif involved in ubiquitin ligase activity and enables BRCA1 to mono- or poly-ubiquitinate cellular proteins. BARD1 (another RING and BRCT domain-containing protein) is the 'permanent' partner of BRCA1 in the formation of the ubiquitine ligase complex. Phosphorylation of specific residues of BRCA1 appears to regulate its participation in transcription regulation and ubiquitination of substrate proteins. As many different BRCA1 species are produced by alternative splicing of its mRNA, the phosphorylated residues each form contains may regulate different functions. Moreover, the balance between full length and spliced forms of BRCA1 may play an important role in tumor suppression (Ouchi, 2006).

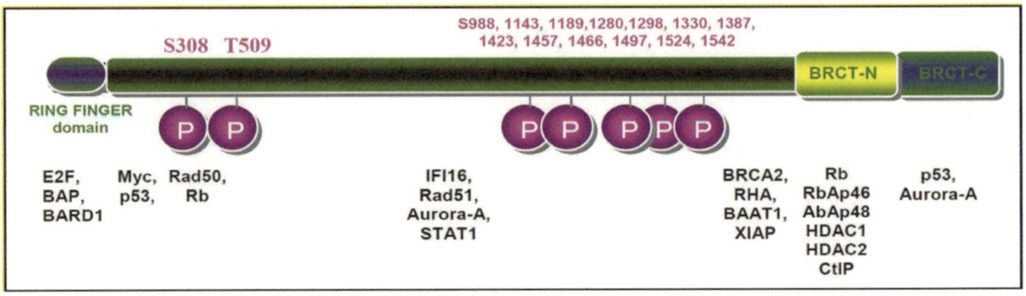

Fig. 1. Primary structure of BRCA1 Tumor Suppressor Protein. The phosphorylation sites and and its binding partners are indicated.

The carboxy-terminal domain of BRCA1 contains two structurally identical BRCT (**BR**CA1 **C-t**erminal) tandem repeats each containing ~90 amino acid residues. BRCT domains are found in proteins involved in DNA repair and maintenance of genomic stability, and more recently, the BRCT repeat has been recognized as a phosphopeptide-binding domain. The structure of each repeat consists of a parallel four-stranded β-sheet located at the central part of the domain surrounded by three α-helices (Fig. 2). The two BRCT repeats fold together in a specific head-to-tail manner, giving rise to the formation of a conserved, almost all-hydrophobic, inter-repeat interface, forming a phosphopeptide binding pocket. BRCT like domains have also been found in BRCA1 interacting proteins such as 53BP1 and BARD1. BRCT repeats are a family of phosphopeptide binding domains implicated in DNA damage response. Therefore, BRCTs are considered as protein-docking modules involved in eukaryotic DNA repair. Although BRCTs are characterized by low sequence homology they retain a generally well-conserved structure organization.

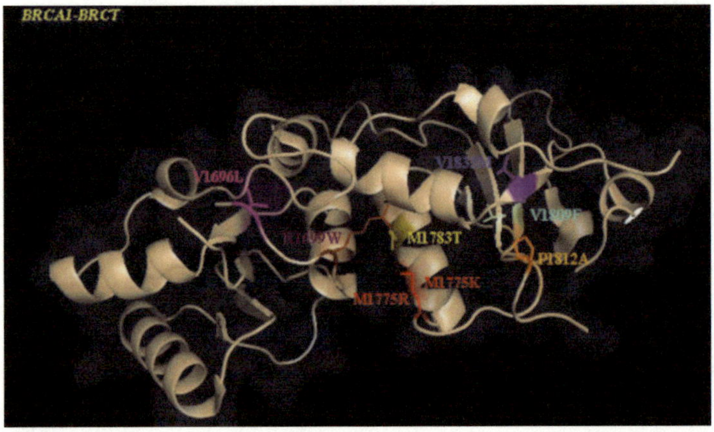

Fig. 2. Ribbon representation of the BRCA1-BRCTstructure. Positions of selected cancer-related mutations are indicated. M1775K and M1783T are located at the inter-BRCT-repeat interface where the BRCA1-BRCT binding groove for Phe 13 is also located. The exposed V1696L is located at the N-terminal BRCTstructural repeat. V1809F, P1812A are found at the C-terminal BRCT repeat. The positions of missense mutations from previously published studies are also depicted. (From Drikos et al., 2009).

Analysis of the BRCA1 mutational database (BIC, http://research.nhgri.nih.gov/bic/) indicates that both RING and BRCT repeats are most frequently mutated in women at risk of cancer, and have been further studied. Many research groups have used structural and biochemical methods to probe the function of BRCA1 and characterize the plethora of unclassified variants identified in breast cancer patients found in BIC database. Among the hundreds of distinct mutations uncovered in BRCA1, for the vast majority, there is insufficient genetic linkage data to determine the cancer risk associated with them (Glover, 2006).

The central region of BRCA1, between the two terminal domains, bears relatively low sequence identity between mammalian BRCA1 homologs, and attempts to define structured domains within this region indicate that this part of BRCA1 is largely unstructured (Glover, 2006; Mark, 2005). This region is extensively phosphorylated by DNA damage-associated kinases like ATM and may serve as a phosphorylation-dependent docking site for other proteins involved in the DNA damage response, or even for damaged DNA itself (Paul et al., 2001; Mark, 2005; Ouchi, 2006).

3.2 BRCA1 structure modifications found in cancer

Mutations in brca1 and brca2 genes have been found in 30-50% of hereditary breast and ovarian cancers. Women carrying BRCA1 mutations are particularly susceptible to the development of breast or ovarian cancer at an age earlier than 35-40 years old with a probability rate of 45-60% and 20-40%, respectively.

Most cancer-associated BRCA1 mutations identified so far, result in the premature translational termination of the protein and influence BRCA1 integrity and function. A large number of missense mutations is located in BRCT tandem repeats of BRCA1, while only few of them may cause loss of the protein's function, abolition of protein interactions and protein miss-localization. Therefore, it seems that the BRCT repeats in BRCA1 are essential for the tumor suppressing function of the protein as protein truncation and missense variants within the BRCT domain have been shown to be associated with human breast and ovarian cancers.

Variants that result in large truncations are deleterious to function and therefore can be classified as disease-associated. In contrast, missense mutations typically remain unclassified. Thus, the BIC database currently contains more than 108 missense mutations in the BRCT domains of BRCA1, but only 7% of them have been classified. These missense mutations may be either polymorphisms or mutations predisposing the carrier to cancer progression. The variants D1692Y, C1697R, R1699W, A1708E, S1715R, P1749R and M1775R all appear to be associated with an increased risk of breast cancer, while M1625I appears to be a benign polymorphism (Williams et al., 2003). Unfortunately, most of the missense mutations could not been assessed for disease association. An attempt to classify these variants by measuring the thermodynamic stability of the BRCA1 BRCT domains resulted in investigation of the effects of 36 missense mutations (Rowling et al., 2010). The mutations show a range of effects. Some do not change the stability, whereas others destabilize the protein by as much as 6 kcal mol−1; one-third of the mutants were considered to destabilize the protein by an even greater amount, as they could not be expressed in soluble form in *Escherichia coli*. Several computer algorithms were used in an attempt to predict the mutant effects. According to these results the variants were grouped into two classes (destabilizing by less than or more than 2.2 kcal mol−1). Importantly, with the exception of the few mutants located in the binding site, none showed a significant reduction in affinity for phosphorylated substrate. These results indicate that despite very large losses in stability, the integrity of the structure is not compromised by the mutations. Thus, the majority of mutations seem to cause loss of function by reducing the proportion of BRCA1 molecules that are in the folded state and increasing the proportion of molecules that are unfolded. The authors predict that small molecule stabilization of the structure could be a generally applicable preventative therapeutic strategy for rescuing many BRCA1 mutations. Another recent approach by Lee et al., 2010, extended in 117 variants, comprehensively shows how functional and structural information can be useful in the development of models to assess cancer risk.

Cancer-associated mutations in the BRCT domain of BRCA1 (BRCA1-BRCT) abolish its tumor suppressor function by disrupting interactions with other proteins such as BACH1. Many cancer-related mutations do not cause sufficient destabilization to lead to global unfolding under physiological conditions, and thus abrogation of function probably is due to localized structural changes. Molecular dynamics simulations on three cancer-associated mutants, A1708E, M1775R, and Y1853ter, and on the wild type and benign M1652I mutant, followed by comparison of the structures and fluctuations showed that only the cancer-associated mutants exhibited significant backbone structure differences from the wild-type crystal structure in BACH1-binding regions, some of which are far from the mutation sites. These BACH1-binding regions of the cancer-associated mutants also exhibited increases in their fluctuation magnitudes compared with the same regions in the wild type and M1562I mutant, as quantified by quasiharmonic analysis. The increased fluctuations in the disease-related mutants suggest an increase in vibrational entropy in the unliganded state that could result in a larger entropy loss in the disease-related mutants upon binding BACH1 than in the wild type. Vibrational entropies of the A1708E and wild type in the free state and bound to a BACH1-derived phosphopeptide, calculated using quasiharmonic analysis, determined the binding entropy difference DeltaDeltaS between the A1708E mutant and the wild type. In overall such biophysical/biochemical studies supported by suited algorithms showed that the observed differences in structure, flexibility, and entropy of binding are likely to be responsible for abolition of BACH1 binding, and illustrate that many disease-related mutations could have very long-range effects. Such methods have potential for identifying correlated motions responsible for other long-range effects of deleterious mutations. (Gough et al., 2007)

The C-terminal BRCT domains are also evidenced to mediate the transcriptional activity of BRCA1. Most of the published mutations within the BRCT domains have been reported to affect BRCA1 nuclear functions including DNA repair and transcriptional activity. The biochemical and biophysical studies of our group have already demonstrated that mutations of the BRCT domain: (i) affected the folding of the domain to a varying degree depending on the induced destabilization and (ii) altered and abolished the affinity of BRCT domain to synthetic phosphopeptides corresponding to BRCT interacting regions of pBACH1/ BRIP1 and pCtIP, by affecting the structural integrity of the BRCT active sites.

BRCA1 is a nuclear-cytoplasmic shuttling protein and its nuclear localization is regulated by the combined action of nuclear localization (NLS) and nuclear export signals (NES). In most cases, however, cellular and ectopically expressed BRCA1 are primarily nuclear due to nuclear import mediated by the two NLSs and interaction with the RING domain binding protein, BARD1, which can carry BRCA1 into the nucleus and trap it there by masking its nuclear export signal.

Despite the structural studies of BRCA1-BRCT protein mutants, the influence of these mutations at protein localization in cellular level has not yet been adequately addressed. Only few of them have already determined to present protein mislocalization. BRCA1 mutations of the BRCT domain altered BRCA1 localization, causing the protein to be excluded from the nucleus. Two of the C-terminal mutations (M1775R and Y1853X) that restricted nuclear localization are identical to mutations that disrupt BRCA1 C-terminal folding, suggesting that the conformational changes they elicit might be deleterious to BRCA1 nuclear transport. This nuclear exclusion was not due to increased nuclear export, but to reduced nuclear import. Similar findings were observed for both the overexpressed and endogenous forms of the BRCT mutant, BRCA1 (5382insC). Also, Chen et al., 1995 have published controversial findings, which claimed that BRCA1 was detected almost exclusively in the cytoplasm in breast cancer tissues, but remained nuclear in normal tissue and in other cancer cell types.

In our laboratory more than fifteen BRCA1-BRCT proteins mutants have already been studied for structural and functional alterations in protein's integrity. The most destabilizing protein mutants such as M1775K, V1809F (Fig3) were collected in order to be examined in cellular level about their impact in BRCA1 subcellular compartmentalization. M1775K is a rare breast cancer-linked mutation and it has been identified only in two unrelated families of European ancestry with a history of breast cancer. Met1775 is strongly involved in the phosphopeptide-binding pocket of the BRCT domain. The mutation of Met1775, namely the mutation M1775R, is much more frequent worldwide among patients with hereditary breast/ovarian cancer, its association with the disease is epidemiologically established and was the first characterized to be linked to cancer. The M1775R mutation has already shown to change the intracellular localization of BRCA1 protein which is less focused into the nucleus. The M1775K missense variant according to our *in vitro* experiments fails to bind to synthetic peptides such pBACH1/BRIP1 or pCtIP. Structural analysis of the interatomic interactions of Lys1775 show a direct clash of its side chain with Phe 13 of either phosphopeptide, a result arising from the disruption of the BRCT-phosphopeptide binding pocket.

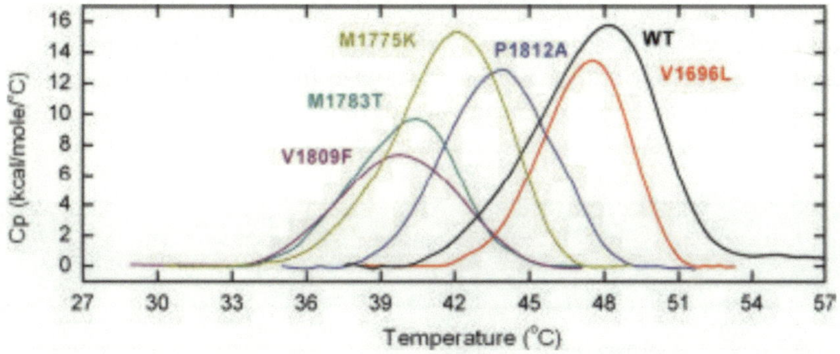

Fig. 3. DSC profiles for the thermally induced denaturation of BRCT-wt and of five missense variants V1809F, M1783T, M1775K, P1812A, and V1696L. (from Drikos et al., 2009).

V1809F is a rare mutation linked to hereditary breast/ ovarian cancer. Only a few cases of the mutation have been submitted to the BIC database with loss of function reported by *in vitro* experiments, regarding the interactions with synthetic phosphopeptides pBACH1/BRIP1 and pCtIP. The residue Val1809 is conserved among species. Val1809 and Met1775 are crucial for the integrity of phosphopeptide binding pocket of the BRCA1 protein and exhibit no binding to either pBACH1/BRIP1 or pCtIP synthetic phosphopeptides. These results, in combination with the fact that V1809F resembles structural destabilization of the native fold similar to M1775R, strongly supports the classification of V1809F as pathogenic.

Additionally, the variant M1652I is located at the first tandem of the BRCT domain and seems to have neutral influence on breast cancer pathogenesis. Based on preliminary structural studies by our laboratory, this variant is less involved in structural alteration of BRCT but further analysis is required. M1652I is classified as low risk mutation. Therefore we decided to include it to our study in order to compare it with more destabilizing mutants such as V1809F and M1775K.

In order to assess how the selected BRCA1-BRCT mutants influence the subcellular localization of BRCA1, we produced BRCA1-GFP fusion proteins with the corresponding mutations introduced at the BRCT domain. The GFP-BRCA1-BRCT mutated proteins were inserted into MCF-7 cells and their subcellular localization was assessed by fluorescent microscopy.

According to our results, destabilizing mutations of the carboxyl terminal region of BRCA1 seem to influence protein localization and presumably DDR. As shown in Fig 4, BRCA1-V1809F-GFP and M17775K are restricted to the cytoplasm in contrast to the nuclear-cytoplasmic localization of BRCA1wt and M1652I. As EGFP-BRCA1-M1652I shows similar subcellular distribution to the BRCA1wt–GFP protein (detected both in the nucleus and the cytoplasm), it is presumed that the structural change caused by replacement of M1652 to Ile has a minor effect of BRCA1 nuclear transport. UV irradiation of cells expressing wt or the mutants mentioned failed to drive M1175K and V1809F to the cell nucleus in contrast to both wt and M1652I which were then detected exclusively in the nucleus and shown to at least in part colocalize with Rad51 foci (data not shown from Drikos et al., submitted). Mutations such as M1775K and V1809F which disrupt BRCA1 C-terminal folding, appears that result to conformational and functional changes which might be restrictive to BRCA1 nuclear transport in contrast to more mild missense variants such as M1652I. These results suggest that structural integrity modifications of the BRCA1-BRCT domain can be reflected to the protein's subcellular localization and therefore can serve for further characterization and classification of the variant, in combination with the structural data (table 1). M1175K and V1809F are located near to the binding site of the inter-repeat region and affect through hydrophobic interactions the structural and functional integrity of the domain.

	Effect of mutation	**Cancer Risk of the mutation**	**Structural Stability**	**Functional Activity with synthetic peptides**	**Subcellular localization (-UV)**	**Subcellular localization (+UV)**
GFP-BRCA1-V1809F	Potential hydrophobic	Deleterious	Destabilizing	Alter binding affinity	Cytoplasmic	Cytoplasmic
GFP-BRCA1-M1775K	Potential hydrophobic	Deleterious	Destabilizing	Alter binding affinity	Cytoplasmic	Cytoplasmic
GFP-BRCA1-M1652I	No effect	Neutral	No effect	Unknown	Nuclear-Cytoplasmic	Nuclear
GFP-BRCA1wt					Nuclear-Cytoplasmic	Nuclear

Table 1. Summary of the impact of BRCA1-BRCT mutants on the structural, functional and cellular levels. Mutations such as M1775K and V1809F, which disrupt BRCA1 C-terminal folding, induce also alterations of the integrity of the BRCA1-BRCT domain and the proteins subcellular localization.

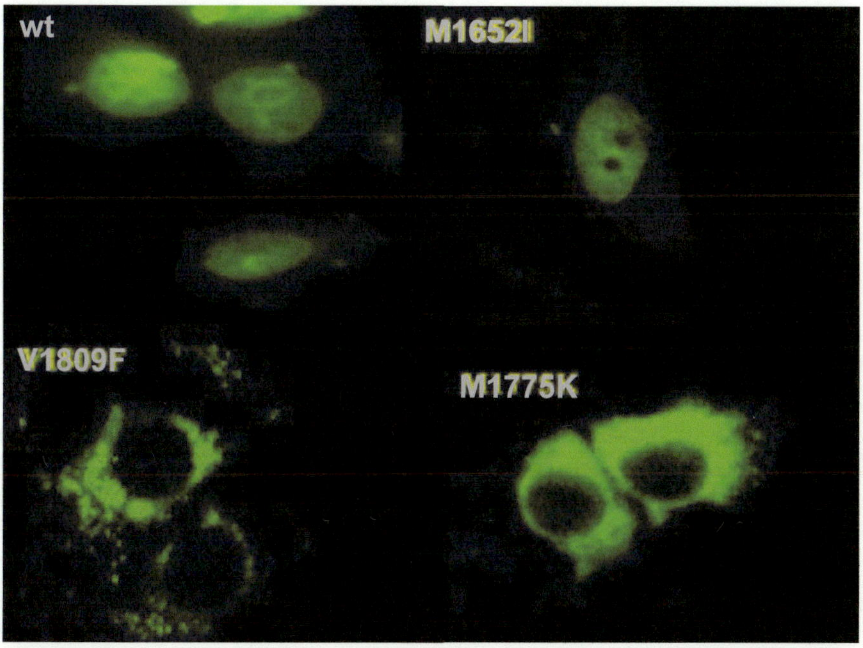

Fig. 4. Subcellular mis-localization of cancer linked GFP-BRCA1-BRCT mutations, M1775K and V1809F in the cytoplasm of MCF-7 cells in contrast to the wild type BRCA1 (wt) and the 'neutral' mutation of BRCT, M1652I which are detected in both the nucleus and the cytoplasm.

A living cell is a dynamic unit with flexible equilibrium between different processes which drive cell fate and determination decisions. The various pathways involved are either activated or suppressed as a result of qualitative and /or quantitative interactions between biomolecules. BRCA1 is an elegant paradigm of both kinds of interactions. Truncated or absent BRCA1 (abolishment of qualitative interactions) leads to impaired DNA repair, carcinogenesis and cancer progression. As indicated by the studies of various missense mutations there are cases where although the mutated BRCA1 seems to function properly, a significant proportion of BRCA1 molecules adopts an unfolding state and only few molecules are found in a given time in proper and functional structure. M1324K, R42573L mutations are good paradigms where biophysical studies of these BRCA1 mutants indicated that although interactions with phosphopeptides were attained, the majority of mutant molecules were detected in improper folding state. Moreover, as many missense variants remain to be characterized, combination of biophysical with cell/molecular biology studies, as in the case of M1775K and V1809F mutations, is expected to substantially contribute in their classification regarding to cancer-relation.

3.3 The RAD51 structure – function relation paradigm

DNA double strand breaks (DSBs), produced by either exogenous causes or in order to restore stalled replication forks during genome replication, are detrimental to cell survival and are mainly restored by either Homologous Recombination Repair (HRR) or Non-Homologous End Joining (NHEJ). The two pathways compete for each other while a number of factors such as cell cycle stage and availability of duplicated DNA regulate the final choice. HRR is the prominent (high fidelity) DSB repair pathway, requiring an homologous DNA sequence present (the identical sister chromatid located in proper distance) and therefore is mainly active during S/G2 phases of cell cycle, while the error prone NHEJ pathway is mainly active during G1 and early S phase, although in certain cases can work in all cell cycle phases. HRR compete NHEJ pathway through a complicated manner, where initial DNA damage signalling factors play important roles. Damage processing and effectiveness of repair are incessantly checked by sensor molecules which through a series of distinct but interconnected pathways prolong cell cycle arrest, induce senescence or apoptosis depending on the information flow and the signals produced (Freeman & Monteiro 2010).

An important early step in HRR is the conversion of double to single stranded DNA in the area of the double strand break, which in turn is coated by the Replication Protein A (RPA) and can be extended up to 4 - 5 Kb on both sides along the break point. Displacement of RPA by RAD51, assembled as a nucleoprotein filament on the ssDNA, is the initial step towards HRR and is highly regulated through interactions with a variety of accessory proteins referred to as the 'recombination mediators' (Essers et al., 2002; Henning & Sturzbecher 2003; Schild & Wiese, 2010; Forget & Kowalczykowski, 2010; West, 2003; San Filippo et al., 2008; Li & Heyer, 2008). The central event in HRR is the synapsis of the single-stranded (ss)DNA molecule - produced along the double strand break point - with homologous duplex DNA. The strand invasion is mediated by the strand transferase RAD51 oligomerized on ssDNA as an active nucleoprotein filament (and the corresponding co-factors needed for filament assembly and function), which initiates the strand exchange that leads to recombination. RAD51, a recombinase essential for cell viability, is one of the most conserved molecules known. RAD51 mediates strand exchange via distinct reactions grouped into the presynaptic, synaptic, and postsynaptic phases (2) (Heyer, 2007; Shivji et al., 2009). The major steps of HRR process are schematically illustrated in Scheme 3.

RAD51 assembly on ssDNA and subsequent catalysis of homology dependent strand invasion is mainly driven by the tumor suppressor protein BRCA2 while during the different phases of HRR RAD51 interacts sequentially with other molecules involved in HRR, cell cycle control and cell fate decisions. RAD51, as part of dynamic structures called DNA damage foci, seems to be a stably associated core component, whereas other co-factors such as Rad52 and Rad54 rapidly and reversibly interact with the structure (Essers et al., 2002). RAD51 function depends on protein re-localization and is mainly regulated by various post-translational modifications, mainly phosphorylation (Slupianek et al., 2001; Venkitaraman, 2001), as well as non-covalent interaction with SUMO (Ouyang et al., 2009). Along evolution recombinase molecules are highly conserved, starting from the prokaryotic orthologue RecA to mammalian RAD51. The fact the RecA seems not to be an ancestor of RAD51 but these two molecules are considered to have evolved by converging evolution, suggests that the structure obtained is crucial for the specific recombination function and cannot afford modifications. This notion is further supported by the absence of RAD51 coding region mutants in any cancer type, while cells or animals that do not express RAD51 eventually are not viable (Tsuzuki et al., 1996; Sonoda et al., 1998). Despite the non-detection of RAD51 mutants itself it is clear that mutations in recombination mediators and co-mediators, which control RAD51 activity and availability, are highly related to cancer susceptibility and particularly breast cancer (Venkitaraman, 2009; Rahan et al., 2007; Seviour & Lin, 2010). Additionally, the 'guardian of the genome' p53, found mutated in more than 50% of cancers, also directly interacts with RAD51 presumably connecting HRR efficiency to cell cycle control and apoptosis (Henning & Sturzbecher, 2003; Gatz & Wiesmuller, 2006; Lazao-Trueba & Silva, 2006).

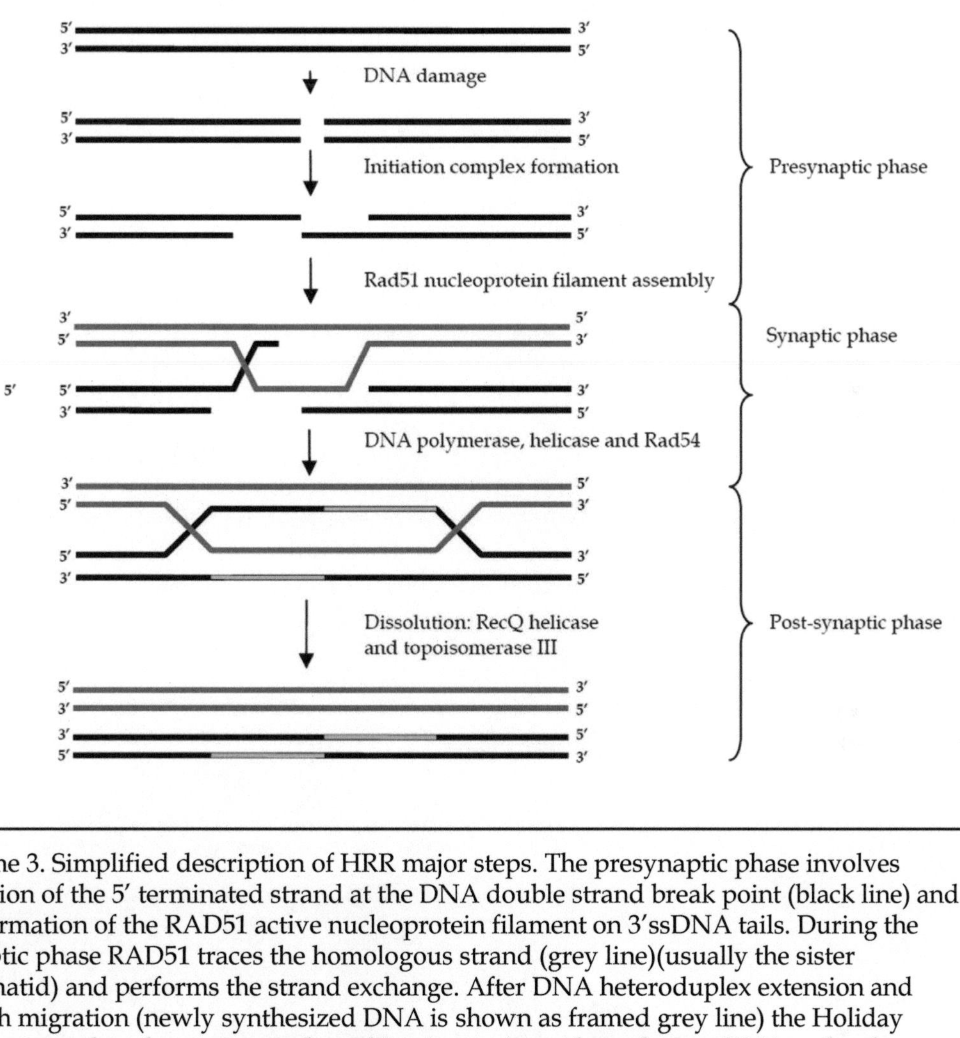

Scheme 3. Simplified description of HRR major steps. The presynaptic phase involves resection of the 5′ terminated strand at the DNA double strand break point (black line) and the formation of the RAD51 active nucleoprotein filament on 3′ssDNA tails. During the synaptic phase RAD51 traces the homologous strand (grey line)(usually the sister chromatid) and performs the strand exchange. After DNA heteroduplex extension and branch migration (newly synthesized DNA is shown as framed grey line) the Holiday junctions produced are separated resulting in two intact homologous DNA molecules. (Resolution or dissolution of holiday junction may also involve crossing over resulting in chimeric but still homologous DNA molecules).

RAD51 function is mainly controlled by the breast cancer susceptibility gene 2 product BRCA2 which acts as a recombination mediator (scheme 4). Briefly, BRCA2 targets RAD51 to ssDNA for assembly into a nucleoprotein filament, stabilizes the ATP-bound form of RAD51 and inhibits RAD51 assembly on dsDNA (Shivji et al., 2009). BRCA2 is an extremely large protein of 3418 residues and essentially contributes to RAD51-mediated HRR through several regions. RAD51 interacts with 8 copies of ~35 residues repeated motifs (BRC repeats) located at exon 11 (Yu et al., 2003), as well as with an unrelated carboxyl-terminal motif in exon 27 (Esashi et al., 2007). The BRC repeats sequence, unlike the C-terminal motif, is evolutionarily conserved. RAD51 replaces RPA in ssDNA, a process regulated by the DNA-binding domain of BRCA2, in cooperation with the BRC repeats and the contribution of other RAD52 epistasis group members as Rad52 and Rad54. BRC repeats of BRCA2 bind to the core of RAD51 by mimicking the structure of an adjacent Rad51 monomer (Pellegrini at al., 2002). RAD51 loading on ssDNA is promoted by the BRCA2[BRC1–8] region while RAD51 assembly on dsDNA is at the same time suppressed. This way the efficiency of RAD51-mediated HRR is further enhanced. RAD51 function can either be stimulated or suppressed by activities of the BRC repeats, depending on the experimental conditions used and the BRC: RAD51 molar ratio used (Galkin et al., 2005; Shivji et al., 2009; Carreira et al., 2009; Rajendra & Venkitaraman, 2010). BRC4 also blocks nucleation of RAD51 onto dsDNA while not disassembling Rad51-dsDNA filaments. (Carreira A, et al., 2009). At lower molar ratios BRC3 or BRC4 actually bind and form stable complexes with RAD51-DNA nucleoprotein filaments. Only at high concentrations of the BRC repeats are filaments disrupted. The specific protein-protein contacts occur in the RAD51 filament by means of the N-terminal domain of RAD51 for BRC3 and the nucleotide-binding core of RAD51 for BRC4 (Galkin et al., 2005; Rajendra & Venkitaraman 2009). These observations show that the BRC repeats bind distinct regions of RAD51 and are nonequivalent in their mode of interaction. These results might explain how disruption of a single RAD51 interaction site in BRCA2 might modulate the ability of RAD51 to promote recombinational repair and lead to an increased risk of breast cancer. Moreover, the dysregulated molar ratio present in a cell may drive hyper-recombination effects leading to abnormal outcome and in part may explain why mutations in BRCA2 predispose individuals to breast cancer, a consequence of the role of BRCA2 in DNA repair.

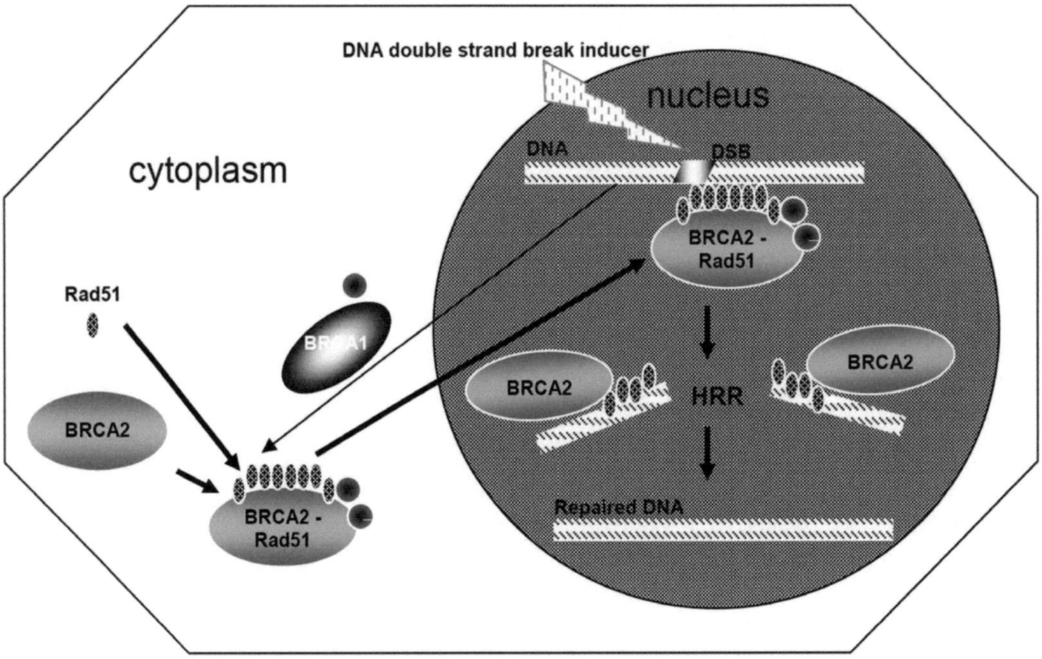

Scheme 4. Simplistic cartoon of the HRR process depicting Rad51 functions.

RAD51 filaments are further stabilized by direct interaction of the BRCA2 C terminus to the interface created by two adjacent RAD51 protomers. This way filaments cannot be dissociated by the BRC repeats. Interaction of the BRCA2 C terminus with the RAD51 filament causes a large movement of the flexible RAD51 N-terminal domain that is important in regulating filament dynamics. RAD51 interaction with the BRCA2 C-terminal region may facilitate efficient nucleation of RAD51 multimers on DNA and thereby stimulate recombination-mediated repair. (Esashi et al., 2007). Data from studies the Caenorhabditis elegans BRCA2 homolog CeBRC-2 support a model where an interaction with RAD-51 alone is likely involved in filament nucleation, whereas a second independent interaction is involved in *in situ* stabilization of RAD51 filaments by BRCA2 and provide further insight into why mutations in many different positions within BRCA2 lead to loss of genomic stability (Petalcorin et al., 2007).

RAD51, the central homology strand search and strand exchange effector in HRR can serve as a nice example to show how unregulated protein levels can abolish normal cell fate decisions and result in premature ageing or malignancies, depending on the mechanisms involved. RAD51 is one of the most conserved proteins known and essential for cell survival (Henning & Sturzbecher, 2003; Sonoda et al., 1998). While no mutations have ever been detected in human cancers, in many tumors significantly up- or downregulated levels of RAD51 have been observed (Maacke et al., 2000; Henning & Sturzbecher 2003; Klein, 2008). Moreover, high-level expression of RAD51 is an independent prognostic marker of survival in non-small-cell lung cancer patients (Qiao et al., 2005). In addition, haematopoietic progenitor cells, when Rad51 is overexpressed showed elevated levels of chromosomal alterations, similar to those observed in tumors of the hematopoietic system (Francis and Richardson, 2007). Notably, both positive and negative regulation of HRR is required in order to maintain genomic stability with precise repair and suppression of deleterious rearrangements. The only tumorigenesis-related variation found in the *rad51* gene is a G->C change in the 5′ untranslated rad51 mRNA region. This variation has been correlated to higher risk for breast cancer in BRCA2 mutation carriers and is possibly involved in mRNA modified translation capability resulting in abnormal RAD51 protein levels (Antoniou et al., 2007).

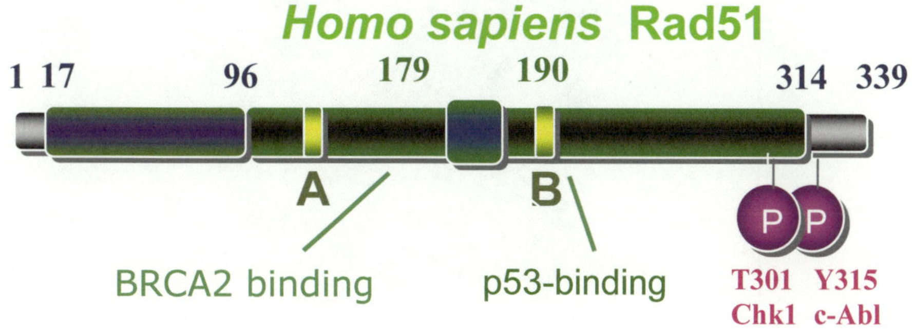

Scheme 5. Scematic representation of human Rad51 protein. The areas responsible for interaction with p53 and BRCA2 are indicated.

Since Rad51 overexpression can compensate for loss of function of other key molecules of DDR, including BRCA1 and BRCA2, experimental evidences from various research groups support two models: 1. Rad51 abnormal levels lead to genomic instability early in cancer development, thereby placing Rad51 modified expression as a leading cause of transformation and 2. Rad51 overexpression can protect cancer cells from DNA damage as more effective repair occurs further stabilizing the neoplastic clone and render it more aggressive and metastatic (Schild & Wiese, 2010). As cancer is an extremely complex set of diseases and can develop by different aetiologies while achieving similar phenotype of independent and uncontrolled growth the two models presented by Schild and Wiese can each adequately explain the neoplastic procedure of different cancer types.

The exact causes of Rad51 overexpression are still poorly explored but there is a number of data indicating both transcriptional regulation and protein stability and turnover modification. p53, the tumor suppressor that is implicated in DNA repair control, is involved in transcriptional regulation of *rad51* (Arias-Lopez et al., 2006). p53 is mutated in about half of human cancers resulting in loss of suppression of rad51 transcriptional regulation. Notably, as p53 directly interacts with Rad51 (Stürzbecher et al., 1996), in cases of p53 mutations inhibition of Rad51 activity could be abolished. Moreover, in cases of either TP53 deletion or some TP53 point mutations Rad51 expression up-regulation is detected. The Transcriptional activator protein 2 (AP2), in combination with p53 suppresses rad51 transcription (Hannay et al., 2007). Abl kinase phosphorylates Rad51 in Tyr315 and in cases of the presence of the oncogenic constituvely active BCR/Abl fusion tyrosine kinase (i.e. in Ph+ leukaemias) Rad 51 expression is increased (Slupianek et al., 2001).

Aiming in further clarifying aspects of structure-function relationship of RAD51, we produced several RAD51 mutants by altering amino acid residue candidates to be involved in RAD51-BRCA2 or RAD51-p53 interaction (fig 5). Exogenous expression the RAD51m6 mutant, fused to EYFP, altered their subcellular localization compared to the wt protein.

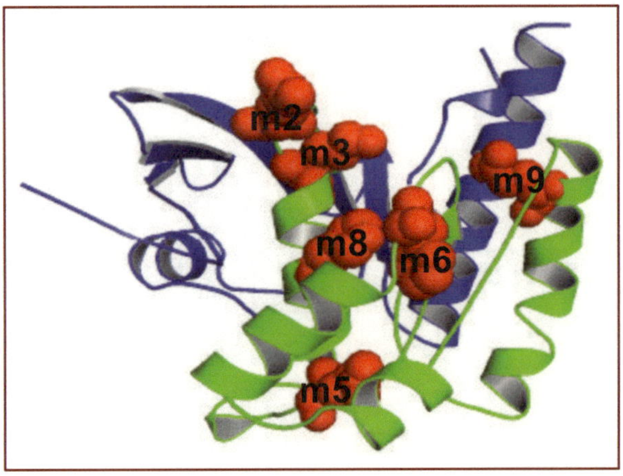

Fig. 5. Solved structure of Rad51-BRC4 complex (adapted from PDB: 1NOW, (Pellegrini et al., 2002)) where candidate residues presumed to alter Rad51-BRCA2/p53 complex interaction are indicated. *In vitro* Site-Directed mutagenesis was employed in order to alter each indicated residue to Ala. Mutant form positions are indicated.

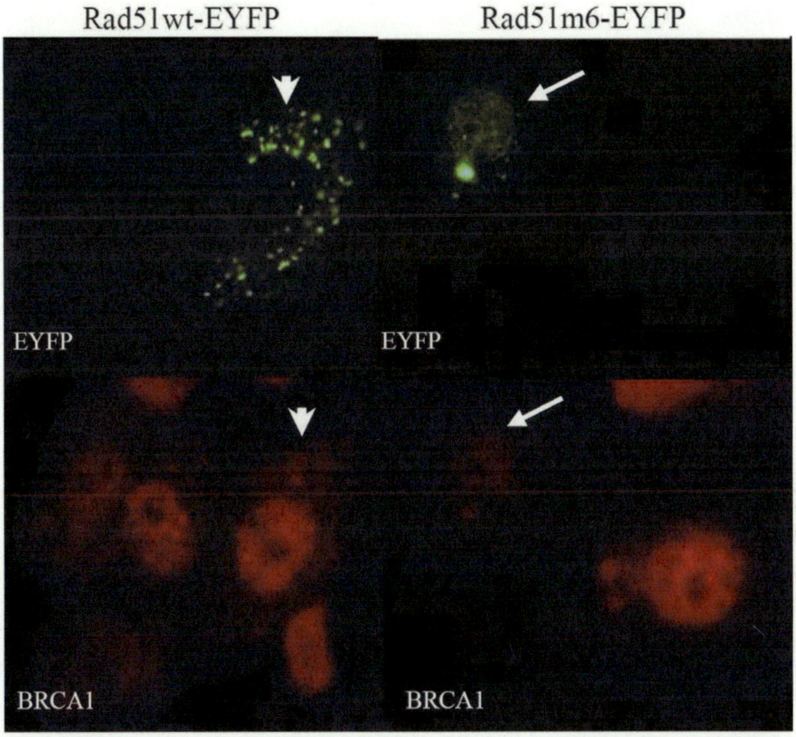

Fig. 6. MCF7 cells expressing exogenous Rad51wt-EYFP and Rad51m6-EYFP as indicated. Endogenous BRCA1 expression, as detected by immunofluoresence, shows a significant reduction in all cells expressing the Rad51m6-EYFP in comparison to both the Rad51wt-EYFP expressing as well as to non-transfected cells (Boutou et al., unpublished data).

Moreover cells expressing RAD51m6 showed a modification in their cell cycle progression (data not shown) accompanied by modifications in expression of BRCA1 (fig 6), p53 and $p21^{waf1}$ (data not shown). Notably, RAD51m6 electively kill certain cancer cell lines as HeLa cells, but do not affect the Caspase 3 defective MCF-7 cells.

Double strand breaks (DSBs) of DNA is the most deleterious damage of the genome since if not repaired accurately can result in ICL, translocations, chromatin rearrangements, LOH and mutation accumulation. HRR restores DNA damage in mitotic cells by gene conversion, where the broken sequence is converted to the sequence of the repair template (original sequence), which remains unaltered. In case of HRR misregulation other templates can be used including homologous chromosomes and repetitive elements on heterologous chromosomes. Such data indicate that single amino acid residue alterations of Rad51 are capable to modify the behaviour of the entire protein, presumably through structural modifications. These results, combined with the fact that RAD51 protein in nature is not mutated, suggest that its proper function is strongly dependent on its high degree of structural conservation throughout evolution. Moreover, the combination of the active peptide of such mutants under the promoter of human RAD51 which in the absence of the N-terminal region of Rad51 enhances expression up to 10 fold in cancer cell lines, could serve as a potential anti-cancer agent, selectively targeting malignant cells.

4. Conclusions

In conclusion maintenance of genome integrity depends on structure-function relationship of the protein molecules involved. Proper response to DNA damage mainly relies on functional components of DDR driving their appropriate complex formation with partner proteins. These processes are regulated by a number of post-translational modifications, distinct protein isoforms and protein availability (stability / degradation). In case these interactions are deregulated due to genetic / epigenetic causes a balanced cell cycle progression and cell fate determination are abolished in favour of cancer/ageing. Structural / biophysical data accompanied by functional experiments of key DNA repair molecules are significant for: (a) elucidating which residues or structural elements are really necessary for proper function at the molecular level, (b) asses/classify variants identified in individuals, (c) enriching diagnostic markers in cancer and (d) designing effective small molecules to target protein molecules essential for cell survival and genome integrity.

Co-operation of various disciplines is a fundamental prerequisite for fulfilling such a vision, and numerous attempts worldwide work on this subject with promising results.

5. References

Arias-Lopez C., Lazaro-Trueba I., Kerr P., Lord C.J., Dexter T., Iravani M., Ashworth A. and Silva A. p53 modulates homologous recombination by transcriptional regulation of the RAD51 gene. *EMBO Rep.* 2006 7: 219-224

Best B.P. Nuclear DNA damage as a direct cause of aging. *Rejuvenation Research* 2009, 12: 199–208.

Buchhop S., Gibson M.K., Wang X.W., Wagner P., Sturzbecher H-W. and Harris C.C. Interaction of p53 with the human Rad51 protein. *Nucleis Acids Res.* 1997 25: 3868-3874.

Carreira A, Hilario J, Amitani I, Baskin RJ, Shivji MK, Venkitaraman AR, Kowalczykowski SC. The BRC repeats of BRCA2 modulate the DNA binding selectivity of RAD51. Cell 2009 136:1032–1043.

Deng C.-X. BRCA1: cell cycle checkpoint, genetic instability, DNA damage response and cancer evolution. *Nucleic Acids Res.*, 2006, 34: 1416–1426

Drikos I. Nounesis G. and Vorgias C.E. Characterization of cancer-linked BRCA1-BRCT missense variants and their interaction with phosphoprotein targets. *Proteins.* 2009 77: 464-76.

Esashi F, Galkin VE, Yu X, Egelman EH, West SC. Stabilization of RAD51 nucleoprotein filaments by the C-terminal region of BRCA2. *Nat Struct Mol Biol.* 2007 14:468-74.

Essers J., Houtsmuller A., van Vielen L., Paulusma C., Nigg A., Pastink A., Vermeulen W., Hoeijmakers J. and Kanaar R. Nuclear dynamics of RAD52 group homologous recombination proteins in response to DNA damage. *EMBO J* 2002 21 2030-37

Feldser D.M., Greider C.W. Short telomeres limit tumor progression in vivo by inducing senescence. *Cancer Cell.* 2007 11:461-9.

Forget A. & Kowalczykowski S.C. Single-molecule imaging brings Rad51 nucleoprotein filaments into focus. *TICS* 2010 20: 269-76

Francis R, Richardson C. Multipotent hematopoietic cells susceptible to alternative double-strand break repair pathways that promote genome rearrangements. *Genes Dev.* 2007 21:1064-74.

Freeman A. and Monteiro A. Phosphatases in the cellular response to DNA damage. *Cell Comm.Signaling* 2010, 8:27-38

Friedberg EC, Walker GC, Siede W, Wood RD, Schultz RA, Ellenberger T. (2006). *DNA Repair and Mutagenesis, part 3.* ASM Press. 2nd edition

Galkin V. E., Esashi F., Yu X. , Yang S., West S. C., and Egelman E. H. BRCA2 BRC motifs bind RAD51–DNA filaments. *PNAS* 2005, 102: 8537–8542

Gatz S.A & Wiesmuller L p53 in recombination and repair. *Cell Death Differ.* 2006 13: 1003-1016

Glover JN, Insights into the molecular basis of human hereditary breast cancer from studies of theBRCA1 BRCT domain. *Familial Cancer* 2006 5: 89-93

Gough CA, Gojobori T, Imanishi T. Cancer-related mutations in BRCA1-BRCT cause long-range structural changes in protein-protein binding sites: a molecular dynamics study. *Proteins,* 2007 66:69-86.

Hannay J.A., Liu J., Zhu Q.S., Bolshakov S.V., Li L., Pisters P.W., Lazar A.J., Yu D., Pollock R.E. and Lev D. Rad51 overexpression contributes to chemoresistance in human soft tissue sarcoma cells: a role for p53/activator protein 2 transcriptional regulation. *Mol. Cancer Ther.* 2007 6: 1650-1660.

Henning W, Sturzbecher HW. 'Homologous recombination and cell cycle checkpoints: Rad51 in tumour progression and therapy resistance'. *Toxicology.* 2003, 193: 91-109.

Heyer W.-D. Biochemistry of eukaryotic homologous recombination. *Top Curr Genet.* 2007, 17: 95–133

Klein H. The consequences of Rad51 overexpression for normal and tumor cells. *DNA Repair (Amst)* 2008 7: 686-693.

Lazao-Trueba I. Arias. C. & Silva A. Double bolt regulation of Rad51 by p53: a role for transcriptional repression. *Cell Cycle* 2006 5: 1062-1065

Lee MS, Green R, Marsillac SM, Coquelle N, Williams RS, Yeung T, Foo D, Hau DD, Hui B, Monteiro AN, Glover JN. Comprehensive analysis of missense variations in the BRCT domain of BRCA1 by structural and functional assays. *Cancer Res.* 2010 70:4880-90.

Li X & Heyer WD. *Cell Res* 2008 Homologous recombination in DNA repair and DNA damage tolerance. 18: 99-113

Lindahl T. Instability and decay of the primary structure of DNA. *Nature.* 1993, 362: 709-715

Lisby M & Rothstein R. Localization of checkpoint and repair proteins in eukaryotes. Biochimie 2005, 87: 579-89.

Lodish H, Berk A, Matsudaira P, Kaiser CA, Krieger M, Scott MP, Zipursky SL, Darnell J. (2004). *Molecular Biology of the Cell,* p963. WH Freeman: New York, NY. 5th ed.

Maacke H, Opitz S, Jost K, Hamdorf W, Henning W, Kruger S, Feller AC, Lopens A, Diedrich K, Schwinger E, Sturzbecher HW. 'Over-expression of wild-type Rad51 correlates with histological grading of invasive ductal breast cancer'. *Int J Cancer.* 2000, 88: 907-13.

Mark W.Y. Liao J.C, Lu Y., Ayed A, Laister R, Szymczyna B, Chakrabartty A, Arrowsmith CH. Characterization of segments from the central region of BRCA1: an intrinsically disordered scaffold for multiple protein-protein and protein-DNA interactions? *J. Mol.Biol.* 2005, 345: 275-87

Morita R, Nakane S, Shimada A, Inoue M, Iino H, Wakamatsu T, Fukui K, Nakagawa N, Masui R, Kuramitsu S. Molecular mechanisms of the whole DNA repair system: a comparison of bacterial and eukaryotic systems. *J Nucleic Acids.* 2010:179594.

Murphy CG, Moynahan ME. BRCA gene structure and function in tumor suppression: a repair-centric perspective. *Cancer J.* 2010 16: 39-47.

Ouchi T. BRCA1 Phosphorylation. Biological Consequences. *Cancer Biol. Ther.* 2006, 5: 470-475

Ouyang KJ, Woo LL, Zhu J, Huo D, Matunis MJ, Ellis NA. 2009 SUMO modification regulates BLM and RAD51 interaction at damaged replication forks. *PLoS Biol.* 7 e1000252

Paull TT, Cortez D, Bowers B, Elledge SJ, Gellert M. 2001, Direct DNA binding by Brca1. *Proc Natl Acad Sci U S A.* 98 6086-91

Pellegrini L, Yu DS, Lo T, Anand S, Lee M, Blundell TL, Venkitaraman AR. Insights into DNA recombination from the structure of a RAD51-BRCA2 complex. *Nature.* 2002 420: 287-93.

Petalcorin MI, Galkin VE, Yu X, Egelman EH, Boulton SJ. 2007 Stabilization of RAD-51-DNA filaments via an interaction domain in Caenorhabditis elegans BRCA2. *Proc Natl Acad Sci U S A*. 104: 8299–8304

Qiao GB, Wu YL, Yang XN, Zhong WZ, Xie D, Guan XY, Fischer D, Kolberg HC, Kruger S, Stuerzbecher HW. High-level expression of Rad51 is an independent prognostic marker of survival in non-small-cell lung cancer patients. *Br J Cancer*. 2005, 93:137-43.

Rahan R et al., Links between DNA double strand break repair and breast cancer: accumulating evidence from both familiar and nonfamilial cases. *Cancer Lett*. 2007 248: 1-17

Rajendra E. and Venkitaraman A. R. Two modules in the BRC repeats of BRCA2 mediate structural and functional interactions with the RAD51 recombinase. *Nucleic Acids Res*. 2010, 38: 82–96

Rogakou E. Megabase chromatin domains involved in DNA double strand breaks *in vivo*. J. Cell Biol. 1999, 146 905-916

Rowling PJ, Cook R, Itzhaki LS. 2010 Toward classification of BRCA1 missense variants using a biophysical approach. *J Biol Chem*. JBC 285(26): 20080–20087

San Filippo J, Sung P, Klein H. Mechanism of eukaryotic homologous recombination. *Annu Rev Biochem*. 2008 77 229

Schild D, Wiese C. Overexpression of RAD51 suppresses recombination defects: a possible mechanism to reverse genomic instability. *Nucleic Acids Res*. 2010 38 1061-70

Seviour E & Lin S-Y 2010 Aging 2 900-907 The DNA damage response: Balancing the scale between cancer and ageing;

Shivji MK, Mukund SR, Rajendra E, Chen S, Short JM, Savill J, Klenerman D, Venkitaraman AR. The BRC repeats of human BRCA2 differentially regulate RAD51 binding on single- versus double-stranded DNA to stimulate strand exchange. *Proc Natl Acad Sci U S A*. 2009 106 13254–13259

Slupianek A. Schmutte C., Tombline G., Nieborowska-Skorska M., Hoser G., Nowicki M.O. Pierce A.J. Fishel R. and Skorski T. BCR/ABL regulates mammalian RecA homologs, resulting in drug resistance. *Mol. Cell* 2001 8: 795-806.

Sonoda E, Sasaki MS, Buerstedde JM, Bezzubova O, Shinohara A, Ogawa H, Takata M, Yamaguchi-Iwai Y, Takeda S. Rad51-deficient vertebrate cells accumulate chromosomal breaks prior to cell death. 1998 EMBO J 17 598-608

Starita LM, Parvin JD. The multiple nuclear functions of BRCA1: transcription, ubiquitination and DNA repair. *Curr Opin Cell Biol* 2003, 15: 345-50

Stürzbecher HW, Donzelmann B, Henning W, Knippschild U, Buchhop S. p53 is linked directly to homologous recombination processes via RAD51/RecA protein interaction. *EMBO J*. 1996 **15:**1992-2002.

Tsuzuki T, Fujii Y, Sakumi K, Tominaga Y, Nakao K, Sekiguchi M, Matsushiro A, Yoshimura Y, MoritaT. Targeted disruption of the Rad51 gene leads to lethality in embryonic mice. *Proc Natl Acad Sci U S A*. 1996 93: 6236-6240

Venkitaraman A.R. Linking the cellular functions of BRCA genes to cancer pathogenesis and treatment. *Ann.Rev. Pathol*. 2009 4: 461-487

Vigneron A, Vousden KH. p53, ROS and senescence in the control of aging. *Aging (Albany NY)*, 2010 2:471-4.

West SC. Molecular views of recombination proteins and their control. *Nat Rev Mol Cell Biol*. 2003 4:435-45.

Williams RS, Chasman DI, Hau DD, Hui B, Lau AY, Glover JN. Detection of protein folding defects caused by BRCA1-BRCT truncation and missense mutations. *J. Biol. Chem*. 2003, 278: 53007-16

8

The Involvement of E2F1 in the Regulation of XRCC1-Dependent Base Excision DNA Repair

Yulin Zhang and Dexi Chen
Department of infectious diseases, Beijing You'an Hospital
Beijing liver disease research institute, Capital Medical University, Beijing
China

1. Introduction

Reactive oxygen species, ionizing radiation and alkylating agents can attack on DNA resulting in single or double strand breaks, generation of abasic sites, base and sugar lesions [1]. Double-strand breaks (ds breaks) are repaired by two different types of mechanism. One type takes advantage of proteins that promote homologous recombination (HR) to obtain instructions from the sister or homologous chromosome for proper repair of breaks. The other type permits joining of ends even if there is no sequence similarity between them. The latter process is called non-homologous end joining (NHEJ).The process by which complex single-strand breaks (those that cannot be directly religated) are repaired (SSBR) in some ways resembles NHEJ. Here we shall mainly discuss the mechanism of base excision repair (BER) of SSBR.

2. Base excision DNA repair

The major pathway to remove damaged DNA bases is Base Excision Repair (BER, *Fig. 1*). BER can be divided into five steps: (i) excision of damaged base by the specific DNA glycosylase and formation of apurinic/apyrimidinic (AP) site; (ii) cleavage of phosphodiester bond at AP site by AP-endonuclease or AP-lyase; (iii) removal of chemical groups interfering with gap filling and ligation; (iv) gap filling; (v) ligation [2].
The first step of the BER pathway is recognition of damaged base by the specific DNA glycosylase, which cleaves N-glycosidic bond leaving behind a free base and an AP site. In humans about 10 DNA glycosylases of different, but partially overlapping substrate specificities are known [3]. Some of them are bifunctional enzymes, which have endowed AP-lyase activity and cleave phosphodiester bonds at 3′ side of AP site either by ß- or ß/δ -elimination. *E. coli* endonuclease III (Nth), its human homolog, hNTH1 and human 8-oxoG DNA glycosylase (OGG1) catalyse reaction of ß- elimination, which creates alpha/ß-unsaturated aldehyde (3′dRP) at the 3′ end of cleaved DNA strand. Bacterial formamidopyrimidine DNA glycosylase (Fpg), endonuclease VIII (Nei) and two human homologs of the latter, NEIL1 and NEIL2 catalyse ß/ δ-elimination and remove deoxyribose residue leaving phosphate at the 3′ end of cleaved DNA strand. Monofunctional DNA glycosylases need the assistance of AP-endonucleases, which hydrolyse phosphodiester bond at the 5′ end of the AP site. This yields DNA single strand break (SSB) with the 5′end

bearing baseless deoxyribose (5′dRP) and the 3′ end with the free hydroxyl group. Both AP sites and SSBs can be formed due to spontaneous hydrolysis of purines, as well as upon DNA damaging agents, like ionizing radiation or oxidation.

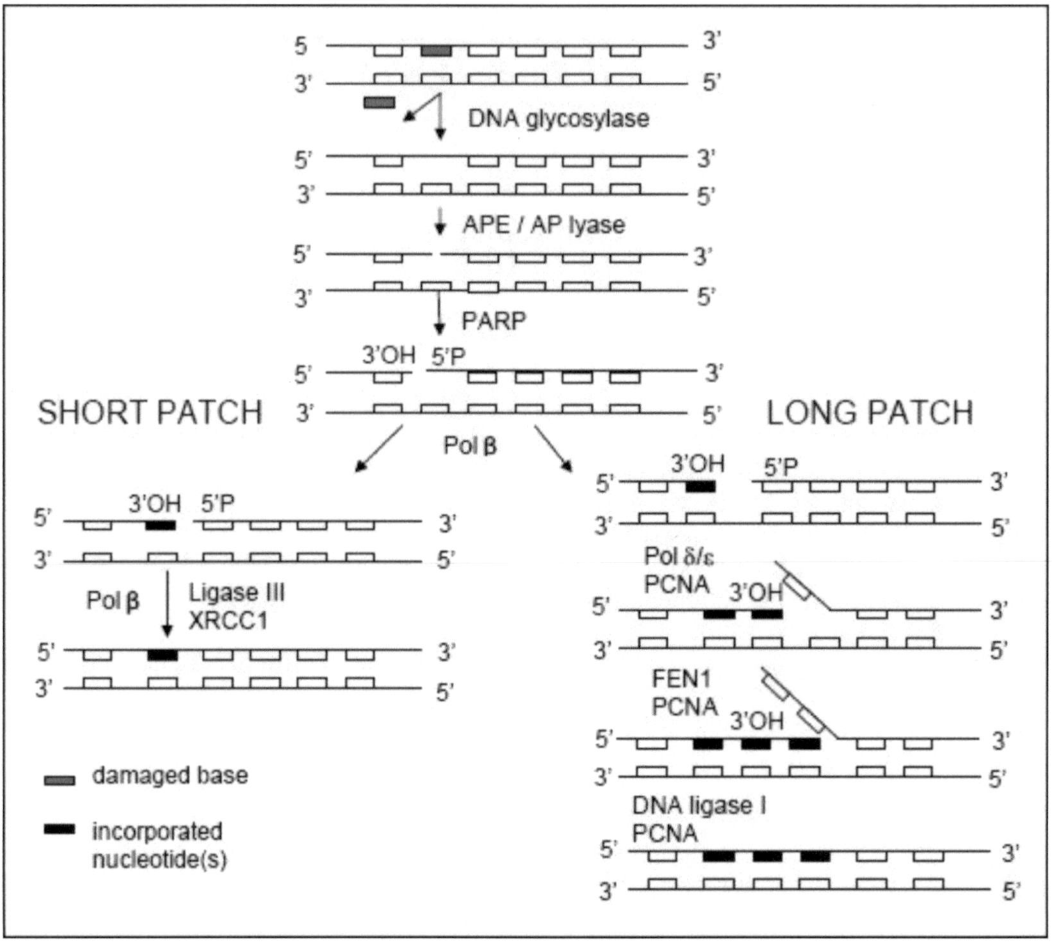

Fig. 1. Base Excision Repair pathway

Before filling the gap by DNA polymerases possible additional chemical groups present on 3′OH end, which may block polymerisation, must be removed. Bacterial enzymes Xth (exonuclease III) and Nfo (Endonuclease IV), besides of cleaving phosphodiester bonds at 5′ AP-site, have as well 3′ phosphatase and 3′ phosphodiesterase activities and remove phosphates and phosphoglycolates from 3′ hydroxyl group of cleaved DNA strand[4]. In contrast, the major mammalian AP-endonuclease, APE1 effciently removes 3′ phosphoglycolate groups, but has a very weak 3′ phosphatase activity [5]. Phosphate groups left e.g. by NEIL1 glycosylase at 3′hydroxyls are most probably removed by polynucleotide kinase[6]. After cleavage of phosphodiester bond, repair may be continued on two alternative pathways (*Fig. 1*): *short-patch* BER (SP-BER) or *long patch* BER (LP-BER). During SP-BER in mammals, only one missing nucleotide is incorporated by DNA polymerase ß (pol ß), which has also endowed 5′dRPase activity and can remove baseless sugar from the

5'site of DNA break. In LP-BER a longer fragment ranging from 2 to 12 nucleotides is excised and re-synthesized [2]. Initially DNA polymerase elongates 3' end by a few nucleotides and moves aside a DNA fragment which contains 5' deoxyribophosphate. Subsequently, such flap structure is cleaved out by specific flap endonuclease, FEN1. It is believed that in LP-BER the first nucleotide is incorporated by DNA polymerase ß, while next ones by DNA polymerases δ or ε [2]. LP-BER demands also other assisting proteins, PCNA (*proliferating cell nuclear antigen*) and RPC (*replication protein C*).

The last stage of BER is ligation of repaired DNA fragments by DNA ligase. Different DNA ligases(LIG) are operating in short and long patch BER, LIG1 in LP-BER and LIG3alpha in SP-BER. LIG3alpha remains in complex with XRCC1 (x-ray repair cross-complementing group 1) protein, which activates ligation of DNA ends by LIG3alpha.

3. The role of XRCC1 protein in base excision DNA repair

X-ray cross-complementing group 1 (XRCC1) is a 70- kDa protein comprising three functional domains; an N-terminal DNA binding domain, a centrally located BRCT I and a C-terminal BRCT II domain. It has no known enzymatic activity. Since it specifically interacts with nicked and gapped DNA *in vitro*[7-9], and rapidly and transiently responds to DNA damage in cells, it may serve as a strand-break sensor [10, 11].

DNA single-strand breaks (SSBs) are one of the most frequent types of DNA damage in cells [12]. SSBs can lead to the accumulation of mutations or can be converted from single to cytotoxic double-strand breaks. Thus, SSBs pose a critical threat to the genetic stability and survival of cells[13]. Various proteins have been identified that are part of the repair machinery for SSBs, including XRCC1 protein. XRCC1 has been shown to be critically involved in DNA SSB repair in studies using XRCC1-mutant cells and XRCC1 knockout mice[14], which have increased sensitivity to alkylating agents, ultraviolet and ionizing radiation [15], as well as elevated levels of sister chromatic exchange. Since XRCC1 interacts with many proteins known to be involved in BER and SSBR, it has been proposed that XRCC1 functions as a scaffold protein able to coordinate and facilitate the steps of various DNA repair pathways[11, 16]. For example, XRCC1 interacts with several DNA glycosylases involved in repair of both oxidative and alkylated base lesions, and stimulates their activity[17, 18]. This protein interacts with DNA ligase III, polymerase beta and poly (ADP-ribose) polymerase to participate in the base excision repair pathway. It is recruited to the site of DNA damage by several DNA glycosylases, e.g. OGG1 or NTH1 and remains at the site of repair till the last stage of ligation (*Fig.* 2), regulating and coordinating the whole process. XRCC1 facilitates exchange of DNA glycosylase with AP-endonuclease at the damaged substrate, which increases the excision rate of modified base, regulates pol ß interactions with APE1, and finally activates ligation step [17]. Binding of XRCC1 to Polynucleotide Kinase (PNK) enhances its capacity for damage discrimination, and binding of XRCC1 to DNA enables displacement of PNK from the phosphorylated product [19] thus accelerating SSBR of damaged DNA[20]. XRCC1 associates with Tyrosyl-DNA phosphodiesterase1(Tdp1) and enhances its activity required for repair of Top1-associated SSBs. It may act to recruit Tdp1 to these damaged sites[21]. Biochemical and nuclear magnetic resonance (NMR) experiments have demonstrated protein-protein interaction between the N-terminal domain of XRCC1 and the polymerase domain of pol β[22-25]. Additionally, stabilization of DNA ligase IIIα is dependent on its interaction with the BRCT II domain of XRCC1[26]. Aprataxin also interacts with XRCC1 and functions to maintain

XRCC1 stability, thus further linking the neurological degeneration associated with ataxia to an inefficiency of SSBR[27-29].

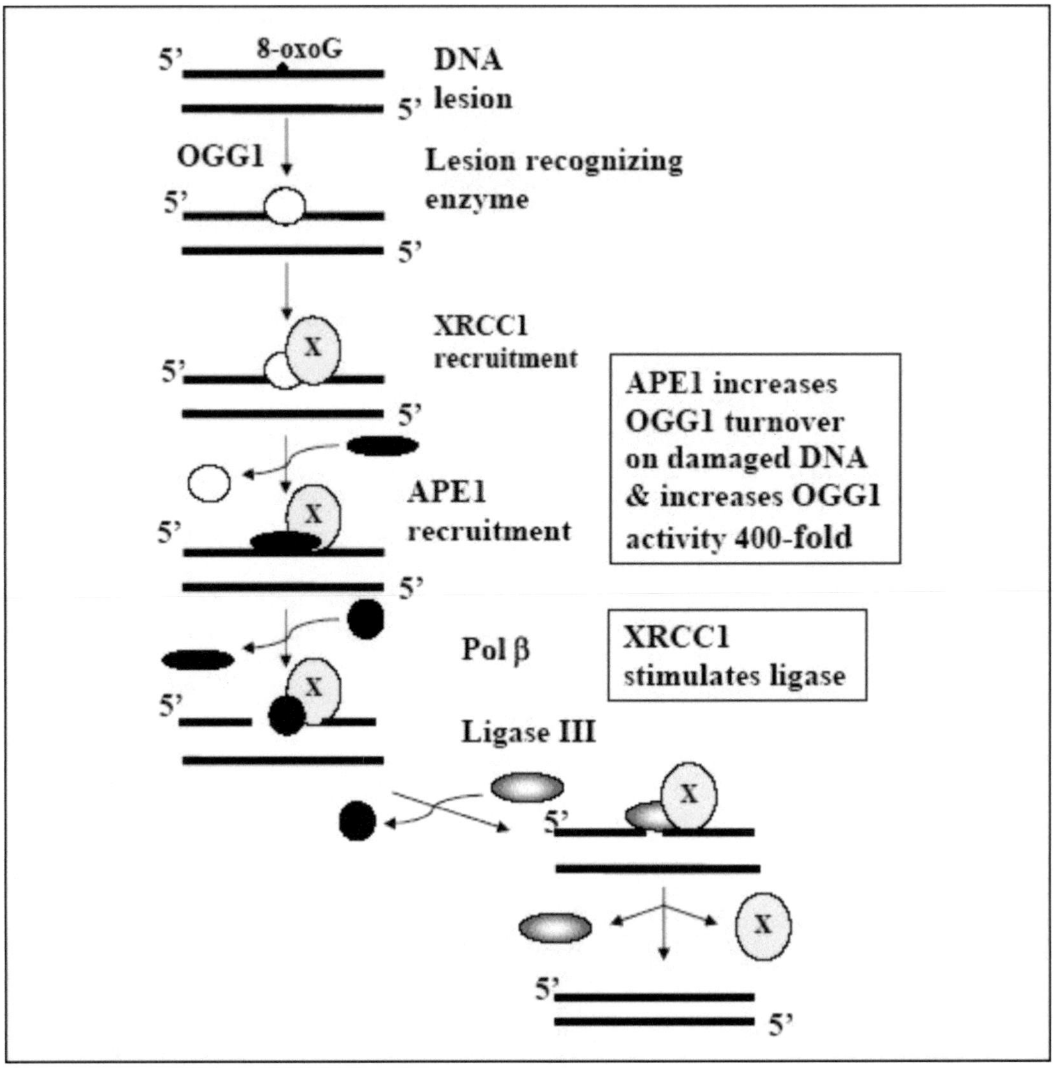

Fig. 2. Coordinative role of XRCC1 protein in BER

Several additional proteins participate in BER and play regulative and coordinative role. The most important proteins are: PARP1 (polyADP ribose polymerase, which binds to free DNA ends and protects them against degradation, participates in chromatin relaxation and probably modulates binding of repair proteins to the site of damage by interaction with poly(ADP-ribose) chains [22, 30, 31], PCNA (proliferating cells nuclear antigen, DNA polymerase processivity subunit in LP-BER), RFC (replication factor C, loading PCNA on DNA), WRN (helicase deficient in Werner syndrome, a premature aging disease) or CSB (helicase deficient in Cockayne syndrome, neurodevelopmental and premature aging disease).

4. The role of E2F1 in XRCC1 associated base excision DNA repair

E2F1 is a member of E2F family of transcription factors which plays an important role in promoting both cellular proliferation and cell death. E2F1 is important for regulating S-phase specific genes as well as promoting apoptosis, just as other "activating" E2F family members [32, 33]. Simultaneously, E2F1 regulates DNA repair through interaction with other factors including RB family proteins, p53 and X-ray repair cross-complementing group 1 (XRCC1) protein.

4.1 E2F family

The E2F transcription factor family consists of at least seven distinct genes divided into two groups. E2F1, E2F2, E2F3, E2F4, and E2F5 constitute one group, while the related DP1 and DP2 genes constitute the other group. Several forms of the DP2 (also referred to as DP3) protein can be produced as the result of alternative splicing, thus providing additional complexity to the E2F family. A functional E2F transcription factor consists of a heterodimer containing an E2F polypeptide and a DP polypeptide. Each of the five E2F polypeptides can heterodimerize with either DP1 or DP2 (DP3). Furthermore, each of these E2F/DP heterodimers (referred to as E2F factors hereafter) can bind consensus E2F sites *in vitro* and stimulate transcription when overexpressed[34].

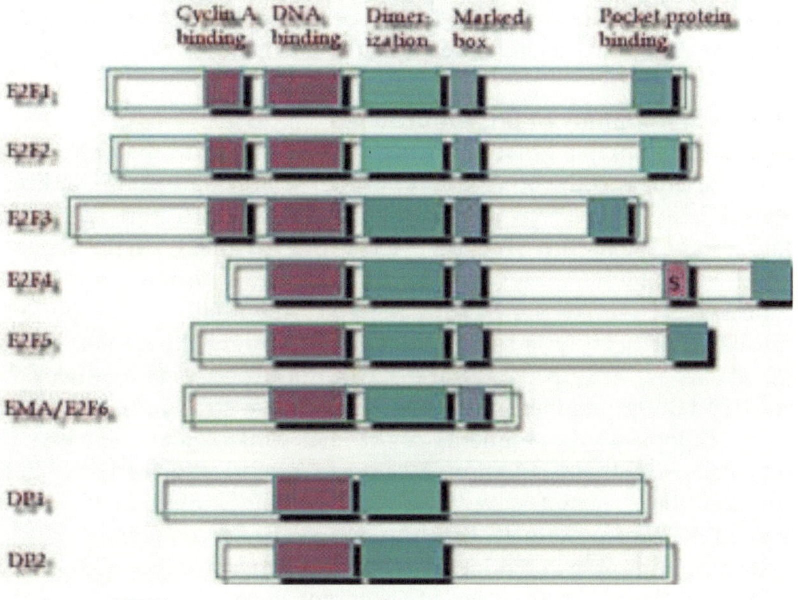

Fig. 3. the members of E2F

All of the E2F subgroup proteins have a similar structure although E2F1, E2F2, and E2F3 are more closely related to each other than to E2F4 and E2F5 (*Fig. 3*). The DNA-binding domain found in the amino terminus represents the area of greatest homology between the five E2F species. Adjacent to the DNA-binding domain is the DP dimerization domain, which contains within it a leucine heptad repeat. The carboxy termini of the five E2F polypeptides contain the defined transcriptional activation domains, which are characterized by an abundance of acidic residues. Embedded within the transactivation domain of each E2F is a region of homology involved in binding to the pocket proteins (Rb, p107, and p130). An additional region of homology, termed the Marked box, lies between the DP dimerization and transcriptional activation domains. Although this Marked box motif is highly conserved between the different E2Fs, its function is unknown. The amino termini of E2F1, E2F2, and E2F3 contain an additional region of homology not found in E2F4 or E2F5. This region has been demonstrated to have several functions, including binding to the cyclin A protein. The E2F4 protein contains a stretch of consecutive serine residues between the Marked box and the pocket protein binding domain not found in other E2F family members. DP1 and DP2 polypeptides contain DNA-binding and dimerization domains related to the E2F proteins but do not contain transcriptional activation domains or regions homologous to the pocket protein binding or Marked box domains.

An additional E2F family member has recently been isolated and termed EMA (E2F-binding site modulating activity) or E2F6[35, 36]. EMA/E2F6 shares homology with the E2F polypeptides in the DNA-binding domain, the DP dimerization domain and the Marked box, but lacks the pocket protein binding domain and acidic transcriptional activation domain found in the carboxy terminus of the other E2F species (figure 1). Like the other E2F polypeptides, EMA/E2F6 dimerizes with DP1 or DP2 and, in conjunction with a DP partner, binds E2F DNA-binding sites with preference for a subset of sites with the core sequence TCCCGCC. EMA/E2F6 appears to function as a repressor of E2F site-dependent transcription independent of pocket protein binding. The mechanism of repression is either through competitive inhibition with other E2F species or through an active transcriptional repression domain located in the amino terminus of EMA/E2F6.

4.2 E2F factors and Rb family of pocket proteins

The activity of E2F factors is regulated through association with the retinoblastoma tumor suppressor protein (Rb) and the other pocket proteins, p107 and p130. Binding of Rb, p107 or p130 converts E2F factors from transcriptional activators to transcriptional repressors. The interplay among G1 cyclins (D-type cyclins and cyclin E), cyclin-dependent kinases (cdk4, 6, and 2), cdk inhibitors, and protein phosphatases determines the phosphorylation state of the pocket proteins which in turn regulates the ability of the pocket proteins to complex with E2F. E2F activity is further regulated through direct interactions with other factors, such cyclin A, Sp1, p53 and the ubiquitin-proteasome pathway. Deregulated expression of E2F family member genes has been shown to induce both inappropriate S phase entry and apoptosis. Experiments show that dimerization between E2F1 and its partner DP1 is stable and that E2F1 stimulates nuclear localization of DP1[37]. E2F1/DP1 is acetylated by the three acetyltransferases P300/CBP-associated factor (PCAF), cAMP-response element-binding protein (CREBBP) and p300 which stabilizes E2F1 protein[38]. The acetylated complex is able to bind to PCAF to form an active dimer. The complex ability to bind to DNA on the promoter sites of its target genes along with its transcriptional activity are increased at the G1/S transition. During G2, the complex is phosphorylated by CycA2/CDK2[39]. The affinity between E2F1 and DP1 is then diminished leading to the dissociation of the complex and the release of PCAF[40]. The proteins undergo further modifications before degradation: E2F1 is deactelylated by histone deacetylase1(HDAC1) [41], dephosphorylated and phosphorylated *de novo* during S phase by Transcription factor II H (TFIIH) kinase for rapid degradation[42].

Upon DNA damage, the complex PCAF/E2F1/DP1 can be phosphorylated and stabilized either by Checkpoint kinases (CHEK1 and CHEK2) through phosphorylation at Ser-364, or by ataxia telangiectasia mutated(ATM) and ATR (ATM and Rad3-related) [43, 44], preventing E2F1 ubiquitination[45]. E2F1 mediates the transcription of many genes involved in apoptosis. However, E2F1 transcriptional activity can also be inhibited when bound to the topoisomerase TopBP1 in order to give time to the cell to repair the damage [46]. Mutations of the RB gene represent the most frequent molecular defect in Osteosarcoma. Studies in animal models and in human cancers have shown that deregulated E2F1 overexpression possesses either "oncogenic" or "oncosuppressor" properties, depending on the cellular context. High E2F1 levels exerted a growth-suppressing effect that relied on the integrity of the DNA damage response network. Surprisingly, induction of p73, an established E2F1 target, was also DNA damage response-dependent. Furthermore, a global proteome analysis associated with bioinformatics revealed novel E2F1-regulated genes and potential E2F1-driven signaling networks that could provide useful targets in challenging this aggressive neoplasm by innovative therapies[47]. Similarly, deregulation of the Rb/E2F pathway in human fibroblasts results in an E2F1-mediated apoptosis dependent on ATM, Nijmegen breakage syndrome 1 (NBS1), CHEK2 and p53. E2F1 expression results in MRN(Mre11-Rad50-Nbs10 foci formation, which is independent of the Nbs1 interacting region and the DNA-binding domain of E2F1. E2F1-induced MRN foci are similar to irradiation-induced foci (IRIF) that result from double-strand DNA breaks because they correlate with 53BP1 and gammaH2AX foci, do not form in NBS cells, do form in AT cells and do not correlate with cell cycle entry. In fact, in human fibroblasts, deregulated E2F1 causes a G1 arrest, blocking serum-induced cell cycle progression, in part through an Nbs1/53BP1/p53/p21(WAF1/CIP1) checkpoint pathway. This checkpoint protects against apoptosis because depletion of 53BP1 or p21(WAF1/CIP1) increases both the rate and extent of apoptosis. Nbs1 and p53 contribute to both checkpoint and apoptosis pathways. These results suggest that E2F1-induced foci generate a cell cycle checkpoint that, with sustained E2F1 activity, eventually yields to apoptosis. Uncontrolled proliferation due to Rb/E2F deregulation as well as inactivation of both checkpoint and apoptosis programs would then be required for transformation of normal cells to tumor cells[48]. ZBRK1 is a zinc finger-containing transcriptional repressor that can modulate the expression of GADD45A, a DNA damage response gene, to induce cell cycle arrest in response to DNA damage. Liao et al found that the ZBRK1 promoter contains an authentic E2F-recognition sequence that specifically binds E2F1, but not E2F4 or E2F6, together with chromatin remodeling proteins CtIP and CtBP to form a repression complex that suppresses zinc finger protein (ZBRK1) transcription. Furthermore, loss of RB-mediated transcriptional repression led to an increase in ZBRK1 transcript levels, correlating with increased sensitivity to ultraviolet (UV) and methyl methanesulfonate-induced DNA damage. Thus, the RB.CtIP (CtBP interacting protein)/CtBP (C terminus-binding protein) /E2F1 complex plays a critical role in ZBRK1 transcriptional repression, and loss of this repression may contribute to cellular sensitivity of DNA damage, ultimately leading to carcinogenesis[49]. One study suggested that E2F1 is also a transcriptional regulator of Xeroderma pigmentosum group C(XPC) and Rb/E2F1 tumor suppressor pathway is involved in the regulation of the DNA lesion recognition step of nucleotide excision repair[50]. Disruption of pRB-E2F interactions by E1A is a key event in the adenoviral life cycle that drives expression of early viral transcription and induces cell cycle progression. This function of E1A is complicated by E2F1. pRB-E2F1 interactions are resistant to E1A-mediated disruption. Using mutant forms of pRB that selectively force E2F1 to bind through only one of the two binding sites on pRB, E1A is unable to disrupt E2F1's unique interaction with pRB. Furthermore, analysis of pRB-E2F complexes during adenoviral infection reveals the selective maintenance of pRB-E2F1 interactions despite the presence of E1A[51].

4.3 E2F1 factors and DNA repair

The E2F1 transcription factor is post-translationally modified and stabilized in response to various forms of DNA damage to regulate the expression of cell cycle and pro-apoptotic genes. E2F1 also forms foci at DNA double-strand breaks (DSBs). The absence of E2F1 leads to spontaneous DNA breaks and impaired recovery following exposure to ionizing radiation. E2F1 deficiency results in defective NBS1 phosphorylation and foci formation in response to DSBs but does not affect NBS1 expression levels. Moreover, an increased association between NBS1 and E2F1 is observed in response to DNA damage, suggesting that E2F1 may promote NBS1 foci formation through a direct or indirect interaction at sites of DNA breaks. E2F1 deficiency also impairs RPA and Rad51 foci formation indicating that E2F1 is important for DNA end resection and the formation of single-stranded DNA at DSBs. These findings establish new roles for E2F1 in the DNA damage response, which may directly contribute to DNA repair and genome maintenance[52]. Chromatin structure is known to be a barrier to DNA repair and a large number of studies have now identified various factors that modify histones and remodel nucleosomes to facilitate repair. In response to ultraviolet (UV) radiation several histones are acetylated and this enhances the repair of DNA photoproducts by the nucleotide excision repair (NER) pathway. The E2F1 transcription factor accumulates at sites of UV-induced DNA damage and directly stimulates NER through a non-transcriptional mechanism. E2F1 associates with the general control nonderepressible(GCN5) acetyltransferase in response to UV radiation and recruits GCN5 to sites of damage. UV radiation induces the acetylation of histone H3 lysine 9 (H3K9) and this requires both GCN5 and E2F1. Moreover, as previously observed for E2F1, knock down of GCN5 results in impaired recruitment of NER factors to sites of damage and inefficient DNA repair. These findings demonstrate a direct role for GCN5 and E2F1 in NER involving H3K9 acetylation and increased accessibility to the NER machinery[53].

Mice lacking E2F1 have increased levels of epidermal apoptosis compared to wild-type mice following exposure to ultraviolet B (UVB) radiation. Moreover, transgenic overexpression of E2F1 in basal layer keratinocytes suppresses apoptosis induced by UVB. Inhibition of UVB-induced apoptosis by E2F1 is unexpected given that most studies have demonstrated a proapoptotic function for E2F1. E2F1-mediated suppression of apoptosis does not involve alterations in mitogen-activated protein kinase activation or B-cell lymphoma (Bcl-2) downregulation in response to UVB and is independent of p53. Instead, inhibition of UVB-induced apoptosis by E2F1 correlates with a stimulation of DNA repair. Mice lacking E2F1 are impaired for the removal of DNA photoproducts, while E2F1 transgenic mice repair UVB-induced DNA damage at an accelerated rate compared to wild-type mice. These findings suggest that E2F1 participates in the response to UVB by promoting DNA repair and suppressing apoptosis[54]. One study showed that E2F1 has a direct, non-transcriptional role in DNA repair involving increased recruitment of NER factors to sites of damage[55].

4.4 The role of E2F1 in the regulation of XRCC1-dependent BER

The exact mechanism of E2F1 regulating XRCC1-dependent base excision DNA repair is still not completely clear. The E2F1 pathway is centrally involved in the highly complex networks coupling cellular proliferation and apoptosis. XRCC1, which plays a critical role in SSBR/BER [15], is a direct E2F1 target gene. E2F1 is upstream of XRCC1 significantly expands on prior observations that E2F plays a role in other repair pathways, such as MMR and NER [56-59]. The BER protein uracil-DNA glycosylase is also E2F-regulated[60]. Intriguingly, although E2F1 is best characterized as a transcription factor, E2F1 protein may have a direct role in DNA repair, as suggested by its localization to repair complexes[46, 61]. Thus, it is likely that multiple E2F-regulated mechanisms function in parallel with XRCC1 to stimulate repair. Chen found that enforced E2F expression stimulated XRCC1 levels and that(methylmethane sulfonate) MMS, which induces predominantly heat-labile DNA damage repaired by an XRCC1-mediated BER pathway[62, 63], causes an E2F1-dependent increase in XRCC1 expression. This is consistent with prior reports demonstrating that cellular stress increases endogenous XRCC1 levels [64-66], although this may be cell type-specific [67]. How MMS-induced stress activates the E2F1-XRCC1 axis remains unknown. Cellular sensitivity to MMS may involve an ATR-dependent pathway, and genetic evidence suggests that MMS-induced damage activates the yeast Rad53 (Chk2 human homologue) pathway [68, 69].

Given that the ATM/ATR and Chk2 pathways phosphorylate and activate E2F1 protein[70-73], it is possible that these kinases stimulate XRCC1 expression through E2F1 activation, although this remains to be demonstrated. Interestingly, Chk2-mediated stabilization of the FoxM1 transcription factor stimulates expression of DNA repair genes, including XRCC1 [74]. Given that XRCC1 function is complex, it is likely that its control involves multiple levels. Indeed, posttranslational mechanisms modulate XRCC1 function, as evidenced by the ability of DNA-dependent protein kinase to phosphorylate XRCC1[75] as well as the requirement of protein kinase CK2 to phosphorylate XRCC1 and enhance SSBR and genetic stability [76]. Consistent with the complex control of XRCC1, serum starvation followed by refeeding stimulated XRCC1 expression. This is consistent with cell conditions of high E2F activity but also suggests that serum/mitogenic factors may be important too. This could be a cell typespecific phenomenon, since density arrest and release does not alter XRCC1 levels in human T24 cells[77]. Nevertheless, the biological importance of E2F1 regulation of XRCC1 is suggested by the attenuated *in vivo* DNA repair in E2F1-/-*versus* E2F1+/+MEFs. Two different methods demonstrated reduced DNA repair after MMS-induced DNA damage, which correlates with the decreased XRCC1 levels observed in E2F1-/-cells. The repair of MMS-damaged DNA still occurs in E2F1-/- cells, suggesting that the E2F1-XRCC1 axis is not an absolute requirement in these systems. This is not surprising, given the complex and overlapping repair pathways involved. However, the significance of even a modestly reduced XRCC1-mediated repair function may have important implications for maintaining genomic stability and cell viability. Consistent with this notion of XRCC1 mediating E2F1 activity is the observation that loss of XRCC1 function resulted in an enhanced E2F1-induced apoptotic response in EM9 cells compared with AA8 cells.

Although E2F1 is a damage response protein, it also plays an important role in promoting the expression of a large number of genes required for replication and proliferation [57, 78-80]. Given the intimate relationship between proliferation and replication/repair, the control of XRCC1 by E2F in undamaged cells further integrates SSBR with cell cycle progression as might be expected if enhanced SSBR were necessary to repair SSBs at replication forks [15, 81-83]. Whether and in what context the other E2F family members play a role, as well as what specific SSBR pathways are utilized (*e.g.* long patch BER), remains to be explored.

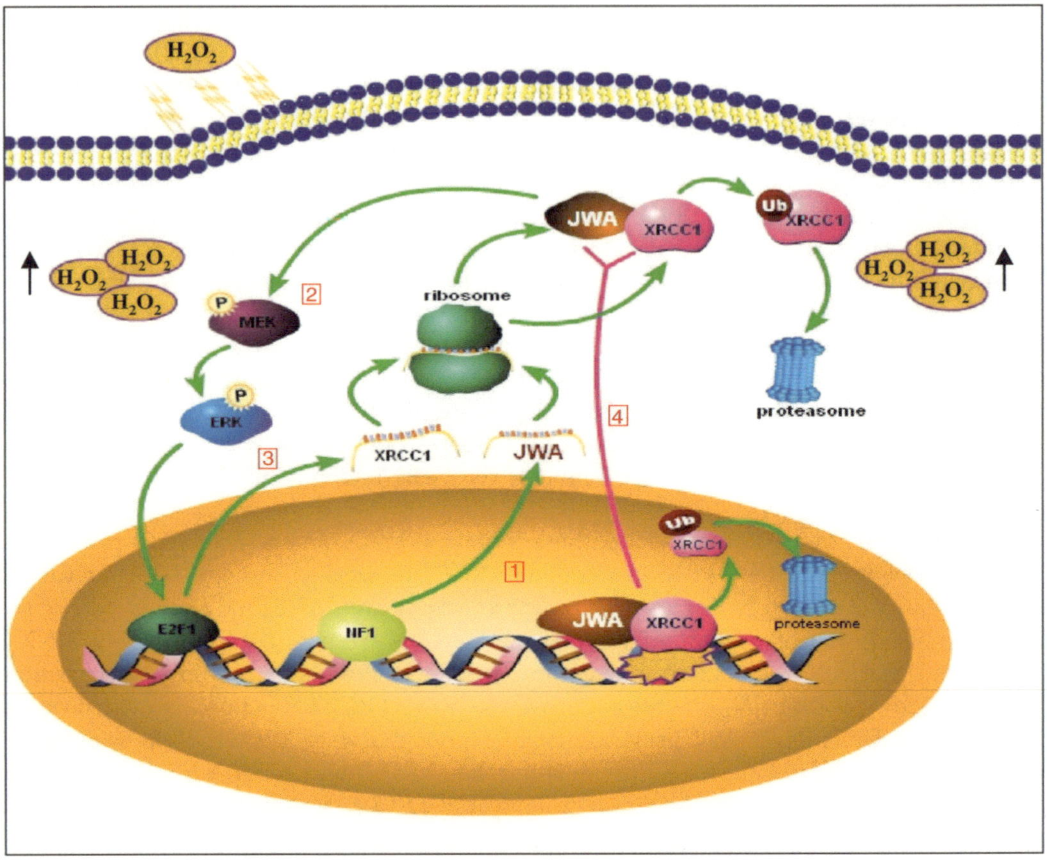

Fig. 4. JWA-E2F1-XRCC1 regulation network in base excision repair

The rapid response of XRCC1-dependent SSBR, especially in S/G2 phase, has been reported [81], and an increased co-localization of XRCC1 with proliferating cell nuclear antigen (PCNA) was observed at sites of replication during S-phase[84]. These results indicate the importance of XRCC1-dependent SSBR and its regulation during the cell cycle. Phosphorylation of E2F1 at serine-31 (S31) in response to DNA damage is required for the activation of ATM-, ATR-and ChK2-dependent DNA damage response pathways [44, 45, 85, 86]. E2F1 has also been suggested to play a potential role in nucleotide excision repair pathway (NER)[54]. Recent reports have shown that XRCC1 is a direct target of E2F1 that is involved in the enhancement of SSBR and BER, which maintain genomic stability and contribute to cell survival[63]. Over-expression of E2F1 has been shown to induce quiescent cells to enter early S-phase and is capable of preventing cells from entering quiescence [87]. Recently, we showed that E2F1 regulates the expression of XRCC1 in response to activation of DNA repair processes, and the exact functional E2F1 binding sites in the XRCC1 promoter region were identified[63]. Certain BER proteins, such as the uracil-DNA glycosylase, have also been demonstrated to be regulated by E2F transcription factors[60]. The fact that enhanced E2F expression stimulates XRCC1-mediated activation of the BER pathway in response to MMS-induced, heat-labile DNA damage suggests it might also be able to promote the expression of a variety of genes involved in DNA replication and cell proliferation.

The p53-E2F network controls and integrates critical functions, such as proliferation, cell cycle checkpoints, apoptosis, and DNA repair [43, 73, 88, 89]. In particular, p53 can promote BER [90, 91], and our discovery that E2F1 may also promote BER expands our understanding of the p53-E2F1 network in regulating DNA repair [63]. Disruption of these cooperative pathways has profound implications for tumorigenesis, as evidenced by enhanced tumor formation in knock-out mouse models for both p53 and E2F1, although intriguingly, both oncogenic and tumor suppressor functions for E2F1 are suggested in compound p53-/- and E2F1-/- mice [73, 92, 93].
The JWA (ARL6IP5)-E2F1-XRCC1 network also plays crucial role in base excision repair [94]. Exposure to oxidative stress increases the generation of intracellular reactive oxygen species, which stimulates NF1 binding to the JWA promoter, enhancing JWA transcription and translation. Then JWA regulates the expression of E2F1, leading to increased transcription of XRCC1. Interactions between JWA and XRCC1 occur in both the cytoplasm and the nucleus when the cells are subjected to oxidative stress (*fig.4*)..

5. References

[1] Tudek, B., et al., *Modulation of oxidative DNA damage repair by the diet, inflammation and neoplastic transformation.* J Physiol Pharmacol, 2006. 57 Suppl 7: p. 33-49

[2] Fortini, P., et al., *The base excision repair: mechanisms and its relevance for cancer susceptibility.* Biochimie, 2003. 85(11): p. 1053-71

[3] Wood, R.D., M. Mitchell, and T. Lindahl, *Human DNA repair genes, 2005.* Mutat Res, 2005. 577(1-2): p. 275-83

[4] Doetsch, P.W. and R.P. Cunningham, *The enzymology of apurinic/apyrimidinic endonucleases.* Mutat Res, 1990. 236(2-3): p. 173-201

[5] Kelley, M.R. and S.H. Parsons, *Redox regulation of the DNA repair function of the human AP endonuclease Ape1/ref-1.* Antioxid Redox Signal, 2001. 3(4): p. 671-83

[6] Wiederhold, L., et al., *AP endonuclease-independent DNA base excision repair in human cells.* Mol Cell, 2004. 15(2): p. 209-20

[7] Marintchev, A., et al., *Solution structure of the single-strand break repair protein XRCC1 N-terminal domain.* Nat Struct Biol, 1999. 6(9): p. 884-93

[8] Mani, R.S., et al., *Biophysical characterization of human XRCC1 and its binding to damaged and undamaged DNA.* Biochemistry, 2004. 43(51): p. 16505-14

[9] Horton, J.K., et al., *XRCC1 and DNA polymerase beta in cellular protection against cytotoxic DNA single-strand breaks.* Cell Res, 2008. 18(1): p. 48-63

[10] Lan, L., et al., *In situ analysis of repair processes for oxidative DNA damage in mammalian cells.* Proc Natl Acad Sci U S A, 2004. 101(38): p. 13738-43

[11] Mortusewicz, O. and H. Leonhardt, *XRCC1 and PCNA are loading platforms with distinct kinetic properties and different capacities to respond to multiple DNA lesions.* BMC Mol Biol, 2007. 8: p. 81

[12] Lindahl, T., *Instability and decay of the primary structure of DNA.* Nature, 1993. 362(6422): p. 709-15

[13] Slupphaug, G., B. Kavli, and H.E. Krokan, *The interacting pathways for prevention and repair of oxidative DNA damage.* Mutat Res, 2003. 531(1-2): p. 231-51

[14] Tebbs, R.S., L.H. Thompson, and J.E. Cleaver, *Rescue of Xrcc1 knockout mouse embryo lethality by transgene-complementation.* DNA Repair (Amst), 2003. 2(12): p. 1405-17

[15] Caldecott, K.W., *XRCC1 and DNA strand break repair.* DNA Repair (Amst), 2003. 2(9): p. 955-69

[16] Wong, H.K. and D.M. Wilson, 3rd, *XRCC1 and DNA polymerase beta interaction contributes to cellular alkylating-agent resistance and single-strand break repair.* J Cell Biochem, 2005. 95(4): p. 794-804

[17] Marsin, S., et al., *Role of XRCC1 in the coordination and stimulation of oxidative DNA damage repair initiated by the DNA glycosylase hOGG1.* J Biol Chem, 2003. 278(45): p. 44068-74

[18] Campalans, A., et al., *XRCC1 interactions with multiple DNA glycosylases: a model for its recruitment to base excision repair.* DNA Repair (Amst), 2005. 4(7): p. 826-35

[19] Mani, R.S., et al., *XRCC1 stimulates polynucleotide kinase by enhancing its damage discrimination and displacement from DNA repair intermediates.* J Biol Chem, 2007. 282(38): p. 28004-13

[20] Whitehouse, C.J., et al., *XRCC1 stimulates human polynucleotide kinase activity at damaged DNA termini and accelerates DNA single-strand break repair.* Cell, 2001. 104(1): p. 107-17

[21] Plo, I., et al., *Association of XRCC1 and tyrosyl DNA phosphodiesterase (Tdp1) for the repair of topoisomerase I-mediated DNA lesions.* DNA Repair (Amst), 2003. 2(10): p. 1087-100

[22] Caldecott, K.W., et al., *XRCC1 polypeptide interacts with DNA polymerase beta and possibly poly (ADP-ribose) polymerase, and DNA ligase III is a novel molecular 'nick-sensor' in vitro.* Nucleic Acids Res, 1996. 24(22): p. 4387-94

[23] Kubota, Y., et al., *Reconstitution of DNA base excision-repair with purified human proteins: interaction between DNA polymerase beta and the XRCC1 protein.* EMBO J, 1996. 15(23): p. 6662-70

[24] Marintchev, A., et al., *Domain specific interaction in the XRCC1-DNA polymerase beta complex.* Nucleic Acids Res, 2000. 28(10): p. 2049-59

[25] Gryk, M.R., et al., *Mapping of the interaction interface of DNA polymerase beta with XRCC1.* Structure, 2002. 10(12): p. 1709-20

[26] Taylor, R.M., et al., *Role of a BRCT domain in the interaction of DNA ligase III-alpha with the DNA repair protein XRCC1.* Curr Biol, 1998. 8(15): p. 877-80

[27] Luo, H., et al., *A new XRCC1-containing complex and its role in cellular survival of methyl methanesulfonate treatment.* Mol Cell Biol, 2004. 24(19): p. 8356-65

[28] Date, H., et al., *The FHA domain of aprataxin interacts with the C-terminal region of XRCC1.* Biochem Biophys Res Commun, 2004. 325(4): p. 1279-85

[29] Clements, P.M., et al., *The ataxia-oculomotor apraxia 1 gene product has a role distinct from ATM and interacts with the DNA strand break repair proteins XRCC1 and XRCC4.* DNA Repair (Amst), 2004. 3(11): p. 1493-502

[30] Schreiber, V., et al., *Poly(ADP-ribose) polymerase-2 (PARP-2) is required for efficient base excision DNA repair in association with PARP-1 and XRCC1.* J Biol Chem, 2002. 277(25): p. 23028-36

[31] Leppard, J.B., et al., *Physical and functional interaction between DNA ligase IIIalpha and poly(ADP-Ribose) polymerase 1 in DNA single-strand break repair.* Mol Cell Biol, 2003. 23(16): p. 5919-27

[32] Sears, R.C. and J.R. Nevins, *Signaling networks that link cell proliferation and cell fate.* J Biol Chem, 2002. 277(14): p. 11617-20

[33] Ginsberg, D., *E2F1 pathways to apoptosis.* FEBS Lett, 2002. 529(1): p. 122-5
[34] Johnson, D.G. and R. Schneider-Broussard, *Role of E2F in cell cycle control and cancer.* Front Biosci, 1998. 3: p. d447-8
[35] Morkel, M., et al., *An E2F-like repressor of transcription.* Nature, 1997. 390(6660): p. 567-8
[36] Cartwright, P., et al., *E2F-6: a novel member of the E2F family is an inhibitor of E2F-dependent transcription.* Oncogene, 1998. 17(5): p. 611-23
[37] Magae, J., et al., *Nuclear localization of DP and E2F transcription factors by heterodimeric partners and retinoblastoma protein family members.* J Cell Sci, 1996. 109 (Pt 7): p. 1717-26
[38] Frolov, M.V. and N.J. Dyson, *Molecular mechanisms of E2F-dependent activation and pRB-mediated repression.* J Cell Sci, 2004. 117(Pt 11): p. 2173-81
[39] He, Y. and W.D. Cress, *E2F-3B is a physiological target of cyclin A.* J Biol Chem, 2002. 277(26): p. 23493-9
[40] Tsantoulis, P.K. and V.G. Gorgoulis, *Involvement of E2F transcription factor family in cancer.* Eur J Cancer, 2005. 41(16): p. 2403-14
[41] Martinez-Balbas, M.A., et al., *Regulation of E2F1 activity by acetylation.* EMBO J, 2000. 19(4): p. 662-71
[42] Ianari, A., et al., *Specific role for p300/CREB-binding protein-associated factor activity in E2F1 stabilization in response to DNA damage.* J Biol Chem, 2004. 279(29): p. 30830-5
[43] Dimova, D.K. and N.J. Dyson, *The E2F transcriptional network: old acquaintances with new faces.* Oncogene, 2005. 24(17): p. 2810-26
[44] Powers, J.T., et al., *E2F1 uses the ATM signaling pathway to induce p53 and Chk2 phosphorylation and apoptosis.* Mol Cancer Res, 2004. 2(4): p. 203-14
[45] Wang, B., et al., *A role for 14-3-3 tau in E2F1 stabilization and DNA damage-induced apoptosis.* J Biol Chem, 2004. 279(52): p. 54140-52
[46] Liu, K., et al., *Regulation of E2F1 by BRCT domain-containing protein TopBP1.* Mol Cell Biol, 2003. 23(9): p. 3287-304
[47] Liontos, M., et al., *Modulation of the E2F1-driven cancer cell fate by the DNA damage response machinery and potential novel E2F1 targets in osteosarcomas.* Am J Pathol, 2009. 175(1): p. 376-91
[48] Frame, F.M., et al., *E2F1 induces MRN foci formation and a cell cycle checkpoint response in human fibroblasts.* Oncogene, 2006. 25(23): p. 3258-66
[49] Liao, C.C., et al., *RB.E2F1 complex mediates DNA damage responses through transcriptional regulation of ZBRK1.* J Biol Chem, 2010. 285(43): p. 33134-43
[50] Lin, P.S., et al., *The role of the retinoblastoma/E2F1 tumor suppressor pathway in the lesion recognition step of nucleotide excision repair.* DNA Repair (Amst), 2009. 8(7): p. 795-802
[51] Seifried, L.A., et al., *pRB-E2F1 complexes are resistant to adenovirus E1A-mediated disruption.* J Virol, 2008. 82(9): p. 4511-20
[52] Chen, J., et al., *E2F1 promotes the recruitment of DNA repair factors to sites of DNA double-strand breaks.* Cell Cycle, 2011. 10(8): p. 1287-94
[53] Guo, R., et al., *GCN5 and E2F1 stimulate nucleotide excision repair by promoting H3K9 acetylation at sites of damage.* Nucleic Acids Res, 2011. 39(4): p. 1390-7

[54] Berton, T.R., et al., *Regulation of epidermal apoptosis and DNA repair by E2F1 in response to ultraviolet B radiation.* Oncogene, 2005. 24(15): p. 2449-60
[55] Guo, R., et al., *E2F1 localizes to sites of UV-induced DNA damage to enhance nucleotide excision repair.* J Biol Chem, 2010. 285(25): p. 19308-15
[56] Youn, C.K., et al., *Bcl-2 expression suppresses mismatch repair activity through inhibition of E2F transcriptional activity.* Nat Cell Biol, 2005. 7(2): p. 137-47
[57] Polager, S., et al., *E2Fs up-regulate expression of genes involved in DNA replication, DNA repair and mitosis.* Oncogene, 2002. 21(3): p. 437-46
[58] Bindra, R.S., et al., *Hypoxia-induced down-regulation of BRCA1 expression by E2Fs.* Cancer Res, 2005. 65(24): p. 11597-604
[59] Prost, S., et al., *E2F regulates DDB2: consequences for DNA repair in Rb-deficient cells.* Oncogene, 2007. 26(24): p. 3572-81
[60] Walsh, M.J., et al., *E2F-1 and a cyclin-like DNA repair enzyme, uracil-DNA glycosylase, provide evidence for an autoregulatory mechanism for transcription.* J Biol Chem, 1995. 270(10): p. 5289-98
[61] Maser, R.S., et al., *Mre11 complex and DNA replication: linkage to E2F and sites of DNA synthesis.* Mol Cell Biol, 2001. 21(17): p. 6006-16
[62] Lundin, C., et al., *Methyl methanesulfonate (MMS) produces heat-labile DNA damage but no detectable in vivo DNA double-strand breaks.* Nucleic Acids Res, 2005. 33(12): p. 3799-811
[63] Chen, D., et al., *E2F1 regulates the base excision repair gene XRCC1 and promotes DNA repair.* J Biol Chem, 2008. 283(22): p. 15381-9
[64] Yacoub, A., et al., *MAPK dependence of DNA damage repair: ionizing radiation and the induction of expression of the DNA repair genes XRCC1 and ERCC1 in DU145 human prostate carcinoma cells in a MEK1/2 dependent fashion.* Int J Radiat Biol, 2001. 77(10): p. 1067-78
[65] Yacoub, A., et al., *Epidermal growth factor and ionizing radiation up-regulate the DNA repair genes XRCC1 and ERCC1 in DU145 and LNCaP prostate carcinoma through MAPK signaling.* Radiat Res, 2003. 159(4): p. 439-52
[66] Shung, B., J. Miyakoshi, and H. Takebe, *X-ray-induced transcriptional activation of c-myc and XRCC1 genes in ataxia telangiectasia cells.* Mutat Res, 1994. 307(1): p. 43-51
[67] Thompson, L.H. and M.G. West, *XRCC1 keeps DNA from getting stranded.* Mutat Res, 2000. 459(1): p. 1-18
[68] Libutti, S.K., et al., *Parathyroid gland-specific deletion of the mouse Men1 gene results in parathyroid neoplasia and hypercalcemic hyperparathyroidism.* Cancer Res, 2003. 63(22): p. 8022-8
[69] Nakada, D., et al., *The ATM-related Tel1 protein of Saccharomyces cerevisiae controls a checkpoint response following phleomycin treatment.* Nucleic Acids Res, 2003. 31(6): p. 1715-24
[70] Lin, W.C., F.T. Lin, and J.R. Nevins, *Selective induction of E2F1 in response to DNA damage, mediated by ATM-dependent phosphorylation.* Genes Dev, 2001. 15(14): p. 1833-44
[71] Stevens, C., L. Smith, and N.B. La Thangue, *Chk2 activates E2F-1 in response to DNA damage.* Nat Cell Biol, 2003. 5(5): p. 401-9
[72] Blattner, C., A. Sparks, and D. Lane, *Transcription factor E2F-1 is upregulated in response to DNA damage in a manner analogous to that of p53.* Mol Cell Biol, 1999. 19(5): p. 3704-13

[73] Stevens, C. and N.B. La Thangue, *The emerging role of E2F-1 in the DNA damage response and checkpoint control.* DNA Repair (Amst), 2004. 3(8-9): p. 1071-9

[74] Tan, Y., P. Raychaudhuri, and R.H. Costa, *Chk2 mediates stabilization of the FoxM1 transcription factor to stimulate expression of DNA repair genes.* Mol Cell Biol, 2007. 27(3): p. 1007-16

[75] Levy, N., et al., *XRCC1 is phosphorylated by DNA-dependent protein kinase in response to DNA damage.* Nucleic Acids Res, 2006. 34(1): p. 32-41

[76] Loizou, J.I., et al., *The protein kinase CK2 facilitates repair of chromosomal DNA single-strand breaks.* Cell, 2004. 117(1): p. 17-28

[77] Dong, Z. and A.E. Tomkinson, *ATM mediates oxidative stress-induced dephosphorylation of DNA ligase IIIalpha.* Nucleic Acids Res, 2006. 34(20): p. 5721-279

[78] Ishida, S., et al., *Role for E2F in control of both DNA replication and mitotic functions as revealed from DNA microarray analysis.* Mol Cell Biol, 2001. 21(14): p. 4684-99

[79] Ren, B., et al., *E2F integrates cell cycle progression with DNA repair, replication, and G(2)/M checkpoints.* Genes Dev, 2002. 16(2): p. 245-56

[80] Weinmann, A.S., et al., *Isolating human transcription factor targets by coupling chromatin immunoprecipitation and CpG island microarray analysis.* Genes Dev, 2002. 16(2): p. 235-44

[81] Fan, J., et al., *XRCC1 co-localizes and physically interacts with PCNA.* Nucleic Acids Res, 2004. 32(7): p. 2193-201

[82] Moore, D.J., et al., *Mutation of a BRCT domain selectively disrupts DNA single-strand break repair in noncycling Chinese hamster ovary cells.* Proc Natl Acad Sci U S A, 2000. 97(25): p. 13649-54

[83] Taylor, R.M., A. Thistlethwaite, and K.W. Caldecott, *Central role for the XRCC1 BRCT I domain in mammalian DNA single-strand break repair.* Mol Cell Biol, 2002. 22(8): p. 2556-63

[84] Taylor, R.M., et al., *A cell cycle-specific requirement for the XRCC1 BRCT II domain during mammalian DNA strand break repair.* Mol Cell Biol, 2000. 20(2): p. 735-40

[85] Inoue, Y., M. Kitagawa, and Y. Taya, *Phosphorylation of pRB at Ser612 by Chk1/2 leads to a complex between pRB and E2F-1 after DNA damage.* EMBO J, 2007. 26(8): p. 2083-93

[86] Pommier, Y., et al., *Targeting chk2 kinase: molecular interaction maps and therapeutic rationale.* Curr Pharm Des, 2005. 11(22): p. 2855-72

[87] Kowalik, T.F., et al., *E2F1 overexpression in quiescent fibroblasts leads to induction of cellular DNA synthesis and apoptosis.* J Virol, 1995. 69(4): p. 2491-500

[88] Harris, S.L. and A.J. Levine, *The p53 pathway: positive and negative feedback loops.* Oncogene, 2005. 24(17): p. 2899-908

[89] Bell, L.A. and K.M. Ryan, *Life and death decisions by E2F-1.* Cell Death Differ, 2004. 11(2): p. 137-42

[90] Sengupta, S. and C.C. Harris, *p53: traffic cop at the crossroads of DNA repair and recombination.* Nat Rev Mol Cell Biol, 2005. 6(1): p. 44-55

[91] Adimoolam, S. and J.M. Ford, *p53 and regulation of DNA damage recognition during nucleotide excision repair.* DNA Repair (Amst), 2003. 2(9): p. 947-54

[92] Yamasaki, L., et al., *Tumor induction and tissue atrophy in mice lacking E2F-1.* Cell, 1996. 85(4): p. 537-48

[93] Field, S.J., et al., *E2F-1 functions in mice to promote apoptosis and suppress proliferation.* Cell, 1996. 85(4): p. 549-61
[94] Wang, S., et al., *JWA regulates XRCC1 and functions as a novel base excision repair protein in oxidative-stress-induced DNA single-strand breaks.* Nucleic Acids Res, 2009. 37(6): p. 1936-50

9

Posttranslational Modifications of Rad51 Protein and Its Direct Partners: Role and Effect on Homologous Recombination – Mediated DNA Repair

Milena Popova*, Sébastien Henry* and Fabrice Fleury
Unité U3B, UMR 6204 CNRS, 2, rue de la Houssinière, University of Nantes France

1. Introduction

Double-strand breaks (DSB) are probably the most deleterious form of DNA alteration in a cell. They may arise from ionizing radiation, free radicals, chemicals, or during replication of single-strand breaks. There are two distinct and complementary mechanisms for DSB repair: non-homologous end-joining (NHEJ) and homologous recombination (HR). Both repair pathways are important for the elimination of DSBs in eukaryotes.

Although the mechanisms of the cellular choice between these two pathways remain unclear, there is evidence that it depends on the cell cycle, as well as on mechanisms such as posttranslational modifications. When an intact DNA copy is available, HR is preferred and it is mainly active during late S and G2 phases of the cell cycle, while NHEJ is predominant during G0 and early S phases. The NHEJ pathway is characterised by a phosphorylation cascade where the first step is the activation of DNA-PKc protein which comprises a catalytic subunit and which is essential to complete the repair process. In contrast to NHEJ, the role of posttranslational modifications of proteins involved in the HR pathway is not clearly defined. Rad51 is a central protein in HR repair and its activity is based on pairing and strand exchange between homologous DNAs. The molecular regulation of Rad51 levels and activity has not been completely established. However, the kinase-induced phosphorylation of this protein modulates its recombinase activity by changing its interface and recognition sites and probably its intracellular distribution. Indeed, Rad51 associates with its paralogues and with other partner proteins, such as Rad52, Rad54, BRCA2 tumour suppressor, BLM helicase (Fig.1). Rad51 forms distinct subnuclear complexes called foci, which represent the functional units in DNA repair by HR. This accumulation of repair proteins to sites of double-strand break repair is closely dependant on protein-protein interactions which can be regulated by posttranslational modification processes including tyrosine, serine and threonine phosphorylations. This underlines the high complexity of HR regulation in mammalian cells.

Regulation of Rad51 recombinase activity and its interactions following DNA damage are poorly understood. In this chapter we have summarized the posttranslational modifications

* M.P. and S.H. contributed equally to this work

of Rad51 and of the proteins interacting physically with Rad51 during HR repair. We then attempt to relate the impact of these modifications on HR DNA repair and on the intracellular distribution of DNA repair proteins.

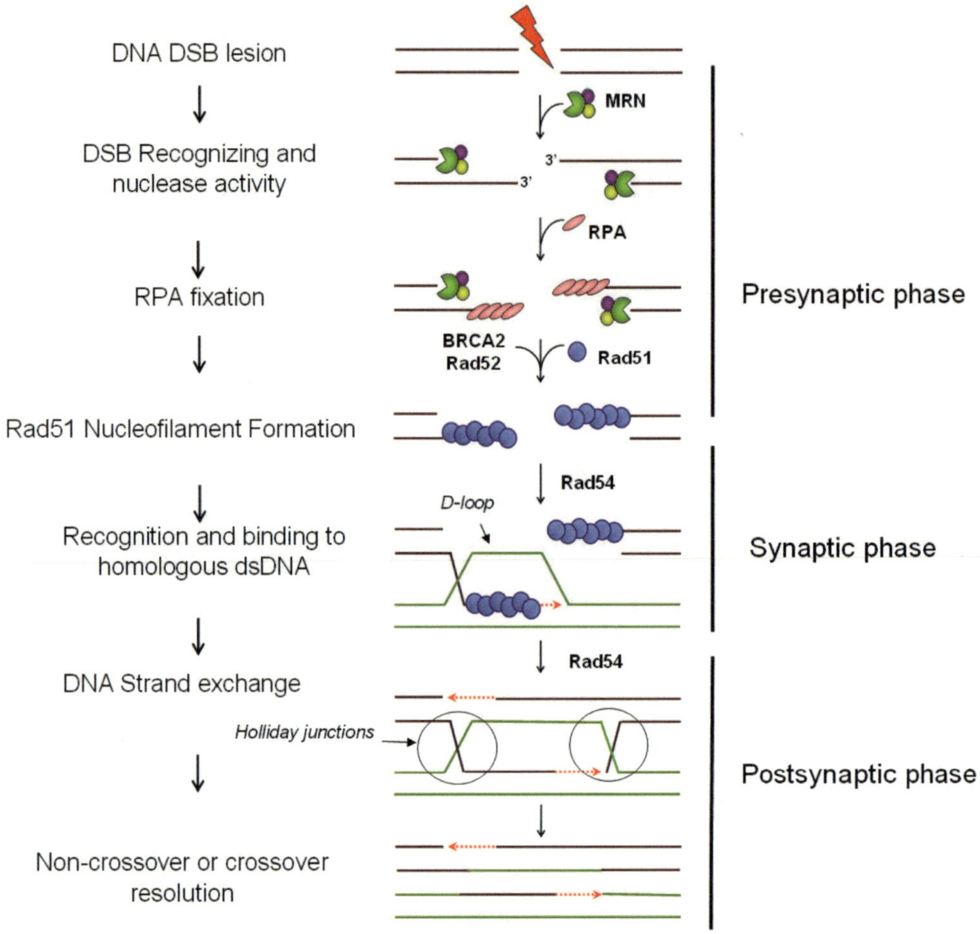

Fig. 1. Schematic representation of the mechanism of DNA DSB repair by homologous recombination.

2. Post-translational modifications of Rad51

2.1 Tyrosine phosphorylation of Rad51 by the c-Abl family of tyrosine kinases

Several studies have shown that Rad51 can be phosphorylated on tyrosine but until recently there were discrepancies on the exact site of phosphorylation. Three studies had shown the phosphorylation of Tyrosine 315 (Y315) and only one the phosphorylation of Tyrosine 54 (Y54). A recent publication demonstrated that both of these tyrosines can be phosphorylated. The kinases which phosphorylate Rad51 belong to the c-Abl family which has two members, c-Abl and Arg. The oncogenic fusion tyrosine kinase BCR/Abl has also been shown to phosphorylate Rad51. However, other tyrosine kinases can also phosphorylate Rad51 at a different site than Tyrosine 315 in MEF cAbl-/- cells (Chen et al., 1999b).

2.1.1 Phosphorylation on Tyrosine 54

The first study showing that Rad51 can be phosphorylated was published in 1998 by Yuan and colleagues. Using co-immunoprecipitation, the authors observed that human Rad51 (hRad51) binds to c-Abl in cells. This association was unaffected by irradiation of the cells and was not dependent on DNA binding. Pull-down assays were performed with a GST-c-Abl fusion protein or a GST-c-Abl SH3 domain fusion peptide. These were incubated with cell lysates or purified hRad51. The results confirmed the association between hRad51 and c-Abl *in vitro* and showed that the binding is direct and is mediated by the SH3 domain of c-Abl.
In vitro phosphorylation assays with purified c-Abl and hRad51 demonstrated that hRad51 is a substrate for this kinase. Immunoprecipitation of Rad51 was performed with lysates from irradiated cells overexpressing hRad51 and c-Abl. The analyses of the immunoprecipitated protein with an anti-phosphoTyrosine antibody confirmed the phosphorylation of Rad51 *in vivo*. The *in vivo* and *in vitro* phosphorylated hRad51 proteins were then purified and analyzed by mass spectroscopy. The detected peaks indicated that the phosphorylation is located on Tyrosine 54 on both *in vivo* and *in vitro* phosphorylated Rad51 (Chen et al., 1999a; Chen et al., 1999b; Chen et al., 1999c; Dong et al., 1999; Yuan et al., 1999; Zhong et al., 1999).

2.1.2 Phosphorylation on Tyrosine 315 by c-Abl

Two years after Yuan and colleagues published their study, another group demonstrated that Rad51 can be phosphorylated. However Chen and colleagues did not observe the phosphorylation of Tyrosine 54 but detected the phosphorylation of another tyrosine residue, in position 315.
The authors used GST pull-down assays and immunoprecipitation to show that Rad51 forms a complex with c-Abl and ATM in cells. The association between the three proteins was independent of irradiation and DNA binding. The level of phosphorylation of Rad51 after irradiation of cells was investigated. The analyses of immunoprecipitated Rad51 with an anti-phosphoTyrosine antibody showed that the level of phosphorylation increases after irradiation. Rad51 was a direct substrate for c-Abl and the phosphorylation was dependent on both c-Abl and ATM. In order to determine which tyrosine residue was phosphorylated, the authors co-expressed c-Abl and wild type or mutated Rad51 in cells. Different tyrosine to phenylalanine Rad51 mutants were performed. Phenylalanine is an amino acid that cannot be phosphorylated. Thus, a signal would no longer be detected by the anti-phosphoTyrosine antibody when the phosphorylated residue is mutated. The mutation of Y315 to phenylalanine abolished Rad51 phosphorylation, indicating that c-Abl phosphorylates Rad51 on this residue (Yuan et al., 1998).

2.1.3 Phosphorylation on Tyrosine 315 by BCR/Abl

Rad51 can also be phosphorylated by the oncogenic fusion tyrosine kinase BCR/Abl. BCR/Abl is expressed in most cases of chronic myeloid leukemia and in some cases of acute myeloid leukemia and possesses constitutive kinase activity.
Slupianek and colleagues suggested that Rad51 and BCR/Abl interact physically since a portion of Rad51 co-localizes with the fusion tyrosine kinase in the cytoplasm of BCR/Abl overexpressing cells. This interaction was confirmed by the co-immunoprecipitation of the two proteins.
Rad51 was immunoprecipitated from cells overexpressing BCR/Abl and its phosphorylation state was examined with an anti-phosphoTyrosine antibody. The interaction between

BCR/Abl and Rad51 resulted in the constitutive phosphorylation of Rad51 on tyrosine. Rad51 was also phosphorylated by c-Abl after treatment of cells with cisplatin and mitomycin C. In order to determine the position of phosphorylation, the authors transiently co-expressed BCR/Abl and wild type or mutated Rad51 in cells. Tyrosine to phenylalanine mutations were performed at Tyrosine 54 or Tyrosine 315. The analysis of the Rad51 immunoprecipitates with an anti-phosphoTyrosine antibody revealed the phosphorylation of the wild type and the Y54F Rad51 protein. A substantial reduction in the phosphorylation level of Rad51 was observed when Y315 was mutated to phenylalanine, indicating that the majority of the phosphorylation of Rad51 occurred on Y315. To further confirm the phosphorylation of the Y315 residue, Slupianek and colleagues prepared an antiserum using a phosphorylated Y315 peptide. Western blots were then performed with lysates from cells overexpressiong Rad51 alone or with BCR/Abl. The antiserum did not recognize Rad51 when the protein was overexpressed in cells alone. In contrast, in cells co-expressing BCR/Abl a strong signal was observed. This confirms that the fusion tyrosine kinase BCR/Abl phosphorylates Rad51 on Tyrosine 315 (Slupianek et al., 2001).

2.1.4 Phosphorylation by Arg

The only other member of the c-Abl family, the kinase Arg, also phosphorylates Rad51. Arg shares considerable structural and sequence homology with c-Abl in the N-terminal SH3 and SH2 domains, as well as in the tyrosine kinase domain (Kruh et al., 1990). Co-immunoprecipitation of Rad51 from cells overexpressing Rad51 and Arg indicated that Arg can interact with Rad51 *in vivo*. An anti-phosphoTyrosine antibody showed that Rad51 is phosphorylated by Arg and this phosphorylation seemed to be more effective than the phosphorylation by c-Abl. However, the position of phosphorylation was not determined (Li et al., 2002).

2.1.5 Phosphorylation of both Tyrosine 54 and Tyrosine 315 by c-Abl

The study conducted by Popova and colleagues has allowed to reconcile the discrepancies on which tyrosine residue is phosphorylated in Rad51. The authors purified specific anti-phosphoTyrosine antibodies for each site of phosphorylation. These antibodies were used to analyze the phosphorylation state of Rad51 by immunoblotting of lysates from cells overexpressing Rad51 and c-Abl. The ability of these specific antibodies to detect distinctively the phosphorylation of the two tyrosine residues has allowed to observe the phosphorylation of both Y54 and Y315 in the same experiment. This confirmed that both Tyrosine 54 and 315 can be phosphorylated (Popova et al., 2009).

In all previous studies the phosphorylation of only one site was observed, either Y54 or Y315. The fact that Yuan and colleagues observed only the phosphorylation of Y54 and did not detect the phosphorylation of Y315 could be due to the technique they used. In their study, the *in vitro* or *in vivo* phosphorylated Rad51 protein, as well as the unphosphorylated protein were digested by trypsin. The obtained fragments were then analyzed by mass spectroscopy and the spectra of the unphosphorylated and the phosphorylated proteins were compared. The lack of a phosphorylation peak in the fragment containing Y315 could be explained by its biophysical characteristics. Following trypsin digestion, the peptide containing Tyrosine 54 is 17 amino acids long and has a pHi of 4,83. On the contrary, the peptide containing Tyrosine 315 is 28 amino acids long and its pHi is 4,03. Thus, the Y315 peptide is longer and more negatively charged compared to the Y54 peptide which could interfere with its detection by mass spectroscopy (Raggiaschi et al., 2005).

Another possible explanation could be the proximity of the digestion and the phosphorylation sites. The presence of phosphorylation near a digestion site may decrease its digestion efficiency (Benore-Parsons et al., 1989; Kjeldsen et al., 2007). Thus the phosphorylated protein would be partially digested resulting in a longer phospho-peptide. A corresponding peptide would not be obtained from the digestion of the unphosphorylated protein. A phosphorylation peak would not be observed in these conditions. In the amino acid sequence of Rad51, only one residue separates the trypsin digestion site from Tyrosine 315. Due to the proximity of the two sites, Rad51 would rather be digested at arginine 310 than on lysine 313. This would result in the generation of a phosphopeptide which would be 3 amino acids longer than the corresponding peptide from the unphosphorylated protein. Consequently, the phosphorylation of Rad51 on Y315 would not be detected by mass spectroscopy.

2.1.6 Model of sequential phosphorylation

Popova and co-authors have established a possible mechanism by which Rad51 is phosphorylated by c-Abl. They co-expressed c-Abl and wild type or mutated hRad51 in cells. In the amino acid sequence of hRad51, Tyrosine 54 or Tyrosine 315 were mutated to phenylalanine, thus rendering the residue at this position nonphosphorylatable. Western blot analysis of the cell lysates, revealed with their specific anti-phosphoTyrosine antibodies, showed a relationship between the phosphorylation of Y54 and Y315. When residue 315 was mutated to phenylalanine and nonphosphorylatable, Tyrosine 54 was no longer phosphorylated. On the contrary, the mutation of residue 54 had no effect on the phosphorylation of Tyrosine 315. The authors hypothesized that the phosphorylation of Tyrosine 315 is needed for the phosphorylation of Tyrosine 54.

The c-Abl kinase possesses a SH3 and a SH2 domain in its N-terminal region. The SH3 domain recognizes and binds preferentially to proline rich regions containing the sequence PXXP. The SH2 domain recognizes pYXXP sequences. hRad51 has two PXXP motifs in its amino acid sequence - between amino acids 283 and 286, and between amino acids 318 and 321. When Tyrosine 315 is phosphorylated, a pYXXP motif is revealed between amino acids 315 and 318. This motif might be recognized by the SH2 domain of c-Abl.

According to this model of sequential phosphorylation, c-Abl recognizes a PXXP motif in the sequence of Rad51 through its SH3 domain and phosphorylates Tyrosine 315. The phosphorylation of this residue reveals the pYXXP binding motif which is recognized by the SH2 domain of c-Abl. This allows the phosphorylation of Tyrosine 54.

To confirm this model, GST pull-down assays were performed. A GST- c-Abl SH2 domain peptide was incubated with lysates from cells overexpressing Rad51 and c-Abl. The results showed that hRad51 binds to the SH2 domain of c-Abl and that this interaction takes place when Rad51 is phosphorylated on Tyrosine 315. Therefore a model of sequential phosphorylation of Rad51, where the phosphorylation of Tyrosine 315 by c-Abl reveals a novel binding site for the kinase thus allowing the phosphorylation of Tyrosine 54, is highly plausible.

2.2 Role of Rad51 phosphorylation

Even though the process of phosphorylation seems to be of considerable importance in the regulation of Rad51 activity, its exact roles and consequences have not been elucidated yet. Moreover, the existing data is contradictory.

In their study, Yuan and colleagues investigated the possible effect of Y54 phosphorylation on Rad51 activity. Strand exchange assays showed that phosphorylation of S. cerevisiae

Rad51 (ScRad51) results in the inhibition of dsDNA conversion to joint molecules and nicked circular dsDNA. An inhibition of the binding of phospho-ScRad51 and phospho-hRad51 to ssDNA was also observed. Because Rad51 exerts its activity by binding to and forming nucleofilaments with ssDNA, the authors concluded that by inhibiting the binding to ssDNA, phosphorylation inhibits Rad51 function (Yuan et al., 1998).

In the search of a possible role for Y315 phosphorylation, Chen and colleagues investigated if the phosphorylation impacts the interaction between Rad51 and Rad52. Rad52 is a protein needed in the presynaptic stage of homologous recombination (Fig. 1). Binding assays with purified *in vitro* phosphorylated Rad51 and Rad52, as well as co-immunoprecipitation of Rad51 and Rad52 from irradiated cells were performed. The results indicated that phosphorylation enhances the interaction between these two proteins *in vitro* and *in vivo*. The authors hypothesized that this irradiation-induced phosphorylation of Rad51 on tyrosine residues and the concomitant increase in association with Rad52 may lead to increased DNA repair efficiency (Chen et al., 1999b). *In vitro* studies with different Y315 mutants suggest that the phosphorylation of this residue is important for the binding of Rad51 to dsDNA and for nucleofilament formation (Takizawa et al., 2004). Moreover, Y315 is located near the polymerisation site of the protein, a region which is essential for the filament formation of Rad51 on DSBs, (Conilleau et al., 2004).

Slupianek and colleagues analyzed the role of Rad51 phosphorylation in the resistance of cells to DNA damaging agents. The resistance of BCR/Abl expressing cells to cisplatin and mitomycin C was decreased upon overexpression of nonphosphorylatable Rad51 Y315F. The mutation of Y54 had no effect on resistance. These results link the phosphorylation of Y315 to the resistance to DNA cross-linking agents and suggest that it has an important impact on DNA repair (Slupianek et al., 2001).

Recently, the same team reported an implication of Y315 phosphorylation in the regulation of BCR/Abl-Rad51 interaction. BCR/Abl-mediated phosphorylation of Y315 appears to be important for the dissociation of Rad51 from BCR/Abl in chronic myeloid leukemia cells (Slupianek et al., 2009). The authors studied the intracellular localization of wild type and mutated Rad51 in response to DSBs induced by genotoxic treatment. The nonphosphorylatable Rad51 Y315F mutant remained mostly in the cytoplasm, while the wild-type protein accumulated in the nucleus in BCR/Abl-positive cells. This indicates that phospho-Y315 stimulates abundant nuclear localization of Rad51 on DSBs.

2.3 Phosphorylation on Threonine 309 by Chk1

Rad51 can also be phosphorylated on threonine. Sorensen and colleagues observed that a Chk1 signal is necessary for efficient homologous recombination. The inhibition of this kinase decreased the level of homologous recombination and of DNA DSB repair. The inhibition of Chk1 also impaired the formation of Rad51 foci which was not due to decreased Rad51 levels. The interaction of Rad51 with chromatin was dependent on Chk1 activity. Using immunoprecipitation, Sorensen and colleagues showed that Chk1 and Rad51 can interact physically in cells. Chk1 phosphorylates Rad51 on Threonine 309 which is located in a Chk1 consensus phosphorylation site. Cells transfected with a nonphosphorylatable Rad51 mutant were more sensitive to hydroxyurea which confirms that Chk1 signaling is required for homologous recombination repair (Sorensen et al., 2005).

2.4 Sumoylation – Ubiquitination of Rad51

Yeast two-hybrid assays have shown that Rad51 can interact with HsUbc9, later named UBE21. HsUbc9/UBE21 is the human homologue of *S. cerevisiae* UBC9 and *S. pombe* Hus5 ubiquitin conjugating enzymes (Kovalenko et al., 1996; Shen et al., 1996). In mammalian cells the downregulation of Ubc9 was associated with defects in cytokinesis and an increased number of apoptotic cells. Furthermore, its gene inactivation is lethal in mouse embryos (Moschos and Mo, 2006). Nuclear depletion of Ubc9 disrupts the intracellular trafficking of Rad51 and thus inhibits the formation of Rad51 nuclear foci following DNA damage (Saitoh et al., 2002).

Rad51 also interacts with UBL1 (ubiquitin like 1), also called PIC1, GMP1, SUMO-1 and Sentrin (Shen et al., 1996). The yeast homologue of UBL1, SMT3, inhibits a centrosome protein involved in centrosome segregation (Shen et al., 1996). UBL1 interacts with HsUBC9/UBE21 (Shen et al., 1996). Studies have shown that HsUbc9/UBE21 is a UBL1-conjugating enzyme, rather than an ubiquitin-conjugating enzyme. Immunoprecipitation essays in HeLa cells and GST pull-down essays have shown that the interaction between Rad51 and Ubl1 is mediated by Rad52 and/or Ubc9. This suggests that Ubc9 can conjugate UBL1 to Rad51. The overexpression of UBL1 in mammalian cells decreases DSB-induced HR and resistance to IR (Li et al., 2000).

3. Rad51-interacting proteins involved in the nuclear translocation of Rad51 and in the HR process

The number and size of Rad51 nuclear foci is a hallmark of the cellular response to genotoxic stress. These nuclear foci characterize the formation of Rad51 filaments. Indeed Rad51 is recruited to sites of DNA DSBs in response to damage where it promotes DNA strand invasion and strand exchange. Impaired formation of Rad51 foci in response to DNA damage has been demonstrated in hamster or chicken cells defective in the Rad51 paralogs XRCC2, XRCC3, Rad51B, Rad51C, and in mammalian BRCA1 or BRCA2-defective cells (Chen et al., 1999c; Takata et al., 2001; Yuan et al., 1999).

The foci formation requires the translocation of Rad51 into the nucleus after DSB induction by genotoxic stress or stalled replication forks (Haaf et al., 1995).) This process is often accompanied by posttranslational modifications of Rad51 partners which cooperate to achieve the fidelity of DNA repair. Several works have shown that these modifications can modulate protein interactions involving Rad51 and can affect Rad51 foci formation.

3.1 Nuclear translocation of Rad51

The first stage of DNA DSB repair by HR requires the delivery of Rad51 at the sites of DNA damage. Since Rad51 does not have a Nuclear Localisation Signal (NLS) sequence, its nuclear entry likely requires the interaction with other proteins containing functional NLS sequences (Gildemeister et al., 2009). BRCA1 and BRCA2 proteins have both been described as primordial recombination mediators for the nuclear translocation of Rad51.

3.1.1 Involvement of BRCA1/Akt1

Several studies have demonstrated that the overexpression of Rad51 results in its cytoplasmic accumulation (Mladenov et al., 2006) but genotoxic stress triggers the translocation of Rad51 from the cytoplasm to the nucleus (Gildemeister et al., 2009). Plo and colleagues have reported that the nuclear translocation of Rad51 was impaired by AKT1 which repressed HR (Plo et al., 2008). In tumour cells with high levels of active AKT1, BRCA1 and Rad51 are retained in the cytoplasm. However, BRCA1 phosphorylation by AKT1 was not required for this retention. Interestingly, 77% of tumours containing high levels of AKT1 exhibited also cytoplasmic retention of Rad51 (Plo et al., 2008). This shows that AKT1 activation strongly favors the cytoplasmic localization of both BRCA1 and Rad51 proteins.

3.1.2 BRCA2-mediated nuclear translocation of Rad51

Like BRCA1, BRCA2 is a tumour suppressor implicated in familial breast cancer. BRCA2 protein contains six highly conserved BRC repeats which are involved in the interaction between BRCA2 and Rad51 (Marmorstein et al., 1998; Mizuta et al., 1997; Wong et al., 1997). It has been proposed that the BRCA2 protein is directly involved in the regulation of the nucleofilament formation and in the nuclear transport of Rad51 (Davies et al., 2001).

Medova and colleagues have demonstrated that the inhibition of the MET receptor tyrosine kinase by a small inhibitor molecule impairs the formation of the Rad51-BRCA2 complex. By targeting MET, the authors have shown the incapacity of tumour cells to repair DNA DSBs through homologous recombination. This was due to the impaired translocation of Rad51 into the nucleus (Medova et al.).

The pancreatic adenocarcinoma cell line CAPAN-1 is the best characterized BRCA2 defective human cell line (Jasin, 2002). CAPAN-1 cells have indeed lost a wild-type BRCA2 allele and presents a 6174delT mutation on the other allele. This mutation causes the premature C-terminal truncation of the protein. This results in the deletion of the BRCA2 domains for DNA repair and the nuclear localization signals (Holt et al., 2008). Rad51 exhibits impaired nuclear translocation in CAPAN-1 cells. Therefore it has been proposed that Rad51 requires BRCA2 for its nuclear translocation and that C-terminally truncated BRCA2 retains Rad51 in the cytoplasm.

Another group has however observed a DNA damage-induced increase in nuclear Rad51 in the BRCA2-defective cell line CAPAN-1. Moreover, chromatin-associated Rad51 levels were found to be increased (2-fold) following IR exposure (Gildemeister et al., 2009).

To analyze a possible BRCA2-independent mechanism for Rad51 nuclear transport, the authors studied two other Rad51-interacting proteins, Rad51C and Xrcc3. Both of these proteins contain a functional NLS. In contrast to Xrcc3, subcellular distribution of Rad51C was affected by DNA damage since nuclear Rad51C was significantly increased following IR exposure. Furthermore, the depletion of Rad51C in HeLa and CAPAN-1 cells by RNA interference resulted in lower levels of nuclear Rad51. These results provide an important overview of the cellular regulation of Rad51 nuclear entry. This data underlines the potential role for Rad51C in the nuclear translocation of Rad51, which suggests a BRCA2-independent mechanism for Rad51 nuclear entry both before and after DNA damage. Other studies have also demonstrated that an interaction between Rad51 and BRCA2 is not required for nuclear transport of Rad51 but it may prevent the formation of Rad51 filaments in the cytoplasm.

3.2 Recruitment of Rad51 at the damage site – Presynaptic phase of HR

Following damage, DSB are recognized by the MRN complex (MRE11-Rad51-NSB1 complex). MRN binds to and resects the extremities of the DSB through its nuclease activity.

This results in the generation of 3′ single-stranded DNA (ssDNA). RPA (Replication Protein A) binds to the 3' overhangs and thus protects them from further resection. This protein also removes secondary structures present on the ssDNA which allows efficient Rad51 nucleofilament formation (McIlwraith et al., 2000).

During the presynaptic phase Rad51 is loaded on the ssDNA ends with the help of BRCA2 (Huen et al., 2010). Rad51 recognizes and binds to the BRC repeats and the TR2 domain of BRCA2 (Fig.2). The Oligonucleotide Binding Folds (OB Folds) in the C-terminal region of the protein are also required for the recruitment of Rad51 (O'Donovan and Livingston, 2010; Wong et al., 1997).

The interaction of BRCA2 with two other proteins, BRCA1 and the bridging factor PALB2, is necessary for its role in the presynaptic phase of HR. These proteins along with other factors form a macro-complex named BRCC whose role in DNA repair has been described elsewhere (Dong et al., 2003).

In addition to its linking function between BRCA1 and BRCA2, PALB2 also interacts with a domain in Rad51 which is comprised between amino acids 184 and 257 (Fig.3) (Buisson et al., 2010). Thus, PALB2 cooperates with BRCA2 to stimulate Rad51 filament assembly during HR. The stimulation of the filament assembly by PALB2 is also mediated by its interaction with another co-factor, Rad51AP1 (Dray et al., 2010).

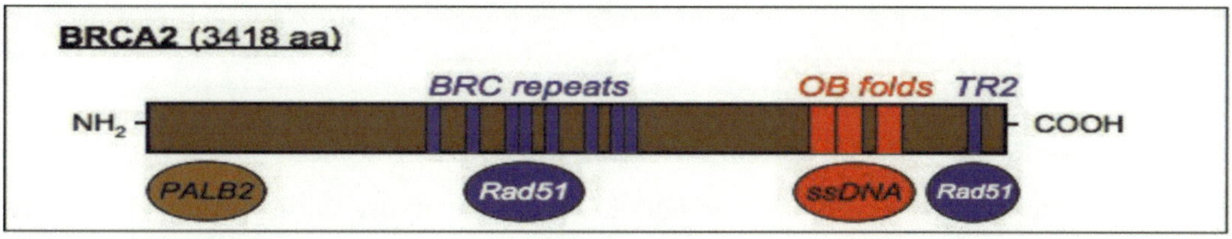

Fig. 2. Domain organization of BRCA2. Schematic drawing indicating the interaction sites with Rad51, PALB2 and DNA.

According to these data, BRCA2 plays an essential role in recruiting and loading Rad51 on sites of DSB and in initiating the HR process.

In order for the Rad51 presynaptic filament to assemble, Rad52 has to displace RPA from the ssDNA (Sugiyama and Kowalczykowski, 2002). RPA is a single-stranded DNA binding protein composed of three subunits, with sizes of respectively 70, 32 and 14 kDa (Wold, 1997). It has previously been shown by co-immunoprecipitation experiments that each of the three subunits of RPA interacts with Rad51, and that the RPA-Rad51 interaction is regulated by the 70kDa subunit (Golub et al., 1998). The co-localization of Rad51 and RPA foci in response to ionizing radiation was observed in a mice fibroblast model and suggests a possible *in vivo* interaction between the two proteins. Furthermore, a recent study has shown that depletion of RPA in mammalian cells leads to the impairment of Rad51 foci formation following DSB induced by hydroxyurea treatment. This confirms the importance of RPA in the presynaptic assembly of Rad51 (Sleeth et al., 2007).

Because RPA binding on ssDNA may prevent Rad51 access to DSB, the presynaptic filament formation needs to be time-regulated by the mediator Rad52. Rad52 is a key member of the RAD52 epistasis group, which includes Rad51, and whose function in HR has been previously described (Symington, 2002). The human Rad52 (hRad52) protein contains 418 amino acids. It has a highly conserved region in its N-terminus, and possesses a ssDNA/dsDNA binding region and a RPA binding site (Kagawa et al., 2002; Park et al., 1996). Shen and colleagues have demonstrated both *in vitro* and *in vivo* that hRad52 physically interacts with hRad51. The Rad51 binding domain on Rad52 has been identified between residues 291 to 330 (Fig.3) located in the C-terminal region of the protein (Shen et al., 1996).

Furthermore, five amino acid residues of hRad51 have been shown to participate in the Rad51-Rad52 interaction. These residues are located in the C-terminal region of hRad51 (Kurumizaka et al., 1999). Interestingly, the Rad52 binding site on Rad51 is not the same in *Homo Sapiens* and *Saccahromyces cerevisiae,* suggesting that this interaction is not conserved among species.

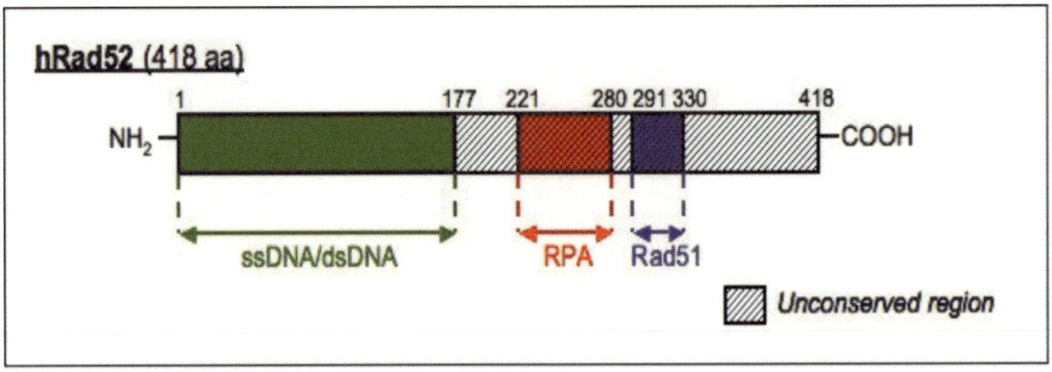

Fig. 3. Human Rad52 (hRad52) domains involved in HR.

The capacity to bind RPA and DNA confers to Rad52 the ability to displace RPA from the ssDNA and thus helps the formation of the Rad51 presynaptic filament (Plate et al., 2008; San Filippo et al., 2008).

The posttranslational modifications of RPA and Rad52 could modulate the formation of the presynaptic filament. Indeed, RPA is phosphorylated on one of its three subunits in a DNA damage-dependent manner and the resulting hyperphosphorylated RPA proteins directly interact with Rad51 (Binz et al., 2004; Wu et al., 2005). More recently, Shi and colleagues demonstrated by mutating the phosphorylation site of RPA that this posttranslational modification is required for Rad51 assembly (Shi et al., 2010). The importance of RPA phosphorylation during the presynaptic phase of HR was confirmed by Deng and colleagues who proposed a model in which RPA phosphorylation promotes Rad52 function and thus prepares DSB to be processed by Rad51 (Deng et al., 2009).

Phosphorylation of the Rad52 mediator in a c-Abl dependant manner has also been described in response to ionizing treatment (Kitao and Yuan, 2002). There is no evidence for the direct effect of Rad52 phosphorylation on Rad51 assembly. However, anterior studies have shown that the phosphorylation of Rad51 by c-Abl has an impact on the interaction between Rad51 and Rad52 (Chen et al., 1999b).

Another important posttranslational modification which plays a role in this stage of the HR process is SUMOylation. SUMOylation is already known to regulate the properties and stability of different proteins (Hay, 2005). It has recently been shown that the 70 kDa subunit of RPA can be SUMOylated and this process may regulate Rad51 presynaptic filament formation (Dou et al., 2010).

3.3 Regulation of Rad51 nucleofilament stability and enhancement of the strand exchange activity - Synaptic phase

Once the Rad51 nucleofilament is assembled, it has to be stabilized before Rad51 strand exchange activity may occur. This is mainly achieved by the Rad54 protein, which interacts both *in vitro* and *in vivo* with Rad51 during the synaptic phase of HR (Golub et al., 1997; Mazin et al., 2010). This protein-protein interaction is mediated by the Rad54 N-terminal region. It can occur either with the free Rad51 protein or with the assembled nucelofilament (Mazin et al., 2003; Raschle et al., 2004). Furthermore, using mouse embryonic stem cells, Tan and colleagues have demonstrated that Rad54 is required for Rad51 IR-induced foci formation (Tan et al., 1999). Rad54 functions in an ATP-independent manner to stabilize the Rad51 nucleofilament (Wolner and Peterson, 2005). However, it can also disrupt the assembled Rad51 complex (Li et al., 2007; Solinger et al., 2002). Thus, Rad54 modulates the stability of the Rad51 filament.

Another important consequence of the Rad51-Rad54 interaction is that Rad54 stimulates the recombinase and strand exchange activities of Rad51 (Mazina and Mazin, 2004; Sigurdsson et al., 2002). An additional protein interacting with Rad51 in the mature synaptic filament has been discovered. First identified as Pir51 (for Protein interacting with Rad51), this cofactor was later renamed Rad51AP1 (Rad51 Associated Protein 1). This protein was first characterized for its DNA crosslink repair activity (Henson et al., 2006; Kovalenko et al., 1997). Modesti and colleagues proposed a model in which Rad51AP1 could stimulate the formation of the D-loop by Rad51, which is the final step of the synaptic phase (Modesti et al., 2007).

To this day, the potential effect of Rad54 posttranslational modifications on Rad51 activity during this late stage of HR has not been demonstrated. Recent results obtained in yeast show that Rad54 phosphorylation leads to a reduction in Rad51-Rad54 complexes (Niu et al., 2009). It is not excluded that a similar mechanism could exist in superior eukaryotes.

3.4 Post-synaptic phase of HR – Resolution of Holliday junction

Following the synaptic phase, D-loops can be eliminated by different subpathways, each requiring different proteins. Here we will present only the pathways involving double Holliday junctions (dHJ) (Bzymek et al., 2010). Double HJ are structural intermediates which are resolved by specific endonucleases and result in either crossover or non-crossover products. The dHJ intermediates can also be resolved by helicases (RecQ helicase family) combined with topoisomerase action. In human cells, this pathway combines BLM helicase and topoisomerase IIIa, both of which catalyze dHJ dissolution (Wu and Hickson, 2003). Interestingly, BLM helicase is phosphorylated by different kinases, such as Chk1, at different stages of the cell cycle or in response to DNA damage. BLM can interact with 53PB1, a signal transducer, and with Topoisomerase IIIa during the presynaptic and the postsynaptic phases of HR respectively. It has been shown that BLM and 53BP1 can interact physically with Rad51 and regulate HR by modulating the assembly of Rad51 filaments. The *in vivo* phosphorylation of both BLM and 53BP1 affects negatively Rad51 foci formation (Tripathi et al., 2007). Concerning Topoisomerase IIIa, Rao and colleagues suggested that the BLM phosphorylation on T99 results in its dissociation from topoisomerase IIIa, thereby modulating the resolution of dHJ (Rao et al., 2005).

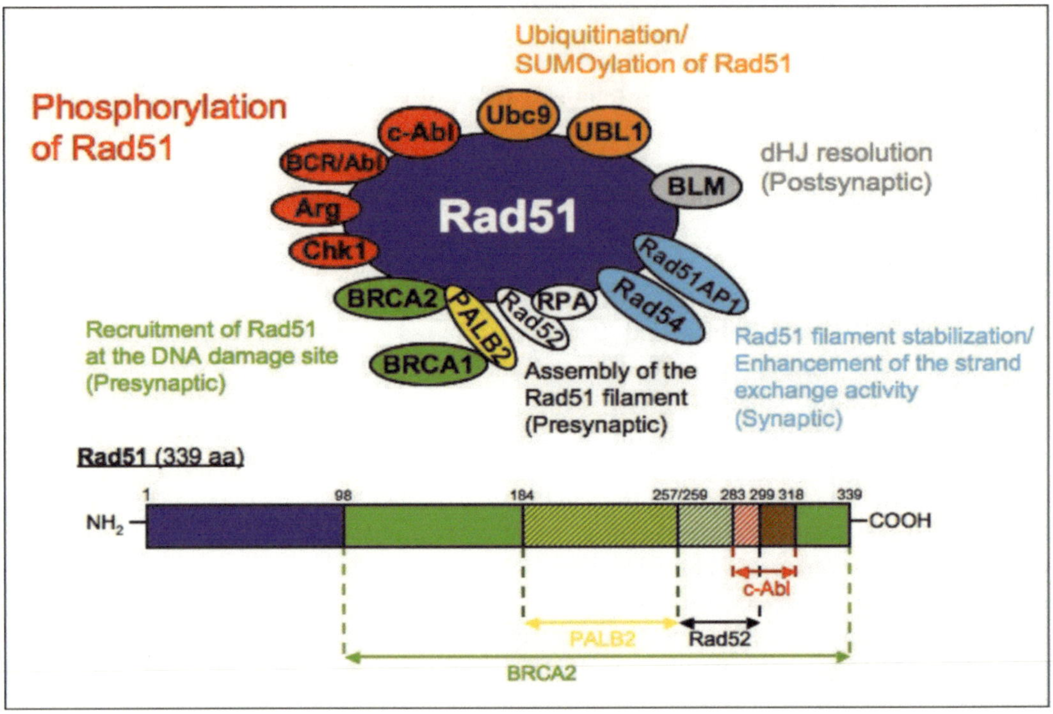

Fig. 4. Schematic representation of Rad51 interactions with its direct partners involved in its posttranslational modification and the steps of HR (top). Localization of binding sites in the hRad51 sequence (bottom).

4. Conclusion

In all living organisms HR is strictly regulated in time and in space to maintain the stability of the genome. Rad51 is the central protein in the HR process. The regulation of HR involves many protein interactions (Fig. 4) which are strongly dependent on posttranslational modifications. Indeed, almost all key mediator proteins of HR are subject to phosphorylation by specific kinases, thereby modulating some stage of this process (e.g. the nucleofilament formation). Hence, these posttranslational reactions underline the complexity of the regulation of HR. Despite of the several studies on the mechanism of Rad51 phosphorylation, its biochemical role in the HR reaction remains unclear.
The impact of phosphorylation on the interactions of Rad51 with its partners still needs to be determined. In order to better understand the regulation of HR, the future challenge will be to identify the complete interaction network of Rad51, the motor protein of HR.

5. Acknowledgment

This work was supported by grants from the Ligue contre le Cancer Comité de Loire Atlantique et du Morbihan. SH is supported by a fellowship from the Region Pays de la Loire (CIMATH2 grant). MP was supported by a fellowship from Conseil Général des Pays de Loire-Atlantique (Atlanthèse grant).

6. References

Benore-Parsons, M., Seidah, N.G., & Wennogle, L.P. (1989). Substrate phosphorylation can inhibit proteolysis by trypsin-like enzymes. Arch Biochem Biophys *272*, 274-280.

Binz, S.K., Sheehan, A.M., & Wold, M.S. (2004). Replication protein A phosphorylation and the cellular response to DNA damage. DNA Repair (Amst) *3*, 1015-1024.

Buisson, R., Dion-Cote, A.M., Coulombe, Y., Launay, H., Cai, H., Stasiak, A.Z., Stasiak, A., Xia, B., & Masson, J.Y. (2010). Cooperation of breast cancer proteins PALB2 and piccolo BRCA2 in stimulating homologous recombination. Nat Struct Mol Biol *17*, 1247-1254.

Bzymek, M., Thayer, N.H., Oh, S.D., Kleckner, N., & Hunter, N. (2010). Double Holliday junctions are intermediates of DNA break repair. Nature *464*, 937-941.

Chen, C.F., Chen, P.L., Zhong, Q., Sharp, Z.D., & Lee, W.H. (1999a). Expression of BRC repeats in breast cancer cells disrupts the BRCA2-Rad51 complex and leads to radiation hypersensitivity and loss of G(2)/M checkpoint control. J Biol Chem *274*, 32931-32935.

Chen, G., Yuan, S.S., Liu, W., Xu, Y., Trujillo, K., Song, B., Cong, F., Goff, S.P., Wu, Y., Arlinghaus, R., *et al.* (1999b). Radiation-induced assembly of Rad51 and Rad52 recombination complex requires ATM and c-Abl. J Biol Chem *274*, 12748-12752.

Chen, J.J., Silver, D., Cantor, S., Livingston, D.M., & Scully, R. (1999c). BRCA1, BRCA2, & Rad51 operate in a common DNA damage response pathway. Cancer Res *59*, 1752s-1756s.

Conilleau, S., Takizawa, Y., Tachiwana, H., Fleury, F., Kurumizaka, H., & Takahashi, M. (2004). Location of tyrosine 315, a target for phosphorylation by cAbl tyrosine kinase, at the edge of the subunit-subunit interface of the human Rad51 filament. J Mol Biol *339*, 797-804.

Davies, A.A., Masson, J.Y., McIlwraith, M.J., Stasiak, A.Z., Stasiak, A., Venkitaraman, A.R., & West, S.C. (2001). Role of BRCA2 in control of the RAD51 recombination and DNA repair protein. Mol Cell *7*, 273-282.

Deng, X., Prakash, A., Dhar, K., Baia, G.S., Kolar, C., Oakley, G.G., & Borgstahl, G.E. (2009). Human replication protein A-Rad52-single-stranded DNA complex: stoichiometry and evidence for strand transfer regulation by phosphorylation. Biochemistry *48*, 6633-6643.

Dong, Y., Hakimi, M.A., Chen, X., Kumaraswamy, E., Cooch, N.S., Godwin, A.K., & Shiekhattar, R. (2003). Regulation of BRCC, a holoenzyme complex containing BRCA1 and BRCA2, by a signalosome-like subunit and its role in DNA repair. Mol Cell *12*, 1087-1099.

Dong, Z., Zhong, Q., & Chen, P.L. (1999). The Nijmegen breakage syndrome protein is essential for Mre11 phosphorylation upon DNA damage. J Biol Chem *274*, 19513-19516.

Dou, H., Huang, C., Singh, M., Carpenter, P.B., & Yeh, E.T. (2010). Regulation of DNA repair through deSUMOylation and SUMOylation of replication protein A complex. Mol Cell *39*, 333-345.

Dray, E., Etchin, J., Wiese, C., Saro, D., Williams, G.J., Hammel, M., Yu, X., Galkin, V.E., Liu, D., Tsai, M.S., *et al.* (2010). Enhancement of RAD51 recombinase activity by the tumor suppressor PALB2. Nat Struct Mol Biol *17*, 1255-1259.

Gildemeister, O.S., Sage, J.M., & Knight, K.L. (2009). Cellular redistribution of Rad51 in response to DNA damage: novel role for Rad51C. J Biol Chem *284*, 31945-31952.

Golub, E.I., Gupta, R.C., Haaf, T., Wold, M.S., & Radding, C.M. (1998). Interaction of human rad51 recombination protein with single-stranded DNA binding protein, RPA. Nucleic Acids Res *26*, 5388-5393.

Golub, E.I., Kovalenko, O.V., Gupta, R.C., Ward, D.C., & Radding, C.M. (1997). Interaction of human recombination proteins Rad51 and Rad54. Nucleic Acids Res *25*, 4106-4110.

Haaf, T., Golub, E.I., Reddy, G., Radding, C.M., and Ward, D.C. (1995). Nuclear foci of mammalian Rad51 recombination protein in somatic cells after DNA damage and its localization in synaptonemal complexes. Proc Natl Acad Sci U S A *92*, 2298-2302.

Hay, R.T. (2005). SUMO: a history of modification. Mol Cell *18*, 1-12.

Henson, S.E., Tsai, S.C., Malone, C.S., Soghomonian, S.V., Ouyang, Y., Wall, R., Marahrens, Y., & Teitell, M.A. (2006). Pir51, a Rad51-interacting protein with high expression in aggressive lymphoma, controls mitomycin C sensitivity and prevents chromosomal breaks. Mutat Res *601*, 113-124.

Holt, J.T., Toole, W.P., Patel, V.R., Hwang, H., & Brown, E.T. (2008). Restoration of CAPAN-1 cells with functional BRCA2 provides insight into the DNA repair activity of individuals who are heterozygous for BRCA2 mutations. Cancer Genet Cytogenet *186*, 85-94.

Huen, M.S., Sy, S.M., & Chen, J. (2010). BRCA1 and its toolbox for the maintenance of genome integrity. Nat Rev Mol Cell Biol *11*, 138-148.

Jasin, M. (2002). Homologous repair of DNA damage and tumorigenesis: the BRCA connection. Oncogene *21*, 8981-8993.

Kagawa, W., Kurumizaka, H., Ishitani, R., Fukai, S., Nureki, O., Shibata, T., & Yokoyama, S. (2002). Crystal structure of the homologous-pairing domain from the human Rad52 recombinase in the undecameric form. Mol Cell *10*, 359-371.

Kitao, H., & Yuan, Z.M. (2002). Regulation of ionizing radiation-induced Rad52 nuclear foci formation by c-Abl-mediated phosphorylation. J Biol Chem *277*, 48944-48948.

Kjeldsen, F., Savitski, M.M., Nielsen, M.L., Shi, L., & Zubarev, R.A. (2007). On studying protein phosphorylation patterns using bottom-up LC-MS/MS: the case of human alpha-casein. Analyst *132*, 768-776.

Kovalenko, O.V., Golub, E.I., Bray-Ward, P., Ward, D.C., & Radding, C.M. (1997). A novel nucleic acid-binding protein that interacts with human rad51 recombinase. Nucleic Acids Res *25*, 4946-4953.

Kovalenko, O.V., Plug, A.W., Haaf, T., Gonda, D.K., Ashley, T., Ward, D.C., Radding, C.M., & Golub, E.I. (1996). Mammalian ubiquitin-conjugating enzyme Ubc9 interacts with Rad51 recombination protein and localizes in synaptonemal complexes. Proc Natl Acad Sci U S A *93*, 2958-2963.

Kruh, G.D., Perego, R., Miki, T., & Aaronson, S.A. (1990). The complete coding sequence of arg defines the Abelson subfamily of cytoplasmic tyrosine kinases. Proc Natl Acad Sci U S A *87*, 5802-5806.

Kurumizaka, H., Aihara, H., Kagawa, W., Shibata, T., & Yokoyama, S. (1999). Human Rad51 amino acid residues required for Rad52 binding. J Mol Biol *291*, 537-548.

Li, W., Hesabi, B., Babbo, A., Pacione, C., Liu, J., Chen, D.J., Nickoloff, J.A., & Shen, Z. (2000). Regulation of double-strand break-induced mammalian homologous recombination by UBL1, a RAD51-interacting protein. Nucleic Acids Res *28*, 1145-1153.

Li, X., Zhang, X.P., Solinger, J.A., Kiianitsa, K., Yu, X., Egelman, E.H., & Heyer, W.D. (2007). Rad51 and Rad54 ATPase activities are both required to modulate Rad51-dsDNA filament dynamics. Nucleic Acids Res *35*, 4124-4140.

Li, Y., Shimizu, H., Xiang, S.L., Maru, Y., Takao, N., & Yamamoto, K. (2002). Arg tyrosine kinase is involved in homologous recombinational DNA repair. Biochem Biophys Res Commun *299*, 697-702.

Marmorstein, L.Y., Ouchi, T., & Aaronson, S.A. (1998). The BRCA2 gene product functionally interacts with p53 and RAD51. Proc Natl Acad Sci U S A *95*, 13869-13874.

Mazin, A.V., Alexeev, A.A., & Kowalczykowski, S.C. (2003). A novel function of Rad54 protein. Stabilization of the Rad51 nucleoprotein filament. J Biol Chem *278*, 14029-14036.

Mazin, A.V., Mazina, O.M., Bugreev, D.V., & Rossi, M.J. (2010). Rad54, the motor of homologous recombination. DNA Repair (Amst) *9*, 286-302.

Mazina, O.M., & Mazin, A.V. (2004). Human Rad54 protein stimulates DNA strand exchange activity of hRad51 protein in the presence of Ca2+. J Biol Chem *279*, 52042-52051.

McIlwraith, M.J., Van Dyck, E., Masson, J.Y., Stasiak, A.Z., Stasiak, A., & West, S.C. (2000). Reconstitution of the strand invasion step of double-strand break repair using human Rad51 Rad52 and RPA proteins. J Mol Biol *304*, 151-164.

Medova, M., Aebersold, D.M., & Zimmer, Y. MET inhibition in tumor cells by PHA665752 impairs homologous recombination repair of DNA double strand breaks. Int J Cancer.

Mizuta, R., LaSalle, J.M., Cheng, H.L., Shinohara, A., Ogawa, H., Copeland, N., Jenkins, N.A., Lalande, M., & Alt, F.W. (1997). RAB22 and RAB163/mouse BRCA2: proteins that specifically interact with the RAD51 protein. Proc Natl Acad Sci U S A *94*, 6927-6932.

Mladenov, E., Anachkova, B., & Tsaneva, I. (2006). Sub-nuclear localization of Rad51 in response to DNA damage. Genes Cells *11*, 513-524.

Modesti, M., Budzowska, M., Baldeyron, C., Demmers, J.A., Ghirlando, R., & Kanaar, R. (2007). RAD51AP1 is a structure-specific DNA binding protein that stimulates joint molecule formation during RAD51-mediated homologous recombination. Mol Cell *28*, 468-481.

Moschos, S.J., & Mo, Y.Y. (2006). Role of SUMO/Ubc9 in DNA damage repair and tumorigenesis. J Mol Histol *37*, 309-319.

Niu, H., Wan, L., Busygina, V., Kwon, Y., Allen, J.A., Li, X., Kunz, R.C., Kubota, K., Wang, B., Sung, P., *et al.* (2009). Regulation of meiotic recombination via Mek1-mediated Rad54 phosphorylation. Mol Cell *36*, 393-404.

O'Donovan, P.J., & Livingston, D.M. (2010). BRCA1 and BRCA2: breast/ovarian cancer susceptibility gene products and participants in DNA double-strand break repair. Carcinogenesis *31*, 961-967.

Park, M.S., Ludwig, D.L., Stigger, E., & Lee, S.H. (1996). Physical interaction between human RAD52 and RPA is required for homologous recombination in mammalian cells. J Biol Chem *271*, 18996-19000.

Plate, I., Hallwyl, S.C., Shi, I., Krejci, L., Muller, C., Albertsen, L., Sung, P., & Mortensen, U.H. (2008). Interaction with RPA is necessary for Rad52 repair center formation and for its mediator activity. J Biol Chem *283*, 29077-29085.

Plo, I., Laulier, C., Gauthier, L., Lebrun, F., Calvo, F., & Lopez, B.S. (2008). AKT1 inhibits homologous recombination by inducing cytoplasmic retention of BRCA1 and RAD51. Cancer Res *68*, 9404-9412.

Popova, M., Shimizu, H., Yamamoto, K., Lebechec, M., Takahashi, M., & Fleury, F. (2009). Detection of c-Abl kinase-promoted phosphorylation of Rad51 by specific antibodies reveals that Y54 phosphorylation is dependent on that of Y315. FEBS Lett *583*, 1867-1872.

Raggiaschi, R., Gotta, S., & Terstappen, G.C. (2005). Phosphoproteome analysis. Biosci Rep *25*, 33-44.

Rao, V.A., Fan, A.M., Meng, L., Doe, C.F., North, P.S., Hickson, I.D., & Pommier, Y. (2005). Phosphorylation of BLM, dissociation from topoisomerase IIIalpha, and colocalization with gamma-H2AX after topoisomerase I-induced replication damage. Mol Cell Biol *25*, 8925-8937.

Raschle, M., Van Komen, S., Chi, P., Ellenberger, T., & Sung, P. (2004). Multiple interactions with the Rad51 recombinase govern the homologous recombination function of Rad54. J Biol Chem *279*, 51973-51980.

Saitoh, H., Pizzi, M.D., & Wang, J. (2002). Perturbation of SUMOlation enzyme Ubc9 by distinct domain within nucleoporin RanBP2/Nup358. J Biol Chem *277*, 4755-4763.

San Filippo, J., Sung, P., & Klein, H. (2008). Mechanism of eukaryotic homologous recombination. Annu Rev Biochem *77*, 229-257.

Shen, Z., Cloud, K.G., Chen, D.J., & Park, M.S. (1996). Specific interactions between the human RAD51 and RAD52 proteins. J Biol Chem *271*, 148-152.

Shi, W., Feng, Z., Zhang, J., Gonzalez-Suarez, I., Vanderwaal, R.P., Wu, X., Powell, S.N., Roti Roti, J.L., & Gonzalo, S. (2010). The role of RPA2 phosphorylation in homologous recombination in response to replication arrest. Carcinogenesis *31*, 994-1002.

Sigurdsson, S., Van Komen, S., Petukhova, G., & Sung, P. (2002). Homologous DNA pairing by human recombination factors Rad51 and Rad54. J Biol Chem *277*, 42790-42794.

Sleeth, K.M., Sorensen, C.S., Issaeva, N., Dziegielewski, J., Bartek, J., & Helleday, T. (2007). RPA mediates recombination repair during replication stress and is displaced from DNA by checkpoint signalling in human cells. J Mol Biol *373*, 38-47.

Slupianek, A., Dasgupta, Y., Ren, S., Cramer, K., & Skorski, T. (2009). Targeting BCR/ABL-RAD51 Interaction to Prevent Unfaithful Homeologous Recombination Repair In 51st ASH Annual Meeting and Exposition.

Slupianek, A., Schmutte, C., Tombline, G., Nieborowska-Skorska, M., Hoser, G., Nowicki, M.O., Pierce, A.J., Fishel, R., & Skorski, T. (2001). BCR/ABL regulates mammalian RecA homologs, resulting in drug resistance. Mol Cell *8*, 795-806.

Solinger, J.A., Kiianitsa, K., & Heyer, W.D. (2002). Rad54, a Swi2/Snf2-like recombinational repair protein, disassembles Rad51:dsDNA filaments. Mol Cell *10*, 1175-1188.

Sorensen, C.S., Hansen, L.T., Dziegielewski, J., Syljuasen, R.G., Lundin, C., Bartek, J., & Helleday, T. (2005). The cell-cycle checkpoint kinase Chk1 is required for mammalian homologous recombination repair. Nat Cell Biol *7*, 195-201.

Sugiyama, T., & Kowalczykowski, S.C. (2002). Rad52 protein associates with replication protein A (RPA)-single-stranded DNA to accelerate Rad51-mediated displacement of RPA and presynaptic complex formation. J Biol Chem *277*, 31663-31672.

Symington, L.S. (2002). Role of RAD52 epistasis group genes in homologous recombination and double-strand break repair. Microbiol Mol Biol Rev *66*, 630-670, table of contents.

Takata, M., Sasaki, M.S., Tachiiri, S., Fukushima, T., Sonoda, E., Schild, D., Thompson, L.H., & Takeda, S. (2001). Chromosome instability and defective recombinational repair in knockout mutants of the five Rad51 paralogs. Mol Cell Biol *21*, 2858-2866.

Takizawa, Y., Kinebuchi, T., Kagawa, W., Yokoyama, S., Shibata, T., & Kurumizaka, H. (2004). Mutational analyses of the human Rad51-Tyr315 residue, a site for phosphorylation in leukaemia cells. Genes Cells *9*, 781-790.

Tan, T.L., Essers, J., Citterio, E., Swagemakers, S.M., de Wit, J., Benson, F.E., Hoeijmakers, J.H., & Kanaar, R. (1999). Mouse Rad54 affects DNA conformation and DNA-damage-induced Rad51 foci formation. Curr Biol *9*, 325-328.

Tripathi, V., Nagarjuna, T., & Sengupta, S. (2007). BLM helicase-dependent and -independent roles of 53BP1 during replication stress-mediated homologous recombination. J Cell Biol *178*, 9-14.

Wold, M.S. (1997). Replication protein A: a heterotrimeric, single-stranded DNA-binding protein required for eukaryotic DNA metabolism. Annu Rev Biochem *66*, 61-92.

Wolner, B., & Peterson, C.L. (2005). ATP-dependent and ATP-independent roles for the Rad54 chromatin remodeling enzyme during recombinational repair of a DNA double strand break. J Biol Chem *280*, 10855-10860.

Wong, A.K., Pero, R., Ormonde, P.A., Tavtigian, S.V., & Bartel, P.L. (1997). RAD51 interacts with the evolutionarily conserved BRC motifs in the human breast cancer susceptibility gene brca2. J Biol Chem *272*, 31941-31944.

Wu, L., & Hickson, I.D. (2003). The Bloom's syndrome helicase suppresses crossing over during homologous recombination. Nature *426*, 870-874.

Wu, X., Yang, Z., Liu, Y., & Zou, Y. (2005). Preferential localization of hyperphosphorylated replication protein A to double-strand break repair and checkpoint complexes upon DNA damage. Biochem J *391*, 473-480.

Yuan, S.S., Lee, S.Y., Chen, G., Song, M., Tomlinson, G.E., & Lee, E.Y. (1999). BRCA2 is required for ionizing radiation-induced assembly of Rad51 complex in vivo. Cancer Res *59*, 3547-3551.

Yuan, Z.M., Huang, Y., Ishiko, T., Nakada, S., Utsugisawa, T., Kharbanda, S., Wang, R., Sung, P., Shinohara, A., Weichselbaum, R., & Kufe, D. (1998). Regulation of Rad51 function by c-Abl in response to DNA damage. J Biol Chem *273*, 3799-3802.

Zhong, Q., Chen, C.F., Li, S., Chen, Y., Wang, C.C., Xiao, J., Chen, P.L., Sharp, Z.D., & Lee, W.H. (1999). Association of BRCA1 with the hRad50-hMre11-p95 complex and the DNA damage response. Science *285*, 747-750.

10

Post-Transcriptional Regulation of E2F Transcription Factors: Fine-Tuning DNA Repair, Cell Cycle Progression and Survival in Development & Disease

Lina Dagnino, Randeep Kaur Singh and David Judah
University of Western Ontario
Canada

1. Introduction

Cells are continually exposed to genotoxic stresses. Upon DNA damage, the cell activates a coordinated and complex series of responses (Levitt and Hickson, 2002). Multiple factors are implicated in each of these responses. Recently, it has become apparent that various transcription factors play important roles in cellular responses to genotoxic stress. In particular, E2F transcription factors are key for the activation of genes involved in these processes.

E2F family comprises two subfamilies, termed E2F and DP, and includes orthologs expressed across many species, from plants to higher vertebrates (McClellan and Slack, 2007). In mammals, multiple E2F (E2F-1 through -8) and DP (DP-1 through -4) genes have been identified. E2F-1, -2 and -3 are associated with DNA synthesis and cell cycle progression, and function as heterodimers with a DP member (McClellan and Slack, 2007). E2F-4 and -5 also require association with a DP protein, but often function to halt cell cycle progression associated with terminal differentiation or reversible entry into quiescence (McClellan and Slack, 2007). E2F-1 through -5 can mediate transcriptional activation when found as "free" E2F/DP dimers, but can also act as transcriptional repressors if they are associated with a member of the retinoblastoma (pRb) family of proteins (Hallstrom and Nevins, 2009). In contrast, E2F-6 lacks both transcriptional activation and pRb-binding domains, and functions as a constitutive transcriptional repressor. The most divergent members of the E2F family are E2F-7 and -8, which bind neither DP nor pRb-family proteins, and also function as transcriptional repressors to mediate cell cycle arrest (Lammens et al., 2009). To regulate gene expression, E2F factors bind GC-rich elements on proximal promoters, which can conform to either a consensus 5' -TTTC[CG]CGC-3' element, or to non-consensus sequences (Judah et al., 2010; Rabinovich et al., 2008). Considerable efforts have been directed to investigate whether different E2F proteins exhibit target selectivity. Genome-wide screens for E2F targets have revealed considerable overlap in the ability of individual E2F proteins to regulate their targets, although a few promoters activated by specific E2F forms have been identified (Cao et al., 2011).

In spite of the vast similarities in the activities of distinct E2F proteins and their ability to bind potential target Genes, to-date E2F1 is the principal E2F member shown to participate in cellular responses to DNA damage (Bracken et al., 2004). The role of E2F-1 upon DNA damage depends on cellular context. E2F-1 can either induce pro-apoptotic or anti-apoptotic outcomes. During the latter, E2F-1 can play roles to induce cell cycle arrest and upregulate DNA repair, by directing expression of multiple genes. These genes are involved in mismatch repair (MSH2, MLH1), nucleotide excision repair (DDB2, RPA), homologous recombination repair (RAD51, RAD54, RECQL), base excision repair (UNG, APE) & non-homologous end joining (Chang et al., 2006; Ishida et al., 2001; Polager and Ginsberg, 2008; Prost et al., 2007).
In humans, E2F-1 is a 437 amino acid protein, which shows constitutive and rapid nucleocytoplasmic shuttling in a variety of cells (Ivanova et al., 2007). E2F-1 stimulates cell proliferation by positively modulating transcription of genes necessary for DNA synthesis and cell cycle progression (Ivanova et al., 2005). In an apparently paradoxical manner, E2F-1 can also induce cell cycle arrest when associated with pRb, or apoptosis, by activating expression of pro-apoptotic genes (Polager and Ginsberg, 2008). The breadth of E2F-1 targets mediates the distinct biological activities of this transcription factor, which encompass both oncogenic and anti-oncogenic properties, as well as positive modulation of tissue regeneration after injury (D'Souza et al., 2002; Field et al., 1996).

2. E2F-1 and the DNA damage response

Genotoxic stress in cells activates the DNA damage response, and can occur as a result of a variety of insults. The latter include DNA double- strand breaks and single-strand damage. DNA damage can result from exogenous agents (e.g. radiation, exposure to reactive and mutagenic chemicals), or from endogenous products of cell metabolism (Shiloh, 2003). In response to DNA damage, cells activate multiple pathways that result in apoptosis or in DNA repair, cell cycle arrest, changes in gene expression, as well as in protein synthesis and degradation.
Cells require efficient response mechanisms to genotoxic stress, as this is a life-threatening event because it can significantly alter their genetic material. Multiple mechanisms have evolved to repair damage induced by genotoxic stress, including activation of a global signalling network termed the DNA damage response (DDR), which is capable of detecting distinct types of DNA damage, coordinating appropriate responses. The latter include transcriptional activation, cell cycle arrest, apoptosis, senescence and DNA repair (Shiloh, 2003). The DNA damage response plays a critical role in cell survival when damage occurs during DNA replication. In addition, there are specialized processes, including base-excision repair (BER), nucleotide-excision repair (NER) & nonhomologous end-joining, which recognize and repair specific types of lesions (Shiloh, 2003). Central to transduce signals that indicate DNA damage and initiate appropriate cellular responses are two related protein kinases, termed ATM (ataxia telangiectasia mutated) and ATR (ATM and Rad3-related). ATM can associate with its regulator, the MRN (Mre11-Rad50-NMS1) complex, when double-strand breaks (DSB) are generated (Levitt and Hickson, 2002). On the other hand, ATR forms complexes with its regulator ATRIP (ATR-interacting protein), which senses single-strand DNA (ssDNA) breaks generated by processing of double-strand breaks, as well as single-strand DNA which arises from stalled replication forks (Shiloh, 2003). These two kinases also phosphorylate E2F-1, thus initiating transcriptional activation of its target DNA repair genes.

2.1 Identification of E2F targets involved in DNA damage repair

Central to understanding the role of the E2F family of transcription factors in DNA repair has been the identification of a large number of putative and demonstrated E2F target genes. Although E2F proteins were originally characterized as important regulators of cell cycle progression, genome-wide screens have demonstrated much broader roles in a variety of primary and immortalized cell types. For example, E2F-1 and E2F-3 bind to the promoters of apurinic/apyrimidinic endonuclease (APE) and other repair enzymes in human primary epidermal keratinocytes, irrespective of their differentiation status (Chang et al., 2006). Similarly, in the GM06990 lymphoblastoid cell line, non-biased genome-wide screening has identified a large number of putative E2F-4 targets involved in responses to DNA damage (Lee et al., 2011). E2F targets important for DNA repair have also been identified in neoplastic cells following therapeutic intervention. For example, treatment of prostate cancer cells with histone deacetylase inhibitors reduces their ability to repair DNA damage induced by radio- and chemotherapy, thus reducing tumour mass (Kachhap et al., 2010). The impaired ability to repair DNA of treated cells was due, at least in part, to decreased recruitment to and activation by E2F-1 to the promoters of key DNA repair genes. Hence, the importance of E2F factors in DNA repair encompasses not only events during carcinogenesis, but also the potential impact of various therapies.

2.2 Role of E2F-1 in responses to DNA damage induced by UV radiation

UV radiation induces severe DNA damage, which is the principal cause of skin carcinogenesis in humans (Brash et al., 1996). UV-B radiation induces formation of cyclobutane pyrimidine dimers (CPD) and pyrimidine (6-4) pyrimidone photoproducts (6-4PP), which would result in loss of DNA integrity and genetic instability if left unrepaired. This type of damage to DNA triggers activation of the nucleotide-excision repair pathway, and can occur *via* one or more streams. Such DNA repair streams include (i) global genome repair (GGR), which repairs damage from the entire genome, (ii) transcription-coupled repair (TCR), which generally repairs damage on actively transcribed DNA strands & (iii) transcription domain-associated repair (DAR), which deals with repairing both strands of actively transcribed regions (Nouspikel, 2009).

Normal responses of the epidermis to UV damage are critically dependent on E2F-1 expression. Indeed, increased levels of epidermal apoptosis upon UV-B irradiation have been reported in E2F-1-null mouse epidermis, whereas repair of UV-B-induced DNA photoproducts is more efficient in keratinocytes that overexpress E2F-1 (Berton et al., 2005). UV-induced DNA damage results in stabilization of E2F-1 protein, which stimulates nucleotide excision repair (Berton et al., 2005; Pediconi et al., 2003; Wikonkal et al., 2003). The mechanisms involved include phosphorylation of E2F-1 on Ser31 by ATR and/or ATM kinases (Lin et al., 2001). This modification facilitates E2F-1 recruitment to sites of double-strand breaks or UV-induced DNA damage. Under these conditions, E2F-1 interacts with two key proteins involved in DNA repair: TopBP1 and GCN5 histone acetyltransferase (Guo et al., 2010a; Guo et al., 2010b). Formation of these E2F-1 complexes is necessary for efficient recruitment of factors involved in nucleotide excision repair. Importantly, the association of E2F-1 with TopBP1 and GCN5 occurs at the expense of the E2F-1-induced expression of pro-apoptotic p73, thus ensuring that DNA repair, rather than apoptosis, takes place (Berton et al., 2005; Pediconi et al., 2003; Wikonkal et al., 2003). In mouse embryo fibroblasts, UV-C irradiation results in the formation of both CPD and 6-4PP. In these cells, nucleotide excision repair is activated through pathways that involve activation of xeroderma pigmentosum

(XPC) gene expression by E2F-1 *via* increased binding to the XPC promoter (Lin et al., 2009). XPC is an essential mediator of DNA damage recognition during global genomic repair, and this phase of repair is actually more efficient in pRB-deficient cells, likely because lack of pRb increases E2F-1 activity.

The importance of E2F in repair of DNA damage induced by UV radiation is further demonstrated by the conservation of this pathway through evolution. For example, in *Arabidopsis* and in maize, MSH2 and MSH6, which are two genes that belong to the mismatch repair system, are targets of E2F transcriptional activation following DNA damage by UV-B radiation (Lario et al., 2011).

2.3 E2F is a key factor to maintain the balance between cell cycle arrest and expression of DNA repair genes following DNA damage

Given the key roles that pRb family proteins play in the regulation of E2F activity, it is not surprising that they also modulate the function of E2F factors following DNA damage. For example, the zinc finger-containing transcriptional repressor ZBRK1 is an important modulator of GADD45A transcription. The latter is involved in induction of cell cycle arrest in response to DNA damage (Siafakas and Richardson, 2009). E2F-1, but not other E2F proteins, binds to the ZBRK1 promoter, together with pRb, CtIP and CtBP, forming repressor complexes that interfere with ZBRK1 expression (Liao et al., 2010). In pRb-deficient cells, increased susceptibility to DNA damage induced by UV radiation or methylating agents occurs, partly as a result of abnormal cell cycle arrest and DNA repair. In a similar manner, E2F-1 is essential for normal expression of XRCC1 (x-ray repair cross-complementation group 1), which participates in the repair of single-strand breaks, thus ensuring efficient repair following DNA damage induced by methylating agents (Chen et al., 2008).

In contrast, loss of pRb can improve DNA repair in other circumstances, such as those involving activation of DDB2. Mutations in the *DDB2* gene, which encodes a protein involved in global genomic repair and repair of CPDs, gives rise to xeroderma pigmentosum, a disorder associated with increased risk of cutaneous and ocular tumours (Bennett and Itoh, 2008). DDB2 expression is positively regulated by E2F-1 and E2F-3. Further, deletion of pRb increases DDB2 mRNA and protein levels, together with ability of these cells to repair DNA damage. The latter is associated with more efficient CPD removal relative to that in pRb-expressing cells (Prost et al., 2007).

Solid tumours frequently exhibit hypoxic cores, which contribute to genetic instability within the tumour microenvironment (Bindra et al., 2005). This is partly due to decreased expression of DNA mismatch genes (MLH1 and MSH2), as well as repair genes (RAD51 and BRCA1). E2F factors can also be involved in the downregulation of some of these repair genes, in apparent contrast to their pro-repair roles in other circumstances. Specifically, hypoxic conditions result in the dephosphorylation of the pRb family member p130, which then associates with E2F-4 in the nucleus. This complex can efficiently bind to E2F sites on the RAD51 and BRCA1 promoters, thus interfering with their transcription (Bindra et al., 2005). Thus, E2F factors can positively or negatively regulate DNA repair, depending on cellular context. Given that E2F-4/p130 complexes are also important for cell cycle exit, a balance must exist between these two outcomes, which is essential to avoid increased genetic instability in transformed cells and their clonal expansion.

2.4 Role of E2F-1 in senescence-associated DNA damage

Senescence is defined as irreversible cell cycle arrest, which occurs both in cultured cells and *in vivo* (Lanigan et al., 2011). Senescence has been recognized as a key mechanism that acts as a barrier to tumour formation and progression. Thus, in spite of any DNA damage that may exist in a long-lived cell, if this cell is senescent it will not undergo clonal expansion to generate daughter cells with altered DNA. A number of molecular mechanisms control cellular senesce, and the E2F/pRb pathway is a key component (Lanigan et al., 2011). Under normal circumstances, the frequency of DNA mutations increases with age. DNA mismatch mutation repair is very efficient in mesenchymal cells from young individuals, as well as in embryonic fibroblasts (Chang et al., 2008). In contrast, these mechanisms are less efficient in senescent cells, in which MSH2 expression is decreased. Associated with these abnormalities is the inhibition of E2F-1 transcriptional activity, which leads to repression of MSH2 gene transcription. Thus, E2F-1 activity is essential to maintain normal capacity of cells to repair mismatch mutations. Whether the reduced activity of E2F-1 also increases the risk of transformation in senescent cells probably depends on cell context, extent of DNA damage, and presence of other oncogenic stimuli.

2.5 Role of E2F/DP interactions in DNA repair

The interactions between E2F-1 through -6 and their partner DP proteins are essential for normal transcriptional activity, and can also contribute to abnormal regulation of DNA repair factors. Again, depending on the exact context, E2F/DP interactions can positively or negatively modulate DNA repair. For example, following DNA damage by a variety of agents, including doxorubicin, etoposide and UV radiation, the abundance of DP-4 protein is substantially increased, replacing other DP proteins in E2F-1-containing complexes (Ingram et al., 2011). As a result, the capacity of E2F-1 to bind target promoters is strongly reduced, which can result in downregulation of cell cycle regulatory and/or DNA repair genes.

A positive modulatory role in DNA nucleotide excision repair through inhibition of repressor E2F complexes has been recently attributed to p14^{Arf} (Dominguez-Brauer et al., 2009). Specifically, DNA damage induces p14^{Arf} expression, which directly binds to DP-1, disrupting its interactions with E2F-4. As a result, repressive E2F-4/p130 complexes lose their ability to bind promoters of genes such as XPC, resulting in upregulation of their expression.

To-date, multiple mechanisms that regulate E2F-1 activity at the post-transcriptional level have been identified, although only a handful has been studied in the context of DNA repair. These forms of regulation of E2F-1 activity can have important consequences on its ability to modulate DNA damage responses, as discussed below.

3. Role of miRNAs in E2F regulation of cell growth and DNA repair

MicroRNAs (miRNAs) are short nucleotide sequences (~21-24nt) that pair with the 3'-untranslated regions of target mRNAs. They negatively regulate gene expression by mediating degradation of the target mRNA, or by inhibition of protein translation (Almeida et al., 2011). Small miRNAs regulate many cellular processes, such as apoptosis, differentiation, and proliferation. They are upregulated in many human disorders, including cancer and neurological diseases (Almeida et al., 2011). To-date, approximately 800 miRNAs have been identified in humans. A single miRNA can target multiple mRNAs (Griffiths-

Jones, 2004). Consistent with their role in cancer, miRNAs control cell proliferation by regulating E2F factors and, thereby, expression of genes that are important for cell cycle progression.
The E2F signalling pathway is regulated by many different types of miRNA clusters, including *miRNA-17-92, miRNA-106b-25, miRNA-34, miRNA330-3p, miRNA-128, miRNA-195, miRNA-37 and miRNA-193a,* as described below.

3.1 Growth-promoting miRNAs

O' Donnell et al. were the first to provide evidence that E2F is a target for miRNAs (O'Donnell et al., 2005). They showed that miRNA-17 and miRNA-20a decrease E2F-1 translation efficiency. This type of regulation prevents uncontrolled activation of E2F-1 during normal cell cycle progression. Disruption of miRNA-17 and miRNA-20a leads to improperly timed expression of E2F-1, resulting in the accumulation of DNA double strand breaks (Pickering et al., 2009).
An auto-regulatory loop between E2F-1 and E2F-3 and the miRNA-17-92 clusters has been demonstrated. E2F-1 and E2F-3 bind to and upregulate the transcription of the miRNA-17-92 cluster. In turn, the miRNA-17-92 cluster downregulates expression of these two transcription factors (Sylvestre et al., 2007; Woods et al., 2007). This negative feedback loop is important to prevent the accumulation of E2F-1 and E2F-3, thereby allowing proper progression of the cell cycle, preventing apoptosis. Another negative feedback loop has been observed between the miRNA-106b-25 clusters and E2F-1 (Petrocca et al., 2008). miRNA106b and miRNA93 downregulate E2F-1 expression. Reciprocally, transcription of these miRNAs is activated by E2F-1. In this manner, properly timed expression of E2F-1 during the G1/S transition is maintained, as the presence of these miRNAs prevents continuous E2F-1 expression throughout the cell cycle, which would induce apoptosis.

3.2 Tumor suppressor miRNAs

The E2F signalling pathway is also regulated by the miRNA-34 family of clusters (Tazawa et al., 2007). miRNA-34b decreases E2F-1 and E2F-3 transcript levels in a p53-dependent manner, inhibiting cell proliferation and inducing senescence in tumour cells. This demonstrates that miRNAs can function as tumor suppressors. A similar role has been suggested for miRNA-195 (Xu et al., 2009), miRNA-128 (Cui et al., 2010), miRNA-330-3p (Lee et al., 2009) and miRNA193a (Kozaki et al., 2008).
Overexpression of miRNA-195 causes cell cycle arrest at the G1/S boundary, by interfering with the expression of cell cycle regulatory proteins, such E2F-3, Cyclin D1 and cyclin-dependent kinase 6 (CDK6). As a result, pRb remains hypophosphorylated, allowing activation of E2F-dependent target genes (Xu et al., 2009). Exogenous expression of miRNA-127 in glioma cells represses E2F-3a translation, thereby decreasing cell proliferation (Cui et al., 2010). Similarly, in oral squamous cell carcinoma, miRNA193a significantly represses cell growth and down-regulates E2F-6 translation (Kozaki et al., 2008).

3.3 Role of miRNAs in modulation of DNA repair by E2F-1

Several miRNA clusters, including *mir17-92, mir-106a-92* and *mir106b-25,* are downregulated by p53 via E2F-dependent mechanisms. This leads to decreased proliferation and/or promotes senescence in normal and transformed cells (Brosh et al., 2008). In addition, in response to mitogenic stimulation, E2F-1 activates transcription of the miRNA clusters *let-*

7a-d, *mir-15b-16-2* and *mir-106b-25* during the G1/S transition (Bueno et al., 2010). These miRNAs, in turn, regulate E2F-1 activity. In their absence, E2F-1 induces entry into S phase, but also DNA damage. Indeed, E2F-1 and other oncogenes can induce stalling and collapsing of DNA replication forks, leading to the formation of DNA double-strand breaks (Halazonetis et al., 2008). Thus, *let-7a-d*, *mir-15b-16-2* and *mir-106b-25* play key roles in prevention of DNA damage and replicative stress associated with abnormal regulation of E2F-1 (Zhang et al., 2011).

4. Regulation of E2F-1 by post-translational modifications

Another mode of E2F regulation that fine-tunes cell cycle progression and DNA repair occurs at the post-translational level. Post-translational modifications identified in E2F-1 include phosphorylation, acetylation, methylation & ubiquitination. These modifications can exert either activating or inhibitory effects on E2F-1 transcriptional activity.

4.1 Acetylation

E2F-1 is acetylated at three highly conserved lysine residues (K117, K120 and K125) by the p300/CREB-binding protein (CBP) or by p300/CBP-associated factor (P/CAF) acetyltransferase (Martinez-Balbas et al., 2000; Marzio et al., 2000). P/CAF directly interacts with E2F-1 through its adenosine deaminase 2 (ADA2) binding domain (Martinez-Balbas et al., 2000). Acetylation of E2F-1 allows for marked stabilization and significant increase in E2F-1 protein levels. This leads to an increase in transcriptional activation of E2F-1 target genes (Farhana et al., 2002; Martinez-Balbas et al., 2000).

Increases in E2F-1 protein levels upon DNA damage are partly due to cell type-specific acetylation (Blattner et al., 1999; Meng et al., 1999; Zhu et al., 1999). For example, adriamycin-mediated treatment induces E2F-1 acetylation in human glioblastoma T98G cells (Pediconi et al., 2003) , but not in HeLa cells (Ozaki et al., 2009). In response to DNA damage, E2F-1 switches to activate pro-apoptotic gene expression, rather than cell cycle progression. This change requires E2F-1 acetylation and recruitment to promoters of pro-apoptotic target genes, such as p73 (Pediconi et al., 2003). P/CAF, but not p300, is required for E2F-1 stabilization upon DNA damage by doxorubicin (Ianari et al., 2004). On the other hand, overexpression of p300 can be sufficient for acetylation and stabilization of E2F-1 in cells treated with camptothecin, a drug that causes double strand break during DNA replication (Galbiati et al., 2005). The distinct actions of these two acetyltransferase can thus determine the outcome of cellular responses by modulating cellular DNA damage checkpoints (p300) or apoptotic events (P/CAF). The stabilization of E2F-1 by acetylation could also allow it to directly interact with activating signal cointegrator-2 (ASC-2), a mitogenic transcription factor co-activator that regulates cellular proliferation and cell cycle progression (Kong et al., 2003).

4.2 Phosphorylation

E2F-1 is phosphorylated on several residues, giving rise to modifications that can alter different functional aspects. E2F-1 was first identified as a substrate for phosphorylation in a cell-free system (Bagchi et al., 1989). This post-translational modification interfered with E2F-1 DNA binding activity. Consistent with these observations, E2F-1 and E2F-3 showed decreased DNA binding capacity upon phosphorylation by cyclin A-activated cyclin-dependent kinase 2 (cdk2) (Dynlacht et al., 1997; Krek et al., 1995). Complexes containing cyclin A, cdk2, E2F-1, and DP-1 are formed during Late S-phase to terminate E2F-dependent DNA binding and transcription, and enable orderly S-phase progression (Krek et al., 1995). In the absence of cyclin A-cdk2 activity, there is decreased E2F-1 phosphorylation and increased DNA binding activity (Li et al., 1997). This results in S-phase delay and/or arrest, by mechanisms that involve transcriptional activation of E2F-dependent cell cycle checkpoint genes. Together, these data demonstrate that E2F-1 phosphorylation is essential for timely activation of E2F-1 function and orderly cell cycle progression and survival. A second proline-directed kinase, c-Jun N-terminal protein kinase (JNK1), can phosphorylate E2F-1 in response to stress stimuli mediated by tumor necrosis factor-alpha, decreasing its ability to bind DNA and activate target gene transcription (Kishore et al., 2003).

Following DNA damage, Chk2 and ATM phosphorylate E2F-1 on Ser364 and Ser31, respectively (Lin et al., 2001). E2F-1 phosphorylated on Ser31 subsequently interacts with 14-3-3τ (Wang et al., 2004). This interaction prevents E2F-1 association with the **S**KP1-**C**ullin-**F**-box/ S-phase kinase-associated protein 2 (SCF^{Skp2}) ubiquitin ligase. As a result, E2F-1 is not ubiquitinated and is protected from degradation. The net result of phosphorylation of E2F-1 at Ser31 and Ser364 after DNA damage is activation of the pro-apoptotic gene p73, as well as accumulation of p53 through upregulation of $p19^{ARF}$ expression. The latter protein inhibits ubiquitination and degradation of p53, inducing apoptosis (Weber et al., 1999). In additon, the ATM and Chk2 promoters are activated by E2F-1, thereby forming a positive feedback pathway that promotes apoptosis (Berkovich and Ginsberg, 2003) .

The phosphorylation of E2F can also affect its ability to interact with other proteins. In *Drosophila melanogaster*, phosphorylation of E2F-1 and E2F-2 enhances their ability to interact with the SCF^{slmb} ubiquitin ligase complex, targetting it for degradation during S phase (Heriche et al., 2003). *In vitro*, E2F-1 is phosphorylated at Ser337 by complexes containing $p34^{cdc2}$ and cyclin B (Dynlacht et al., 1997). The significance of this finding is not clear, as E2F-1 phosphorylation on these residues occurs during late G1 phase, and is mediated by cyclin D-cdk4 complexes (Mann and Jones, 1996). Phosphorylation of E2F-1 at Ser332 and Ser337 enhances E2F-1 interactions with the adenovirus E4 protein, simultaneously attenuating its ability to bind pRb (Fagan et al., 1994). Upon adenovirus infection, the enhanced interaction between E2F-1 and E4 increases the efficiency of E2A transcription, which is required for viral DNA replication (Hardy et al., 1989).

Changes in phosphorylation status also modulate the activity and subcellular localization of E2F-4 and E2F-5, although these changes are unlikely to be mediated by cyclin A-dependent cdk activity (Dynlacht et al., 1997). Regulation of E2F-4 and E2F-5 by phosphorylation is important during entry into quiescence associated with cell differentiation, but varies depending on the cell type. For example, hypophosphorylated forms of E3F-4 efficiently associate with p130 in the nucleus, forming transcriptional repressor complexes associated with growth arrest in muscle cells (Shin et al., 1995). In contrast, in human intestinal crypt cells, hypophosphorylated E2F-4 is imported into the nucleus in response to mitogenic stimuli or inhibition of p38 MAP kinase, where it activate genes necessary for S phase entry (Deschenes et al., 2004).

E2F-5 is phosphorylated by cyclin E/cdk2 complexes on Thr251 in the transcriptional activation domain, stimulating cell cycle progression (Morris et al., 2000). This modification stabilizes E2F-5 interaction with the co-activator p300/CBP, resulting in transcription of genes required for DNA synthesis. Significantly, phosphorylation of E2F-5 at Thr251 does not affect its DNA binding activity, intracellular localization or ability to interact with pRb family proteins.

In epidermal keratinocytes, E2F-1 is tightly regulated during normal proliferation and differentiation (Ivanova and Dagnino, 2007; Ivanova et al., 2009; Wong et al., 2003). E2F-1 is localized in the nucleus in undifferentiated keratinocytes, but differentiation induces its export to the cytoplasm, where it is degraded. The signaling pathways involved in E2F-1 turnover in differentiating keratinocytes involve activation by Ca^{2+} of protein kinase C eta and delta, followed by activation of p38β. The latter appears to phosphorylate E2F-1 at Ser403 and Thr433. Once E2F-1 is phosphorylated, it is exported from the nucleus in a CRM1-dependent fashion, and degraded in the proteasome. This sequence of events involving E2F-1 phosphorylation, ubiquitination, nuclear export and subsequent degradation is required for proper keratinocyte differentiation (Ivanova et al., 2006; Ivanova and Dagnino, 2007; Ivanova et al., 2009).

E2F-1 degradation subsequent to phosphorylation also occurs in HeLa cells. Specifically, phosphorylation of E2F-1 at Ser403 and Thr433 by TFIIH-cdk7 targets E2F-1 for degradation during S phase (Vandel and Kouzarides, 1999). Phosphorylation at Ser403 is also induced upon DNA damage (Real et al., 2010). Ser403 and Thr433 in E2F-1 are also phosphorylated by glycogen synthase kinase-3β (GSK3β) in HEK293T cells (Garcia-Alvarez et al., 2007). In U2OS osteosarcoma cells treated with doxorubicin, Ser403 is phosphorylated, but is not a substrate of either p38 MAP or GSK3β kinases (Real et al., 2010). Under these conditions, phosphorylation of Ser403 results in changes in E2F-1 target selectivity. Thus, the mechanisms and consequences of E2F-1 phosphorylation on Ser403 appear to be cell-type and context dependent (Ivanova et al., 2009).

4.3 Methylation

Lysine methylation plays critical regulatory roles for histones and non-histone proteins (Huang et al., 2008). The consequences of methylation on E2F-1 activity are controversial at present. E2F-1 is methylated by Set9, a histone H3 methyltransferase, at Lys185, both *in vitro* and in cultured cells (Kontaki et al., 2010, Xie et al., 2011). It has been reported that DNA damage in p53-deficent H1299 lung carcinoma cells is associated with loss of E2F-1 methylation by the lysine-specific demethylase 1(LSD1). Demethylation stabilizes E2F-1, allowing its upregulation of p73. Importantly, methylation of E2F-1 at Lys185 impairs its acetylation and phosphorylation on Ser364, targeting E2F-1 for ubiquitination and degradation in doxorubicin-treated cells (Kontaki et al., 2010). In stark contrast, methylation of E2F-1 at Lys185 by Set9 in U2OS and HCT116 cells treated with adriamycin resulted in E2F-1 stabilization and cell apoptosis (Xie et al., 2011). The reasons for these pronounced discrepancies are not clear.

4.4 Ubiquitination

Many studies have shown that the expression of E2F-1 is regulated by the ubiquitin proteasome pathway, and that E2F-1 is protected from degradation by binding to pRb (Campanero and Flemington, 1997; Hateboer et al., 1996; Hofmann et al., 1996). In mammalian and plant cells, E2F-1 is regulated at the S/G2 phases of the cell cycle through ubiquitination by the SCF^{SKP2}-dependent pathway (del Pozo et al., 2002; Marti et al., 1999). *In vitro*, ROC-cullin ligase ubiquitinates E2F-1 in a Skp2-independent manner. Further, phosphorylation of E2F-1 by cyclin A/cdk complexes does not affect E2F-1 ubiquitination (Ohta and Xiong, 2001). Another E3 ubiquitin ligase complex, the anaphase-promoting complex or cyclosome (ACPC/C), also regulates E2F-1 stability during late S phase (Peart et al., 2010). The presence of multiple E3 ligases that interact with and mediate degradation of E2F-1 enables orderly control of E2F-1 expression under multiple circumstances.

5. Regulation of E2F activity by protein-protein interactions

The first type of protein-protein interactions shown to modulate E2F transcriptional activity included association with the retinoblastoma family of proteins (pRB, p107 and p130). pRB is a key regulator of E2F-1, -2 and -3 activity and G1/S-phase transition (Weintraub et al., 1995). The importance of pRb regulation of E2F is evidenced by the fact that a majority of human tumours exhibit inactivating alterations in the pRb pathway (Nevins, 2001). Subsequent studies have revealed thet E2F forms complexes with a multitude of additional proteins, underlining the levels of complexity of E2F regulation.

Protein-protein interactions also appear to assist or provide target specificity to E2F under certain conditions. This effects appear to involve cooperative interactions between E2F and other transcription factors, mediated by binding to neighbouring consensus sites on target promoters. Consensus binding sites for various transcription factors have been identified in the promoters of a subset of E2F target genes. These sites are generally adjacent to the E2F binding sites, and include recognition sequences for YY1, TFE3, and C/EBPα (Schlisio et al., 2002; van Ginkel et al., 1997). These sites possess biological significance, and assist E2F in binding to its consensus sequence. This determines the specific phase of the cell cycle in which E2F activates such promoters. In addition, as these other transcription factors do not interact equally well with all E2F members, they constitute a mechanism of activation of individual E2F factors (Giangrande et al., 2003; Schlisio et al., 2002).

5.1 Retinoblastoma family proteins

pRb binds predominantly to E2F-1, E2F-2, and E2F-3, blocking their transactivation domains (Flemington et al., 1993; Xiao et al., 2003). Under certain circumstances, such as during responses to transforming growth factor-beta in certain cell lines, pRb also binds E2F-4 and represses transcription (Yang, et al. 2008). The pRb family of proteins can also repress transcription of E2F target genes by recruiting other factors, such as histone deacetylases, thus creating transcriptional repressor complexes (Dick, 2007; Morrison et al., 2002; Herrera et al., 1996). pRb is, in turn, regulated by cyclin and cyclin-dependent kinases (Cdk),which deactivate pRb through phosphorylation. Specifically, Cyclin D/Cdk4 and Cyclin E/Cdk2 complexes phosphorylate pRb in the G1 phase of the cell cycle, allowing E2F-1, E2F-2 and E2F-3 to activate target genes (Connell-Crowley et al., 1997; Smith et al., 1996). The other pRb family proteins, p107 and p130, generally bind to E2F-4 and E2F-5, and function to modulate their nucleocytoplasmic shuttling during different periods of the cell cycle. Specifically, E2F-4 and E2F-5 translocate into the nucleus outside of the G1 and S-phases, and act as transcriptional repressors in complexes containing p107 and p130 (Ginsberg et al., 1994; Moberg et al., 1996) (Hijmans et al., 1995) (Guo et al., 2009).

5.2 DP proteins

Optimal binding of E2F to DNA requires cooperative interactions with a member of the other subfamily of E2F proteins, the DP (Dimerization Partner) family. In fact, with the exception of E2F-7 and -8, all functional E2F complexes identified contain a member of the E2F family associated with a DP protein. The DP family is composed of three known members, DP-1 (with isoforms DP-1α and DP-1β), DP-2 (and its mouse orthologue DP-3), and DP-4 (Helin and Harlow, 1994; Milton et al., 2006; Ormondroyd et al., 1995). Different DP proteins have distinct modulatory effects on E2F. For example, DP-1β can mediate E2F translocation to the nucleus, whereas DP-1α, which shows reduced affinity for E2F, participates in E2F nuclear export and translocation to the cytoplasm. In this manner, DP-1α indirectly represses the ability of E2F-1 to activate transcription (Ishida et al., 2005). DP-4 can mediate transcriptional repression as well (Milton et al., 2006). Furthermore, a growing body of evidence shows that other proteins that interact with DP factors, such as C/EBP, TRIP-Br and SOCS3, can modulate E2F activation of gene transcription (Masuhiro et al., 2008; Zaragoza et al., 2010).

5.3 C/EBP

CCAAT/Enhancer Binding Protein (C/EBP) factors are generally characterized as effectors of cellular growth arrest. Within the C/EBP family, C/EBPα has been shown to associate with and repress E2F-1 (Wang et al., 2007). This interaction has been demonstrated through co-immunoprecipitation assays and is independent of pRb family proteins. Rather, it requires the presence of DP-1 or DP-2 (Zaragoza et al., 2010).

The effect of C/EBP repression on E2F activity has been demonstrated in multiple tissues. In primary murine keratinocytes, C/EBPα and β are upregulated as these cells differentiate and move from the basal to the suprabasal layers of the epidermis. Further, the repression of E2F target genes via the action C/EBP is necessary for proper differentiation (Lopez et al., 2009). Interactions between C/EBP and E2F also play important roles during senescence. Indeed, C/EBPα and HDAC1 are recruited to hepatic DNA from older, but not young, mice (Wang et al., 2008). Recruitment of these two factors is accompanied by decreased transcription of E2F target genes.

In mouse 3T3-L1 preadipocytes, C/EBPα, but not C/EBPβ, disrupts E2F-p107 and induces E2F-p130 complexes, leading to decreased proliferation, likely involved in preadipocyte differentiation (Timchenko et al., 1999).

In mouse hepatocytes devoid of C/EBPβ, E2F target genes are repressed and DNA synthesis is severely impaired. In these cells, C/EBP β interacts with E2F-1, facilitating recruitment of CBP and p300 to E2F target genes. The recruitment of these multiprotein complexes results in upregulation of E2F targets involved in cell proliferation (Wang et al., 2007). C/EBPβ is also required for expression of E2F-3 and S-phase progression in uterine epithelial cells (Ramathal et al., 2010). In primary epidermal keratinocytes, C/EBPα interferes with DNA synthesis in response to DNA damage (Johnson, 2005). However, the mechanisms involved are not fully undertood. It has been proposed that C/EBPα functions with E2F/pRb complexes to repress transcription of S-phase genes. In neuroblastoma cells, C/EBP is involved in induction of apoptotic gene transcription by E2F-1 (Marabese et al., 2003).

5.4 SOCS3

The Suppressor of Cytokine Signaling (SOCS) family of proteins act as negative feedback regulators of the JAK-STAT pathway. Recently, SOCS factors have also been shown to associate with DP-1 and DP-3. SOCS3 inhibits transcriptional activation of E2F target genes and cell cycle progression. The mechanisms involved in this repression include SOCS3 inhibition of E2F/DP dimerization, thus preventing the formation of the E2F DNA-binding complexes (Masuhiro et al., 2008).

5.5 TRIP-BR1

The Transcriptional Regulator Interacting with the PHD zinc finger and/or the Bromodomain-1 (TRIP-Br1) protein (also known as p34) is a transcriptional modulator that directly interacts with DP-1, as well as with the co-activators p300/CBP and KRIP1(Hsu et al., 2001). As such, TRIP-Br co-activates E2F responsive genes, such as B-myb, in U2OS osteosarcoma cells, an ability potentiated by KRIP1. This effect is impaired by pRb. TRIP-Br1 also interferes with deactivation of Cyclin D/Cdk4 complex by $p16^{INK4}$, effectively activating E2F by inhibiting pRb (Sim et al., 2004).

5.6 p110 CUX1

Cut homeobox 1 (CUX1) proteins are transcription factors that can either activate or repress transcription. In particular, the CUX1 isoform p110 can stably interact with DNA and promote entry into the S-phase of the cell cycle (Truscott et al., 2008). P110 CUX1 interacts with E2F-1 or E2F-2, stimulating their recruitment to the DNA polymerase α gene promoter, in a manner that requires ability of E2F to bind DNA. Further, common targets for E2F and p110 CUX1 include genes involved in cell cycle progression, DNA repair and replication (Truscott et al., 2008).

5.7 YY1

The transcriptional repressor YY1 can bind to target sites adjacent to E2F binding elements in the promoters of genes such as *Cdc6* (Schlisio et al., 2002). In addition, the YY1 accessory protein Ring1 and YY1 binding protein (RYBP) can interact with E2F-2, -3 and -4 to synergistically enhance binding of E2F-2 and -3 (but not of E2F-1). In this manner, YY1 and RYBP not only enhance the binding and transcription of E2F to certain promoters, but also add specificity.

5.8 TFE3

Studies of the p68 promoter have shown that transcription factor E3 (TFE3) operates in a similar manner to YY1. Thus, the E Box bound by TFE3 and the E2F consensus sequence occur in close proximity in the *p68* promoter. TFE3 and E2F-3 bind to those sites cooperatively (Giangrande et al., 2003; Giangrande et al., 2004). This interaction requires E2F-3, but not TFE3 binding to DNA. Although a direct interaction between these two proteins was not be demonstrated, these two factors likely work together in a larger protein complex, or interact temporarily to recruit one another to the *p68* promoter.

6. Regulation of E2F activity by viral oncoproteins

Viruses work by hijacking the cellular machinery of their host cell, to facilitate their replication. Hence, it is not surprising that constitutive activation of E2F, which induces cell transition into a state of DNA replication (S-phase), is a critical step in the viral modification of infected cell functions.

6.1 Human papillomavirus protein E7

The human papillomaviruses (HPV) are commonly known oncoviruses. This notoriety is due to their ability to activate E2F proteins, causing rapid and unregulated progression through the cell cycle (Lee et al., 1998). HPV couples this action with deactivation of pathways that act as fail-safe mechanisms for E2F activity, such as p53-mediated apoptosis (Moody and Laimins, 2010). The key HPV viral protein involved in activating E2Fs is E7. This protein carries an LXCXE domain characteristic of proteins that associate with pRb family proteins (Lee et al., 1998). In this manner, E7 proteins bind to pRb, p107 and p130, dissociating them from E2F factors. The mechanisms involved in this effect include blockade by E7 of the pRb-E2F binding domain (Lee et al., 1998). As a result, E2F species bind to and activate target genes without the possibility of repression. E7 also induces pRb proteasomal degradation, by increasing its ubiquitination (Moody and Laimins). Furthermore, there is evidence to indicate that E7 also binds to p300/CBP, allowing this acetyltransferase to facilitate and rapidly increase the transcription of E2F target genes (Bernat et al., 2003).

6.2 SV40 large-T antigen

The simian virus 40 (SV40) genome encodes a protein that shares some characteristics with HPV E7, termed large T-antigen. Similar to HPV E7, large-T antigen has a LXCXE domain, which can bind all three pRb family proteins, leading to release of free E2F and expression of its target genes (DeCaprio, 2009). In addition, large-T antigen binds preferentially to the hypophosphorylated form of pRb, present during the G1-phase of the cell cycle (Ludlow et al., 1989). The characterization of the interactions between large-T antigen and complexes containing p130 or p107 and E2F-4 has been central to understanding the mechanisms involved in deactivation of pRb family proteins by this viral factor (Sullivan et al., 2000). Dissociation of p107 or p130 from E2F also requires Large-T antigen interactions with the J type of chaperone protein Hsc70 and ATP.

Similar to HPV E7, large-T antigen binds to p300/CBP through its C-terminus (Eckner et al., 1996). This interaction is likely involved in histone acetylation and transcriptional activation of E2F target genes. Significantly, mutations in the C-termimus of large-T antigen impair its ability to bind p300/CBP, but are without effect on its capacity to disrupt pRb binding to E2F (Nemethova et al., 2004).

6.3 Adenovirus E1A

Adenovirus protein E1A functions in a similar manner to HPV E7 and SV40 large-T antigen. E1A interacts with multiple cellular proteins, including the pRb family and p300/CBP (Raychaudhuri, 1991; Liu, 2007). X-ray crystallographic characterization of E1A has revealed that its N-terminal domain competes with the transactivation domain of E2F for binding to pRb. This induces a decrease in E2F binding to pRb by competition (Liu, 2007). Similar to other viral oncoproteins, E1A also has an LXCXE domain that binds to pRb, p107 and p130 (Dyson, 1992). E1A also binds the 400-kDa protein p400, which mediates further interactions with TRRAP/PAF400, along with the DNA helicase TAP54α/β). Together, these proteins form a chromatin remodeling complex, which contributes to cell transformation and activation of E2F target genes that mediate viral DNA replication (Liu, 2007).

6.4 Human parvovirus NS1

Human parvovirus B19 (B19V) is the only pathogenic human parvovirus, and it targets cells of the erythroid lineage, expecially erythroid progenitors (Wan et al., 2010). The B19V protein NS1 (nonstructural protein 1) interacts with E2F-4 and E2F-5, inducing their nuclear accumulation and G2 arrest, necessary for viral replication (Wan et al., 2010). Simultaneously, NS1 also decreases expression of E2F-1, E2F-2, and E2F-3, resulting in transcriptional repression of genes necessary for the G2/M transition. Thus, B19V targets cells for arrest in the G2 phase by altering E2F activity, indicating the importance of this family of transcription factors in all phases of the cell cycle and multiple aspects of cell cycle progression and DNA replication and repair.

7. Conclusions

A large body of work has been focused on identifying the mechanisms that regulate E2F activity and its consequences on induction of DNA repair. As a result, it has become apparent that E2F activity is complex, and is regulated at multiple levels, including transcription, post-translational modifications and protein-protein interactions. However, understanding of how different post-translational modifications modulate E2F interactions with other proteins, allowing it to form transcriptional activator or repressor complexes is in its infancy.

The biological roles of the various modes of E2F modulation go well beyond normal development and cell differentiation, implicate mechanisms of DNA repair as a central function, and are involved in the genesis of multiple pathologies.

Although pRb family proteins form the central backbone of E2F regulation, they are only one component. Studies of HPV proteins have shown that, in addition to E7, the proteins E5 and E6 are critical for the functional transformation of a cell. In the case of HPV, these proteins serve to deactivate the p53 pathway, preventing the pro-apoptotic responses normally switched on with abnormal activation of E2F. Other viruses encode proteins that serve a similar function. The identification and study of these proteins may provide key insights into the function of these viruses and the pathways that regulate E2F during normal tissue development and homeostasis, and affect DNA repair mechanisms to ensure viral replication.

8. Acknowledgement

Work in the author's laboratory was supported with funds from the Canadian Institutes of Health Research.

9. References

Almeida, M.I., Reis, R.M., and Calin, G.A. (2011). MicroRNA history: Discovery, recent applications, and next frontiers. *Mutat Res.*

Bagchi, S., Raychaudhuri, P., and Nevins, J.R. (1989). Phosphorylation-dependent activation of the adenovirus-inducible E2F transcription factor in a cell-free system. *Proc Natl Acad Sci U S A* 86, 12.(4352-4356).

Bennett, D., and Itoh, T. (2008). The XPE gene of xeroderma pigmentosum, its product and biological roles. *Adv Exp Med Biol* 63757-64).

Berkovich, E., and Ginsberg, D. (2003). ATM is a target for positive regulation by E2F-1. *Oncogene* 22, 2.(161-167).

Bernat, A., Avvakumov, N., Mymryk, J.S., and Banks, L. (2003). Interaction between the HPV E7 oncoprotein and the transcriptional coactivator p300. *Oncogene* 22, 39.(7871-7881).

Berton, T.R., Mitchell, D.L., Guo, R., and Johnson, D.G. (2005). Regulation of epidermal apoptosis and DNA repair by E2F1 in response to ultraviolet B radiation. *Oncogene* 242449-2460).

Bindra, R.S., Gibson, S.L., Ment, A., Westermark, U., Jasin, M., Pierce, A.J., Bristow, R.G., Classon, M.K., and Glazer, P.M. (2005). Hypoxia-induced down regulation of BRCA1 expression by E2Fs. *Cancer Res* 6511597-11604).

Blattner, C., Sparks, A., and Lane, D. (1999). Transcription factor E2F-1 is upregulated in response to DNA damage in a manner analogous to that of p53. *Mol Cell Biol* 193704-3713).

Bracken, A.P., Ciro, M., Cocito, A., and Helin, K. (2004). E2F target genes: unraveling the biology. *Trends Biochem Sci* 29409-417).

Brash, D.E., Ziegler, A., Jonason, A.S., Simon, J.A., Kunala, S., and Leffell, D.J. (1996). Sunlight and sunburn in human skin cancer: p53, apoptosis and tumor promotion. *J Invest Dermatol Symp Proc* 1136-142).

Brosh, R., Shalgi, R., Liran, A., Landan, G., Korotayev, K., Nguyen, G.H., Enerly, E., Johnsen, H., Buganim, Y., Solomon, H., *et al.* (2008). p53-Repressed miRNAs are involved with E2F in a feed-forward loop promoting proliferation. *Mol Syst Biol* 4229).

Bueno, M.J., Gomez de Cedron, M., Laresgoiti, U., Fernandez-Piqueras, J., Zubiaga, A.M., and Malumbres, M. (2010). Multiple E2F-induced microRNAs prevent replicative stress in response to mitogenic signaling. *Mol Cell Biol* 30, 12.(2983-2995).

Campanero, M.R., and Flemington, E.K. (1997). Regulation of E2F through ubiquitin-proteasome-dependent degradation: stabilization by the pRB tumor suppressor protein. *Proc Natl Acad Sci U S A* 94, 6.(2221-2226).

Cao, A.R., Rabinovich, R., Xu, M., Xu, X., Jin, V.X., and Farnham, P.J. (2011). Genome-wide Analysis of Transcription Factor E2F1 Mutant Proteins Reveals That N- and C-terminal Protein Interaction Domains Do Not Participate in Targeting E2F1 to the Human Genome. *J Biol Chem* 286, 14.(11985-11996).

Chang, I.Y., Jin, M., Yoon, S.P., Youn, C.K., Yoon, Y., Moon, S.P., Hyun, J.W., Jun, J.Y., and You, H.J. (2008). Senescence-dependent MutS alpha dysfunction attenuates mismatch repair. *Mol Cancer Res* 6, 6.(978-989).

Chang, W.Y., Andrews, J., Carter, D.E., and Dagnino, L. (2006). Differentiation and injury-repair signals modulate the interaction of E2F and pRB proteins with novel target genes in keratinocytes. *Cell Cycle* 51872-1879).

Chang, W.Y., Bryce, D.M., D'Souza, S.J.A., and Dagnino, L. (2004). The DP-1 transcription factor is required for keratinocyte growth and epidermal stratification. *J Biol Chem* 27951343-51353).

Chen, D., Yu, Z., Zhu, Z., and Lopez, C.D. (2008). E2F1 regulates the base excision repair gene XRCC1 and promotes DNA repair. *J Biol Chem* 283, 22.(15381-15389).

Connell-Crowley, L., Harper, J.W., and Goodrich, D.W. (1997). Cyclin D1/Cdk4 regulates retinoblastoma protein-mediated cell cycle arrest by site-specific phosphorylation. *Mol Biol Cell* 8, 2.(287-301).

Cui, J.G., Zhao, Y., Sethi, P., Li, Y.Y., Mahta, A., Culicchia, F., and Lukiw, W.J. (2010). Micro-RNA-128 (miRNA-128) down-regulation in glioblastoma targets ARP5 (ANGPTL6), Bmi-1 and E2F-3a, key regulators of brain cell proliferation. *J Neurooncol* 98, 3.(297-304).

D'Souza, S.J.A., Vespa, A., Murkherjee, S., Maher, A., Pajak, S., and Dagnino, L. (2002). E2F-1 is essential for normal epidermal wound repair. *J Biol Chem* 27710626-10632).

DeCaprio, J.A. (2009). How the Rb tumor suppressor structure and function was revealed by the study of Adenovirus and SV40. *Virology* 384, 2.(274-284).

del Pozo, J.C., Boniotti, M.B., and Gutierrez, C. (2002). Arabidopsis E2Fc functions in cell division and is degraded by the ubiquitin-SCF(AtSKP2) pathway in response to light. *Plant Cell* 14, 12.(3057-3071).

Deschenes, C., Alvarez, L., Lizotte, M.E., Vezina, A., and Rivard, N. (2004). The nucleocytoplasmic shuttling of E2F4 is involved in the regulation of human intestinal epithelial cell proliferation and differentiation. *J Cell Physiol* 199, 2.(262-273).

Dick, F.A. (2007). Structure-function analysis of the retinoblastoma tumor suppressor protein - is the whole a sum of its parts? *Cell Div* 226).

Dominguez-Brauer, C., Chen, Y.J., Brauer, P.M., Pimkina, J., and Raychaudhuri, P. (2009). ARF stimulates XPC to trigger nucleotide excision repair by regulating the repressor complex of E2F4. *EMBO Rep* 10, 9.(1036-1042).

Dynlacht, B.D., Moberg, K., Lees, J.A., Harlow, E., and Zhu, L. (1997). Specific regulation of E2F family members by cyclin-dependent kinases. *Mol Cell Biol* 17, 7.(3867-3875).

Dyson, N and Harlow, E. (1992). Adenovirus E1A targets key regulators of cell proliferation. *Cancer Surveys* 12.(161-195).

Eckner, R., Ludlow, J.W., Lill, N.L., Oldread, E., Arany, Z., Modjtahedi, N., DeCaprio, J.A., Livingston, D.M., and Morgan, J.A. (1996). Association of p300 and CBP with simian virus 40 large T antigen. *Mol Cell Biol* 16, 7.(3454-3464).

Fagan, R., Flint, K.J., and Jones, N. (1994). Phosphorylation of E2F-1 modulates its interaction with the retinoblastoma gene product and the adenoviral E4 19 kDa protein. *Cell* 78799-811).

Farhana, L., Dawson, M., Rishi, A.K., Zhang, Y., Van Buren, E., Trivedi, C., Reichert, U., Fang, G., Kirschner, M.W., and Fontana, J.A. (2002). Cyclin B and E2F-1 expression in prostate carcinoma cells treated with the novel retinoid CD437 are regulated by the ubiquitin-mediated pathway. *Cancer Res* 623842-3849).

Field, S.J., Tsai, F.Y., Kuo, F., Zubiaga, A.M., Kaelin, W.G., Jr., Livingston, D.M., Orkin, S.H., and Greenberg, M.E. (1996). E2F-1 functions in mice to promote apoptosis and suppress proliferation. *Cell* 85, 4.(549-561).

Flemington, E.K., Speck, S.H., and Kaelin, W.J. (1993). E2F-1 mediated transactivation is inhibited by complex formation with the retinoblastoma susceptibility gene product. *Proc Natl Acad Sci USA*, 90.(

Galbiati, L., Mendoza-Maldonado, R., Gutierrez, M.I., and Giacca, M. (2005). Regulation of E2F1 after DNA damage by p300-mediated acetylation and ubiquitination. *Cell Cycle* 4930-939).

Garcia-Alvarez, G., Ventura, V., Ros, O., Gil, J., and Tauler, A. (2007). Glycogen synthase kinase-3beta binds to E2F1 and regulates its transcriptional activity. *Biochim Biophys Acta* 1773375-382).

Giangrande, P., Hallstrom, T.C., Tunyaplin, C., Calame, K., and Nevins, J.R. (2003). Identification of E-box factor TFE3 as a functional partner for the E2F3 transcription factor. *Mol Cell Biol* 233707-3720).

Giangrande, P., Zhu, W., Rempel, R. E., Laasko, N., and Nevins, J.R. (2004). Combinatorial gene control involving E2F and E box family members. *EMBO J* 231336-1347).

Ginsberg, D., Vairo, G., Chittenden, T., Xiao, Z.X., Xu, G., Wydner, K.L., DeCaprio, J.A., Lawrence, J.B., and Livingston, D.M. (1994). E2F-4, a new member of the E2F transcription factor family, interacts with p107. *Genes Dev* 8, 22.(2665-2679).

Griffiths-Jones, S. (2004). The microRNA Registry. *Nucleic Acids Res* 32, Database issue.(D109-111).

Guo, J., Longshore, S., Nair, R., and Warner, B.W. (2009). Retinoblastoma protein (pRb), but not p107 or p130, is required for maintenance of enterocyte quiescence and differentiation in small intestine. *J Biol Chem* 284, 1.(134-140).

Guo, R., Chen, J., Mitchell, D.L., and Johnson, D.G. (2010a). GCN5 and E2F1 stimulate nucleotide excision repair by promoting H3K9 acetylation at sites of damage. *Nucleic Acids Res*.

Guo, R., Chen, J., Zhu, F., Biswas, A.K., Berton, T.R., Mitchell, D.L., and Johnson, D.G. (2010b). E2F1 localizes to sites of UV-induced DNA damage to enhance nucleotide excision repair. *J Biol Chem* 285, 25.(19308-19315).

Halazonetis, T.D., Gorgoulis, V.G., and Bartek, J. (2008). An oncogene-induced DNA damage model for cancer development. *Science* 319, 5868.(1352-1355).

Hallstrom, T.C., and Nevins, J.R. (2009). Balancing the decision of cell proliferation and cell fate. *Cell Cycle* 8, 4.(532-535).

Hardy, S., Engel, D.A., and Shenk, T. (1989). An adenovirus early region 4 gene product is required for induction of the infection-specific form of cellular E2F activity. *Genes Dev* 3, 7.(1062-1074).

Hateboer, G., Kerkhoven, R.M., Shvarts, A., Bernards, R., and Beijersbergen, R.L. (1996). Degradation of E2F by the ubiquitin-proteasome pathway: regulation by retinoblastoma family proteins and adenovirus transforming proteins. *Genes Dev* 10, 23.(2960-2970).

Helin, K., and Harlow, E. (1994). Heterodimerization of the transcription factors E2F-1 and DP-1 is required for binding to the adenovirus E4 (ORF6/7) protein. *J Virol* 68, 8.(5027-5035).

Heriche, J.K., Ang, D., Bier, E., and O'Farrell, P.H. (2003). Involvement of an SCFSlmb complex in timely elimination of E2F upon initiation of DNA replication in Drosophila. *BMC Genet* 49).

Herrera, R.E., Chen, F., and Weinberg, R.A. (1996). Increased histone H1 phosphorylation and relaxed chromatin structure in Rb-deficient fibroblasts. *Proc Natl Acad Sci U S A* 93, 21.(11510-11515).

Hijmans, E.M., Voorhoeve, P.M., Beijersbergen, R.L., van 't Veer, L.J., and Bernards, R. (1995). E2F-5, a new E2F family member that interacts with p130 in vivo. *Mol Cell Biol* 15, 6.(3082-3089).

Hofmann, F., Martelli, F., Livingston, D.M., and Wang, Z. (1996). The retinoblastoma gene product protects E2F-1 from degradation by the ubiquitin-proteasome pathway. *Genes Dev* 10, 23.(2949-2959).

Hsu, S.I.-H., Yang, C.M., Sim, K.G., Hentschel, D.M., O'Leary, E., and Bonventre, J.V. (2001). Trip-Br: a novel family of PHD zing finger- and bromodomain-interacting proteins that regulate the transcriptional activity of E2F-1/DP-1. *EMBO J* 202273-2285).

Huang, Y.C., Misquitta, S., Blond, S.Y., Adams, E., and Colman, R.F. (2008). Catalytically active monomer of glutathione S-transferase pi and key residues involved in the electrostatic interaction between subunits. *J Biol Chem* 283, 47.(32880-32888).

Ianari, A., Gallo, R., Palma, M., Alesse, E., and Gulino, A. (2004). Specific role for p300/CREB-binding protein-associated factor activity in E2F1 stabilization in response to DNA damage. *J Biol Chem* 27930830-30835).

Ingram, L., Munro, S., Coutts, A.S., and La Thangue, N.B. (2011). E2F-1 regulation by an unusual DNA damage-responsive DP partner subunit. *Cell Death Differ* 18, 1.(122-132).

Ishida, H., Masuhiro, Y., Fukushima, A., Argueta, J.G., Yamaguchi, N., Shiota, S., and Hanazawa, S. (2005). Identification and characterization of novel isoforms of human DP-1: DP-1{alpha} regulates the transcriptional activity of E2F1 as well as cell cycle progression in a dominant-negative manner. *J Biol Chem* 280, 26.(24642-24648).

Ishida, S., Huang, E., Zuzan, H., Spang, R., Leone, G., West, M., and Nevins, J.R. (2001). Role for E2F in control of both DNA replication and mitotic functions as revealed from DNA microarrays. *Mol Cell Biol* 214684-4699).

Ivanova, I.A., D'Souza, S.J.A., and Dagnino, L. (2005). Signalling in the epidermis: The E2F cell cycle regulatory pathway in epidermal morphogenesis, regeneration and transformation. *Int J Biol Sci* 187-95).

Ivanova, I.A., D'Souza, S.J.A., and Dagnino, L. (2006). E2F stability is regulated by a novel-PKC/p38® MAP kinase signalling pathway during keratinocyte differentiation. *Oncogene* 25430-437).

Ivanova, I.A., and Dagnino, L. (2007). Activation of p38- and CRM1-dependent nuclear export promotes E2F1 degradation during keratinocyte differentiation. *Oncogene* 261147-1154).

Ivanova, I.A., Nakrieko, K.A., and Dagnino, L. (2009). Phosphorylation by p38 MAP kinase is required for E2F1 degradation and keratinocyte differentiation. *Oncogene* 2852-63).

Ivanova, I.A., Vespa, A., and Dagnino, L. (2007). A novel mechanism of E2F1 regulation via nucleocytoplasmic shuttling: determinants of nuclear import and export. *Cell Cycle* 62186-2195).

Johnson, P.F. (2005). Molecular stop signs: regulation of cell-cycle arrest by C/EBP transcription factors. *J Cell Sci* 118, Pt 12.(2545-2555).

Judah, D., Chang, W.Y., and Dagnino, L. (2010). EBP1 is a novel E2F target gene regulated by transforming growth factor-beta. *PLoS One* 5, 11.(e13941).

Kachhap, S.K., Rosmus, N., Collis, S.J., Kortenhorst, M.S., Wissing, M.D., Hedayati, M., Shabbeer, S., Mendonca, J., Deangelis, J., Marchionni, L., *et al.* (2010). Downregulation of homologous recombination DNA repair genes by HDAC inhibition in prostate cancer is mediated through the E2F1 transcription factor. *PLoS One* 5, 6.(e11208).

Kontaki, H., and Talianidis, I. (2010). Lysine methylation regulates E2F1-induced cell death. *Molec Cell* 39, 2. (152-160)

Kishore, R., Luedemann, C., Bord, E., Goukassian, D., and Losordo, D.W. (2003). Tumor necrosis factor-mediated E2F1 suppression in endothelial cells: differential requirement of c-Jun N-terminal kinase and p38 mitogen-activated protein kinase signal transduction pathways. *Circ Res* 93, 10.(932-940).

Kong, H.J., Yu, H.J., Hong, S., Park, M.J., Choi, Y.H., An, W.G., Lee, J.W., and Cheong, J. (2003). Interaction and functional cooperation of the cancer-amplified transcriptional coactivator activating signal cointegrator-2 and E2F-1 in cell proliferation. *Mol Cancer Res* 1, 13.(948-958).

Kozaki, K., Imoto, I., Mogi, S., Omura, K., and Inazawa, J. (2008). Exploration of tumor-suppressive microRNAs silenced by DNA hypermethylation in oral cancer. *Cancer Res* 68, 7.(2094-2105).

Krek, W., Xu, G., and Livingston, D.M. (1995). Cyclin A-kinase regulation of E2F-1 DNA binding function underlies suppression of an S phase checkpoint. *Cell* 83, 7.(1149-1158).

Lammens, T., Li, J., Leone, G., and De Veylder, L. (2009). Atypical E2Fs: new players in the E2F transcription factor family. *Trends Cell Biol* 19, 3.(111-118).

Lanigan, F., Geraghty, J.G., and Bracken, A.P. (2011). Transcriptional regulation of cellular senescence. *Oncogene*.

Lario, L.D., Ramirez-Parra, E., Gutierrez, C., Casati, P., and Spampinato, C.P. (2011). Regulation of plant MSH2 and MSH6 genes in the UV-B-induced DNA damage response. *J Exp Bot*.

Lee, B.K., Bhinge, A.A., and Iyer, V.R. (2011). Wide-ranging functions of E2F4 in transcriptional activation and repression revealed by genome-wide analysis. *Nucleic Acids Res*.

Lee, J.O., Russo, A.A., and Pavletich, N.P. (1998). Structure of the retinoblastoma tumour-suppressor pocket domain bound to a peptide from HPV E7. *Nature* 391, 6670.(859-865).

Lee, K.H., Chen, Y.L., Yeh, S.D., Hsiao, M., Lin, J.T., Goan, Y.G., and Lu, P.J. (2009). MicroRNA-330 acts as tumor suppressor and induces apoptosis of prostate cancer cells through E2F1-mediated suppression of Akt phosphorylation. *Oncogene* 28, 38.(3360-3370).

Levitt, N.C., and Hickson, I.D. (2002). Caretaker tumour suppressor genes that defend genome integrity. *Trends Mol Med* 8, 4.(179-186).

Li, W.W., Fan, J., Hochhauser, D., and Bertino, J.R. (1997). Overexpression of p21waf1 leads to increased inhibition of E2F-1 phosphorylation and sensitivity to anticancer drugs in retinoblastoma-negative human sarcoma cells. *Cancer Res* 57, 11.(2193-2199).

Liao, C.C., Tsai, C.Y., Chang, W.C., Lee, W.H., and Wang, J.M. (2010). RB.E2F1 complex mediates DNA damage responses through transcriptional regulation of ZBRK1. *J Biol Chem* 285, 43.(33134-33143).

Lin, P.S., McPherson, L.A., Chen, A.Y., Sage, J., and Ford, J.M. (2009). The role of the retinoblastoma/E2F1 tumor suppressor pathway in the lesion recognition step of nucleotide excision repair. *DNA Repair (Amst)* 8, 7.(795-802).

Lin, W.-C., Lin, F.-T., and Nevins, J.R. (2001). Selective induction of E2F1 in response to DNA damage, mediated by ATM-dependent phosphorylation. *Genes Dev* 151833-1844).

Liu, X. and R. Marmorstein (2007). Structure of the retinoblastoma protein bound to adenovirus E1A reveals the molecular basis for viral oncoprotein inactivation of a tumor suppressor. *Genes Dev* 21,21. (2711-2716).

Lopez, R.G., Garcia-Silva, S., Moore, S.J., Bereshchenko, O., Martinez-Cruz, A.B., Ermakova, O., Kurz, E., Paramio, J.M., and Nerlov, C. (2009). C/EBPalpha and beta couple interfollicular keratinocyte proliferation arrest to commitment and terminal differentiation. *Nat Cell Biol* 11, 10.(1181-1190).

Ludlow, J.W., DeCaprio, J.A., Huang, C.M., Lee, W.H., Paucha, E., and Livingston, D.M. (1989). SV40 large T antigen binds preferentially to an underphosphorylated member of the retinoblastoma susceptibility gene product family. *Cell* 56, 1. (57-65).

Mann, D.J., and Jones, N.C. (1996). E2F-1 but not E2F-4 can overcome p16-induced G1 cell-cycle arrest. *Curr Biol* 6, 4.(474-483).

Marabese, M., Vikhanskaya, F., Rainelli, C., Sakai, T., and Broggini, M. (2003). DNA damage induces transcriptional activation of p73 by removing C-EBPalpha repression on E2F1. *Nucleic Acids Res* 31, 22.(6624-6632).

Marti, A., Wirbelauer, C., Scheffner, M., and Krek, W. (1999). Interaction between ubiquitin-protein ligase SCF^{SKP2} and E2F-1 underlies the regulation of E2F-1 degradation. *Nature Cell Biol* 114-19).

Martinez-Balbas, M.A., Bauer, U.M., Nielsen, S.J., Brehm, A., and Kouzarides, T. (2000). Regulation of E2F1 activity by acetylation. *Embo J* 19, 4.(662-671).

Marzio, G., Wagener, C., Gutierrez, M.I., Cartwright, P., Helin, K., and Giacca, M. (2000). E2F family members are differentially regulated by reversible acetylation. *J Biol Chem* 275, 15.(10887-10892).

Masuhiro, Y., Kayama, K., Fukushima, A., Baba, K., Soutsu, M., Kamiya, Y., Gotoh, M., Yamaguchi, N., and Hanazawa, S. (2008). SOCS-3 inhibits E2F/DP-1 transcriptional activity and cell cycle progression via interaction with DP-1. *J Biol Chem* 283, 46.(31575-31583).

McClellan, K.A., and Slack, R.S. (2007). Specific in vivo roles for E2Fs in differentiation and development. *Cell Cycle* 6, 23.(2917-2927).

Meng, R.D., Phillips, P., and El-Deiry, W.S. (1999). p53-independent increase in E2F-1 expression enhances the cytotoxic effects of etoposide and of adriamycin. *Int J Oncol* 14, 1.(5-14).

Milton, A., Luoto, K., Ingram, L., Munro, S., Logan, N., Graham, A.L., Brummelkamp, T.R., Hijmans, E.M., Bernards, R., and La Thangue, N.B. (2006). A functionally distinct member of the DP family of E2F subunits. *Oncogene* 25, 22.(3212-3218).

Moberg, K., Starz, M.A., and Lees, J.A. (1996). E2F-4 switches from p130 to p107 and pRB in response to cell cycle reentry. *Mol Cell Biol* 161436-1449).

Moody, C.A., and Laimins, L.A. (2010). Human papillomavirus oncoproteins: pathways to transformation. *Nat Rev Cancer* 10, 8.(550-560).

Morris, L., Allen, K.E., and La Thangue, N.B. (2000). Regulation of E2F transcription by cyclin E-Cdk2 kinase mediated through p300/CBP co-activators. *Nat Cell Biol* 2, 4.(232-239).

Morrison, A.J., Sardet, C., and Herrera, R.E. (2002). Retinoblastoma protein transcriptional repression through histone deacetylation of a single nucleosome. *Mol Cell Biol* 22, 3.(856-865).

Nemethova, M., Smutny, M., and Wintersberger, E. (2004). Transactivation of E2F-regulated genes by polyomavirus large T antigen: evidence for a two-step mechanism. *Mol Cell Biol* 24, 24.(10986-10994).

Nevins, J.R. (2001). The Rb/E2F pathway and cancer. *Human Mole Genet* 10699-703).

Nouspikel, T. (2009). DNA repair in mammalian cells : Nucleotide excision repair: variations on versatility. *Cell Mol Life Sci* 66, 6.(994-1009).

O'Donnell, K.A., Wentzel, E.A., Zeller, K.I., Dang, C.V., and Mendell, J.T. (2005). c-Myc-regulated microRNAs modulate E2F1 expression. *Nature* 435, 7043.(839-843).

Ohta, T., and Xiong, Y. (2001). Phosphorylation- and SKP1-independent in vitro ubiquitination of E2F1 by multiple ROC-Cullin ligases. *Cancer Res* 611347-1353).

Ormondroyd, E., de la Luna, S., and La Thangue, N.B. (1995). A new member of the DP family, DP-3, with distinct protein products suggests a regulatory role for alternative splicing in the cell cycle transcription factor DRTF1/E2F. *Oncogene* 11, 8.(1437-1446).

Ozaki, T., Okoshi, R., Sang, M., Kubo, N., and Nakagawara, A. (2009). Acetylation status of E2F-1 has an important role in the regulation of E2F-1-mediated transactivation of tumor suppressor p73. *Biochem Biophys Res Commun* 386, 1.(207-211).

Peart, M.J., Poyurovsky, M.V., Kass, E.M., Urist, M., Verschuren, E.W., Summers, M.K., Jackson, P.K., and Prives, C. (2010). APC/C(Cdc20) targets E2F1 for degradation in prometaphase. *Cell Cycle* 9, 19.(3956-3964).

Pediconi, N., Ianari, A., Costanzo, A., Belloni, L., Gallo, R., Cimino, L., Porcellini, A., Screpanti, I., Balsano, C., Alesse, E., *et al.* (2003). Differential regulation of E2F1 apoptotic target genes in response to DNA damage. *Nat Cell Biol* 5552-558).

Petrocca, F., Visone, R., Onelli, M.R., Shah, M.H., Nicoloso, M.S., de Martino, I., Iliopoulos, D., Pilozzi, E., Liu, C.G., Negrini, M., *et al.* (2008). E2F1-regulated microRNAs impair TGFbeta-dependent cell-cycle arrest and apoptosis in gastric cancer. *Cancer Cell* 13, 3.(272-286).

Pickering, M.T., Stadler, B.M., and Kowalik, T.F. (2009). miR-17 and miR-20a temper an E2F1-induced G1 checkpoint to regulate cell cycle progression. *Oncogene* 28, 1.(140-145).

Polager, S., and Ginsberg, D. (2008). E2F - at the crossroads of life and death. *Trends Cell Biol* 18, 11.(528-535).

Prost, S., Lu, P., Caldwell, H., and Harrison, D. (2007). E2F regulates DDB2: consequences for DNA repair in Rb-deficient cells. *Oncogene* 26, 24.(3572-3581).

Rabinovich, A., Jin, V.X., Rabinovich, R., Xu, X., and Farnham, P.J. (2008). E2F in vivo binding specificity: comparison of consensus versus nonconsensus binding sites. *Genome Res* 18, 11.(1763-1777).

Raychaudhuri, P., Bagchi, S., Devoto, S.H., Knaus, V. B., Moran, E. and Nevins, J. R. (1991). Domains of the adenovirus E1A protein required for oncogenenic activity are also required for dissociation of E2F transcription factor complexes. *Genes Dev* 5, 7.(1200-1211).

Ramathal, C., Bagchi, I.C., and Bagchi, M.K. (2010). Lack of CCAAT enhancer binding protein beta (C/EBPbeta) in uterine epithelial cells impairs estrogen-induced DNA replication, induces DNA damage response pathways, and promotes apoptosis. *Mol Cell Biol* 30, 7.(1607-1619).

Real, S., Espada, L., Espinet, C., Santidrian, A.F., and Tauler, A. (2010). Study of the in vivo phosphorylation of E2F1 on Ser403. *Biochim Biophys Acta* 1803, 8.(912-918).

Schlisio, S., Halperin, T., Vidal, M., and Nevins, J.R. (2002). Interaction of YY1 with E2Fs, mediated by RYBP, provides a mechanism for specificity of E2F function. *EMBO J* 21, 21.(5775-5786).

Shiloh, Y. (2003). ATM and related protein kinases: safeguarding genome integrity. *Nat Rev Cancer* 3, 3.(155-168).

Shin, E.K., Shin, A., Paulding, C., Schaffhausen, B., and Yee, A.S. (1995). Multiple change in E2F function and regulation occur upon muscle differentiation. *Mol Cell Biol* 15, 4.(2252-2262).

Siafakas, R., and Richardson, D.R. (2009). Growth arrest and DNA damage-45 alpha (GADD45alpha). *Int J Biochem Cell Biol* 41986-989).

Sim, K.G., Zang, Z., Yang, C.M., Bonventre, J.V., and Hsu, S.I. (2004). TRIP-Br links E2F to novel functions in the regulation of cyclin E expression during cell cycle progression and in the maintenance of genomic stability. *Cell Cycle* 3, 10.(1296-1304).

Smith, E.J., Leone, G., DeGregori, J., Jakoi, L., and Nevins, J.R. (1996). The accumulation of an E2F-p130 transcriptional repressor distinguishes a G0 cell state from a G1 cell state. *Mol Cell Biol* 16, 12.(6965-6976).

Sullivan, C.S., Cantalupo, P., and Pipas, J.M. (2000). The molecular chaperone activity of simian virus 40 large T antigen is required to disrupt Rb-E2F family complexes by an ATP-dependent mechanism. *Mol Cell Biol* 20, 17.(6233-6243).

Sylvestre, Y., De Guire, V., Querido, E., Mukhopadhyay, U.K., Bourdeau, V., Major, F., Ferbeyre, G., and Chartrand, P. (2007). An E2F/miR-20a autoregulatory feedback loop. *J Biol Chem* 282, 4.(2135-2143).

Tazawa, H., Tsuchiya, N., Izumiya, M., and Nakagama, H. (2007). Tumor-suppressive miR-34a induces senescence-like growth arrest through modulation of the E2F pathway in human colon cancer cells. *Proc Natl Acad Sci U S A* 104, 39.(15472-15477).

Timchenko, N.A., Wilde, M., Iakova, P., Albrecht, J.H., and Darlington, G.J. (1999). E2F/p107 and E2F/p130 complexes are regulated by C/EBPalpha in 3T3-L1 adipocytes. *Nucleic Acids Res* 27, 17.(3621-3630).

Truscott, M., Harada, R., Vadnais, C., Robert, F., and Nepveu, A. (2008). p110 CUX1 cooperates with E2F transcription factors in the transcriptional activation of cell cycle-regulated genes. *Mol Cell Biol* 28, 10.(3127-3138).

van Ginkel, P.R., Hsiao, K.M., Schjerven, H., and Farnham, P.J. (1997). E2F-mediated growth regulation requires transcription factor cooperation. *J Biol Chem* 272, 29.(18367-18374).

Vandel, L., and Kouzarides, T. (1999). Residues phosphorylated by TFIIH are required fpr E2F-1 degradation during S-phase. *EMBO J* 184280-4291).

Wang, B., Liu, K., Lin, F.T., and Lin, W.C. (2004). A role for 14-3-3 tau in E2F1 stabilization and DNA damage-induced apoptosis. *J Biol Chem* 279, 52.(54140-54152).

Wang, G.L., Salisbury, E., Shi, X., Timchenko, L., Medrano, E.E., and Timchenko, N.A. (2008). HDAC1 cooperates with C/EBPalpha in the inhibition of liver proliferation in old mice. *J Biol Chem* 283, 38.(26169-26178).

Wang, H., Larris, B., Peiris, T.H., Zhang, L., Le Lay, J., Gao, Y., and Greenbaum, L.E. (2007). C/EBPbeta activates E2F-regulated genes in vivo via recruitment of the coactivator CREB-binding protein/P300. *J Biol Chem* 282, 34.(24679-24688).

Wan, Z., Zhi, N., Wong, S., Keyvanfar, K., Liu, D., Raghvachari, N., Munson, P. J., Su, S. Malide, D., Kajigaya, S., and Young, N. S.(2010). Human parvovirus B19 cauyses cell cycle arrest of human erythroid progenitors via deregulation of the E2F family of transcription factors. *J Clin Invest* 120, 10.(3530-3544).

Weber, J.D., Taylor, L.J., Roussel, M.F., Sherr, C.J., and Bar-Sagi, D. (1999). Nucleolar Arf sequesters Mdm2 and activates p53. *Nat Cell Biol* 1, 1.(20-26).

Weintraub, S.J., Chow, K.N., Luo, R.X., Zhang, S.H., He, D., and Dean, D.C. (1995). Mechanism of active transcriptional repression by the retinoblastoma protein. *Nature* 375812-815).

Wikonkal, N.M., Remenyik, E., Knezevic, D., Zhang, W., Liu, M., Zhao, H., Berton, T.R., and Johnson, D.G. (2003). Inactivating E2f1 reverts apoptosis resistance and cancer sensitivity in Trp53-deficient mice. *Nat Cell Biol* 5655-660).

Wong, C.F., Barnes, L.M., Dahler, A.L., Smith, L., Serewko-Auret, M.M., Popa, C., Abdul-Jabbar, I., and Saunders, N.A. (2003). E2F modulates keratinocyte squamous differentiation: Implications for E2F inhibition in squamous cell carcinoma. *J Biol Chem* 27828516-28522).

Woods, K., Thomson, J.M., and Hammond, S.M. (2007). Direct regulation of an oncogenic micro-RNA cluster by E2F transcription factors. *J Biol Chem* 282, 4.(2130-2134).

Xiao, B., Spencer, J., Clements, A., Ali-Khan, N., Mittnacht, S., Broceno, C., Burghammer, M., Perrakis, A., Marmorstein, R., and Gamblin, S.J. (2003). Crystal structure of the retinoblastoma tumor suppressor protein bound to E2F and the molecular basis of its regulation. *Proc Natl Acad Sci U S A* 100, 5.(2363-2368).

Xie, Q., Bai, Y., Wu, J., Sun, Y., Wang, Y., Zhang, Y., Mei. P., and Yuan, Z. (2011) Methylation-mediated regulation of E2F1 in DANN damage-induced cell death. *J Recept Signal Transduct Res* 31, 2. (139-146).

Xu, T., Zhu, Y., Xiong, Y., Ge, Y.Y., Yun, J.P., and Zhuang, S.M. (2009). MicroRNA-195 suppresses tumorigenicity and regulates G1/S transition of human hepatocellular carcinoma cells. *Hepatology* 50, 1.(113-121).

Yang, J., Song, K., Krebs, T. L., Jackson, M. W., and Danielpour, D. (2008). Rb/E2F4 and Smad2/3 link survivin to TGF-beta-induced apoptosis and tumor progression. *Oncogene* 27, 40.(5226-5238).

Zaragoza, K., Begay, V., Schuetz, A., Heinemann, U., and Leutz, A. (2010). Repression of transcriptional activity of C/EBPalpha by E2F-dimerization partner complexes. *Mol Cell Biol* 30, 9.(2293-2304).

Zhang, X., Wan, G., Berger, F.G., He, X., and Lu, X. (2011). The ATM Kinase Induces MicroRNA Biogenesis in the DNA Damage Response. *Mol Cell* 41, 4.(371-383).

Zhu, J.W., DeRyckere, D., Li, F.X., Wan, Y.Y., and DeGregori, J. (1999). A role for E2F1 in the induction of ARF, p53, and apoptosis during thymic negative selection. *Cell Growth Differ* 10, 12.(829-838).

11

Eidetic Analysis of the Premature Chromosome Condensation Process

Dorota Rybaczek
Department of Cytophysiology, University of Łódź
Poland

'Why does this written doe bound through these written woods?
(…) Perched on four slim legs borrowed from the truth,
She pricks up her ears beneath my fingertips (…)'
(Szymborska, 1993)

1. Introduction

An exact transfer of genetic information depends on the accuracy of mechanisms duplicating DNA molecules in the S-phase and the precise division sister chromosomes during mitosis. The regulation systems of these processes (checkpoints) not only control the activation course of the factors imposing different metabolic specificity on each of the cell cycle phases, but first of all - supervising the proper chronology of events - they condition the behavior of the structural and functional genome integrity. Checkpoints receive signals of all abnormalities or structural damages to DNA and in response evoke reactions inhibiting successive transitions through the cell cycle to enable the expression of specific genes and activation of DNA repair factors. One of the easily perceptible effects of disorders in this signaling system is the induction of premature chromosome condensation (PCC).
The present chapter is a review of the ways and mode of the induction of PCC. The term 'PCC' is inseparably associated with Johnson & Rao (1970) and their experiments on the premature mitosis induced by fusion of interphase and mitotic HeLa cells (G1/M, S/M and G2/M) which were originally carried out using Sendai virus. PCC process can be also induced by chemical signals. Drug-induced PCC provides the new knowledge that DNA replication is tightly coupled with the premature chromosome condensation and that the genome stability results first of all from the alternation of the S-phase and mitosis. The main objective of this review is to show that the PCC induction is possible from various subperiods of cell cycle. Moreover, it has been shown that there are cause-and-effect relationships between the chromosome structure defining 'PCC phenotype' and subperiods, e.g. of the S-phase, initiating the biosynthesis of 'early' or 'late' replicons. Attempts have been made to find answers to questions such as: How to force cells to break out of the rules being developed by Nature for billions of years? How - despite the interrupted, still unterminated process of genome replication - to force a cell to initiate its division? What mechanisms annihilate the subordination principle verified in the course of evolution: first create (DNA-duplicating S-phase) and then divide (mitosis - a stage of DNA condensation and formation of sister

descendant nuclei)? Interference in the regulatory systems of cell cycle is not a simple matter. The gene pool, whose products participate in the creation of these systems, is constantly changing with time to continually form new systems and new interactions. Huge difficulties in the development of effective and selective methods that would arrest the proliferation of cancer cells result from their multiplicity and complication degree, as well as from the possibilities of starting the mechanisms of substitutive and biochemical emergency systems. Studies on the mechanisms inhibiting cell divisions seem to be the shortest way to reach the desired end. This chapter shows the usefulness of attempts to force divisions in cells, simultaneously taking into account the strategy of anticancer therapy.

Therefore the PCC phenomenon constitutes in reality not only a significant fundamental problem in the biology of cell cycle, but it is also an issue of paramount importance in view of practical applications. The radio- and chemotherapy methods used in the treatment of malignant diseases lead to extensive damages to DNA, arresting the replication process of genetic material. Despite this fact, the inhibition of cancer cell proliferation most often is of temporary character or it comprises only part of their population. Drug-induced PCC gives a novel tool to characterize the role of the chromosome instability in cancer development. In this chapter, an attempt is also made to explain the molecular base of PCC induction, for which the starting-point is the biochemical organization of the S-phase checkpoints that block mitosis initiation and the mechanisms which make it possible to suppress their restrictive interactions.

2. Discovery of the premature chromosome condensation (PCC)

The process of separate mitotic chromosome formation from chromatin of an interphase cell nucleus is associated with the construction of giant complexes or macromolecules this consequence being a specific expression of molecular morphogenesis. Simultaneously, it results from action of a complicated regulatory system, causing long, replicated DNA molecules to assume a form adapted to the biomechanical processes of mitosis. Control over these processes is provided on many planes of molecular chromatin organization, e.g. by the association of their components with the nuclear matrix, by specific phosphorylations and dephosphorylations conditioned by changes in the activity of protein kinases and phosphatases or by translocations of some molecules along the length of the fibrils of condensing chromatin or along the arms of existing chromosomes. The degree of packing achieved by chromatin throughout its domain organization before the G2→M transition falls short of the culminant metaphase condensation, the concomitant structural changes always resulting from biochemical modifications that proceed in the protein scaffold of the chromosome under formation.

Attentiveness to the integrity of genome determines the fundamental principles governing the regulation of cell cycle: the replication of each DNA molecule during S-phase can take place only once. The second condition involves the initiation of mitosis: this cannot begin before the complete termination of DNA replication. Control over the course of successive phases of cell cycle is extraordinarily precise and rigorous since initiation of the S-phase is restricted exclusively to unreplicated post-mitotic chromatin. Meanwhile, it is known that competence to initiate mitosis is not always conditioned by the replicated state of chromatin (this does not mean however that control over this process is not precise; simply, it results from the closely specified timing involved in setting-up factors liberating the activity of MPF [i.e. Cdk1 kinase and cyclin B complex or maturation/mitosis promoting factor] and its co-operation with aspects of the activators' and inhibitors' character).

Carefully designed experiments by Johnson & Rao (1970) have resulted in the first correct interpretation of the phenomenon of premature chromosome condensation (PCC). The term PCC appeared in the description of phenomena observed during the fusion of interphase and mitotic malignant HeLa cells. It has been shown that the PCC phenomenon is accompanied by disappearance of the nuclear envelope, chromatin condensation and the formation of mitotic spindle. Subsequent investigations have shown that the induction of PCC is inseparably connected with the activity of MPF complex. The experiments, involving fusion of interphase and mitotic cells have clearly shown that the cells in all the subperiods of interphase are characterized by capability to induce PCC. Thus: (i) if the fusion took place between a mitotic cell and an interphase cell in G1 phase, then PCC resulted in the formation of chromosomes consisting of a single chromatid only (univalent chromosomes); (ii) if the fusion took place between a mitotic cell and an interphase cell in S-phase, strongly fragmented chromosomes were formed in the PCC process, and their morphology constituted a specific reminder of the nucleoplasm organization in the period of the activity of the cell replication apparatus (a 'pulverized' appearance that consisted of univalent and bivalent chromosomes); (iii) if a mitotic cell and interphase cell in G2-phase participated in the combination, PCC resulted in the formation of chromosomes consisting of two chromatids apparently non-differentiated morphologically as compared to normal chromosomes, although probably less condensed (bivalent chromosomes). Despite the fact that the first observation of PCC was reported by Kato & Sandberg (1967) in virus mediated multinucleated fused cells of interphase and mitotic cells, it was Johnson & Rao who in 1970 properly defined the observed phenomenon as 'premature chromosome condensation' (PCC), and the condensed interphase chromatin as 'prematurely condensed chromosomes' (PCCs) (Gotoh & Durante, 2006). Generally, the PCC method facilitates the visualization of interphase chromatin as a condensed form of chromosome structure (Gotoh, 2007). Nowadays, the efficiency and scope of PCC induction have been proved by combining techniques.

Premature chromosome condensation became a method used to: (1) distinguish a cell cycle stage (Cadwell et al., 2011) and the Rabl-orientation of interphase chromosomes, e.g. G1-PCCs and G2-PCCs (Cremer et al., 1982); (2) investigations in chromosome dynamics, also that in interphase chromatin, chromosome replication studies and DNA repair analysis (Gotoh & Durante, 2006, as cited in Cornforth & Bedford, 1983; Hittelman & Pollard, 1982; Hittelman & Rao, 1974; Mullinger & Johnson, 1983; Schor et al., 1975); (3) perform mutagenic assay (Gotoh, 2009, as cited in Cornforth & Bedford, 1983; Durante et al., 1996); (4) chromosome instability analysis (Bezrookove et al., 2003); (5) prenatal diagnosis (Gotoh & Durante, 2006, as cited in Srebniak et al., 2005); (6) karyotyping of chromosomes (Kowalska et al., 2003); and (6) cytogenetic analysis of cancers (Darroudi et al., 2010).

2.1 Induction of PCC in historical and methodological terms

Virus-mediated PCC was first reported more than 40 years ago. In 1983, cell fusion could be achieved by means of polyethylene glycol (PEG-induced or chemically-mediated; Pantelias & Maillie, 1983). This allowed the external MPF to migrate from the inducing mitotic cell to the interphase recipient. A few years later it was possible to obtain chemically-induced PCC (drug-induced PCC): initially from synchronized cells and later still from each phase of the cell cycle (Gotoh & Durante, 2006, as cited in Schlegel & Pardee, 1986, Schlegel et al., 1990; Yamashita et al., 1990). Detailed data concerning PCC induction reported so far in the world literature are presented in Table 1.

The way of induction of PCC	References
A. Fusion-induced PCC Exploits the action of external MPF	
A1. Virus-induced fusion	
(a) UV inactivated Sendai virus-induced PCC	Kato & Sandberg, 1967 *The first observation of PCC* Johnson & Rao, 1970 *The first correct interpretation of PCC*
(b) PCC-type remodeling of the donor nucleus after somatic cell nuclear transfer (SCNT)	Le Bourhis et al., 2010
A2. Chemically-induced fusion	
(a) (PEG)-induced fusion	Pantelias & Maillie, 1983 *The first successfully applied polyethylene glycol (PEG)-induced fusion just before PCC induction*
B. Drug-induced PCC Exploits the activation of endogenous MPF	
B1. With synchronization Cells had to be synchronized in G1- or S- or G2-phase before PCC induction	
B1.1. Induced by protein phosphatase inhibitors	
(a) Okadaic acid	Schlegel & Pardee, 1986 *The first one successfully applied in chemically-induced PCC in S phase cells* Ghosh et al., 1998; Schlegel et al., 1990; Yamashita et al., 1990
(b) Sodium metavanadate	Ghosh et al., 1998; Rybaczek & Kowalewicz-Kulbat, 2011;
B1.2. Induced by protein kinase inhibitors	
(a) Caffeine	Schlegel & Pardee, 1986 *The first one successfully applied in chemically-induced PCC in S phase cells* Schlegel et al., 1990; Yamashita et al., 1990; Nghiem et al., 2001
(b) Caffeine 2-aminopurine Staurosporine 6-dimethylaminopurine	Sen & Ghosh, 1998; Rybaczek et al., 2008; Rybaczek & Kowalewicz-Kulbat, 2011; Steinmann et al., 1991
B2. Without synchronization PCC induction occurs without synchronization (in any phase of cell cycle)	
B2.1. Induced by protein phosphatase inhibitors	
(a) Okadaic acid Calyculin A	Bialojan & Takai, 1988; Cohen et al., 1990; Gotoh et al., 1995; Gotoh & Tanno, 2007; Ishihara et al., 1989; Prasanna et al., 2000
B2.2. Adriamycin (Doxorubicin)	Hittelman & Rao, 1975
C. Spontaneous PCC (SPCC)	
(a) In the ontogenesis of generative cells and during the development of endosperm	cited by Tam & Schlegel, 1995
(b) During heat exposure	Mackey et al., 1988; Swanson et al., 1995;
(c) In normal and transformed mammal cells	Kovaleva et al., 2007
(d) After X-irradiation of HeLa cells	Ianzini & Mackey, 1997

Table 1. Data concerning PCC induction reported in the word literature

A specific change occurred when the preliminary cell-free cytoplasmic extracts (obtained by the centrifugation of *Xenopus* egg cells) were used *in vitro* to study the assembly of 'synthetic nuclei' involving the conversion of chromatin sperms into mitotic chromosomes. The resulting expansion of knowledge concerning the action of inhibitors and/or activators used for PCC induction has created new opportunities and perspectives for researchers (Prokhorova et al., 2003). In cells with disturbed DNA structure or those blocked during DNA biosynthesis, PCC-type processes can be induced by various chemical compounds such as: (i) inhibitors of protein kinases, e.g. 2-aminopurine (Herbig et al., 2004), caffeine (Wang et al., 1999, Gabrielli et al., 2007), staurosporine, 7-hydroxystaurosporine (UCN-01), CEP-3891 (Kohn et al., 2002; Syljuåsen et al., 2005), wortmannin (WORT) (Liu et al., 2007) and Gö6976 (Jia et al., 2008) as well as (ii) inhibitors of protein phosphatases, e.g. calyculin A (CalA), okadaic acid (OA) and sodium metavanadate (Van) (Hosseini & Mozdarani, 2004; Rybaczek & Kowalewicz-Kulbat, 2011). In order to induce the PCC phenomenon, an incubation with a strong inhibitor, e.g. of a given kinase or phosphatase or alternating incubation in two different inhibitors, of which the former slows down the course of S phase (e.g. hydroxyurea or aphidicolin) and the latter specifically influences the activity of selected kinases or phosphatases is a frequently used approach. Such substances restore the activity of protein kinases and control the phosphorylation of subordinate proteins in the regulatory pathways of cell cycle simultaneously creating conditions necessary for the initiation of prophase chromosome condensation, thereby fulfilling the role of the inductors of Cdk1-cyclin B complexes and realising mitotic phosphorylations (Sturgeon et al., 2008).

Disturbance of the efficiency of cell cycle checkpoints can result from the action of many factors followed by overriding or breakage of control over genome integrity and the course of various interphase subperiods and finally PCC induction. The premature mitosis induced in meristems of *V. faba* roots by prolonged incubation with a mixture of hydroxyurea and caffeine is characterized by strong differentiation between the morphological forms of chromosomes, which allows one to separate several different cell classes. The degree of chromosome fragmentation (number of sections lost in anaphase) probably determines the level of genetic material disintegration in cells blocked by hydroxyurea in S-phase. Such observations suggest that there is a relationship between the chromosome structure determining 'PCC phenotype' and S-phase subperiod (initiating the biosynthesis of 'early' or 'late' replicons), in which replication block has taken place. This assumes that the period of time elapsing between the beginning of PCC induction and the appearance of first cells with symptoms of premature mitosis depends on the number of replication units in which the biosynthesis processes of complementary DNA strands have been initiated but not terminated. The same mechanism may also explain the considerable differentiation between cells showing morphological features of premature mitosis (Figure 1A).

Modern models assume that phosphorylation of the N-terminal fragments of H3 histones constitutes a preliminary molecular signal which makes initiation of chromosome condensation possible by creating conditions for the assembly of other proteins directly engaged in the structural metamorphoses of chromatin (e.g. condesin complexes). Therefore, the post-translation modifications of H3 molecules are only one of the symptoms reflecting the action of complicated regulatory system which leads to the increase in chromatin packing during prophase chromosome condensation. This view is consistent with observations pointing to considerable asynchrony of the period of intensified H3 histone phosphorylation and the initial stages of mitotic condensation among various organisms, as well as to the phosphorylation of H3 molecules in plant cells taking place in condensed

chromosomes. Meanwhile, S10 phosphorylation of H3 histone has turned out to be an excellent marker in phenotyping PCC from various subperiods of e.g. S-phase (Figure 1B).
The G2→M transition is a period of an increased sensitivity of cells also to the action of factors that directly do not lead DNA damage. For example, when cells entering the early stages of prophase are subjected to hypothermia, anoxia, osmotic shock or other stresses, their chromosomes are decondensed followed by a return to late G2 phase. This phenomenon usually is reversible following a period of stress adaptation or regression of mitosis (Mikhailov & Rieder, 2002). So, the question - what is the beginning of mitosis? – is not trivial, especially in the context of its irreversibility. It is known that almost always the very fact of initiation of S phase determines future mitosis. On the other hand, the fact of DNA replication involving a successful transition through the cell cycle checkpoints gives the process of genetic material segregation to two daughter cells the status of authority or even necessity. It helps when seeking the answer to the question 'what is the beginning of mitosis?' to recall the term 'antephase', historically associated with the paper by Furlough & Johnson published in 1951 (Pines & Rieder, 2001, as cited in Furlough & Johnson, 1951).
The term 'antephase' is used to describe the final stage of G2 phase directly preceding the first perceptible symptoms of prophase chromosome condensation. Cells in the middle stages of prophase (cf. neuroblasts of grasshopper, cells of newt or PtK_1 cell line) subjected to ionizing radiation gradually decondense the chromosomes under formation, their proteins are dephosphorylated and the course of cell cycle is arrested. The same cells irradiated during late stages of prophase, despite strong chromosome fragmentation, initiate further mitosis stages. A similar process – gradual chromosome decondensation – is also observed when the disassembly of microtubules by nocodazole takes place before cell transition through the middle stage of prophase. The action of nocodazole in later periods of prophase induces colcemid-mitoses – the division of chromosomes deprived of communication with the microtubular spindle apparatus leading to the formation of polyploid nuclei. Thus there is a specified point, i.e. the final period of 'antephase', after which a cell is unable to return to the interphase condition. In the cells of many animal species (vertebrates), 'the point of the last chance to return to G2 phase' occurs during the final stages of prophase, the border here between interphase and mitosis being set considerably later than usual (Pines & Rieder, 2001).
Thus, there are cells in which advanced stages of chromosome condensation are an easily recognizable indicator of G2 phase termination ('antephase'), whence they become convenient subjects for studying the transient G2→M period at a molecular level. The activity of kinase Cdk1-cyclin A complexes increases during the G2 phase and reaches its maximum at the moment of nuclear envelope decomposition. The microinjection of these complexes into G2 cells induces a violent chromosome condensation but inhibitors of Cdk1 kinase (such as $p21^{Waf1/Cip1}$) block the transition to mitosis and then the early-prophase cells return to the interphase state. This is a period during which inactive Cdk1-cyclin B complexes remain in the area of cytoplasm (Furuno et al., 1999). Thus, it seems that preparation for the entry into mitosis taking place in vertebrate cells during 'antephase' is mainly controlled by Cdk1-cyclin A complex and not by the association of Cdk1 with cyclin B. An important role is also played by Plk1 kinase, which controls organization of the cell centrosomal apparatus and, while phosphorylating Cdc25 phosphatase, indirectly activates Cdk1-cyclin B complexes (Kumagai & Dunphy, 1996). Another protein kinase, Aurora B (animals) or its homologue in yeast cells (Ipl1) induces chromosome condensation via phosphorylation of S10 in H3 histone (Hsu et al., 2000). In many types of cells, changes occur at the level of chromosome condensation causing centrosomes to interact with a

growing number of γ-tubulin molecules. Meanwhile, normal cells (and not the transformed ones) are subjected to the control mechanisms of G2 phase which, by the intervention of ATM/ATR kinases, monitor the condition of DNA structure and make it possible to arrest the cell cycle just before the initiation of mitosis.

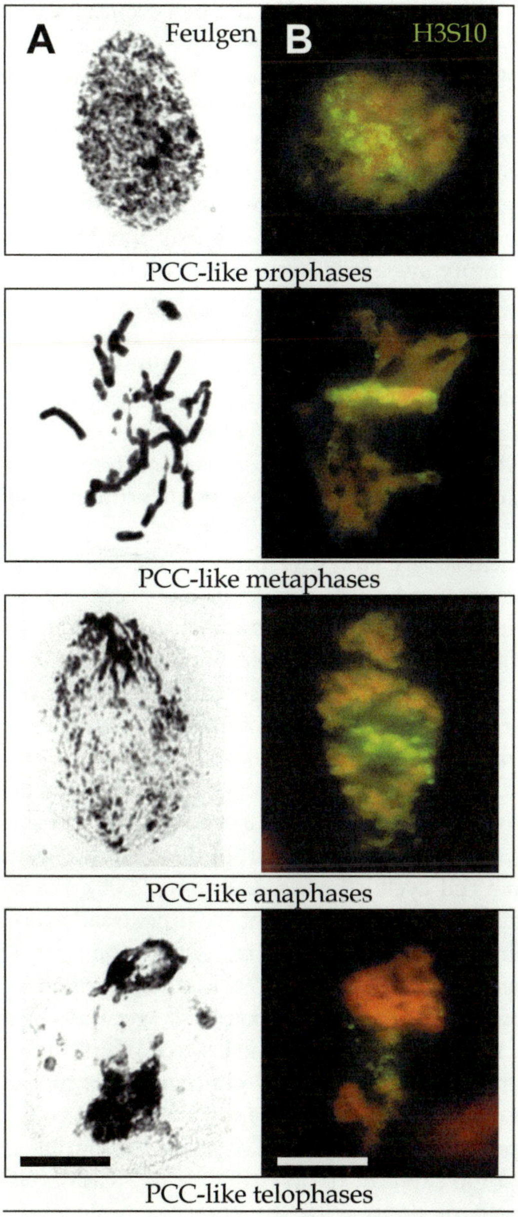

Fig. 1. A. Caffeine-induced PCC in Feulgen-stained root meristem cells of *Vicia faba*. The full array of aberrations included: chromosomal breaks and gaps, lost and lagging chromatids and chromosomes, acentric fragments and micronuclei. B. Immunofluorescence of phospho-H3 (S10; Cell Signaling) after caffeine-induced PCC in root meristem cells of *Vicia faba*. *Bar* 20 μm

3. Molecular origin of PCC induction

Hypotheses describing the mechanism of PCC induction are based on the results of genetic and biochemical analyses of yeast cells and human and animal cells *in vitro*. Among plants, the induction of premature chromosome condensation sometimes spontaneously occurs in the ontogenesis of generative cells and during the development of endosperm (cited by Tam & Schlegel, 1995). The special nature of these phenomena, the role played in them by phytohormonal factors and conditioning connected with the specificity of plant cell mitotic divisions have not yet been recognized. Neither have the organization of checkpoints blocking the initiation of mitosis, nor the mechanism that could overcome their restrictive interactions, been explained.

During the cell cycle, there are mechanisms governing transition 'to' and 'from' proliferation and coordinating of the complexes responsible for the successive stages of cell cycle transition. The first regulatory system is connected with the transition from G0 phase to cell cycle, which results in the transcription of appropriate genes, this being realization of the program responsible for leaving the resting condition. This leads to the commencement of DNA synthesis and consequently the initiation of mitotic division. The action of the second regulatory system involves arresting the course of G1 phase - before the start of DNA replication - or G2 phase - before the initiation of mitosis.

In cell cycles of the G1-S-G2-M type, the function of two main checkpoints is directly associated with the coordination of transient stages determining the maintenance of genetic identity. The G1 phase checkpoint monitors the metabolic conditions of cells in the G1 phase, the integrity of the nuclear DNA structure prior to the beginning of the synthesis of the complementary chromosome set and the level of necessary substrates, enzymes and replication factors. In plant cytology, it is known as the 'Principal Control Point 1' (PCP1), being the counterpart of the START point in yeast and of the Restriction Point in animal cells. The second checkpoint, PCP2, of a more conservative character, plays a similar role in G2 phase. Its functions are connected with the assessment of internal and external conditions of the cell environment during mitosis and cytokinesis. PCP2 controls if the replication of DNA is properly terminated and also monitors the integrity of chromatin structure before its mitotic condensation (Del Campo et al., 2003). The checkpoint pathways functioning in G1 and G2 phases of cell cycle constitute however only part of the complex system formed by checkpoint mechanisms of the whole cell cycle (Bucher & Britten, 2008). For example, the mechanisms determining S-phase initiation and development are functionally connected with the system of three S-phase checkpoints: (i) the intra-S-phase checkpoint or DSB-induced replication-independent intra-S-phase checkpoint which block mitosis initiation in the case of structural DNA damage; (ii) the replication checkpoint or replication-dependent intra-S-phase checkpoint which block mitosis initiation in the case of inhibition of DNA biosynthesis; and (iii) the replication-dependent S-M checkpoint which ensures that the G2 phase and mitosis can begin after complete genome replication (Bartek et al., 2004).

In many respects, the control mechanisms of G2 phase are similar to the regulatory systems that protect a cell against too rapid initiation of DNA replication. Still more analogies can be found by comparing both of them with the complex molecular systems of the S phase checkpoints. Admitting some simplification, it can be assumed that this continual repetition is not unusual: if monitoring of the DNA structure integrity is the basic aim of complicated biochemical mechanisms, the means serving that end do not have to be adapted for the realization of many targets, but just one – the most important. On the other hand, their molecular construction must take into account the specificity of the successive phases of the cell cycle.

The mentioned analogies have probably contributed to the fact that the best known function of checkpoints in G2 phase consists in blocking the initiation of mitosis in case of DNA damage. Detection of structural anomalies liberates the action of two complementary and partly convergent molecular pathways centred on ATM/ATR kinases and a common purpose - maintenance the Cdk1 kinase complexes with cyclin B inactive (Mikhailov & Rieder, 2002; Paulsen & Cimprich, 2007). In one pathway, ATM directly (or indirectly) activates part of the regulatory system, with a key factor p53. This protein induces the synthesis of inhibitors of cyclin-dependent kinases, e.g. $p21^{Waf1/Cip1}$. In the other pathway, independent of p53, ATM activates effector kinases Chk1 and Chk2 that, in turn, prevent the activation of Cdc25C phosphatase (sometimes by Plk1 kinase). Undoubtedly, we have here an excellent example of two coincident regulatory systems that mutually intensify the effectiveness of their individual interactions, while at the same time providing an example of 'economical' use of the same metabolic networks in three different cell cycle phases (Brown & Baltimore, 2007; Matthews et al., 2007; Peddibhotla et al., 2009).

Mitosis is the most dramatic and potentially most 'dangerous' cell cycle phase - involving the condensation of replicated chromosomes, their association with the kinetochores and finally the segregation of sister chromatids to opposite poles. Not only chromosomes replicated in S phase are divided (karyokinesis) but also all organelles (cytokinesis). Thus the checkpoints of mitosis monitor all the transient stages of this complicated process but primarily they control the condition of mitotic spindle by detecting abnormalities in its structural and functional organization (Cortez & Elledge, 2000). Chromatin condensation forming mitotic chromosomes under physiological conditions takes place only during mitosis. Condensins are the key elements in this process. Condensin I and II occur among vertebrates. Condensin I obtains access to chromosomes always after the nuclear envelope breakdown (NEBD) and then, in cooperation with condensin II responsible for the initial stages of condensation in prophase nuclei, promotes the assembly of metaphase chromosomes. Condensins are regulated by phosphorylation dependent on Cdk1, which was demonstrated in the studies utilizing *Xenopus* egg extract. Active MPF initiates the nuclear envelope breakdown to allow condensin I to acquire chromosomes. Hypothetically, it is assumed that Cdk1-cyclin A complex phosphorylates and activates condensin II to initiate the early stage of chromosome condensation inside the prophase nucleus. Next, directly after the nuclear envelope breakdown, Cdk1-cyclin B complex phosphorylates and activates condensin I (Hirano, 2005).

Cell cycle checkpoints act via the principle of establishing a cause-effect relationship between separate biochemical processes (Hartwell & Weinert, 1989) involving feedback loops (Elledge, 1996). The term 'checkpoint' refers to a definite subset of internal and external regulatory mechanisms that link further processes to the realization of earlier ones. At the same time, one has to remember to always take into account the existence of hysteresis in the molecular interaction of the control network in the cell cycle system. Hysteresis means that it takes more to push a system from point A to point B than it does to keep the system at stage B (Sha et al., 2003; Solomon, 2003). Generally, there are two classes of regulatory systems in the cell cycle: (i) intrinsic systems of a constitutive character sorting out the events directly connected with the cell cycle, and (ii) extrinsic systems that are revealed under the influence of inducing factors and are engaged only when DNA damage is detected (Elledge, 1996).

Each of the cell cycle checkpoints comprises three essential parts: (i) capability of sensing that a cell cycle event is aberrant or incomplete, (ii) means by which this signal is transmitted, and finally, (iii) effectors that delay or block the cell cycle transitions until the problem is resolved. The position of arrest within the cell cycle varies depending on the phase during which the damage is sensed. Since the main role of all these checkpoints is to make a decision whether or not the cell division cycle can be continued, their particular elements deserve special attention as promising targets for pharmacological treatment of cancer (Deckert et al., 2009). The action of checkpoints of cell cycle crucially depends on the effectiveness of the system transmitting signals released by the cell sensory apparatus. The activation of mitotic protein kinases (M-Cdk) is then blocked which makes it possible to effect repairs or to terminate DNA replication or apoptosis induction (Khanna & Jackson, 2001; Zhou & Elledge, 2000).

The PCC phenomenon results from the overriding of S-M checkpoint. It blocks the ability of cells to make mitotic divisions after extensive DNA damage or under conditions of unfinished replication. DNA damage activates in the first place sensor kinases from the PIKK family, ATM and/or ATR which subsequently inhibit the formation of active MPFs by the phosphorylation of Chk2 and Chk1 kinases, which blocks the onset of mitosis. The initiated cascade of signals simultaneously activates repair factors including DNA-PK kinase which is essential for the repair of DNA suffering NHEJ-type damage. Blocking of the function of sensor ATM and/or ATR kinases can bring about avoidance of the restrictive interactions of S phase checkpoints causing premature mitosis (Block et al., 2004).

Knowledge of PCC mechanisms and S-M checkpoint action goes hand in hand with studies of malignant diseases and eagerness to maximize the beneficial effects of radio- and chemotherapy (Erenpreisa & Cragg, 2007). Despite evidence that overexpression of Cdk1-cyclin B complexes can promote PCC, it is not clear if these complexes initiate PCC in human cells. Studies of the import of cyclin B1 in human beings and in asteroid oocytes have shown that it is imported within the period of last several minutes of prophase, just after the initiation of chromosome condensation. These observations suggest that normal chromosome condensation is not initiated by Cdk1-cyclin B1 complexes. On the other hand, there is evidence indicating that the chromosome condensation and other phenomena occurring in the early prophase are initiated by Cdk2-cyclin A complexes present in this period within the cell nucleus. The initiation of cytoplasmic phenomena of mitotic character such as reorganization of Golgi apparatus and microtubular changes probably requires no import of Cdk1-cyclin B1 complexes into the nucleus (Takizawa & Morgan, 2000). On the other hand, the initiation of mitotic division occurs once Cdc25 phosphatase has dephosphorylated phosphate groups (both Y15 and T14) from the area of exposed pocket binding ATP within kinase $p34^{cdc2}$. Thus Cdc25 phosphatase is the activator of mitosis.

Dysfunctions of S phase checkpoints also occur in mutated cells (Krause et al., 2001). Deletions of *wee1* and *mik1* genes cause disappearance of proteins transmitting signals about DNA structure damage or blocked replication. Such cells initiate mitosis, but underreplications result in broken chromosomes being lost in the central spindle zone. Similar results follow from changes in the activity balance of protein kinases and phosphatases caused by overexpression of *cdc25* genes. Disappearance of intra-S-phase checkpoint function, caused e.g. by the lack (or mutation) of *atr*, also brings about the initiation of mitosis by cells that contain partly replicated genetic material (as opposed to normal cells in which replication forks activate ATR if they meet a defect impeding the biosynthesis of DNA which leads to the activation of S phase checkpoints and cell cycle inhibition). In the embryonic evolution of *Drosophila melanogaster*, grapes (*grp*) - whose product is a homolog of Chk1 kinase - is one of the genes of checkpoints functioning in this period of morphogenesis. Grapes mutants show a shortened course of interphase, a defective chromosome condensation and delayed metaphase initiation (Yu et al., 2000). In this case, premature mitosis is caused firstly by overriding of function of S phase checkpoints (then chromosome condensation is not dependent on the termination of S phase) and secondly, by the moment of initiation of chromosome condensation (ICC) occurring with no delay. Thus, only the period between ICC and metaphase is shortened, which seems to be the direct cause of incomplete chromosome condensation. To sum up, in *D. melanogaster* the delay in *grp* embryo entry into metaphase is caused by chromatin condensation defects rather than by partial DNA replication (Royou et al., 2005).

The facts presented above that barely outline extensive problems connected with the cellular control mechanisms show a huge complexity of both stimulating and inhibiting biochemical systems. The associated regulatory network comprises processes that activate the expression of genes at the moment desired for the cell and block the course of chemical reactions when their products could accumulate in excessive amount or prematurely encourage cell cycle transitions. It seems that all eukaryotic cells are equipped with sensory factors, signal transmitting systems and effector factors. The significance of these consists in the fact that they make DNA replication and chromosome division possible without endangering the whole information contained in them which is indispensable for the organism development and maintenance of species continuity.

4. PCC and DNA damages

The successive phases of prematurely initiated mitosis follow an aberrated course. The loss of relatively large chromosome sections suggests that disturbances of post-replication repair processes in the G2 (G2-PCC) are responsible for this. On the other hand, much higher disintegration of genetic material in some chromosomes leads to the conclusion that this is symptomatic of mitosis initiated from cell subpopulations that have not yet finished the DNA replication process (S-PCC; Rybaczek et al., 2008). Some influence on the degree of DNA fragmentation can be exerted by chemical compounds used in studies of PCC induction, e.g. caffeine which additionally intensifies chromosome destruction during their individualization. It is certain that the losses or breaks in the chromosome continuity: (i) either illustrate the unreplicated areas of genome; (ii) or result from physical stresses created during the mitotic condensation and segregation of chromosomes; (iii) or originate from relative fragility of single-stranded DNA sections generated during retardation of replication forks under the conditions of nucleotide triphosphate deficiency (i.e. after the use of replication inhibitors, e.g. hydroxyurea) (Cimprich, 2003; El Achkar et al., 2005).

The appearance of double strand breaks (DSBs) in DNA molecules is connected with the formation of immunofluorescence foci associated with the phosphorylated form of H2AX histones at S139 (DSB marker). The family of lysine-like H2A histones includes three subfamilies of proteins (H2A1-H2A2, H2AZ and H2AX). In mammalian cells, H2AX amounts to about 2 to 25% (probably almost 100% in *S. cerevisiae*) (Rogakou et al., 1998). The C-terminal motif of AQ(D/E)(I/L/Y) is the sequence distinguishing H2AX among H2A histones, while S139, ahead of it, is the site of γ-phosphorylation. Formation of γ-H2AX molecules resulting from the exposure of mammalian cells (or living mice) to the action of ionizing radiation (in sublethal or lethal doses) is an extremely violent process (Kurose et al.,

2006). Half of the γ-H2AX histones appears after a 1-minute period of irradiation, while the maximal level is reached within 3 to 10 minutes of exposure (per 1 Gy of radiation about 1% of H2AX histone molecules undergoes γ-phosphorylation, which corresponds to about $2x10^6$ bp DNA in the area of the double-strand break of its structure) (Paull et al., 2000; Rogakou et al., 1998). It is assumed that each group of these molecules indicates a single DSB region, therefore the formation of H2AX foci phosphorylated at S139 constitutes a sensitive test revealing the presence of structural genome damage (Friesner et al., 2005). Literature reports in recent years show the occurrence of fluorescence foci of H2AX molecules within the area of S139 during PCC induction (Huang et al., 2006; Rybaczek et al., 2007; Rybaczek & Kowalewicz-Kulbat, 2011). On the other hand, Stevens and his co-workers (2010) clearly indicate that PCC is γ-H2AX negative, and that γ-H2AX phosphorylation is only a hallmark of a chromosome fragmentation phenomenon. However, simultaneously they define PCC as occurring in interphase cells exposed to active MPF vs that occurring during mitosis chromosome fragmentation. According to other investigations, however, the actual definition of drug-induced PCC involves both the described phenomena, i.e. PCC and chromosome fragmentation (Riesterer et al., 2009; Rybaczek et al., 2008; Terzoudi et al., 2010).

To protect against disturbances during DNA biosynthesis, cells have developed a network of biochemical reactions known as DNA-replication-stress-response. The basic strategy of this response is retardation of processes, whose continuation would result, among other things, in the transfer of affected DNA molecules to a new cell generation. Therefore under the conditions of replication stress, the DNA biosynthesis rate is slowed down and onset of mitosis is - most frequently - completely blocked. This continues until the expression of specific genes and activation of repair factors (Deckert et al., 2009; Mosesso et al., 2010). Each structural disturbance (e.g. DSB) causes the rate of production of replication forks to slow down. Additionally, any limitation of the replication apparatus effectiveness (resulting, e.g. from the deficiency of nucleotide triphosphate or polymerase dysfunction) can facilitate DNA damage. In such a situation, the action of checkpoint sensory factors releases a cascade of signals supplied to various effector proteins through intermediary elements.

The detection of double-strand breaks in DNA molecules activates the biochemical pathway in which ATM kinase is the superior element. The processes proceeding with its contribution are triggered in all the phases of cell cycle, while the factors participating here may also assist the second pathway going in parallel. ATR is also activated by damage resulting in disruption of continuity in both DNA strands, but here the induction process occurs more slowly (Scott & Pandita, 2006). The pathway subordinated to ATR kinase is specialized first of all in reacting to disturbance of the replication fork function. These disturbances can results from endogenous interactions, chemotherapy or experimental procedures leading to the inhibition or disturbance of replication processes caused by hydroxyurea (HU) or ultraviolet radiation (UV). In both biochemical pathways, Cdc25 phosphatase is the target substrate.

Mec1 and Tel1 kinases in *S. cerevisiae* and Rad3 and Tel1 kinases in humans are homologues of both conservative signaling ATM and ATR kinases (Garber et al., 2005). Their substrates, kinases of the CHK family, are subordinate factors activated by ATM/ATR/Mec1/Rad3. Such groups jointly form the central pathway module of response to replication stress, which both records incoming information on the DNA condition and sends signals to replication forks. In human and *Xenopus* cells, ATR kinase is indispensable in the phosphorylation of Chk1 kinase and it occurs in stable combination with ATR-interacting protein (ATRIP), there complexes being concentrated in those areas of cell nucleus showing DNA damage. The activator of ATR-ATRIP complexes in vertebrate cells consists of TopBP1 protein. Investigations utilizing cytoplasmic extracts of *Xenopus* egg cells have also shown that the association of ATR with chromatin takes place during the period of DNA replication, whereas it disappears after the termination of replication (Freire et al., 2006; Harper & Elledge, 2007).

It is uncertain whether disturbances of DNA replication are detected by means of only one, universal, sensory mechanism. Maybe, regardless of the type of the factor blocking S phase, the DNA structure generated by replication forks is identical at the damage site. However, one cannot exclude the possibility that each type of the DNA structure disturbance exerts different, specific influence on replication forks and that the factors associated with particular types of damage are also different.

5. Consequences of PCC induction

Literature shows that proper functioning of all multicellular organisms, including *Homo sapiens*, depends not only on their ability to produce new cells but also on the ability of each cell to annihilate itself when it becomes unwanted or damaged. This takes place also when the control mechanisms of the cell cycle have been overridden during a simultaneous strong and/or long-lasting action of stress stimulus. Thus, among cells induced to enter premature, unauthorized division, there are also those that choose the apoptosis pathway (Sahu et al., 2009). Therefore premature mitoses/PCC are described as a mitotic catastrophe, abortive or suicidal. During the induction of apoptosis - following PCC induction - chromatin undergoes drastic changes: previously usually dispersed, it suddenly begins to condense into one or more aggregates in the vicinity of a nuclear membrane (Figure 2A). Changes connected with the initial phase of apoptosis also involve formation of intranuclear membranous structures (sometimes strongly developed and multi-layered) adhering to the nuclear envelope (Figure 2B-D).

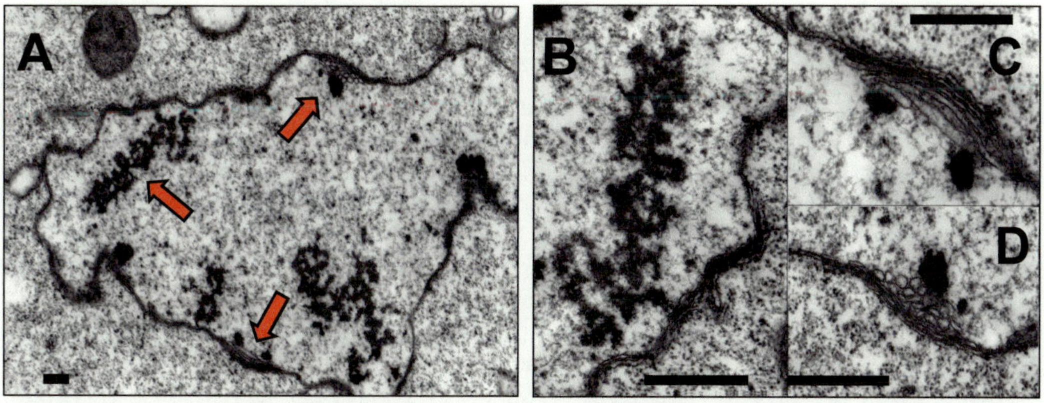

Fig. 2. Ultrastructure of an apoptotic cell of *V. faba* root meristem (after PCC induction caused by 5 mM caffeine). Selected fragments of the above micro-photography (marked with arrows) at magnification. *Bar* 1μm

Among unicellular organisms, irregularities in the organization of cell cycle control systems result in a decreased reproduction potential, while among multicellular mechanisms they cause uncontrolled proliferation, cancer development and genetic disease transfer (Hartwell & Weinert, 1989; Russell, 1998).

6. Conclusion

What are the practical implications and prospects of PCC induction? Could PCC induction serve as a novel anti-cancer approach? Undoubtedly, the phenomenon of premature mitosis is an essential characteristic of cell biology, therefore an important issue in respect of potential medical applications. It is so because, according to many researchers, the chemotherapy commonly used for the treatment of malignancy leads to extensive DNA damage, whereas PCC induction (resulting from the stimulation of biochemical mechanisms overriding the action of S-M checkpoint) can intensify therapeutic effects. Recently, drug-induced PCC was optimized to assist analysis of the behavior of cancer cells with minimal side effects. However, PCC will also contribute to the understanding of normal cellular processes.

7. Acknowledgement

The author expresses her cordial thanks to Professor Joanna Deckert for her support and inspiration, to Anna Pastucha for her assistance with immunocytochemical assays employing anti-H3S10, and to Małgorzata Fronczak M.Sc. for her help in preparing this manuscript in English. This work was funded by the Ministry of Science and Higher Education, grant N N303 355935 (contract no. 3559/B/P01/2008/25).

8. References

Bartek, J., Lukas, C. & Lukas, J. (2004) Checking on DNA damage in S phase. *Nat Rev Mol Cell Biol* 5, 792-804.

Bezrookove, V., Smits, R., Moeslein, G., Fodde, R., Tanke, H.J., Raap, A.K. & Darroudi, F. (2003) Premature chromosome condensation revisited: a novel chemical approach permits efficient cytogenetic analysis of cancers. *Genes Chromosomes Cancer* 38, 177-186.

Bialojan, C. & Takai, A. (1988) Inhibitory effect of a marine-sponge toxin, okadaic acid, on protein phosphatases. Specificity and kinetics. *Biochem J* 256, 283-290.

Block, W.D., Merkle, D., Meek, K. & Lees-Miller, S.P. (2004) Selective inhibition of the DNA-dependent protein kinase (DNA-PK) by the radiosensitizing agent caffeine. *Nucleic Acids Res* 32, 1967-1972.

Brown, E.J. & Baltimore, D. (2007) Essential and dispensable roles of ATR in cell cycle arrest and genome maintenance. *Genes Dev* 17, 615-628.

Bucher, N. & Britten, C.D. (2008) G2 treatment abrogation and checkpoint kinase-I targeting in the treatment of cancer. *Br J Cancer* 98, 532-528.

Cadwell, K.K., Curwen, G.B., Tawn, E.J., Winther, J.F., Boice, J.D. Jr. (2011) G2 checkpoint control and G2 chromosomal radiosensitivity in cancer survivors and their families. *Mutagenesis* 26, 291-294.

Cimprich, K.A. (2003) Fragile sites: Breaking up over a slowdown. *Curr Biol* 13, R231–R233.

Cohen, P., Holmes, C.F. & Tsukitani, Y. (1990) Okadaic acid: A new probe for the study of cellular regulation. *Trends Biochem Sci* 15, 98-102.

Cortez, D. & Elledge, S.J. (2000) Conducting the mitotic symphony. *Nature* 406, 354-356.

Cremer, T., Cremer, C., Baumann, H., Luedtke, E-K., Sperling, K., Teuber, V. & Zorn, C. (1982) Rabl's model of the interphase chromosome arrangement tested in Chinese hamster cells by premature chromosome condensation and laser-UV-microbeam experiments. *Hum Genet* 60, 46-56.

Darroudi, F., Bergs, J.W.J., Bezrookove, V., Buist, M.R., Stalpers, L.J. & Franken, N.A.P. (2010) PCC and COBRA-FISH a new tool to characterize primary cervical carcinomas: To asses hall-marks and stage specificity. *Cancer Lett* 287, 67-74.

Deckert, J., Pawlak, S. & Rybaczek, D. (2009) The nucleus as a 'headquarters' and target in plant cell stress reactions, In: *Compartmentation of Responses to Stresses in Higher Plants, True or False,* Waldemar Maksymiec, pp. 61-90, Transworld Research Network, ISBN: 978-81-7895-422-6, Kerala, India.

Del Campo, A., Samaniego, R., Giménez-Abián, J.F., Giménez-Martín, G., López-Sáez, J.F., Moreno Díaz de la Espina, S. & De la Torre C. (2003) G2 checkpoint targets late replicating DNA. *Biology of the Cell* 95, 521-526.

El Achkar, E., Gerbault-Seureau, M., Muleris, M., Dutrillaux, B. & Debatisse, M. (2005) Premature condensation induces breaks at the interface of early and late replicating chromosome bands bearing common fragile sites. *Proc Natl Acad Sci USA* 102, 18069-18074.

Elledge, S.J. (1996) Cell cycle checkpoint: preventing an identity crisis. *Science* 274, 1664-1672.

Erenpreisa, J. & Cragg, M.S. (2007) Cancer: A matter of life cycle? *Cell Biol Int* 31, 1507-1510.

Freire, R., van Vugt, M.A.T.M., Mamely, I. & Medema R.H. (2006) Claspin. Timing the cell cycle arrest when the genome is damaged. *Cell Cycle* 5, 2831-2834.

Friesner, J.D., Liu, B., Culligan, K. & Britt, A.B. (2005) Ionizing radiation-dependent γ-H2AX focus formation requires ataxia telangiectasia mutated and ataxia telangiectasia mutated and Rad3-related. *Mol Biol Cell* 16, 2566-2576.

Furuno, N., den Elzen, N. & Pines, J. (1999) Human cyclin A is required for mitosis until mid-prophase. *J Cell Biol* 147, 295-306.

Gabrielli, B., Chau, Y.Q., Giles, N., Harding, A., Stevens, F. & Beamish, H. (2007) Caffeine promotes apoptosis in mitotic spindle checkpoint-arrested cells. *J Biol Chem* 10, 6954-6964.

Garber, P.M., Vidanes, G.M. & Toczyski, D.P. (2005) Damage in transition, *Trends Biochem Sci* 30, 63-66.

Ghosh, S., Paweletz, N. & Schroeter, D. (1998) Cdc2-independent induction of premature mitosis by okadaic acid in HeLa cells. *Exp Cell Res* 242, 1-9.

Gotoh, E. & Durante, M. (2006) Chromosome condensation outside of mitosis: mechanisms and new tools. *J Cell Physiol* 209, 297-304.

Gotoh, E. & Tanno, Y. (2007) Simple biodosimetry method for cases of high-dose radiation exposure using the ratio of the longest/shortest length of Giemsa-stained drug-induced prematurely condensed chromosomes (PCC). *Int J Radiat Biol* 81, 379-385.

Gotoh, E. (2007) Visualizing the dynamics of chromosome structure formation coupled with DNA replication. *Chromosoma* 116, 453-462.

Gotoh, E. (2009) Drug-induced premature chromosome condensation (PCC) protocols : cytogenetic approaches in mitotic chromosome and interphase chromatin, In : *Chromatin Protocols: Second Edition, series: Methods in Molecular Biology*, Srikumar P. Chellappan, 523, 83-92, Humana Press, 523, 83-92.

Gotoh, E., Asakawa, Y. & Kosaka, H. (1995) Inhibition of protein serine/threonine phosphatases directly induces premature chromosome condensation in mammalian somatic cells. *Biomed Res* 16, 63-68.

Harper, J.W. & Elledge, S.J. (2007) The DNA damage response: ten years after. *Mol Cell* 28, 739-745

Hartwell, L.H. & Weinert, T.A. (1989) Checkpoints: controls that ensure the order of cell cycle events. *Science* 246, 629-634.

Herbig, U., Jobling, W.A., Chen, B.P.C., Chen, D.J. & Sedivy, J.M. (2004) Telomere shortening triggers senescence of human cells through a pathway involving ATM, p53, and $p21^{CIP1}$, but not $p16^{INK4a}$. *Mol Cell* 4, 501-513.

Hirano, T. (2005) Condensins: organizing and segregating the genome. *Curr Biol* 15, 265-275.

Hittelman, W.N. & Rao, P.N. (1975) The nature of adriamycin-induced cytotoxicity in Chinese hamster cells as revealed by premature chromosome condensation. *Cancer Res* 35, 27-35.

Hosseini, S. & Mozdarani, H. (2004) Induction of premature chromosome condensation (PCC) by calyculin A for biodosimetry. *Iran J Radiat Res* 1, 1-6.

Hsu, J-Y., Sun, Z-W., Li, X., Reuben, M., Tatchell, K., Bishop, D.K., Grushcow, J.M., Brame, C.J., Caldwell, J.A. & Hunt, D.F. (2000) Mitotic phosphorylation of histone H3 is governed by Ipl1/aurora kinase and glc7/PP1 phosphatase in budding yeast and nematodes. *Cell* 102, 279-291.

Huang, X., Kurose, A., Tanaka, T., Traganos, F., Dai, W. & Darzynkiewicz, Z. (2006) Sequential phosphorylation of *Ser*-10 on histone H3 and *Ser*-139 on histone H2AX and ATM activation during premature chromosome condensation: relationship to cell-cycle phase and apoptosis. *Cytometry Part A* 69A, 222-229.

Ianzini, F. & Mackey, M.A. (1997) Spontaneous premature chromosome condensation and mitotic catastrophe following irradiation of HeLa S3 cells. *Int J Radiat Biol* 72, 409-421.

Ishihara, H., Martin, B.L., Brautigan, D.L., Karaki, H., Ozaki, H., Kato, Y., Fusetani, N., Watabe, S., Hashimoto, K., Uemura, D., et al. (1989) Calyculin A and okadaic acid: Inhibitors of protein phosphatase activity. *Biochem Biophys Res Commun* 159, 871-877.

Jia, X.Z., Yang, S.Y., Zhou, J., Li, S.L., Ni, J.H., An, G.S. & Jia, H.T. (2008) Inhibition of CHK1 kinase by Gö6976 converts 8-chloro-adenosine-induced G2/M arrest into S arrest in human myelocytic leukemia K562 cells. *Biochem Pharmacol* 5, 770-780.

Johnson, R.T. & Rao, P.N. (1970) Mammalian cell fusion: Induction of premature chromosome condensation in interphase nuclei. *Nature* 226, 717-722.

Kato, H. & Sandberg, A. (1967) Chromosome pulverization in human binucleate cells following colcemid treatment. *J Cell Biol* 34, 35-46.

Khanna, K.K. & Jackson, S.P. (2001) DNA double-strand breaks: signaling, repair and the cancer connection. *Nat Genet* 27, 247-254.

Kohn, E.A., Ruth, N.D., Brown, M.K., Livingstone, M. & Eastman, A. (2002) Abrogation of the S phase damage checkpoint results in S phase progression or premature mitosis depending on the concentration of 7-hydroxystaurosporine and the kinetics of Cdc25C activation. *J Biol Chem* 277, 26553-26564.

Kovaleva, O.A., Glazko, T.T., Kochubey, T.P., Lukash, L.L. & Kudryavets, Y.I. (2007) Spontaneous premature condensation of chromosomes in normal and transformed mammal cells. *Exp Oncol* 29, 18-22.

Kowalska, A., Srebniak, M., Wawrzkiewicz, A. & Kaminski, K. (2003) The influence of calyculin A on lymphocytes in vitro. *J Appl Genet* 44, 413-418.

Krause, S.A., Loupert, M.-L., Vass. S., Schoefelder, S., Harrison, S. & Heck, M.M.S. (2001) Loss of cell cycle checkpoint control in *Drosophila* RFC4 mutants. *Mol Cell Biol* 21, 5156-5168.

Kumagai, A. & Dunphy, W.G. (1996) Purification and molecular cloning of Plx1, a Cdc25-regulatory kinase from *Xenopus* egg extracts. *Science* 273, 1377-1380.

Kurose, A., Tanaka, T., Huang, X., Traganos, F. & Darzynkiewicz, Z. (2006) Synchronization in the cell cycle by inhibitors of DNA replication induces histone H2AX phosphorylation : an induction of DNA damage. *Cell Prolif* 39, 231-240.

Le Bourhis, D., Beaujean, N., Ruffini, S., Vignon, X. & Gall, L. (2010) Nuclear remodeling in bovine somatic cell nuclear transfer embryos using MG132-treated recipient oocytes. *Cell Reprogram* 12, 729-738.

Liu, Y., Jiang, N., Wu, J., Dai, W. & Rosenblum, J.S. (2007) Polo-like kinases inhibited by wortmannin: labeling site and downstream effects. *J Biol Chem* 4, 2505-2511.

Mackey, M.A., Morgan, W.F. & Dewey, W.C. (1988) Nuclear fragmentation and premature chromosome condensation induced by heat shock in S-phase Chinese hamster ovary cells. *Cancer Res* 48, 6478-6483.

Matthews, D.J., Yakes, F.M., Chen, J., Tadano, M., Bornheim, L., Clary, D.O., Tai, A., Wagner, J.M., Miller, N., Kim, Y.D., Robertson, S., Murray, L. & Karnitz, L.M. (2007) Pharmacological abrogation of S-phase checkpoint enhances the anti-tumor activity of gemcitabine in vivo. *Cell Cycle* 6, 104-110.

Mikhailov, A. & Rieder, C.L. (2002) Cell cycle: stressed out of mitosis. *Curr Biol* 12, R331-R333.

Mosesso, P., Palitti, F., Pepe, G., Pinero, J., Bellacima, R., Ahnstrom, G. & Natarajan, A.T. (2010) Relationship between chromatin structure, DNA damage and repair following X-irradiation of human leukocytes. *Mutat Res* 701, 86-91.

Nghiem, P., Park, P.K., Kim, Y-S, Vaziri, C. & Schreiber, S.L. (2001) ATR inhibition selectively sensitizes G_1 checkpoint-deficient cells to lethal premature chromatin condensation. *Proc Natl Acad Sci USA* 98, 9092-9097.

Pantelias, G.E. & Maillie, H.D. (1983) A simple method for premature chromosome condensation induction in primary human and rodent cells using polyethylene glycol. *Somatic Cell Genet* 9, 533-547.

Paull, T.T., Rogakou, E.P., Yamazaki, V., Kirchgessner, C.U., Gellert, M. & Bonner, W.M. (2000) A critical role for histone H2AX in recruitment of repair factors to nuclear foci after DNA damage. *Curr Biol* 10, 886-895.

Paulsen, R.D. & Cimprich, K.A. (2007) The ATR pathway: Fine-tuning the fork. *DNA Repair* 6, 953-966.

Peddibhotla, S., Lam, M.H., Gonzalez-Rimbau , M. & Rosen J.M. (2009) The DNA-damage effector checkpoint kinase 1 is essential for chromosome segregation and cytokinesis. *Proc Natl Acad Sci USA* 106, 5159-5164.

Pines, J. & Rieder, C.L. (2001) Re-staging mitosis: a contemporary view of mitotic progression. *Nat Cell Biol* 3, E3-E6.

Prasanna, P.G.S., Escalada, N.D. & Blakely, W.F. (2000) Induction of premature chromosome condensation by a phosphatase inhibitor and a protein kinase in unstimulated human peripheral blood lymphocytes: a simple and rapid technique to study chromosome aberrations using specific whole-chromosome DNA hybridization probes for biological dosimetry. *Mutation Res* 466, 131-141.

Prokhorova, T.A., Mowrer, K., Gilbert, C.H. & Walter, J.C. (2003) DNA replication of mitotic chromatin in Xenopus egg extracts. *Proc Natl Acad Sci USA* 100, 13241-13246.

Riesterer, O., Matsumoto, F., Wang, L., Pickett, J., Molkentine, D., Giri, U., Milas, L. & Raju, U. (2009) A novel Chk inhibitor, XL-844, increases human cancer cell rediosensitivity through promotion of mitotic catastrophe. *Invest New Drugs* 29, 514-522.

Rogakou, E.P., Pilch, D.R., Orr, A.H., Ivanova, V.S. & Bonner, W.M. (1998) DNA double-stranded breaks induce histone H2AX phosphorylation on serine 139. *J Biol Chem* 273, 5858–5868.

Royou, A., Macias, H. & Sullivan, W. (2005) The Drosophila Grp/Chk1 DNA damage checkpoint controls entry into anaphase. *Curr Biol* 15, 334-339.

Russell, P. (1998) Checkpoint on the road to mitosis. *Trends Biol Sci* 23, 399-402.

Rybaczek, D. & Kowalewicz-Kulbat, M. (2011) Premature chromosome condensation induced by caffeine, 2-aminopurine, staurosporine and sodium metavanadate in S-phase arrested HeLa cells is associated with a decrease in Chk1 phosphorylation, formation of phospho-H2AX and minor cytoskeletal rearrangements. *Histochem Cell Biol 135*, 263-280.

Rybaczek, D., Bodys, A., Maszewski, J. (2007) H2AX foci in late S/G2- and M-phase cells after hydroxyurea- and aphidicolin-induced DNA replication stress in *Vicia*. *Histochem Cell Biol* 128, 227-241.

Rybaczek, D., Żabka, A., Pastucha, A. & Maszewski, J. (2008) Various chemical agents can induce premature chromosome condensation in *Vicia faba*. *Acta Physiol Plant* 30, 663-672.

Sahu, R.P., Batra, S. & Srivastava, S.K. (2009) Activation of ATM/Chk1 by cucrumin causes cell cycle arrest and apoptosis in human pancreatic cancer cells. *Br J Cancer* 100, 1425-1433.

Schlegel, R. & Pardee A.B. (1986) Caffeine-induced uncoupling of mitosis from the completion of DNA replication in mammalian cells. *Science* 232, 1264-1266.

Schlegel, R., Belinsky, G.S., Harris, MO. (1990) Premature mitosis induced by mammalian cells by the protein kinase inhibitors 2-aminopurine and 6-dimentylaminopurine. *Cell Growth Differ* 1, 171-178.

Scott, S.P. & Pandita, T.K. (2006) The cellular control of DNA double-strand breaks. *J Biol Chem* 99, 1463-1475.

Sen, R. & Ghosh, S. (1998) Induction of premature mitosis in S-blocked onion cells. *Cell Biol Int* 22, 867-874.

Sha,W., Moore, J., Chen, K., Lassaletta, A.D., Yi, C-S. & Tyson, J.J., (2003) Hysteresis drives cell-cycle transitions in *Xenopus laevis* egg extracts. *Proc Natl Acad Sci USA* 100, 975-980.

Solomon, M.J. (2003) Hysteresis meets the cell cycle. *Proc Natl Acad Sci USA* 100, 771-772.

Steinmann, K.E., Belinsky, G.S., Lee, D. & Schlegel, R. (1991) Chemically induced premature mitosis: Differential response in rodent and human cells and the relationship to cyclin B synthesis and $p34^{cdc2}$/cyclin B complex formation. *Cell Biology* 88, 6843-6847.

Stevens, J.B., Abdallah, b.Y., Regan, S.M., Liu, G., Bremer, S.W., Ye, C.J. & Heng, H.H. (2010) Comparison of mitotic cell death by chromosome fragmentation to premature chromosome condensation. *Molecular Cytogenetics* 3, 20-30.

Sturgeon, C.M., Cinel, B., Díaz-Marrero, A.R., McHardy, L.M., Ngo, M., Andersen, R.J. & Roberge, M. (2008) Abrogation and inhibition of nuclear export by *Cryptocarya* pyrones. *Cancer Chemother Pharmacol* 3, 407-413.

Swanson, P.E., Carroll, S.B., Zhang, X.F. & Mackey, M.A. (1995) Spontaneous premature chromosome condensation, micronucleus formation, and non-apoptotic cell death in heated HeLa S3 cells. *Am J Pathol* 146, 963-971.

Syljuåsen, R.G., Sørennsen, C.S., Hansen, L.T., Fugger, K., Lundin, C., Johansson, F., Helleday, T., Sehested, M., Lukas, J. & Bartek, J. (2005) Inhibition of human Chk1 causes increased initiation of DNA replication, phosphorylation of ATR targets, and DNA breakage. *Mol Cell Biol* 9, 3553-3562.

Szymborska, W. (1993). *Poems New and Collected*. English translation by Barańczak S. & Cavanagh C. (1998), Harcourt Inc., ISBN 0-15-601146-8, Orlando, Florida, USA

Takizawa, C.G. & Morgan D.O. (2000) Control of mitosis by changes in the subcellular location of cyclin-B1-Cdk1 and Cdc25. *Curr Op Cell Biol* 12, 658-665.

Tam, S.W. & Schlegel, R. (1995) Quantification of premature and normal mitosis, In: *Cell Cycle - Materials and Methods*, Michele Pagano, pp. 93-99, Springer-Verlag, ISBN 3-540-58066-2, Berlin-Heidelberg-New York.

Terzoudi, G.I., Hatzi, V.I., Donta-Bakoyianni D. & Pantelias G.E. (2010) Chromatin dynamics during cell cycle mediate conversion of DNA damage into chromatin breaks and affect formation of chromosomal aberrations: Biological and clinical significance. *Mutation Res* 711, 174-186.

Waldren, C.A. & Johnson, R.T. (1974) Analysis of interphase chromosome damage by means of premature chromosome condensation after X- and ultraviolet-irradiation. *Proc Nat Acad Sci USA* 71, 1137-1141.

Wang, S.-W., Norbury, C., Harris, A.L. & Toda, T. (1999) Caffeine can override the S-M checkpoint in fission yeast. *J Cell Sci* 112, 927-937.

Yamashita, K., Yasuda, H., Pines, J., Yasumoto, K., Nishitani, H., Ohtsubo, M., Hunter, T., Sugimura, T. & Nishimoto, T. (1990) Okadaic acid, a potent inhibitor of type 1 and type 2A protein phosphatases, activates cdc2/H1 kinase and transciently induces a premature mitosis-like state in BHK21 cells. *EMBO J* 9, 4331-4338.

Yu, K.R., Saint, R.B. & Sullivan, W. (2000) The Grapes checkpoint coordinates nuclear envelope breakdown and chromosome condensation. *Nat Cell Biol* 2, 609-615.

Zhou B.-B.S. & Elledge S.J. (2000) The DNA damage response: putting checkpoints in perspective. *Nature* 408, 433-439.

12

A DNA Repair Protein BRCA1 as a Potentially Molecular Target for the Anticancer Platinum Drug Cisplatin

Adisorn Ratanaphan
Prince of Songkla University
Thailand

1. Introduction

Cancer is a leading cause of death in the world. The incidence of cancers is related to environmental factors, behavioral patterns, and genetic disorders. Cancer therapy usually aims to selectively destroy cancer cells while sparing normal tissue. Most chemotherapeutic agents function by damaging cancer cell DNA. The cellular responses to DNA damage are thus critical factors for determining the effectiveness of most cancer therapies (Ashworth, 2008). When normal cells are exposed to damage, DNA repair mechanism is induced. The DNA repair processes are the cellular responses associated with the restoration of the normal DNA nucleotide sequences. The DNA repair activity of the cell is an important determinant of a cells sensitivity to chemotherapeutic agents. It is known that resistance to DNA-damaging agents can be associated with increased cellular repair activities, while defects in DNA repair pathways result in hypersensitivity to damage (Kelley & Fishel, 2008; Quinn et al., 2003, 2009). Several studies have clearly demonstrated that the impairment or absence of genes or proteins responsible for DNA damage repair, frequently causes genomic instability, cell cycle arrest and apoptosis. The importance of these repair pathways is highlighted by the fact that more than 100 genes have been found in mammalian cells that are involved in some way in DNA damage repair pathways. The breast cancer susceptibility gene 1 (*BRCA1*) is a tumor suppressor gene involved in maintaining genomic integrity through multiple functions in DNA damage repair, transcriptional regulation, a cell cycle checkpoint and protein ubiquitination (Brzovic et al., 2001; Hashizume et al., 2001; Mark et al., 2005; Varma et al., 2005; Williams et al., 2004). In cancer cells, damage to *BRCA1* by the anticancer platinum drug cisplatin may lead to a loss of such functions and ultimately results in cancer cell death. In addition, preclinical and clinical studies have recently revealed that inactivation of the BRCA1 protein in cancer cells leads to chemosensitivity. Therefore, approaching the BRCA1 protein as a potential therapeutic target for cisplatin or other such platinum based drugs might be of interest for molecular-targeted cancer therapy. In this chapter, the biophysical characterization and functional consequences of the human *BRCA1* gene and the BRCA1 RING protein induced by cisplatin are described.

2. Breast cancer susceptibility gene 1 (*BRCA1*) and its encoded protein

In 1990, chromosome 17q21 was identified by linkage analysis as the location of a breast cancer susceptibility gene 1 or *BRCA1* (Hall et al., 1990). The entire gene covers approximately 100 kb of genomic sequence, and was subsequently cloned four years later (Miki et al., 1994). BRCA1 is a tumor suppressor gene composed of 24 exons, with an mRNA that is 7.8 kb in length, and 22 coding exons that translate into a protein of 1863 amino acids (Fig. 1) with a molecular weight of 220 kDa (Brzovic et al., 1998). It has 3 major domains, including (1) the N-terminal RING finger domain (BRCA1 RING domain), (2) the large central segment with the nuclear localization signal (NLS), and (3) the BRCA1 C-terminal domain (BRCT). The BRCA1 protein plays an essential role in maintaining genomic stability associated with a number of cellular processes, including DNA repair, a cell cycle checkpoint, transcriptional regulation, and protein ubiquitination (Huen et al., 2010; O'Donovan & Livingston, 2010).

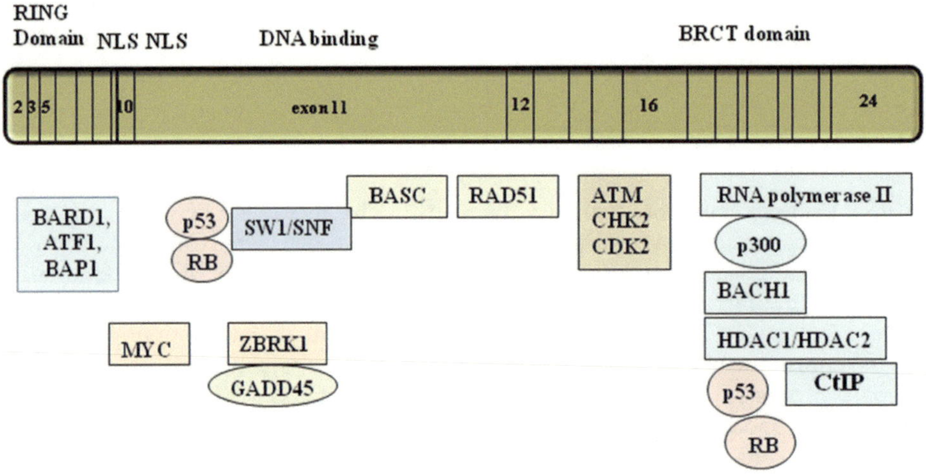

Fig. 1. Scheme of BRCA1 mRNA and sites of protein interaction

2.1 The BRCA1 RING domain

The N-terminal RING finger domain contains the conservative sequences of cysteine and histidine residues (C_3HC_4) necessary for specific coordination with two Zn^{2+} ions. The first 109 amino acids of BRCA1 protein constitute a protease-resistance domain. The solution structure of the BRCA1 RING domain revealed the existence of antiparallel α-helices at both ends, flanking the central RING motif (residues 24-64) and was characterized by a short antiparallel three-stranded β-sheet, and two large Zn^{2+}-binding loops, and a central α-helix (Brzovic et al., 2001)The two Zn^{2+}-binding sites are formed in an interleaved fashion in which the first and third pairs of cysteines (Cys24, Cys27, Cys44, and Cys47) form site I, and the second and fourth pairs of cysteines and a histidine (Cys39, His41, Cys61, and Cys64) form site II. It is an important domain since it might mediate a central role in macromolecular interactions to exert the tumor suppression functions. The solution structure together with yeast-two-hybrid studies revealed that the BRCA1 RING domain preferentially formed a heterodimeric complex with another RING domain BARD1 (BRCA1-associated RING domain 1) through an extensive four-helix-bundle interface (Brzovic et al., 2001; Wu et al., 1996). The binding interface is composed of residues 8-22 and 81-96 of BRCA1, and residues 36-48 and 101-116 of BARD1. The BRCA1-BARD1 complex requires each other for their mutual stabilities, and they are co-localized in nuclear dots during S phase but not the G phase of the cell cycle and in nuclear foci (Hashizume et al., 2001). The progression to S phase by aggregation of nuclear BRCA1 and BARD1 implied the importance of both proteins for a DNA repair function (Jin et al., 1997). The BRCA1-BARD1 complex also exhibits enzymatic activity of an E3 ubiquitin ligase that specifically transfers ubiquitin to protein substrates that are essential for cellular viability (Hashizume et al., 2001; Xia et al., 2003). Cancer-predisposing mutations in the Zn^{2+}-binding sites were demonstrated not only to alter the affinity for Zn^{2+} and the native BRCA1 RING structure but also abolished the interaction with BARD1 and the E3 ligase activity (Morris et al., 2006). The results supported the importance of Zn^{2+} as a structural component, as it obviously played a critical role in the stabilization of the structure and function of the BRCA1 RING domain.

2.2 The large central segment of BRCA1

The central segment of BRCA1 covers exon 11 (approximately 3500 bp) and constitutes approximately 60 percent of the coding region of the gene. Deletion of exon 11 results in removal of the nuclear localization signal of BRCA1. Biophysical characterization revealed that this domain was intrinsically disordered or natively unfolded under physiological conditions. This might potentially allow the BRCA1 central region to act as a long flexible scaffold, to mediate interactions with DNA, and perhaps a number of other proteins involved in the DNA damage response and repair (Mark et al., 2005). The reported binding partners to the central region were c-Myc, RB, p53, FANCA, RAD50, RAD51, JunB, and BRCA2 (Rosen et al., 2003). Recently, the BRCA1 central region has been shown to efficiently interact with p53, and stimulate p53-mediated DNA binding and transcriptional activities (Buck, 2008). This result indicated that the BRCA1 central segment facilitated the induction of cell cycle arrest and apoptosis in response to DNA damage. Furthermore, the association between the central region of BRCA1 and PALB2 (partner and localizer of BRCA2, also known as FANCN) was observed primarily through apolar bonding between their respective coiled-coil domains (Sy et al., 2009). PALB2 binds directly to BRCA1, and serves as the molecular scaffold for the formation of the BRCA1-PALB2-BRCA2 complex. BRCA1 mutations (L1407P and M1411T) identified in cancer patients were shown to disrupt the specific interaction between BRCA1 and PALB2, resulting in a defective homologous recombination (HR) repair and a compromised cell survival after DNA damage (Sy et al., 2009).

2.3 The BRCA1 C-terminal domain

The C-terminal region (residues 1646-1863) of BRCA1 contains two BRCT (BRCA1 C-terminal) domains in tandem (motif 1: amino acids 1653-1736; motif 2: amino acids 1760-1855). Each BRCT domain is characterized by a central, parallel four-stranded β-sheet with a pair of α-helices (α1 and α3) packed against one face, and a single α-helix (α2) packed against the opposite face of the sheet (Williams et al., 2001). The two BRCA1-BRCT repeats interact in a head-to-tail fashion. This domain serves as a multipurpose protein-protein interaction module that binds to other BRCT repeats or other protein domains with apparently unrelated structures (Watts & Brissett, 2010). Based on its physical interactions with other proteins, BRCA1 has been implicated in a wide array of cellular functions, including cell cycle regulation, DNA damage response, transcriptional regulation, replication and recombination, and higher chromatin hierarchical control (Starita & Parvin, 2003). The BRCA1-BRCT domain has been identified as a phosphopeptide recognition module, and is demonstrated to bind to the phosphorylated protein partners (BACH1 and

CtIP, containing the consensus sequence pSer-X-X-Phe) that is involved mainly in the control of the G2/M phase checkpoint and DNA damage repair (Varma et al., 2005; Williams et al., 2004). Several cancer-predisposing mutations in the BRCA1-BRCT domain resulted in destabilization of the structural integrity at the BRCT active sites, and abolished their affinities to synthetic BACH1 and CtIP phosphopeptides (Rowling et al., 2010). These findings provide a better understanding of the pathogenic BRCA1 mutations on functional mechanisms and tumorigenesis.

3. BRCA1 and DNA damage repair

A substantial amount of evidence that has implicated BRCA1 in the DNA damage repair pathways has been documented. BRCA1 co-localizes with RAD51 and BARD1 to nuclear foci (sites associated with repair of DNA caused by the damaging agents or γ-irradiation) (Hashizume et al., 2001; Scully et al., 1997). The nuclear foci is marked by the histone variant H2AX that was phosphorylated on Ser139 (known as γH2AX) (Rogakou et al., 1998). γH2AX is one of the initial recruiting factors for various checkpoints and DNA repair proteins, including Abraxas, RAP80, and BRCA1, at sites of DNA breaks (Foulkes, 2010). The H2AX signaling cascade begins to emerge with the finding that MDC1 (mediator of DNA damage checkpoint 1) is the main downstream factor in the pathway, and is required for the damage-induced focal accumulation of a number of DNA damage repair factors at the DNA breaks (Stucki et al., 2005).

BRCA1 plays a role in maintaining genome integrity through its role in DNA damage repair. Several observations have implicated BRCA1 in homologous recombination (HR), non-homologous end-joining (NHEJ and nucleotide excision repair (NER). A role for BRCA1 in HR-mediated repair is involved through its stable complex formation with BRCA2, which has a well-defined role in HR through its direct interaction with RAD51 (Bhattacharyya et al., 2000). RAD51 (the mammalian homolog of the Escherichia coli RecA protein) is a DNA recombinase that catalyzes strand exchange in an early step of HR (Baumann et al., 1996). PALB2 (the partner and localizer of BRCA2) has recently been identified as the bridging factor required for the BRCA1-BRCA2 association (Rahman et al., 2007). The BRCA1-PALB2 interaction was mediated by their respective coiled-coil domains, and was found to promote HR-mediated repair (Rahman et al., 2007). Importantly, missense mutations identified in the PALB2-binding region on BRCA1 disrupted the specific interaction of BRCA1 with PALB2, and compromised DNA repair in a gene conversion assay (Sy et al., 2009). Although these studies have revealed a molecular link between BRCA1 function and HR-mediated repair, the mechanism by which BRCA1 promotes HR through the PALB2-BRCA2-RAD51 axis remains unclear.

As an alternative to HR, there is a growing body of evidences, to indicate that a component of NHEJ is regulated by BRCA1. The exact role of BRCA1 in NHEJ, however, has not been well defined (Zhang & Powell, 2005). In the NHEJ pathway, the DNA-dependent protein kinase catalytic subunit (DNA-PKcs) and a Ku heterodimer of Ku80 and Ku70 are recruited to the sites of DNA DSBs for preparing the DNA ends before ligation by the XRCC4 ligase IV. The most possible explanation for BRCA1 being involved in NHEJ is its association with a NHEJ factor Ku80 (Chiba & Parvin, 2001; Wei et al., 2008). Many studies have provided strong evidences that the NHEJ pathway was impaired, both in vivo and in vitro, in BRCA1-deficient mouse embryonic fibroblasts and in the human breast cancer cell line HCC1937 which carries a homozygous mutation in the BRCA1 gene (Bau et al., 2004; Zhong et al., 2002).

4. BRCA1 and transcriptional regulation

As described earlier, BRCA1 contains a C-terminal transactivation domain as was first defined using the yeast two-hybrid system (Chapman & Verma, 1996; Monteiro et al., 1996). The transactivation domain was mapped to the region of the protein encoded by exons 21-24 using deletion constructs of BRCA1 fused to the GAL4 DNA binding domain. The BRCA1-BRCT domain has been implicated in the regulation of transcription of several genes responsible for DNA damage. The ability of BRCA1 to act as either a co-activator or a co-repressor of transcription may involve its ability to recruit the basal transcriptional machinery and other proteins that have been implicated in chromatin remodeling (Mullan et al., 2006). BRCA1 was capable of activating the p21 promoter (Somasundaram et al., 1997). One report claimed that BRCA1 participated in the stabilization of p53 in response to DNA damage, and served as a co-activator for p53 (Zhang et al., 1998). The interaction of BRCA1 and p53 potentially resulted in the redirection of p53-mediated transactivation from a pro-apoptotic target to genes involved in DNA repair and cell cycle arrest (Zhang et al., 1998). In addition, BRCA1 has been shown to interact with the RNA polymerase II holoenzyme (Scully et al., 1997). However, BRCA1 could repress the transcription of an estrogen receptor α (ERα) and its downstream estrogen responsive genes (Fan et al., 1999). The transcriptional repression activity of BRCA1 for ERα occurs by the association of the N-terminus of BRCA1 (residues 1-300) with the C-terminal activation function (AF-2) of ERα. Breast cancer-associated mutations of BRCA1 were found to abolish its ability to inhibit ERα activity (Fan et al., 2001). The repression activity exerted by BRCA1 involved the ability of BRCA1 to down-regulate levels of the transcriptional coactivator p300, which has also been shown to interact with the AF-2 domain of ERα (Fan et al., 2002). Further investigations revealed that overexpression of BRCA1 could inhibit the recruitment of the co-activators [steroid receptor co-activator 1 (SRC1), and amplified breast cancer 1 (AIB1)], and enhanced the recruitment of a co-repressor [histone deacetylase 1 (HDAC1)] to the progesterone response elements (PRE) of c-Myc.

5. BRCA1 and protein ubiquitination

The BRCA1 protein displays an E3 ubiquitin ligase activity through its RING domain, and this activity is enhanced when it exists as a heterodimer with the BARD1 RING domain (Xia et al., 2003). In vitro and in vivo studies have indicated that the BRCA1-BARD1 complex was capable of autoubiquitination that paradoxically stabilized the protein complex, and that also activated its in vitro E3 ligase activity with other proteins (Chen et al., 2002; Wu-Baer et al., 2010). However, the substrate specificity of the BRCA1 E3 ligase activity and its biological relevance to tumor suppression function are still unknown. Putative substrates for ubiquitination by the BRCA1-BARD1 RING complexes have recently emerged from in vitro and in vivo studies such as the nucleosomal histones H2A and its variant H2AX, RNA polymerase II, γ-tubulin, nucleophosmin/B23, and estrogen receptor α (ERα) (Eakin et al., 2007; Horwitz et al., 2007; Parvin, 2009; Sato et al., 2004; Starita et al., 2005; Thakar et al., 2010). BRCA1 can form a RING heterodimer E3 ligase activity with BARD1, and this is required for the recruitment of BRCA2 and RAD51 to damaged sites for HR repair (Ransburgh et al., 2010). Many cancer-predisposing mutations in the BRCA1 RING domain, that inhibited the E3 ligase activity and its ability to accumulate at damaged sites, were defective in homologous recombination that is critical for tumor suppression (Morris et al.,

2006, 2009; Ransburgh et al., 2010). Moreover, BRCA1 accumulation at the sites of DSBs occurred rapidly (within 20 s), and the RING structure was required (residue 1-200 of BRCA1) for the rapid recruitment with Ku80 at damaged sites in response to non-homologous end joining (Wei et al., 2008). Missense mutations in the BRCA1 RING domain significantly reduced their accumulations at DSBs, and abolished the association with Ku80. Therefore, the loss of the BRCA1 E3 ligase activity rendered cancerous cells hypersensitive to DNA-damaging agents,and clearly demonstrated a significant role for ubiquitnation in the DNA damage response and DNA repair activity (Ransburgh et al., 2010; Ruffner et al., 2001). Thus ubiquitination is involved in key steps that properly conduct the DNA repair process after DSBs.

Several reports have shown that the BRCA1 E3 ligase was capable of in vitro monoubiquitination of histones H2A and its variant H2AX (Thakar et al., 2010). This implied a BRCA1 function in regulating chromatin structure in the context of transcriptional regulation and DNA repair. Hyperphosphorylated RNA polymerase II (RNAPII) at its carboxyl terminal domain (CTD), consists of multiple repeats of the heptapeptide (YSPTSPS), involved in a generalized response to UV irradiation. It also served as a substrate for the BRCA1-dependent ubiquitination that was proposed to facilitate BRCA1 function in DNA repair by inhibiting DNA transcription, and then recruiting other DNA repair proteins at a lesion (Starita et al., 2005). Recently, It was found that the BRCA1-mediated ubiquitination of RNAPII prevented a stable association of some transcription factors (TFIIE and TFIIH) in the transcriptional preinitiation complex, and thus blocked the initiation of mRNA synthesis (Horwitz et al., 2007). Ubiquitination of the preinitiation complex was not targeting proteins for degradation by proteasome but rather the ubiquitin moiety itself interfered with the assembly of basal transcription factors at the promoter (Horwitz et al., 2007). Nucleoplasmin B23 and γ-tubulin were found to be the candidate substrates of the BRCA1 E3 ligase activity in vivo (Parvin, 2009; Sato et al., 2004). Both proteins were present in centrosomes, and apparently were not targeted for degradation by BRCA1-mediated modifications. The results indicated that ubiquitination of nucleoplasmin B23 and γ-tubulin played a vital role in regulating the centrosome number and maintenance of genomic stability by unknown mechanisms. Recently, the BRCA1 protein has been shown to inhibit ERα transcriptional activity, and to induce repression of estrogen response genes and cell proliferation (Xu et al., 2005). A potential explanation for the regulation of estrogen signaling by BRCA1 was the ERα ubiquitination and degradation mediated by the BRCA1 E3 ligase activity (Dizin & Irminger-Finger, 2010; Eakin et al., 2007). Conversely, the BRCA1-associated protein 1 (BAP1) is a deubiquitinating enzyme that can interact with the BRCA1 RING domain (Jensen et al., 1998). It was shown that BAP1 inhibited the BRCA1 autoubiquitination, and the nucleophosmin/B23 ubiquitination mediated by the BRCA1 E3 ligase activity (Nishikawa et al., 2009). Down-regulation of BAP1 in cells also resulted in the retardation of the S phase and ionizing irradiation hypersensitivity, a phenotype similar to BRCA1 deficiency. This again indicated that the BRCA1-BARD1 complex and the BAP1 protein coordinately regulated ubiquitination during a DNA damage response and the cell cycle.

6. Cisplatin

Cisplatin [*cis*-diamminedichloroplatinum(II)] is the platinum-based anticancer drug and is most effective in the treatment of metastatic testiscular cancers, ovarian, head, neck, bladder, cervical and lung cancers (Kelland, 2007). Although widely used as a well established anticancer drug in cancer chemotherapy, cisplatin displays major toxic side effects, such as nephrotoxicity, nausea and vomiting and neurotoxicity. In addition to its toxic side effects, a major limitation of cisplatin chemotherapy is the development of genetic mechanisms of resistance. The effectiveness of cisplatin depends on the drug uptake, and the actual amount that reacts with cellular targets.

6.1 Cisplatin-DNA adducts

It is generally accepted that DNA is the most important intracellular target of cisplatin. When cisplatin is dissolved in aqueous solution, chloride ions are displaced to allow the formation of aquated species, which are the reactive forms of the compound (Pinto and Lippard, 1985). The concentration of chloride ions influences the reactivity of cisplatin. After intravenous administration it is relatively less reactive in the extracellular space where the physiological chloride concentration is about 100 mM, but on crossing the plasma membrane, it is activated in the intracellular space where the chloride concentration drops to 2-3 mM. Chlorine groups of cisplatin are easily replaced by water molecules to allow the formation of aqauted species in a stepwise manner. Activated cisplatin is a potent electrophile that will react with any nucleophile, including the sulfhydryl groups on proteins and nucleophilic groups on nucleic acids. DNA is attacked by activated cisplatin at guanine residues in position N7, in double stranded DNA from the side of the major groove. The attack is apparently preceeded by an electrostatic attraction between the positively charged platinum (II) complex and the negatively charged phosphodeoxyribose DNA backbone and facilitated by bidirectional diffusion along the backbone. The initial attack of DNA by activated cisplatin is followed by the replacement of the remaining chloro ligand before the adduct forms an intramolecular attack on a second purine residue (either guanine or adenine). The hydration rate constant of the monoaqua form was faster than that of diaqua form ($2.38 \times 10^{-5}\ s^{-1}$ compared to $1.4 \times 10^{-5}\ s^{-1}$) (Cubo et al., 2009).
The anticancer activity of cisplatin potentially results from the modification of DNA through a covalent cross-link or platinum (Pt)-DNA adduct (Fig. 2). The DNA adducts interfere with DNA replication and transcription, and ultimately lead to cell death by cancer (Ahmad, 2010; Wang & Lippard, 2005). The predominant adducts formed by cisplatin in vitro are 1,2-intrastrand crosslinks. Quantitative studies show that the 1,2-intrastrand d(GpG), and d(ApG) crosslinks account for 65% and 25%, respectively (Fichtinger-Schepman et al., 1985; Eastman, 1986). They alter the DNA structure, block replication and transcription and activate a programmed cell death (apoptosis). X-ray diffraction of the crosslinked dinucleotide *cis*-$Pt(NH_3)_2$[d(pGpG)] reveals that the intrastrand cisplatin crosslink produces a severe local distortion in the DNA double helix, leading to unwinding and kinking. These crosslinks bend and unwind the duplex. The altered structure is recognized by high-mobility-group (HMG) proteins and other proteins. The binding of HMG proteins to cisplatin-modified DNA has been postulated to potentiate the anticancer activity of the drug.

6.2 Cisplatin-protein adducts

The interaction of cisplatin with proteins is of particular significance, and is believed to play an important role in distribution of the drug and the inactivation responsible for determining its efficacy and toxicity (Casini et al., 2008; Sun et al., 2009; Timerbaev et al., 2006). It is intriguing, that protein adducts affect some crucial aspects of protein structure

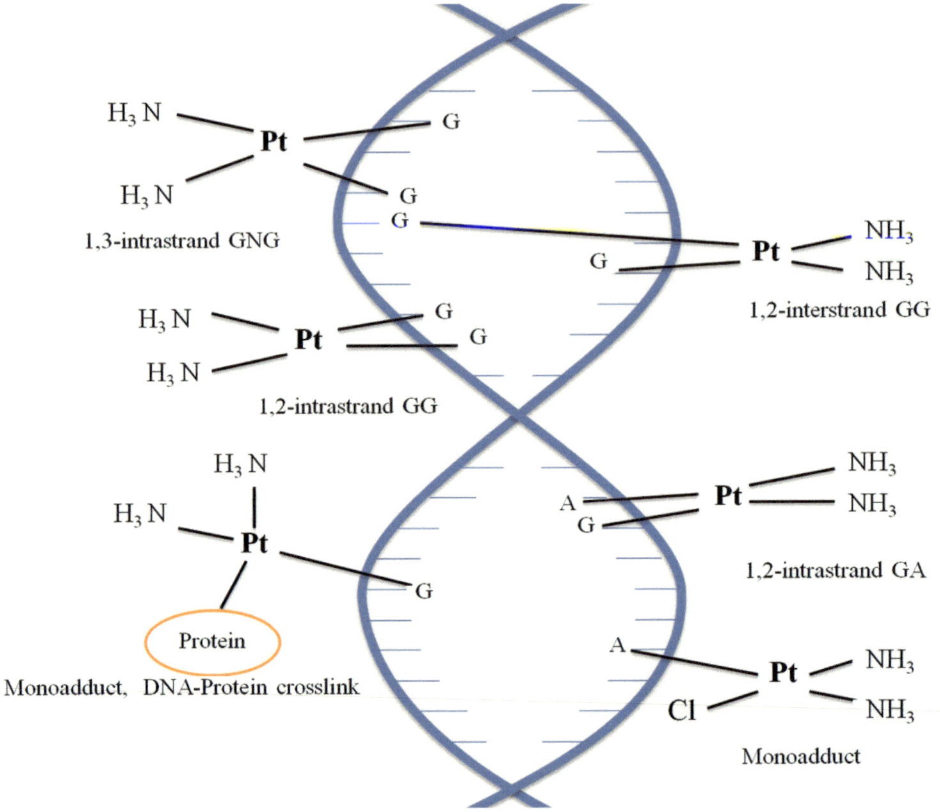

Fig. 2. Common cisplatin-DNA adducts

and functions. For instance, the platination of human serum albumin caused partial unfolding of the protein structure at a high drug concentration, and induced intermolecular crosslinks possibly at Cys34 and/or Met298 via bifunctional adducts or via NH_3 release (Ivanov et al., 1998; Neault & Tajmir-Riahi, 1998). Myoglobin, a small protein, containing a heme group required for the transport of oxygen in skeletal muscles and myocardial cells, formed intramolecular mono- and bi-functional adducts with cisplatin. Its putative platinum-binding sites were His116 and His119 (Zhao & King, 2010). A number of intramolecular crosslinks also occurred with ubiquitin adducts (Casini et al., 2009). The loss of activity of the C-terminal heat shock protein 90 after protein aggregation was reported to be a consequence of cisplatin binding but it did not exhibit any conformational change (Ishidaa et al., 2008). It is intriguing, that cisplatin can cause a structural perturbation of a synthetic peptide containing a Zn^{2+} finger domain. The platinum coordinates to Zn^{2+}-binding sites to induce Zn^{2+} ejection and subsequently the loss of the protein tertiary structure. This implies that cisplatin can inhibit critical biological functions regulated by Zn^{2+} finger proteins. Such a mechanism has been discussed in the apoptosis process mediated by the interaction of cisplatin and platinum-based compounds with Zn^{2+} finger transcriptional factors (Bose et al., 2005). Likewise, the nucleocapsid Zn^{2+} finger NCp7 protein, a protein required for the recognition and packaging of viral RNA, became attached to some platinum compounds, when its ability to bind nucleic acid was changed and prevented viral infectivity (de Paula et al., 2009; Musah, 2004).

7. ***BRCA1*** and its encoded product as potentially molecular targets for cisplatin for cancer therapy

In recent years, there has been significant progress made in evaluating what happens when BRCA1 is inactivated so it cannot respond to DNA damage in cancer cells, in other words, taking advantage of the inherent weakness of the BRCA1 dysfunction in cancer cells. These cells have increased sensitivity to DNA-damaging agents that eventually result in major genomic instability and cell death (Amir et al., 2010; Ashworth, 2008; Helleday et al., 2008; Lieberman, 2008; Powell & Bindra, 2009; Quinn et al., 2009; Tassone et al., 2009; Zhu et al., 2009). Cancerous cells with inactivated BRCA1 had defects in DNA repair of double strand breaks (DSBs) (Farmer et al., 2005; Kennedy et al., 2004; Litman et al., 2008). Moreover, extensive investigations have revealed the relevance of the BRCA1-mediated ubiquitination to DNA repair functions. Mutations in the BRCA1 RING domain resulted in the loss of the E3 ubiquitin ligase activity, and conferred hypersensitivity of the cancerous cells to DNA-damaged chemotherapy and γ-irradiation (Ransburgh et al., 2010; Ruffer et al., 2001; Wei et al., 2008).

It was initially reported that overexpression of BRCA1 in the human breast cancer MCF7 cell line resulted in an increased resistance to cisplatin (Husain et al., 1998). Furthermore, antisense or siRNA-based inhibition of endogenous BRCA1 expression promoted the increased sensitivity to cisplatin that was associated with the decreased DNA repair by NER and an increased apoptosis (Lafarge et al., 2001; Quinn et al., 2003). This indicates that the reduced BRCA1 expression observed in sporadic cancers may also be exploited for DNA damage-based chemotherapy (James et al., 2007; Quinn et al., 2009). In a similar situation, BRCA1-deficient mouse embryonic stem cells displayed defective DNA repair and a 100-fold increased sensitivity to the alkylating agent mitomycin C and cisplatin than those containing wild-type BRCA1 (Bhattacharyya et al., 2000; Moynahan et al., 2001). This sensitivity was reversed upon correction of the BRCA1 mutation in mouse embryonic fibroblast cells with a disrupted BRCA1 (Fedier et al., 2003). Reconstitution of BRCA1 in the cells via transfection meant that BRCA1 functions were regained, and resulted in a reduced level of cancer cell death, following treatment with cisplatin or other DNA damaging agents (Quinn et al., 2003). Moreover, more recent evidence has revealed the implication of BRCA1 in cisplatin-resistant breast and ovarian cancer cell lines. These cells that acquired resistance to DNA-damaging agents was mediated by a secondary mutation in BRCA1. This mutation restored the BRCA1 protein expression and function for DNA repair, causing the cancer cells to become more tolerant to cisplatin (Swisher et al., 2008; Tassone et al., 2003; Wang & Figg, 2008). Recently, a number of clinical studies have examined the utilization of this BRCA1 dysfunction in response to the DNA-damaging drug cisplatin. A pathological complete response (pCR) with excellent compliance was observed in cancer patients with BRCA1 mutations (Byrski et al., 2009; Font et al., 2010; Quinn et al., 2007; Silver et al., 2010; Taron et al., 2004). This indicates that patients with BRCA1 dysfunction gain more benefit from treatments that exert their effects by causing DNA damage.

Therefore, it is important to continue elucidating *BRCA1*/BRCA1-dependent pathways to design molecular-targeted therapy for the platinum treatment of cancer cells by taking advantage of their impairment of the *BRCA1*/BRCA1 repair capacity and BRCA1-dependent ubiquitination inactivated by cisplatin.

7.1 Cellular repair of cisplatin-damaged *BRCA1*

Preliminary results from our laboratory have indicated that the cisplatin-modified *BRCA1* gene sequence was resistant to restriction endonuclease cleavage, and indicated that cisplatin preferentially formed 1,2-intrastrand d(GpG) cross-links (Ratanaphan et al., 2009). The drug inhibited *BRCA1* amplification in a dose-dependent manner. It has been found that cisplatin-treated, *BRCA1* exon 11, of adenocarcinoma MCF-7 cells exhibited a time dependent recovery after drug exposure to the cells at 37°C for 6 h, with an initial low level of lesion removal during the first 4 h (Fig. 3). A more complete lesion removal was observed with over 90% of 50 µM cisplatin after 18 h of repair time. However, only 30% of the lesion repair was observed at a higher cisplatin concentration of 200 µM (Ratanaphan et al., 2009). From a host cell reactivation assay, the result indicated that a reduction in cellular reactivation of the drug-damaged reporter gene encoding plasmid was a consequence of an increase in platination levels within the transcribed reporter gene. This indicated that the cellular response to cisplatin reflected its intrinsically low capacity for removal of cisplatin-*BRCA1* adducts. Following cisplatin-induced *BRCA1* adducts, a number of cellular repair proteins, excluding BRCA1, are responsible for recognizing and processing the removal of DNA damage. NER is a major process for removing platinum-damaged DNA. This process requires an ATP-dependent multiple protein complex that recognizes the bending induced on DNA by cisplatin. The NER complex has a dual role that can unwind the DNA strands (helicase), and excise the damage strand (endonuclease) of about 24-32 nucleotides in length, containing a platinum lesion. DNA resynthesis factors are recruited at the site of the incised DNA, and employ the opposite strand as template to fill in the gap in concert with DNA ligases. Two distinct sub-pathways of NER that may be involved, are transcription-coupled repair (TCR) and/or global genomic repair (GGR). TCR preferentially repairs transcribed strands of the RNA polymerase II-transcribed active gene, while GGR repairs throughout the genome (Shuck et al., 2008). Recently, the suppression of ERCC1 expression in a HeLa S3 cell line by small interfering RNA (siRNA) led to a decrease in the repair activity of cisplatin-induced DNA damage along with a decrease in cell viability against platinum-

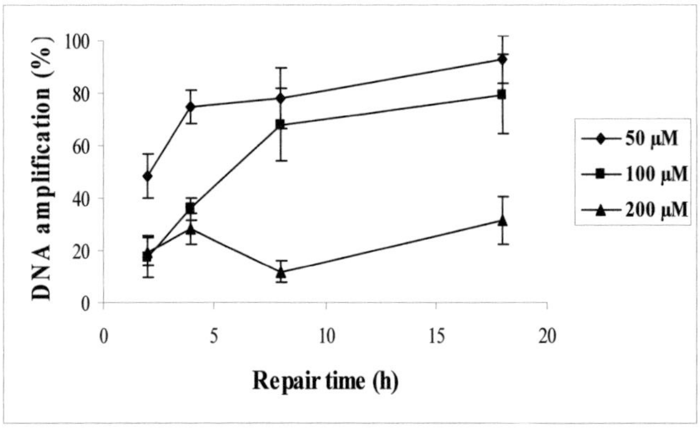

Fig. 3. Cellular repair of cisplatin-damaged 3,426-bp *BRCA1* exon 11. MCF-7 cells were incubated with medium plus cisplatin at various concentrations (50–200 µM) for 6 h. The cells were washed twice with PBS and fresh medium was added. The genomic DNA was then extracted at 2, 4, 8 and 18 h and used as the template for the QPCR assay (Ratanaphan et al., 2005, 2009).

based drugs (Chang et al., 2005). Recombination pathways can also be involved as repair systems responsible for DNA damage induced by the anticancer drug cisplatin. Recombination-deficient *E. coli* mutants were sensitive to cisplatin and exhibited a decreased survival by four orders of magnitude in comparison with the parental strain at a cisplatin concentration of 75-80 μM (Zdraveski et al., 2000). Many recombination-deficient strains showed a sensitivity to the drug equal to that of the NER-deficient strains. Double mutations in recombination and NER proteins were approximately 4-fold more sensitive to cisplatin than the corresponding single mutants. This indicates that recombination and NER pathways play roles that are independent of each other in protecting cells from cisplatin-induced damage. Impaired recombination DNA repair in yeast and prostate cancer cell lines also showed an increased sensitivity to cisplatin (Wang et al., 2005).

7.2 Inhibition of *BRCA1* transcriptional transactivation

The one hybrid GAL4 transcription assay is used to study the effect of cisplatin on transcriptional transactivation. The level of transcriptional transactivation is inversely proportional to the amount of platinum-*BRCA1* adducts. The results are most likely due to inhibition of transcription of the reporter plasmid that resulted from interstrand crosslinks (Ratanaphan et al., 2009). The transcriptional transactivation activity of *BRCA1* has previously been reported by fusing the C-terminal domain of *BRCA1* to a heterogenous DNA-binding domain (Chapman and Verma, 1996). The BRCT domain (amino acids 1380-1863) of human *BRCA1* scores positively in transcriptional activation trap experiments using various forms of so-called "one hybrid assay".The *BRCA1*-fused DNA-binding domain activates transcription in a cell-free system to a similar extent as a dose of the powerful activator, VP16 (Scully et al., 1997). A *GAL4:BRCA1* has also been introduced in yeast- and mammalian-based transcription assays to characterize the deleterious mutations in the 3/ -terminal region of the *BRCA1* (Vallon-Christersson et al., 2001). The transcriptional activity reflects a tumor-suppressing function of the BRCA1 protein.

In order to investigate whether the drug-damaged *BRCA1* is able to transactivate the expression of a firefly luciferase gene, DNA repair-proficient MCF-7 cells were transiently transfected with the cisplatin-damaged pBIND-BRCT along with the reporter plasmid pG5Luc. The firefly luciferase activity was significantly decreased at a cisplatin concentration of 12.5 μM (Fig. 4).

It has been hypothesized that the BRCT domain could transactivate the expression of another reporter gene. The reporter gene pSV-β-galactosidase was used for this purpose. It was of interest, that the level of transactivation was significantly higher when co-transfected with the pBIND-BRCT than with the parental pBIND (Fig. 5). This indicated that the GAL4-BRCT domain may stimulate the pSV-β-galactosidase. However, the expression of β-galactosidase was decreased to the level of β-galactosidase alone when co-transfected with the platinated pBIND-BRCT. It was again of interest that, β-galactosidase expression was dramatically diminished when both the pSV-β-galactosidase and the pBIND-BRCT were platinated (Fig. 6). Expression of β-galactosidase from the pSV-β-galactosidase can be transactivated both by the GAL4 domain of the pBIND and pBIND-BRCT. Acting upon the GAL4 DNA sequence similarity, the GAL4 protein alone can stimulate the expression of β-galactosidase. However, the degree of transactivation was slightly higher by the pBIND-BRCT. This indicates that the BRCT domain on the fusion protein is able to transactivate the β-galactosidase gene-bearing pSV-β-galactosidase. When platinated pSV-β-galactosidase is co-transfected with the pBIND or the pBIND-BRCT, a relatively lower expression of β-galactosidase was observed. The transcription level of β-galactosidase expression was reduced from 2-2.5 fold to 1.3 fold in both plasmids. Considering the data from the proficiency in repairing cisplatin-*BRCA1* adducts, it demonstrated that over 80% of the DNA lesion was repaired 8 h after cisplatin removal. Thus, it is possible that, during the repair time, RNA polymerase II or other transcriptional machineries may be blocked at any lesion on DNA (Jung & Lippard, 2003, 2006; Tornaletti et al., 2003).

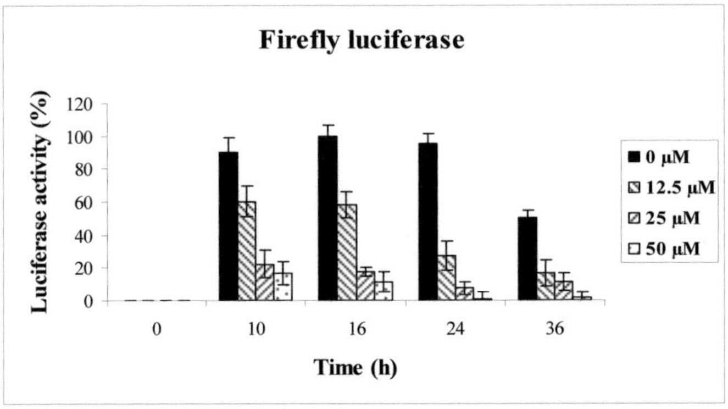

Fig. 4. Time course of firefly luciferase expression. The pBIND-BRCT was incubated with cisplatin at concentrations of 0, 12.5, 25 and 50 μM and then co-transfected with the pG5Luc plasmid into MCF-7 cells. A cell lysate was prepared at 10, 16, 24 and 36 h after transfection. Firefly luciferase expression is detected by the Dual-Luciferase® Reporter Assay System. The data were derived from four independent experiments ± standard deviations (SD) (Ratanaphan et al., 2009).

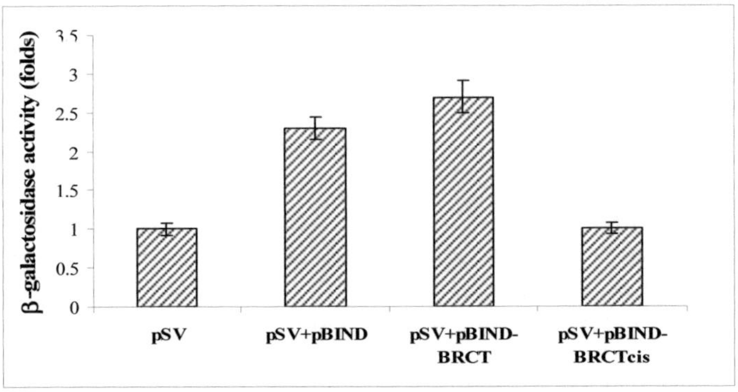

Fig. 5. Transcriptional transactivation. The pBIND or pBIND-BRCT was co-transfected with pSV-β-galactosidase. Cell lysates were prepared at 16 h after transfection. β-galactosidase activity was detected using the β-galactosidase assay. The data were derived from four independent experiments ± standard deviations (SD) (Ratanaphan et al., 2009).

Several investigations have revealed transcriptional inhibition on DNA templates, containing the site-specific Pt-DNA adducts. The mammalian RNA polymerase II and *E. coli* RNA polymerase did not catalyze the transcriptional reactions when the DNA template strands carried the 1,2-intrastrand d(GpG) and d(ApG) adducts, whereas those polymerases

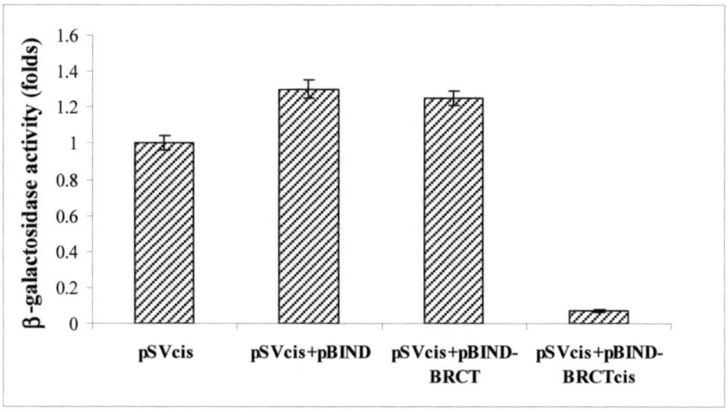

Fig. 6. Transcriptional transactivation of platinated pBIND-BRCT on platinated pSV-β-galactosidase. The platinated pSV-β-galactosidase (with cisplatin at a concentration of 12.5 μM) was co-transfected with non-platinated pBIND and pBIND-BRCT or platinated pBIND-BRCT. Cell lysates were prepared at 16 h after transfection. β-galactosidase expression was detected using the β-galactosidase assay. The data were derived from four independent experiments ± standard deviations (SD) (Ratanaphan et al., 2009).

could transcribe the complementary templates which had no DNA lesions on the template strands (Corda et al., 1991). Transcription of globally platinated DNA templates by SP6 and T7 RNA polymerases were also blocked primarily at 1,2-d(GpG) and d(ApG) Pt adducts, and to a lesser extent at the interstrand crosslink (Tornaletti, 2005). Bifunctional Pt-DNA adducts were much more effective at impeding transcription progression than monofunctional DNA adducts (Tornaletti, 2005). Moreover, cisplatin caused a dose-dependent inhibition of mRNA synthesis. Treatment of human fibroblast cells with 50 μM cisplatin for 24 h resulted in a 55% decrease in mRNA level and a reduced expression of $p21^{WAF1}$ protein. This indicated that cisplatin inhibited the transcription of the $p21^{WAF1}$ gene (Ljungman et al., 1999). Recently, the processing of site-specific Pt-DNA crosslinks in mammalian cells was investigated (Ang et al., 2010). Site-specific platinated oligonucleotides, containing 1,2-d(GpG) and 1,3-d(GpTpG) adducts, were inserted into an expression vector between its promoter and a luciferase reporter gene. Transcription inhibitions that occurred by blocking passage of the RNA polymerase complex through the 1,2-d(GpG) and 1,3-d(GpTpG) adducts were 50% and 37.7% of the unplatinated controls for vectors, repectively. An X-ray crystal structure of RNA polymerase II showed stalling at the 1,2-intrastrand d(GpG) crosslink to explain the physical block of transcription by the cisplatin-DNA adduct (Damsma et al., 2007). Disruption of chromatin remodeling was another mechanism by which a cisplatin adduct could interfere with transcription. Nucleosomal DNA, containing the 1,2-d(GpG) or 1,3-d(GpTpG) intrastrand crosslinks, enforced a characteristic rotational positioning of the DNA around the histone octamer such that the Pt adduct faced inward towards the histone core (Ober and Lippard, 2008). Increased solvent accessibility of the platinated DNA strand was observed, and this indicated it might be caused by a structural perturbation in proximity of the DNA lesion. In addition, the nucleosomes treated with cisplatin exhibited a significant decrease in heat-induced mobility (Wu et al., 2008). These effects also indicated that a cisplatin assault could inhibit transcription by altering the native nucleosomal organization, and limiting the nucleosomal sliding that protected access of the RNA polymerase to the DNA template.

It has been suggested that inhibition of transcription by cisplatin was a critical determinant of cell-cycle arrest in the G2 phase because cells could not synthesize the mRNA necessary to pass into mitosis, and this eventually led to apoptosis. Possible mechanisms to explain this inhibitory process can be divided into three categories; (1) hijack of transcription factors (2) physical block of RNA polymerase, and (3) inhibition of chromatin remodeling (Todd & Lippard, 2009). A number of proteins have been identified that specifically recognize the distorted Pt-DNA adducts, including transcription factors. The upstream binding factor (UBF), a member of the HMG-domain proteins, is a ribosomal RNA transcription factor. hUBF can bind the 1,2-intrastrand adducts with a high K_d of 60 pM (Jordan & Carmo-Fonseca, 1998). Treatment of DNA with cisplatin inhibited ribosomal RNA synthesis by competing with hUBF for its natural binding site in an in vitro transcription assay (Zhai et al., 1998). The TATA-binding protein (TBP) is a critical transcription factor for all three mammalian RNA polymerases (pol I, II, and III). TBP binding to the DNA duplex, containing the 1,2-intrastrand d(GpG) crosslinks of cisplatin, was similar to that of the TATA-promoter binding in terms of structural and affinity aspects with a K_d of 0.3 nM (Jung et al., 2001). It was shown that TBP interacted directly with cisplatin-damaged DNA, and the introduction of exogenous cisplatin-modified DNA into the HeLa whole cell extract could sequester TBP and inhibit transcription 3-to 4-fold more than undamaged DNA (Vichi et al., 1997). Collectively, the failure of RNA synthesis resulted from the hijack of transcription factors by Pt-DNA adducts, that prevented the assembly of transcriptional elongation complexes at their normal promoter sequence and inhibited the transcriptional process. Significant reduction in transcriptional transactivation of cisplatin-modified *BRCA1* in the presence of a second expression vector containing multiple cisplatin-damaged sites could address the lack of or the unavailability of cellular transcription factors at cisplatin-*BRCA1* lesions. Damage of *BRCA1*, if not properly repaired, may lead to its functional impairment in cancerous cells which ultimately induce programed cell death.

7.3 Cisplatin binding to the BRCA1 RING domain

The types of adduct formed with cisplatin are distinctive and dependent on the accessibility of the platinum center and protein side-chains (Ivanov et al., 1998; Peleg-Shulman et al., 2002). The BRCA1 RING domain has been found to form favourable intramolecular and intermolecular cross-links caused by cisplatin (Atipairin et al., 2010). Although cisplatin has been demonstrated to induce protein dimerization and has caused perturbations in some protein structures, the secondary structure of the BRCA1 RING domain in the apo-form was maintained and underwent more folded structural rearrangement after increasing cisplatin concentrations as judged by an increase in the negative CD spectra at 208 and 220 nm. It was possible that cisplatin might bind to the unoccupied Zn^{2+}-binding sites and caused the structural changes. The binding constant of the in vitro platination was $3.00 \pm 0.11 \times 10^6$ M^{-1}, and the free energy of binding (ΔG) was -8.68 kcal Mol^{-1}. In addition, the CD spectra of BRCA1 pre-incubated with Zn^{2+} gave identical profiles to indicate that cisplatin could interact with other residues rather than the Zn^{2+}-binding sites and barely affected the overall conformation of the Zn^{2+}-bound BRCA1. In order to locate the binding site of cisplatin on the BRCA1 (1-139) protein, in-gel tryptic digestion of the free BRCA1 and the cisplatin-BRCA1 adducts (molar ratio 1:1) were subjected to analysis by LC-MS. A unique fragment ion of 656.29^{2+} was obtained from the cisplatin-BRCA1 adduct digests. Tandem mass spectrometric analyses of this fragment ion indicated that the ion arose from

$[Pt(NH_3)_2(OH)]^+$ that was attached to a BRCA1 peptide [111]ENNSPEHLK[119] (Fig. 7) (Berners-Price et al., 1992).

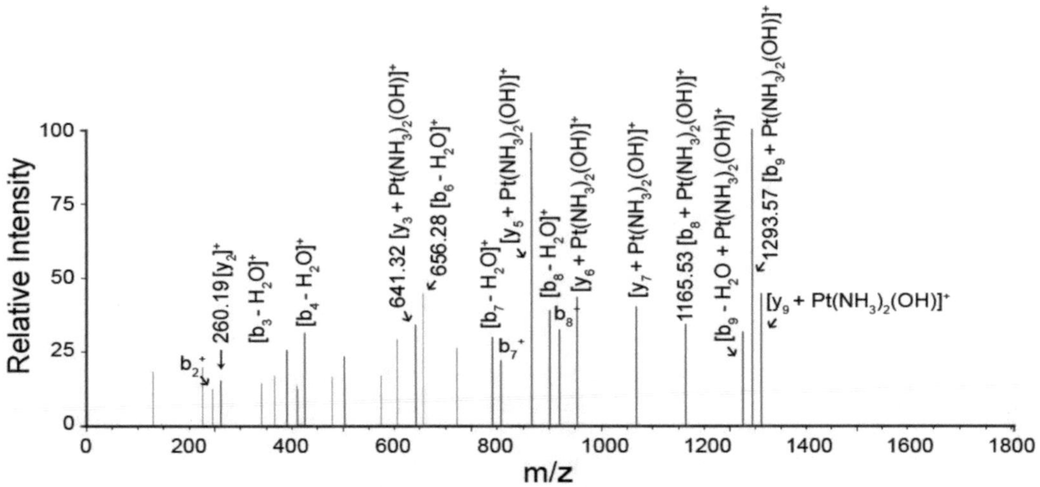

Fig. 7. The product-ion spectrum of the MS/MS analysis for the 656.29^{2+} ion. It indicated that $[Pt(NH_3)_2(OH)]^+$ is attached to a peptide [111]ENNSPEHLK[119] of BRCA1 (Atipairin et al., 2010).

7.4 Thermal stability of the cisplatin-BRCA1 adducts

Thermal denaturation was monitored by circular dichroism (CD) to follow heat-induced unfolding which determined the effect of cisplatin binding on the stability of the BRCA1 RING domain. The BRCA1(1-139) protein pre-incubated with or without Zn^{2+} was incubated with cisplatin, and the CD spectra showed identical changes with an increase in ellipticity when the temperature was raised from 15°C to 95°C (Fig. 8). It indicated that the folded proteins gradually lost their ordered structures. When cooling to 20°C after being heated at 95°C, the CD spectrum partially recovered. This indicated that the reversibility of the unfolding/refolding process was incomplete. The melting temperatures of the BRCA1(1-139) proteins were about 74°C and 83°C in the absence and presence of Zn^{2+}, respectively (Fig. 9). This indicated that the BRCA1 RING domain was more thermostable by about 9°C upon Zn^{2+}-binding. Thus, it supported the important role of Zn^{2+} in the determination and stabilization of the local secondary structure in the RING domain. It was notable that cisplatin at a concentration of 10 μM had similar melting temperatures to those observed for Zn^{2+} binding to the BRCA1 RING domain. However, higher melting temperatures were observed at a 10-fold concentration of cisplatin (100 μM). These data indicated that cisplatin binding to the BRCA1 RING domain conferred an enhanced thermostability by 13°C. Resistance to thermal denaturation of the cisplatin-modifed BRCA1 RING domain might result from the favourably intramolecular and intermolecular crosslinks driven by the free energy (Atipairin et al., 2010).

7.5 Inactivation of BRCA1 E3 ligase activity by cisplatin

To gain further insights into the functional consequences of cisplatin-induced BRCA1, the BRCA1 RING protein was platinated in vitro by cisplatin at various concentrations. The results showed that the relative E3 ligase activity was inversely proportional to the

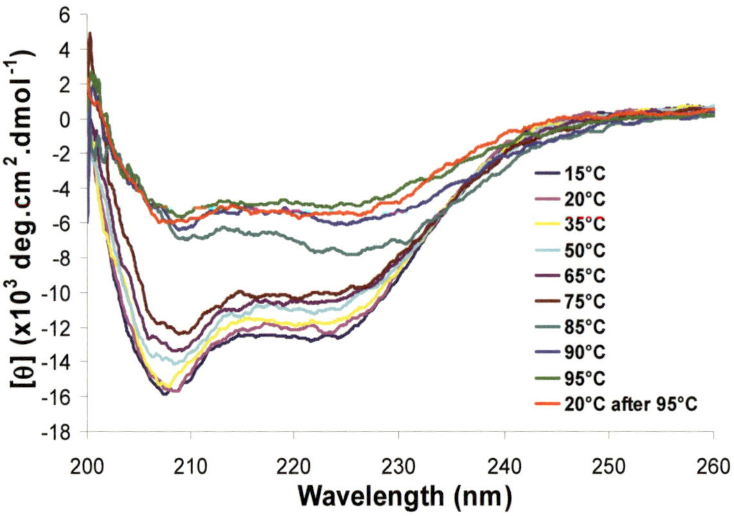

Fig. 8. Thermal transition of the cisplatin-BRCA1 adducts in the presence of Zn^{2+}. The BRCA1(1-139) proteins (10 μM) after pre-incubation with a 3 molar equivalent ratio of Zn^{2+} to protein were mixed with cisplatin concentrations of 10 μM. Samples were incubated in the dark at ambient temperature for 24 h. The measurements were performed from 15°C to 95°C with a heating rate of 1°C/min. After heating to 95°C, the measurement at 20°C was also performed. The CD spectra were plotted between the mean residue ellipticity and wavelength (Atipairin et al., 2010).

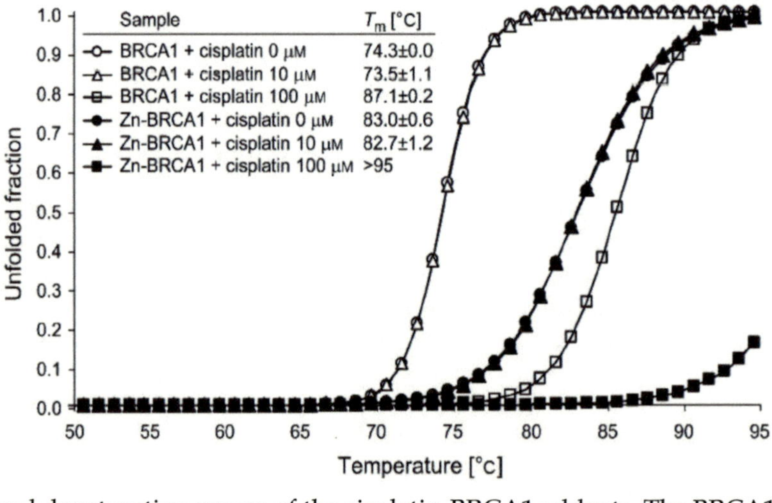

Fig. 9. Thermal denaturation curves of the cisplatin-BRCA1 adducts. The BRCA1(1-139) protein (10 μM) without Zn^{2+} and after pre-incubation with a 3 molar equivalent ratio of Zn^{2+} to protein were mixed with various concentrations of cisplatin (0, 10, and 100 μM). Samples were incubated in the dark at ambient temperature for 24 h before CD measurements. The CD signals at 208 nm were measured, and the unfolded fraction as a function of temperature was plotted (Atipairin et al., 2010).

concentration of the drug (Fig. 10). An increase in platinum concentration was accompanied by a high amount of BRCA1 adducts and a low amount of native BRCA1 protein. To address whether the inhibition of the E3 ligase activity resulted from the formation of BRCA1 adducts or a reduced amount of the BRCA1 subunit, a ten-fold excess amount of the platinated BRCA1 was assayed for the E3 ligase activity. The result demonstrated that platination of BRCA1 was indeed involved in the inhibition of the E3 ligase activity (Atipairin et al., 2011a).

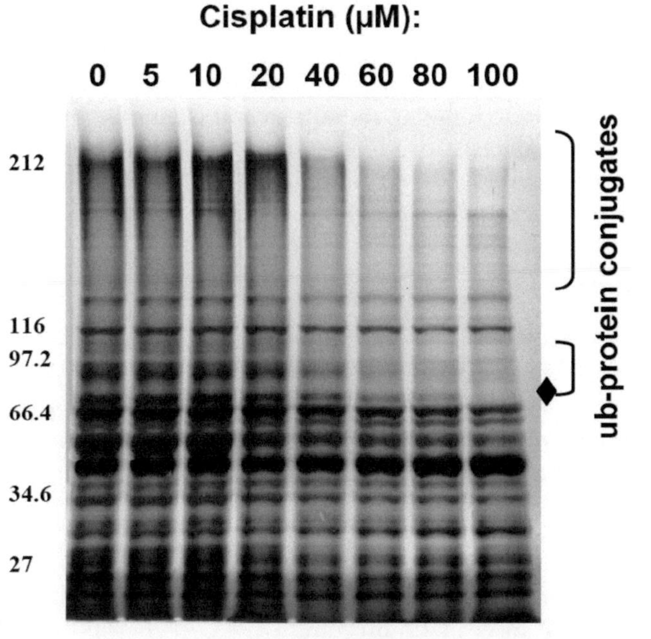

Fig. 10. *In vitro* ubiquitin ligase activity of cisplatin-BRCA1 complexes. Two μg of the drug-BRCA1 adducts with a number of defined concentrations of cisplatin was assayed for the ubiquitin ligase activitiy. An apparent ubiquitinated product (as indicated by the filled diamond) was markedly reduced as the concentration of platinum increased (Atipairin et al., 2011a).

8. Conclusion

We have demonstrated an in vitro inactivation of *BRCA1*/BRCA1 by the anticancer platinum drug cisplatin. The transcriptional activation of cisplatin-modified *BRCA1*, when tested in a "one-hybrid GAL4 transcriptional assay", was inversely proportional to cisplatin doses and was dramatically diminished in the presence of a second expression vector containing multiple cisplatin-damaged sites. This indicates a repair-mediated transcriptional transactivation of cisplatin-damaged *BRCA1* as well as the lack or unavailability of cellular transcription factors at cisplatin-*BRCA1* lesions. The BRCA1 protein contained a preformed structure in the apo-form with structural changes and more resistance to limited proteolysis after Zn^{2+} binding. Cisplatin-bound protein exhibited an enhanced thermostability, resulting from the favourable intermolecular crosslinks driven by the free energy. Only the apo-form, not the holo-form, of BRCA1 underwent a more folded structural rearrangement with the retention of protein structure upon cisplatin binding with the preferential His117 site of the BRCA1 peptide ^{111}Glu-Asn-Asn-Ser-Pro-Glu-His-Leu-Lys^{119}. BRCA1 E3 ubiquitin ligase activity was also inactivated by the drug. These data could raise the possibility of selectively targeting the BRCA1 DNA repair for cisplatin in cancer chemotherapy.

As mentioned earlier, the BRCA1-BARD1 RING complex has an E3 ubiquitin ligase function that plays essential roles in response to DNA damage and DNA repair. Evidence from several preclinical and clinical studies have provided data showing that many cancer-predisposing mutations within the BRCA1 RING domain demonstrated a loss of ubiquitin ligase and repair of DNA double-strand break activities (Atipairin, et al., 2011a, 2011b; Morris et al., 2006, 2009; Ransburgh et al., 2010). Furthermore, the BRCA1-associated cancers conferred a hypersensitivity to ionizing radiations and chemotherapeutic agents. Therefore, it would be of great interest to identify a relationship between BRCA1-mediated ubiquitination and chemosensitivity by approaching the BRCA1 RING domain as a potentially molecular target or predictor with cisplatin.

9. Acknowledgments

The author would like to thank all the members of BRCA1 lab for discussion and comments. This work was financial supported by grants of the Synchrotron Light Research Institute (Public organization) (1-2548/LS01), the National Research Council of Thailand (02011420-0003, PHA530097S), Prince of Songkla University (PHA530188S), and Dr. Brian Hodgson for the proof reading and assistance with the English.

10. References

Ahmad, S. (2010). Platinum-DNA interactions and subsequent cellular processes controlling sensitivity to anticancer platinum complexes. *Chem Biodivers.* 7 (3): 543-566.

Amir, E., Seruga, B., Serrano, R. & Ocana A. (2010). Targeting DNA repair in breast cancer: A clinical and translational update. *Cancer Treat Rev.* 36 (7): 557-565.

Ang, W.H., Myint, M. & Lippard, S.J. (2010). Transcription inhibition by platinum-DNA cross-links in live mammalian cells. *J Am Chem Soc.* 132 (21): 7429-7435.

Ashworth, A. (2008). A synthetic lethal therapeutic approach: poly(ADP) ribose polymerase inhibitors for the treatment of cancers deficient in DNA double-strand break repair. *J Clin Oncol.* 26 (22): 3785-3790.

Atipairin, A., Canyuk, B. & Ratanaphan, A. (2010). Cisplatin affects the conformation of apo-form, not holo-form, of BRCA1 RING finger domain and confers thermal stability. *Chem Biodivers.* 7 (8): 1949-1967.

Atipairin, A., Canyuk, B. & Ratanaphan, A. (2011a). The RING heterodimer BRCA1-BARD1 is a ubiquitin ligase inactivated by the platinum-based anticancer drugs. *Breast Cancer Res Treat.* 126 (1): 203-209.

Atipairin, A., Canyuk, B. & Ratanaphan, A. (2011b). Substitution of aspartic acid with glutamic acid at position 67 of BRCA1 RING domain retains ubiquitin ligase activity and zinc(II)-binding with a reduced transition temperature. *J Biol Inorg Chem.* 16 (2): 217-226.

Bau, D.T., Fu, Y.P., Chen, S.T., Cheng, T.C., Yu, J.C., Wu, P.E., et al. (2004). Breast cancer risk and the DNA double-strand break end-joining capacity of nonhomologous end-joining genes are affected by BRCA1. *Cancer Res.* 64 (14): 5013-5019.

Baumann, P., Benson, F.E. & West, S.C. (1996). Human Rad51 protein promotes ATP-dependent homologous pairing and strand transfer reactions *in vitro*. *Cell.* 87 (4): 757-766.

Berners-Price, S.J., Frenkiel, T.A., Frey, U., Ranford, J.D. & Sadler, P.J. (1992). Hydrolysis products of cisplatin: pKa determinations via [^{1}H,^{15}N] NMR spectroscopy. *J Chem Soc., Chem Commun.* 789-791.

Bhattacharyya, A., Ear, U.S., Koller, B.H., Weichselbaum, R.R. & Bishop, D.K. (2000). The breast cancer susceptibility gene *BRCA1* is required for subnuclear assembly of Rad51 and survival following treatment with the DNA cross-linking agent cisplatin. *J Biol Chem.* 275 (31): 23899-23903.

Bose, R.N., Yang, W.W. & Evanics, F. (2005). Structural perturbation of a C4 zinc-finger module by *cis*-diamminedichloroplatinum(II): insights into the inhibition of transcription processes by the antitumor drug. *Inorg Chim Acta.* 358 (10): 2844-2854.

Brzovic, P.S., Meza, J., King, M.C. & Klevit, R.E. (1998). The cancer-predisposing mutation C61G disrupts homodimer formation in the NH2-terminal BRCA1 RING finger domain. *J Biol Chem.* 273(14): 7795-7799.

Brzovic, P.S., Rajagopal, P., Hoyt, D.W., King, M.C. & Klevit, R.E. (2001). Structure of a BRCA1-BARD1 heterodimeric RING-RING complex. *Nat Struct Biol.* 8(10): 833-837.

Byrski, T., Huzarski, T., Dent, R., Gronwald, J., Zuziak, D., Cybulski, C., et al. (2009) Response to neoadjuvant therapy with cisplatin in BRCA1-positive breast cancer patients. *Breast Cancer Res Treat.* 115(2): 359-363.

Casini, A., Gabbiani, C., Michelucci, E., Pieraccini, G., Moneti, G., Dyson, P.J., et al. (2009). Exploring metallodrug-protein interactions by mass spectrometry: comparisons between platinum coordination complexes and an organometallic ruthenium compound. *J Biol Inorg Chem.* 14(5): 761-770.

Casini, A., Guerri, A., Gabbiani, C. & Messori, L. (2008). Biophysical characterisation of adducts formed between anticancer metallodrugs and selected proteins: New insights from X-ray diffraction and mass spectrometry studies. *J Inorg Biochem.* 102(5-6): 995-1006.

Chang, I.Y., Kim, M.H., Kim, H.B., Lee, D.Y., Kim, S.H., Kim, H.Y,, et al., (2005). Small interfering RNA-induced suppression of ERCC1 enhances sensitivity of human cancer cells to cisplatin. *Biochem Biophys Res Commun.* 327(1): 225-233.

Chapman, M.S. & Verma, I.M. (1996). Transcriptional activation by BRCA1. *Nature.* 382 (6593): 678-679.

Chen, A., Kleiman, F.E., Manley, J.L., Ouchi, T. & Pan, Z.Q. (2002). Autoubiquitination of the BRCA1-BARD1 RING ubiquitin ligase. *J Biol Chem.* 277(24): 22085-22092.

Chiba, N. & Parvin, J.D. (2001). Redistribution of BRCA1 among four different protein complexes following replication blockage. *J Biol Chem.* 276(42): 38549-38554.

Corda, Y., Job, C., Anin, M-F, Leng, M. & Job, D. (1991). Transcription by eukaryotic and prokaryotic RNA polymerases of DNA modified at a d(GG) or a d(AG) site by the antitumor drug *cis*-diamminedichloroplatinum(II). *Biochemistry.* 30(1): 222-230.

Cubo, L., Thomas, D.S., Zhang, J., Quiroga, A.G., Navarro-Ranninger, C. & Berners-Price, S.J. (2009). [^{1}H,^{15}N] NMR studies of the aquation of *cis*-diamine platinum(II) complexes. *Inorg Chim Acta.* 362(3): 1022-1026.

Damsma, G.E., Alt, A., Brueckner, F., Carell, T. & Cramer, P. (2007). Mechanism of transcriptional stalling at cisplatin-damaged DNA. *Nat Struc Mol Biol.* 14(12): 1127-1133.

de Paula, Q.A., Mangrum, J.B. & Farrell, N.P. (2009). Zinc finger proteins as templates for metal ion exchange: Substitution effects on the C-finger of HIV nucleocapsid NCp7 using M(chelate) species (M=Pt, Pd, Au). *J Inorg Biochem.* 103(10): 1347-1354.

Dizin, E. & Irminger-Finger, I. (2010). Negative feedback loop of BRCA1-BARD1 ubiquitin ligase on estrogen receptor α stability and activity antagonized by cancer-associated isoform of BARD1. *Int J Biochem Cell Biol.* 42(5): 693-700.

Eakin, C.M., Maccoss, M.J., Finney, G.L. & Klevit, R.E. (2007). Estrogen receptor α is a putative substrate for the BRCA1 ubiquitin ligase. *Proc Natl Acad Sci USA.* 104(14): 5794-5799.

Eastman, A. (1986). Reevaluation of interaction of cis-dichloro(ethylenediamine)platinum(II) with DNA. *Biochemistry.* 25 (13): 3912-3915.

Fan, S., Ma, Y.X., Wang, C., Yuan, R.Q., Meng, Q., Wang, J.A., et al. (2002). p300 Modulates the BRCA1 inhibition of estrogen receptor activity. *Cancer Res.* 62(1): 141-151.

Fan, S., Ma, Y.X., Wang, C., Yuan, R.Q., Meng, Q., Wang, J-N., et al. (2001). Role of direct interaction in BRCA1 inhibition of estrogen receptor activity. *Oncogene.* 20(1): 77-87.

Fan, S., Wang, J., Yuan, R., Ma, Y., Meng, Q., Erdos, M.R., et al. (1999). BRCA1 inhibition of estrogen receptor signaling in transfected cells. *Science.* 284(5418): 1354-1356.

Farmer, H., McCabe, N., Lord, C.J., Tutt, A.N., Johnson, D.A., Richardson, T.B., et al. (2005). Targeting the DNA repair defect in BRCA mutant cells as a therapeutic strategy. *Nature.* 434(7035): 917-921.

Fedier, A., Steiner, R.A., Schwarz, V.A., Lenherr, L., Haller, U. & Fink, D. (2003). The effect of loss of Brca1 on the sensitivity to anticancer agents in p53-deficient cells. *Int J Oncol.* 22(5): 1169-1173.

Fichtinger-Schepman, A.M., Van der Veer, J.L., den Hartog, J.H., Lohman, P.H. & Reedijk, J. (1985). Adducts of the antitumor drug cis-diamminedichloroplatinum(II) with DNA: formation, identification, and quantitation. *Biochemistry.* 24 (3): 707-713.

Font, A., Taron, M., Gago, J.L., Costa, C., Sánchez, J.J., Carrato, C., et al. (2010). BRCA1 mRNA expression and outcome to neoadjuvant cisplatin-based chemotherapy in bladder cancer. Ann Oncol. doi:10.1093/annonc/mdq333

Hall, J.M., Lee, M.K., Newman, B., Morrow, J.E., Anderson, L.A., Huey, B., et al. (1990). Linkage of early onset familial breast cancer to chromosome 17q21. *Science.* 250(4988): 1684-1689.

Hashizume, R., Fukuda, M., Maeda, I., Nishikawa, H., Oyake, D., Yabuki, Y., et al. (2001). The RING heterodimer BRCA1-BARD1 is a ubiquitin ligase inactivated by a breast cancer-derived mutation. *J Biol Chem.* 276(18): 14537-14540.

Helleday, T., Petermann, E., Lundin, C., Hodgson, B. & Sharma, R.A. (2008). DNA repair pathways as targets for cancer therapy. *Nat Rev Cancer.* 8(3): 193-204.

Horwitz, A.A., Affar, E.B., Heine, G.F., Shi, Y. & Parvin, J.D. (2007). A mechanism for transcriptional repression dependent on the BRCA1 E3 ubiquitin ligase. *Proc Natl Acad Sci USA.* 104(16): 6614-6619.

Huen, M.S.Y., Sy, S.M.H. & Chen, J. (2010). BRCA1 and its toolbox for the maintenance of genome integrity. *Nat Rev Mol Cell Biol.* 11(2): 138-148.

Husain, A., He, G., Venkatraman, E.S. & Spriggs, D.R. (1998). BRCA1 up-regulation is associated with repair-mediated resistance to cis-diamminedichloroplatinum(II). *Cancer Res.* 58(6): 1120-1123.

Ishidaa, R., Takaokaa, Y., Yamamotoa, S., Miyazakia, T., Otakab, M., Watanabeb, S., et al. (2008). Cisplatin differently affects amino terminal and carboxyl terminal domains of HSP90. *FEBS Lett.* 582(28): 3879-3883.

Ivanov, A.I., Christodoulou, J., Parkinson, J.A., Barnham, K.J., Tucker, A., Woodrow, J., et al. (1998). Cisplatin binding sites on human albumin. *J Biol Chem.* 273(24): 14721-14730.

James, C.R., Quinn, J.E.,Mullan, P.B., Johnston, P.G. & Harkin, D.P. (2007). BRCA1, a potential predictive biomarker in the treatment of breast cancer. *Oncologist.* 12(2): 142-150.

Jensen, D.E., Proctor, M., Marquis, S.T., Gardner, H.P., Ha, S.I., Chodosh, L.A., et al. (1998). BAP1: a novel ubiquitin hydrolase which binds to the BRCA1 RING finger and enhances BRCA1-mediated cell growth suppression. *Oncogene.* 16(9): 1097-1112.

Jin, Y., Xu, X.L., Yang, M.C., Wei, F., Ayi, T.C., Bowcock, A.M. et al., (1997). Cell cycle-dependent colocalization of BARD1 and BRCA1 proteins in discrete nuclear domains. *Proc Natl Acad Sci USA* 94 (22): 12075-12080.

Jordan, P. & Carmo-Fonseca, M. (1998). Cisplatin inhibits synthesis of ribosomal RNA *in vivo*. *Nucleic Acids Res.* 26(12): 2831-2836.

Jung, Y. & Lippard, S.J. (2003). Multiple states of stalled T7 RNA polymerase at DNA lesions generated by platinum anticancer agents. *J Biol Chem.* 278(52): 52084-52092.

Jung, Y., Mikata, Y. & Lippard, S.J. (2001). Kinetic studies of the TATA-binding protein interaction with cisplatin-modified DNA. *J Biol Chem.* 276(47): 43589-43596.

Kelland, L. (2007). The resurgence of platinum-based cancer chemotherapy. *Nat Rev Cancer.* 7(8): 573-584.

Kelley, M.R., & Fishel, M.L. (2008). DNA repair proteins as molecular targets for cancer therapeutics. *Anticancer Agents Med Chem.* 8(4): 417-425.

Kennedy, R.D., Quinn, J.E., Mullan, P.B., Johnston, P.G. & Harkin, D.P. (2004). The role of BRCA1 in the cellular response to chemotherapy. *J Natl Cancer Inst.* 96(22): 1659-1668.

Lafarge, S., Sylvain, V., Ferrara, M. & Bignon, Y.J. (2001). Inhibition of BRCA1 leads to increased chemoresistance to microtubule-interfering agents, an effect that involves the JNK pathway. *Oncogene.* 20(45): 6597-6606.

Lieberman, H.B. (2008). DNA damage repair and response proteins as targets for cancer therapy. *Curr Med Chem.* 15(4): 360-367.

Litman, R., Gupta, R., Brosh, Jr R.M. & Cantor, S.B. (2008). BRCA-FA pathway as a target for anti-tumor drugs. *Anticancer Agents Med Chem.* 8(4): 426-430.

Ljungman, M., Zhang, F., Chen, F., Rainbow, A.J. & McKay, B.C. (1999). Inhibition of RNA polymerase II as a trigger for the p53 response. *Oncogene.* 18(3): 583-592.

Mark, W.Y., Liao, J.C., Lu, Y., Ayed, A., Laister, R., Szymczyna, B., et al. (2005). Characterization of segments from the central region of BRCA1: an intrinsically disordered scaffold for multiple protein-protein and protein-DNA interactions? *J Mol Biol.* 345(2): 275-287.

Miki, Y., Swensen, J., Shattuck-Eidens, D., Futreal, P.A., Harshman, K., Tavtigian, S., et al. (1994). A strong candidate for the breast and ovarian cancer susceptibility gene BRCA1. *Science.* 266(5182): 66-71.

Monteiro, A.N., August, A. & Hanafusa, H. (1996). Evidence for a transcriptional activation function of BRCA1 C-terminal region. *Proc Natl Acad Sci USA* 93(24): 13595-13599.

Morris, J.R., Boutell, C., Keppler, M., Densham, R., Weekes, D., Alamshah, A., et al. (2009). The SUMO modification pathway is involved in the BRCA1 response to genotoxic stress. *Nature.* 462(7275): 886-890.

Morris, J.R., Pangon, L., Boutell, C., Katagiri, T., Keep, N.H. & Solomon, E. (2006). Genetic analysis of BRCA1 ubiquitin ligase activity and its relationship to breast cancer susceptibility. *Hum Mol Genet.* 15(4): 599-606.

Moynahan, M.E., Cui, T.Y. & Jasin, M. (2001). Homology-directed dna repair, mitomycin c resistance, and chromosome stability is restored with correction of a Brca1 mutation. *Cancer Res.* 61(12): 4842-4850.

Mullan, P.B., Quinn, J.E. & Harkin, D.P. (2006). The role of BRCA1 in transcriptional regulation and cell cycle control. *Oncogene.* 25(43): 5854-5863.

Musah, R.A. (2004). The HIV-1 nucleocapsid zinc finger protein as a target of antiretroviral therapy. *Curr Top Med Chem.* 4(15): 1605-1622.

Neault, J.F. & Tajmir-Riahi, H.A. (1998). Interaction of cisplatin with human serum albumin. Drug binding mode and protein secondary structure. *Biochim Biophys Acta.* 1384(1): 153-159.

Nishikawa, H., Wu, W., Koike, A., Kojima, R., Gomi, H., Fukuda, M., et al. (2009). BRCA1-associated protein 1 interferes with BRCA1/BARD1 RING heterodimer activity. *Cancer Res.* 69(1): 111-119.

Ober, M. & Lippard, S.J. (2008). A 1,2-d(GpG) cisplatin intrastrand cross-link influences the rotational and translational setting of DNA in nucleosomes. *J Am Chem Soc.* 130 (9): 2851-2861.

O'Donovan, P.J. & Livingston, D.M. (2010). BRCA1 and BRCA2: breast/ovarian cancer susceptibility gene products and participants in DNA double-strand break repair. *Carcinogenesis.* 31(6): 961-967.

Parvin, J.D. (2009). The BRCA1-dependent ubiquitin ligase, gamma-tubulin, and centrosomes. *Environ Mol Mutagen.* 50(8): 649-653.

Peleg-Shulman, T., Najajreh, Y. & Gibson, D. (2002). Interactions of cisplatin and transplatin with proteins: Comparison of binding kinetics, binding sites and reactivity of the Pt-protein adducts of cisplatin and transplatin towards biological nucleophiles. *J Inorg Biochem.* 91(1): 306-311.

Pinto, A.L. & Lippard, S.J. (1985). Sequence-dependent termination of in vitro DNA synthesis by cis- and trans-diamminedichloroplatinum(II). *Proc Natl Acad Sci USA* 82(14): 4616-4619.

Powell, S.N. & Bindra, R.S. (2009). Targeting the DNA damage response for cancer therapy. *DNA Repair.* 8(9): 1153-1165.

Quinn, J.E., Carser, J.E., James, C.R., Kennedy, R.D. & Harkin, D.P. (2009). BRCA1 and implications for response to chemotherapy in ovarian cancer. *Gynecol Oncol.* 113(1): 134-142.

Quinn, J.E., James, C,R., Stewart, G.E., Mulligan, J.M., White, P., Chang, G.K., et al. (2007). BRCA1 mRNA expression levels predict for overall survival in ovarian cancer after chemotherapy. *Clin Cancer Res.* 13(24): 7413-7420.

Quinn, J.E., Kennedy, R.E., Mullan, P.B., Gilmore, P.M., Carty, M., Johnston, P.G., et al. (2003). BRCA1 functions as a differential modulator of chemotherapy-induced apoptosis. *Cancer Res.* 63(19): 6221-6228.

Rahman, N., Seal, S., Thompson, D., Kelly, P., Renwick, A., Elliott, A., et al. (2007). PALB2, which encodes a BRCA2-interacting protein, is a breast cancer susceptibility gene. *Nature Genet.* 39(2): 165-167.

Ransburgh, D.J., Chiba, N., Ishioka, C., Toland, A.E. & Parvin, J.D. (2010). Identification of breast tumor mutations in BRCA1 that abolish its function in homologous DNA recombination. *Cancer Res.* 70(3): 988-995.

Ratanaphan, A., Canyuk, B., Wasiksiri, S. & Mahasawat, P. (2005). In vitro platination of human breast cancer suppressor gene 1 (BRCA1) by the anticancer drug carboplatin. Biochim Biophys Acta. 1725(2): 145-151.

Ratanaphan, A., Wasiksiri, S., Canyuk, B. & Prasertsan, P. (2009). Cisplatin-damaged BRCA1 exhibits altered thermostability and transcriptional transctivation. *Cancer Biol Ther.* 8(10): 890-898.

Rogakou, E.P., Pilch, D.R., Orr, A.H., Ivanova, V.S. & Bonner, W.M. (1998). DNA double-stranded breaks induce histone H2AX phosphorylation on serine 139. *J Biol Chem.* 273(10): 5858-5868.

Rosen, E.M., Fan, S., Pestell, R.G. & Goldberg, I.D. (2003). BRCA1 gene in breast cancer. *J Cell Physiol.* 196(1): 19-41.

Rowling, P.J.E., Cook, R. & Itzhaki, L.S. (2010). Toward classification of BRCA1 missense variants using a biophysical approach. *J Biol Chem.* 285(26): 20080-20087.

Ruffner, H., Joazeiro, C.A., Hemmati, D., Hunter, T. & Verma, I.M. (2001). Cancer-predisposing mutations within the RING domain of BRCA1: loss of ubiquitin protein ligase activity and protection from radiation hypersensitivity. *Proc Natl Acad Sci USA.* 98(9): 5134-5139.

Sato, K., Hayami, R., Wu, W., Nishikawa, T., Nishikawa, H., Okuda, Y., et al. (2004). Nucleophosmin/B23 is a candidate substrate for the BRCA1-BARD1 ubiquitin ligase. *J Biol Chem.* 279(30): 30919-30922.

Scully, R., Chen, J., Plug, A., Xiao, Y., Weaver, D., Feunteun, J., et al. (1997). Association of BRCA1 with Rad51 in mitotic and meiotic cells. *Cell.* 88(2): 265-275.

Shuck, S.C., Short, E.A. & Turchi, J.J. (2008). Eukaryotic nucleotide excision repair: from understanding mechanisms to influencing biology. *Cell Res.* 18(1): 64-72.

Silver, D.P., Richardson, A.L., Eklund, A.C., Wang, Z.C., Szallasi, Z., Li, O., et al. (2010). Efficacy of neoadjuvant cisplatin in triple-negative breast cancer. *J Clin Oncol.* 28(7): 1145-1153.

Somasundaram, K., Zhang, H., Zeng, Y.X., Houvras, Y., Peng, Y., Zhang, H. et al., (1997). Arrest of the cell cycle by the tumour-suppressor BRCA1 requires the CDK-inhibitor p21WAF1/CiP1. *Nature.* 389 (6647): 187-190.

Starita, L.M., Horwitz, A.A., Keogh, M.C., Ishioka, C., Parvin, J.D. & Chiba, N. (2005). BRCA1/BARD1 ubiquitinate phosphorylated RNA polymerase II. *J Biol Chem.* 280(26): 24498-24505.

Starita, L.M. & Parvin, J.D. (2003). The multiple nuclear functions of BRCA1: transcription, ubiquitination and DNA repair. *Curr Opin Cell Biol.* 15(3): 345-350.

Stucki, M., Clapperton, J.A., Mohammad, D., Yaffe, M.B., Smerdon, S.J. & Jackson, S.P. (2005). MDC1 directly binds phosphorylated histone H2AX to regulate cellular responses to DNA double-strand breaks. *Cell.* 123(7): 1213-1226.

Sun, X., Tsang, C-N. & Sun, H. (2009). Identification and characterization of metallodrug binding proteins by (metallo)proteomics. *Metallomics.* 1(1): 25-31.

Swisher, E.M., Sakai, W., Karlan, B.Y., Wurz, K., Urban, N. & Taniguchi, T. (2008). Secondary BRCA1 mutations in BRCA1-mutated ovarian carcinomas with platinum resistance. *Cancer Res.* 68(8): 2581-2586.

Sy, S.M.H., Huen, M.S.Y. & Chen, J. (2009). PALB2 is an integral component of the BRCA complex required for homologous recombination repair. *Proc Natl Acad Sci USA.* 106(17): 7155-7160.

Taron, M., Rosell, R., Felip, E., Mendez, P., Souglakos, J., Ronco, M.S., et al. (2004). BRCA1 mRNA expression as an indicator of chemoresistance in lung cancer. *Hum Mol Genet.* 13(20): 2443-2449.

Tassone, P., Martino, M.T.D., Ventura, M., Pietragalla, A., Cucinotto, I., Calimeri, T., et al. (2009). Loss of BRCA1 function increases the antitumor activity of cisplatin against human breast cancer xenografts in vivo. *Cancer Biol Ther.* 8(7): 648-653.

Tassone, P., Tagliaferri, P., Perricelli, A., Blotta, S., Quaresima, B., Martelli, M.L., et al. (2003). BRCA1 expression modulates chemosensitivity of BRCA1-defective HCC1937 human breast cancer cells. *Br J Cancer.* 88(8): 1285-1291.

Thakar, A., Parvin, J.D. & Zlatanova, J. (2010). BRCA1/BARD1 E3 ubiquitin ligase can modify histones H2A and H2B in the nucleosome particle. *J Biomol Struct Dyn.* 27(4): 399-406.

Timerbaev, A.R., Hartinger, C.G., Aleksenko, S.S. & Keppler, B.K. (2006). Interactions of antitumor metallodrugs with serum proteins: advances in characterization using modern analytical methodology. *Chem Rev.* 106(6): 2224-2248.

Todd, R.C. & Lippard, S.J. (2009). Inhibition of transcription by platinum antitumor compounds. *Metallomics.* 1(4): 280-291.

Tornaletti, S. (2005). Transcription arrest at DNA damage sites. *Mutat Res.* 577(1-2): 131-145.

Vallon-Christersson, J., Cayanan, C., Haraldsson, K., Loman, N., Bergthorsson, J.T., Brondum-Nielsen, K. et al. (2001). Functional analysis of BRCA1 C-terminal missense mutations identified in breast and ovarian cancer families. *Hum Mol Genet* 10(4): 353-360.

Varma, A.K., Brown, R.S., Birrane, G. & Ladias, J.A. (2005). Structural basis for cell cycle checkpoint control by the BRCA1-CtIP complex. *Biochemistry.* 44(33): 10941-10946.

Vichi, P., Coin, F., Renaud, J-P., Vermeulen, W., Hoeijmakers, J.H.J., Moras, D., et al. (1997). Cisplatin- and UV-damaged DNA lure the basal transcription factor TFIID/TBP. *EMBO J.* 16(24): 7444-7456.

Wang, D., & Lippard, S. (2005). Cellular processing of platinum anticancer drugs. *Nat Rev Drug Discov.* 4(4): 307-320.

Wang, W. & Figg, W.D. (2008). Secondary BRCA1 and BRCA2 alterations and acquired chemoresistance. *Cancer Biol Ther.* 7(7): 1004-1005.

Wei, L., Lan, L., Hong, Z., Yasui, A., Ishioka, C. & Chiba, N. (2008). Rapid recruitment of BRCA1 to DNA double-strand breaks is dependent on its association with Ku80. *Mol Cell Biol.* 28(24): 7380-7393.

Williams, R.S., Green, R. & Glover, J.N. (2001). Crystal structure of the BRCT repeat region from the breast cancer-associated protein BRCA1. *Nat Struct Biol.* 8(10): 838-42.

Williams, R.S., Lee, M.S., Hau, D.D. & Glover, J.N. (2004). Structural basis of phosphopeptide recognition by the BRCT domain of BRCA1. *Nat Struct Mol Biol.* 11(6): 519-525.

Wu, B., Dröge, P. & Davey, C.A. (2008). Site selectivity of platinum anticancer therapeutics. *Nat Chem Biol.* 4(2): 110-112.

Wu, L.C., Wang, Z.W., Tsan, J.T., Spillman, M.A., Phung, A., Xu, X.L., et al. (1996). Identification of a RING protein that can interact in vivo with the *BRCA1* gene product. *Nat Genet.* 14(4): 430-440.

Wu-Baer, F., Ludwig, T. & Baer, R. (2010). The UBXN1 protein associates with autoubiquitinated forms of the BRCA1 tumor suppressor and inhibits its enzymatic function. *Mol Cell Biol.* 30(11): 2787-2798.

Xia, Y., Pao, G.M., Chen, H-W., Verma, I.M. & Hunter, T. (2003). Enhancement of BRCA1 E3 ubiquitin ligase activity through direct interaction with the BARD1 protein. *J Biol Chem.* 278(7): 5255-5263.

Xu, J., Fan, S. & Rosen, E.M. (2005). Regulation of the estrogen-inducible gene expression profile by the breast cancer susceptibility gene BRCA1. *Endocrinology.* 146(4): 2031-2047.

Zdraveski, Z.Z., Mello, J.A., Marinus, M.G. & Essigmann, J.M. (2000). Multiple pathways of recombination define cellular responses to cisplatin. *Chem Biol.* 7(1): 39-50.

Zhai, X., Beckmann, H., Jantzen, H-M. & Essigmann, J.M. (1998). Cisplatin-DNA adducts inhibit ribosomal RNA synthesis by hijacking the transcription factor human upstream binding factor. *Biochemistry.* 37(46): 16307-16315.

Zhang, H., Somasundaram, K., Peng, Y., Tian, H., Bi, D., Weber, B.L., et al. (1998) BRCA1 physically associates with p53 and stimulates its transcriptional activity. *Oncogene.* 16(13): 1713-1721.

Zhang, J. & Powell, S.N. (2005). The role of the BRCA1 tumor suppressor in DNA double-strand break repair. *Mol Cancer Res.* 3(10): 531-539.

Zhao, T. & King, F.L. (2010). A mass spectrometric comparison of the interactions of cisplatin and transplatin with myoglobin. *J Inorg Biochem.* 104(2): 186-192.

Zhong, Q., Boyer, T.G., Chen, P.L. & Lee, W.H. (2002). Deficient nonhomologous end-joining activity in cell-free extracts from Brca1-null fibroblasts. *Cancer Res.* 62(14): 3966-3970.

Zhu, Y., Hub, J., Hu, Y. & Liu, W. (2009). Targeting DNA repair pathways: a novel approach to reduce cancer therapeutic resistance. *Cancer Treat Rev.* 35(7): 590-596.

13

Saccharomyces cerevisiae as a Model System to Study the Role of Human DDB2 in Chromatin Repair

Kristi L. Jones, Ling Zhang and Feng Gong
Department of Biochemistry and Molecular Biology, University of Miami
USA

1. Introduction

Genetic and biochemical studies in *Saccharomyces cerevisiae* have made major contributions in elucidating the mechanism of several DNA repair pathways, including the nucleotide excision repair (NER) pathway that remove bulky DNA damage from the genome. Although NER is conserved from yeast to humans, there are differences in NER between yeast and humans. For example, no homolog of the human NER factor DNA damage-binding protein 2 (DDB2) has been identified in the budding yeast *S. cerevisiae*. Here, we present evidence suggesting that *S. cerevisiae* can be used to dissect the roles of DDB2 in initiating NER in chromatin.

Ultraviolet light (UV) is a well studied genotoxic stress that induces bulky DNA damage. These UV lesions are repaired by the NER pathway (Hanawalt, 2002; Sancar & Reardon, 2004). The particular lesions induced by UV irradiation have been characterized, namely, cyclobutane pyrimidine dimers (CPDs) and 6-4 photoproducts (6-4PPs). Both lesions result in the distortion of the DNA double helix, but 6-4PPs result in a greater distortion. Additionally, there are other minor differences between the two types of lesions. CPDs have been consistently shown to have higher incidence than 6-4PPs (Douki & Cadet, 2001). CPDs are induced both in nucleosome core and linker DNA, whereas 6-4PPs are formed with 6-fold greater frequency in linker DNA. In addition, 6-4PPs are repaired much faster than CPDs, as reviewed by Smerdon (Smerdon, 1991).

In humans, a defect in NER results in xeroderma pigmentosum (XP) and several other rare diseases (Kraemer et al., 2007). XP patients are extremely sensitive to UV light and have about 2000-fold higher incidence of sunlight induced skin cancers than the general population. NER lesion recognition is via protein interaction with the structural DNA changes that are induced. Other bulky DNA lesions repaired by NER include those induced by cigarette smoke, cisplatin treatment and a newly identified form of bulky oxidative DNA damage (Zamble et al., 1996; Setlow, 2001; Wang, 2008).

NER has been extensively studied and the basic mechanism is understood. It consists of three main steps: 1) lesion detection, 2) dual incision to remove an oligonucleotide containing the lesion and 3) repair synthesis to fill the gap. There are two sub-pathways of NER, termed transcription coupled repair (TC-NER) and global genome repair (GG-NER) (Hanawalt, 2002). TC-NER is responsible for repair of damage on the actively transcribed strand; while GG-NER is responsible for repair in the remainder of the genome, including lesions on the non-transcribed strand of actively transcribed genes, as well as those in repressed or silent chromatin regions. Both TC-NER and GG-NER consist of all three steps, but, they differ in the lesion recognition step. In TC-NER the lesion is thought to be detected by pausing of RNA polymerase I or II (Conconi et al., 2002; Hanawalt, 2002; Fousteri & Mullenders, 2008). GG-NER, on the other hand, requires a specific lesion recognition hetero-dimeric protein complex, XPC-hRad23 (Xeroderma Pigmentosum complementation group C-human Rad23) in humans and Rad4-Rad23 (RADiation sensitive) in budding yeast (Wood 2010; Guzder et al., 1998; Jansen et al., 1998; Sugasawa, 2009). However, under certain *in vivo* circumstances, DDB2 is the pioneering damage recognition factor during GG-NER (Hwang et al., 1999; Nichols et al., 2000; Sugasawa, 2009). So far, no DDB2 homolog has been identified in the budding yeast (Fig. 1). Of note, the Rad16-Rad7 heterodimer, without a known human homolog, is required for GG-NER in the budding yeast.

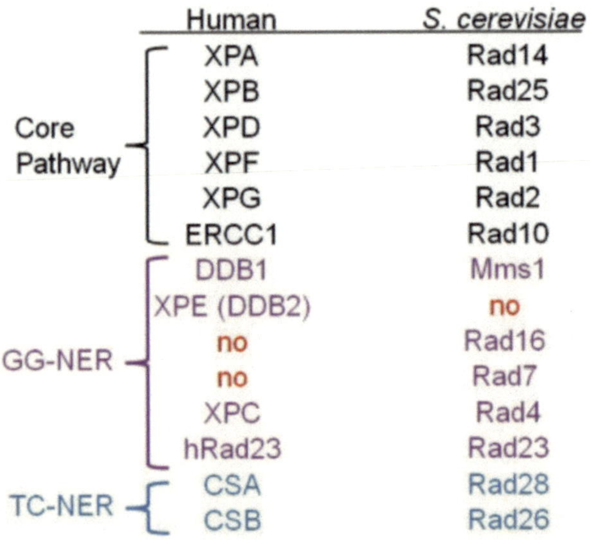

Fig. 1. Conservation of NER pathway between humans and the budding yeast *S. cerevisiae*. Of note, no DDB2 counterpart has been identified in *S. cerevisiae*. Likewise, humans don't have a homolog of the Rad16-Rad7 heterodimer that is essential for GG-NER in *S. cerevisiae*.

Several lines of evidence suggest that DDB2 plays a key role in **chromatin repair** of UV damage. It has been shown that DDB2 is responsible for the lesion detection by directly interacting with the damaged DNA (Tang, et al., 2000; Scrima et al., 2008). Additionally, DDB2 binds the lesion independent of XPC (Wakasugi et al., 2002). DDB2 can co-localize with both CPDs and 6-4 PPs *in vivo*, while XPC seems to bind 6-4 PPs efficiently, but not CPDs. This suggests the necessity of DDB2 in GG-NER is specific for CPD repair (Fitch et al., 2003). Importantly, it has been suggested that the observed high affinity of DDB2 for 6-4PPs aids in the targeting of XPC to 6-4PPs when low levels of damage are present (Nishi et al., 2009).

Additionally, DDB2 is in complex with the E3 ubiquitin ligase complex consisting of DDB1, Cul4 (CULlin 4) and ROC (Ring Of Cullins) (Jackson & Xiong, 2009). E3 ubiquitin ligases transfer ubiquitin to the target protein. DDB2 is thought to be the substrate receptor targeting the E3 ubiquitin ligase complex to DNA lesion sites to facilitate GG-NER. Of note, DDB1 and Cul4 have been shown to be in complex with other proteins, including CSA, a TC-NER specific protein (Jackson & Xiong, 2009). Consistent with its classification as an E3 ubiquitin ligase, XPC, histone H2A, H3, H4, and DDB2 itself have been identified as UV-dependent ubiquitination targets of the DDB1-DDB2 E3 ligase complex (Chen et al., 2001; Nag et al., 2001; Matsuda et al., 2005; Sugasawa et al., 2005; Kapetanaki et al., 2006; Wang et al., 2006). The UV-dependent mono-ubiquitination of histone H2A has been suggested to be involved in both chromatin relaxation and restoration (Kapetanaki et al., 2006; Zhu et al., 2009). Clearly, understanding the role of DDB2 in NER will yield important insights into the mechanisms of NER operation in the context of chromatin.

Chromatin is a hierarchal structure composed of DNA and protein. The core component is the nucleosome. It is a complex of 147 base pairs of DNA wrapped around the core histone octamer. The core histone octamer consists of four subunits, H2A, H2B, H3 and H4 in a 2:2:2:2 ratio (Luger et al., 1997; Kornberg & Lorch, 1999). The innate structure of chromatin restricts DNA protein interactions. ATP-dependent chromatin reconfiguration is an important mechanism to alleviate this tight association. Several groups have demonstrated a requirement for the ATP-dependent chromatin remodeling in chromatin repair (Jiang et al., 2010; Gong et al. 2006; Zhang et al. 2009a; Zhang et al. 2009b; Zhao et al. 2009; Lans et al. 2010; Sarkar et al. 2010). How DNA repair occurs in chromatin is an emerging question and has been discussed in several recent review articles (Osley et al., 2007; Nag & Smerdon, 2009; Waters et al., 2009; Zhang et al., 2009a; Jones et al., 2010).

2. *S. cerevisiae* as a model system to study DDB2-mediated GG-NER in chromatin

It has been demonstrated that DDB2 is the initial lesion detection factor in GG-NER (Tang et al., 2000; Wakasugi et al., 2002; Fitch et al., 2003b; Pines et al., 2009). Although it has been implicated in the recruitment of XPC to CPD sites (Fitch et al., 2003b); how DDB2 transfers these identified lesions to XPC remains controversial. It is believed that ubiquitination of DDB2 leads to its degradation at damage sites and this degradation is required for CPD repair. However, there are several lines of evidence disputing this model, including: 1) inhibition of ubiquitination-mediated DDB2 degradation in mouse via Cul4a ablation enhances CPD repair (Liu et al., 2009), 2) DDB2 degradation is not stimulated by either DNA binding or XPC association (Luijsterburg et al., 2007), and 3) crystal structures suggest that DDB2 and XPC can co-localize on the lesion (Min & Pavletich, 2007; Scrima et al., 2008). Therefore, we try to explore the budding yeast as a simplified, alternative model system to begin to dissect the role(s) of ubiquitination in DDB2-mediated GG-NER.

2.1 Galactose induced expression of DDB2 in *S. cerevisiae*

As discussed in the introduction, DDB2 has no homolog in budding yeast. However, conservation of the GG-NER pathway and interacting partners such as DDB1 are known (Zaidi et al., 2008). Therefore, we hypothesized that DDB2 would act in a physiological relevant manner in budding yeast GG-NER. We first cloned the DDB2 gene into a low copy number, galactose inducible yeast expression vector. The cloning results in a fusion protein;

DDB2 fused with V5His6 tag (Fig. 2A). Both the empty plasmid vector and the DDB2 containing plasmid were transformed into *S. cerevisiae*. As expected, when cells were grown in the presence of galactose, DDB2 protein was produced as identified by Western blot using both V5 and DDB2 antibodies (Fig. 2B and data not shown). No protein was detectable at the calculated molecular weight of DDB2 in the empty vector control using the same Western blot technique (Fig. 2B).

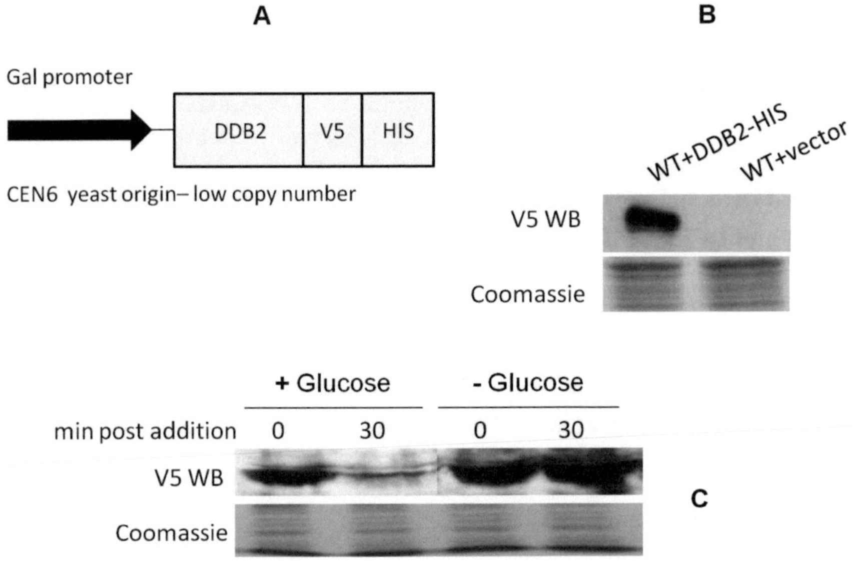

Fig. 2. Expression of DDB2-HIS in S. cerevisiae. (A) Schematic of DDB2 fusion cloned into pYCT/C2 expression vector. (B). Western blot (WB) using V5 antibody to detect expression of DDB2 containing or empty vector. (C) Glucose addition (4%) stops production of DDB2 detected by Western blot using V5 antibody, equal amount of total protein was verified using coomassie blue staining. BY4741 is the wild type (WT) strain used in these experiments.

To access the efficacy of the galactose induction 4% glucose was added to the media. Rapid shut down of the galactose inducible promoter is presumed due to the significant decrease in DDB2 protein levels 30 min post addition of glucose (Fig. 2C). This observed decrease in DDB2 protein levels is likely due to normal protein turnover in the absence of nascent DDB2 transcription and subsequent translation. These data confirm that DDB2 is expressed in *S. cerevisiae* cells under the control of the galactose promoter.

2.2 DDB2 suppresses UV sensitivity of Δ*rad26* cells

Next we identified genetic background in which a DDB2-dependent phenotype could be observed. We screened several yeast strains in which various NER proteins were deleted. The strains tested were Δ*rad7* and Δ*rad16* in which only TC-NER is active, Δ*rad26* in which only GG-NER is active, and Δ*rad1* in which the core pathway is defective and therefore there is no active NER. The spotting assay was used to determine DDB2 dependent suppression of UV sensitivity. Clearly, DDB2 expression suppresses the UV sensitive phenotype of Δ*rad26* cells (Fig. 3A). Survival curve experiments verified these findings (Data not shown).

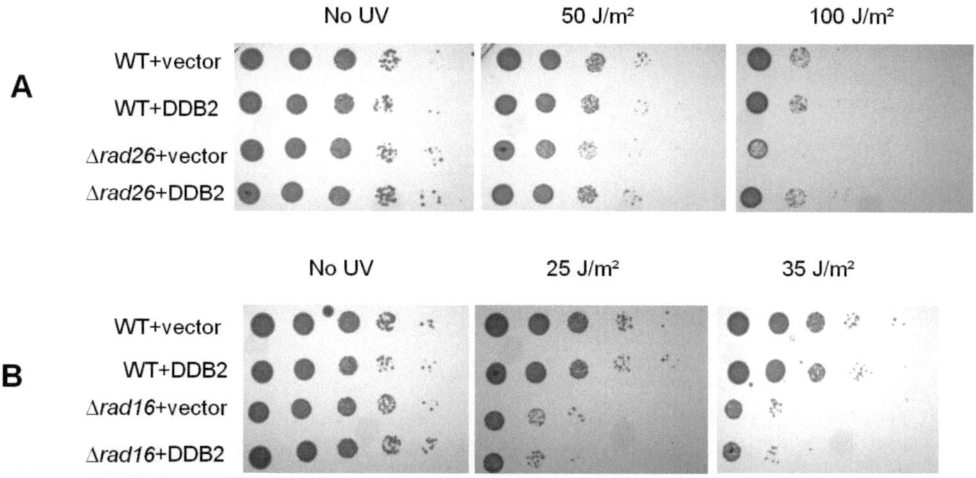

Fig. 3. DDB2 expression suppresses UV sensitivity of Δ*rad26* mutant, but not Δ*rad16* mutant. BY4741 (WT) cells expressing DDB2 or empty vector were diluted 1/10 and plated on galactose media. Cells were exposed to UV irradiation at dose indicated and grown in dark at 30 °C for 48 hours. Δ*rad26* (A). Δ*rad16* (B).

As discussed in the introduction, both DDB2 and Rad16 are necessary for lesion identification *in vivo* and are part of E3 ubiquitin ligase complexes (Verhage et al., 1994; Mueller & Smerdon, 1995; Shiyanov et al., 1999; Tang et al., 2000; Wakasugi et al., 2002; Fitch et al., 2003b; Groisman et al., 2003; Ramsey et al., 2004; Pines et al., 2009). Therefore, it was surprising that DDB2 was unable to suppress the Δ*rad16* UV sensitive (Fig. 3B). Our data suggest that despite similarities in their biochemical properties, on a gross functional level DDB2 and Rad16 are not analogs. It should be noted that Rad16 has also been implicated in post-incision processes (Reed et al., 1998) while DDB2 has not. It is therefore plausible that DDB2 and Rad16 have analogus functions in the lesion identification step of GG-NER, but this post-incision function of Rad16 is unable to be rescued by DDB2 expression.
In addition, we found that DDB2 was not able to significantly suppress UV sensitivity of any other knockout strains, including Δ*rad7* cells (data not shown). These data are consistent with no known DDB2 homolog in budding yeast. The observed DDB2-dependent suppression of TC-NER deficient UV sensitivity is consistent with reported DDB2 stimulation of GG-NER (Wakasugi et al., 2001; Wakasugi et al., 2002).

2.3 DDB2 mutations abrogate its ability to suppress Δ*rad26* UV sensitivity

To assess if DDB2 is functioning in a physiologically relevant manner, we first examined the phenotypic effects of mutant DDB2 on DDB2-dependnet suppression of Δ*rad26* UV sensitive phenotype. Several DDB2 mutations identified in XPE patients are known to interfere with its ability to function properly in GG-NER. It has been reported that a point mutation changing lysine 244 to glutamic acid (DDB2 K244E) results in inability of DDB2 to make contact with DNA lesions (Scrima et al., 2008) (Fig. 4A). However, this mutation does not alter the ability of DDB2 to interact with DDB1 in the Cul4a E3 ubiquitin ligase complex, therefore its role in ubiquitination is not altered. When this damage recognition deficient mutant DDB2 was introduced into Δ*rad26* cells, it was unable to suppress Δ*rad26* UV sensitivity (Fig. 5). This suggests that the observed DDB2-conferred UV resistance is linked to its function in DNA damage detection.

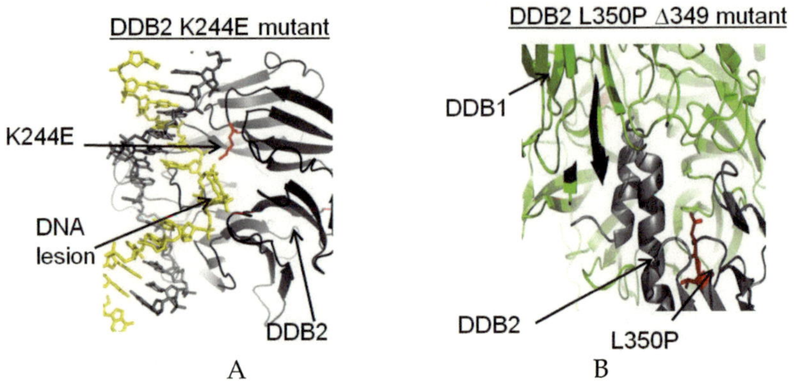

Fig. 4. Crystal structure of DDB2 mutations modified from crystal structure solved by Scrima et al. (A) Lysine to glutamic acid substitution at aa 244 predicted to effect DDB2 DNA interaction. Red residue indicates site of mutation. Yellow indicates damaged DNA strand. (B) Deletion of aa 349 and substitution of proline for leucine at aa 350. This mutation is predicted to effect the DDB2 DDB1 interaction. Red indicates site of mutation. Mutant DDB2 was constructed by site directed mutagenesis.

Another mutation that affects DDB2's function prevents the interaction with its in vivo partner DDB1 (Nichols et al. 2000). This mutation was also constructed and is a complex mutation, consisting of both a deletion of amino acid 349 and a proline substitution for leucine at amino acid 350 (DDB2 L350P) (Fig. 4B). Like DDB2 K244E, this mutation also abrogated DDB2's ability to suppress UV sensitivity in *Δrad26* cells (Fig. 5). These data suggest DDB2-conferred UV resistance is dependent on a conserved interacting partner.

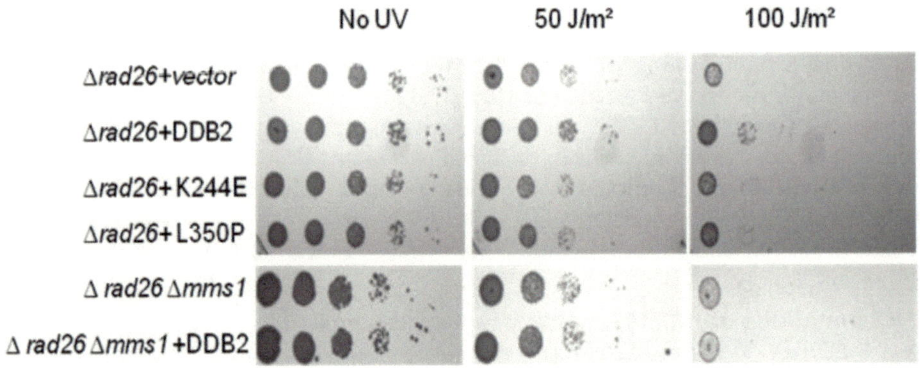

Fig. 5. DDB2 mutations and deletion of Mms1 (DDB1 homolog) abrogate suppression of UV sensitivity in *Δrad26* cells.

Although Mms1 has been identified as the budding yeast DDB1 homolog (Zaidi et al., 2008), there are no reports of it being involved in NER. However, our previous observation suggesting DDB2 function requires a conserved interacting partner prompted us to test DDB2 function in the absence of Mms1. To test this, wild type DDB2 was expressed in the *Δrad26Δmms1* double mutant and UV sensitivity was accessed by spotting assays. Indeed, this reciprocal experiment verified that Mms1 is necessary for DDB2-dependent suppression of UV sensitivity (Fig. 5).

Taken together, these data suggest that exogenously expressed DDB2 is acting in a physiologically relevant manner. Additionally, our findings indicate that the DNA damage recognition function of DDB2 is essential for the observed suppression of UV sensitivity. We also found that DDB2 function is dependent on interaction with Mms1, a subunit of an E3 ubiquitin ligase. These observations are consistent with what is reported for DDB2 function in human cells.

3. Conclusion

Studies in *Saccharomyces cerevisiae* have made major contributions to our understanding of NER. Here, we present evidence suggesting that *S. cerevisiae* can be used to dissect the roles of human DDB2 in initiating NER in chromatin. Since DDB2 functions are regulated by the ubiquitin pathway and DDB2 itself is a component of an E3 ligase, it will be interesting to explore the regulation of DDB2 functions by ubiquitination, using yeast mutants with defects in various steps of the ubiquitin pathway.

Ubiquitination is a well studied post-translational modification and recent data suggest multiple fates of ubiquitin modified proteins (Sadowski & Sarcevic, 2010). It will be important to determine if ubiquitination of DDB2 promotes its degradation or controls DDB2 association with chromatin. The budding yeast system described here will also provide an alternative system to screen the effect(s) of various DDB2 lysine mutations to determine which amino acid residue(s) is modified. Additionally, as reviewed by Kirkin et al., ubiquitin signaling is altered in many cancers (Kirkin and Dikic 2010), suggesting a potential role of ubiquitination in regulating DNA binding proteins such as transcription factors and repair proteins. Therefore, it will be interesting to determine what, if any, role ubiquitination plays in the chromatin association of other DNA binding proteins, specifically transcription factors and repair proteins. The utilization of the budding yeast model system will facilitate deciphering such questions.

4. Acknowledgment

The project described in this article was supported by Award R01ES017784 from the National Institute of Environmental Health Sciences and by a young investigator award from the Concern Foundation.

5. References

Chen, X., Zhang, Y., Douglas, L., and Zhou, P. 2001. UV-damaged DNA-binding proteins are targets of CUL-4A-mediated ubiquitination and degradation. J Biol Chem 276(51): 48175-48182.

Conconi, A., Bespalov, V.A., and Smerdon, M.J. 2002. Transcription-coupled repair in RNA polymerase I-transcribed genes of yeast. Proc Natl Acad Sci U S A 99(2): 649-654.

Douki, T. and Cadet, J. 2001. Individual determination of the yield of the main UV-induced dimeric pyrimidine photoproducts in DNA suggests a high mutagenicity of CC photolesions. Biochemistry 40(8): 2495-2501.

Fitch, M.E., Cross, I.V., Turner, S.J., Adimoolam, S., Lin, C.X., Williams, K.G., and Ford, J.M. 2003a. The DDB2 nucleotide excision repair gene product p48 enhances global genomic repair in p53 deficient human fibroblasts. DNA Repair (Amst) 2(7): 819-826.

Fitch, M.E., Nakajima, S., Yasui, A., and Ford, J.M. 2003b. In vivo recruitment of XPC to UV-induced cyclobutane pyrimidine dimers by the DDB2 gene product. J Biol Chem 278(47): 46906-46910.

Fousteri, M. and Mullenders, L.H. 2008. Transcription-coupled nucleotide excision repair in mammalian cells: molecular mechanisms and biological effects. Cell Res 18(1): 73-84.

Gong, F., Fahy, D., and Smerdon, M.J. 2006. Rad4-Rad23 interaction with SWI/SNF links ATP-dependent chromatin remodeling with nucleotide excision repair. Nat Struct Mol Biol 13(10): 902-907.

Gong, F., Kwon, Y., and Smerdon, M.J. 2005. Nucleotide excision repair in chromatin and the right of entry. DNA Repair (Amst) 4(8): 884-896.

Groisman, R., Polanowska, J., Kuraoka, I., Sawada, J., Saijo, M., Drapkin, R., Kisselev, A.F., Tanaka, K., and Nakatani, Y. 2003. The ubiquitin ligase activity in the DDB2 and CSA complexes is differentially regulated by the COP9 signalosome in response to DNA damage. Cell 113(3): 357-367.

Guzder, S.N., Sung, P., Prakash, L., and Prakash, S. 1999. Synergistic interaction between yeast nucleotide excision repair factors NEF2 and NEF4 in the binding of ultraviolet-damaged DNA. J Biol Chem 274(34): 24257-24262.

Hanawalt, P.C. 2002. Subpathways of nucleotide excision repair and their regulation. Oncogene 21(58): 8949-8956.

Hwang, B.J., Ford, J.M., Hanawalt, P.C., and Chu, G. 1999. Expression of the p48 xeroderma pigmentosum gene is p53-dependent and is involved in global genomic repair. Proc Natl Acad Sci U S A 96(2): 424-428.

Jackson, S. and Xiong, Y. 2009. CRL4s: the CUL4-RING E3 ubiquitin ligases. Trends Biochem Sci 34(11): 562-570.

Jansen, L.E., Verhage, R.A., and Brouwer, J. 1998. Preferential binding of yeast Rad4.Rad23 complex to damaged DNA. J Biol Chem 273(50): 33111-33114.

Jiang, Y., Wang, X., Bao, S., Guo, R., Johnson, D.G., Shen, X., and Li, L. 2010. INO80 chromatin remodeling complex promotes the removal of UV lesions by the nucleotide excision repair pathway. *Proc Natl Acad Sci U S A* 107(40): 17274-17279.

Jones, K.L., Zhang, L., Seldeen, K.L., and Gong, F. 2010. Detection of bulky DNA lesions: DDB2 at the interface of chromatin and DNA repair in eukaryotes. *IUBMB Life* 62(11): 803-811.

Kapetanaki, M.G., Guerrero-Santoro, J., Bisi, D.C., Hsieh, C.L., Rapic-Otrin, V., and Levine, A.S. 2006. The DDB1-CUL4ADDB2 ubiquitin ligase is deficient in xeroderma pigmentosum group E and targets histone H2A at UV-damaged DNA sites. Proc Natl Acad Sci U S A 103(8): 2588-2593.

Kirkin, V. and Dikic, I. 2010. Ubiquitin networks in cancer. *Curr Opin Genet Dev* 21(1): 21-28.

Kornberg, R.D. and Lorch, Y. 1999. Twenty-five years of the nucleosome, fundamental particle of the eukaryote chromosome. Cell 98(3): 285-294.

Kraemer, K.H., Patronas, N.J., Schiffmann, R., Brooks, B.P., Tamura, D., and DiGiovanna, J.J. 2007. Xeroderma pigmentosum, trichothiodystrophy and Cockayne syndrome: a complex genotype-phenotype relationship. Neuroscience 145(4): 1388-1396.

Lans, H., Marteijn, J.A., Schumacher, B., Hoeijmakers, J.H., Jansen, G., and Vermeulen, W. 2010. Involvement of global genome repair, transcription coupled repair, and chromatin remodeling in UV DNA damage response changes during development. *PLoS Genet* 6(5): e1000941.

Liu, L., Lee, S., Zhang, J., Peters, S.B., Hannah, J., Zhang, Y., Yin, Y., Koff, A., Ma, L., and Zhou, P. 2009. CUL4A abrogation augments DNA damage response and protection against skin carcinogenesis. Mol Cell 34(4): 451-460.

Luger, K., Mader, A.W., Richmond, R.K., Sargent, D.F., and Richmond, T.J. 1997. Crystal structure of the nucleosome core particle at 2.8 A resolution. Nature 389(6648): 251-260.

Luijsterburg, M.S., Goedhart, J., Moser, J., Kool, H., Geverts, B., Houtsmuller, A.B., Mullenders, L.H., Vermeulen, W., and van Driel, R. 2007. Dynamic in vivo interaction of DDB2 E3 ubiquitin ligase with UV-damaged DNA is independent of damage-recognition protein XPC. J Cell Sci 120(Pt 15): 2706-2716.

Matsuda, N., Azuma, K., Saijo, M., Iemura, S., Hioki, Y., Natsume, T., Chiba, T., and Tanaka, K. 2005. DDB2, the xeroderma pigmentosum group E gene product, is directly ubiquitylated by Cullin 4A-based ubiquitin ligase complex. DNA Repair (Amst) 4(5): 537-545.

Min, J.H. and Pavletich, N.P. 2007. Recognition of DNA damage by the Rad4 nucleotide excision repair protein. Nature 449(7162): 570-575.

Mueller, J.P. and Smerdon, M.J. 1995. Repair of plasmid and genomic DNA in a rad7 delta mutant of yeast. Nucleic Acids Res 23(17): 3457-3464.

Nag, A., Bondar, T., Shiv, S., and Raychaudhuri, P. 2001. The xeroderma pigmentosum group E gene product DDB2 is a specific target of cullin 4A in mammalian cells. Mol Cell Biol 21(20): 6738-6747.

Nag, R. and Smerdon, M.J. 2009. Altering the chromatin landscape for nucleotide excision repair. Mutat Res 682(1): 13-20.

Nichols, A.F., Itoh, T., Graham, J.A., Liu, W., Yamaizumi, M., and Linn, S. 2000. Human damage-specific DNA-binding protein p48. Characterization of XPE mutations and regulation following UV irradiation. J Biol Chem 275(28): 21422-21428.

Osley, M.A., Tsukuda, T., and Nickoloff, J.A. 2007. ATP-dependent chromatin remodeling factors and DNA damage repair. *Mutat Res* 618(1-2): 65-80.

Pines, A., Backendorf, C., Alekseev, S., Jansen, J.G., de Gruijl, F.R., Vrieling, H., and Mullenders, L.H. 2009. Differential activity of UV-DDB in mouse keratinocytes and fibroblasts: impact on DNA repair and UV-induced skin cancer. DNA Repair (Amst) 8(2): 153-161.

Ramsey, K.L., Smith, J.J., Dasgupta, A., Maqani, N., Grant, P., and Auble, D.T. 2004. The NEF4 complex regulates Rad4 levels and utilizes Snf2/Swi2-related ATPase activity for nucleotide excision repair. Mol Cell Biol 24(14): 6362-6378.

Reed, S.H., You, Z., and Friedberg, E.C. 1998. The yeast RAD7 and RAD16 genes are required for postincision events during nucleotide excision repair. In vitro and in vivo studies with rad7 and rad16 mutants and purification of a Rad7/Rad16-containing protein complex. J Biol Chem 273(45): 29481-29488.

Sadowski, M. and Sarcevic, B. 2010. Mechanisms of mono- and poly-ubiquitination: Ubiquitination specificity depends on compatibility between the E2 catalytic core and amino acid residues proximal to the lysine. Cell Div 5: 19.

Sancar, A. and Reardon, J.T. 2004. Nucleotide excision repair in E. coli and man. Adv Protein Chem 69: 43-71.

Sarkar, S., Kiely, R., and McHugh, P.J. 2010. The Ino80 chromatin-remodeling complex restores chromatin structure during UV DNA damage repair. *J Cell Biol* 191(6): 1061-1068.

Scrima, A., Konickova, R., Czyzewski, B.K., Kawasaki, Y., Jeffrey, P.D., Groisman, R., Nakatani, Y., Iwai, S., Pavletich, N.P., and Thoma, N.H. 2008. Structural basis of UV DNA-damage recognition by the DDB1-DDB2 complex. Cell 135(7): 1213-1223.

Setlow, R.B. 2001. Human cancer: etiologic agents/dose responses/DNA repair/cellular and animal models. Mutat Res 477(1-2): 1-6.

Shiyanov, P., Nag, A., and Raychaudhuri, P. 1999. Cullin 4A associates with the UV-damaged DNA-binding protein DDB. J Biol Chem 274(50): 35309-35312.

Smerdon, M.J. 1991. DNA repair and the role of chromatin structure. Curr Opin Cell Biol 3(3): 422-428.

Sugasawa, K. 2009. UV-DDB: A molecular machine linking DNA repair with ubiquitination. DNA Repair (Amst).

Sugasawa, K., Okuda, Y., Saijo, M., Nishi, R., Matsuda, N., Chu, G., Mori, T., Iwai, S., Tanaka, K., and Hanaoka, F. 2005. UV-induced ubiquitylation of XPC protein mediated by UV-DDB-ubiquitin ligase complex. Cell 121(3): 387-400.

Tang, J. and Chu, G. 2002. Xeroderma pigmentosum complementation group E and UV-damaged DNA-binding protein. DNA Repair (Amst) 1(8): 601-616.

Tang, J.Y., Hwang, B.J., Ford, J.M., Hanawalt, P.C., and Chu, G. 2000. Xeroderma pigmentosum p48 gene enhances global genomic repair and suppresses UV-induced mutagenesis. Mol Cell 5(4): 737-744.

Verhage, R., Zeeman, A.M., de Groot, N., Gleig, F., Bang, D.D., van de Putte, P., and Brouwer, J. 1994. The RAD7 and RAD16 genes, which are essential for pyrimidine dimer removal from the silent mating type loci, are also required for repair of the nontranscribed strand of an active gene in Saccharomyces cerevisiae. Mol Cell Biol 14(9): 6135-6142.

Wakasugi, M., Kawashima, A., Morioka, H., Linn, S., Sancar, A., Mori, T., Nikaido, O., and Matsunaga, T. 2002. DDB accumulates at DNA damage sites immediately after UV irradiation and directly stimulates nucleotide excision repair. J Biol Chem 277(3): 1637-1640.

Wang, H., Zhai, L., Xu, J., Joo, H.Y., Jackson, S., Erdjument-Bromage, H., Tempst, P., Xiong, Y., and Zhang, Y. 2006. Histone H3 and H4 ubiquitylation by the CUL4-DDB-ROC1 ubiquitin ligase facilitates cellular response to DNA damage. Mol Cell 22(3): 383-394.

Wang, Y. 2008. Bulky DNA lesions induced by reactive oxygen species. Chem Res Toxicol 21(2): 276-281.

Waters, R., Teng, Y., Yu, Y., Yu, S., and Reed, S.H. 2009. Tilting at windmills? The nucleotide excision repair of chromosomal DNA. DNA Repair (Amst) 8(2): 146-152.

Wood, R.D. 2010. Mammalian nucleotide excision repair proteins and interstrand crosslink repair. Environ Mol Mutagen 51(6): 520-526.

Zaidi, I.W., Rabut, G., Poveda, A., Scheel, H., Malmstrom, J., Ulrich, H., Hofmann, K., Pasero, P., Peter, M., and Luke, B. 2008. Rtt101 and Mms1 in budding yeast form a CUL4(DDB1)-like ubiquitin ligase that promotes replication through damaged DNA. EMBO Rep 9(10): 1034-1040.

Zamble, D.B., Mu, D., Reardon, J.T., Sancar, A., and Lippard, S.J. 1996. Repair of cisplatin--DNA adducts by the mammalian excision nuclease. Biochemistry 35(31): 10004-10013.

Zhang, L., Jones, K., and Gong, F. 2009a. The molecular basis of chromatin dynamics during nucleotide excision repair. Biochem Cell Biol 87(1): 265-272.

Zhang, L., Zhang, Q., Jones, K., Patel, M., and Gong, F. 2009b. The chromatin remodeling factor BRG1 stimulates nucleotide excision repair by facilitating recruitment of XPC to sites of DNA damage. Cell Cycle 8(23): 3953-3959.

Zhao, Q., Wang, Q.E., Ray, A., Wani, G., Han, C., Milum, K., and Wani, A.A. 2009. Modulation of nucleotide excision repair by mammalian SWI/SNF chromatin-remodeling complex. J Biol Chem 284(44): 30424-30432.

Zhu, Q., Wani, G., Arab, H.H., El-Mahdy, M.A., Ray, A., and Wani, A.A. 2009. Chromatin restoration following nucleotide excision repair involves the incorporation of ubiquitinated H2A at damaged genomic sites. DNA Repair (Amst) 8(2): 262-273.

14

Cell Cycle and DNA Damage Response in Postmitotic Neurons

Inna I. Kruman
Texas Tech University Health Sciences Center
USA

1. Introduction

Cellular DNA copes with constant exposure to different hazards, environmental and intrinsic. This leads to DNA lesions which interfere with transcription and replication and if not repaired or repaired incorrectly, can produce mutations or large-scale genome aberrations that may lead to cell malfunction or cell death and contribute to different pathologies (Jackson, 2009; Sancar et al., 2004). For this reason, virtually every organism is equipped with highly conserved genome surveillance network known as the DNA damage response (DDR) whose function is to sense genome damage and activate several downstream pathways, including cell cycle checkpoints, DNA repair and apoptotic signaling (Rouse & Jackson, 2002; Zhou & Elledge., 2000). The DDR has been investigated mainly in mitotic cells, in which the cell cycle checkpoints are a major contributor to the DDR, required for DNA repair (Stracker et al., 2008). Not much is known about the DDR in postmitotic neurons. It is known, however, that all eukaryotic DNA repair systems operating in proliferating cells also operate in neurons (Fishel et al., 2007; Lee & McKinnon, 2007; Sharma, 2007; Weissman et al., 2007; Wilson, & McNeill, 2007) and that dysfunctional DDR plays an important role in neurodegeneration and is associated with syndromes (e.g. ataxia telangiectasia) characterized by neurological abnormalities (Barzilai, 2010; Rass et al., 2007; Shiloh, 2003, 2006). This suggests the importance of DDR for postmitotic neurons. While the cell cycle checkpoints are part of DDR involved in DNA repair, apoptotic signaling, and cell fate decisions in mitotic cells, their contribution to the DDR of postmitotic neurons remains unclear. Nonetheless, evidence accumulates that DNA damage-initiated apoptosis of postmitotic neurons is associated with cell cycle signaling. Recently, we have demonstrated the importance of the cell cycle activation for DNA repair in postmitotic neurons (Tomashevski et al., 2010). This suggests that the expression of cell-cycle markers (Schmetsdorf et al., 2007, 2009) and DNA repair activity (Sharma, 2007) observed in the brain under physiological conditions may contribute to DNA repair. The involvement of the cell cycle machinery to both DNA repair and DNA damage-initiated apoptosis in postmitotic neurons suggests a potential function of cell cycle checkpoints in the DDR of these postmitotic cells.

This review focuses on the DDR of postmitotic neurons in the context of what is known about the DDR of mitotic cells.

2. DNA damage response in mitotic cells

The genome of eukaryotic cells is continuously exposed to chemicals, ultraviolet (UV) or ionizing radiation (IR), as well as to by-products of intracellular metabolism (e.g.

oxyradicals). The resulting DNA lesions can block genome replication and transcription and result in loss or incorrect transmission of genetic information. If left unrepaired or are repaired incorrectly, DNA lesions lead to mutations or cell death resulting in different abnormalities, including tumorigenesis and neurodegeneration. To maintain genomic integrity during cell division, cells are equipped with highly efficient defense mechanism, the DDR (Reinhardt & Yaffe, 2009) which functions to recognize and remove DNA lesions by DNA repair and eliminate the irreparably damaged cells by apoptosis (Ciccia & Elledge, 2010; Jackson, 2009; Jackson & Bartek 2009). The DDR cascade senses genome damage and activates several pathways, including cell cycle checkpoints, DNA repair and apoptotic programs. Defects in DDR or DNA repair contribute to aging and various disorders, including neurodegenerative diseases and cancer (Jackson & Bartek 2009). This underlines the critical importance of DDR as a regulator of both cell death and survival processes.

2.1 Formation of DDR foci

The earliest events of the DDR involve alterations in chromatin structure (Berkovich et al., 2007; Downs et al., 2007; Smerdon et al., 1978) and the formation of DDR foci. The biochemical details of these processes are poorly understood. Since DDR foci are the sites where DDR signaling originates, the understanding of their formation and functioning is crucial to understanding how DDR activities are exerted. Among the first events of the DDR is recruitment of a mediator complex MRN consisting of Mre11, Rad50, and Nbs1, and phosphorylation of a variant H2A histone - H2AX - near the break, extending for distances up to several megabases (Fernandez-Capetillo et al., 2004). Working together, MRN and phosphorylated H2AX (γH2AX) act as a signal amplifier that recruits additional signaling molecules to the DSB lesion. The MRN complex serves as an initial DSB sensor, at least one component of which (Nbs1) localizes to the break in an H2AX-independent manner (Celeste et al., 2002, 2003) and facilitates the recruitment and activation of the apical DDR phosphoinositide-3-kinase related kinase (PIKK) ataxia telangiectasia mutated (ATM) (Falck et al., 2005; Lee & Paull 2005; Uziel et al., 2003). This is an important step in the DDR. ATM phosphorylates a number of proteins essential in the control of cell-cycle checkpoints, DNA repair and, in the case of excessive DNA damage, cell death (Khanna et al., 2001; Shiloh, 2003). The widely accepted model of ATM activation is its autophosphorylation at Ser 1981 which releases it from the inhibitory homodimer structure, leading to its recruitment to sites of DNA double-strand breaks (DSBs) (Dupre et al., 2006; Lavin & Kozlov, 2007). Among the first proteins recruited to DNA breaks are direct sensors of DNA breaks such as PARP-1 and PARP-2 whose catalytic activity is triggered by their binding to single-strand breaks (SSBs) and DSBs (D'Amours et al. 1999; de Murcia & Ménissier de Murcia, 1994). The Ku70–Ku80 heterodimer and the MRN complex, DSB sensors, directly bind to DSBs (de Jager et al., 2001; Kim et al., 2005; Lisby et al., 2004; Mimori & Hardin, 1986). Ku heterodimer possibly competes with MRN and PARP-1 for binding to DSBs (Clerici et al., 2008; Wang et al., 2006; Zhang et al., 2007). The direct binding of DNA breaks by factors such as Ku and MRN is crucial for the DDR. The recruitment and activation of the apical DDR kinases ATM, ATM rad3-related (ATR), and DNA-dependent protein kinase (DNA-PK) have also well-known significance at sites of DNA breaks and in DDR foci formation (Polo & Jackson, 2011). The functional importance of downstream DDR factors is not well understood which can be explained by complexity and diversity of downstream DDR events, and the fact that multiple systems appear to cooperate to control the formation of DDR foci. However, it is clear the DDR foci formation is critical for the maintenance of genome integrity.

Downstream from direct sensors of DNA breaks, mediator of DNA damage checkpoint protein1 (MDC1) is recruited. This DDR component serves as a binding platform for DNA damage checkpoint and repair proteins (Jungmichel & Stucki, 2010). For example, ATM-dependent phosphorylation of MDC1 creates binding sites for the FHA domain of the ubiquitin E3 ligase RNF8, which in turn promotes the focal accumulation of another mediator of the DNA damage checkpoint, 53BP1 and breast cancer 1 (BRCA1) at DSB sites (Huen et al., 2008; Kolas et al., 2007; Mailand et al. 2006). Constitutive phosphorylation of MDC1 by casein kinase 2 (CK2) mediates DSB focus formation by MRN (Chapman & Jackson, 2008; Melander et al. 2008; Spycher et al., 2008).

The building of multiprotein DDR foci at DNA breaks is tightly controlled by posttranslational protein modifications, including phosphorylation, ubiquitylation, sumoylation, methylation, acetylation, and PARylation (Polo & Jackson, 2011).

ATM, ATR, and DNA-PK phosphorylate H2AX (Burma et al., 2001; Downs et al., 2000; Rogakou et al., 1998; Stiff et al. 2004; Ward & Chen 2001) which is followed by the recruitment of downstream DDR components, including checkpoint mediators such as MDC1 (Hammet et al., 2007; Nakamura et al., 2004; Sanders et al., 2010; Sofueva et al., 2010; Stucki et al., 2005). Phosphorylated H2AX also promotes the recruitment of chromatin modifying complexes, such as p400 (Downs et al., 2004; Kusch et al., 2004; van Attikum et al., 2004, 2007; Xu et al., 2010). In some cases, phosphorylation promotes the dissociation of proteins from sites of DNA breaks. For example, autophosphorylation of DNA-PK catalytic subunit (DNA-PKcs) induces its dissociation from Ku (Chan & Lees-Miller, 1996; Merkle et al., 2002). Recent studies have revealed the critical importance of ubiquitylation, the process whereby ubiquitin (monoubiquitylation) or polyubiquitin (polyubiquitylation) is covalently attached to proteins in the assembly of DDR proteins at DSB sites (Al-Hakim et al., 2010; Messick & Greenberg, 2009; Pickart, 2001). Another critical modification involved in control of DDR foci is histone acetylation near DSBs. Acetylation of histones H3 and H4 is essential for DNA repair (Averbeck & Durante, 2011). The importance of this modification is underlined by the recruitment of several histone acetyltransferases including Hat1, and NuA4 and deacetylases such as Sir2 and Hst1 in budding yeast (Downs et al., 2004; Qin & Parthun, 2006; Tamburini & Tyler 2005) and the Tip60 acetyltransferase and deacetylases (HDAC1, HDAC2, HDAC4, SIRT1 and SIRT6) in mammalian cells (Kaidi et al., 2010; Miller et al., 2010; Murr et al., 2006; O'Hagan et al., 2008; Oberdoerffer et al., 2008). SIRT1 binding in the DSB area has been found to promote the recruitment of NBS1 and RAD51 (Oberdoerffer et al., 2008). Histone H3K56 deacetylation by HDAC1 and HDAC2 regulates recruiting DNA repair factors of nonhomologous end-joining pathway to DSB regions (Miller et al., 2010). Additionally, MOF (males absent on the first)-dependent acetylation of histone H4K16 is important for IR-induced focus formation of MDC1, 53BP1, and BRCA1 in mammalian cells (Li et al., 2010; Sharma et al., 2010). H2AX acetylation by Tip60 promotes H2AX eviction from damaged chromatin, as shown in both Drosophila and mammalian cells (Ikura et al., 2007; Kusch et al., 2004). The acetylation of histone proteins in the DNA break area can regulate the assembly of DDR factors indirectly by modulating chromatin compaction (Lee et al., 2010).

The covalent protein modification process of binding with ADP-ribose polymers, known as PARylation, is one of the earliest events in the DDR. The PARylation is catalyzed by PARP enzymes (Hakme et al. 2008) comprising a large family of proteins, several members of which have clearly identified DDR functions (Citarelli et al., 2010). PARylation is quickly suppressed by PARG (PARG) (Gagne et al., 2006; Hakme et al. 2008; Krishnakumar & Kraus, 2010). It is involved in buildup of the chromatin remodeling factors ALC1 and CHD4 (Ahel et al., 2009; Chou et al., 2010; Gottschalk et al., 2009; Polo et al., 2010), the Polycomb histone-modifying complex (Chou et al., 2010), and the histone variant macro H2A (Timinszky et al., 2009). A contribution of PARylation to the early recruitment of MRN has also been reported (Haince et al., 2008). PARylation can also promote protein dissociation from DNA damage, as shown for the histone chaperone FACT which facilitates chromatin transcription (Heo et al., 2008; Huang et al., 2006).

The mobilization of DDR factors to SSBs or DSBs is very rapid and transient (Gagne et al. 2006; Hakme et al., 2008; Lieber, 2010; Mahaney et al., 2009; Mortusewicz et al., 2007). Responses to DSBs can be markedly influenced by cell cycle status. While accumulation of DDR factors such as γH2AX, MRN, and MDC1 occurs regardless of the cell cycle phase, others - including BRCA1 and RAD51 accumulate effectively only in S/G2 cells (Bekker-Jensen et al., 2006; Jazayeri et al., 2006; Lisby et al., 2004; Sartori et al., 2007). Studies in yeast and mammalian systems have demonstrated that colocalization of DDR proteins rather than DNA damage per se is critical for DNA damage signaling (Bonilla et al., 2008; Soutoglou & Misteli, 2008). One of important regulatory functions of DDR foci is to contribute to the proper coordination of DNA damage signaling and repair with other DNA metabolic activities by inhibiting replication and transcription. In this regard, DNA and histone modifications at sites of DNA breaks have been proposed to contribute to silencing of damaged chromatin (O'Hagan et al., 2008; Shanbhag et al., 2010).

It is now clear that chromatin modifications are an important component DDR network (van Attikum & Gasser, 2009). Recent electron microscopy studies revealed that generation of DSB leads to a rapid, ATP-dependent, local decondensation of chromatin that occurs in the absence of ATM activation. ATM activation itself leads to chromatin relaxation at DSB sites (Ziv et al., 2006). The local and global changes in chromatin organization facilitate recruitment of damage-response proteins and remodeling factors, which further modify chromatin in the vicinity of the DSB and propagate the DNA damage response, thereby providing functional crosstalk between chromatin modification and proteins involved in DDR (Peterson & Cote, 2004; van Attikum & Gasser, 2005).

2.2 DNA repair

DNA repair is essential for maintaining the integrity of the genome. The complicated network of DNA repair mechanisms functions to remove DNA damage by DNA repair pathways. This network include base excision repair (BER), mismatch repair (MMR) and nucleotide excision repair (NER) (Hakem, 2008). One of the most powerful activators of the DDR are DSBs, the most cytotoxic DNA lesions which potentially induce gross chromosomal aberrations, often linked to cell death or cancer (Hopfner, 2009). It has been estimated that a single unrepaired DSB is sufficient for cell lethality (Khanna & Jackson, 2001). DSBs in eukaryotic cells are repaired by two major mechanisms: nonhomologous end-joining (NHEJ), an error-prone ligation mechanism, and a high-fidelity process based on homologous recombination (HR) between sister chromatids that operate in the S and G2 phases of the cell cycle (Pardo et al., 2009; van Gent & der Burg, 2007). DNA damage-induced recruitment of the protein MDC1 dramatically enhances activation of ATM which in turn recruits 53BP1 and BRCA (Bekker-Jensen et al., 2005; Stewart et al., 2003; Stucki et al., 2005). 53BP1 facilitates DNA repair by NHEJ pathway, predominant in mammalian cells

(Moynahan et al., 1999). Several proteins are required for efficient repair of DSB by NHEJ. The core complex consists of the DNA-PK and the ligase IV/XRCC4/XLF complexes. NHEJ initiates upon the binding of two ring-shaped Ku70/Ku80 heterodimers to both DNA broken ends within seconds of the creation of the DNA damage (Lieber, 2010; Mahaney et al., 2009). DNA-PKcs is also recruited to this DNA-Ku scaffold and probably enables the formation of a synaptic complex. In the synaptic complex, the DNA broken ends are positioned next to each other. Depending on the properties of the lesion, some DNA ends must be processed before the final ligation step. For example, a damaged DNA end can contain an aberrant 5' hydroxyl group, aberrant 3' phosphate, damaged base and/or damaged backbone sugar residue. Several enzymes can process such lesions (Chappell et al., 2002; Koch et al., 2004). Werner helicase, associated with Ku70 and Artemis, a structure-specific nuclease, which can cleave DNA hairpin structures and remove 3' overhang DNA may prepare DNA ends (Perry et al., 2006). When the end processing has been accomplished, ligase IV/XRCC4 can catalyze the final ligation reaction. For NHEJ, the Ku70–Ku80 heterodimer plays a central role in recruiting other NHEJ components. In particular, Ku recruits the protein kinase DNA-PKcs (Dvir et al., 1992; Gottlieb & Jackson, 1993) via a specific interaction between DNA-PKcs and the Ku80 C terminus (Gell & Jackson, 1999; Singleton et al., 1999), as well as the downstream NHEJ complex XLF–XRCC4–LigaseIV and the nuclease Artemis (Calsou et al., 2003; Yano et al., 2008).

2.3 Cell cycle checkpoints

Checkpoints are complex kinase signaling pathways that prevent further progression through the cell cycle and coordinate DNA repair with chromosome metabolism and cell-cycle transitions (Houtgraaf et al., 2006; Poehlmann & Roessner, 2010). In response to DNA damage, the checkpoints delay or stop the cell cycle at critical points before or during DNA replication (G1/S and intra-S checkpoints) and before cell division (G2/M checkpoint), thereby preventing replication and segregation of damaged DNA. The critical importance of the cell cycle checkpoint pathways in maintaining genomic integrity is highlighted by the observation that loss or mutation of checkpoint genes is frequently observed in cancer (Kastan & Bartek, 2004). Recent evidence suggests mutually integrated roles of the checkpoint machinery in the activation of DNA repair, chromatin remodelling, modulation of transcriptional programmes and the optional triggering of permanent cell cycle withdrawal by cellular senescence or apoptosis (Bartek & Lukas, 2001; Shiloh, 2003; Zhou & Elledge, 2000). The canonical DDR network has traditionally been divided into two major kinase signaling branches utilizing the upstream kineses ATM and ATR. These kinases control the G1/S, intra-S, and G2/M checkpoints through activating their downstream effector kinases Chk2 and Chk1, respectively (Reinhardt & Yaffe, 2009). The ATM/Chk2 module is activated after DNA DSBs and the ATR/Chk1 pathway responds primarily to DNA SSBs or bulky lesions. Both pathways converge on cell division cycle 25 homolog **A** (Cdc25A), a positive regulator of cell cycle progression, which is inhibited by Chk1- or Chk2-mediated phosphorylation (Poehlmann & Roessner, 2010). Post-translational modifications, such as checkpoint- and cyclin-dependent kinase (CDK)-dependent phosphorylation, ubiquitylation and sumoylation were shown to be crucial for regulation of stability and activity of important components of the checkpoint machinery, thereby regulating important cell cycle events. These post-translational modifications may affect the recruitment of repair proteins to damaged DNA or tune the efficiency or the specificity of the repair machinery towards a certain type of DNA damage and facilitate repair in a specific cell-cycle phase (Branzei & Foiani, 2008). Chromatin structure and compaction is also regulated throughout the cell cycle, and can be influenced by checkpoints and post-translational modifications (Groth et al., 2007; Karagiannis & El-Osta, 2007; Kouzarides, 2007). Thus, cell cycle checkpoints induce G1, S, and G2 cell cycle arrest, recruit repair machinery to the sites of damage, and target irreversibly damaged cells for apoptosis (Kastan & Bartek, 2004; Reinhardt & Yaffe, 2009). ATM and DNA-PK respond mainly to DSBs, whereas ATR is activated in response to incomplete DNA replication due to stalled replication forks (Bartek, & Lukas, 2007; Reinhardt & Yaffe, 2009). During replication, single-stranded DNA becomes opsonized by the replication protein A, which recruits ATR via the ATR-interacting protein to the DNA lesions exposed by stalled forks and orchestrates DNA-topoisomerase II beta-binding protein (TopBP1)-dependent ATR- (Kumagai & Dunphy, 2006) and checkpoint activation (Elledge, 1996). Following activation, the checkpoint transducers transmit and amplify the checkpoint signal to downstream targets such as the DNA-repair apparatus and the cell-cycle machinery (Branzei & Foiani, 2008). DNA synthesis is frequently associated with nucleotide misincorporation, accumulation of nicks and gaps, slippage at repetitive sequences, fork collapse at DNA breaks and aberrant transitions at collapsed forks that cause reversed and/or resected forks. Replication-fork collapse during S phase can often induce DSBs (Branzei & Foiani, 2008). ATR activation by DSBs requires ATM and MRN (Jazayeri et al., 2006; Sartori et al., 2007). It is possible that activation of the tumor suppressor protein, p53, following this replication fork collapse could be detrimental per se, taking into account its implication in apoptosis (Brady & Attardi, 2010). However, there are mechanisms that operate in the S phase to prevent p53 from a death-related activation of p53 transcription programme. It has been speculated that induction of such program within S phase, when the E2F-1 transcription factor (known to cooperate with p53 to induce apoptosis) is highly active, could promote unwanted cell death (Gottifredi et al., 2001).

A major target of ATM in checkpoint pathways is the effector kinase Chk2 that functions to arrest the cell cycle after DSBs by inactivating phosphatases of the Cdc25 family through catalytic inactivation, nuclear exclusion, and/or proteasomal degradation (Aressy & Ducommun, 2008; Busino et al., 2004). This, in turn, prevents Cdc25 family members from dephosphorylating and activating cyclin-CDK complexes, thereby initiating G1/S and G2/M cell cycle checkpoints. In contrast to G1/S or G2/M arrest, cells that experience genotoxic stress during DNA replication only delay their progression through S phase in a transient manner, and if damage is not repaired during this delay they exit S phase and are arrested later when reaching the G2 checkpoint (Bartek et al., 2004).

Following DNA repair, cells must extinguish the DNA damage signal to allow the cells to reenter the cell cycle, but the mechanisms through which this occurs, particularly with respect to the ATM-Chk2 pathway, are poorly understood. Since DNA damage checkpoints respond to as little as a single DNA DSB (Lobrich &, Jeggo, 2007), it has long been assumed that human cells also maintain the G2/M checkpoint until all of the breaks are repaired. Recent evidence, however, shows that the G2 checkpoint in immortalized human cells in culture displays a defined threshold of approximately 10–20 DSBs (Deckbar et al., 2007). Limited checkpoint control was not only apparent in response to IR doses that cause very few DNA DSBs, but also in response to more extensive amounts of DNA damage where checkpoint release occurred at fewer than 10–20 unrepaired DSBs (Deckbar et al., 2007).

Although the fate of cells that continue proliferating in the presence of unrepaired DNA breaks is unclear, and the identity of the rate-limiting DNA damage checkpoint components has yet to be revealed, accumulating evidence suggests that the DNA damage checkpoint machinery can be overridden. G2 checkpoint escape in the presence of unrepaired DNA damage may be particularly common during the evolution of cancer cells (Bartek & Lukas, 2007; Bartkova et al., 2005; Gorgoulis et al., 2005; Kastan & Bartek 2004; Shiloh, 2003).

In mammalian cells, p53 is an important player of the cell cycle checkpoint machinery (Polager & Ginsberg, 2009). During checkpoint control following DNA damage, p53 can either be phosphorylated directly by ATM or ATR (Banin et al., 1998; Hammond et al., 2002; Tibbetts et al., 1999), or indirectly via Chk1 and Chk2 (Hirao et al., 2000, Shieh et al., 2000). Certain cancer-related mutations in the *Chk2* gene can prevent phosphorylation of p53 (Falck et al., 2001; Jazayeri et al., 2006). The effects of Chk1 and Chk2 in the regulation of p53 also depend on the site where p53 is phosphorylated (Polo & Jackson, 2011). A target of p53 in cell cycle checkpoints is the CDK inhibitor p21 (Deng et al., 1995; el-Deiry et al., 1993; Gu et al., 1993; Xiong et al., 1993). P21 functions by inhibiting several CDKs, including CDK4/6, and CDK2 (Harper et al., 1993; Xiong et al., 1993). The silencing of cyclin E - CDK2 activity in late G1 occurs even in cells lacking p53 or p21 (Bartek & Lukas, 2001). These facts argue for a two-wave model of the G1 checkpoint response in mammalian cells, in which the initial, rapid, transient and p53-independent response (Chk2 - Cdc25A – CDK2 axis) is followed by the delayed but more sustained G1 arrest imposed by the Chk1/Chk2–p53–p21-CDK pathway centered on p53 (Bartek & Lukas, 2001; Polager & Ginsberg, 2009). G2 arrest following DNA damage is dependent on the actions of several proteins such as 14-3-3δ which is strongly induced by DNA damage (Chan et al., 1999; Laronga et al., 2000). It acts by sequestering CDK1 -cyclin B complex to prevent entry into mitosis and by modulating the p53-Mdm2 axis (Chan et al., 1999; Yang et al., 2008). *14-3-3δ* is a valid tumor suppressor gene that is frequently inactivated in a number of human malignancies (Ferguson et al., 2000; Henrique et al., 2005; Kuroda et al., 2007). P21 and 14-3-3δ cooperate to maintain G2 arrest following DNA damage. CDK1-cyclin B is subsequently inactivated by p21 in the nucleus (Chan et al., 2000).

The G1/S checkpoint generated through the Chk1/Chk2 - Cdc25A - CDK2 pathway is executed by the active unphosphorylated Cdc25A phosphatase through dephosphorylation of the CDK2–cyclin E complex (Poehlmann & Roessner, 2010). As a consequence, the CDK2 - cyclin E complex is kept in its active form, which causes G1-S transition. Following DNA damage, Chk1 and Chk2 phosphorylate Cdc25A, inducing its degradation. Due to the degradation of the Cdc25A phosphatase, the CDK2-Cyclin E complex remains in its hyperphosphorylated inactive form, culminating in G1/S arrest. P21 potentially participates in the G1/S checkpoint by blocking directly DNA synthesis due to its ability to bind the central region of proliferating cell nuclear antigen (PCNA), a protein that acts as a processivity factor for DNA synthesis in eukaryotic cells (Oku et al., 1998). *In vitro* studies showed that the C-terminal domain of p21 is sufficient to displace DNA replication enzymes from PCNA, thereby blocking DNA synthesis (Chen et al., 1996; Warbrick et al., 1995). The main role of p21 in the G1 checkpoint lies in its ability to inhibit the activity of cyclin E- and cyclin A-CDK2 compexes required for the G1-S transition (Brugarolas et al., 1999). Consequently, pRb remains hypophosphorylated thereby sequestering the transcription factor E2F, whose activity is required for S-phase entry (Ewen et al., 1993).

The G2/M checkpoint generated through the Chk1/Chk2 - Cdc25C - CDK1 pathway is executed by Cdc25C through. dephosphorylation of CDK1-Cyclin B1 complex (Reagan-Shaw et al., 2005; Roshak et al., 2000). Since activating dephosphorylation of only a small amount of CDK1- Cyclin B1 complex is the initiating step for mitotic entry (Hoffmann et al., 1993), and the maintenance of the Cdk1–Cyclin B1 complex in its inactive state blocks entry into mitosis (Poehlmann and Roessner, 2010), CDK1 is the ultimate target of the G2 checkpoint regulation. CDK1 is phosphorylated at two positions by protein kinases Wee1 and Myt1, and is dephosphorylated by Cdc25C phosphatase. G2/M DNA damage checkpoint arrest may be induced by increased phosphorylation of CDK1 by Wee1/Myt1 or by preventing CDK1 dephosphorylation by Cdc25C phosphatase triggered by activated Chk1.

In response to DNA damage, p53 can be phosphorylated at multiple sites by several different protein kinases such as ATM, ATR, DNA-PK, and Chk1/Chk2 (Meek et al., 1994; Milczarek et al., 1997). Phosphorylation impairs the ability of Mdm2 to bind p53, promoting p53 accumulation and activation (Shieh et al., 1997, Tibbetts et al., 1999). Activated p53 upregulates a number of target genes, such as Gadd45 and p21. The accumulation of p21 inhibits CDK2–cyclin E kinase activity, which results in G1 arrest (Bartek et al., 2007). Thus, G1 arrest is a consequence of preventing pRb phosphorylation via inhibition of CDK2. P53 also has functions in the G2/M checkpoint via activating by Chk1/Chk2 which may trigger induction of p21 and by blocking the activity of the mitotic CDK1-Cyclin B1 complex (Stark & Taylor, 2006; Stewart et al., 1995; Taylor & Stark, 2001). In general, one key function of Chk1 and Chk2 activated by ATR and ATM, respectively, manifests in the inactivation of different members of the Cdc25 family by phosphorylation, resulting in a stop of cell cycle progression after DNA damage in the G1/S - or G2/M phases of the cell cycle.

In order for cells to survive following DNA damage, it is important that cell cycle arrest is not only initiated but also maintained for the duration of time necessary for DNA repair (Van Vugt et al., 2010). Mechanisms governing checkpoint initiation versus maintenance appear to be molecularly distinct. This was initially demonstrated by the observation that interference with specific checkpoint components can leave checkpoint initiation intact but disrupt checkpoint maintenance, leading to premature cell cycle reentry accompanied by death by mitotic catastrophe (Bekker-Jensen et al., 2005; Castedo et al., 2004; Deckbar et al., 2007; Lal et al., 2006; Lobrich & Jeggo, 2007). Although the process of checkpoint termination and cell cycle reentry has not been studied extensively, the existing data suggest that inactivation of a checkpoint response is an active process that requires dedicated signaling pathways, such as the the polo-like kinase 1 (Plk1) pathway (Bartek & Lukas, 2007; van Vugt & Medema, 2004). Interestingly, a number of proteins involved in terminating the maintenance phase of a DNA damage checkpoint also play critical roles in later mitotic events, suggesting the existence of a positive feedback in which the earliest events of mitosis involve the DNA damage checkpoint through unclear mechanism(s). Resumption of cell cycle progression following DNA repair involves switching off the DDR, including disassembly of DDR foci (Bartek & Lukas, 2007. This occurs mainly by reversing the posttranslational modifications associated with focal DDR protein assembly such as PARG-induced erasing PARylation (Gagne et al., 2006) or γH2AX dephosphorylation which plays an important role in terminating checkpoint signaling (Bazzi et al. 2010; Cha et al. 2010; Chowdhury et al., 2008; Macurek et al. 2010; Nakada et al. 2008). Deubiquitylating enzymes have also been implicated in terminating DDR processes (Nicassio et al., 2007; Shao et al. 2009). Deubiquitylation of histone H2A was shown to relieve the inhibition of RNA polymerase II transcription at DSBs (Shanbhag et al., 2010). Automodification is coupled to its dissociation from DNA damage sites, such as DNA-PKcs autophosphorylation and its dissociation from Ku (Chan & Lees-Miller 1996; Hammel et al. 2010; Merkle et al., 2002) and auto-PARylation of PARP-1 and its dissociation from DNA damage sites (Mortusewicz et al. 2007). Checkpoint silencing has been best studied in the budding yeast S. cerevisiae (Leroy et al., 2003; Toczyski et al., 1997; Vaze et al., 2002). The Plk Cdc5 is required for silencing checkpoint signaling, and this requirement appears to be widely conserved, since S. cerevisiae, and human cells all depend on Plks for silencing of the S- or G2 checkpoints, respectively (Syljuasen et al., 2006; Toczyski et al., 1997; van Vugt et al., 2004; Yoo et al., 2004). The activity of Plks has been shown to be required for inactivation of the ATR-Chk1 pathway and the Wee1 axis of checkpoint signaling (Mailand et al., 2006; Mamely et al., 2006; van Vugt et al., 2004; Yoo et al., 2004). DSBs primarily trigger a checkpoint arrest through the ATM-Chk2 signaling pathway. The CDK- and Plk1-dependent phosphorylation of 53BP1 and Chk2 are critical checkpoint-inactivating events in the sensor and effector arms of the G2/M checkpoint pathway, important for checkpoint termination and cell cycle reentry (Van Vugt et al., 2010). This inactivation can take place on chromatin, as reported in human cells (Chowdhury et al., 2008; Nakada et al., 2008). The reversal of H2AX phosphorylation also involves Tip60-dependent histone acetylation and subsequent histone eviction from damaged chromatin in Drosophila and human cells (Jha et al., 2008; Kusch et al. 2004). This is particularly relevant if one considers that DNA damage checkpoints are to respond to very small numbers of DSBs, with some experimental data indicating that 10 -20 DSBs are enough to elicit G2 arrest in human cells (Deckbar et al., 2007), while very few or even a single unrepaired DSB can be sufficient to trigger p53-dependent G1 arrest in human cells (Huang et al., 1996) or cell death in yeast (Bennett et al., 1993).

2.4 DNA damage-induced apoptosis

Programmed cell death, or apoptosis, is a natural process of removing unnecessary or damaged cells, and is required for the proper execution of the organism's life cycle (Chowdhury et al., 2006; Zimmermann et al., 2001). Apoptosis was shown to be involved in numerous processes including embryonic development, response to cellular damage, aging and as a mechanism of tumor suppression (Blank &, Shiloh, 2007; Cohen et al., 2004; Lee et al., 2007; Mazumder et al., 2007; Rich et al., 2000; Subramanian et al., 2005). Two pathways were shown to induce apoptosis: an extrinsic and an intrinsic pathways. The difference between these two pathways is the mechanism by which the death signal is transduced (Chowdhury et al., 2006). Whereas the extrinsic pathway is activated by binding of ligands to a death receptor, the intrinsic pathway is activated by cellular stress, for example DNA damage. The intrinsic pathway involves the release of cytochrome *c* from the intermembrane space of the mitochondria. Together with apoptotic protease activating factor 1 (APAF1), cytochrome *c* activates caspase 9, leading to activation of downstream caspases and the induction of the death response (Bitomsky & Hofmann, 2009). Key players in the regulation of the intrinsic pathway include the Bcl2 protein family, which can influence the permeability of the outer mitochondrial membrane (Reed, 2006). Members of the Bcl2 protein family are divided into proapoptotic proteins such as Bax, Bak and Bok, and antiapoptotic ones including Bcl2, Bcl-X, Bcl-w and Mcl-1. Proteins of a third subfamily, known as the BH3-only proteins, are thought to be initiators of apoptosis, and probably function by regulating Bcl2-like proteins from the other two subfamilies. In healthy cells,

Bax exists as a monomer, either in the cytosol or weakly bound to the outer mitochondrial membrane. Upon stimulation of apoptosis, Bax translocates to the mitochondria, where it becomes anchored into the mitochondrial membrane. Following its translocation, Bax oligomerizes into large complexes, which are essential for the permeabilization of the mitochondrial membrane (Antignani & Youle, 2006; Bitomsky & Hofmann, 2009; Reed, 2006). Given its central role in mediating apoptosis, several mechanisms have been proposed for Bax regulation and retention in the cytosol, both by binding to other proteins and through posttranslational modifications. One of the first proteins that were shown to sequester Bax away from the mitochondria was Ku70 (Cohen et al., 2004; Lee et al., 2007; Mazumder et al., 2007; Subramanian et al., 2005). Thus, in addition to its role in regulating NHEJ DNA-repair, Ku70 functions in regulating Bax-mediated apoptosis. Overexpression of Ku70 lowered levels of cell death after apoptotic stimuli, while reducing Ku70 levels increased sensitivity to Bax-mediated apoptosis (Amsel et al., 2008). Taken together, these results suggest that Ku70 has anti-apoptotic activity. Such activity is associated with its ability to be acetylated (Cohen et al., 2004). Apoptotic stimuli lead to dissociation of the Ku70-Bax complex, resulting in cell death following Bax translocation to the mitochondria. It was suggested that under normal conditions, Bax undergoes ubiquitylation, which negatively regulates its proapoptotic function by labeling it for proteasomal degradation. The association with Ku70 mediates and promotes Bax deubiquitylation. Upon apoptotic stimulus, Ku70 is acetylated and releases Bax which translocates to the mitochondria where induces apoptosis. These findings suggest a complex role for Ku70 with both pro-apoptotic (maintaining an active pool of Bax) and anti-apoptotic (sequestering Bax away from the mitochondria) elements.

In response to DNA damage, deacetylase SIRT1 binds to and deacetylates specific lysine residue of substrate proteins, the modification of which leads to the repression of their transcriptional activities (Luo et al., 2001; Picard et al., 2004; Vaziri et al., 2001). SIRT1 has been suggested to suppress apoptotic responses (Luo et al., 2001; Vaziri et al., 2001). It has been demonstrated that, when exposed to IR, SIRT1 enhances DNA repair activity by binding to Ku70 and subsequently deacetylating this protein. This could facilitate one possible mechanism of cell survival (Jeong et al., 2007).

Another mechanism of cell fate regulation involves p21 (Abbas &. Dutta, 2009; Garner & Raj, 2008; Liu et al., 2003). Under some circumstances (i.e., enforced overexpression), p21 may promote apoptotic signaling that ultimately leads to cell death (Liu et al., 2003). However, DNA-damaged cells can undergo cell cycle arrest followed by apoptosis in the absence of p21 (Waldman et al., 1996, 1997). The mechanism by which p21 negatively regulates DNA damage-induced death machinery relies on its binding to key apoptotic regulatory proteins (Liu et al., 2003). P21 physically interacts, through its first N-terminal 33 aminoacids, with procaspase-3, i.e. the inactive precursor of the apoptotic executioner caspase-3 (Suzuki et al., 1998, 1999). When bound to p21, the inactive pro-caspase cannot be converted into the active protease, and apoptosis is impeded (Suzuki et al.,1999). Caspase 2, which acts upstream of caspase 3, is also kept in a repressed status by p21 (Baptiste-Okoh et al., 2008). The strict interaction between p21 and caspases is supported also by the observation that p21 itself is cleaved by caspases early during DNA damage- induced apoptosis (Jin et al., 2000; Levkau et al., 1998). The anti- or pro-apoptotic role of p21 could depend on the nature of the apoptotic stimulus. For example, apoptosis was enhanced or inhibited by p21, according to whether cells were treated with cisplatin, or methotrexate (Kraljevic Pavelic et al., 2008).

Functions of p21 in response to DNA damage could be also modulated by the extent of genotoxic lesions, through either stabilization or degradation of the protein. Low levels of DNA lesions will allow p21 stabilization and induce cell cycle arrest (thus having anti-apoptotic activity). In contrast, after extensive DNA damage, p21 down-modulation will allow cells to go to apoptosis (Lee et al., 2009; Martinez et al., 2002).

It is well established that p53 is capable of inducing apoptosis by transcription-dependent and transcription-independent mechanisms (Caelles et al., 1994). It has been demonstrated that recombinant p53 is capable of triggering mitochondrial membrane permeabilization in cell-free systems (Ding et al., 1998; Schuler et al., 2000). Later on, p53 has been reported to translocate to the cytoplasm in response to numerous stress signals, including DNA damage, where it drives mitochondrial outer membrane permeabilization and caspase activation (Marchenko et al., 2000; Mihara et al., 2003). Modifications of p53 may affect its transcriptional activity. For example, acetylation at p53 carboxyl-terminal lysine residues enhances its transcriptional activity associated with cell cycle arrest and apoptosis (Yamaguchi et al., 2009). The interaction between p53 and Ku70 is independent of p53 acetylation. However, p53 acetylation at its carboxyl terminus is required for p53 to prevent and/or displace Bax from its inhibitory interaction with Ku70, thus allowing this key proapoptotic protein to target mitochondria and initiate apoptosis (Yamaguchi et al., 2009).

P53 has powerful apoptotic effects, and consequently is a subject to tight regulatory control. Normally, p53 protein is maintained at a low level through the Mdm2-mediated ubiquitination and degradation pathway. However, when cells are exposed to stress including genotoxic one, p53 protein is rapidly accumulated and activated for downstream biological functions. The regulatory events that affect the amount, stability and activity of p53 are in part associated with a variety of post-translational modifications, including phosphorylation, ubiquitination and acetylation. In fact, p53 is the first functional non-histone substrate identified for the histone acetyltransferases (HATs) (Yi & Luo, 2010).

Another key molecule critically involved in DNA damage-induced cell death signaling is the p53-related tumour suppressor and transcription factor p73 (Melino et al., 2003). In unstressed cells, p73 forms a complex with the E3 ubiquitin ligase Itch, which marks it for degradation by the ubiquitin-proteasome system. Upon DNA damage, the levels of Itch become reduced and allow the accumulation of p73 (Rossi et al., 2005). Many of p73 pro-apoptotic target genes such as Puma, caspase-6 or CD95, overlap with those of p53 (Dobbelstein et al., 2005). Post-translational modifications of p73 by acetylation through p300 and by phosphorylation by the DNA damage-activated, nonreceptor tyrosine kinase c-Abl were found to be crucial for transactivation of its pro-apoptotic target genes (Costanzo et al., 2002).

The E2F1 transcription factor, which was originally identified as a cell-cycle initiator, mediates apoptosis in response to DNA damage (Iaquinta & Lees, 2007; Polager & Ginsberg, 2008; Yamasaki et al., 1996). Under certain conditions, deregulated E2F1 triggers apoptosis via both p53-dependent and p53-independent mechanisms. To induce p53-dependent apoptosis, E2F1 activates the expression of p14/p19ARF tumor suppressor gene to stabilize p53 (Phillips & Vousden, 2001). Alternatively, E2F1 directly activates various proapoptotic genes or inactivates several antiapoptotic genes (Iaquinta & Lees, 2007; Polager & Ginsberg, 2008). In support of the importance of E2F1 for apoptotic signaling, germline deletion of E2F1 in mice leads to the formation of various tumors, presumably resulting from the lack of E2F1-induced apoptosis (Field et al., 1996; Yamasaki et al., 1996).

2.5 Cell fate decision

Depending on the amount of damage, the DDR activates one of two alternatives: a prosurvival network that includes the damage-induced cell cycle checkpoints and DNA repair or programmed cell death (Barzilai et al., 2008). The mechanistic aspects of this critical choice remain unclear. Activation of p53 in response to DNA damage results in either cell cycle arrest or apoptosis. Although genes that regulate these cellular processes are essentially p53 targets, activation of p53 always results in specific and selective transcription of p53-regulated genes (Riley et al, 2008). Thus, it is likely that unique sets of p53-regulated genes operate in tandem to bring about a desired outcome in response to specific stimuli. How p53 executes these two distinct functions remains largely unclear. Recent reports suggest that activation of specific promoters by p53 is achieved through its interaction with heterologous transcription factors such as Hzf and ASPP family proteins (Das et al, 2007; Tanaka et al, 2007). P53 modifications following stress such as phosphorylation and acetylation stabilize p53, enhancing its sequence-specific DNA binding and transcriptional activity (Sakaguchi et al, 1998). The phosphorylation at amino-terminus is required for p53 stability, while acetylation at carboxyl-terminus is indispensable for p53 transcriptional activation (Tang et al., 2008). The p53 target gene SMAR1 modulates the cellular response to genotoxic stress by a dual mechanism. First, SMAR1 interacts with p53 and facilitates p53 deacetylation through recruitment of deacetylase HDAC1. Then SMAR1 represses the transcription of Bax and Puma by binding to an identical 25 bp MAR element in their promoters (Sinha et al., 2010). A mild DNA damage induces SMAR1-generated anti-apoptotic response by promoting p53 deacetylation and specifically repressing Bax and Puma expression. Reducing the expression of SMAR1 by shRNA leads to significant increase in p53-dependent apoptosis (Sinha et al., 2010). Severe DNA damage results in sequestration of SMAR1, p53 acetylation and transactivation of Bax and Puma leading to apoptosis. Thus, sequestration of SMAR1 into the PML-NBs acts as a molecular switch to p53-dependent cell arrest and apoptosis in response to DNA damage (Sinha et al., 2010). The mechanisms by which moderate damage resulting from mild stress leads to repair, while severe damage results in the 'decision' to kill a cell, remains unclear. Every single cell is therefore continuously confronted with the choice: repair and live or die. Irreparable damage triggers p53's killer functions to eliminate genetically-altered cells. The killer functions of p53 are tightly regulated and balanced against protector functions that promote damage repair and support survival in response to mild damage (Schlereth et al., 2010). In molecular terms, these p53-based cell fate decisions involve protein interactions with factors, which modulate the activation of distinct sets of p53 target genes. The induction of a transient cell cycle arrest that allows for damage repair depends critically on the genes *p21*, *14-3-3σ* and *GADD45A*, with *p21* being crucial for cell cycle arrest in the G1 phase, while *14-3-3σ* and *GADD45A* - for arrest in G2 (Levine & Oren, 2009). In the case of prolonged damage, p53-mediated transactivation of the sestrins (*SESN1*and *SESN2*) causes inhibition of the mammalian target of rapamycin (mTOR) signaling and helps to maintain the arrest reversible, while activation of mTOR under these conditions triggers a shift to irreversible cell cycle exit (senescence) (Demidenko et al., 2010; Korotchkina et al., 2010; Steelman & McCubrey, 2009). Another way for p53 to permanently stop cell proliferation without compromising cell viability is induction of differentiation (Schlereth, 2010). Only when cells have irrepairable DNA damage that is incompatible with further survival, p53 shifts to the most extreme and irrevocable antiproliferative response - apoptosis (Aylon & Oren, 2007). p53-induced apoptosis does not only require activation of proapoptotic target genes such as *Bax* and *Noxa* but may also involve transcription-independent functions of p53 in the cytoplasm (Green & Kroemer, 2009; Morselli et al., 2009; Vaseva et al., 2009). Discriminatory effects on target can also be exerted by interacting proteins that modulate p53's DNA binding properties via covalent post-translational modifications including phosphorylation, acetylation, methylation, ubiquitylation, and sumoylation. Among the phosphorylation sites, serine 46 (S46) has clear discriminatory function for p53 as a transcriptional activator (Okoshi et al., 2008; Rinaldo et al., 2007). P53 is phosphorylated at this residue by homeodomain interacting protein kinase 2 (HIPK2), dual-specificity tyrosine-phosphorylation-regulated kinase 2 (DYRK2), AMPK, protein kinase C delta or p38 mitogen activated protein kinase in response to severe cellular damage (Okoshi et al., 2008; Rinaldo et al., 2007). While numerous studies have implicated acetylation of lysine residues in the C-terminus of p53 as being important for p53's transcriptional activity in general, acetylation of lysine 120 (K120) in the DNA binding domain by the MYST family histone acetyl transferases, hMOF and Tip60 specifically results in increased binding to proapoptotic targets like *Bax* and *Puma,* while the nonapoptotic targets *p21* and *Mdm2* remain unaffected (Sykes et al., 2006; Tang et al., 2006). On the other hand, acetylation of lysine 320 (K320) by the transcriptional coactivator p300/CBP-associated factor (PCAF) predisposes p53 to activate *p21* and decreases its ability to induce proapoptotic genes. Cells ectopically expressing a mutant p53 where K320 is mutated to glutamine (K320Q) to mimic acetylation, display reduced apoptosis after some forms of DNA damage (Knights et al., 2006). In contrast, K317R knockin mice, where K317 acetylation is missing, consistently display increased apoptosis and higher expression of relevant target genes in several cell types (Chao et al., 2006). However, K320 is not only a target for acetylation but it is also ubiquitylated by the zincfinger protein E4F1 (Le Cam et al., 2006). This modification facilitates p53-dependent activation of *p21* and *Cyclin G1* expression without affecting the expression of the proapoptotic gene *Noxa,* overall resulting in reduced p53-mediated cell death in response to UV. P53-mediated cell cycle arrest is also favored following methylation of at least two arginine residues (R333 and R335) by the arginine methyltransferase PRMT5. Consistently, depletion of PRMT5 by siRNA leads to increased apoptosis following p53 activation (Durant et al., 2009; Jansson et al., 2008).

Another factor which can impact cell fate decision is Chk2. Following DNA damage, Chk2 functions by suppressing apoptosis. In cells that express cell cycle inhibitors such as p21 and 14-3-3δ, cell cycle arrest appears to prevent or slow the onset of cell death. Without these proteins, Chk2-regulated apoptosis is much more apparent. Thus, it seems that the balance between cell cycle inhibitors and Chk2 dictates the outcome following DNA damage (Antoni et al., 2007). The finding that loss of both p21 and 14-3-3δ but not each alone is required to unmask the effect of Chk2 can be understood in the context of how each functions to effect cell cycle arrest. 14-3-3δ is a cytoplasmic protein which in response to DNA damage accumulates and acts by sequestering CDK1 and CDK2 in the cytoplasm and preventing cytokinesis (Chan et al., 1999; Laronga et al., 2000; Wilker et al., 2007). P21 is a nuclear cyclin-dependent kinase inhibitor that directly binds and inactivates cyclin-CDK complexes (el-Deiry et al., 1993; Harper et al., 1993; Xiong et al., 1993). Cooperative effects between these two factors have been shown to dictate the biological response to apoptotic stimuli (Jazayeri et al., 2006; Meng et al., 2009). This implies that the ultimate outcome of

Chk2 activation may depend on the particular cellular context and on molecular determinants of Chk2 function, 14-3-3δ and p21.

3. DNA damage response in postmitotic neurons

Neurons are extremely active cells (Barzilai, 2010; Fishel et al., 2007) and generally exhibit high mitochondrial respiration and production of reactive oxygen species (ROS) that can damage mitochondrial and nuclear DNA (Weissman et al., 2007). For this reason, neurons are particularly susceptible to genotoxic effects generated by ROS (Barzilai et al., 2008). ROS induce the formation of various DNA lesions including oxidative DNA base modifications, SSBs and DSBs (Martin, 2008). DNA damage plays an important role in brain damage (Nagayama et al., 2000). This damage is a common feature of neurodegenerative diseases (Kraemer et al., 2007; Trushina, & McMurray, 2007). The importance of DNA damage in pathogenesis of neurodegenerative diseases is illustrated by the observation that defective DNA repair in various human syndromes such as ataxia telangiectasia is accompanied by neurological abnormalities (Rolig, & McKinnon, 2000). There is a growing interest in the role of DNA damage in neurological dysfunctions associated with cancer treatments (Wefel et al., 2004). Significant evidence points to the critical role of cumulative DNA damage in the aging process of neurons in the central nervous system (CNS) (Coppede` & Migliore, 2010; Fishel et al., 2007; Weissman et al., 2007).

3.1 Cell cycle and neuronal apoptosis

Although accumulating evidence suggests the importance of proper DDR for the nervous system, most of the work to elucidate DDR components has been carried out in proliferating cells. The signal transduction mechanisms in neurons that link DNA damage to apoptosis are not well characterized, and the sensors of DNA damage in neurons are largely unknown (Martin et al., 2009). However, some observations suggest that DDR in postmitotic neurons may have survival checkpoint that serves to eliminate neurons with excessive DNA damage. A loss of function of DDR proteins such as ATM leads to genomic instability and human hereditary diseases, characterized by neurodegeneration (Rass et al, 2007). ATM has a pro-apoptotic function in the developing mouse CNS (Herzog et al., 1998; Lee et al., 2001) and operates similarly to how it operates in proliferating cells (Biton et al., 2006, 2007; Gorodetsky et al., 2007). In addition, neurons in ATM-/- mice are resistant to DNA damage-induced apoptosis (Herzog et al., 1998; Kruman et al., 2004; Lee & McKinnon, 2000; McKinnon, 2001). However, ascribing to ATM and cell cycle checkpoints in neurons the same functions they have in proliferating cells poses certain conceptual difficulties, given the postmitotic nature of these cells.

Another indication of possible cell cycle checkpoint functioning in neurons is extensively documented cell cycle reentry of these postmitotic cells following genotoxic stress. The neurons undergo full or partial DNA replication, showing that they reenter the S phase (Kruman et al., 2004; Yang et al., 2001). This attempt to enter the cell cycle is abortive and does not result in actual division (Athanasiou et al., 1998; Becker & Bonni, 2004; Feddersen et al., 1992) but culminates in apoptotic cell death (Becker & Bonni, 2004; Kruman, 2004; Yang & Herrup, 2001). Cell cycle activation is a common feature of neuronal apoptosis during development and in neurodegenerative disorders (Becker & Bonni, 2004; Herrup et al., 2004; Kruman, 2004; Kruman et al., 2004; Park et al., 1997, 1998). On the other hand, forced cell cycle entry mediated by targeted disruption of the pRb or ectopic E2F1 expression also results in apoptosis of postmitotic neurons (Becker & Bonni, 2004; Feddersen et al., 1995; Johnson et al., 1993; Smith et al., 2000), while preventing cell cycle entry is protective against neurotoxic insults, such as ischemia and kainate-induced excitotoxicity (Kim & Tsai, 2009; Kruman et al., 2004; Zhang et al., 2006). Exposure of mice or mesencephalic neuronal cultures to the dopaminergic cell neurotoxins 1-methyl-4-phenyl-1,2,3,6-tertahydropyridine (MPTP) results in cell cycle activation in post-mitotic neurons prior to their subsequent death, while E2F1 deficiency leads to a significant resistance to MPTP-induced dopaminergic cell death (Hoglinger et al., 2007).

Our recent findings demonstrate the particular role of S phase entry and DNA replication in DNA damage-induced neuronal apoptosis (Kruman et al., 2004; Tomashevski et al., 2010). Expression of S-phase markers was reported in post-mitotic neurons following hypoxia-ischemia (Kuan et al., 2004), in neurons in Alzheimer's disease (Yang et al., 2001) and in neurons ectopically expressing E2F1 (Smith et al., 2000). The special role of S phase might be linked to DNA replication errors which are usually accompanied by DNA damage and activation of cell cycle checkpoints (Elledge, 1996; Kumagai & Dunphy, 2006). Activation of Chk2 following DSB formation was observed in primary neurons exposed to DSB inducer producing repairable DSBs (Sordet et al., 2009). This is consistent with previous finding demonstrating that Chk2, in contrast to Chk1, is expressed and activatable in quiescent cells. This may suggest the survival mechanism by which S phase entry is prevented in postmitotic cells. Since differentiated neurons which enter S phase prior apoptosis predominantly express a highly error prone DNA polymerase β (Copani et al., 2002), the DNA replication might produce additional DNA damage. This may amplify DNA damage and generate apoptotic signaling. The functional link between neuronal cell cycle reentry, DDR, cell cycle checkpoints and apoptosis is supported by data demonstrating that both cell cycle activation and apoptosis in postmitotic neurons exposed to DSB-inducing agents are ATM-dependent (Alvira et al., 2007; Kruman et al., 2004; Otsuka et al., 2004). There is no evidence of entry of neurons under conditions of DNA damage-induced apoptosis into mitosis, although they may progress through DNA synthesis and G2 (Athanasiou et al., 1998; Becker & Bonni, 2004; Feddersen et al., 1992; Yang et al., 2001). This may be explained by activation of G2/M checkpoint induced by replication stress which prevents entry into mitosis. Indeed, expression of G2/M checkpoint markers has been reported in vascular dementia (McShea et al., 1999), and several other neurodegenerative diseases (Husseman et al., 2000).

3.2 Cell cycle and DNA repair in neurons

Terminally differentiated neurons are highly susceptible to oxidative DNA damage (Fishel et al., 2007), and DNA repair is very important for these cells (Biton et al., 2008; Fishel et al., 2007; Lavin & Kozlov, 2007). All eukaryotic DNA repair systems operating in proliferating cells also operate in neurons (Fishel et al., 2007; Lee, & McKinnon, 2007; Sharma, 2007; Weissman et al., 2007; Wilson, & McNeill, 2007). It is believed that most of the lesions inflicted in neuronal genomic and mitochondrial DNA are produced by ROS. These lesions are repaired mainly via the BER pathway, although other types of DNA repair are involved (Fishel et al., 2007; Weissman et al., 2007; Wilson & McNeill, 2007). Although DNA repair activity exists in neurons, it was found that this repair is not as effective as in dividing cells, suggesting that lesions are likely to accumulate (Gobbel et al., 1998; McMurray, 2005; Nouspikel, & Hanawalt, 2000, 2002). Indeed, following cellular differentiation, the levels of many repair factors are reduced (Bill et al., 1992; Nouspikel, & Hanawalt, 2000, 2002).

However, in contrast to global genomic repair (GGR), the repair of transcribed genes is more vigorous (Nouspikel, & Hanawalt, 2000). Thus, DNA repair in the nonessential bulk of the genome of postmitotic neurons is dispensable, and they repair only DNA needed for neuronal functioning (Nouspikel, 2007; Nouspikel, & Hanawalt, 2002). Since neurons are very active and the repair process carries a high energy cost, it is reasonable that these cells preferentially repair transcribed genes. This is important to avoid harming the fidelity of information transcribed to proteins (Fishel et al., 2007; Lu et al., 2004).

It is commonly believed that neurons remain in G0 phase of the cell cycle indefinitely. Cell-cycle reentry, however, is coupled with DNA damage-induced apoptosis of postmitotic neurons (Becker & Bonni, 2004; Herrup et al., 2004; Kruman, 2004; Kruman et al., 2004; Park et al., 1997, 1998). Moreover, recent evidence demonstrates the expression of cell-cycle proteins in differentiated neurons at physiological conditions (Schmetsdorf et al., 2007, 2009). The functional roles of such expression remain unclear. Since DNA repair is generally attenuated by differentiation in most cell types (McMurray, 2005; Narciso et al., 2007), the cell-cycle-associated events in postmitotic cells may reflect the need to reenter the cell cycle to activate DNA repair. Recently, we have demonstrated that the NHEJ activation in postmitotic neurons is associated with G0-G1 transition, driven by cyclin-C-associated pRb-kinase activity, while preventing cell cycle entry attenuated DNA repair (Tomashevski et al., 2010). This suggests the importance of cell cycle entry for DNA repair in postmitotic cells. Previously, quiescent cells, including differentiated cells, were shown to be able to reenter the cell cycle simply by removing appropriate cell cycle inhibitors such as p21. Interference with p21 was sufficient to reactivate the cell cycle and DNA synthesis in terminally differentiated skeletal muscle cells, quiescent fibroblasts and primary cortical neurons (Pajalunga et al., 2007; Tomashevski et al., 2010). Reactivation of cell cycle and DNA replication has also been documented in quiescent cells overexpressing E2F1 and Cdc25A (Pajalunga et al., 2007; Rogoff & Kowalik, 2004; Smith et al., 2000; Zhang et al., 2006). Such reactivation of cell cycle and DNA replication were sufficient to promote neuronal death even in the absence of DNA damage (O'Hare et al., 2000). However, preventing S phase entry, attenuated apoptotic signaling (Tomashevski et al., 2010), suggesting a decisive role of G1-S transition for activation of the apoptotic machinery. Thus, cell cycle activation occurs in response to DNA damage and is involved in both DNA repair and apoptosis in postmitotic neurons. These findings may imply that cell cycle checkpoints may orchestrate both DNA repair and apoptosis of postmitotic neurons, as it occurs in proliferating cells (Bartek & Lukas, 2001; Shiloh, 2003; Zhou & Elledge, 2000).

4. Conclusion and future perspectives

The way that cells react to DNA damage constantly produced by exogenous and endogenous factors is to trigger a complex and coordinated set of events termed the DDR (Reinhardt & Yaffe, 2009). The function of such response is to sense genome damage and activate several downstream pathways, including cell cycle checkpoints, DNA repair and apoptotic programs (Jackson, 2009; Zhou & Elledge, 2000). The earliest events of the DDR are associated with alterations in chromatin structure and the formation of DDR foci facilitating recruitment of proteins involved in DDR propagation (Berkovich et al., 2007; Downs et al., 2007; Smerdon et al., 1978). The biochemical details of these processes are poorly understood. However, studies in yeast and mammalian systems have demonstrated that colocalization of DDR proteins rather than DNA damage per se is critical for DNA damage signaling (Bonilla et al., 2008; Soutoglou & Misteli, 2008). Another important component of DDR network is the cell cycle checkpoint pathway which plays roles in the activation of DNA repair, modulation of transcriptional programmes and the optional triggering apoptosis (Bartek & Lukas, 2001; Shiloh, 2003; Zhou & Elledge, 2000). In response to DNA damage, the checkpoints delay or stop the cell cycle at critical points before or during DNA replication (G1/S and intra-S checkpoints) and before cell division (G2/M checkpoint). This prevents replication and segregation of damaged DNA (Houtgraaf et al., 2006; Poehlmann & Roessner, 2010). DDR is involved in two alternatives: activation of a prosurvival network associated with DNA repair or initiation of programmed cell death removing cells with irrepairable DNA (Barzilai et al., 2008; Kruman, 2004). The checkpoints play important roles in both processes (Bartek & Lukas, 2001; Shiloh, 2003; Zhou & Elledge, 2000). The importance of DDR is illustrated by various pathologies associated with defects in DDR proteins. Mutations in key DDR regulators such as ATM, ATR, MRE11, NBS1 are associated with severe genome instability disorders (Ciccia & Elledge, 2010; Jackson & Bartek 2009).

Due to a high rate of oxygen metabolism and the low levels of antioxidant enzymes compared to other cells, the DNA of postmitotic neurons is under increased risk of damage from free radicals. (Barzilai, 2010; Kruman, 2004). For this reason, DNA repair is critical for the nervous system. While all eukaryotic DNA repair systems operating in proliferating cells also operate in neurons (Fishel et al., 2007; Lee, & McKinnon, 2007; Sharma, 2007; Weissman et al., 2007; Wilson, & McNeill, 2007), differentiation is associated with a decrease in levels of many repair enzymes (Bill et al., 1992; Nouspikel, & Hanawalt, 2000, 2002; Tofilon & Meyn, 1988), and DNA repair in neurons, is not as effective as in dividing cells (Gobbel et al., 1998; McMurray, 2005; Nouspikel, & Hanawalt, 2000, 2002). It raises the question whether DDR in postmitotic neurons is similar to the DDR of mitotic cells. Some evidence such as a contribution of ATM to apoptosis of postmitotic neurons (Herzog et al., 1998; Kruman et al., 2004; Lee & McKinnon, 2000; McKinnon, 2001) points to such similarity. Although postmitotic neurons are quiescent cells, they are capable to reenter the cell cycle before apoptosis induced by genotoxic stress, as was extensively documented (Barzilai, 2010; Kim & Tsai, 2009; Kruman et al., 2004; Yang et al., 2001). Moreover, we recently demonstrated that DNA repair is also depends on cell cycle activation, driven by cyclin-C-associated pRb-kinase activity (Tomashevski et al., 2010). These findings together with observation that Chk2 is expressed and activated in postmitotic neurons and other postmitotic cells following genotoxic stress (Lukas et al., 2001; Sordet et al., 2009), are indications of cell cycle checkpoint functioning in neurons.

Compelling evidence points to similarities in the DDR of proliferating cells and postmitotic neurons. However, neurons are quiescent cells which requires adaptation of the DDR. The major future challenge is to understand the mechanisms by which cell cycle checkpoint machinery operates in postmitotic neurons and involves in DNA repair, apoptosis and cell fate decisions. Further investigation of the DDR in human genomic instability syndromes, neurodegenerative pathologies, and animal models of these conditions, will help to disclose these mechanisms. Clarification of the mechanisms at work will help guide the search for novel treatment modalities for a variety of neurodegenerative conditions.

5. Acknowledgments

This work was supported by Texas Tech University Health Sciences Center grant.

6. References

Abbas, T. & Dutta, A. (2009). p21 in cancer: intricate networks and multiple activities. *Nat Rev Cancer*, Vol.9, No.6, (June 2009), pp.400-414, ISSN 1944-0234

Ahel, D.; Horejsí, Z.; Wiechens, N.; Polo, S.E.; Garcia-Wilson, E.; Ahel, I.; Flynn, H.; Skehel, M.; West, S.C.; Jackson S.P.; Owen-Hughes, T. & Boulton, S.J. (2009). Poly(ADP-ribose)-dependent regulation of DNA repair by the chromatin remodeling enzyme ALC1. *Science*, Vol.325, No.5945, (August 2010), pp.1240-1243, ISSN 1966-1379

Al-Hakim, A.; Escribano-Diaz, C.; Landry, M.C.; O'Donnell, L.; Panier, S.; Szilard, R.K. & Durocher, D. (2010). The ubiquitous role of ubiquitin in the DNA damage response. *DNA Repair (Amst)*, Vol.9, No.12, (November 2010), pp.1229-1240, ISSN 2105-6014

Alvira, D.; Yeste-Velasco, M.; Folch, J.; Casadesús, G.; Smith, M.A.; Pallàs, M. & Camins, A. (2007). Neuroprotective effects of caffeine against complex I inhibition-induced apoptosis are mediated by inhibition of the Atm/p53/E2F-1 path in cerebellar granule neurons. *J Neurosci Res*, Vol.85, No.14, (November 2007), pp.3079-3088, ISSN 1763-8302

Amsel, A.D.; Rathaus, M.; Kronman, N. & Cohen, H.Y. (2008). Regulation of the proapoptotic factor Bax by Ku70-dependent deubiquitylation. *Proc Natl Acad Sci U S A*, Vol.105, No.13, (March 2008), pp. 5117-5122, ISSN 1836-2350

Antignani, A. & Youle, R.J. (2006). How do Bax and Bak lead to permeabilization of the outer mitochondrial membrane? *Curr Opin Cell Biol*, Vol.18, No.6, (October 2006), pp. 685-689, ISSN 1704-6225

Antoni, L.; Sodha, N.; Collins, I. & Garrett, M.D. (2007). CHK2 kinase: cancer susceptibility and cancer therapy-two sides of the same coin? *Nat Rev Cancer*, Vol.7, No.12, (December 2007), pp.925-936, ISSN 1800-4398

Aressy, B. & Ducommun, B. (2008) Cell cycle control by the CDC25 phosphatases. *Anticancer Agents Med Chem*, Vol.8, No.8, (December 2008), pp.818-824, ISSN 1907-5563

Athanasiou, M.C.; Yunis, W.; Coleman, N.; Ehlenfeldt, R.; Clark, H.B.; Orr, H.T. & Feddersen, R.M. (1998). The transcription factor E2F-1 in SV40 T antigen-induced cerebellar Purkinje cell degeneration. *Mol Cell Neurosci*, Vol.12, No.1-2, (September 1998), pp.16-28, ISSN 977-0337

Averbeck, N.B. & Durante, M. (2011). Protein acetylation within the cellular response to radiation. *J Cell Physiol*, Vol.226, No.4, (April 2011), pp.962-967, ISSN 2094-5393

Aylon, Y. & Oren, M. (2007). Living with p53, dying of p53. *Cell*, Vol.130, No.4, (August 2007), pp. 597-600, ISSN 1771-9538

Banin, S.; Moyal, L.; Shieh, S.; Taya, Y.; Anderson, C.W.; Chessa, L.; Smorodinsky, N.I.; Prives, C.; Reiss, Y.; Shiloh, Y.& Ziv, Y. (1998). Enhanced phosphorylation of p53 by ATM in response to DNA damage. *Science*, Vol.281, No.5383, (September 1998), pp. 1674–1677, ISSN 973-3514

Baptiste-Okoh, N.; Barsotti, A.M. & Prives, C. (2008). Caspase 2 is both required for p53-mediated apoptosis and downregulated by p53 in a p21-dependent manner. *Cell Cycle*, Vol.7, No.9, (February 2008), pp.1133-1138, ISSN 1841-8048

Bartek, J. & Lukas, J. (2001). Mammalian G1- and S-phase checkpoints in response to DNA damage. *Curr Opin Cell Biol*, Vol.13, No.6, (December 2001), pp.738-747, ISSN 1169-8191

Bartek, J.; Lukas, C. & Lukas, J. (2004). Checking on DNA damage in S phase. *Nat Rev Mol Cell Biol*, Vol.5, No.10, (October 2007), pp. 792-804, ISSN1545-9660

Bartek, J. & Lukas, J. (2007). DNA damage checkpoints: from initiation to recovery or adaptation. *Curr Opin Cell Biol*, Vol.19, No.2, (February 2007), pp.238-245. ISSN 1730-3408

Bartek, J.; Lukas, J. & Bartkova, J. (2007). DNA damage response as an anti-cancer barrier: damage threshold and the concept of 'conditional haploinsufficiency'. *Cell Cycle*, Vol.6, No.19, (July 2007), pp. 2344–2347, ISSN 1770-0066

Bartkova, J.; Horejsí, Z.; Koed, K.; Krämer, A.; Tort, F.; Zieger, K.; Guldberg, P.; Sehested, M.; Nesland, J.M.; Lukas, C.; Ørntoft, T.; Lukas, J. & Bartek, J. (2005). DNA damage response as a candidate anti-cancer barrier in early human tumorigenesis. *Nature*, Vol.434, No.7035, (April 2005), pp. 864-870. ISSN 1582-9956

Barzilai, A.; Biton, S. & Shiloh, Y. (2008). The role of the DNA damage response in neuronal development, organization and maintenance. *DNA Repair (Amst)*, Vol.7, No.7, (May 2008), pp. 1010-1027. ISSN 1845-8000

Barzilai A. (2010). DNA damage, neuronal and glial cell death and neurodegeneration. *Apoptosis*, Vol.15, No.11, (November 2010), pp.1371-1381. ISSN 2043-7103

Bazzi, M.; Mantiero, D.; Trovesi, C.; Lucchini, G. & Longhese, M.P. (2010). Dephosphorylation of gamma H2A by

Glc7/protein phosphatase 1 promotes recovery from inhibition of DNA replication. *Mol Cell Biol*, Vol.30, No.1, (January 2010), pp.131-145, ISSN 1988-4341

Becker, E.B. & Bonni, A. (2004). Cell cycle regulation of neuronal apoptosis in development and disease. *Prog Neurobiol*, Vol.72, No.1, (January 2004), pp.1-25, ISSN 1501-9174

Bekker-Jensen, S.; Lukas, C.; Melander, F.; Bartek, J. & Lukas, J. (2005). Dynamic assembly and sustained retention of 53BP1 at the sites of DNA damage are controlled by Mdc1/NFBD1. *J Cell Biol*, Vol.170, No.2, (July 2005), pp.201–211, ISSN 1600-9723

Bekker-Jensen, S.; Lukas, C.; Kitagawa, R.; Melander, F.; Kastan, M.B.; Bartek, J. & Lukas, J. (2006). Spatial organization of the mammalian genome surveillance machinery in response to DNA strand breaks. *J Cell Biol*, Vol.173, No.2, (April 2006), pp.195-206, ISSN 1661-8811

Bennett, C.B.; Lewis, A.L.; Baldwin, K.K. & Resnick, M.A. (1993). Lethality induced by a single site-specific double-strand break in a dispensable yeast plasmid. *Proc Natl Acad Sci U S A*, Vol.90, No.12, (June 1993), pp. 5613-5617, ISSN 851- 6308

Berkovich, E.; Monnat, R.J. Jr. & Kastan, M.B. (2007). Roles of ATM and NBS1 in chromatin structure modulation and DNA double-strand break repair. *Nat Cell Biol*, Vol.9, No.6, (May 2007), pp.683–690, ISSN 1748-6112

Bill, C.A.; Grochan, B.M.; Vrdoljak, E.; Mendoza, E.A. & Tofilon, P.J. (1992). Decreased repair of radiation-induced DNA double-strand breaks with cellular differentiation. *Radiat Res*, Vol.132, No.2, (November 1992), pp.254–258, ISSN 143- 8708

Bitomsky, N. & Hofmann, T.G. (2009). Apoptosis and autophagy: Regulation of apoptosis by DNA damage signalling - roles of p53, p73 and HIPK2. *FEBS J*, Vol.276, No.21, (September 2007), pp. 6074-6083, ISSN 1978-8416

Biton, S.; Dar, I.; Mittelman, L;. Pereg, Y.; Barzilai, A. & Shiloh, Y. (2006). Nuclear ataxia-telangiectasia mutated (ATM) mediates the cellular response to DNA double strand breaks in human neuron-like cells, *J Biol Chem*, Vol.281, No.25, (April 2006), pp.17482-17491, ISSN 1662-7474

Biton, S.; Gropp, M.; Itsykson, P.; Pereg, Y.; Mittelman, L.; Johe, K.; Reubinoff, B. & Shiloh, Y. (2007). ATM-mediated response to DNA double strand breaks in human neurons derived from stem cells. *DNA Repair (Amst),* Vol.6, No.1, (December 2006), pp.128-134, ISSN 1717-8256

Biton, S.; Barzilai, A. & Shiloh, Y. (2008). The neurological phenotype of ataxia-telangiectasia: solving a persistent puzzle. *DNA Repair (Amst),* Vol.7, No.7, (May 2008), pp.1028-1038, ISSN 1845-6574

Blank, M. & Shiloh, Y. (2007). Programs for cell death: apoptosis is only one way to go. *Cell Cycle,* Vol.6, No.6, (March 2007), pp. 686-95, ISSN 1736-1099

Bonilla, C.Y.; Melo, J.A. & Toczyski, D.P. (2008). Colocalization of sensors is sufficient to activate the DNA damage checkpoint in the absence of damage. *Mol Cell,* Vol.30, No.3, (May 2008), pp.267–276, ISSN 1847-1973

Brady, C.A. & Attardi, L.D. (2010). p53 at a glance. *J Cell Sci,* Vol.123, Pt.15, (August 2010), pp.2527-2532, ISSN 2094-0128

Branzei, D. & Foiani, M. (2008). Regulation of DNA repair throughout the cell cycle. *Nat Rev Mol Cell Biol,* Vol.9, No.4, (February 2008), pp.297–308, ISSN 1828-5803

Brugarolas, J.; Moberg, K.; Boyd, S.D.; Taya, Y.; Jacks, T. & Lees, J.A. (1999). Inhibition of cyclindependent kinase 2 by p21 is necessary for retinoblastoma protein-mediated G1arrest after gamma-irradiation. *Proc Natl Acad Sci USA,* Vol.96, No.3, (February 1999), pp.1002–1007, ISSN 992-7683

Burma, S.; Chen, B.P.; Murphy, M.; Kurimasa, A. & Chen, D.J. (2001). ATM phosphorylates histone H2AX in response to DNA double-strand breaks. *J Biol Chem,* Vol.276, No.45, (September 2001), pp.42462-42467, ISSN 1157-1274

Busino, L.; Chiesa, M.; Draetta, G.F. & Donzelli, M. (2004) Cdc25A phosphatase:combinatorial phosphorylation, ubiquitylation and proteolysis. *Oncogene,* Vol.23, No.11, (March 2004), pp. 2050-2056, ISSN 1502-1892

Caelles, C.; Helmberg, A. & Karin, M. (1994) p53-dependentapoptosis in the absence of transcriptional activation of p53- target genes. *Nature,* Vol.370, No.6486, (July 1994), pp. 220-223, ISSN 802-8670

Calsou, P.; Delteil, C.; Frit, P.; Drouet, J. & Salles, B. (2003). Coordinated assembly of Ku and p460 subunits of the DNA- dependent protein kinase on DNA ends is necessary for XRCC4-ligase IV recruitment. *J Mol Biol,* Vol.326, No.1, (February 2003), pp.93-103, ISSN 1254-7193

Castedo, M.; Perfettini, J.L.; Roumier, T.; Andreau, K.; Medema, R. & Kroemer, G. (2004). Cell death by mitotic catastrophe: a molecular definition. *Oncogene,* Vol.23, No.16, (April 2004), pp. 2825-2837, ISSN 1507-7146

Celeste, A.; Petersen, S.; Romanienko, P.J.; Fernandez-Capetillo, O.; Chen, H.T.; Sedelnikova, O.A.; Reina-San-Martin, B.; Coppola, V.; Meffre, E.; Difilippantonio, M.J.; Redon, C.; Pilch, D.R.; Olaru, A.; Eckhaus, M.; Camerini-Otero, R.D.; Tessarollo, L.; Livak, F.; Manova, K.; Bonner ,W.M.; Nussenzweig, M.C. & Nussenzweig, A. (2002). Genomic instability in mice lacking histone H2AX. *Science,* Vol.296, No.5569, (May 2002) pp.922–927, ISSN 1193-4988

Celeste, A.; Fernandez-Capetillo, O.; Kruhlak, M.J.; Pilch, D.R.; Staudt, D.W.; Lee, A.; Bonner, R.F.; Bonner,W.M. & Nussenzweig, A. (2003). Histone H2AX phosphorylation is dispensable for the initial recognition of DNA breaks. *Nat Cell Biol,* Vol.5, No7, (July 2003), pp.675–679, ISSN 1279-2649

Cha, H.; Lowe, J.M.; Li, H.; Lee, .;, Belova, G.;, Bulavin, D.V. & Fornace, A.J. Jr. (2010). Wip1 directly dephosphorylates gamma-H2AX and attenuates the DNA damage response. *Cancer Res*, Vol.70, No.10, (May 2010), pp.4112-2412, ISSN 204-60517

Chan, D.W. & Lees-Miller, S.P. (1996). The DNA-dependent protein kinase is inactivated by autophosphorylation of the catalytic subunit. *J Biol Chem*, Vol.271, No.15, (April 1996), pp.8936-8941, ISSN 86-21537

Chan, T.A.; Hermeking, H.; Lengauer, C.; Kinzler, K.W. & Vogelstein, B. (1999). 14-3-3Sigma is required to prevent mitotic catastrophe after DNA damage. *Nature*, Vol.401, No. 6753, (October 1999), pp. 616-620, ISSN 1052-4633

Chan, T.A.; Hwang, P.M.; Hermeking, H.; Kinzler, K.W. & Vogelstein, B. (2000). Cooperative effects of genes controlling the G(2)/M checkpoint. *Genes Dev*, Vol.14, No.13, (July 2000), pp.1584-1588, ISSN 1088-7152

Chao, C.; Wu, Z.; Mazur, S.J.; Borges, H.; Rossi, M.; Lin, T.; Wang, J.Y.; Anderson, C.W.; Appella, E. & Xu, Y. (2006). Acetylation of mouse p53 at lysine 317 negatively regulates p53 apoptotic activities after DNA damage. *Mol Cell Biol*, Vol.26, No.18, (September 2006), pp. 6859-6869, ISSN 1694-3427

Chapman, J.R. & Jackson, S.P. (2008). Phospho-dependent interactions between NBS1 and MDC1 mediate chromatin retention of the MRN complex at sites of DNA damage. *EMBO Rep*, Vol.9, No.8, (June 2008), pp.795-801, ISSN 1858- 3988

Chappell, C.; Hanakahi, L.A.; Karimi-Busheri, F.; Weinfeld, M. & West, S.C. (2002). Involvement of human polynucleotide kinase in double-strand break repair by non-homologous end joining. *EMBO J*, Vol.21, No.11, (June 2002), pp. 2827- 2832, ISSN 1203-2095

Chen, J.; Peters, R.; Saha, P.; Lee, P.; Theodoras, A.; Pagano, M.; Wagner, G. & Dutta, A. (1996). A 39 amino acid fragment of the cell cycle regulator p21 is sufficient to bind PCNA and partially inhibit DNA replication in vivo. *Nucleic Acids Res*, Vol.24, No.9, (May 1996), pp.1727–1733, ISSN 864-9992

Chou, D.M., Adamson, B, Dephoure, N.E., Tan, X., Nottke, A.C., Hurov, K.E., Gygi, S.P., Colaiácovo, M.P., Elledge, S.J. (2010). A chromatin localization screen reveals poly (ADP ribose)-regulated recruitment of the repressive polycomb and NuRD complexes to sites of DNA damage. *Proc Natl Acad Sci U S A*, Vol.107, No.43, (October 2010), pp. 18475- 18480, ISSN 2093-7877

Chowdhury, I.; Tharakan, B. & Bhat, G.K. (2006). Current concepts in apoptosis: The physiological suicide program revisited. *Cell Mol Biol Lett*, Vol.11, No.4, (September 2006), pp. 506-525, ISSN 1697-7376

Chowdhury, D.; Xu, X.; Zhong, X.; Ahmed, F.; Zhong, J.; Liao, J.; Dykxhoorn, D.M.; Weinstock, D.M.; Pfeifer, G.P. & Lieberman, J. (2008). A PP4-phosphatase complex dephosphorylates gamma-H2AX generated during DNA replication. *Mol Cell*, Vol.31, No.1, (July 2008), pp. 33-46, ISSN 1861-4045

Ciccia, A. & Elledge, S.J. (2010). The DNA damage response: making it safe to play with knives. *Mol Cell*, Vol.40, No.2, (October 2010), pp.179-204, ISSN 2096-5415

Citarelli, M.; Teotia, S. & Lamb, R.S. (2010). Evolutionary history of the poly(ADP-ribose) polymerase gene family in eukaryotes. *BMC Evol Biol*, Vol.10, (October 2010), pp.308-334, ISSN 2094-2953

Clerici, M.; Mantiero, D.; Guerini, I.; Lucchini, G. & Longhese, M.P. (2008). The Yku70-Yku80 complex contributes to regulate double-strand break processing and checkpoint activation during the cell cycle. *EMBO Rep,* Vol.9, No.8, (July 2008), pp.810-818, ISSN 1860-0234

Cohen, H.Y.; Lavu, S.; Bitterman, K.J.; Hekking, B.; Imahiyerobo, T.A.; Miller, C.; Frye, R.; Ploegh, H.; Kessler, B.M. & Sinclair, D.A. (2004). Acetylation of the C terminus of Ku70 by CBP and PCAF controls Bax-mediated apoptosis. *Mol Cell,* Vol.13, No.5, (March 2004), pp. 627-638, ISSN 1502-3334

Copani, A.; Sortino, M.A.; Caricasole, A.; Chiechio, S.; Chisari, M.; Battaglia, G.; Giuffrida-Stella, A.M.; Vancheri, C. & Nicoletti, F. (2002). Erratic expression of DNA polymerases by beta-amyloid causes neuronal death. *FASEB J,* Vol.16, No.14, (October 2002), pp. 2006-2008, ISSN 1239-7084

Coppede, F & Migliore, L. (2010). DNA repair in premature aging disorders and neurodegeneration. *Curr Aging Sci,* Vol.3, No.1, (February 2010), pp.3-19, ISSN 2029-8165

Costanzo, A.; Merlo, P.; Pediconi, N.; Fulco, M.; Sartorelli, V.; Cole, P.A.; Fontemaggi, G.; Fanciulli, M.; Schiltz, L.;

Blandino, G.; Balsano, C. & Levrero, M. (2002). DNA damage-dependent acetylation of p73 dictates the selective activation of apoptotic target genes. *Mol Cell,* Vol.9, No.1, (January 2002), pp.175–186, ISSN 1180-4596

Elledge, S. J. (1996). Cell cycle checkpoints: preventing an identity crisis. *Science,* Vol.274, No.5293, (December 1996), pp. 1664-1672, ISSN 893-9848

D'Amours, D.; Desnoyers, S.; D'Silva, I. & Poirier, G.G. (1999). Poly(ADP-ribosyl)ation reactions in the regulation of nuclear functions. *Biochem J,* Vol.342, Pt. 2, (September 1999), pp.249-268, ISSN 1045-5009

Das, S.; Boswell, S.A.; Aaronson, S.A. & Lee, S.W. (2008). P53 promoter selection: choosing between life and death. *Cell Cycle,* Vol.7, No.2, (October 2007), pp.154-157, ISSN 1821-2532

Deckbar, D.; Birraux, J.; Krempler, A.; Tchouandong, L.; Beucher, A.; Walker, S.; Stiff, T.; Jeggo, P. & Löbrich, M. (2007). Chromosome breakage after G2 checkpoint release. *J Cell Biol,* Vol.176, No.6, (March 2007), pp.749-755, ISSN 1735- 3355

de Jager, M.; van Noort, J.; van Gent, D.C.; Dekker, C.; Kanaar, R. & Wyman, C. (2001). *Mol Cell,* 2001 Nov;Vol.8, No.5, (November 2001), pp.1129-1135, ISSN 1174-1547

de Murcia, G. & Ménissier de Murcia, J. (1994). Poly(ADP-ribose) polymerase: a molecular nick-sensor. *Trends Biochem Sci,* Vol.19, No.4 (April 1994), pp172-176, ISSN 8016-868

Demidenko, Z.N.; Korotchkina, L.G.; Gudkov, A.V. & Blagosklonny, M.V. (2010). Paradoxical suppression of cellular senescence by p53. *Proc Natl Acad Sci USA,* Vol.107, No.21 (May 2010), pp.9660-9664, ISSN 2045-7898

Deng, C.; Zhang, P.; Harper, J.; Elledge, S.J. & Leder, P. (1995). Mice lacking p21CIP1/WAF1 undergo normal development, but are defective in G1 checkpoint control. *Cell,* Vol.82, No.4 (August 1995), pp. 675-684, ISSN 766-4346

Ding, H.F.; McGill, G.; Rowan, S.; Schmaltz, C.; Shimamura, A. & Fisher, D.E. (1998). Oncogene-dependent regulation

of caspase activation by p53 protein in a cell-free system. *J Biol Chem,* Vol.273, No.43 (October 1998), pp.28378-28383, ISSN 977-4464

Dobbelstein, M.; Strano, S.; Roth, J. & Blandino, G. (2005). p73-induced apoptosis: a question of compartments and cooperation. *Biochem Biophys Res Commun,* Vol.331, No.3 (June 2005), pp. 688-693, ISSN 1586-5923

Downs, J.A.; Lowndes, N.F. & Jackson, S.P. (2000). A role for Saccharomyces cerevisiae histone H2A in DNA repair. *Nature*, Vol.408, No.6815, (Decemeber 2000), pp.1001-1004, ISSN 1114-0636

Downs, J.A.; Allard, S.; Jobin-Robitaille, O.; Javaheri, A.; Auger, A.; Bouchard, N.; Kron, S.J.; Jackson, S.P. & Côté, J. (2004). *Mol Cell,* Vol.16, No.6, (December 2004), pp.979-990,ISSN 1561-0740

Downs, J.A.; Allard, S.; Jobin-Robitaille, O.; Javaheri, A.; Auger, A.; Bouchard, N.; Kron, S.J.; Jackson, S.P. & Côté J. (2004). Binding of chromatin-modifying activities to phosphorylated histone H2A at DNA damage sites. *Mol Cell*, 2004 Dec 22;Vol.16, No.6, (December 2004), pp.979-990, ISSN 15610740

Downs, J.A.; Nussenzweig, M.C. & Nussenzweig, A. (2007). Chromatin dynamics and the preservation of genetic information. *Nature,* Vol.447, No.7147, (June 2007), pp.951-958, ISSN 1758-1578

Dupre, A.; Boyer-Chatenet, L. & Gautier, J. (2006). Two-step activation of ATM by DNA and the Mre11-Rad50-Nbs1 complex. *Nature Struct Mol Biol,* Vol. 13, No.5, (May 2006), pp.451–457, ISSN 1662-2404

Durant S.T.; Cho, E.C. & La Thangue, N.B. (2009).p53 methylation—the argument is clear. *Cell Cycle,* Vol.8, No.6, (March 2009), pp. 801-802, ISSN 1922-1494

Dvir, A.; Peterson, S.R.; Knuth, M.W.; Lu, H. & Dynan, W.S. (1992). Ku autoantigen is the regulatory component of a template-associated protein kinase that phosphorylates RNA polymerase II. *Proc Natl Acad Sci U S A,* Vol.89, No.24, (December 1992), pp.11920-11924, ISSN 146-5419

el-Deiry, W.S.; Tokino, T.; Velculescu, V.E.; Levy, D.B.; Parsons, R.; Trent, J.M.; Lin, D.; Mercer, W.E.; Kinzler, K.W. & Vogelstein, B. (1993). WAF1, a potential mediator of p53 tumor suppression. *Cell,* Vol.75, No.4, (September 1993), pp.817-825, ISSN 824-2752

Ewen, M.E.; Sluss, H.K.; Sherr, C.J.; Matsushime, H.; Kato, J. & Livingston, D.M. (1993). Functional interactions of the retinoblastoma protein with mammalian D-type cyclins. *Cell,* Vol.73, No.3, (May 1993), pp. 487–497, ISSN 834-3202

Falck, J.; Lukas, C.; Protopopova, M.; Lukas, J.; Selivanova, G. & Bartek, J. (2001). Functional impact of concomitant versus alternative defects in the Chk2–p53 tumour suppressor pathway. *Oncogene,* Vol.20, No.39, (September 2001), pp.5503- 5510, ISSN 1157-1648.

Falck, J.; Coates, J. & Jackson, S.P. (2005). Conserved modes of recruitment of ATM, ATR and DNA-PKcs to sites of DNA damage. *Nature,* Vol.434, No.7033, (March 2005), pp.605–611, ISSN 1575-8953

Feddersen, R.M.; Ehlenfeldt, R.; Yunis, W.S.; Clark, H.B. & Orr, H.T. (1992). Disrupted cerebellar cortical development and progressive degeneration of Purkinje cells in SV40 T antigen transgenic mice. *Neuron,* Vol.9, No.5, (November 1992),

Feddersen, R.M.; Clark, H.B.; Yunis, W.S. & Orr, H.T. (1995). In vivo viability of postmitotic Purkinje neurons requires pRb family member function. *Mol Cell Neurosci.* Vol.6, No.2, (April 1995), pp.153-167, ISSN 755-1567

Ferguson, A.T.; Evron, E.; Umbricht, C.B.; Pandita, T.; Chan, T.A.; Hermeking, H.; Marks, J.R.; Lambers, A.R.; Futreal, P.A.; Stampfer, M.R. & Sukumar, S. (2000). High frequency of hypermethylation at the 14-3-3sigma locus leads to gene silencing in breast cancer. *Proc Natl Acad Sci USA*, Vol.97, No.22, (May 2000), pp. 6049-6054, ISSN 1081-1911

Fernandez-Capetillo, O.; Lee, A.; Nussenzweig, M.; & Nussenzweig, A. (2004). H2AX: the histone guardian of the genome. *DNA Repair (Amst)*, Vol.3, No.8-9, (Aug-Sep 2004), pp.959–967, ISSN 1527-9782

Field, S.J.; Tsai, F.; Kuo, F.; Zubiaga, A.M.; Kaelin, Jr. W.G.; Livingston, D.M.; Orkin, S.H. & Greenberg, M.E. (1996). E2F-1 functions in mice to promote apoptosis and suppress proliferation. *Cell*, Vol.85, No.4, (May 1996), pp. 549–561, ISSN 865-3790

Fishel, M.L.; Vasko, M.R. & Kelley, M.R. (2007). DNA repair in neurons: so if they don't divide what's to repair? *Mutat Res*, Vol.614, No.1-2, (August 2006), pp.24–36, ISSN 1687-9837

Gagné, J.P.; Hendzel, M.J.; Droit, A. & Poirier, G.G. (2006). The expanding role of poly(ADP-ribose) metabolism: current challenges and new perspectives. *Curr Opin Cell Biol*, Vol.18, No.2, (April 2006), pp.145-151, ISSN 1651-6457

Garner, E. & Raj, K. (2008). Protective mechanisms of p53–p21–pRb proteins against DNA damage-induced cell death. *Cell Cycle*, Vol.7, No.3, (November 2008), pp.277–282, ISSN 1823-5223

Gell, D. & Jackson SP. (1999). Mapping of protein-protein interactions within the DNA-dependent protein kinase complex. *Nucleic Acids Res*, Vol.27, No.17, (September 1999), pp. 3494-3502, ISSN 1044-6239

Gobbel, G.T.; Bellinzona, M.; Vogt, A.R.; Gupta, N.; Fike, J.R. & Chan, P.H. (1998). Response of postmitotic neurons to X- irradiation: implications for the role of DNA damage in neuronal apoptosis. *J Neurosci*, Vol.18, No.1, (January 1998), pp.147–155, ISSN, 941-2495

Gorgoulis, V.; Vassiliou, L.V.; Karakaidos, P.; Zacharatos, P.; Kotsinas, A.; Liloglou, T.; Venere, M.; Ditullio, R.A. Jr.; Kastrinakis, N.G.; Levy, B.; Kletsas, D.; Yoneta, A.; Herlyn, M.; Kittas, C. & Halazonetis, T.D. (2005). Activation of the DNA damage checkpoint and genomic instability in human precancerous lesions. *Nature*, Vol.434, No.7035, (April 2005), pp. 907-913, ISSN 1582-9965

Gorodetsky, E.; Calkins, S.; Ahn, J. & Brooks, P.J. (2007). ATM, the Mre11/Rad50/Nbs1 complex, and topoisomerase I are concentrated in the nucleus of Purkinje neurons in the juvenile human brain. *DNA Repair (Amst)*, Vol.6, No.11, (August 2007), pp.1698-1707, ISSN 1770-6468

Gottlieb, T.M. & Jackson, S.P. (1993). The DNA-dependent protein kinase: requirement for DNA ends and association with Ku antigen. *Cell*, Vol.72, No.1, (January 1993), pp. 131-142, ISSN 842-2676

Gottschalk, A.J.; Timinszky, G.; Kong, S.E.; Jin, J.; Cai, Y.; Swanson, S.K.; Washburn, M.P.; Florens, L.; Ladurner, A.G.; Conaway, J.W. & Conaway, R.C. (2009). Poly(ADP-ribosyl)ation directs recruitment and activation of an ATP- dependent chromatin remodeler. *Proc Natl Acad Sci U S A*, Vol.106, No.33, (August 2009), pp. 13770-13774, ISSN 1966- 6485

Gottifredi, V.; Shieh, S.Y.; Taya, Y. & Prives, C. (2001). p53 accumulates but is functionally impaired when DNA synthesis is blocked. *Proc Natl Acad Sci USA*, Vol.98, No.3, (January 2001), pp.1036-1041, ISSN 1115-8590

Green, D.R. & Kroemer, G. (2009). Cytoplasmic functions of the tumour suppressor p53. *Nature*, Vol.458, No.7242, (April 2009), pp.1127-1130, ISSN 1940-7794

Groth, A.; Rocha, W.; Verreault, A. & Almouzni, G. (2007). Chromatin challenges during DNA replication and repair. *Cell*, Vol.128, (February 2007), pp. 721-733, ISSN 173-20509

Gu, Y.; Turck, C.W. & Morgan, D.O. (1993). Inhibition of CDK2 activity in vivo by an associated 20K regulatory subunit. *Nature*, Vol.366, No.6456, (December 1993), pp.707–710, ISSN 825-9216

Haince, J.F.; McDonald, D.; Rodrigue, A.; Déry, U.; Masson, J.Y.; Hendzel, M.J. & Poirier, G.G. (2008). PARP1-dependent kinetics of recruitment of MRE11 and NBS1 proteins to multiple DNA damage sites. *J Biol Chem*, Vol.283, No.21, (November 2008), pp.1197-1208, ISSN 1802-5084

Hakem, R. (2008). DNA-damage repair; the good, the bad, and the ugly. *EMBO J*, Vol.27, No.4, (February 2008), pp.589-605, ISSN 1828-5820

Hakmé, A.; Wong, H.K.; Dantzer, F. & Schreiber, V. (2008). The expanding field of poly(ADP-ribosyl)ation reactions. 'Protein Modifications: Beyond the Usual Suspects' Review Series. *EMBO Rep*, Vol.9, No.11, (October 2008), pp.1094-100, ISSN 1892-7583

Hammel, M.; Yu, Y.; Mahaney, B.L.; Cai, B.; Ye, R.; Phipps, B.M.; Rambo, R.P.; Hura, G.L.; Pelikan, M.; So, S.; Abolfath, R.M.; Chen, D.J.; Lees-Miller, S.P. & Tainer, J.A. (2009). Ku and DNA-dependent protein kinase dynamic conformations and assembly regulate DNA binding and the initial non-homologous end joining complex. *J Biol Chem*, Vol.285, No.2, (November 2009), pp.1414-1423, ISSN 1989-3054

Hammet, A.; Magill, C.; Heierhorst, J. & Jackson, S.P. (2007). Rad9 BRCT domain interaction with phosphorylated H2AX regulates the G1 checkpoint in budding yeast. *EMBO Rep*, Vol.8, No.9, (August 2007), pp.851-857, ISSN 1772-1446

Hammond, E.M.; Denko, N.C.; Dorie, M.J.; Abraham, R.T. & Giaccia, A.J. (2002). Hypoxia links ATR and p53 through replication arrest. *Mol Cell Biol*, Vol.22, No.6, (March 2002), pp.1834-1843, ISSN 1186-5061

Harper, J.W.; Adami, G.R.; Wei, N.; Keyomarsi, K. & Elledge, S.J. (1993). The p21 Cdk-interacting protein Cip1 is a potent inhibitor of G1 cyclin-dependent kinases. *Cell*, Vol.75, No.4, (November 1993), pp.805-816, ISSN 824-2751

Henrique, R.; Jeronimo, C.; Hoque, M.O.; Carvalho, A.L.; Oliveira, J.; Teixeira, M.R.; Lopes, C. & Sidransky, D. (2005). Frequent 14-3-3sigma promoter methylation in benign and malignant prostate lesions. *DNA Cell Biol*, Vol.24, No.4, (April 2005), pp.264-269, ISSN 1581-2243

Heo, K.; Kim, H.; Choi, S.H.; Choi, J.; Kim, K.; Gu, J.; Lieber, M.R.; Yang, A.S. & An, W. (2008). FACT-mediated exchange of histone variant H2AX regulated by phosphorylation of H2AX and ADP-ribosylation of Spt16. *Mol Cell*, Vol.30, No.1, (April 2008), pp.86-97, ISSN 1840-6329

Herrup, K.; Neve, R.; Ackerman, S.L. & Copani, A. (2004). Divide and die: cell cycle events as triggers of nerve cell death. *J Neurosci*, Vol.24, No.42, (October 2004), pp.9232-9239, ISSN 1549-6657

Herzog, K.H.; Chong, M.J.; Kapsetaki, M.; Morgan, J.I. & McKinnon, P.J. (1998). Requirement for Atm in ionizing radiation- induced cell death in the developing central nervous system. *Science*, Vol.280, No.55366, (May 1998), pp.1089–1091, ISSN 9582124

Hirao, A.; Kong, Y.Y.; Matsuoka, S.; Wakeham, A.; Ruland, J.; Yoshida, H.; Liu, D.; Elledge, S.J. & Mak, T.W. (2000). DNA damage-induced activation of p53 by the checkpoint kinase Chk2. *Science*, Vol.287, No.5459, (March 2000), pp.1824- 1827, ISSN 1071-0310

Hoffmann, I.; Clarke, P.R.; Marcote, M.J.; Karsenti, E. & Draetta, G. (1993). Phosphorylation and activation of human cdc25-C by cdc2–cyclin B and its involvement in the self-amplification ofMPFatmitosis. *EMBOJ*, Vol.12, No.1, (January 1993), pp.53-63, ISSN 842-8594

Höglinger, G.U.; Breunig, J.J.; Depboylu, C.; Rouaux, C.; Michel, P.P.; Alvarez-Fischer, D.; Boutillier, A.L.; Degregori, J.; Oertel, W.H.; Rakic, P.; Hirsch, E.C. & Hunot, S. (2007). The pRb/E2F cell-cycle pathway mediates cell death in Parkinson's disease. *Proc Natl Acad Sci USA*, Vol.104, No.9, (February 2007), pp.25-27, ISSN 1736-0686

Hopfner, K.P. (2009). DNA double-strand breaks come into focus. *Cell*, Vol.139, No.1, (October 2009), pp.25-27, ISSN 1980- 4750

Houtgraaf, J.H.; Versmissen, J. & van der Giessen, W.J. (2006). A concise review of DNA damage checkpoints and repair in mammalian cells. *Cardiovasc Revasc Med*, Vol.7, No.3, (July-September 2006), pp.165-172, ISSN 1694-5824

Huang, J.Y.; Chen, W.H.; Chang, Y.L.; Wang, H.T.; Chuang, W.T & Lee SC. (2006). Modulation of nucleosome-binding activity of FACT by poly(ADP-ribosyl)ation. *Nucleic Acids Res*, Vol.34, No.8, (May 2006), pp.2398-2407, ISSN 1668- 2447

Huen, M.S. & Chen, J. (2008). The DNA damage response pathways: at the crossroad of protein modifications. *Cell Res*, Vol.18, No.1, (January 2008), pp.8-16, ISSN 1808-7291

Husseman, J.W.; D. Nochlin, D. & Vincent, I. (2000). Mitotic activation: a convergent mechanism for a cohort of neurodegenerative diseases. *Neurobiol Aging*, Vol.21, No.6, (November 2000), pp.815-828, ISSN 1112-4425

Iaquinta, P.J. & Lees, J.A. (2007). Life and death decisions by the E2F transcription factors. *Curr Opin Cell Biol*, Vol.19, No.6, (November 2007), pp. 649–657, ISSN 1803-2011

Ikura, T.; Tashiro, S.; Kakino, A.; Shima, H.; Jacob, N.; Amunugama, R.; Yoder, K.; Izumi, S.; Kuraoka, I.; Tanaka, K.; Kimura, H.; Ikura, M.; Nishikubo, S.; Ito, T.; Muto, A.; Miyagawa, K.; Takeda, S.; Fishel, R.; Igarashi, K. & Kamiya, K. (2007). DNA damage-dependent acetylation and ubiquitination of H2AX enhances chromatin dynamics. *Mol Cell Biol*, Vol.27, No.20, August 2007), pp.7028-7040, ISSN 1770-9392

Jackson, S.P. (2009). The DNA-damage response: new molecular insights and new approaches to cancer therapy. *Biochem Soc Trans*, Vol.37, Pt.3, (June 2009), pp. 483–494, ISSN 1984-7258

Jackson, S.P. & Bartek, J. (2009). The DNA-damage response in human biology and disease. *Nature*, Vol.461, No.7267, (October 2009), pp.1071-1078, ISSN 1984-7258

Jansson, M.; Durant, S.T.; Cho, E.C.; Sheahan, S.; Edelmann, M.; Kessler, B. & La Thangue, N.B. (2008). Arginine methylation regulates the p53 response. *Nat Cell Biol*, Vol.10, No.12, (November 2008), pp. 1431-1439, ISSN 1901-1621

Jazayeri, A.; Falck, J.; Lukas, C.; Bartek, J.; Smith, G.C.; Lukas, J. & Jackson, S.P. (2006). ATM- and cell cycle-dependent regulation of ATR in response to DNA double-strand breaks *Nat Cell Biol*, Vol.8, No.1, (December 2005), pp.37-45, ISSN 1632-7781

Jeong, J.; Juhn, K.; Lee, H.; Kim, S.H.; Min, B.H.; Lee, K.M.; Cho, M.H.; Park, G.H. & Lee, K.H. (2007). SIRT1 promotes DNA repair activity and deacetylation of Ku70. *Exp Mol Med*, Vol.39, No.1, (February 2007), pp.8-13, ISSN 1733-4224

Jha, S.; Shibata, E. & Dutta, A. (2008). Human Rvb1/Tip49 is required for the histone acetyltransferase activity of Tip60/NuA4 and for the downregulation of phosphorylation on H2AX after DNA damage. *Mol Cell Biol*, Vol.28, No.8, (February 2008), pp. 2690-2700, ISSN 1828-5460

Jin, Y.H.; Yoo, K.J.; Lee, Y.H. & Lee SK. (2000). Caspase 3-mediated cleavage of p21WAF1/CIP1 associated with the cyclin A- cyclin-dependent kinase 2 complex is a prerequisite for apoptosis in SK-HEP-1 cells. *J Biol Chem*, Vol.275, No.39, (September 2000), pp.30256-30263, ISSN 1088-4382

Johnson, D.G.; Schwarz, J.K.; Cress, W.D. & Nevins, J.R. (1993). Expression of transcription factor E2F1 induces quiescent cells to enter S phase. *Nature*, Vol.365, No.6444, (September, 1993), pp.349-352. ISSN 837-7827

Jungmichel, S. & Stucki, M. (2010). MDC1: The art of keeping things in focus. *Chromosoma*, Vol.119, No.4, (March, 2010), pp.337-349. ISSN 2022-4865

Kaidi, A.; Weinert, B.T.; Choudhary, C. & Jackson, S.P. (2010). Human SIRT6 promotes DNA end resection through CtIP deacetylation. *Science*, Vol.329, No.5997, (September 2010), pp.1348-1353, ISSN 2082-9486

Karagiannis, T. C. & El-Osta, A. (2007). Chromatin modifications and DNA double-strand breaks: the current state of play. *Leukemia*, Vol.21, No.2, (December 2006), pp.195–200, ISSN 1715-1702

Kastan, M.B. & Bartek, J. (2004). Cell-cycle checkpoints and cancer. *Nature*, Vol. 432, No. 7015, (November 2004), pp.316– 323, ISSN 1554-9093

Khanna, K.K. & Jackson, S.P. (2001). DNA double-strand breaks: signaling, repair and the cancer connection. *Nat Genet*, Vol. 27, No.3, (March 2001), pp.247–254, ISSN 1124-2102

Khanna, K. K.; Lavin, M. F., Jackson, S. P. & Mulhern, T. D. (2001). ATM, a central controller of cellular responses to DNA damage. *Cell Death Differ*, Vol. 8, No. 11, (November 2001), pp.1052–1065, ISSN 1168-7884

Kim, D. & Tsai, L.H. (2009). Linking cell cycle reentry and DNA damage in neurodegeneration. *Ann N Y Acad Sci*, Vol. 1170, (July 2009), pp. 674-679, ISSN 1968-6210

Kim, M.Y.; Zhang, T. & Kraus, W.L. (2005). Poly(ADP-ribosyl)ation by PARP-1: 'PAR-laying' NAD+ into a nuclear signal. *Genes Dev*, Vol.19, No.17, (September 2005), pp.1951-1967, ISSN 1614-0981

Knights, C.D.; Catania, J.; Di Giovanni, S.; Muratoglu, S.; Perez, R.; Swartzbeck, A.; Quong, A.A.; Zhang, X.; Beerman, T.; Pestell, R.G. & Avantaggiati, M.L. (2006). Distinct p53 acetylation cassettes differentially influence gene-expression patterns and cell fate. *J Cell Biol*, Vol.173, No.4, (May 2006), pp.533-544, ISSN 1671-7128

Koch, C.A.; Agyei, R.; Galicia, S.; Metalnikov, P.; O'Donnell, P.; Starostine, A.; Weinfeld, M. & Durocher, D. (2004).Xrcc4 physically links DNA end processing by polynucleotide kinase to DNA ligation by DNA ligase IV. *EMBO J*, Vol. 23, No.19, (September 2004), pp. 3874–3885, ISSN 1538-5968

Kolas, N.K.; Chapman, J.R.; Nakada, S.; Ylanko, J.; Chahwan, R.; Sweeney, F.D.; Panier, S.; Mendez, M.; Wildenhain, J.; Thomson, T.M.; Pelletier, L.; Jackson, S.P. & Durocher, D. (2007). Orchestration of the DNA-damage response by the RNF8 ubiquitin ligase. *Science*, Vol.318, No.5856, (November 2007), pp.1637-1640, ISSN 1800-6705

Korotchkina, L.G.; Leontieva, O.V.; Bukreeva, E.I.; Demidenko, Z.N.; Gudkov, A.V. & Blagosklonny, M.V. (2010).The choice between p53-induced senescence and quiescence is determined in part by the mTOR pathway. *Aging (Albany NY)*, Vol.2, No.6, (June 2010), pp. 344-352, ISSN 2060-6252

Kraemer, K.H.; Sander, M. & Bohr, V.A. (2007). New areas of focus at workshop on human diseases involving DNA repair deficiency and premature aging. *Mech Ageing Dev*, Vol.128, No.2, (February 2007), pp.229-235, ISSN 1736-1460

Kraljevic Pavelic, S.; Cacev, T. & Kralj, M. (2008). A dual role of p21waf1/cip1 gene in apoptosis of HEp-2 treated with cisplatin or methotrexate. *Cancer Gene Ther*, Vol.15, No.9, (May 2008), pp. 576-590, ISSN 1848-3502

Krishnakumar, R. & Kraus, W.L. (2010). The PARP side of the nucleus: molecular actions, physiological outcomes, and clinical targets. *Mol Cell*, Vol.39, No.1, (July 2010), pp.8-24, ISSN 2060-3072

Kouzarides, T. (2007).Chromatin modifications and their function. *Cell*, Vol.128, No.4, (February 2007), pp.693–705, ISSN 1732-0507

Kruman, I.I. (2004). Why do neurons enter the cell cycle? *Cell Cycle*, Vol.3, No.6, (June 2004), pp. 769-773, ISSN 1513-6759

Kruman, I.I., Wersto, R.P.; Cardozo-Pelaez, F.; Smilenov, L.; Chan, S.; Chrest, F.; Emokpae, R. Jr.; Gorospe, M. & Mattson, M.P. (2004). Cell cycle activation linked to neuronal cell death initiated by DNA damage. *Neuron*, Vol.41, No.4, (February 2004), pp.549–561, ISSN 1498-0204

Kuan, C.Y.; Schloemer, A.J.; Lu, A.; Burns, K.A.; Weng, W.L.; Williams, M.T.; Strauss, K.I.; Vorhees, C.V.; Flavell, R.A.; Davis, R.J.; Sharp, F.R. & Rakic, P. (2004). Hypoxia-ischemia induces DNA synthesis without cell proliferation in dying neurons in adult rodent brain. *J Neurosci*, Vol.24, No.47, (November 2004), pp. 10763-10772, ISSN 1556-4594

Kumagai, A. & Dunphy, W.G. (2006) How cells activate ATR. *Cell Cycle*, Vol.5, No.12, (June 2006), pp. 1265-1268, ISSN 1676- 0665

Kuroda, Y.; Aishima, S.; Taketomi, A.; Nishihara, Y.; Iguchi, T.; Taguchi, K.; Maehara, Y. & Tsuneyoshi, M. (2007). 14-3- 3sigma negatively regulates the cell cycle, and its downregulation is associated with poor outcome in intrahepatic cholangiocarcinoma. *Hum Pathol*, Vol.38, No.7, (March 2007), pp. 1014-1022, ISSN 1739-1729

Kusch, T.; Florens, L.; Macdonald, W.H.; Swanson, S.K.; Glaser, R.L.; Yates, J.R. 3rd.; Abmayr, S.M.; Washburn, M.P. & Workman, J.L. (2004). Acetylation by Tip60 is required for selective histone variant exchange at DNA lesions. *Science*, Vol.306, No.5704, (November 2004), pp.2084-2087, ISSN 1552-8408

Lal, A.; Abdelmohsen, K.; Pullmann, R.; Kawai, T.; Galban, S.; Yang, X.; Brewer, G. & Gorospe, M. (2006). Posttranscriptional derepression of GADD45alpha by genotoxic stress. *Mol Cell*, Vol.22, No.1, (April 2006), pp.117-128, ISSN 1660-0875

Laronga, C.; Yang, H.Y.; Neal, C. & Lee, M.H. (2000). Association of the cyclin-dependent kinases and 14-3-3sigma negatively regulates cell cycle progression. *J Biol Chem*, Vol. 275, No.30, (July 2000), pp. 23106-23112, ISSN 1076-7298

Lavin, M.F. & Kozlov, S. (2007). DNA damage-induced signalling in ataxia–telangiectasia and related syndromes. *Radiother Oncol*, Vol. 83, No.3, (May 2007), pp.231–237, ISSN 1751-2070

Le Cam, L.; Linares, L.K.; Paul, C.; Julien, E.; Lacroix, M.; Hatchi, E.; Triboulet, R.; Bossis, G.; Shmueli, A.; Rodriguez, M.S.; Coux, O. & Sardet, C. (2006). E4F1 is an atypical ubiquitin ligase that modulates p53 effector functions independently of degradation. *Cell*, Vol.127, No.4, (November 2006), pp. 775-788, ISSN 1711-0336

Lee, E.W.; Lee, M.S.; Camus, S.; Ghim, J.; Yang, M.R.; Oh, W.; Ha, N.C.; Lane, D.P. & Song, J. (2009).Differential regulation of p53 and p21 by MKRN1 E3 ligase controls cell cyclearrest and apoptosis, *EMBO J,*. Vol.28, No.14, (June 2009), pp.2100–2113, ISSN 1953-6131

Lee, J.H. & Paull, T.T. (2005). ATM activation by DNA double-strand breaks through the Mre11-Rad50-Nbs1 complex. *Science,* Vol.308, No. 5721, (March 2005), pp.551-554, ISSN 1579-0808

Lee, J.H., Choy, M.L., Ngo, L., Foster, S.S., Marks, P.A. (2010). Histone deacetylase inhibitor induces DNA damage, which normal but not transformed cells can repair. *Proc Natl Acad Sci U S A,* Vol.107, No.33, (August 2010), pp.14639-14644, ISSN 2067-9231

Lee, S.M.; Bae, J.H.; Kim, M.J.; Lee, H.S.; Lee, M.K.;Chung, B.S.; Kim, D.W.; Kang, C.D. & Kim, S.H. (2007). Bcr-Abl- independent imatinib-resistant K562 cells show aberrant protein acetylation and increased sensitivity to histone deacetylase inhibitors. *J Pharmacol Exp Ther,* Vol.322, No.3, (June 2007), pp.1084-1092, ISSN 1756-9822

Lee, Y. & McKinnon, P.J. (2000). ATM dependent apoptosis in the nervous system. *Apoptosis* Vol.5, No.6, (December 2000), pp.523–529, ISSN 1130-3911

Lee, Y.; Chong, M.J. & McKinnon PJ. (2001). Ataxia telangiectasia mutated–dependent apoptosis after genotoxic stress in the developing nervous system is determined by cellular differentiation status. *J Neurosci,* Vol.21, No.17, (September 2001), pp.6687–6693, ISSN 1151-7258

Lee, Y. & McKinnon, P.J. (2007). Responding to DNA double strand breaks in the nervous system. *Neuroscience,* Vol.145, No.4, (April 2007), pp.1365-1374, ISSN 16934412

Leroy, C.; Lee, S.E.; Vaze, M.B.; Ochsenbien, F.; Guerois, R.; Haber, J.E. & Marsolier-Kergoat, M.C. (2003). PP2C phosphatases Ptc2 and Ptc3 are required for DNA checkpoint inactivation after a double-strand break. *Mol Cell,* Vol.285, No.2, (November 2003), pp.1414-1423, ISSN 1989-3054

Levine, A.J. & Oren, M. (2009). The first 30 years of p53: growing ever more complex. *Nat Rev Cancer,* Vol.9, No.10, (October 2009), pp.749-758, ISSN 1977-6744

Levkau, B.; Koyama, H.; Raines, E.W.; Clurman, B.; Herren, B.; Orth, K.; Roberts, J.M. & Ross, R. (1998). Cleavage of p21Cip1/Waf1 and p27Kip1 mediates apoptosis in endothelial cells through activation of Cdk2: role of a caspase cascade. *Mol Cell,* Vol.1, No.4, (March 1998), pp.553-563, ISSN 966-0939

Li, X.; Corsa, C.A.; Pan, P.W.; Wu, L.; Ferguson, D.; Yu, X.; Min, J. & Dou, Y. (2010). MOF and H4 K16 acetylation play important roles in DNA damage repair by modulating recruitment of DNA damage repair protein Mdc1. *Mol Cell Biol,* Vol.30, No.22, (September 2010), pp.5335-5347, ISSN 2083-7706

Lieber MR. (2010). The mechanism of double-strand DNA break repair by the nonhomologous DNA end-joining pathway. *Annu Rev Biochem,* Vol.79, pp. 181-211, ISSN 2019-2759

Lisby, M; Barlow, J.H.; Burgess, R.C. & Rothstein, R. (2004). *Cell,* Vol.118, No.6, (September 2004), pp.699-713, ISSN 1536- 9670

Liu, Z.M.; Chen, G.G.; Ng, E.K.; Leung, W.K.; Sung, J.J. & Chung, S.C. (2004). Upregulation of heme oxygenase-1 and p21 confers resistance to apoptosis in human gastric cancer cells. *Oncogene*, Vol.23, No.2, (January 2004), pp.503-13, ISSN 1464-7439

Lobrich, M. & Jeggo, P.A. (2007). The impact of a negligent G2/M checkpoint on genomic instability and cancer induction. *Nat Rev Cancer*, Vol. 7, No.11, (November 2007), pp.861–869, ISSN 1794-3134

Lu, T.; Pan, Y.; Kao, S.Y.; Li, C.; Kohane, I.; Chan, J. & Yankner, B.A. (2004). Gene regulation and DNA damage in the ageing human brain. *Nature*, Vol.429, No.6994, (June 2004), pp.883-891, ISSN 1519-0254

Lukas, C.; Bartkova, J.; Latella, L.; Falck, J.; Mailand, N.; Schroeder, T.; Sehested, M.; Lukas, J. & Bartek, J. (2001). DNA damage-activated kinase Chk2 is independent of proliferation or differentiation yet correlates with tissue biology. *Cancer Res*, Vol.61, No.13, (July 2001), pp.4990-4903, ISSN 1143-1331

Luo, J.; Nikolaev, A.Y.; Imai, S.; Chen, D.; Su, F.; Shiloh, A.; Guarente, L. & Gu, W. (2001). Negative control of p53 by Sir2alpha promotes cell survival under stress. *Cell*, Vol.107, No.2, (October 2001), pp. 137-148, ISSN 1167-2522

Macůrek, L.; Lindqvist, A.; Voets, O.; Kool, J.; Vos, H.R. & Medema, R.H. (2010). Wip1 phosphatase is associated with chromatin and dephosphorylates gammaH2AX to promote checkpoint inhibition. *Oncogene*, Vol.29, No.15, (January 2010), pp.2281-2291, ISSN 2010-1220

Mahaney, B.L.; Meek, K. & Lees-Miller, S.P. (2009). Repair of ionizing radiation-induced DNA double-strand breaks by non- homologous end-joining. *Biochem*, Vol.417, No.3, (February 2009), pp.639–650, ISSN 1913-3841

Mailand, N.; Bekker-Jensen,S.; Bartek, J. & Lukas, J. (2006). Destruction of Claspin by SCFbetaTrCP restrains Chk1 activation and facilitates recovery from genotoxic stress. *Mol Cell*, Vol.23, No.3, (August 2006), pp.307–318, ISSN 1688-5021

Mamely, I., van Vugt, M.A., Smits, V.A., Semple, J.I., Lemmens, B., Perrakis, A., Medema, R.H, & Freire, R. (2006). Pololike kinase-1 controls proteasome-dependent degradation of claspin during checkpoint recovery. *Curr Biol*, Vol.16, No.19, (August 2006), pp. 1950-1955, ISSN 1693-4469

Marchenko. N.D.; Zaika, A. & Moll, U.M. (2000) Death signal-induced localization of p53 protein to mitochondria. A potential role in apoptotic signaling. *J Biol Chem*, Vol.275, No.21, (May 2000), pp.16202–16212, ISSN 1082-1866

Martin, L.J. (2008). DNA damage and repair: relevance to mechanisms of neurodegeneration. *J Neuropathol Exp Neurol*, Vol.67, No.5, (May 2008), pp.377-387, ISSN 1843-1258

Martin, L.J.; Liu, Z.; Pipino, J.; Chestnut, B. & Landek, M.A. (2009). Molecular regulation of DNA damage-induced apoptosis of neurons in cerebral cortex. *Cerebral Cortex*, Vol.19, No.6, (September 2008), pp. 1273-1293, ISSN 1882-0287

Martinez, L.A.; Yang, J.; Vazquez, E.S.; Rodriguez-Vargas Mdel, C.; Olive, M.; Hsieh, J.T.; Logothetis, C.J. & Navone, N.M. (2002).p21 modulates threshold of apoptosis induced by DNA-damage and growth factor withdrawal in prostate cancer cells. *Carcinogenesis*, Vol.23, No.8, (August 2002), pp.1289–1296, ISSN 1215-1346

Mazumder, S.; Plesca, D.; Kinter, M. & Almasan, A. (2007). Interaction of a cyclin e fragment with Ku70 regulates bax- mediated apoptosis. *Mol Cell Biol*, Vol.27, No.9, (February 2007), pp.3511-3520, ISSN 1732-5036

McKinnon, P.J. (2001). Ataxia telangiectasia: new neurons and ATM. *Trends Mol Med*, Vol.7, No.6, (June 2001), pp.233-234, ISSN 1137-8498

McMurray, C.T. (2005). To die or not to die: DNA repair in neurons. *Mutat Res*, Vol.577, No.1-2, (September 2005), pp.260– 274, ISSN 1592-1706

McShea, A.; Wahl, A.F. & Smith, M.A. (1999). Re-entry into the cell cycle: a mechanism for neurodegeneration in Alzheimer disease. *Med Hypotheses*, Vol.52, No.6, (June 1999), pp. 525–527, ISSN 1045-9833

Meek, D.W. (1994). Post-translational modification of p53. *Semin Cancer Biol*, Vol.5, No.3, (June 1994), pp.203-210, ISSN 794- 8948

Melander, F.; Bekker-Jensen, S.; Falck, J.; Bartek, J.; Mailand, N. & Lukas, J. (2008). Phosphorylation of SDT repeats in the MDC1 N terminus triggers retention of NBS1 at the DNA damage-modified chromatin. *J Cell Biol*, Vol.181, No.2, (April 2008), pp.213-226, ISSN 1841-1307

Melino, G. (2003) p73, the ''assistant'' guardian of the genome? *Ann N Y Acad Sci*, Vol.1010, pp.9-15, ISSN 1503-3688

Meng, S.; Arbit, T.; Veeriah, S.; Mellinghoff, I.K.; Fang, F.; Vivanco, I.; Rohle, D. & Chan, T.A. (2009). 14-3-3sigma and p21 synergize to determine DNA damage response following Chk2 inhibition. *Cell Cycle*, Vol.8, No.14, (July 2009), pp. 2238- 2246, ISSN 1950-2805

Merkle, D.; Douglas, P.; Moorhead, G.B.; Leonenko, Z.; Yu, Y.; Cramb, D.; Bazett-Jones, D.P. & Lees-Miller, S.P. (2002). The DNA-dependent protein kinase interacts with DNA to form a protein-DNA complex that is disrupted by phosphorylation. *Biochemistry*, Vol.41, No.42, (October 2002), pp.12706-12714, ISSN 1237-9113

Milczarek, G.J.; Martinez, J. & Bowden, G.T. (1997). p53 Phosphorylation: biochemical and functional consequences. *Life Sci*, Vol.60, No.1, pp.1-11, ISSN 899-5526

Messick TE, Greenberg RA. (2009). The ubiquitin landscape at DNA double-strand breaks. *J Cell Biol*, Vol.187, No.3, (November 2009), pp.319-326. ISSN 1994-8475

Mihara, M.; Erster, S.; Zaika, A.; Petrenko, O.; Chittenden, T.; Pancoska, P. & Moll, U.M. (2003) p53 has a direct apoptogenic role at the mitochondria. *Mol Cell*, Vol.11, No.3, (March 2003), pp. 577-590. ISSN 1266-7443

Miller, S.A.; Mohn, S.E. & Weinmann, A.S. (2010). Jmjd3 and UTX play a demethylase-independent role in chromatin remodeling to regulate T-box family member-dependent gene expression. *Mol Cell*, Vol.40, No.4, (November 2010), pp.594-605, ISSN 2109-5589

Mimori, T. & Hardin, J.A.(1986). Mechanism of interaction between Ku protein and DNA. *J Biol Chem*, Vol.261, No,22, (August 1986), pp.10375-10379, ISSN 301-5926

Morselli, E.; Galluzzi, L.; Kepp, O. & Kroemer, G. (2009). Nutlin kills cancer cells via mitochondrial p53. *Cell Cycle*, Vol.8, No.11, (June 2009), pp. 1647-1648, ISSN 1944-8434

Mortusewicz, O.; Amé, J.C.; Schreiber, V. & Leonhardt, H. (2007). Feedback-regulated poly(ADP-ribosyl)ation by PARP-1 is required for rapid response to DNA damage in living cells. *Nucleic Acids Res*, Vol.35, No.22, (November 2007), pp.7665- 7675, ISSN 1798-2172

Moynahan, M.E.; Chiu, J.W.; Koller, B.H. & Jasin, M. (1999). Brca1 controls homology-directed DNA repair. *Mol Cell*, Vol. 4, No.4, (October 1999), pp.511-518, ISSN 1054-9283

Murr, R.; Loizou, J.I.; Yang, Y.G.; Cuenin, C.; Li, H.; Wang, Z.Q. & Herceg, Z. (2006). Histone acetylation by Trrap-Tip60 modulates loading of repair proteins and repair of DNA double-strand breaks. *Nat Cell Biol,* Vol.8, No.1, (Dec 2006), pp.91–99, ISSN 1634-1205

Nagayama, T.; Lan, J.; Henshall, D.C.; Chen, D.; O'Horo, C.; Simon, R.P. & Chen, J. (2000). Induction of oxidative DNA damage in the peri-infarct region after permanent focal cerebral ischemia. *J Neurochem,* Vol.75, No.4, (October 2000), pp.1716-1728, ISSN 1098-7855

Nakada, S.; Chen, G.I.; Gingras, A.C. & Durocher, D. (2008). PP4 is a gamma H2AX phosphatase required for recovery from the DNA damage checkpoint. *EMBO Rep,* Vol.9, No.10, (August 2008), pp.1019-1026, ISSN 1875-8438

Nakamura, T.M.; Du, L.L.; Redon, C. & Russell, P. (2004). Histone H2A phosphorylation controls Crb2 recruitment at DNA breaks, maintains checkpoint arrest, and influences DNA repair in fission yeast. *Mol Cell Biol,* Vol.24, No.1,14, (July 2004), pp.6215-6230, ISSN 1522-6425

Narciso, L.; Fortini, P.; Pajalunga, D.; Franchitto, A.; Liu, P.; Degan, P.; Frechet, M.; Demple, B.; Crescenzi, M. & Dogliotti, E. (2007). Terminally differentiated muscle cells are defective in base excision DNA repair and hypersensitive to oxygen injury. *Proc Natl Acad Sci U S A,* Vol.104, No.43, (October 2007), pp.17010-17015, ISSN 1794-0040

Nicassio, F.; Corrado, N.; Vissers, J.H.; Areces, L.B.; Bergink, S.; Marteijn, J.A.; Geverts, B.; Houtsmuller, A.B.; Vermeulen, W.; Di Fiore, P.P. & Citterio, E. (2007). Human USP3 is a chromatin modifier required for S phase progression and genome stability. *Curr Biol,* Vol.17, No.22, (November 2007), pp.1972-1977, ISSN 1798-0597

Nouspikel, T. & Hanawalt, P.C. (2000). Terminally differentiatedhuman neurons repair transcribed genes but display attenuated global DNA repair and modulation of repair gene expression.*Mol Cell Biol,* Vol.20, No.5, (March 2000), pp.1562–1570, ISSN 1066-9734

Nouspikel, T. & Hanawalt, P.C. (2002). DNA repair in terminally differentiated cells. *DNA Repair (Amst),* Vol.1, No.1, (January 2002), pp.59-75, ISSN 1250-9297

Nouspikel, T. (2007). DNA repair in differentiated cells: some new answers to old questions. *Neuroscience,* Vol.145, No.4, (August 2006), pp.1213-1221, ISSN 1692-0273

Oberdoerffer, P.; Michan, S.; McVay, M.; Mostoslavsky, R.; Vann, J.; Park, S.K.; Hartlerode, A.; Stegmuller, J.; Hafner, A.; Loerch, P.; Wright, S.M.; Mills, K.D.; Bonni, A.; Yankner, B.A.; Scully, R.; Prolla, T.A.; Alt, F.W. & Sinclair, D.A. (2008). SIRT1 redistribution on chromatin promotes genomic stability but alters gene expression during aging. *Cell,* Vol.135, No.5, (November 2008), pp.907-918, ISSN 1904-1753

O'Hagan, H.M.; Mohammad, H.P. & Baylin, S.B. (2008). Double strand breaks can initiate gene silencing and SIRT1- dependent onset of DNA methylation in an exogenous promoter CpG island. *PLoS Genet,* Vol.4, No.8, (August 2008), pp.e1000155, ISSN 1870-4159

O'Hare, M.J.; Hou, S.T.; Morris, E.J.; Cregan, S.P.; Xu, Q.; Slack, R.S. & Park, D.S. (2000). Induction and modulation of cerebellar granule neuron death by E2F-1. *J Biol Chem,* Vol.275, No.33, (August 2000), pp. 25358–25364, ISSN 1085- 1232

Okoshi, R.; Ozaki, T.; Yamamoto, H.; Ando, K.; Koida, N.; Ono, S.; Koda, T.; Kamijo, T.; Nakagawara, A. & Kizaki, H. (2008). Activation of AMP-activated protein kinase induces p53-dependent apoptotic cell death in response to energetic stress. *J Biol Chem,* Vol.283, No.7, (December 2007), pp. 3979-3987, ISSN 1805-6705

Oku, T.; Ikeda, S.; Sasaki, H.; Fukuda, K.; Morioka, H.; Ohtsuka, E.; Yoshikawa, H. & Tsurimoto, T. (1998). Functional sites of human PCNA which interact with p21 (Cip1/Waf1), DNA polymerase delta and replication factor C. *Gene Cells*, Vol.3, No.6, (June 1998), pp. 357-369, ISSN 973-4782

Otsuka, Y.; Tanaka, T.; Uchida, D.; Noguchi, Y.; Saeki, N.; Saito, Y. & Tatsuno, I. (2004). Roles of cyclin-dependent kinase 4 and p53 in neuronal cell death induced by doxorubicin on cerebellar granule neurons in mouse. *Neurosci Lett*, Vol.365, No.3, (July 2004), pp. 180-185, ISSN 1524-6544

Pajalunga, D.; Mazzola, A.; Salzano, A.M.; Biferi, M.G.; De Luca, G. & Crescenzi, M. (2007). Critical requirement for cell cycle inhibitors in sustaining nonproliferative states. *J Cell Biol*, Vol.176, No.6, (March 2007), pp.1039-1056, ISSN 1735-3358

Pardo, B.; Gómez-González, B. & Aguilera, A. (2009). DNA repair in mammalian cells: DNA double-strand break repair: how to fix a broken relationship. *Cell Mol Life Sci*, Vol.66, No.6, (March 2009), pp.1039-1056, ISSN 1915-3654

Park, D.S.; Morris, E.J.; Greene, L.A. & Geller, H.M. (1997). G1/S cell cycle blockers and inhibitors of cyclin-dependent kinases suppress camptothecin-induced neuronal apoptosis. *J Neurosci*, Vol.17, No.4, (February 1997), pp. 1256–1270, ISSN 900- 6970

Park, D.S.; Morris, E.J.; Padmanabhan, J.; Shelanski, M.L.; Geller, H.M. & Greene, L.A. (1998). Cyclin-dependent kinases participate in death of neurons evoked by DNA-damaging agents. *J Cell Biol*, Vol.143, No.2, (October 1998), pp.457–467, ISSN 978-6955

Perry, J.J.; Yannone, S.M.; Holden, L.G.; Hitomi, C.; Asaithamby, A.; Han, S.; Cooper, P.K.; Chen, D.J. & Tainer, J.A. (2006). WRN exonuclease structure and molecular mechanism imply an editing role in DNA end processing. *Nat Struct Mol Biol*, Vol.13, No.5, (April 2006), pp.414-422. ISSN 1662-2405

Peterson, C.L. & Cote, J. (2004) Cellular machineries for chromosomal DNA repair. *Genes Dev*, Vol.18, No.6, (March 2004), pp.602-616. ISSN 1507-5289

Phillips, A.C. & Vousden, K.H. (2001). E2F-1 induced apoptosis. *Apoptosis*, Vol.6, No.3, (June 2001), pp.173–182. ISSN 1138- 8666

Pickart, C.M. (2001). Ubiquitin enters the new millennium. *Mol Cell*, Vol.8, No.3, (September 2001), pp.499-504. ISSN 1158- 3613

Picard, F.; Kurtev, M.; Chung, N.; Topark-Ngarm, A.; Senawong, T.; Machado De Oliveira, R.; Leid, M.; McBurney, M.W. & Guarente, L. (2004). Sirt1 promotes fat mobilization in white adipocytes by repressing PPAR-gamma. *Nature,* Vol.429, No.6993, (June 2004), pp. 771-776, ISSN 1517-5761

Poehlmann, A. & Roessner, A. (2010). Importance of DNA damage checkpoints in the pathogenesis of human cancers. *Pathol Res Pract*, Vol.206, No.9, (August 2010), pp. 591-601, ISSN 2067-4189

Polager, S. & Ginsberg, D. (2008). E2F - at the crossroads of life and death. *Trends Cell Biol*, Vol.18, No.11, (September 2008), pp. 528-535, ISSN 1880-5009

Polager, S. & Ginsberg, D. (2009). p53 and E2f: partners in life and death. *Nat Rev Cancer*, Vol.9, No.10, (October 2009), pp.738-748, ISSN 1977-6743

Polo, S.E.; Kaidi, A.; Baskcomb, L.; Galanty, Y.& Jackson, S.P. (2010). Regulation of DNA-damage responses and cell-cycle progression by the chromatin remodelling factor CHD4. *EMBO J*, Vol.29, No.18, (August 2010), pp.3130-3139, ISSN 2069-3977

Polo, S.E. & Jackson, S.P. (2011). Dynamics of DNA damage response proteins at DNA breaks: a focus on protein modifications. *Genes Dev*, Vol.25, No.5, (March, 2011), pp.409-33, ISSN 2136-3960

Qin, S. & Parthun, M.R. (2006). Recruitment of the type B histone acetyltransferase Hat1p to chromatin is linked to DNA double-strand breaks. *Mol Cell Biol*, Vol.26, No.9, (May 2006), pp.3649-3658, ISSN 1661-2003

Rass, U.; Ahel, I. & West, S.C. (2007). Defective DNA repair and neurodegenerative disease. *Cell*, Vol.130, No.6, (September 2007), pp.991-1004, ISSN 1788-9645

Reagan-Shaw, S. & Ahmad, N. (2005). Silencing of polo-like kinase (Plk) 1 via siRNA causes induction of apoptosis and impairment of mitosis machinery in human prostate cancer cells: implications for the treatment of prostate cancer. *FASEB J*, Vol.19, No.6, (January 2005), pp.611-613, ISSN 1566-1849

Reed, J.C. (2006). Proapoptotic multidomain Bcl-2/Bax-family proteins: mechanisms, physiological roles and therapeutic opportunities. *Cell Death Differ*, Vol.13, No.8, (June 2006), pp.1378-1386, ISSN 1672-9025

Reinhardt, H.C. & Yaffe, M.B. (2009). Kinases that control the cell cycle in response to DNA damage: Chk1, Chk2, and MK2. *Curr Opin Cell Biol*, Vol.21, No.2, (February 2009), pp.245-255, ISSN 1923-0643

Rich, T.; Allen, R.L. & Wyllie, A.H. (2000). Defying death after DNA damage. *Nature*, Vol.407, No.6805, (October 2000), pp.777-783, ISSN 1104-8728

Riley, T.; Sontag, E.; Chen, P. & Levine, A. (2008). Transcriptional control of human p53-regulated genes. *Nat Rev Mol Cell Biol*, Vol.9, No.5, (May 2008), pp.402-412, ISSN 1843-1400

Rinaldo, C.; Prodosmo, A.; Mancini, F.; Iacovelli, S.; Sacchi, A.; Moretti, F. & Soddu, S. (2007). MDM2-regulated degradation of HIPK2 prevents p53Ser46 phosphorylation and DNA damage-induced apoptosis. *Mol Cell*, Vol.25, No.5, (March 2007), pp.739-750, ISSN 1734-9959

Rogakou, E.P.; Pilch, D.R.; Orr, A.H.; Ivanova, V.S. & Bonner, W.M. (1998). DNA double-stranded breaks induce histone H2AX phosphorylation on serine 139. *J Biol Chem*, 1998 Mar 6;Vol.273, No.10, (March 1998), pp.5858-5868, ISSN 9488723

Rogoff, H.A. & Kowalik, T.F. (2004). Life, death and E2F: linking proliferation control and DNA damage signaling via E2F1. *Cell Cycle*, Vol.3, No.7, (July 2004), pp. 845-846, ISSN 1519-0206

Rolig, R.L. & McKinnon, P.J. (2000). Linking DNA damage and neurodegeneration. *Trends Neuroscie*, Vol.23, No.9, (September 2000), pp. 417-424, ISSN 1094-1191

Roshak, A.K.; Capper, E.A.; Imburgia, C.; Fornwald, J.; Scott, G. & Marshall, L.A. (2000). The human polo-like kinase PLK, regulates cdc2/cyclin B through phosphorylation and activation of the cdc25C phosphatase, *Cell Signal*, Vol.12, No.6, (June 2000), pp. 405-411, ISSN 1120-2906

Rossi, M.; De Laurenzi, V.; Munarriz, E.; Green, D.R.; Liu, Y.C.; Vousden, K.H.; Cesareni, G. & Melino, G. (2005) The ubiquitin-protein ligase Itch regulates p73 stability. *EMBO J*, Vol.24, No.4, (February 2005), pp. 836-848, ISSN 1567- 8106

Rouse, J. & Jackson SP. (2002). Interfaces between the detection, signaling, and repair of DNA damage. *Science*, Vol.297, No.5581, (July, 2002), pp. 547-551, ISSN 1214-2523]

Sakaguchi, K.; Herrera, J.E.; Saito, S.; Miki, T.; Bustin, M.; Vassilev, A.; Anderson, C.W. & Appella, E. (1998). DNA damage activates p53 through a phosphorylation-acetylation cascade. *Genes Dev*, Vol.12, N0.18, (September 1998), pp.2831-2841, ISSN 9744-860

Sancar, A.; Lindsey-Boltz, L.A.; Unsal-Kacmaz, K. & Linn, S. (July 2004). Molecular mechanisms of mammalian DNA repair and the DNA damage checkpoints. *Annu Rev Biochem, Vol.* 73, No. , (January, 2004), pp.39–85, ISSN 1518-9136

Sanders, S.L.; Arida, A.R. & Phan, F.P. (2010). Requirement for the phospho-H2AX binding module of Crb2 in double-strand break targeting and checkpoint activation. *Mol Cell Biol*, Vol.30, N0.19, (August 2010), pp.4722-4731, ISSN 2067-9488

Sartori, A.A.; Lukas, C.; Coates, J.; Mistrik, M.; Fu, S.; Bartek, J.; Baer, R.; Lukas, J. & Jackson, S.P. (2007). Human CtIP promotes DNA end resection. Nature, Vol.450, No.7169, (October 2007), pp.509–514, ISSN 1796-5729

Schlereth, K.; Beinoraviciute-Kellner, R.; Zeitlinger, M.K.; Bretz, A.C.; Sauer, M.; Charles, J.P.; Vogiatzi, F.; Leich, E.; Samans, B.; Eilers, M.; Kisker, C.; Rosenwald, A. & Stiewe, T. (2010). DNA binding cooperativity of p53 modulates the decision between cell cycle arrest and apoptosis. *Mol Cell*, Vol.38, No.3, (May 2010), pp.356-368, ISSN 2047-1942

Schmetsdorf, S.; Gartner, U. & Arendt, T. (2007). Constitutive expression of functionally active cyclin dependent kinases and their binding partners suggests noncanonical functions of cell cycle regulators in differentiated neurons. *Cereb Cortex,* Vol.17, No.8, (October 2006), pp.1821–1829, ISSN 1705-0646

Schmetsdorf, S.; Arnold, E.; Holzer, M.; Arendt, T.& Gartner, U. (2009). A putative role for cell cycle-related proteins in microtubule-based neuroplasticity. *Eur J Neurosci* , Vol.29, No.6, (March 2009), pp.1096–10107, ISSN 1930-2146

Schuler, M.; Bossy-Wetzel, E.; Goldstein, J.C.; Fitzgerald, P. & Green, D,R. (2000) p53 induces apoptosis by caspase activation through mitochondrial cytochrome c release. *J Biol Chem*, Vol.275, No.10, (March 2000), pp. 7337-7342, ISSN 1070-2305

Shanbhag, N.M.; Rafalska-Metcalf, I.U.; Balane-Bolivar, C.; Janicki, S.M. & Greenberg, R.A. (2010). ATM-dependent chromatin changes silence transcription in cis to DNA double-strand breaks. *Cell*, Vol.1413, No.6, (June 2010), pp.970– 981. ISSN 2055-0933

Shao, G.; Lilli, D.R.; Patterson-Fortin, J.; Coleman, K.A.; Morrissey, D.E. & Greenberg, R.A. (2009). The Rap80-BRCC36 de- ubiquitinating enzyme complex antagonizes RNF8-Ubc13-dependent ubiquitination events at DNA double strand breaks. *Proc Natl Acad Sci U S A*, Vol.106, No.9, (February 2009), pp. 3166-3171, ISSN 1920-2061

Sharma, S. (2007). Age-related nonhomologous end joining activity in rat neurons. *Brain Res Bull*, Vol.73, No1-3, (June 2007), pp.48–54. ISSN 1749-9636

Sharma, G.; Mirza, S.; Parshad, R.; Srivastava, A.; Gupta, S.D.; Pandya, P. & Ralhan, R. (2010). Clinical significance of promoter hypermethylation of DNA repair genes in tumor and serum DNA in invasive ductal breast carcinoma patients. *Life Sci*, Vol.87, No.3-4, (May 2010), pp.83-91, ISSN 2047-0789

Shieh, S-Y.; Ikeda, M.; Taya, Y. & Prives, C. (1997). DNA damage-induced phosphorylation of p53 alleviates inhibition by MDM2. *Cell*, Vol.91, No.3, (October, 2003), pp. 325-334, ISSN 936-3941

Shieh, S.Y.; Ahn, J.; Tamai, K.; Taya, Y. & Prives, C. (2000). The human homologs of checkpoint kinases Chk1 and Cds1 (Chk2) phosphorylate p53 at multiple DNA damage-inducible sites. *Genes Dev*, Vol.14, No.3, (February, 2000), pp. 289- 300, ISSN 1067-3501

Shiloh, Y. (2003). ATM and related protein kinases: safeguarding genome integrity. *Nat Rev Cancer*, 2003; Vol.3, No.3, (March, 2003), pp.155-168, ISSN 1261-2651

Shiloh, Y. (2006). The ATM-mediated DNA-damage response: taking shape. *Trends Biochem Sci*, Vol.31, No.7 (June 2006), pp.402-10. ISSN 1677-4833

Singleton, B.K.; Torres-Arzayus, M.I.; Rottinghaus, S.T.; Taccioli, G.E. & Jeggo, P.A. (1999). The C terminus of Ku80 activates the DNA-dependent protein kinase catalytic subunit. *Mol Cell Biol*, Vol.19, No.15, (May 1999), pp. 3267-3277, ISSN1020- 7052

Sinha, S.; Malonia, S.K.; Mittal, S.P.; Singh, K.; Kadreppa, S.; Kamat, R.; Mukhopadhyaya, R.; Pal, J.K. & Chattopadhyay, S. (2010). Coordinated regulation of p53 apoptotic targets Bax and Puma by SMAR1 through an identical MAR element. *EMBO J*, Vol.29, No.4, (January 2010), pp.830-842, ISSN 2007-5864

Smerdon MJ, Tlsty TD, Lieberman MW. (1978). Distribution of ultraviolet-induced DNA repair synthesis in nuclease sensitive and resistant regions of human chromatin. *Biochemistry*, Vol.17, No.12, (June 1978), pp.2377–2386, ISSN 678515

Smith, D.S.; Leone, G.; DeGregori, J.; Ahmed, M.N.; Qumsiyeh, M.B. & Nevins, J.R. (2000). Induction of DNA replication in adult rat neurons by deregulation of the retinoblastoma/E2F G1 cell cycle pathway. *Cell Growth Differ*, Vol.11, No.12, (December 2000), pp. 625-633, ISSN 1114-9597

Sofueva S, Du LL, Limbo O, Williams JS, Russell P. (2010). BRCT domain interactions with phospho-histone H2A target Crb2 to chromatin at double-strand breaks and maintain the DNA damage checkpoint. *Mol Cell Biol*, Vol.30, No.19, (August 2010), pp.4732-4743, ISSN 2067-9485

Sordet, O.; Redon, C.E.; Guirouilh-Barbat, J.; Smith, S.; Solier, S.; Douarre, C.; Conti, C.; Nakamura, A.J.; Das, B.B.; Nicolas, E.; Kohn, K.; Bonner, W.M. & Pommier, Y. (2009). Ataxia telangiectasia mutated activation by transcription- and topoisomerase I-induced DNA double-strand breaks. *EMBO Rep*, Vol.10, No.8, (June 2009), pp.887-893, ISSN 1955-7000

Soutoglou, E. & Misteli, T. (2008). Activation of the cellular DNA damage response in the absence of DNA lesions. *Science*, Vol.320, No.5882, (May 2008), pp.1507-1510, ISSN 1848-3401

Spycher, C.; Miller, E.S.; Townsend, K.; Pavic, L.; Morrice, N.A.; Janscak, P.; Stewart, G.S. & Stucki, M. (2008). Constitutive phosphorylation of MDC1 physically links the MRE11-RAD50-NBS1 complex to damaged chromatin. *J Cell Biol*, Vol.181, No.2, (April 2008), pp.227-240, ISSN 1841-1308

Stark, G.R. & Taylor, W.R. (2006). Control of the G2/M transition. *Mol. Biotechnol*, Vol.32, No.3, (March 2006), pp.227-248, ISSN 1663-2889

Steelman, L.S. & McCubrey, J.A. (2010). Intriguing novel abilities of Nutlin-3A: induction of cellular quiescence as opposed to cellular senescence - implications for chemotherapy. *Cell Cycle*, Vol.8, No.22, (November 2010), pp. 3634-3635, ISSN 1987-5921

Stewart, G.S.; Wang, B.; Bignell, C.R.; Taylor, A.M. & Elledge, S.J. (2003). MDC1 is a mediator of the mammalian DNA damage checkpoint. *Nature*, Vol.421, No.6926, (February 2003), pp. 961–966, ISSN1260-7005

Stewart, N.; Hicks, G.G.; Paraskevas, F. & Mowat, M. (1995). Evidence for a second cell cycle block at G2/M by p53. *Oncogene*, Vol. 10, No.1, (January 1995), pp. 109-115, ISSN 7529-916

Stiff, T.; O'Driscoll, M.; Rief, N.; Iwabuchi, K.; Löbrich, M. & Jeggo, P.A. (2004). ATM and DNA-PK function redundantly to phosphorylate H2AX after exposure to ionizing radiation. *Cancer Res*, Vol.64, No.7, (April 2004), pp.2390-2396, ISSN 1505-9890

Stracker, T.H.; Couto, S.S.; Cordon-Cardo, C.; Matos, T. & Petrini, J.H. (2008). Chk2 suppresses the oncogenic potential of DNA replication-associated DNA damage. *Mol Cell* Vol.31, No.1, (July 2008), pp.21-32, ISSN 1861-4044

Stucki, M.; Clapperton, J.A.; Mohammad, D.; Yaffe, M.B.; Smerdon, S.J. & Jackson SP. (2005). MDC1 directly binds phosphorylated histone H2AX to regulate cellular responses to DNA double-strand breaks. *Cell*, Vol.123, No.7, (December 2005), pp.1213–1226, ISSN 1637-7563

Subramanian, C.; Opipari, A.W. Jr.; Bian, X.; Castle, V.P. & Kwok, R.P. (2005). Ku70 acetylation mediates neuroblastoma cell death induced by histone deacetylase inhibitors. *Proc Natl Acad SciUSA*, Vol.102, No.13, (March 2005), pp. 4842-4847, ISSN 1577-8293

Suzuki, A.; Tsutomi, Y.; Akahane, K.; Araki, T. & Miura, M. (1998). Resistance to Fas-mediated apoptosis: activation of caspase 3 is regulated by cell cycle regulator p21WAF1 and IAP gene family ILP. *Oncogene*, Vol.17, No.8, (August 1998), pp. 931-939, ISSN 974-7872

Suzuki, A.; Tsutomi, Y.; Miura, M. & Akahane, K. (1999). Caspase 3 inactivation to suppress Fas-mediated apoptosis: identification of binding domain with p21 and ILP and inactivation machinery by p21. *Oncogene*, Vol.18, No.5, (February 1999), pp. 1239-1244, ISSN 1002-2130

Sykes, S.M.; Mellert, H.S.; Holbert, M.A.; Li, K.; Marmorstein, R.; Lane, W.S. & McMahon, S.B. (2006). Acetylation of the p53 DNA-binding domain regulates apoptosis induction. *Mol Cell*, Vol.24, No.6, (December 2006), pp.841-851, ISSN 1718- 9187

Syljuasen, R.G.; Jensen, S.; Bartek, J. & Lukas, J. (2006) Adaptation to the ionizing radiation-induced G2 checkpoint occurs in human cells and depends on checkpoint kinase 1 and Polo-like kinase 1 kinases. *Cancer Res*, Vol.66, No.21, (November 2006), pp.10253–10257, ISSN 1707-9442

Tanaka, T.; Ohkubo, S.; Tatsuno, I. & Prives, C. (2007). hCAS/CSE1L associates with chromatin and regulates expression of select p53 target genes. *Cell*, Vol.130, No.4, (August 2007), pp.638-650, ISSN 1771-9542

Tang, Y.; Luo, J.; Zhang, W. & Gu, W. (2006). Tip60-dependent acetylation of p53 modulates the decision between cell cycle arrest and apoptosis. *Mol Cell*, Vol.24, No.6, (December 2006), pp.827-839, ISSN 1718-9186

Tamburini, B.A. & Tyler, J.K. (2005). Localized histone acetylation and deacetylation triggered by the homologous recombination pathway of double-strand DNA repair. *Mol Cell Biol*, 2005 Jun;Vol.25, No.12, (June 2005), pp.4903-4913, ISSN 1592-3609

Taylor, W.R. & Stark, G.R. (2001). Regulation of the G2/M transition by p53. *Oncogene*, Vol.20, No.15, (April 2001), pp.1803- 1815, ISSN1131-3928

Tibbetts, R.S.; Brumbaugh, K.M.; Williams, J.M.; Sarkaria, J.N.; Cliby, W.A.; Shieh, S.Y.; Taya, Y.; Prives, C. & Abraham, R.T. (1999). A role for ATR in the DNA damageinduced phosphorylation of p53. *Genes Dev*, Vol.13, No.2, (January 1999), pp. 152-157, ISSN 992-5639

Timinszky, G.; Till, S.; Hassa, P.O.; Hothorn, M.; Kustatscher, G.; Nijmeijer, B.; Colombelli, J.; Altmeyer, M.; Stelzer, E.H.; Scheffzek, K.; Hottiger, M.O. & Ladurner, A.G.

(2009). A macrodomain-containing histone rearranges chromatin upon sensing PARP1 activation. *Nat Struct Mol Biol*, Vol.16, No.9, (August 2009), pp.923-929, ISSN 1968-0243

Toczyski, D.P.; Galgoczy, D.J. & Hartwell, L.H. (1997) CDC5 and CKII control adaptation to the yeast DNA damage checkpoint. *Cell*, Vol.90, No.6, (September 1997), pp.1097-10106, ISSN 932-3137

Tofilon, P.J. & Meyn, E. (1988). Reduction in DNA repair capacity following differentiation of murine proadipocytes. *Exp. Cell Res*, Vol.174, No.2, (February 1988), pp.502–510, ISSN 333-8499

Tomashevski, A.; Webster, D.R.; Grammas, P.; Gorospe, M. & Kruman, I.I. (2010). Cyclin-C-dependent cell-cycle entry is required for activation of non-homologous end joining DNA repair in postmitotic neurons. *Cell Death Differ*. Vol.17, No.7 (January 2010), pp.1189-1198, ISSN 2011-1042

Trushina, E. &C McMurray, C.T. (2007). Oxidative stress and mitochondrial dysfunction in neurodegenerative diseases. *Neuroscience*, Vol.145, No.4 (February 2007), pp.1233–1248, ISSN 1730-3344

Uziel T, Lerenthal Y, Moyal L, Andegeko Y, Mittelman L, Shiloh Y. (2003). Requirement of the MRN complex for ATM activation by DNA damage. *EMBO J*, Vol.22, No20, (October 2003), pp.5612-5621, ISSN 1453-2133

van Attikum, H.; Fritsch, O.; Hohn, B. & Gasser, S.M.(2004). Recruitment of the INO80 complex by H2A phosphorylation links ATP-dependent chromatin remodeling with DNA double-strand break repair. *Cell*, Vol.119, No.6,(December 2004), pp.777-788, ISSN 1560-7975

van Attikum, H.; Fritsch, O. & Gasser, S.M. (2007). Distinct roles for SWR1 and INO80 chromatin remodeling complexes at chromosomal double-strand breaks. *EMBO J*, Vol.26, No.18, (August 2007), pp.4113-4125. ISSN 1776-2868

Van Attikum, H. & Gasser, S.M. (2005) The histone code at DNA breaks: a guide to repair? *Nat Rev Mol Cell Biol*, Vol. 6, No.10, (October 2005), pp.757-765, ISSN 1616-7054

van Attikum, H. & Gasser, S.M. (2009). Crosstalk between histone modifications during the DNA damage response. *Trends Cell Biol*, Vol.19, No.5, (April 2009), pp.207-217, ISSN 1934-2239

van Gent, D.C. & van der Burg, M. (2007). Non-homologous end-joining, a sticky affair. *Oncogene*, Vol. 26, No.56, (December 2007), pp. 7731–7740, ISSN 1806-6085

van Vugt, M.A. & Medema, R.H. (2004). Checkpoint adaptation and recovery: back with Polo after the break. *Cell Cycle*, Vol.3, No.11, (November 2004), pp. 1383-1386, ISSN 1549-2511

van Vugt, M.A.; Bras, A. & Medema, R.H. (2004). Polo-like kinase-1 controls recovery from a G2 DNA damage-induced arrest in mammalian cells. *Mol Cell*, Vol. 15, No.5, (September 2004), pp.799-811, ISSN 1535-0223

van Vugt, M.A.; Gardino, A.K.; Linding, R.; Ostheimer, G.J.; Reinhardt, H.C.; Ong, S.E.; Tan, C.S.; Miao, H.; Keezer, S.M.; Li, J.; Pawson, T.; Lewis, T.A.; Carr, S.A.; Smerdon, S.J.; Brummelkamp, T.R. & Yaffe, M.B. (2010). A mitotic phosphorylation feedback network connects Cdk1, Plk1, 53BP1, and Chk2 to inactivate the G(2)/M DNA damage checkpoint. *PLoS Biol*, Vol. 8, No.1, (January 2010), pp.e1000287, ISSN 2012-6263

Vaseva, A.V.; Marchenko, N.D. & Moll, U.M. (2009). The transcription-independent mitochondrial p53 program is a major contributor to nutlin-induced apoptosis in tumor cells. *Cell Cycle*, Vol.8, No.11, (June 2009), pp.1711-1719, ISSN 1941- 1846

Vaze, M.B.; Pellicioli, A.; Lee, S.E.; Ira, G.; Liberi, G.; Arbel-Eden, A.; Foiani, M. & Haber JE. (2002) Recovery from checkpoint-mediated arrest after repair of a double-strand break requires Srs2 helicase. *Mol Cell*, Vol. 10, No.2, (August 2002), pp. 373–385, ISSN 1219-1482

Vaziri, H.; Dessain, S.K.; Ng Eaton, E.; Imai, S.;, Frye, R.A.; Pandita, T.K.; Guarente, L. & Weinberg, R.A. (2001). hSIR2(SIRT1) functions as an NAD-dependent p53 deacetylase. *Cell*, Vol.107, No.2, (October 2001), pp. 149-159, ISSN 1167-2523

Waldman, T.; Lengauer, C.; Kinzler, K.W. & Vogelstein, B. (1996). Uncoupling of S phase and mitosis induced by anticancer agents in cells lacking p21. *Nature*, Vol.381, No.6584, (June 1996), pp.713-716, ISSN 864-9519

Waldman, T.; Zhang, Y.; Dillehay, L.; Yu, J.; Kinzler, K.; Vogelstein, B. & Williams, J. (1997). *Cell cycle*, arrest versus cell death in cancer therapy. *Nat Med*, Vol.3, No.9, (September 1997), pp. 1034-1036, ISSN 928-8734

Wang, M.; Wu, W.; Wu, W.; Rosidi,B.; Zhang,L.; Wang, H. & Iliakis, G. (2006). PARP-1 and Ku compete for repair of DNA double strand breaks by distinct NHEJ pathways. *Nucleic Acids Res*, 2006;Vol.34, No.21, (November 2006), pp.6170- 6182, ISSN 1708-8286

Ward, I.M. & Chen, J. (2001). Histone H2AX is phosphorylated in an ATR-dependent manner in response to replicational stress. *J Biol Chem*, Vol.276, No.51, (October 2001), pp.47759-47762, ISSN 1167-3449

Warbrick, E.; Lane, D.P.; Glover, D.M. & Cox, L.S. (1995). A small peptide inhibitor of DNA replication defines the site of interaction between the cyclin-dependent kinase inhibitor p21WAF1 and proliferating cell nuclear antigen. *Curr Biol*, Vol.5, No.3, (March 1995), pp.275-282, ISSN 778-0738

Wefel, J.S.; Kayl, A.E. & Meyers, C.A. (2004). Neuropsychological dysfunction associated with cancer and cancer therapies: a conceptual review of an emerging target. *Br J Cancer*, Vol. 90, No.9 (May, 2004), pp.1691-1696, ISSN 1515-0608

Weissman, L.; de Souza-Pinto, N.C.; Stevnsner, T. & Bohr, V.A. (2007). DNA repair, mitochondria, and neurodegeneration. *Neuroscience*, Vol. 145, No.4 (November, 2006), pp.1318–1329, ISSN 1709-2652

Wilker, E.W.; van Vugt, M.A.; Artim, S.A.; Huang, P.H.; Petersen, C.P.; Reinhardt, H.C.; Feng, Y.; Sharp, P.A.; Sonenberg, N.; White, F.M. & Yaffe, M.B. (2007). 14-3-3sigma controls mitotic translation to facilitate cytokinesis. *Nature*, Vol.446, No.7133 (March 2007), pp.329-332, ISSN 1736-1185

Wilson, D. M. 3rd. & McNeill, D. R. (2007). Base excision repair and the central nervous system. *Neuroscience*, Vol.145, No.4 (August 2006), pp.1187–1200, ISSN 1693-4943

Xiong, Y.; Hannon, G.J.; Zhang, H.; Casso, D.; Kobayashi, R. & Beach, D. (1993). p21 is a universal inhibitor of cyclin kinases. *Nature*, Vol.366, No.6456, (December 1993), pp.701-704, ISSN 825-9214

Xu Y, Sun Y, Jiang X, Ayrapetov MK, Moskwa P, Yang S, Weinstock DM, Price BD. (2010). The p400 ATPase regulates nucleosome stability and chromatin ubiquitination during DNA repair. *J Cell Biol*, Vol.191, No.1, (September 2010), pp.31-43, ISSN 2087-6283

Yamaguchi, H.; Woods, N.T.; Piluso, L.G.; Lee, H.H.; Chen, J.; Bhalla, K.N.; Monteiro, A.; Liu, X.; Hung, M.C. & Wang, H.G. (2009). p53 acetylation is crucial for Its transcription-independentproapoptotic functions. *J Biol Chem*, Vol.284, No.17, (March 2009), pp. 11171-11183, ISSN 1926-5193

Yamasaki, L.; Jacks, T.; Bronson, R.; Goillot, E.; Harlow, E. & Dyson, N.J. (1996). Tumor induction and tissue atrophy in mice lacking E2F-1. *Cell*, Vol.85, No.4, (May 1996), pp.537–548, ISSN 865-3789

Yang, W.; Dicker, D.T.; Chen, J. & El-Deiry, W.S. (2008). CARPs enhance p53 turnover by degrading 14-3-3sigma and stabilizing MDM2. *Cell Cycle*, Vol.7, No.5, (January 2008), pp. 670-682, ISSN 1838-2127

Yang, Y. & Herrup, K. (2001). Loss of neuronal cell cycle control in ataxia-telangiectasia: a unified disease mechanism, *J Neurosci*, Vol.21, No.8, (April 2001), pp. 2661–2668 , ISSN 1130-6619

Yang, Y.; Geldmacher, D.S. & Herrup, K. (2001) DNA replication precedes neuronal cell death in Alzheimer's disease. *J Neurosci*, Vol.21, No.7, (April 2001), pp. 2661–2668 , ISSN1130-6619

Yano, K.; Morotomi-Yano, K.; Wang, S.Y.; Uematsu, N.; Lee, K.J.; Asaithamby, A.; Weterings, E. & Chen, D.J. (2008). Ku recruits XLF to DNA double-strand breaks. *EMBO Rep*, Vol.9, No.1, (January 2008), pp.91-96, ISSN 1806-4046

Yi, J. & Luo, J. (2010). SIRT1 and p53, effect on cancer, senescence and beyond. *Biochim Biophys Acta*, Vol.1804, No.8, (May 2008), pp. 1684-1689, ISSN 2047-1503

Yoo, H.Y.; Kumagai, A.; Shevchenko, A.; Shevchenko, A. & Dunphy, W.G. (2004). Adaptation of a DNA replication checkpoint response depends upon inactivation of Claspin by the Polo-like kinase. *Cell*, Vol.117, No.5, (May 2004), pp. 575-588, ISSN 1516-3406

Zhang, Y.; Qu, D.; Morris, E.J.; O'Hare, M.J.; Callaghan, S.M.; Slack, R.S.; Geller, H.M. & Park, D.S. (2006). The Chk1/Cdc25A pathway as activators of the cell cycle in neuronal death induced by camptothecin. *J Neurosci*, Vol.26, No.34, (August 2006), pp. 8819–8828, ISSN 1692-8871

Zhang, Y.; Hefferin, M.L.; Chen, L.; Shim, E.Y.; Tseng, H.M.; Kwon, Y.; Sung, P.; Lee, S.E. & Tomkinson, A.E. (2007). Role of Dnl4-Lif1 in nonhomologous end-joining repair complex assembly and suppression of homologous recombination. *Nat Struct Mol Biol*, Vol.14, No.7, (June 2007), pp.639-46, ISSN 1758-9524

Zhou, B.B. & Elledge, S.J. (2000). The DNA damage response: putting checkpoints in perspective. *Nature*, Vol.408, No.6811, (November 2000), pp. 433–439, ISSN 1110-0718

Zimmermann, K.C.; Bonzon, C. & Green, D.R. (2001). The machinery of programmed cell death. *Pharmacol Ther*, Vol.92, No.1, (October 2001), pp.57-70, ISSN 1175-0036

Ziv, Y.; Bielopolski, D.; Galanty, Y.; Lukas, C.; Taya, Y.; Schultz, D.C.; Lukas, J.; Bekker-Jensen, S.; Bartek, J. & Shiloh, Y. (2006). Chromatin relaxation in response to DNA double-strand breaks is modulated by a novel ATM- and KAP-1 dependent pathway. *Nat Cell Biol*, Vol. 8, No.8, (July 2006), pp. 870–876, ISSN 1686-2143

15

TopBP1 in DNA Damage Response

Ewa Forma, Magdalena Brys and Wanda M. Krajewska
Department of Cytobiochemistry, University of Lodz
Poland

1. Introduction

DNA, the genetic material of cells, is constantly exposed to a range of endogenous and environmental damaging agents (Jungmichel & Stucki, 2010). DNA molecule is the target of endogenous cellular metabolites such as reactive oxygen species (ROS) (Ciccia & Elledge, 2010; Poehlmann & Roessner, 2010). ROS may cause different alterations in a genome, e.g. simple DNA mutations, DNA single and double strand breaks (SSBs and DSBs, respectively), or more complex changes, including deletions, translocations and fusions (Poehlmann & Roessner, 2010). Alterations may be generated spontaneously due to dNTP misincorporation during DNA replication, interconversion between DNA bases caused by deamination, loss of DNA bases following DNA depurination or depyrimidination and modification of DNA bases by alkylation. Hydrolytic deamination (loss of an amino group) can directly convert one base to another. For example, deamination of cytosine results in uracil and with much lower frequency converts adenine to hypoxanthine. In depurination or depyrimidination, purine or pyrimidine bases are completely removed, leaving deoxyribose sugar depurinated or depyrimidinated that may cause breakage in the DNA backbone (Ciccia & Elledge, 2010; Rastogi et al., 2010). Altogether, it has been estimated that every cell could experience up to 10^5 spontaneous DNA lesions per day (Ciccia & Elledge, 2010). Environmental DNA damage can be produced by physical or chemical sources, such as ionizing radiation (IR), ultraviolet (UV) light from sunlight and organic and inorganic chemical substances (Muniandy et al., 2010; Rastogi et al., 2010; Su et al., 2010). Exposure to ionizing radiation from, e.g. cosmic radiation and medical treatments employing X-rays or radiotherapy inflicts DNA single and double strand breaks, oxidation of DNA bases and DNA-protein crosslinks in the genomic DNA (Ciccia & Elledge, 2010; Su et al., 2010). Ionizing radiation provokes DNA damage directly by energy deposit on the DNA double helix and indirectly by reactive oxygen/nitrogen species (ROS/RNS) (Corre et al., 2010). Ultraviolet radiation (mainly UV-B) is a powerful agent that may lead to the formation of three major classes of DNA lesions, such as cyclobutane pyrimidine dimmers (CPDs), pyrimidine 6-4 pyrimidone photoproducts (6-4 PPs) and their Devar isomers (Rastogi et al., 2010). Cells may become transiently exposed to external sources of DNA damage, such as cigarette smoke or various toxic chemical compounds (Jungmichel & Stucki, 2010). Many antineoplastic drugs currently used in cancer treatment express their cytotoxic effects through their ability to directly or indirectly damage DNA and thus resulting in cell death. Major types of DNA damage induced by anticancer treatment include single and double strand breaks, interstrand, intrastrand and DNA-protein crosslinks, as well as interference with nucleotide metabolism and DNA synthesis (Pallis & Karamouzis, 2010). Alkylating agents, such as methyl methanesulphonate (MMS), tenozalamide, streptozotocin, procarbazine, dacarbazine, ethylnitrosourea, diethylnitrosamine and nitrosoureas attach alkyl groups to DNA bases, while crosslinking agents such as mitomycin (MMC), cisplatin, psoralen and nitrogen mustard induce covalent links between bases of the same DNA strand (intrastrand crosslinks) or of different DNA strands (interstrands crosslinks) (Ciccia & Elledge, 2010; Muniandy et al., 2010; Pallis & Karamouzis, 2010). Other chemical agents, such as topoisomerase inhibitors induce the formation of single or double strand breaks by trapping topoisomerase-DNA covalent complexes (Ciccia & Elledge, 2010). Camptothecin and novel noncamptothecins in clinical development target eukaryotic IB type topoisomerase (Topo I), whereas human IIA type topoisomerases (Topo IIα and Topo IIβ) are the targets of widely used anticancer agents, such as etoposide, anthracyclines (doxorubicin, daunorubicin) and mitoxantrone (Pommier et al., 2010).

The biochemical consequences of DNA lesions are diverse and range from obstruction of fundamental cellular pathways like transcription and replication to fixation of mutations. Cellular misfunctioning, cell death, aging and cancer are the phenotypical consequences of DNA damage accumulation in the genome. To counteract DNA damage, repair mechanisms specific for many types of lesions have evolved. Mispaired DNA bases are replaced with correct bases by mismatch repair (MMR) (Ciccia & Elledge, 2010). The bases excision repair (BER) exerts its biological role by removing bases that have been damaged by alkylation, oxidation, ring saturation, as well as a short strand that contains the damaged bases. BER also plays an important role in the repair of DNA single strand breaks generated spontaneously or induced by exogenous DNA-damaging factors such as cytotoxic anticancer agents (Pallis & Karamouzis, 2010). DNA single strand breaks may be also repaired by single strand break repair (SSBR) (Ciccia & Elledge, 2010). Nucleotide excision repair (NER) is a highly conserved pathway that repairs DNA damage caused by UV radiation, mutagenic chemicals or chemotherapeutic drugs that form bulky DNA adducts (Pallis & Karamouzis, 2010). The most toxic lesions in DNA are double strand breaks where the phosphate backbones of the two complementary DNA strands are broken simultaneously (Hiom, 2010). Double strand breaks are repaired by two major repair pathways depending on the context of DNA damage, i.e. homologous recombination (HR) and nonhomologous end-joining (NHEJ) (Hiom, 2010; Pallis & Karamouzis, 2010). While NHEJ promotes potential inaccurate relegation of double strand breaks, HR precisely restores genomic sequence of the broken DNA ends by using sister chromatids as template for repair (Ciccia & Elledge, 2010). Additionally, some specialized polymerases can temporarily take over lesion-arrested DNA polymerases during S phase, in a mutagenic mechanism called translesion synthesis (TLS). Such polymerases only work if a more reliable system, such as homologous recombination, cannot avoid stumbled DNA replication (Essers et al., 2006).

DNA repair is carried out by the plethora of enzymatic activities that chemically modify DNA to repair DNA damage, including nucleases, helicases, polymerases, topoisomerases, recombinases, ligases, glycosylases, demethylases, kinases and phosphatases. These repair tools must be precisely regulated, because each in its own right can wreak havoc on the integrity of DNA if misused or allowed to gain access to DNA at the inappropriate time or place (Ciccia & Elledge, 2010). The DNA repair mechanisms function in conjunction with an intricate machinery of damage sensors, responsible of a series of phosphorylations and chromatin modifications that signal to the rest of the cell the presence of lesions on DNA.

Together DNA repair mechanisms and DNA damage signaling system form a molecular shield against genomic instability.

2. DNA damage checkpoints

To maintain genomic integrity and faithful transmission of fully replicated and undamaged DNA during cell division, eukaryotic organisms evolved a complex DNA surveillance program (Reihardt & Yaffe, 2009). Apart from DNA repair mechanisms mentioned above, DNA damage response represents a complex network of multiple signaling pathways involving cell cycle checkpoints, transcriptional regulation, chromatin remodeling and apoptosis (Dai & Grant, 2010; Danielsen et al., 2009). In response to DNA damage, eukaryotic cells activate a complex protein kinase-based signaling network to arrest progression through the cell cycle. Activation of signaling cascade recruits repair machinery to the site of DNA damage, provides time for repair or if the genotoxic insult exceeds repair capacity, additional signaling pathways leading to cell death, presumably *via* apoptosis, are activated (Reinhardt et al., 2010; Reinhardt & Yaffe, 2009). When DNA damage occurs, distinct, albeit overlapping and cooperating checkpoint pathways are activated, which block S phase entry (the G1/S phase checkpoint), delay S phase progression (the S phase checkpoints) or prevent mitotic entry (the G2/M phase checkpoint). The primary G1/S cell cycle checkpoint controls the commitment of eukaryotic cells to transition through G1 phase and enter DNA synthesis phase. In G1 phase, cells have to make a decision between continuing proliferation or exiting the cell cycle to become quiescent differentiated, senescent or apoptotic (Dijkstra et al., 2009). The S phase checkpoints are activated when DNA damage occurs during DNA synthesis, or when DNA replication intermediates accumulate. Depending on the type and magnitude of damage, cells activate one of three distinct S phase checkpoint pathways: an intra-S phase checkpoint induced by double strand breaks, a replication checkpoint by the stalled replication fork and the S/M checkpoint blocking premature mitosis. The S/M checkpoint differs from the well-defined G2/M checkpoint. The S/M checkpoint is ATM-independent, it is measurable only several hours after DNA damage and is initiated in cells that were in S phase at the time of insult (Hurley & Bunz, 2009; Rodriguez-Bravo et al., 2007). When cells encounter DNA damage in G2, the G2/M checkpoint stops the cell cycle to prevent the cell from entering mitosis. Defects in cell cycle arrest at the respective checkpoint are associated with genome instability and oncogenesis (Houtgraaf et al., 2006).

3. Checkpoint signaling cascade

Proteins of checkpoint signaling pathways are classified as sensors, transducers and effectors (Fig. 1). Following DNA damage, sensor multiprotein complexes, e.g. MRN (MRE11-Rad50-NBS1) or 9-1-1 (Rad9-Rad1-Hus1) recognize damage and recruit proximal transducers, i.e. ATM (ataxia telangiectasia mutated) and ATR (ATM and Rad3-related) kinases to lesions where they are initially activated. ATM and ATR transduce signals to distal transducer, i.e. checkpoint kinases Chk1 and Chk2 (Dai & Grant, 2010; Niida & Nakanishi, 2006). Chk1 and Chk2 kinases, distal transducers, transfer the signal of DNA damage to effectors, such as Cdks (cyclin-dependent kinases), Cdc25 (cell division cycle 25) and p53 (Dai & Grant, 2010; Houtgraaf et al., 2006; Nakanishi, 2009; Nakanishi et al., 2009). The key difference between ATM and ATR is the signal that activates them. ATM is activated exclusively by DSBs, which can arise from endogenous (ROS, eroded telomeres, intermediates of immune and meiotic recombination) or exogenous (IR, genotoxic drugs) sources (Lopez-Contreras & Fernandez-Capetillo, 2010). In contrast, ATR responds to many types of DNA damage and replication stress including breaks, crosslinks and base adducts. ATR senses abnormally long stretches of single strand DNA that arise from the functional uncoupling of helicase and polymerase activities at replication forks or from the processing of DNA lesions such as the resection of DSBs (Mordes & Cortez, 2008). ATR but not ATM is essential for viability. The early embryonic death in ATR knockout mice shows that ATR is essential for cell growth and differentiation at an early stage of development (Smits et al., 2010). In addition, disruption of ATR in mouse or human cells results in cell cycle arrest or death, even without exogenous DNA damage (Cortez et al., 2001; Smits et al., 2010). Although complete inactivation of ATR is lethal, a hypomorphic mutation was found in humans suffering from the rare autosomal recessive disorder, Seckel syndrome, characterized by growth retardation and microcephaly. In homozygosity, that mutation affects ATR splicing which results in the reduction of ATR protein levels to almost undetectable, yet the remaining protein is sufficient for viability (Kerzendorfer & O'Driscoll, 2009; O'Driscoll et al., 2004; Smits et al., 2010).

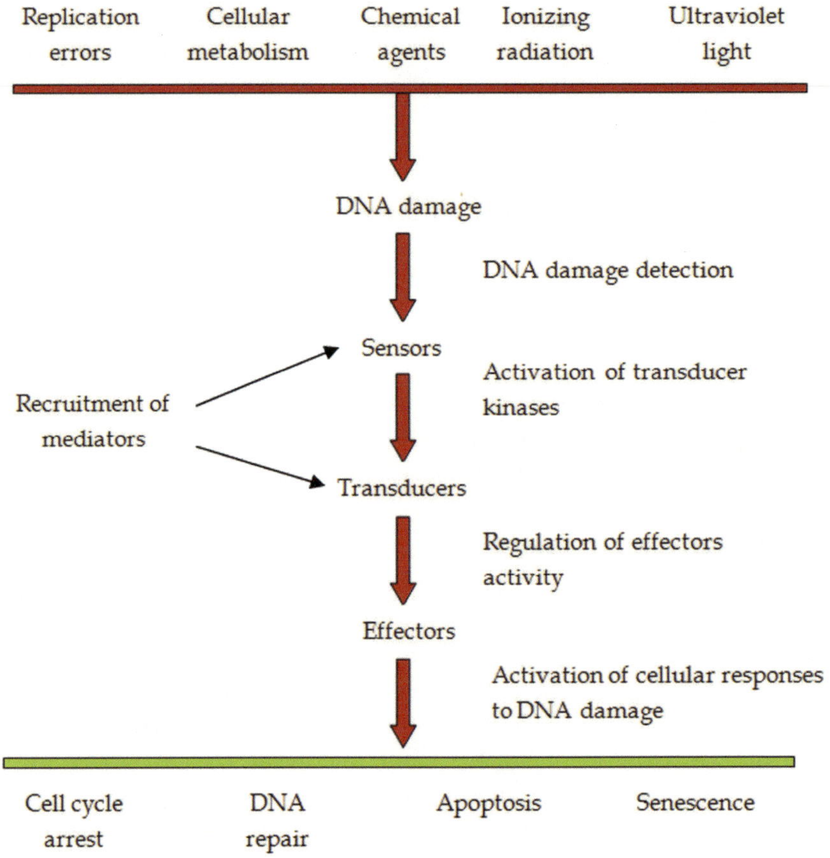

Fig. 1. Signal transduction of DNA damage response (DDR)

In addition to damage sensors and signal transducers, many other proteins called mediators are involved in DNA damage response. Mediators are mostly cell cycle specific proteins associated with damage sensors and signal transducers at particular phases of the cell cycle and, as a consequence, help provide signal transduction specificity. ATM and ATR phosphorylate most of these mediators. Well-known examples of mediators are 53BP1 (p53 binding protein 1), MDC1 (mediator of DNA damage checkpoint 1), BRCA1 (breast cancer 1), SMC1 (structural maintenance of chromosomes 1), FANCD2 (Fanconi anemia, complementation group D2), Claspin, Timeless, Tipin and histone H2AX (Dai & Grant, 2010; Houtgraaf et al., 2006; Yang et al., 2010). This group of regulators involves also TopBP1 protein (topoisomerase IIβ binding protein 1) (Cimprich & Cortez, 2008). Certain molecules may have multiple functions in this signal transduction pathway. For example ATM and ATR can simultaneously act as a sensor and a transducer. Consequently, signal transduction in DNA damage response is not one-dimensional but a complex network of interacting molecules (Poehlmann & Roessner, 2010).

4. Structure of TopBP1 and its similarity to BRCA1

Topoisomerase IIβ binding protein 1 (TopBP1) has been identified as a protein interacting with topoisomerase IIβ in a yeast two-hybrid screen (Morishima et al., 2007; Yamane et al., 1997). Interaction with topoisomerase IIβ is mediated by carboxyl-terminal region (aa 862-1522) of TopBP1 *in vitro* (Honda et al., 2002; Yamane et al., 1997). TopBP1 shares sequence and structural homologies with *Saccharomyces cerevisiae* Dpb11, *Schizosaccharomyces pombe* Cut5/Rad4, *Drosophila melanogaster* Mus101 and *Xenopus levis* Xmus101 (Araki et al., 1995; Garcia et al., 2005; Morishima et al., 2007; Ogiwara et al., 2006; Parrilla-Castellar & Karnitz, 2003; Taricani & Wand, 2006; van Hatten et al., 2002).

TopBP1 protein seems to be essential for maintenance of chromosomal integrity and cell proliferation. This protein appeared to be involved in DNA damage response, DNA replication checkpoint, chromosome replication and regulation of transcription (Bang et al., 2011; Garcia et al., 2005; Jeon et al., 2011). TopBP1 knockout mouse exhibits early embryonic lethality at the peri-implantation stage and TopBP1 deficiency induces cellular senescence in primary cells (Bang et al., 2011; Jeon et al., 2011).

TopBP1 gene comprising 28 exons is located on chromosome 3q22.1 and encodes a 1522 amino acid protein (180 kDa) (Karppinen et al., 2006; Xu & Leffak, 2010; Yan & Michael, 2009a,b). The structure of protein is characterized by the presence of interspersed throughout the whole molecule eight copies of the BRCT domain (C-terminal domain of BRCA1), originally identified as a tandemly repeated sequence motif in carboxyl-terminal region of BRCA1 (Fig. 2) (Glover, 2006; Lelung et al., 2010; Wright et al., 2006; Yamane et al., 1997; Yamane & Tsuruo, 1999). BRCT domains, about 90 amino acids in length, are hydrophobic and are involved in an interaction with other proteins and phosphorylated peptides, as well as in an interaction with single- and double-stranded DNA (Glover, 2006; Rodriquez et al., 2003; Wright et al., 2006). A sequence analysis has shown that BRCT repeats are present in a large family of proteins that are implicated in the cellular response to DNA damage. Next to BRCA1 and TopBP1, members of this family include several proteins that are directly linked to DNA repair and cell cycle checkpoints, such as XRCC1 (X-ray cross complementing protein 1), DNA ligase III and IV, MDC1, BARD1 (BRCA1 associated RING domain protein 1), Rad9, MCPH1 (microcephalin 1) (Glover, 2006; Glover et al., 2004; Hou et al., 2010; Yamane et al., 2002; Yamane & Tsuruo, 1999; Yang et al., 2008).

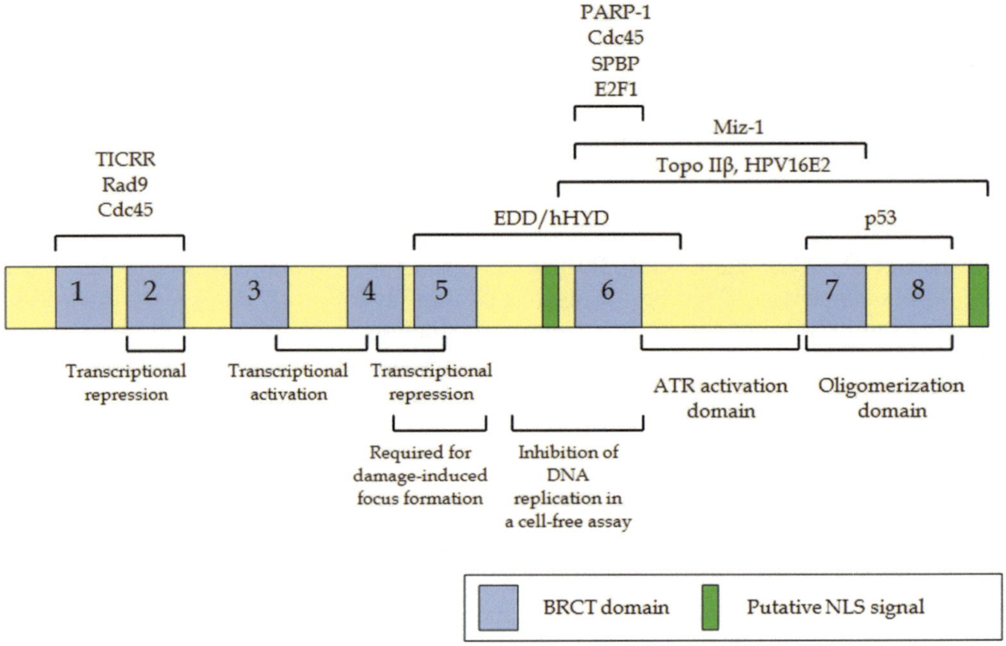

Fig. 2. TopBP1 functional domains and sites of interacting proteins

The carboxyl-terminal region of TopBP1 containing two BRCT domains shows considerable similarity to the corresponding part of BRCA1 (Going et al., 2007; Karppinen et al., 2006; Makiniemi et al., 2001; Morris et al., 2009; Yamane et al., 1997, 2003). Apart from structural similarity TopBP1 shares many other common features with BRCA1. The expression of both proteins is the highest in S phase cells. TopBP1 and BRCA1 are phosphorylated by ATM in response to DNA damage and DNA replication stress and they both colocalize with PCNA (proliferating cell nuclear antigen) at stalled replication forks (Makiniemi et al., 2001; Yamane et al., 2003). The localization patterns of TopBP1 and BRCA1 have similarities also during late mitosis, as well as in meiotic prophase I (Karppinen et al., 2006; Reini et al., 2004). Furthermore, the two proteins have been shown to possess overlapping functions in G2/M checkpoint regulation (Karppinen et al., 2006). Yamane et al. (2003) demonstrated that a BRCA1-mutant or a TopBP1-reduced background results in only partial abrogation at G2/M checkpoint, whereas the combined TopBP1-reduced and BRCA-mutant background result in the nearly complete abrogation. In response to ionizing radiation TopBP1 and BRAC1 colocalize with Rad50, ATM, Rad9, BLM (Bloom syndrome protein), PCNA, NBS1 (Nijmegen breakage syndrome 1) and γH2AX in IR-induced nuclear foci (Germann et al., 2010; Xu et al., 2003).

TopBP1 protein possesses transcriptional-activation domain and two surrounding repressor domains and can play a role in regulating transcription directly (Fig. 2). A transcriptional-activation domain is located between amino acids 460 - 591 and partly contains BRCT4 domain. This region essential for transactivation is rich in hydrophobic amino acids interspersed with acidic residues, typical of identified transcriptional domains. On amino-terminal side of the transcriptional activation domain, Wright et al., (2006) identified a repressor domain involving BRCT2 that is able to repress the TopBP1 transcriptional activation domain. Additionally, another repressor domain exists on the C terminus of the activation domain, which requires amino acids 586 - 675. TopBP1 protein exerts its function in the nucleus and the carboxyl-terminal region of TopBP1 contains two putative nuclear localization signals (Going et al., 2007; Liu et al., 2003; Sokka et al., 2010). Liu et al. (2003) showed that deletion of the BRCT7-8 and NLS region of TopBP1 induces cytoplasmic localization of the protein. Aberrant expression and intracellular localization of TopBP1 is observed immunohistochemically in breast cancer (Going et al., 2007).

5. TopBP1 as multifunctional protein

TopBP1 protein has been proposed as a transcriptional repressor of E2F1 and transcriptional co-activator with HPV16 E2 (Liu et al., 2004; Wright et al., 2006; Yoshida & Inoue, 2004). The E2F transcription factors E2F1 to E2F6 bind to E2F sites in promoters and regulate the expression of a large array of genes that encode proteins important for DNA replication and cell cycle progression. In response to growth signals, activated G1 cycline-dependent kinase phosphorylate retinoblastoma protein (Rb) and release E2F from Rb binding. This event is critical in controlling G1/S transition. Among the E2F family members, E2F1, E2F2 and E2F3 are transcriptional activators and are induced in response to growth stimulation, with peak accumulation at G1/S. Together, they are essential for cellular proliferation since a combined mutation of E2F1, E2F2 and E2F3 completely blocks cellular proliferation. In contrary, E2F4 and E2F5 act mainly as transcriptional repressors (Chen et al., 2009; Liu et al., 2003; Poznic, 2009). TopBP1 protein interacts with E2F1 through the sixth BRCT motif of TopBP1 and N terminus of E2F1 (Fig. 2) (Lelung et al., 2010; Liu et al., 2003). This interaction is induced by ATM-mediated phosphorylation of E2F1 at Ser31 during DNA damage. By this interaction, the transcriptional activity of E2F1 is repressed and E2F1 is recruited to DNA damage induced nuclear foci (Liu et al., 2003). Moreover, the interaction between TopBP1 protein and E2F1, as well as the repression of E2F1 activity, are specific for E2F1 but are not seen in E2F2, E2F3 and E2F4, suggesting that TopBP1 is E2F1 exclusive regulator (Liu et al., 2004). Liu et al. (2004) showed that E2F1 is also regulated by a novel Rb-independent mechanism, in which TopBP1 protein recruits Brg1/BRM (Brahma-related gene 1/Brahma protein), a central subunit of the SWI/SNF (SWItch/sucrose nonfermentable) chromatin modeling complex, to specifically inhibit E2F1 transcriptional activity. This regulation appeared to be critical for E2F1-dependent apoptosis control during S phase and DNA damage. On the other hand, TopBP1 is induced by E2F1 and interacts with E2F1 during G1/S transition. Thus, E2F1 and TopBP1 form a feedback regulation to prevent apoptosis during DNA replication (Liu et al., 2003).

Human papillomaviruses (HPVs) are causative agents in a number of human diseases the most common of which is cervical cancer. More than 95% of cervical carcinomas harbor HPV sequences and HPV16 is most frequently detected. The HPV16 E2 protein is a 43 kDa phosphoprotein that binds as a homodimer to 12 bp palindromic DNA sequences in the transcriptional control region of the viral genome. After binding, E2 can either upregulate or repress transcription from the adjacent promoter depending on cell type and protein levels and this regulation controls the expression of viral oncoproteins E6 and E7. The carboxyl-terminal portion of TopBP1 interacts with E2 and TopBP1 protein can enhance the ability of E2 to activate transcription and replication (Fig. 2) (Boner et al., 2002).

TopBP1 protein also interacts with SPBP (stromelysin-1 platelet-derived growth factor (PDGF) responsive element binding protein) and enhances the transcriptional activity of Ets1 on the *Myc* and *MMP-3* promoters *in vitro* and *in vivo* (Sjottem et al., 2007). This interaction is mediated by ePHD (extended plant homeodomain) domain of SPBP and the BRCT6 domain of TopBP1 (Sjottem et al., 2007). SPBP a 220 kDa ubiquitously expressed nuclear protein is shown to intensify or repress the transcriptional activity. Originally SPBP was identified as a protein involved in transcriptional activation of matrix metalloproteinase-3 (MMP3), stromelysin-1 promoter *via* the specific sequence element SPRE (stromelysin-1 PDGF responsive element) (Rekdal et al., 2000; Sonz et al., 1995). Later SPBP was found to act as a transcriptional coactivator since it enhanced the transcriptional activity of the positive cofactor and RING finger protein SNURF/RNF4 (small nuclear RING finger protein/RING finger protein 4) and of certain transcription factors, such as Sp1 (specificity protein 1), Ets (E-twenty-six specific), Pax6 (paired box gene 6) and Jun (Lyngso et al., 2000; Rekdal et al., 2000; Sjottem et al., 2007). On the other hand, SPBP appears to act as phosphoserine-specific repressor of estrogen receptor α (ERα) (Gburick et al., 2005; Sjottem et al., 2007).

In unstressed cells TopBP1 protein associates with Miz-1 (Myc interacting zinc finger protein 1). BRCT6 and BRCT7 of TopBP1 are required and largely sufficient to mediate the interaction with Miz-1 (Fig. 2) (Herold et al., 2002, 2008; Wenzel et al., 2003). This zinc finger protein that contains an amino-terminal POZ (poxvirus and zinc finger) was initially described as a protein that interacts with C terminus of Myc oncoprotein (Courapied et al., 2010; Herold et al., 2008). Miz-1 protein activates transcription of genes encoding the cell cycle inhibitors $p15^{INK46}$ and $p21^{Cip1}$, leading to cell cycle arrest. Miz-1 can also repress transcription when it forms complexes with Myc and other transcription factors (Herold et al., 2002, 2008; Wenzel et al., 2003). In response to UV irradiation Miz-1 is released from an inhibitory complex formed with TopBP1 and binds to the start site of $p21^{Cip1}$ promoter. Thus the dissociation of TopBP1 from Miz-1 may facilitate the induction of $p21^{Cip1}$ (Herold et al., 2002, 2008; Wenzel et al., 2003). On the other hand, Miz-1 is required for the binding of TopBP1 to chromatin and to protect TopBP1 from proteasomal degradation. TopBP1 protein that is not bound to chromatin is ubiquitilated by HECTH9 (HUWE1) ligase. Expression of Myc leads to dissociation of TopBP1 from chromatin and reduces the amount of total TopBP1 (Herold et al., 2008). Furthermore, TopBP1 has been shown to be ubiquitilated by ubiquitin ligase EDD/hHYD (E3 identified by differential display/ human hyperplastic discs), another HECT (homologous to E6-AP C-terminus) domain E3 enzymes. The HECT E3 ubiquitin-protein ligases have been found from yeast to humans. They are characterized by the HECT domain. EDD/hHYD interacts with the minimal region of the amino acids 661 - 1080 including BRCT5 and BRCT6 of TopBP1 protein. TopBP1 was found to be usually ubiqitilated and degraded by the proteasome in intact cells. X-irradiation seems to abolish TopBP1 degradation and induce the stable complex formation of TopBP1 with other molecules in DNA double strand breaks (Honda et al., 2002; Scheffrer & Staub, 2007). Binding of the transcription factor Miz-1 and TopBP1 protein is also regulated by TopBP1 ADP-ribosylation (Table 1). ADP-ribosylation is one of the post-translational protein modifications. Polymers of ADP-ribose are formed from donor NAD^+ molecules and covalently attached to glutamic acid, aspartic acid or lysine residues of a target protein. The process is catalyzed by the poly(ADP-ribose) polymerase (PARP) family of proteins. The best known of these proteins is PARP1 which is implicated in transcription, chromatin remodeling, apoptosis and DNA repair (Sokka et al., 2010; Woodhouse & Dainov, 2008). TopBP1 and PARP-1 interact both *in vitro* and *in vivo*. The interaction depends on sixth BRCT domain of TopBP1 and on the fact that this domain is ADP-ribosylated by PARP-1. The post-translational ADP-ribosylation of TopBP1 by PARP1 may support the release of

Miz-1 from the complex with TopBP1 (Wollmann et al., 2007; Yamane et al., 1997; Yamane & Tsuruo, 1999).

Site(s)	Modification	Enzyme	Reference
Y in BRCT1-4 region	phosphorylation	c-Abl	Zeng et al., 2005
S214	phosphorylation	ATM/ATR	Matsuoka et al., 2007
S492	phosphorylation	ATM	Sokka et al., 2010
S405	phosphorylation	ATM/ATR	Matsuoka et al., 2007
S409	phosphorylation	ATM/ATR	Matsuoka et al., 2007
S554	phosphorylation	ATM	Sokka et al., 2010
K581	acetylation	N/D	Choudhary et al., 2010
S766	phosphorylation	ATM	Sokka et al., 2010
S805	phosphorylation	N/D	Beausoleil et al., 2006; Wang et al., 2008
T848	phosphorylation	N/D	Dephoure et al., 2008
S860	phosphorylation	N/D	Dephoure et al., 2008
S861	phosphorylation	N/D	Dephoure et al., 2008
S864	phosphorylation	N/D	Dephoure et al., 2008
S888	phosphorylation	N/D	Beausoleil et al., 2006; Dephoure et al., 2008; Wang et al., 2008
900-991 (BRCT6)	ADP-ribosylation	PARP-1	Wollmann et al., 2007; Yamane et al., 1997; Yamane & Tsuruo, 1999
T975	phosphorylation	ATM/ATR	Matsuoka et al., 2007
S1002	phosphorylation	N/D	Dephoure et al., 2008; Wang et al., 2008
S1051	phosphorylation	ATM/ATR	Matsuoka et al., 2007
T1062	phosphorylation	ATM	Sokka et al., 2010
T1086	phosphorylation	ATM/ATR	Matsuoka et al., 2007
S1138	phosphorylation	ATM	Yoo et al., 2007
S1159	phosphorylation	Akt	Liu et al., 2006

Table 1. Post-translation modifications of the human TopBP1 protein (N/D – not determined)

Apart from the mentioned above ADP-ribosylation, TopBP1 undergoes other post-translational modifications, such as acetylation and phosphorylation (Table 1). Lysine acetylation is a reversible post-translational modification, which neutralizes the positive charge of this amino acid changing protein function. Lysine acetylation preferentially targets large macromolecular complexes involved in diverse cellular processes, such as chromatin remodeling, cell cycle, splicing, nuclear transport and actin nucleation. Acetylation of TopBP1 protein occurs at position 581 but the exact role of this modification remains to be resolved (Choudhary et al., 2010).

TopBP1 is a phosphoprotein and is phosphorylated in response to DNA damage (Makiniemi et al., 2001; Yamane et al., 2003). After DNA damage, TopBP1 protein localizes at IR-induced nuclear foci and is phosphorylated by ATM kinase (Yamane et al.,

2003). Human TopBP1 is phosphorylated at several S/TQ sites, which are consensus sequences of PIKK (phosphatidylinositol 3-kinase-related kinase) targets (Hashimoto et al., 2006; Matsuoka et al., 2007). However, the phosphorylation of TopBP1 protein occurs mostly on serine and to a lesser extent on threonine (Makiniemi et al., 2001). TopBP1 protein is also phosphorylated by Akt *in vitro* and *in vivo* on Ser1159. Phosphorylation by Akt kinase induces oligomerization of TopBP1 through its seventh and eighth BRCT domains. The Akt-dependent oligomerization is crucial for TopBP1 to interact with E2F1 and repress its activity. TopBP1 phosphorylation by Akt is also required for interaction between TopBP1 and Miz-1 or HPV16 E2 and repression of Miz-1 transcriptional activity, suggesting a general role for TopBP1 oligomerization in the control of transcription factors (Liu et al., 2006a).

The other TopBP1 interacting proteins are PML (promyelocytic leukemia protein), TICRR (TopBP1-interacting, checkpoint and replication regulator) and p53. PML is a multifunctional protein that plays essential roles in cell growth regulation, apoptosis, transcriptional regulation and genome stability. PML tumor suppressor gene is consistently disrupted by t(15;17) in patients with acute promyelocytic leukemia. PML colocalizes and associates *in vivo* with TopBP1 in response to ionizing radiation and both proteins colocalize with Rad50, BRCA1, ATM, Rad9 and BLM. PML plays a role in regulation of TopBP1 functions by association and stabilization of the protein in response to IR-induced DNA damage (Xu et al., 2003). TICRR is required to prevent mitotic entry after treatment with ionizing radiation. TICRR deficiency is embryonic-lethal in the absence of exogenous DNA damage because it is essential for normal cell cycle progression. Specifically, the loss of TICRR impairs DNA replication and disrupts the S/M checkpoint, leading to premature mitotic entry and mitotic catastrophe. TICRR associates with TopBP1 *in vivo* and this interaction requires the two N-terminal BRCT domains. Sansam et al. (2010) showed that interaction between TICRR and TopBP1 is essential for replication preinitiation complex. TopBP1 is also involved in regulation of p53 activity. The regulation is mediated by an interaction between the seventh and eighth BRCT domains of TopBP1 and the DNA binding domain of p53, leading to inhibition of p53 promoter binding activity. Thus, TopBP1 may inhibit expression of several canonic p53 target genes including GADD45 (growth arrest and DNA damage protein 45), $p21^{Cip1}$, PUMA (p53 upregulated modulator of apoptosis), NOXA, BAX (Bcl-2 associated X protein), IGFBP3 (insulin-like growth factor binding protein 3). The repression of p53 proapoptotic genes such as NOXA, PUMA and BAX suggests that TopBP1 can inhibit p53-mediated apoptosis during DNA damage. Deregulation of this control may have pathological consequences (Liu et al., 2009).

TopBP1 also plays a role in DNA replication and S phase progression. Expression of TopBP1 mRNA and protein is induced concomitantly with S phase entry (Makiniemi et al., 2001). Neutralizing TopBP1 with a polyclonal antiserum raised against the sixth BRCT domain inhibits replicative DNA synthesis in HeLa cell nuclei *in vitro*. This may indicate that the sixth BRCT domain is critical for replication activity, possibly *via* interaction with crucial replication factors (Makiniemi et al., 2001; Schmidt et al., 2008). The physical interaction between TopBP1 and polymerase ε also implies an involvement of TopBP1 in replication (Makiniemi et al., 2001). The loading of Cdc45 (cell division cycle 45) onto chromatin is critical for loading various replication proteins, including DNA polymerase α, DNA polymerase ε, RPA (replication protein A) and PCNA. Human TopBP1 recruits Cdc45 to origins of DNA replication and is required for the formation of the initiation complex of replication in human cells. The first, second and sixth BRCT domains of TopBP1 interact with Cdc45 and this interaction inhibits transcriptional activity of TopBP1 (Schmidt et al., 2008; Sokka et al., 2010). Both proteins interact exclusively at the G1/S boundary of cell cycle. Only weak interaction could be found at the G2/M boundary (Schmidt et al., 2008).

6. TopBP1 and activation of ATR pathway

The major regulators of DNA damage response are the phosphoinositide 3-kinase (PI3K)-related proteins kinases (PIKKs), including ataxia telangiectasia mutated (ATM) and ATM and Rad3-related (ATR) (Cimprich & Cortez, 2008; Lopez-Contreras & Fernandez-Capetillo, 2010; Takeishi et al., 2010). Other members of this family comprise mTOR (mammalian target of rapamycin), which coordinates protein synthesis and cell growth, DNA-PKcs (DNA-dependent protein kinase catalytic subunit), which promotes DNA double strand break repair by nonhomologous end-joining and SMG1, which regulates nonsense-mediated mRNA decay (Cimprich & Cortez, 2008; Mordes et al., 2008). PIKKs are large proteins (2549 - 4128 amino acids) with common domain architecture. All of them contain a large region of repeated HEAT (Huntington, elongation factor 3, PR65/A, TOR) domains in the N terminus, highly conserved C-terminal kinase domain flanked by FAT (FRAP, ATM, TRAP /FKBP-rapamycin associated protein, ATM, *trp* RNA binding attenuation protein) and FATC (FAT C terminus) and PIKK regulatory domain (PRD) between the kinase and FATC domains (Cimprich & Cortez, 2008; Lopez-Contreras & Fernandez-Capetillo, 2010; Mordes et al., 2008). PRD, poorly conserved between family members but highly conserved within orthologous present in different organisms, is not essential for basal kinase activity but plays a regulatory role in at least ATM, ATR and mTOR (Cimprich & Cortez, 2008). PRD of ATM and mTOR is targeted for post-translational modifications that regulate their activity (Cimprich & Cortez, 2008; Mordes et al., 2008). The N-terminal regions of the kinases mediate interaction with the protein cofactors (Cimprich & Cortez, 2008). ATM and ATR are proteins of about 300 kDa, with a conserved C-terminal catalytic domain that preferably phosphorylates serine or threonine residues followed by a glutamine, i.e. SQ or TQ motif (Choi et al., 2009; Smits et al., 2010).
The initial step in ATR activation is recognition of DNA structures that are induced by the damaging agents (Smits et al., 2010). As mentioned, ATR responds to a wide variety of DNA damage that results in the generation of single-stranded DNA (ssDNA) (Takeishi et al., 2010). In eukaryotes, DNA damage-induced ssDNA is first detected by ssDNA binding protein complex RPA (Fig. 3) (Smits et al., 2010). RPA is a heterotrimeric protein complex composed of three subunits with a size of 70, 30 and 14 kDa, which are known as RPA70, RPA32 and RPA14 or alternatively RPA1, RPA2 and RPA3, respectively (Binz et al., 2004; Broderick et al., 2010; Fanning et al., 2006). RPA is identified to be a crucial component in DNA replication, DNA recombination and DNA repair (Ball et al., 2007; Broderick et al., 2010; Cimprich & Cortez, 2008). After binding to ssDNA either during DNA replication or in response to DNA damage, RPA is phosphorylated and this is thought to be an important event in DNA damage response (Binz et al., 2004; Broderick et al., 2010). Recent observations have shown the involvement of ATR in the RPA2 phosphorylation in response to stalled replication fork in S phase generated by genotoxic agents such as UV (Broderick et al., 2010; Olson et al., 2006).
RPA-coated ssDNA is necessary for ATR activation, but it is not sufficient, as at least several additional factors are also required. This kinase forms a stable complex with ATRIP (ATR-interacting protein) which regulates the localization of ATR to sites of replication stress and

DNA damage. Apart from ATRIP, activation of ATR requires the activator protein TopBP1 which plays dual role in the initiation of DNA replication and DNA damage response (Mordes & Cortez, 2008). ATRIP was identified as a 85 kDa an ATR binding partner that interacts directly with RPA to dock the ATR-ATRIP complex onto ssDNA (Ball et al., 2007; Choi et al., 2010; Kim et al., 2005; Warmerdam & Kanaar, 2010; Yan & Michael, 2009a,b). Independently, the Rad17-RFC complex is loaded onto these sites of damage in RPA-dependent manner (Burrows & Elledge, 2008; Lee & Dunphy, 2010). The Rad17-RFC complex consists of the Rad17 subunit and four additional subunits of replication factor C named from RFC2 to RFC5. During normal replication the RFC complex, containing RFC1 instead of Rad17, plays a role in the loading of PCNA onto DNA. PCNA is a processivity factor for DNA polymerases. Both the Rad17 and RFC complexes require RPA for their loading onto DNA (Majka et al., 2006; Medhurst et al., 2008; Warmerdam & Kanaar, 2010). However, Rad17-RFC requires 5′ dsDNA-ssDNA junctions, rather than the 3′ ended junctions preferred by PCNA. These types of structures are specifically created by the resection of DSBs, stalled replication forks and UV-induced ssDNA gaps. The Rad17-RFC protein complex facilitates the loading of the Rad9-Rad1-Hus1 (9-1-1) sliding clamp onto the DNA (Choi et al., 2010; Lopez-Contreras & Fernandez-Capetillo, 2010; Van et al., 2010; Warmerdam & Kanaar, 2010; Yan & Michael, 2009a). The necessity of the 9-1-1 complex in the ATR branch was explained by showing that Rad9 recruits the ATR-activator TopBP1 protein near sites of DNA damage, which was consistent with earlier reports showing interaction between Rad9 and TopBP1 protein (Greer et al., 2003; Makiniemi et al., 2001; Smits et al., 2010). The amino-terminal region of TopBP1 protein comprising BRCT1 and BRCT2 binds the C terminus of Rad9. More precisely, the interaction between Rad9 and TopBP1 depends on Ser373 phosphorylation in the C-terminal tail of Rad9 (Delacroix et al., 2007; Kumagai et al., 2006; Lee et al., 2007; Rappas et al., 2011; Smits et al., 2010; Takeishi et al., 2010). Then, TopBP1 protein binds ATR through its ATR activation domain (AAD), located between the sixth and seventh BRCT repeats, in an ATRIP-dependent manner and this interaction is required for ATR stimulation (Kumagai et al, 2006; Mordes et al., 2008; Smits et al., 2010; Takeishi et al., 2010). ATRIP contains a conserved TopBP1 interacting region, required for the association of TopBP1 and ATR and the subsequent TopBP1-mediated triggering of ATR activity (Mordes et al., 2008; Smits et al., 2010).

ATR-mediated activation of Chk1 in response to genotoxic stress requires another protein that binds independently of ATR or Rad17/9-1-1 named Claspin (Kumagai et al., 2004; Liu et al., 2006b; Scorah & McGowan, 2009; Smits et al., 2010). Claspin is proposed to function as adaptor molecule bringing ATR and Chk1 together (Kumagai & Dunphy, 2000; Smits et al., 2010). The Claspin-Chk1 interaction depends on ATR-mediated phosphorylation of Claspin and is required for Chk1 phosphorylation by ATR. Subsequent studies identified repeated phosphopeptide motifs in Claspin, which are required for association with phosphate binding sites in the N-terminal kinase domain of Chk1, resulting in full activation of Chk1 (Smits et al., 2010). In response to DNA damage or replication stress activated ATR and its effectors such as Chk1 ultimately slow origin firing and induce cell cycle arrest, as well as stabilize and restart stalled replication forks (Cimprich & Cortez, 2008).

The mechanism by which TopBP1 binding activates ATR is poorly defined. The primary binding site for the activation domain of TopBP1 on the ATR complex is within ATRIP and mutations in this region of ATRIP block activation (Cimprich & Cortez, 2008; Mordes et al., 2008). In addition, activation involves amino acids that are located between the ATR kinase domain and the FATC domain, of PIKK regulatory domain - PRD of ATR. Mutations in this region have no effect on the basal activity of ATR, although they prevent ATR activation by TopBP1 protein and cause checkpoint defects and mimic a complete deletion of ATR in human somatic cells (Cimprich & Cortez, 2008; Mordes et al., 2008). Thus, efficient activation of ATR by TopBP1 protein may be required to achieve sufficient signal amplification for the proper execution of cellular response to DNA damage (Sokka et al., 2010).

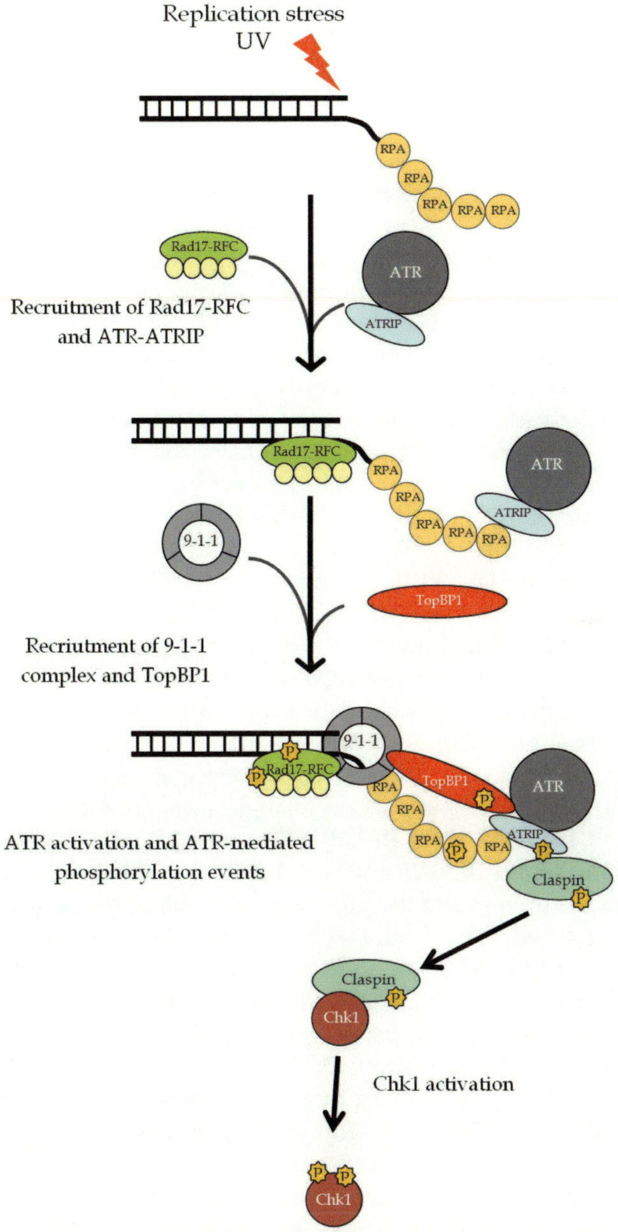

Fig. 3. Role of TopBP1 in activation of ATR pathway in response to replication stress and UV-induced DNA damage

7. Role of TopBP1 in DSB repair

TopBP1 protein also plays a direct and essential role in the pathway that connects ATM to ATR, specifically in response to the occurrence of DSBs in a genome (Yoo et al., 2007). DNA double strand breaks are among the most deleterious DNA lesions that threaten genomic integrity. DSBs are generated not only by exogenous DNA-damaging agents, but also by normal cellular processes, such as V(D)J recombination, meiosis and DNA replication. Furthermore, increased amounts of DSBs are induced by oncogenic stresses during the early stage at tumorigenesis (O'Driscoll & Jeggo, 2005; Shiotani & Zou, 2009; Williams et al., 2007). Two major forms of DSB repair are found within eukaryotic cells: nonhomologous end-joining (NHEJ) and homologous recombination (HR). NHEJ requires several complementary bases for repair and is the predominant form of DSB repair in G0/G1 cells. During NHEJ DNA ends are minimally processed to reveal short stretches of complementarity on either side of the break. NHEJ pathway is inherently mutagenic. In contrast, HR pathway predominates during S and G2 phases and repairs DNA with high fidelity by employing homologous chromosomal or sister chromatid DNA as a template to synthesize new error-free DNA (Williams et al., 2007). The main PIKK that responds to DSBs is ATM, the protein that is defective in the hereditary disorder ataxia telangiectasia (O'Driscoll & Jeggo, 2005). DSBs are recognized by the MRE11-RAD50-NBS1 complex, which promotes the activation of ATM and the preparation of DNA ends for homologous recombination (Fig. 4) (Ciccia & Elledge, 2010; O'Driscoll & Jeggo, 2005; Williams et al., 2007). RAD50 contains ATPase domains that interact with MRE11 (meiotic recombination 11) and associates with the DNA ends. MRE11 has endonuclease and exonuclease activities important for the initial step of DNA end resection that is essential for homologous recombination (Ciccia & Elledge, 2010; Williams et al., 2007). The third subunit of the MRN complex, NBS1, interacts with MRE11 and contains additional protein-protein interaction domains important for MRN function in DNA damage response. NBS1 associates with ATM *via* its C-terminal region, which promotes the recruitment of ATM to DSBs, where ATM is activated by the MRN complex (Ciccia & Elledge, 2010; Jazayeri et al., 2008; Kanaar & Wyman, 2008; Rupnik et al., 2010). Mutations in the human *NBS1* gene result in Nijmegen breakage syndrome (NBS), a rare disorder with abnormal responses to ionizing radiation that resemble those in patients with ataxia telangiectasia (Horton et al., 2011). DNA end resection is regulated by ATM through CtIP (C-terminal binding protein/CtBP interacting protein), which interacts with BRCA1 and MRN (Ciccia & Elledge, 2010). In addition, Exo1 (exonuclease 1), which is involved in the processive stage of DSB resection together with BLM following the initial resection carried out by CtIP, is also stimulated by ATM phosphorylation (Bolderson et al., 2010; Ciccia & Elledge, 2010; Shiotani et al., 2009; Smits et al., 2010). DSB resection and formation of 3′ ssDNA ends leads to RPA accumulation. RPA-ssDNA complexes play a critical role in activation of ATR pathway, as described in detail above.

TopBP1 protein appeared to be involved in ATR-dependent DSB repair. In human cells, DSB induces formation of distinct TopBP1 foci that colocalize with BRCA1, PCNA, NBS1, 53BP1 and γH2AX (Germann et al., 2011). *In vitro* studies showed that in nuclear foci, TopBP1 protein physically associates with NBS1. Several of TopBP1 foci increased and colocalized with NBS1 after ionizing radiation, whereas these nuclear foci were not observed in Nijmegen breakage syndrome cells. The association between TopBP1 and NBS1 involves the first pair of BRCT repeats in TopBP1. In addition the two tandem BRCT repeats of NBS1 are required for this binding. Functional studies with mutated forms of TopBP1 and NBS1

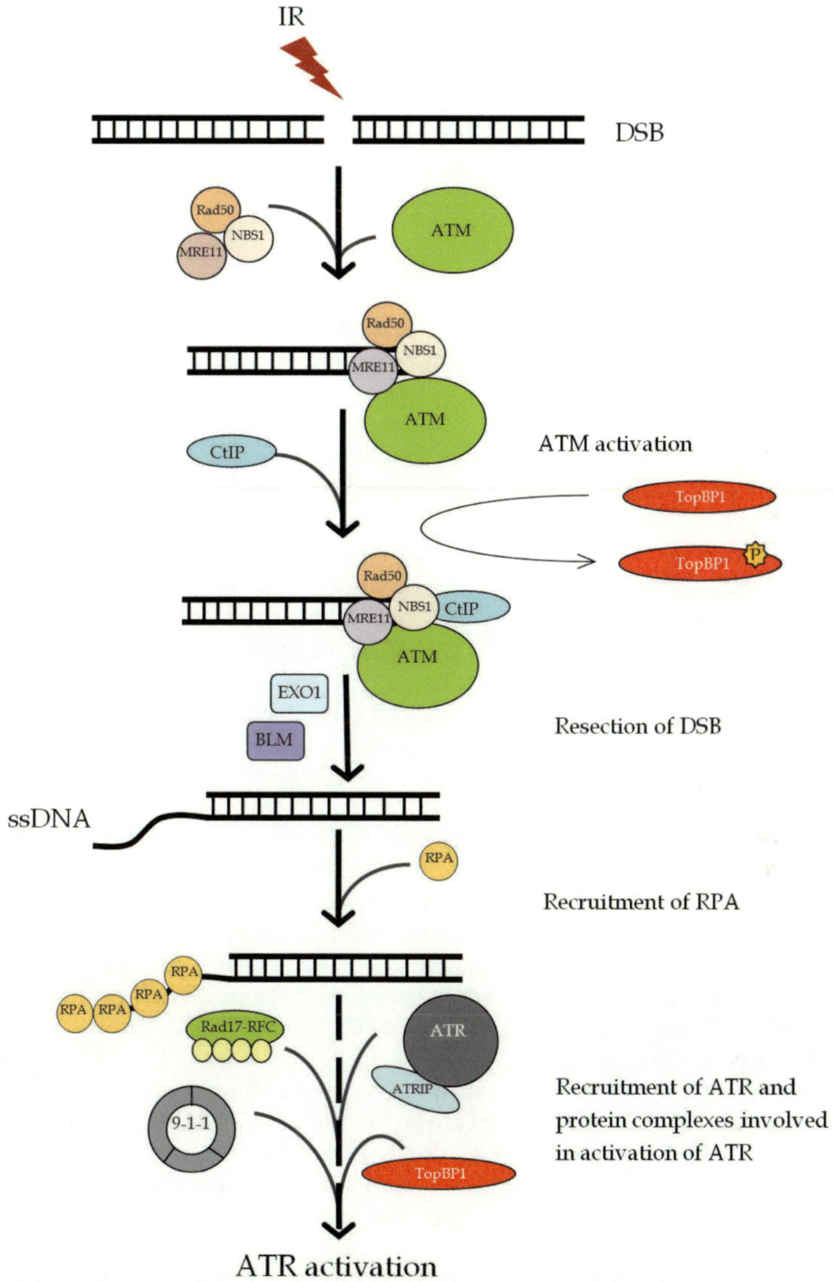

Fig. 4. Role of TopBP1 in ATR activation in response to DNA double strand breaks

suggest that the BRCT-dependent association of these proteins is critical for normal checkpoint response to DSB (Morishima et al., 2007; Yoo et al., 2009). The MRN complex is a crucial mediator in the process whereby ATM promotes the TopBP1-dependent activation of ATR-ATRIP in response to DSBs (Morishima et al., 2007; Yoo et al., 2009). In *Xenopus* egg extracts, ATM associates with TopBP1 protein and phosphorylates it on Ser1131. This phosphorylation enhances the capacity for TopBP1 protein to activate ATR-ATRIP (Yoo et al., 2009). Yoo et al. (2009) showed that ATM can no longer interact with TopBP1 protein in NBS1-depleted egg extracts. Thus, the MRN complex helps to bridge ATM and TopBP1 together. ATM contributes to the activation of ATR through two collaborating mechanisms. First, ATM helps to create appropriate DNA structures that trigger activation of ATR. Second, ATM strongly stimulates the function of TopBP1 protein *via* its phosphorylation that directly carries out the ATR activation (Yoo et al., 2007).

8. Conclusion

DNA is continuously exposed to a range of damaging agents, including reactive cellular metabolites, environmental chemicals, ionizing radiation and UV light. To prevent loss or incorrect transmission of genetic information and development of abnormalities and tumorigenesis all cells have evolved DNA damage response pathways to maintain their genome integrity. The DNA damage response involves the sensing of DNA damage signal to a network of cellular pathways, including cell cycle checkpoint, DNA repair and apoptosis. TopBP1 protein was first identified as an interacting partner for topoisomerase IIβ. This protein shares structural and functional similarities with BRCA1 and plays a critical role in the DNA damage response and checkpoint control. TopBP1 is essential for ATR activation in response to replication stress and UV-induced damage and also plays a direct role in the pathway that connects ATM to ATR in response to DSBs. The biological functions of TopBP1 protein, as well as its close relation with BRCA1 suggest a crucial role of TopBP1 in the maintenance of genome integrity and cell cycle regulation.

9. References

Araki H., Leem S.H., Phongdara A. & Sugino A. (1995). Dpb11, which interacts with DNA polymerase II (ε) in *Sacharomyces cerevisiae*, has a dual role in S-phase progression and at a cell cycle checkpoint. *Proceedings of the National Academy of Sciences of the United States of America*, Vol. 92, No. 25, (December 1995), pp. 11791-11795, ISSN: 0027-8424

Ball H.L., Ehrhardt M.R., Mordes D.A., Glick G.G., Chazin W.J. & Cortez D. (2007). Function of a conserved checkpoint recruitment domain in ATRIP proteins. *Molecular and Cellular Biology*, Vol. 27, No. 9, (May 2007), pp. 3367-3377, ISSN: 0270-7306

Bang S.W., Ko M.J., Kang S., Kim G.S., Kang D., Lee J.H. & Hwang D.S. (2011). Human TopBP1 localization to the mitotic centrosome mediates mitotic progression. *Experimental Cell Research*, Vol. 317, No. 7, (April 2011), pp. 994-1004, ISSN: 0014-4827

Beausoleil S.A., Villen J., Gerber S.A., Rush J. & Gygi S.P. (2006). A probability-based approach for high-throughput protein phosphorylation analysis and site localization. *Nature Biotechnology*, Vol. 24, No. 10, (October 2006), pp. 1285-1292, ISSN: 1087-0156

Binz S.K., Sheehan A.M. & Wold M.S. (2004). Replication protein A phosphorylation and the cellular response to DNA damage. *DNA Repair*, Vol. 3, No. 8-9, (August-September 2004), pp. 1015-1024, ISSN: 1568-7856

Bolderson E., Tomimatsu N., Richard D.J., Boucher D., Kumar R., Pandita T.K., Burma S. & Khanna K.K. (2009). Phosphorylation of Exo1 modulates homologous recombination repair of DNA double-strand breaks. *Nucleic Acids Research*, Vol. 38, No. 6, (December 2009), pp. 1821-1831, ISSN: 0305-1048

Boner W., Taylor E.R., Tsirimonaki E., Yamane K., Campo M.S. & Morgan I.M. (2002). A functional interaction between the human papillomavirus 16 transcription/replication factor E2 and the DNA damage response protein TopBP1. *The Journal of Biological Chemistry*, Vol. 277, No. 25, (June 2002), pp. 22297-22303, ISSN: 0021-9258

Broderic S., Rehmet K., Concannon C. & Nasheuer H.P. (2010), In: *Genome stability and human diseases*, Nasheuer H.P., pp. 143-164, Springer, ISBN: 978-90-481-3470-0, Dordrecht, Holland

Burrows A.E. & Elledge S.J. (2008). How ATR turns on: TopBP1 goes on ATRIP with ATR. *Genes and Development*, Vol. 22, No. 11, (June 2008), pp. 1416-1421, ISSN 0890-9369

Chen H.Z., Tsai S.Y. & Leone G. (2009). Emerging roles of E2Fs in cancer: an exit from cell cycle control. *Nature Reviews Cancer*, Vol. 9, No. 11, (November 2009), pp. 785-797, ISSN: 1474-175X

Choi J.H., Lindsey-Boltz L.A., Kemp M., Mason A.C., Wold M.S. & Sancar A. (2010). Reconsititution of RPA-covered single-stranded DNA activated ATR-Chk1 signaling. *Proceedings of the National Academy of Science of the United States of America*, Vol. 107, No. 31, (August 2010), pp. 13660-13665, ISSN: 0027-8424

Choi J.H., Sancar A., Lindsey-Boltz L.A. (2009). The human ATR-mediated DNA damage checkpoint in a reconstituted system. *Methods*, Vol. 48, No. 1, (May 2009), pp. 3-7, ISSN: 1046-2023

Choudhary C., Kumar C., Gnad F., Nielsen M.L., Rehman M., Walther T.C., Olsen J.V. & Mann M. (2009). Lysine acetylation targets protein complexes and co-regulates major cellular functions. *Science*, Vol. 325. No. 5942, (August 2009), pp. 834-840, ISSN: 0036-8075

Ciccia A. & Elledge S.J. (2010). The DNA damage response: making it safe to play with knives. *Molecular Cell*, Vol. 40, No. 2, (October 2010), pp. 179-204, ISSN: 1097-2765

Cimprich K.A. & Cortez D. (2008). ATR: an essential regulator of genome integrity. *Nature Reviews Molecular Cell Biology*, Vol. 9, No. 8, (August 2008), pp. 616-627, ISSN: 1471-0072

Corre I., Niaudet C. & Paris F. (2010). Plasma membrane signaling induced by ionizing radiation. *Mutation Research*, Vol. 704, No. 1-3, (April-June 2010), pp. 61-67, ISSN: 0027-5107

Cortez D., Gutunku S., Qin J. & Elledge S.J. (2001). ATR and ATRIP: partners in checkpoint signaling. *Science*, Vol. 294, No. 5547, (November 2001), pp. 1713-1716, ISSN: 0193-4511

Courapied S., Cherier J., Vigneron A., Troadec M.B., Giraud S., Valo I., Prigent C., Gamelin E., Coqueret O. & Barre B. (2010). Regulation of the Aurora-A gene following topoisomerase I inhibition: implication of the Myc transcription factor. *Molecular Cancer*, Vol. 9, No. 1, (August 2010), pp. 205, ISSN: 1476-4598

Dai Y. & Grant S. (2010). New insights into Checkpoint kinase 1 (Chk1) in the DNA damage response (DDR) signaling network: rationale for employing Chk1 inhibitors in cancer therapeutics. *Clinical Cancer Research*, Vol. 16, No. 2, (January 2010), pp. 376-383, ISSN: 1078-0432

Danielsen J.M.R., Larsen D.H., Schou K.B., Freire R., Falck J., Bartek J. & Lukas J. (2009). HCLK2 is required for activity of the DNA damage response kinase ATR. *The Journal of Biological Chemistry*, Vol. 284, No. 7, (February 2009), pp. 4140-4147, ISSN: 0021-9258

Delacroix S., Wagner J.M., Kobayashi M., Yamamoto K. & Karnitz L.M. (2007). The Rad9-Hus1-Rad1 (9-1-1) clamp activates checkpoint signaling *via* TopBP1. *Genes and Development*, Vol. 21, No. 12, (June 2007), pp. 1472-1477, ISSN: 0890-9369

Dephoure N., Zhou C., Villen J., Beausoleil S.A., Bakalarski C.E., Elledge S.J. & Gygi S.P.(2008). A quantitative atlas of mitotic phosphorylation. *Proceedings of the National Academy of Science of the United States of America*, Vol. 105, No. 31, (August 2008), pp. 10762-10767, ISSN: 0027-8424

Dijkstra K.K., Blanchetot C. & Boonstra J. (2009). Evasion of G1 checkpoint in cancer, In: *Checkpoint Controls and Targets in Cancer Therapy*, Siddik Z.H., pp. 3-26, Humana Press, ISBN: 978-1-60761-177-6, Totowa, New Jersey, USA

Essers J., Vermeulen W. & Houtsmeller A.B. (2006). DNA damage repair: anytime, anywhere? *Current Opinion in Cell Biology*, Vol. 18, No. 3, (June 2006), pp. 240-246, ISSN: 0955-0674

Fannig E., Klimovich V. & Nager A.R. (2006). A dynamic model for replication protein A (RPA) function in DNA processing pathways. *Nucleic Acids Research*, Vol. 34, No. 15, (August 2006), pp. 4126-4137, ISSN: 0305-1048

Garcia V., Furuya K. & Carr A.M. (2005). Identification and functional analysis of TopBP1 and its homologs. *DNA Repair*, Vol. 4, No. 11, (November 2005), pp. 1227-1239, ISSN: 1568-7856

Gburcik V., Bot N., Maggiolini M. & Picard D. (2005). SPBP is a phosphoserine-specific repressor of estrogen receptor α. *Molecular and Cellular Biology*, Vol. 25, No. 9, (May 2005), pp. 3421-3430, ISSN: 0270-7306

Germann S.M., Oestergaard V.H., Haas C., Salis P., Motegi A. & Lisby M. (2011). Dpb11/TopBP1 plays distinct roles in DNA replication, checkpoint response and homologous recombination. *DNA Repair*, Vol. 10, No. 2, (February 2011), pp. 210-224, ISSN: 1568-7856

Glover J.N.M. (2006). Insights into the molecular basis of human hereditary breast cancer from studies of the BRCA1 BRCT domain. *Familial Cancer*, Vol. 5, No. 1, (March 2006), pp. 89-93, ISSN: 1389-9600

Glover J.N.M., Williams R.S. & Lee M.S. (2004). Interactions between BRCT repeats and phosphoproteins: tangled up in two. *Trends in Biochemical Sciences*, Vol. 29, No. 11, (November 2004), pp. 579-585, ISSN: 0968-0004

Going J.J., Nixon C., Dornan E.S., Boner W., Donaldson M.M. & Morgan I.M. (2007). Aberrant expression of TopBP1 in breast cancer. *Histopathology*, Vol. 50, No. 4, (March 2007), pp. 418-424, ISSN: 0309-0167

Greer D.A., Besley B.D.A., Kennedy K.B. & Davey S. (2003). hRad9 rapidly binds DNA containing double-strand breaks and is required for damage-dependent topoisomerase IIβ binding protein 1 focus formation. *Cancer Research*, Vol. 63, No. 16, (August 2003), pp. 4829-4835, ISSN: 0008-5472

Hashimoto Y., Tsujimura T., Sugino A. & Takisawa H. (2006). The phosphorylated C-terminal domain of *Xenopus* Cut5 directly mediates ATR-dependent activation of Chk1. *Genes to Cells*, Vol. 11, No. 9, (September 2006), pp. 993-1007, ISSN: 1356-9597

Herold S., Hock A., Herkert B., Berns K., Mullenders J., Beijersbergen R., Bernards R. & Eilers M. (2008). Miz1 and HectH9 regulate the stability of the checkpoint protein, TopBP1. *EMBO Journal*, Vol. 27, No. 21, (November 2008), pp. 2851-2861, ISSN: 0261-4189

Herold S., Wenzel M., Beuger V., Frohme C., Beul D., Hillukkala T., Syvaoja J., Saluz H.P., Haenel F. & Eilers M. (2002). Negative regulation of the mammalian UV response by Myc through association with Miz-1. *Molecular Cell*, Vol. 10, No. 3, (September 2002), pp. 509-521, ISSN: 1097-2765

Hiom K. (2010). Coping with DNA double strand breaks. *DNA Repair*, Vol. 9, No. 12, (December 2010), pp. 1256-1263, ISSN: 1568-7856

Honda Y., Tojo M., Matsuzaki K., Anan T., Matsumoto M., Ando M., Saya H. & Nakao M. (2002). Cooperation of HECT-domain ubiquitin ligase hHYD and DNA topoisomerase II-binding protein for DNA damage response. *The Journal of Biological Chemistry*, Vol. 277, No. 5, (February 2002), pp. 3599-3605, ISSN: 0021-9258

Horton J.K., Stefanick D.F., Zeng J.Y., Carrozza M.J. & Wilson S.H. (2011). Requirement for NBS1 in the S phase checkpoint response to DNA methylation combined with PARP inhibition. *DNA Repair*, Vol. 10, No. 2, (February 2011), pp. 225-234, ISSN: 1568-7856

Houtgraaf J.H., Versmissen J. & van der Giessen W.J. (2006). A concise review of DNA damage checkpoints and repair in mammalian cells. *Cardiovascular Revascularization Medicine*, Vol. 7, No. 3, (July-September 2006), pp. 165-172, ISSN: 1553-8389

Huo Y., Bai L., Xu M. & Jiang T. (2010). Crystal structure of the N-terminal region of human Topoisomerase IIβ binding protein 1. *Biochemical and Biophysical Research Communications*, Vol. 401, No. 3, (October 2010), pp. 401-405, ISSN: 0006-291X

Hurley P.J. & Bunz F. (2009). Distinct pathways involved in S-phase checkpoint control, In: *Checkpoint Controls and Targets in Cancer Therapy*, Siddik Z.H., pp. 27-36, Humana Press, ISBN: 978-1-60761-177-6, Totowa, New Jersey, USA

Jazayeri A., Balestrini A., Garner E., Haber J.E. & Costanzo V. (2008). Mre11-Rad50-Nbs1-dependent processing of DNA breaks generates oligonucleotides that stimulate ATM activity. *EMBO Journal*, Vol. 27, No. 14, (July 2008), pp. 1953-1962, ISSN: 0261-4189

Jeon Y., Ko E., Lee K.Y., Ko M.J, Park S.Y., Kang J., Jeon C.H., Lee H. & Hwang D.S. (2011). TopBP1 deficiency causes an early embryonic lethality and induces cellular senescence in primary cells. *The Journal of Biological Chemistry*, Vol. 286, No. 7, (February 2011), pp. 5414-5422, ISSN: 0021-9258

Jungmichel S. & Stucki M. (2010). MDC1: The art of keeping things in focus. *Chromosoma*, Vol. 119, No. 4, (August 2010), pp. 337-349, ISSN: 0009-5915

Kanaar R. & Wyman C. (2008). DNA repair by the MRN complex: break it to make it. *Cell*, Vol. 135, No. 1, (October 2008), pp. 14-16, ISSN: 0092-8674

Karppinen S.M., Erkko H., Reini K., Pospiech H., Heikkinen K., Rapakko K., Syvaoja J.E. & Winqvist R. (2006). Identification of a common polymorphism in the TopBP1 gene associated with hereditary susceptibility to breast and ovarian cancer. *European Journal of Cancer*, Vol. 42, No. 15, (October 2006), pp. 2647-2652, ISSN: 0959-8049

Kerzendorfer C. & O'Driscoll M. (2009). Human DNA damage response and repair deficiency syndromes: Linking genomic instability and cell cycle checkpoint proficiency. *DNA Repair*, Vol. 8, No. 9, (September 2009), pp. 1139-1152, ISSN: 1568-7856

Kim J.E., McAvoy S.A., Smith D.I. & Chen J. (2005). Human TopBP1 ensures genome integrity during normal S phase. *Molecular and Cellular Biology*, Vol. 25, No. 24, (December 2005), pp. 10907-10915, ISSN: 0270-7306

Kumagai A., Kim S.M. & Dunphy W.G. (2004). Claspin and the activated from of ATR-ATRIP collaborate in the activation of Chk1. *The Journal of Biological Chemistry*, Vol. 279, No. 48, (November 2004), pp. 49599-49608, ISSN: 0021-9258

Kumagai A., Lee J., Yoo H.Y. & Dunphy W.G. (2006). TopBP1 activates the ATR-ATRIP complex. *Cell*, Vol. 124, No. 5, (March 2006), pp. 943-955, ISSN: 0092-8674

Lee J. & Dunphy W.G. (2010). Rad17 plays a central role in establishment of the interaction between TopBP1 and the Rad9-Hus1-Rad1 complex at stalled replication forks. *Molecular Biology of the Cell*, Vol. 21, No. 6, (March 2010), pp. 926-935, ISSN: 1059-1524

Lee J., Kumagai A. & Dunphy W.G. (2007). The Rad9-Hus1-Rad1 checkpoint clamp regulates interaction of TopBP1 with ATR. *The Journal of Biological Chemistry*, Vol. 282, No. 38, (September 2007), pp. 28036-28044, ISSN: 0021-9258

Lelung C.C.Y., Kellogg E., Kuhnert A., Hanel F., Baker D. & Glover J.N.M. (2010). Insights from the crystal structure of the sixth BRCT domain of topoisomerase IIβ binding protein 1. *Protein Science*, Vo. 19, No. 1, (January 2010), pp. 162-167, ISSN: 0961-8368

Liu K., Bellam N., Lin H.Y., Wang B., Stockard C.R., Grizzle W.E. & Lin W.C. (2009). Regulation of p53 by TopBP1: a potential mechanism for p53 inactivation in cancer, *Molecular and Cellular Biology*, Vol. 29, No. 10, (May 2009), pp. 2673-2693, ISSN: 0270-7306

Liu K., Paik J.C., Wang B., Lin F.T. & Lin W.C. (2006a). Regulation of TopBP1 oligomerization by Akt/PKB for cell survival. *EMBO Journal*, Vol. 25, No. 20, (October 2006), pp. 4795-4807, ISSN: 0261-4189

Liu S., Bekker-Jensen S., Mailand N., Lukas C., Bartek J. & Lukas J. (2006b). Claspin operates downstream of TopBP1 to direct ATR signaling towards Chk1 activation. *Molecular and Cellular Biology*, Vol. 26, No. 16, (August 2006), pp. 6056-6064, ISSN: 0270-7306

Liu K., Luo Y., Lin F.T. & Lin W.C. (2004). TopBP1 recruits Brg1/Brm to repress E2F1-induced apoptosis, a novel pRb-independent and E2F1-specific control for cell survival. *Genes and Development*, Vol. 18, No. 6, (March 2004), pp. 673-686, ISSN: 0890-9369

Liu K., Lin F.T., Ruppert J.M. & Lin W.C. (2003). Regulation of E2F1 by BRCT domain-containing protein TopBP1. *Molecular and Cellular Biology*, Vol. 23, No. 9, (May 2003), pp. 3287-3304, ISSN: 0270-7306

Lopez-Contreras A.J. & Fernandez-Capetillo O. (2010). The ATR barrier to replication-born DNA damage. *DNA Repair*, Vol. 9, No. 12, (December 2010), pp. 1249-1255, ISSN: 1568-7856

Lyngso C., Bouteiller G., Damgaard C.K., Ryom D., Sanchez-Munoz S., Norby P.L., Bonven B.J. & Jorgensen P. (2000). Interaction between the transcription factor SPBP and the positive cofactor RNF4. *The Journal of Biological Chemistry*, Vol. 275, No. 34, (August 2000), pp. 26144-26149, ISSN: 0021-9258

Majka J., Binz S.K., Wold M.S. & Burgers P.M. (2006). Replication protein A directs loading of the DNA damage checkpoint clamp to 5'-DNA junctions. *The Journal of Biological Chemistry*, Vol. 281, No. 38, (September 2006), pp. 27855-27861, ISSN: 0021-9258

Makiniemi M., Hillukkala T., Tuusa J., Reini K., Vaara M., Huang D., Pospiech H., Majuri I., Westerling T., Makela T.P. & Syvaoja J.E. (2001). BRCT domain-containing protein TopBP1 functions in DNA replication and damage response. *The Journal of Biological Chemistry*, Vol. 276, No. 32, (August 2001), pp. 30399-30406, ISSN: 0021-9258

Matsuoka S., Ballif B.A., Smogorzewska A., McDonald III E.R., Hurov K.E., Luo J., Bakalarski C.E., Zhao Z., Solimini N., Lerenthal Y., Shiloh Y., Gygi S.P. & Elledge

S.J. (2007). ATM and ATR substrate analysis reveals extensive protein networks responsive to DNA damage. *Science,* Vo. 316, No. 5828, (May 2007), pp. 1160-1166, ISSN: 0193-4511

Medhurst A.L., Warmerdam D.O., Akerman I., Verwayen E.H., Kanaar R., Smits V.A.J. & Lakin N.D. (2008). ATR and Rad17 collaborate in modulating Rad9 localisation at sites of DNA damage. *Journal of Cell Science,* Vol. 121, No. 23, (December 2008), pp. 3933-3940, ISSN: 0021-9533

Mordes D.A. & Cortez D. (2008). Activation of ATR and related PIKKs. *Cell Cycle,* Vol. 7, No. 18, (September 2008), pp. 2809-2812, ISSN: 1551-4005

Mordes D.A., Glick G.G., Zhao R. & Cortez D. (2008). TopBP1 activates ATR through ATRIP and a PIKK regulatory domain. *Genes and Development,* Vol. 22, No. 11, (June 2008), pp. 1478-1489, ISSN: 0890-9369

Morishima K., Sakamoto S., Kobayashi J., Izumi H., Suda T., Matsumoto Y., Tauchi H., Ide H., Komatsu K. & Matsuura S. (2007). TopBP1 associates with NBS1 and is involved in homologous recombination repair. *Biochemical and Biophysical Research Communications,* Vol. 362, No. 4, (November 2007), pp. 872-879, ISSN: 0006-291X

Morris J.S., Nixon C., King O.J.A., Morgan I.M. & Philbey A.W. (2009). Expression of TopBP1 in canine mammary neoplasia in relation to histological type, Ki67, ERα and p53. *The Veterinary Journal,* Vol. 179, No. 3, (March 2009), pp. 422-429, ISSN: 1090-0233

Muniandy P., Liu J., Majumdar A., Liu S. & Seidman M.M. (2010). DNA interstrand cross link repair in mammalian cells: step by step. *Critical Reviews in Biochemistry and Molecular Biology,* Vol. 45, No. 1, (February 2010), pp. 23-49, ISSN: 1040-9238

Nakanishi M. (2009). Chromatin modifications and orchestration of checkpoint response in cancer, In: *Checkpoint Controls and Targets in Cancer Therapy,* Siddik Z.H., pp. 83-94, Humana Press, ISBN: 978-1-60761-177-6, Totowa, New Jersey, USA

Nakanishi M., Niida H., Murakami H. & Shimada M. (2009). DNA damage responses in skin biology - Implication in tumor prevention and aging acceleration. *Journal of Dermatological Science,* Vol. 56, No. 2, (November 2009), pp. 76-81, ISSN: 0923-1811

Niida H. & Nakanishi M. (2006). DNA damage checkpoints in mammals. *Mutagenesis,* Vol. 21, No. 1, (January 2006), pp. 3-9, ISSN: 0267-8357

O'Driscoll M. & Jeggo P.A. (2006). The role of double-strand break repair - insights from human genetics. *Nature Reviews Genetics,* Vol. 7, No. 1, (January 2006), pp. 45-54, ISSN: 1471-0056

Ogiwara H., Ui A., Onoda F., Tada S., Enomoto T. & Seki M. (2006). Dpb11, the pudding yeast homolog of TopBP1, functions with the checkpoint clamp in recombination repair. *Nucleic Acids Research,* Vol. 34, No. 11, (July 2006), pp. 3389-3398, ISSN: 0305-1048

Olson E., Nievera C.J., Klimovivh V., Fanning E. & Wu X. (2006). RPA2 is a direct downstream target for ATR to regulate the S-phase checkpoint. *The Journal of Biological Chemistry,* Vol. 281, No. 51, (December 2006), pp. 39517-39533, ISSN: 0021-9258

Pallis A.G. & Karamouzis M.V. (2010). DNA repair pathways and their implication in cancer treatment. *Cancer and Metastasis Reviews,* Vol. 29, No. 4, (September 2010), pp. 677-685, ISSN: 0167-7659

Parrilla-Castellar E.R. & Karnitz L.M. (2003). Cut5 is required for the binding of Atr and DNA polymerase α to genotoxin-damaged chromatin. *The Journal of Biological Chemistry,* Vol. 278, No. 46, (November 2003), pp. 45507-45511, ISSN: 0021-9258

Poehlmann A. & Roessner A. (2010). Importance of DNA damage checkpoints in the pathogenesis of human cancers. *Pathology Research and Practice,* Vol. 206, No. 9, (September 2010), pp. 591-601, ISSN: 0344-0338

Pommier Y., Leo E., Zhang H.L. & Marchand C. (2010). DNA topoisomerases and their poisoning by anticancer and antibacterial drugs. *Chemistry and Biology*, Vol. 17, No. 5, (May 2010), pp. 421-433, ISSN: 1074-5521

Poznic M. (2009). Retinoblastoma protein: a central processing unit. *Journal of Biosciences*, Vol. 34, No. 2, (June 2009), pp. 305-312, ISSN: 0250-5991

Rappas M., Oliver A.W. & Pearl L.H. (2011). Structure and function of the Rad9-binding region of the DNA-damage checkpoint adaptor TopBP1. *Nucleic Acids Research*, Vol. 39, No. 1, (January 2011), pp. 313-324, ISSN: 0305-1048

Rastogi R.P., Richa, Kumar A., Tyagi M.B. & Sinha R.P. (2010). Molecular mechanisms of ultraviolet radiation-induced DNA damage and repair. *Journal of Nucleic Acids*, Vol. 2010:592980, (December 2010), ISSN: 2090-0201

Reinhardt H.C. & Yaffe M.B. (2009). Kinases that control the cell cycle in response to DNA damage: Chk1, Chk2, and MK2. *Current Opinion in Cell Biology*, Vol. 21, No. 2, (April 2009), pp. 245-255, ISSN: 0955-0674

Reinhardt H.C., Hasskamp P., Schmedding I., Morandell S., van Vugt M.A.T.M., Wang X.Z., Linding R., Ong S.E., Weaver D., Carr S.A. & Yaffe M.B. (2010). DNA damage activates a spatially distinct late cytoplasmic cell-cycle checkpoint network controlled by MK2-mediated RNA stabilization. *Molecular Cell*, Vol. 40, No. 1, (October 2010), pp. 34-49, ISSN: 1097-2765

Reini K., Uitto L., Perera D., Moens P.B., Freire R. & Syvaoja J.E. (2004). TopBP1 localises to centrosomes in mitosis and to chromosome cores in meiosis. *Chromosoma*, Vol. 112, No. 7, (May 2004), pp. 323-330, ISSN: 0009-5915

Rekdal C., Sjottem E. & Johansen T. (2000). The nuclear factor SPBP contains different functional domains and stimulates the activity of various transcriptional activators. *The Journal of Biological Chemistry*, Vol. 275, No. 51, (December 200), pp. 40288-40300, ISSN: 0021-9258

Rodriguez-Bravo V., Guaita-Esteruelas S., Salvador N., Bachs O. & Agell N. (2007). Different S/M checkpoint responses of tumor and non-tumor cell lines to DNA replication inhibition. *Cancer Research*, Vol. 67, No. 24, (December 2007), pp. 11648-11656, ISSN: 0008-5472

Rogriguez M., Yu X., Chen J. & Songyang Z. (2003). Phosphopeptide binding specificities of BRCA1 COOH-terminal (BRCT) domains. *The Journal of Biological Chemistry*, Vol. 278, No. 52, (December 2003), pp. 52914-52918, ISSN: 0021-9258

Rupnik A., Lownde N. & Grenon M. (2010). MRN and the race to the break. *Chromosoma*, Vol. 119, No. 2, (April 2010), pp. 115-135, ISSN: 0009-5915

Sansam C.L., Cruz N.M., Danielian P.S., Amsterdam A., Lau M.L., Hopkins N. & Lees J.A. (2010). A vertebrate gene, *ticrr*, is an essential checkpoint and replication regulator. *Genes and Development*, Vol. 24, No. 2, (January 2010), pp. 183-194, ISSN: 0890-9369

Sanz L., Moscat J. & Diaz-Meco M. (1995). Molecular characterization of a novel transcription factor that controls stromelysin expression. *Molecular and Cellular Biology*, Vol. 15, No. 6, (June 1995), pp. 3164-3170, ISSN: 0270-7306

Scheffner M. & Staub O. (2007). HECT E3s and human disease. *BioMed Central Biochemistry*, Vol. 8, Suppl. 1, (November 2007), pp. S6, ISSN: 1471-2091

Schmidt U., Wollmann Y., Franke C., Grosse F., Saluz H.P. & Hanel F. (2008). Characterization of the interaction between the human DNA topoisomerase IIβ-binding protein (TopBP1) and the cell division cycle 45 (Cdc45) protein. *The Biochemical Journal*, Vol. 409, No. 1, (January 2008), pp. 169-177, ISSN: 0264-6021

Scorah J. & McGowan C.H. (2009). Claspin and Chk1 regulate replication fork stability by different mechanisms. *Cell Cycle*, Vol. 8, No. 7, (April 2009), pp. 1036-1043, ISSN: 1551-4005

Shiotani B. & Zou L. (2009). Single-stranded DNA orchestrates an ATM-to-ATR switch at DNA breaks. *Molecular Cell*, Vol. 33, No. 5, (March 2009), pp. 547-558, ISSN: 1097-2765

Sjottem E., Rekdal C., Svineng G., Johansen S.S., Klenow H., Uglehus R.D. & Johansen T. (2007). The ePHD protein SPBP interacts with TopBP1 and together they co-operate to stimulate Ets1-mediated transcription. *Nucleic Acids Research*, Vol. 35, No. 19, (October 2007), pp. 6648-6662, ISSN: 0305-1048

Smits V.A.J., Warmerdam D.O., Martin Y. & Freire R. (2010). Mechanisms of ATR-mediated checkpoint signaling. *Frontiers in Bioscience*, Vol. 15, No. 3, (June 2010), pp. 840-853, ISSN: 1093-4715

Sokka M., Parkkinen S., Pospiech H. & Syvaoja J.E. (2010), Function of TopBP1 in genome stability, In: *Genome stability and human diseases*, Nasheuer H.P., pp. 119-141, Springer, ISBN: 978-90-481-3470-0, Dordrecht, Holland

Su Y., Meador J.A., Geard C.R. & Balajee A.S. (2010). Analysis of ionizing radiation-induced DNA damage and repair in three-dimensional human skin model system. *Experimental Dermatology*, Vol. 19, No. 8, (August 2010), pp. e16-22, ISSN: 0906-6705

Takeishi Y., Ohashi E., Ogawa K., Masai H., Obuse C. & Tsurimoto T. (2010). Casein kinase 2-dependent phosphorylation of human Rad9 mediates the interaction between human Rad9-Hus1-Rad1 complex and TopBP1. *Genes to Cells*, Vol. 15, No. 7, (June 2010), pp. 761-771, ISSN: 1356-9597

Taricani L. & Wang T.S.F. (2006). $Rad4^{TopBP1}$, a scaffold protein, plays separate roles in DNA damage and replication checkpoints and DNA replication. *Molecular Biology of the Cell*, Vol. 17, No. 8, (August 2006), pp. 3456-3468, ISSN: 1059-1524

Van C., Yan S., Michael W.M., Waga S. & Cimprich K.A. (2010). Continued primer synthesis at stalled replication forks contributes to checkpoint activation. *The Journal of Cell Biology*, Vol. 189, No. 2, (April 2010), pp. 233-246, ISSN: 0021-9525

Van Hatten R.A., Tutter A.V., Holway A.H., Khederian A.M., Walter J.C. & Michael W.M. (2002). The *Xenopus* Xmus101 protein is required for the recruitment of Cdc45 to origins of DNA replication. *The Journal of Cell Biology*, Vol. 159, No. 4, (November 2002), pp. 541-547, IISN: 0021-9525

Wang B., Malik R., Nigg E.A. & Korner R. (2008). Evaluation of the low-specificity protease elastase for large-scale phosphoproteome analysis. *Analytical Chemistry*, Vol. 80, No. 24, (December 2008), pp. 9536-9533, ISSN: 0003-2700

Wanzel M., Herold S. & Eilers M. (2003). Transcriptional repression by Myc. *Trends in Cell Biology*, Vol. 13, No. 3, (March 2003), pp. 146-150, ISSN: 0962-8924

Warmerdam D.O. & Kanaar R. (2010). Dealing with DNA damage: Relationships between checkpoint and repair pathways. *Mutation Research*, Vol. 704, No. 1-3, (April-June 2010), pp. 2-11, ISSN: 0027-5107

Williams R.S., Williams J.S. & Tainer J.A. (2007). Mre11-Rad50-Nbs1 is a keystone complex connecting DNA repair machinery, double-strand break signaling, and the chromatin template. *Biochemistry and Cell Biology*, Vol. 85, No. 4, (August 2007), pp. 509-520, ISSN: 0829-8211

Wollmann Y., Schmidt U., Wieland G.D., Zipfel P.F., Saluz H.P. & Hanel F. (2007). The DNA topoisomerase IIβ binding protein 1 (TopBP1) interacts with poly (ADP-ribose) polymerase (PARP-1). *Journal of Cellular Biochemistry*, Vol. 102, No. 1, (September 2007), pp. 171-182, ISSN: 0730-2312

Woodhouse B.C. & Dianov G.L. (2008). Poly ADP-ribose polymerase-1: An international molecule of mystery. *DNA Repair*, Vol. 7, No. 7, (July 2008), pp. 1077-1086, ISSN: 1568-7856

Wright R.H.G., Dornan E.S., Donaldson M.M. & Morgan I.M. (2006). TopBP1 contains a transcriptional activation domain suppressed by two adjacent BRCT domains. *The Biochemical Journal*, Vol. 400, No. 3, (December 2006), pp. 573-582, ISSN: 0264-6021

Xu Y. & Leffak M. (2010). ATRIP from TopBP1 to ATR – *in vitro* activation of a DNA damage checkpoint. *Proceedings of the National Academy of Science of the United States of America*, Vol. 107, No. 31, (August 2010), pp. 13561-13562

Xu Z.X., Timanova-Atanasova A., Zhao R.X. & Chang K.S. (2003). PML colocalizes with and stabilizes the DNA damage response protein TopBP1. *Molecular and Cellular Biology*, Vol. 23, No. 12, (June 2003), pp. 4247-4256, ISSN: 0270-7306

Yamane K., Chen J. & Kinsella T.J. (2003). Both DNA topoisomerase II-binding protein 1 and BRCA1 regulate the G2-M cell cycle checkpoint. *Cancer Research*, Vol. 63, No. 12, (June 2003), pp. 3049-3053, ISSN: 0008-5472

Yamane K., Wu X. & Chen J. (2002). A DNA damage-regulated BRCT-containing protein, TopBP1, is required for cell survival. *Molecular and Cellular Biology*, Vol. 22, No. 2, (January 2002), pp. 555-566, ISSN: 0270-7306

Yamane K. & Tsuruo T. (1999). Conserved BRCT regions of TopBP1 and of the tumor suppressor BRCA1 bind strand breaks and termini of DNA. *Oncogene*, Vol. 18, No. 37, (September 1999), pp. 5194-5203, ISSN: 0950-9232

Yamane K., Kawabata M. & Tsuruo T. (1997). A DNA-topoisomerase-II – binding protein with eight repeating regions similar to DNA-repair enzymes and to a cell-cycle regulator. *European Journal of Biochemistry*, Vol. 250, No. 3, (December 1997), pp. 794-799, ISSN: 0014-2956

Yan S. & Michael W.M. (2009). TopBP1 and DNA polymerase α-mediated recruitment of the 9-1-1 complex to stalled replication forks. *Cell Cycle*, Vol. 8, No. 18, (September 2009), pp. 2877-2884, ISSN: 1551-4005

Yan S. & Michael W.M. (2009). TopBP1 and DNA polymerase-α directly recruit the 9-1-1 complex to stalled DNA replication forks. *The Journal of Cell Biology*, Vol. 184, No. 6, (March 2009), pp. 793-804, ISSN: 0021-9525

Yang X., Wood P.A. & Hrushesky W.J.M. (2010). Mammalian TIMELESS is required for ATM-dependent CHK2 activation and G_2/M checkpoint control. *The Journal of Biological Chemistry*, Vol. 285, No. 5, (January 2010), pp. 3030-3034, ISSN: 0021-9258

Yang S.Z., Lin F.T. & Lin W.C. (2008). MCPH1/BRIT1 cooperates with E2F1 in the activation of checkpoint, DNA repair and apoptosis. *EMBO Journal*, Vol. 9. No. 9, (September 2008), pp. 907-915, ISSN: 1469-221X

Yoo H.Y., Kumagai A., Shevchenko A., Schevchenko A. & Dunphy W.G. (2009). The Mre11-Rad50-Nbs1 complex mediates activation of TopBP1 by ATM. *Molecular Biology of the Cell*, Vol. 20, No. 9, (May 2009), pp. 2351-2360, ISSN: 1059-1524

Yoo H.Y., Kumagai A., Schevchenko A., Schevchenko A. & Dunphy W.G. (2007). Ataxia-telangiectasia mutated (ATM)-dependent activation of ATR occurs through phosphorylation of TopBP1 by ATM. *The Journal of Biological Chemistry*, Vol. 282, No. 24, (June 2007), pp. 17501-17506, ISSN: 0021-9258

Yoshida K. & Inoue I. (2004). Expression of MCM10 and TopBP1 is regulated by cell proliferation and UV irradiation *via* E2F transcription factor. *Oncogene*, Vol. 23, No. 37, (August 2004), pp. 6250-6260, ISSN: 0950-9232

Zeng L., Hu Y. & Li B. (2005). Identification of TopBP1 as a c-Abl-interacting protein and a repressor for c-Abl expression. *The Journal of Biological Chemistry*, Vol. 280, No. 32, (August 2005), pp. 29374-29380, ISSN: 0021-9258

16

Post-Meiotic DNA Damage and Response in Male Germ Cells

Guylain Boissonneault et al.*
Department of Biochemistry, Faculty of Medicine and Health Sciences
Université de Sherbrooke
Canada

1. Introduction

Spermatids are haploid cells that differentiate into spermatozoa and may be considered as an interesting model of DNA damage response and repair. Key features, such a unique set of chromosomes, radioresistance to apoptosis, the presence of known end-joining DNA repair pathways and an underlying prerogative to limit the transmission of any mutation to the next generation, make them a unique cell type to provide new insights on similar pathways in somatic cells. Although DNA damage signaling and repair mechanisms have been extensively studied during meiosis, the contribution of post-meiotic germ cells to the genetic integrity of the male gamete have been overlooked. In this chapter we present clear evidences that the haploid phase of spermatogenesis, termed spermiogenesis, may represent an even greater challenge for the maintenance of the genetic integrity of the male gamete. Since transient DNA strand breaks are intrinsic to the differentiation program of spermatids (Leduc et al., 2008a; Marcon and Boissonneault, 2004), a better understanding of DNA repair pathways involved may shed some light on their potential contribution to male-driven *de novo* mutations and eventually to some unresolved cases of male infertility. This chapter will mainly focus on DNA breaks occurring in the post-meiotic phase of the spermatogenesis and how germ cells deal with it.

2. Spermatogenesis

In most mammals, testes are found in the scrotum and are maintained at lower temperature (2-8°C) than the core body (Harrison and Weiner, 1949; Setchell, 1998). In fact, spermatogenesis is known to work better at lower temperature and it was shown that fertility declines with scrotal hyperthermia. For example, higher scrotal temperature due to fever or lifestyle correlates with decreased semen quality in humans (reviewed in Jung and Schuppe, 2007).
To support germ cells in their development, Sertoli cells are located at the basal lamina, throughout the seminiferous tubules (Russell, 1990). They provide nutrients and essential

---

* Frédéric Leduc, Geneviève Acteau, Marie-Chantal Grégoire, Olivier Simard, Jessica Leroux, Audrey Carrier-Leclerc and Mélina Arguin
Department of biochemistry, Faculty of medicine and health sciences, Université de Sherbrooke, Canada

molecules to the differentiating germ cells and regulate the seminiferous tubular fluid (Griswold, 1998; Rato et al., 2010). The Sertoli cells are interconnected by different junctions, creating a unique barrier between surrounding blood vessels and differentiating germ cells that is known as the "blood-testis barrier" (Cheng and Mruk, 2002; Dym and Fawcett, 1970; Setchell, 1969; Vogl et al., 2008). This barrier restricts molecules to enter or exit the adluminal compartment, creating a microenvironment with diverse transporters and preventing immunological response against germ cells (reviewed in Mital et al., 2011).

Spermatogenesis is the cellular differentiation pathway leading to the production of male gametes. This process takes place in seminiferous tubules in the testis, which is a unique environment regulated by follicle-stimulating and luteinizing hormones, secreted by the pituitary gland (Russell, 1990). From birth to puberty, seminiferous tubules are composed of spermatogonia, the precursor stem cell of the germinal cells, and Sertoli cells. At the onset of puberty, spermatogonia undergo mitosis and commit to the differentiation pathway leading to male germ cells. As the germ cells differentiate, they migrate towards the lumen of the tubule, creating an organized stratified structure. Spermatogenesis can be divided in two phases, spermatocytogenesis and spermiogenesis.

Spermatocytogenesis is the process by which a spermatogonium differentiates into primary spermatocytes, which duplicate their DNA to undergo meiosis and become haploid spermatids. This meiotic division is important to create genetic variations by meiotic crossovers and random segregation of parental chromosomes. Spermiogenesis is characterized by the radical metamorphosis of the haploid spermatid into spermatozoa, requiring the reorganization of their organelles. The acrosome, a cap-like structure needed for enzymatic digestion of the oocyte outer membrane, is formed from the Golgi apparatus. At the opposite nuclear pole, the flagellum begins to grow from the centrioles and mitochondria groups at the mid-piece of the emerging flagellum to produce the required energy for its later motion. Finally, the spermatid is stripped of most of its cytoplasm and ultimately released in the lumen of the seminiferous tubule. Most interestingly, the nucleus of spermatids is also remodeled and condensed to protect the paternal genome as well as providing a more hydrodynamic shape. However, this nuclear reorganization is characterized by transient DNA strand breaks that may be necessary to relieve the torsional stress as outlined below.

2.1 Chromatin remodeling process

Through the chromatin remodeling process of spermatids, the paternal genome is condensed tenfold compared to somatic cells, forming a nucleus with an hydrodynamic-shape (Balhorn et al., 1984). To achieve such a high degree of compaction, chromatin must first rely on a set of abundant transition proteins (TPs) subsequently replaced by the protamines (PRMs) (Balhorn et al., 1984; Braun, 2001). The arginine-rich PRMs bind DNA and neutralize the phosphodiester backbone of the double helix (Balhorn, 1982), allowing for a tight compaction of the DNA into torroids (Ward, 1993). Although the onset of chromatin remodeling is poorly understood, incorporation of testis-specific histone variants (Churikov et al., 2004; Govin et al., 2007; Lu et al., 2009; Martianov et al., 2005; Yan et al., 2003) and regulated post-translational modifications of histones, such as acetylation (Christensen et al., 1984; Grimes and Henderson, 1984; Marcon and Boissonneault, 2004; Meistrich et al., 1992), ubiquitination (Baarends et al., 1999; Chen et al., 1998), methylation (Godmann et al., 2007; van der Heijden et al., 2006) and phosphorylation (Blanco-Rodríguez,

2009; Krishnamoorthy et al., 2006; Leduc et al., 2008a; Meyer-Ficca et al., 2005) are known to initiate and participate in the exchange from histones to the more basic proteins such as TPs and PRMs during the transition from the round to the elongated spermatids. These modifications are known to modulate the affinity of histones for DNA, but also the affinity of other proteins for histones, such as chromatin remodelers, DNA repair proteins or the transcription machinery. After spermiation, this unique protamine-based chromatin is further stabilized by the creation of intraprotamine disulfide bonds during the transit through the epididymis (Golan et al., 1996). Therefore, protamination provides both chemical and mechanical protection to the male haploid genome. Interestingly, protamination of the male genome is not complete and varies across species. In the mouse spermatozoon, about 1-2% of the genome remains organized by histones (Balhorn et al., 1977), whereas up to 15% of histones are still found in humans spermatozoa (Gatewood et al., 1990; Gusse et al., 1986; Tanphaichitr et al., 1978). This observation lead to hypothesize that these nucleosomes could serve as epigenetic markers for embryonic development (Arpanahi et al., 2009; Zalenskaya et al., 2000) (for a more detailed review on the sperm chromatin organization, see Johnson et al., 2011)

3. Nature of endogenous DNA damages during spermiogenesis

3.1 Single strand damage and repair

Depending on the type of damage, specific pathways achieve single strand damage repair (see Table 1). Mispaired DNA bases that primarily arise during replication are corrected by mismatch repair (MMR), while small chemical alterations of DNA bases such as alkylation, deamination and oxidative damage are repaired by base excision repair (BER) (Mukherjee et al., 2010; Robertson et al., 2009). More complex lesions such as those induced by UV (pyrimidine dimers and helix-distorting lesions) are corrected by nucleotide excision repair (NER), a multistep pathway that involves more than 30 proteins (Hoeijmakers, 2009; Nouspikel, 2009). DNA nicks are repaired by single-strand break repair (SSBR). These DNA repair pathways are known to be present and active during spermiogenesis (Olsen et al., 2001; Schultz et al., 2003). To our knowledge, single-strand damages do not present a major threat to spermatids. With the exception of exposures to toxicant that could challenge these pathways, in normal conditions, single-strand DNA damage during spermiogenesis is likely attributed to the massive transcription that is taking place at these steps and is efficiently resolved by spermatids (Olsen et al., 2001). DNA double-strand breaks were reported as part of the normal differentiation program of spermatids during spermiogenesis which may represent an important source of genetic instability and therefore we will focus on these pathways.

3.2 Double-strand breaks in spermatids

3.2.1 Possible origin of DNA breaks

Several hypotheses have been formulated to elucidate the origin and role of DNA strand breaks in spermatids. Sakkas and colleagues suggested that "abortive apoptosis" may be the cause since abnormal human spermatozoa presented some apoptotic-like features (Sakkas et al., 1999). Further investigation led to the demonstration that other biomarkers of apoptosis in sperm cells were present such as BCL-X, TP53, caspases, in addition to diverse structural defects (Baccetti et al., 1997; Donnelly et al., 2000; Gandini et al., 2000; Sakkas et al., 2002; Weng et al., 2002). Due to technical limitations at the time, DNA breaks were only observed

DNA repair pathways		DNA damages	Implicated proteins
Mismatch repair (MMR)		Mispaired DNA bases	MSH1-6, MLH1, MLH3, PMS1, PMS2, EXO1, RPA, PCNA, RFC
Base excision repair (BER)	Short-patch	Small DNA bases chemical alteration arising from alkylation, deamination and oxidative damage	UNG, APEX1, POL β, XRCC1, LIG3
	Long-patch		UNG, APEX1, POL β / δ, FEN1, PCNA, LIG1
Nucleotide excision repair (NER)	Transcription -coupled or not	Pyrimidine dimer	XPC complex, DDB complex, ERCC3 (TFIIH), XPA-RPA complex, ERCC5 (XPG), ERCC1-ERCC4 (XPF), LIG3, DNA polymerase δ
Single strand break repair (SSBR)	Short-patch or long-patch	Single strand break (SSB)	APE1, PNKP, APTX, TDP1, POL β/δ/ε, PCNA, XRCC1, LIG1/3, FENI, PARP

Table 1. Summary of the single strand DNA repair pathways in mammalian cells (Ciccia and Elledge, 2010; Hoeijmakers, 2009; Martin et al., 2010; Mukherjee et al., 2010; Nouspikel, 2009; Robertson et al., 2009).

in a subset of the whole population of elongating spermatids and therefore abortive apoptosis could represent a sound explanation. However, some studies demonstrated that round spermatids are radioresistant to apoptosis and may not have the proper machinery and checkpoints to trigger such process (Ahmed et al., 2010; Oakberg and Diminno, 1960). Furthermore, our group have demonstrated that transient DNA breaks were present in the whole population of elongating spermatids of fertile mice and humans during chromatin remodeling and were therefore part of the normal differentiation program of these cells (Marcon and Boissonneault, 2004). The persistence of these breaks beyond the chromatin remodeling steps in pathological conditions may explain the presence of DNA fragmentation found in spermatozoa of infertile men (Leduc et al., 2008b).

Generation of controlled DNA breaks either single- or double-stranded may be important to relieve the torsional stress induced by the withdrawal of histones (Boissonneault, 2002). The simple mechanical stress resulting from the accumulation of free supercoils could induce non-B DNA structures and possibly DNA breaks as the chromatin remodeling is extensive and takes place within many differentiation steps. However, enzymatic induction of DNA strand breaks is more likely, as their free ends can be end-labeled with polymerases that require a 3'OH as substrate, such as the terminal deoxynucleotidyl transferase (TdT) used in TUNEL labeling. Specific nucleases could be involved in this process, and it is not excluded that retrotransposon nucleases could play a role as they are expressed throughout spermatogenesis, including in the nucleus of spermatids (Branciforte and Martin, 1994; Ergün et al., 2004; Gasior et al., 2006). However, topoisomerases have long been considered likely candidates to support chromatin remodeling from bulky histone-bound chromatin to compact and transcriptionally inert protamine-bound DNA because of their ubiquitous role in chromosome dynamics during the somatic cell cycle (McPherson and Longo, 1993).

3.2.2 Topoisomerases as candidates to supercoiling removal

Change in DNA topology can be achieved by single-strand breaks (SSBs) generated by type I topoisomerase, which modifies the linking number in steps of one. Single-strand breaks would be considered a much smaller threat for the genome's integrity of spermatids than a DSB that could be generated by type II topoisomerases. However, chromatin remodeling in spermatids was clearly shown to be associated with an increase in type II topoisomerase (Chen and Longo, 1996; Laberge and Boissonneault, 2005; Leduc et al., 2008a; McPherson and Longo, 1992, 1993; Meyer-Ficca et al., 2011b; Roca and Mezquita, 1989). A possible link between type II topoisomerases and DNA breaks found in elongating spermatids was suggested by the elimination of DNA breaks in spermatids nuclei incubated with type II topoisomerase inhibitors such as suramin and etoposide (Laberge and Boissonneault, 2005). In mammal cells, the α and β isoforms of topoisomerase share more than 80% of homology and are differentially expressed. Topoisomerase IIα (TOP2A) is mostly found in replicating cells whereas topoisomerase IIβ (TOP2B) predominates in quiescent cells (Morse-Gaudio and Risley, 1994; Turley et al., 1997). Using immunofluorescence on mouse testis sections, we have observed TOP2B foci in nuclei of elongating spermatids whereas TOP2A remained undetected in these cells but highly present in spermatocytes (see Figure 1) (Leduc et al., 2008a). Detection of TOP2B in elongating spermatids is not surprising, as spermatids are non-replicative cells. Recent studies confirmed the involvement of TOP2B in elongating spermatids (Meyer-Ficca et al., 2011b) and also observed its presence further downstream of the male germ cells differentiation program as part of the nuclear matrix of sperm cells, supporting its earlier role in the chromatin remodeling of spermatids (Shaman et al., 2006).

3.2.3 Topoisomerases and DNA repair

Type II topoisomerase activity may be modulated by post-translational modifications, such as phosphorylation by kinases and poly (ADP-ribosyl)ation by poly (ADP-ribose) polymerases (PARPs), a well-known family of proteins involved in a multitude of nuclear events, such as DNA repair and chromatin remodeling. This complementary interaction between TOP2B and PARPs may be involved in numerous cellular processes. For example, TOP2B and PARP1 are known to modulate transcription in somatic cells (Ju et al., 2006). Furthermore, these proteins may be important constituents of the nuclear matrix; Zaalishvili and coworkers observed the stimulation of cleavage of nuclear matrix associated DNA loops of neuron and leukocyte nucleoids when incubated in buffer supporting topoisomerase and PARP activity (Zaalishvili et al., 2005). This stimulation was reversed by the addition of thymidine, a PARP inhibitor. The authors suggested that a PARP-modified topoisomerase II may cut efficiently but the (ADP-ribosyl)ation could inhibit the religation. Recently, Meyer-Ficca and colleagues demonstrated a possible modulation of TOP2B activity by PARP and PARG *in vitro* using recombinant proteins as well as *in vivo* during mouse spermiogenesis through the use of inhibitors and knockout mouse models (Meyer-Ficca et al., 2011b). According to their findings, there is a functional relationship between the DNA strand break activity of TOP2B and the DNA strand break-dependent activation of

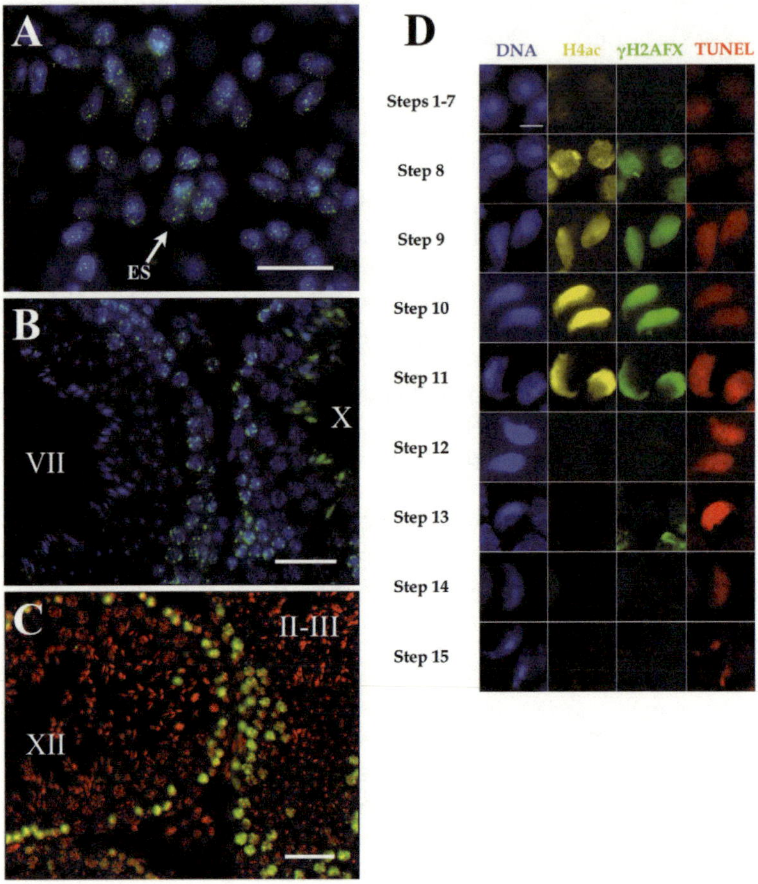

Fig. 1. Presence of type II topoisomerases, hyperacetylated histone H4, γH2AFX and DNA breaks during mouse spermiogenesis. (A) Overlay of TOP2B immunofluorescence (green) and DAPI nuclear staining (blue) of a stage IX tubule demonstrating the presence of TOP2B in nuclei of elongating spermatids (ES) at the onset of chromatin remodeling. (B) Overlay of TOP2B immunofluorescence (green) and DAPI (blue) nuclear staining of stages VII and X tubules. (C) Overlay of immunofluorescence of TOP2A (green) and TO-PRO3 (red) nuclear staining of stages XII and II-III demonstrating the nuclear presence of TOP2A in zygotene and pachytene spermatocytes but complete absence in spermatids. (D) Detection of hyperacetylated histone H4 and γH2AFX by immunofluorescence and DNA breaks by TUNEL during mouse spermiogenesis. DNA was counterstained by TO-PRO3. (A-C) Immunofluoresence on Bouin-fixed testis sections was done as previously described(Leduc et al., 2008a). (D) Squash preparation were done as previously described (Kotaja et al., 2004; Leduc et al., 2008a), fixed with ice-cold ethanol and processed for TUNEL and immunofluorescence. Bars = 10 µm (A and B), 20 µm (C) and 5µm (D).

PARP enzymes. Moreover, alteration in the PAR metabolism leads to a greater retention of histones in spermatozoa (Meyer-Ficca et al., 2011a). Whether PARP1 is involved directly in chromatin remodeling, DNA repair or combination of both in spermatids remains to be determined and will be discussed further in section 4.

4. DNA damage response and DNA repair of double-strand breaks

4.1 DNA damage signaling pathways

The first step following a DSB is the detection of the DNA damage by sensors (Lamarche et al., 2010). At least four independent sensors can detect DSBs: PARPs in all cases of SSBs and, to a lesser extent, DSBs, Ku70/80 in D-NHEJ, MRE11-RAD50-NBS1 (MRN) complex in all cases of DSBs and replication protein A1 (RPA) in HR (Ciccia and Elledge, 2010; Lamarche et al., 2010).

As previously stated in section 3.2.3, the presence and activity of PARP1 and PARP2 have been recently investigated during spermiogenesis of mouse and rat (Ahmed et al., 2010; Dantzer et al., 2006; Meyer-Ficca et al., 2005; Meyer-Ficca et al., 2011a; Meyer-Ficca et al., 2009; Meyer-Ficca et al., 2011b). Although the individual absence of these proteins leads only to subfertility in male, it is believed that they play a key role in the maintenance of genomic integrity of spermatids. As discussed previously, PARPs may be involved in DNA repair and signaling, in the drastic chromatin remodeling of spermatids and even in the repackaging of their genome with protamines (Quénet et al., 2009). However, the embryonic lethal phenotype of double knockout mouse prevent a better assessment of their critical role during spermiogenesis, as the absence of one can be compensated for by the other. The Ku heterodimer binds to DSB ends and is required for the non-homologous end-joining pathway (NHEJ). In addition to its role in DNA repair, Ku proteins are also required for the maintenance of telomeres and subtelomeric gene silencing (Celli et al., 2006; Lamarche et al., 2010). KU70 is present during the spermiogenesis of mouse (Goedecke et al., 1999; Hamer et al., 2003), human (Leduc *et al.*, unpublished observations), and grasshoppers (Cabrero et al., 2007), but seems to decrease as spermiogenesis proceeds, most notably after the expulsion of histones. Although initial analyses of the implication of MRN complex as sensor in non-homologous end-joining pathways produced conflicting results (Di Virgilio and Gautier, 2005; Huang and Dynan, 2002), recent studies showed that siRNA mediated knockdown of Mre11 results in reduced end-joining efficiency in both D-NHEJ and B-NHEJ pathways (Rass et al., 2009; Xie et al., 2009) and should be considered a good candidate for DNA breaks detection and signaling in spermatids. As for Ku proteins, Mre11 is also present during spermiogenesis (Goedecke et al., 1999). Contrary to these DNA break sensor proteins, RPA may not play such an important role during spermiogenesis as spermatids, being haploid, cannot rely on HR repair processes.

The detection of DNA damage by sensors activates proteins of the phosphatidylinositol 3-kinase-like protein kinase (PIKKs) family such as ATM, ATR, and DNA PKcs and members of the PARP family. These proteins post-translationnally modify key protein targets triggering a signal transduction cascades that forms the DNA damage response (DDR) (Lamarche et al., 2010). During mouse spermiogenesis, ATM and DNA PKcs are present and active (Ahmed et al., 2010; Scherthan et al., 2000). These kinases are responsible for the phosphorylation of the histone H2A variant, H2AFX, at serine 139 (γH2AFX, previously referred to as γH2AX), which quickly occurs after a DSB. This modification can spread up to a 2 Mbp region flanking all DSBs (Kinner et al., 2008) and it could help the recruitment of other proteins of the DDR (Celeste et al., 2003). Within minutes following DNA damage, γH2AFX appears at discrete nuclear foci that dissolve after the completion of DNA repair. It remains unclear whether γH2AFX is replaced completely with new H2AFX histones, or simply dephosphorylated, but strong evidences suggest that the latter mechanism is prominent (Chowdhury et al., 2005; Rogakou et al., 1999). Therefore, the implication of γH2AFX in all cases of DSBs makes it a novel biomarker for DSBs detection by immunoflorescence (Mah et al., 2010; Mah et al., 2011). Upon γH2AFX signaling, specific pathways are recruited according to cell type or the cell cycle phase (Shrivastav et al., 2008). The presence of γH2AFX during spermiogenesis has been first shown in rats (Meyer-Ficca et al., 2005) and we confirmed its presence at the corresponding steps during mouse spermiogenesis (Leduc et al., 2008a) (see Figure 1). As shown in Figure 1, the presence of γH2AFX and hyperacetylated histone H4, a biomarker of chromatin remodeling coincides with the presence of TOP2B. These results confirm the previously published strong TUNEL labeling of elongating spermatids during chromatin remodeling (Laberge and Boissonneault, 2005; Marcon and Boissonneault, 2004).

Therefore, spermatids undergo multiple transient DSBs, inducing a classic DDR signaling. In addition, as seen by immunofluorescence in Figure 1, γH2AFX is present in all spermatids throughout chromatin remodeling as part of the normal process of maturation of spermatids. The pattern of γH2AFX in spermatids as seen in Figures 1 and 2 is dependent on fixation and tissue processing; ethanol fixation provides a better context for TUNEL labeling but alters nuclear distribution of proteins. Furthermore, we have also found the presence of γH2AFX and DNA breaks during human spermiogenesis (see Figure 2), while other groups subsequently demonstrated similar DDR signaling in grasshoppers (Cabrero et al., 2007) and even in the algae *Charas vulgaris* (Wojtczak et al., 2008). Moreover, the presence of DNA breaks has also been found during spermiogenesis of drosophila (Rathke et al., 2007). Altogether, these results suggest that the DDR triggered by endogenous breaks in spermatids is evolutionary conserved and could represent a new source of male-driven genetic instability in species where gametogenesis requires condensation of the genetic material.

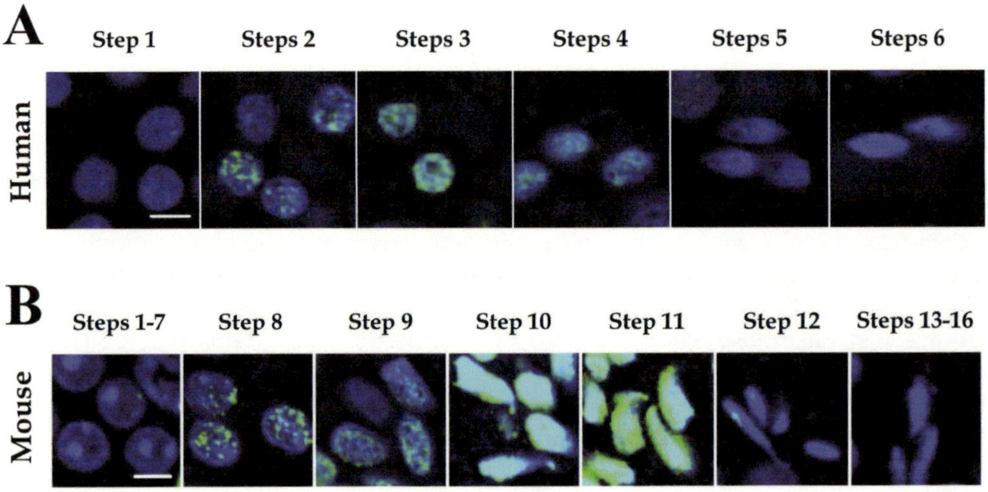

Fig. 2. Detection of γH2AFX during spermiogenesis of human (upper panel), and mouse (lower panel). DNA was counterstained by TO-PRO3. Bars = 5μm. Immunofluoresence on paraformaldehyde-fixed testis sections was done as previously described (Leduc et al., 2008a).

4.2 Evidences of an active DNA repair system during spermiogenesis

Although these DSBs are considered the most harmful genetic damage for a cell, we know from experimental data (Marcon and Boissonneault, 2004) that these breaks are repaired by the end of spermiogenesis in fertile animals. The disappearance of γH2AFX in mouse spermatids (step 13 to 16) shown in Figure 1 cannot be associated with completion of DNA repair or dephosphorylation as a majority of histones are expulsed from the nucleus to be replaced by PRMs. However, we obtained other evidences of an active DNA repair system at these steps by demonstrating incorporation of dNTPs *in situ* that is sustained through all the chromatin remodeling steps (see Figure 3) (Leduc et al., 2008a). Furthermore, as seen in Figure 1, the appearance and disappearance of TUNEL labeling is coincident with γH2AFX fluorescence. To confirm that the loss of TUNEL labeling was associated with DNA repair and not with the lack of penetrability of the TdT in the nuclei of condensed spermatids, we decondensed spermatids prior to TUNEL with similar results (Marcon and Boissonneault, 2004) (Acteau et al., unpublished observations). Therefore, DNA breaks are properly repaired by the end of the spermatids differentiation program. As previously stated, mammalian cells can rely on four DNA DSBs repair pathways, each of which having different degree of fidelity. As spermatids differentiate to spermatozoa with fertilizing potential, any errors due to faulty or incomplete DNA repair may be transmitted to the next generation. Severe alteration in the repair process may cause infertility or possibly be incompatible with embryonic development (Leduc et al., 2008b).

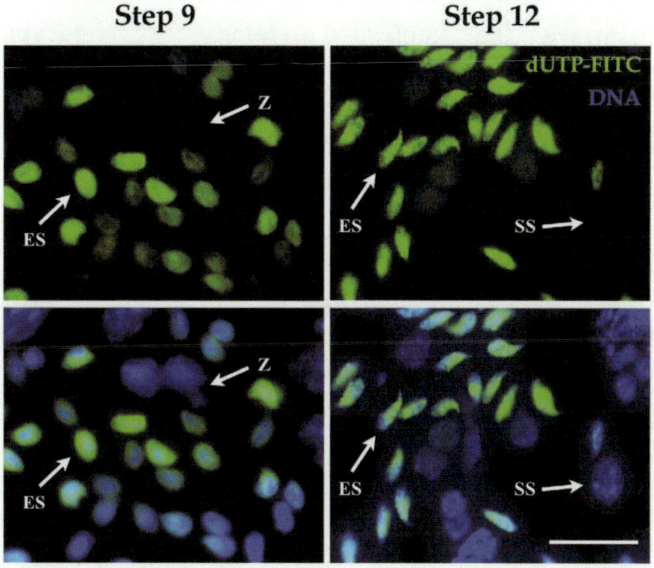

Fig. 3. In situ endogenous DNA polymerase activity assay (Leduc et al., 2008a) on squash preparation of stage IX and XII tubules. DNA was counterstained by DAPI. Bar = 10 μm

4.3 Towards identification of DNA repair pathways

Double-strand breaks are processed either by homologous recombination, single-strand annealing (SSA) or non-homologous end-joining (Caldecott, 2008). Two types of NHEJ are available to mammalian cells: the pathway that is dependent of DNA PKcs (referred to as D-

NHEJ) and the alternative (or "back-up") pathway (referred to as B-NHEJ), which is also known as microhomology-mediated end-joining (MMEJ) (Ciccia and Elledge, 2010; West, 2003). Therefore, we will discuss known somatic DNA repair pathways and their potential role in spermatids when supported by published data.

4.3.1 Homologous recombination and single-strand annealing

Given the haploid character spermatids, HR could not take place as sister chromatids or homologous chromosomes are not available for recombination. Considering that HR precisely restores the genomic sequence of the broken DNA ends by utilizing sister chromatids as template for DNA repair, HR usually occurs in late S2 and G phase of the cycle in mammals (Kass and Jasin, 2010), whereas spermatids are considered to be in a G1-like phase (Ahmed et al., 2010). Upon resection at DNA breaks by the MRN complex, two different pathways are usually possible: HR or SSA (Wold, 1997). The SSA pathway could use repetitive DNA sequences to promote the DNA repair of DSBs in spermatids (Hartlerode and Scully, 2009; Motycka et al., 2004). This pathway is known to introduce errors such as deletions, insertions and even be a substrate for chromosomal translocations (Griffin and Thacker, 2004). There is currently no evidence that spermatids use SSA rather than NHEJ to repair DSBs, but some key proteins of this pathway, although also part of the NER pathway (see Table 1 and Table 2), are present during spermiogenesis including ERCC1 (Hsia et al., 2003; Paul et al., 2007) as well as XPF (Shannon, 1999).

DNA repair pathways	Implicated proteins	Typical error
Homologous recombination (HR)	BRCA1/2, Rad51, XRCC2, LIG1, RPA	Error free
Single strand annealing (SSA)	ERCC1, ERCC4 (XPF), Rad52	Indels (++) Chromosomal translocation (++)
Non-homologous end-joining DNA PK dependant (D-NHEJ)	DNA PKcs, Ku70, ARTEMIS, XRCC4, LIG4, XLF (NHEJ1)	Indels (+) Chromosomal translocation (+)
Alternative non-homologous end joining (B-NHEJ)	PARP, XRCC1, LIG3	Indels (+) Chromosomal translocation (+)

Table 2. DNA double-strand break repair pathways and their typical error. (+) Occasional, (++) frequent (Ciccia and Elledge, 2010; Griffin and Thacker, 2004).

4.3.2 Non-homologous end joining

Besides SSA, B-NHEJ and D-NHEJ are potentially available for the repair of double-strand breaks during spermiogenesis (Leduc et al., 2008a; Leduc et al., 2008b). In somatic cells, NHEJ pathways promote the religation of DSBs, introducing small insertions and deletions. NHEJ pathways operates throughout the cell cycle but are most active during G1 phase because HR cannot proceed during that time (Daley et al., 2005). Spermatids provide a similar cellular context as G1 phase of somatic cells. However, dynamics of DNA repair by NHEJ pathways, as illustrated in irradiated round spermatids, are much slower (Ahmed et al., 2010). According to Ahmed and colleagues both pathways are present and active during mouse spermiogenesis: spermatids of SCID mice, lacking the D-NHEJ because of the absence of DNA PKcs, displayed slower repair than those from wild type mice (Ahmed et al., 2010). Further studies on the end-joining pathways in elongating spermatids will be required as these are known to be error-prone in somatic cells. This may also be the case in spermatids. Although an attenuation of the frequency of mutations may be found in the germ line (Walter et al., 1998), the chromatin remodeling in spermatids may still be the key differentiation steps where most of the new mutations repertoire is being produced for the transmission to the next generation.

5. Possible consequences on fertility and genetic integrity

5.1 Incomplete DNA repair

High level of sperm DNA fragmentation, sperm DNA damages and chromatin alterations decrease pregnancy rates in natural fertilization, intrauterine insemination and *in vitro* fertilization (Bungum et al., 2007; Duran, 2002; Evenson et al., 1999; Evenson and Wixon, 2006; Spano et al., 2000; Zini, 2011). Moreover, pregnancy loss following *in vitro* fertilization (IVF) or intracytoplasmic sperm injection (ICSI) treatments has also been attributed to poor sperm DNA integrity (Zini et al., 2008). Although sperm DNA fragmentation is more frequent in infertile men, sperm of fertile men display DNA fragmentation but to a lesser extent (Bellver et al., 2010; Brahem et al., 2011; Perrin et al., 2009; Rybar et al., 2009; Venkatesh et al., 2011; Watanabe et al., 2011). After fertilization, the oocyte can efficiently repair some paternal DNA damages (Brandriff and Pedersen, 1981; Marchetti et al., 2007), but in the case of highly damaged sperm DNA, this could exceed the DNA repair capacity of the oocyte leading to some genetic aberrations, developmental arrest or pregnancy loss.

5.2 Faulty repair

Structural aberrations

Chromosomal structural aberrations such as translocations, deletions and inversions, may originate from meiotic recombination involving non-allelic repeated DNA sequences (Heyer et al., 2010). However, since about 80% of chromosomal rearrangements are reported to be of paternal origin (Buwe et al., 2005; Thomas et al., 2006) and that male and female meiosis involves similar genetic mechanisms (Gu et al., 2008; Thomas et al., 2006), one can surmise that yet another process unique to male gametogenesis may be involved. We therefore hypothesize that the chromatin remodeling process in spermatids, generating transient double-strand breaks, may provide the proper context for faulty repair and induction of transgenerational polymorphism. In addition, it is tempting to speculate that, because chromatin condensation occurs, free DNA ends are brought in juxtaposition, increasing the chance of NHEJ repair involving two different chromosomes, which may lead to translocations. Interestingly, chromosomes possess their own territory within the nucleus of somatic cells and in sperm cells (Hazzouri et al., 2000; Manvelyan et al., 2008; Mudrak et al., 2005; Zalenskaya et al., 2000). Moreover, chromosomes known to have higher translocation rates have close chromosomal territories in somatic cells (Branco and Pombo, 2006; Brianna

Caddle et al., 2007; Manoj S Gandhi and Nikiforov, 2009). Thus, chromosomes with close chromosomal territories in spermatids could be more prone to interchromosomal translocation during chromatin remodeling. In addition, the potential for the spermatidal chromatin remodeling to produce non-B DNA structure may exacerbate the propensity for spermatids to produce translocation (Hidehito Inagaki and Kurahashi, 2009; Raghavan and Lieber, 2004). Further investigation is needed on the mechanism and potential involvement of chromatin remodeling in such events.

Insertions and deletions

As outlined above, NHEJ repair pathways are known to create insertions and deletions (indels) as they use microhomology to join the two DNA ends. This type of mutations may be particularly harmful in coding sequences as it may cause codon frameshifts or alteration of mRNA splicing. Moreover, Y chromosomes microdeletions, associated with increased male infertility, may exhibit the classical signature of micro-homology based DNA repair pathways such as SSA and B-NHEJ as the deletion occurs between repetitive, often palindromic sequences (Paulo Navarro-Costa and Plancha; Yen, 1998). Although SSA is available during most of spermatogenesis, the B-NHEJ signature on the highly repetitive Y chromosome may be indicative of a faulty DNA repair in spermatids as this pathway is inhibited during meiosis.

Dynamic mutations

Several diseases with dynamic mutation, characterized by the expansion over generation of a trinucleotidic repeat (TNRs), are associated with a paternal bias of expansion, such as Huntington disease (HD), spinocerebellar ataxia type 2 and 7 (Cancel et al., 1997; Stevanin et al., 1998; Zühlke et al., 1993). TNRs are microsatellites sequences in coding or non-coding region of the genome. Their stability, which is relative to the chance of adopting a secondary structure, is dependent of the nature of the sequence and the length of the TNR (Kovtun et al.; Tóth et al., 2000). The exact mechanism of TNR expansion or contraction is still not clear. However, studies show strong evidences that TNR expansion in the huntingtin gene occurs during spermiogenesis; in a transgenic mouse model carrying the mutated human gene, an increased length of the CAG repetition was observed in mature spermatozoa but not in early haploid spermatids and other tissues. Kovtun and McMurray also demonstrated the involvement of MSH2, a protein involved in the gap repair and mismatch repair pathways, as this expansion was absent in HD mice MSH2-/- (Albin and Tagle, 1995; Kovtun and McMurray, 2001). The remodeling chromatin of spermatids may promote secondary structure formation at TNRs, providing an ideal context for such mutations.

6. Conclusion

The chromatin remodeling in spermatids involves transient DNA-strand breaks. Our group has generated evidences that a significant number of double-strand breaks are generated. These DSBs seemingly trigger a damage response as H2AFX is phosphorylated and a DNA repair pathway yet to be identified. As a result, no such DSBs are found in the mature sperm unless a pathological condition prevails. The non-templated DNA repair of these transient DSBs are expected to introduce small mutations likely distributed randomly across the haploid genome although their distribution remains to be established. Meiosis is well known to produce new combination of alleles but is not a primary driver of sequence divergence (Noor, 2008). Potential new gene function must arise through point mutations or indels and the present review suggests chromatin remodeling of spermatids as an appropriate context for such induction of new polymorphism and possible translocations. Although the frequency of mutation may be lower in germ cells than in somatic cells (Walter et al., 1998), we hypothesize that most of the new mutations generated during spermatogenesis may be through the process of endogenous strand breaks and repair during spermiogenesis. Owing to the 1% chance for a random mutation to occur within genes due to exonic representation in the genome, most mutations are expected to be silent but, if within coding sequences, potential alteration of gene function may be transmitted. In summary, repair of the endogenous DSBs in spermatids may represent a new male-driven source of genetic variation.

7. References

Ahmed, E.A., de Boer, P., Philippens, M.E.P., Kal, H.B., and de Rooij, D.G. (2010). Parp1–XRCC1 and the repair of DNA double strand breaks in mouse round spermatids. Mutation Research *683*, 84-90.

Albin, R.L., and Tagle, D.A. (1995). Genetics and molecular biology of Huntington's disease. Trends in Neurosciences *18*, 11-14.

Arpanahi, A., Brinkworth, M., Iles, D., Krawetz, S., Paradowska, A., Platts, A., Saida, M., Steger, K., Tedder, P., and Miller, D. (2009). Endonuclease-sensitive regions of human spermatozoal chromatin are highly enriched in promoter and CTCF binding sequences. Genome Res.

Baarends, W., Hoogerbrugge, J., Roest, H., Ooms, M., Vreeburg, J., Hoeijmakers, J., and Grootegoed, J. (1999). Histone ubiquitination and chromatin remodeling in mouse spermatogenesis. Dev Biol *207*, 322-333.

Baccetti, B., Strehler, E., Capitani, S., Collodel, G., De Santo, M., Moretti, E., Piomboni, P., Wiedeman, R., and Sterzik, K. (1997). The effect of follicle stimulating hormone therapy on human sperm structure. Hum Reprod *12*, 1955-1968.

Balhorn, R. (1982). A model for the structure of chromatin in mammalian sperm. J Cell Biol *93*, 298-305.

Balhorn, R., Gledhill, B.L., and Wyrobek, A.J. (1977). Mouse sperm chromatin proteins: quantitative isolation and partial characterization. Biochemistry *16*, 4074-4080.

Balhorn, R., Weston, S., Thomas, C., and Wyrobek, A. (1984). DNA packaging in mouse spermatids. Synthesis of protamine variants and four transition proteins. Exp Cell Res *150*, 298-308.

Bellver, J., Meseguer, M., Muriel, L., García-Herrero, S., Barreto, M.A.M., Garda, A.L., Remohí, J., Pellicer, A., and Garrido, N. (2010). Y chromosome microdeletions, sperm DNA fragmentation and sperm oxidative stress as causes of recurrent spontaneous abortion of unknown etiology. Human Reproduction *25*, 1713-1721.

Blanco-Rodríguez, J. (2009). gammaH2AX marks the main events of the spermatogenic process. Microsc Res Tech.

Boissonneault, G. (2002). Chromatin remodeling during spermiogenesis: a possible role for the transition proteins in DNA strand break repair. FEBS Lett *514*, 111-114.

Brahem, S., Mehdi, M., Elghezal, H., and Saad, A. (2011). Analysis of Sperm Aneuploidies and DNA Fragmentation in Patients With Globozoospermia or With Abnormal Acrosomes. Urology.

Branciforte, D., and Martin, S.L. (1994). Developmental and cell type specificity of LINE-1 expression in mouse testis: implications for transposition. Mol Cell Biol *14*, 2584-2592.

Branco, M.R., and Pombo, A. (2006). Intermingling of Chromosome Territories in Interphase Suggests Role in Translocations and Transcription-Dependent Associations. PLoS biology *4*, e138.

Brandriff, B., and Pedersen, R. (1981). Repair of the ultraviolet-irradiated male genome in fertilized mouse eggs. Science *211*, 1431-1433.

Braun, R.E. (2001). Packaging paternal chromosomes with protamine. Nat Genet *28*, 10-12.

Brianna Caddle, L., Grant, J.L., Szatkiewicz, J., Hase, J., Shirley, B.-J., Bewersdorf, J., Cremer, C., Arneodo, A., Khalil, A., and Mills, K.D. (2007). Chromosome neighborhood composition determines translocation outcomes after exposure to high-dose radiation in primary cells. Chromosome research *15*, 1061-1073.

Bungum, M., Humaidan, P., Axmon, A., Spano, M., Bungum, L., Erenpreiss, J., and Giwercman, A. (2007). Sperm DNA integrity assessment in prediction of assisted reproduction technology outcome. Human reproduction *22*, 174-179.

Buwe, A., Guttenbach, M., and Schmid, M. (2005). Effect of paternal age on the frequency of cytogenetic abnormalities in human spermatozoa. Cytogenet Gen Res *111*, 213-228.

Cabrero, J., Palomino-Morales, R.J., and Camacho, J.P.M. (2007). The DNA-repair Ku70 protein is located in the nucleus and tail of elongating spermatids in grasshoppers. Chromosome Res *15*, 1093-1100.

Caldecott, K.W. (2008). Single-strand break repair and genetic disease. Nature Reviews Genetics *9*, 619-631.

Cancel, G., Dürr, A., Didierjean, O., Imbert, G., Bürk, K., Lezin, A., Belal, S., Benomar, A., Abada-Bendib, M., Vial, C., *et al.* (1997). Molecular and clinical correlations in spinocerebellar ataxia 2: a study of 32 families. Human Molecular Genetics *6*, 709-715.

Celeste, A., Fernandez-Capetillo, O., Kruhlak, M.J., Pilch, D.R., Staudt, D.W., Lee, A., Bonner, R.F., Bonner, W.M., and Nussenzweig, A. (2003). Histone H2AX phosphorylation is dispensable for the initial recognition of DNA breaks. Nature Cell Biology *5*, 675-679.

Celli, G.B., Denchi, E.L., and de Lange, T. (2006). Ku70 stimulates fusion of dysfunctional telomeres yet protects chromosome ends from homologous recombination. Nat Cell Biol *8*, 885-890.

Chen, H., Sun, J., Zhang, Y., Davie, J., and Meistrich, M. (1998). Ubiquitination of histone H3 in elongating spermatids of rat testes. J Biol Chem *273*, 13165-13169.

Chen, J., and Longo, F. (1996). Expression and localization of DNA topoisomerase II during rat spermatogenesis. Mol Reprod Dev *45*, 61-71.

Cheng, C.Y., and Mruk, D.D. (2002). Cell junction dynamics in the testis: Sertoli-germ cell interactions and male contraceptive development. Physiol rev *82*, 825-874.

Chowdhury, D., Keogh, M.-C., Ishii, H., Peterson, C.L., Buratowski, S., and Lieberman, J. (2005). gamma-H2AX dephosphorylation by protein phosphatase 2A facilitates DNA double-strand break repair. Molecular cell *20*, 801-809.

Christensen, M., Rattner, J., and Dixon, G. (1984). Hyperacetylation of histone H4 promotes chromatin decondensation prior to histone replacement by protamines during spermatogenesis in rainbow trout. Nucleic Acids Res *12*, 4575-4592.

Churikov, D., Siino, J., Svetlova, M., Zhang, K., Gineitis, A., Morton Bradbury, E., and Zalensky, A. (2004). Novel human testis-specific histone H2B encoded by the interrupted gene on the X chromosome. Genomics *84*, 745-756.

Ciccia, A., and Elledge, S.J. (2010). The DNA Damage Response: Making It Safe to Play with Knives. Molecular cell *40*, 179-204.

Daley, J.M., Laan, R.L.V., Suresh, A., and Wilson, T.E. (2005). DNA joint dependence of pol X family polymerase action in nonhomologous end joining. The Journal of biological chemistry *280*, 29030-29037.

Dantzer, F., Mark, M., Quenet, D., Scherthan, H., Huber, A., Liebe, B., Monaco, L., Chicheportiche, A., Sassone-Corsi, P., de Murcia, G., *et al.* (2006). Poly(ADP-ribose) polymerase-2 contributes to the fidelity of male meiosis I and spermiogenesis. Proc Natl Acad Sci USA *103*, 14854-14859.

Di Virgilio, M., and Gautier, J. (2005). Repair of double-strand breaks by nonhomologous end joining in the absence of Mre11. The Journal of cell biology *171*, 765-771.

Donnelly, E.T., O'Connell, M., McClure, N., and Lewis, S.E. (2000). Differences in nuclear DNA fragmentation and mitochondrial integrity of semen and prepared human spermatozoa. Hum Reprod *15*, 1552-1561.

Duran, E.H. (2002). Sperm DNA quality predicts intrauterine insemination outcome: a prospective cohort study. Human Reproduction *17*, 3122-3128.

Dym, M., and Fawcett, D.W. (1970). The blood-testis barrier in the rat and the physiological compartmentation of the seminiferous epithelium. Biol Reprod *3*, 308-326.

Ergün, S., Buschmann, C., Heukeshoven, J., Dammann, K., Schnieders, F., Lauke, H., Chalajour, F., Kilic, N., Strätling, W.H., and Schumann, G.G. (2004). Cell type-specific expression of LINE-1 open reading frames 1 and 2 in fetal and adult human tissues. J Biol Chem *279*, 27753-27763.

Evenson, D., Jost, L., Marshall, D., Zinaman, M., Clegg, E., Purvis, K., de Angelis, P., and Claussen, O. (1999). Utility of the sperm chromatin structure assay as a diagnostic and prognostic tool in the human fertility clinic. Hum Reprod *14*, 1039-1049.

Evenson, D., and Wixon, R. (2006). Clinical aspects of sperm DNA fragmentation detection and male infertility. Theriogenology *65*, 979-991.

Gandini, L., Lombardo, F., Paoli, D., Caponecchia, L., Familiari, G., Verlengia, C., Dondero, F., and Lenzi, A. (2000). Study of apoptotic DNA fragmentation in human spermatozoa. Hum Reprod *15*, 830-839.

Gasior, S.L., Wakeman, T.P., Xu, B., and Deininger, P.L. (2006). The human LINE-1 retrotransposon creates DNA double-strand breaks. J Mol Biol *357*, 1383-1393.

Gatewood, J.M., Cook, G.R., Balhorn, R., Schmid, C.W., and Bradbury, E.M. (1990). Isolation of four core histones from human sperm chromatin representing a minor subset of somatic histones. J Biol Chem *265*, 20662-20666.

Godmann, Auger, Ferraroni-Aguiar, Sauro, D., Sette, Behr, and Kimmins (2007). Dynamic Regulation of Histone H3 Methylation at Lysine 4 in Mammalian Spermatogenesis. Biol Reprod.

Goedecke, W., Eijpe, M., Offenberg, H., van Aalderen, M., and Heyting, C. (1999). Mre11 and Ku70 interact in somatic cells, but are differentially expressed in early meiosis. Nat Genet *23*, 194-198.

Golan, R., Cooper, T.G., Oschry, Y., Oberpenning, F., Schulze, H., Shochat, L., and Lewin, L.M. (1996). Changes in chromatin condensation of human spermatozoa during epididymal transit as determined by flow cytometry. Hum Reprod *11*, 1457-1462.

Govin, J., Escoffier, E., Rousseaux, S., Kuhn, L., Ferro, M., Thévenon, J., Catena, R., Davidson, I., Garin, J., Khochbin, S., *et al.* (2007). Pericentric heterochromatin reprogramming by new histone variants during mouse spermiogenesis. J Cell Biol *176*, 283-294.

Griffin, C.S., and Thacker, J. (2004). The role of homologous recombination repair in the formation of chromosome aberrations. Cytogenet Genome Res *104*, 21-27.

Grimes, S., and Henderson, N. (1984). Hyperacetylation of histone H4 in rat testis spermatids. Exp Cell Res *152*, 91-97.

Griswold, M.D. (1998). The central role of Sertoli cells in spermatogenesis. Seminars in cell & developmental biology *9*, 411-416.

Gu, W., Zhang, F., and Lupski, J. (2008). Mechanisms for human genomic rearrangements. Patho Genetics *1*, 4.

Gusse, M., Sautière, P., Bélaiche, D., Martinage, A., Roux, C., Dadoune, J.P., and Chevaillier, P. (1986). Purification and characterization of nuclear basic proteins of human sperm. Biochim Biophys Acta *884*, 124-134.

Hamer, G., Roepers-Gajadien, H.L., van Duyn-Goedhart, A., Gademan, I.S., Kal, H.B., van Buul, P.P.W., Ashley, T., and de Rooij, D.G. (2003). Function of DNA-protein kinase catalytic subunit during the early meiotic prophase without Ku70 and Ku86. Biol Reprod *68*, 717-721.

Harrison, R.G., and Weiner, J.S. (1949). Vascular patterns of the mammalian testis and their functional significance. The Journal of experimental biology *26*, 304-316, 302 pl.

Hartlerode, A.J., and Scully, R. (2009). Mechanisms of double-strand break repair in somatic mammalian cells. The Biochemical journal *423*, 157-168.

Hazzouri, M., Pivot-Pajot, C., Faure, A., Usson, Y., Pelletier, R., Sele, B., Khochbin, S., and Rousseaux, S. (2000). Regulated hyperacetylation of core histones during mouse spermatogenesis: involvement of histone deacetylases. Eur J Cell Biol *79*, 950-960.

Heyer, W.-D., Ehmsen, K.T., and Liu, J. (2010). Regulation of homologous recombination in eukaryotes. Annual review of genetics *44*, 113-139.

Inagaki H, Ohye T, Kogo H, Kato T, Bolor H, Taniguchi M, Shaikh TH, Emanuel BS and Kurahashi H (2009). Chromosomal instability mediated by non-B DNA: Cruciform conformation and not DNA sequence is responsible for recurrent translocation in humans. Genome research *19*, 191.

Hoeijmakers, J.H.J. (2009). DNA damage, aging, and cancer. The New England journal of medicine *361*, 1475-1485.

Hsia, K., Millar, M., King, S., Selfridge, J., Redhead, N., Melton, D., and Saunders, P. (2003). DNA repair gene Ercc1 is essential for normal spermatogenesis and oogenesis and for functional integrity of germ cell DNA in the mouse. Development *130*, 369-378.

Huang, J., and Dynan, W.S. (2002). Reconstitution of the mammalian DNA double-strand break end-joining reaction reveals a requirement for an Mre11/Rad50/NBS1-containing fraction. Nucleic acids research *30*, 667-674.

Johnson, G.D., Lalancette, C., Linnemann, A.K., Leduc, F., Boissonneault, G., and Krawetz, S.A. (2011). The sperm nucleus: chromatin, RNA, and the nuclear matrix. Reproduction *141*, 21-36.

Ju, B., Lunyak, V., Perissi, V., Garcia-Bassets, I., Rose, D., Glass, C., and Rosenfeld, M. (2006). A topoisomerase IIbeta-mediated dsDNA break required for regulated transcription. Science *312*, 1798-1802.

Jung, A., and Schuppe, H.-C. (2007). Influence of genital heat stress on semen quality in humans. Andrologia *39*, 203-215.

Kass, E.M., and Jasin, M. (2010). Collaboration and competition between DNA double-strand break repair pathways. FEBS letters *584*, 3703-3708.

Kinner, A., Wu, W., Staudt, C., and Iliakis, G. (2008). Gamma-H2AX in recognition and signaling of DNA double-strand breaks in the context of chromatin. Nucleic acids research *36*, 5678-5694.

Kotaja, N., Kimmins, S., Brancorsini, S., Hentsch, D., Vonesch, J., Davidson, I., Parvinen, M., and Sassone-Corsi, P. (2004). Preparation, isolation and characterization of stage-specific spermatogenic cells for cellular and molecular analysis. Nat Methods *1*, 249-254.

Kovtun, I., and McMurray, C. (2001). Trinucleotide expansion in haploid germ cells by gap repair. Nat Genet *27*, 407-411.

Kovtun, I.V., Goellner, G., and McMurray, C.T. Structural features of trinucleotide repeats associated with DNA expansion. Biochem Cell Biol. *79*, 325-36.

Krishnamoorthy, T., Chen, X., Govin, J., Cheung, W., Dorsey, J., Schindler, K., Winter, E., Allis, C., Guacci, V., and Khochbin, S. (2006). Phosphorylation of histone H4 Ser1 regulates sporulation in yeast and is conserved in fly and mouse spermatogenesis. Genes & development *20*, 2580.

Laberge, R.-M., and Boissonneault, G. (2005). On the nature and origin of DNA strand breaks in elongating spermatids. Biol Reprod *73*, 289-296.

Lamarche, B.J., Orazio, N.I., and Weitzman, M.D. (2010). The MRN complex in double-strand break repair and telomere maintenance. FEBS letters *584*, 3682-3695.

Leduc, F., Maquennehan, V., Nkoma, G.B., and Boissonneault, G. (2008a). DNA damage response during chromatin remodeling in elongating spermatids of mice. Biol Reprod *78*, 324-332.

Leduc, F., Nkoma, G.B., and Boissonneault, G. (2008b). Spermiogenesis and DNA repair: a possible etiology of human infertility and genetic disorders. Syst Biol Reprod Med *54*, 3-10.

Loonie D. Russell, A.P.S.H., Robert Ettlin (1990). Histological and histopathological evaluation of the testis (Cache River Press).

Lu, S., Xie, Y.M., Li, X., Luo, J., Shi, X.Q., Hong, X., Pan, Y.H., and Ma, X. (2009). Mass spectrometry analysis of dynamic post-translational modifications of TH2B during spermatogenesis. Mol Hum Reprod *15*, 373-378.

Mah, L.-J., El-Osta, A., and Karagiannis, T.C. (2010). gammaH2AX: a sensitive molecular marker of DNA damage and repair. Leukemia : official journal of the Leukemia Society of America, Leukemia Research Fund, UK *24*, 679-686.

Mah, L.-J., Orlowski, C., Ververis, K., Vasireddy, R.S., El-Osta, A., and Karagiannis, T.C. (2011). Evaluation of the efficacy of radiation-modifying compounds using γH2AX as a molecular marker of DNA double-strand breaks. Genome integrity *2*, 3.

Gandhi MS, Stringer JR, Nikiforova MN, Medvedovic M and Nikiforov YE.. (2009). Gene position within chromosome territories correlates with their involvment in distinct rearrangement types in thyroid cancer cells. Genes Chromosomes Cancer *48*, 222.

Manvelyan, M., Hunstig, F., Bhatt, S., Mrasek, K., Pellestor, F., Weise, A., Simonyan, I., Aroutiounian, R., and Liehr, T. (2008). Chromosome distribution in human sperm - a 3D multicolor banding-study. Molecular cytogenetics *1*, 25.

Marchetti, F., Essers, J., Kanaar, R., and Wyrobek, A.J. (2007). Disruption of maternal DNA repair increases sperm-derived chromosomal aberrations. Proc Natl Acad Sci USA *104*, 17725-17729.

Marcon, L., and Boissonneault, G. (2004). Transient DNA strand breaks during mouse and human spermiogenesis new insights in stage specificity and link to chromatin remodeling. Biol Reprod *70*, 910-918.

Martianov, I., Brancorsini, S., Catena, R., Gansmuller, A., Kotaja, N., Parvinen, M., Sassone-Corsi, P., and Davidson, I. (2005). Polar nuclear localization of H1T2, a histone H1 variant, required for spermatid elongation and DNA condensation during spermiogenesis. Proc Natl Acad Sci USA *102*, 2808-2813.

Martin, L.M., Marples, B., Coffey, M., Lawler, M., Lynch, T.H., Hollywood, D., and Marignol, L. (2010). DNA mismatch repair and the DNA damage response to ionizing radiation: making sense of apparently conflicting data. Cancer treatment reviews *36*, 518-527.

McPherson, S., and Longo, F. (1992). Localization of DNase I-hypersensitive regions during rat spermatogenesis: stage-dependent patterns and unique sensitivity of elongating spermatids. Mol Reprod Dev *31*, 268-279.

McPherson, S., and Longo, F. (1993). Nicking of rat spermatid and spermatozoa DNA: possible involvement of DNA topoisomerase II. Dev Biol *158*, 122-130.

Meistrich, M.L., Trostle-Weige, P.K., Lin, R., Bhatnagar, Y.M., and Allis, C.D. (1992). Highly acetylated H4 is associated with histone displacement in rat spermatids. Mol Reprod Dev *31*, 170-181.

Meyer-Ficca, M., Scherthan, H., Burkle, A., and Meyer, R. (2005). Poly(ADP-ribosyl)ation during chromatin remodeling steps in rat spermiogenesis. Chromosoma *114*, 67-74.

Meyer-Ficca, M.L., Ihara, M., Lonchar, J.D., Meistrich, M.L., Austin, C.A., Min, W., Wang, Z.-Q., and Meyer, R.G. (2011a). Poly(ADP-ribose) metabolism is essential for proper nucleoprotein exchange during mouse spermiogenesis. Biol Reprod *84*, 218-228.

Meyer-Ficca, M.L., Lonchar, J., Credidio, C., Ihara, M., Li, Y., Wang, Z.-Q., and Meyer, R.G. (2009). Disruption of poly(ADP-ribose) homeostasis affects spermiogenesis and sperm chromatin integrity in mice. Biol Reprod *81*, 46-55.

Meyer-Ficca, M.L., Lonchar, J.D., Ihara, M., Meistrich, M.L., Austin, C.A., and Meyer, R.G. (2011b). Poly(ADP-Ribose) Polymerases PARP1 and PARP2 Modulate Topoisomerase II Beta (TOP2B) Function During Chromatin Condensation in Mouse Spermiogenesis. Biology of reproduction.

Mital, P., Hinton, B.T., and Dufour, J.M. (2011). The Blood-Testis and Blood-Epididymis Barriers Are More Than Just Their Tight Junctions. Biology of reproduction.

Morse-Gaudio, M., and Risley, M.S. (1994). Topoisomerase II expression and VM-26 induction of DNA breaks during spermatogenesis in Xenopus laevis. J Cell Sci *107 (Pt 10)*, 2887-2898.

Motycka, T.A., Bessho, T., Post, S.M., Sung, P., and Tomkinson, A.E. (2004). Physical and functional interaction between the XPF/ERCC1 endonuclease and hRad52. The Journal of biological chemistry *279*, 13634-13639.

Mudrak, O., Tomilin, N., and Zalensky, A. (2005). Chromosome architecture in the decondensing human sperm nucleus. Journal of Cell Science *118*, 4541-4550.

Mukherjee, S., Ridgeway, A.D., and Lamb, D.J. (2010). DNA mismatch repair and infertility. Current Opinion in Urology *20*, 525-532.

Noor, M.A.F. (2008). Mutagenesis from Meiotic Recombination Is Not a Primary Driver of Sequence Divergence between Saccharomyces Species. Molecular biology and evolution *25*, 2439-2444.

Nouspikel, T. (2009). DNA repair in mammalian cells : Nucleotide excision repair: variations on versatility. Cellular and molecular life sciences : CMLS *66*, 994-1009.

Oakberg, E.F., and Diminno, R.L. (1960). X-ray sensitivity of primary spermatocytes of the mouse.int. Int J Radiat Biol *2*, 196-209.

Olsen, A., Bjørtuft, H., Wiger, R., Holme, J., Seeberg, E., Bjørås, M., and Brunborg, G. (2001). Highly efficient base excision repair (BER) in human and rat male germ cells. Nucleic Acids Res *29*, 1781-1790.

Paul, C., Povey, J.E., Lawrence, N.J., Selfridge, J., Melton, D.W., and Saunders, P.T.K. (2007). Deletion of Genes Implicated in Protecting the Integrity of Male Germ Cells Has Differential Effects on the Incidence of DNA Breaks and Germ Cell Loss. PLoS ONE *2*, e989.

Paulo Navarro-Costa, J.G., and Plancha, C.E. The AZFc region of the Y chromosome: at the crossroads between genetic diversity and male infertility. Human Reproduction Update *16*, 525.

Perrin, A., Caer, E., Oliver-Bonet, M., Navarro, J., Benet, J., Amice, V., De Braekeleer, M., and Morel, F. (2009). DNA fragmentation and meiotic segregation in sperm of carriers of a chromosomal structural abnormality. Fertility and sterility *92*, 583-589.

Quénet, D., Mark, M., Govin, J., van Dorsselear, A., Schreiber, V., Khochbin, S., and Dantzer, F. (2009). Parp2 is required for the differentiation of post-meiotic germ cells: identification of a spermatid-specific complex containing Parp1, Parp2, TP2 and HSPA2. Exp Cell Res *315*, 2824-2834.

Raghavan, S.C., and Lieber, M.R. (2004). Chromosomal Translocations and Non-B DNA Structures in the Human Genome. Cell cycle *3*, 760-766.

Rass, E., Grabarz, A., Plo, I., Gautier, J., Bertrand, P., and Lopez, B.S. (2009). Role of Mre11 in chromosomal nonhomologous end joining in mammalian cells. Nature structural molecular biology *16*, 819-824.

Rathke, C., Baarends, W.M., Jayaramaiah-Raja, S., Bartkuhn, M., Renkawitz, R., and Renkawitz-Pohl, R. (2007). Transition from a nucleosome-based to a protamine-based chromatin configuration during spermiogenesis in Drosophila. J Cell Sci *120*, 1689-1700.

Rato, L., Socorro, S., Cavaco, J.E.B., and Oliveira, P.F. (2010). Tubular fluid secretion in the seminiferous epithelium: ion transporters and aquaporins in Sertoli cells. The Journal of membrane biology *236*, 215-224.

Robertson, A.B., Klungland, A., Rognes, T., and Leiros, I. (2009). DNA repair in mammalian cells: Base excision repair: the long and short of it. Cellular and molecular life sciences *66*, 981-993.

Roca, J., and Mezquita, C. (1989). DNA topoisomerase II activity in nonreplicating, transcriptionally inactive, chicken late spermatids. Embo J *8*, 1855-1860.

Rogakou, E.P., Boon, C., Redon, C., and Bonner, W.M. (1999). Megabase chromatin domains involved in DNA double-strand breaks in vivo. The Journal of cell biology *146*, 905-916.

Rybar, R., Markova, P., Veznik, Z., Faldikova, L., Kunetkova, M., Zajicova, A., Kopecka, V., and Rubes, J. (2009). Sperm chromatin integrity in young men with no experiences of infertility and men from idiopathic infertility couples. Andrologia *41*, 141-149.

Sakkas, D., Mariethoz, E., Manicardi, G., Bizzaro, D., Bianchi, P.G., and Bianchi, U. (1999). Origin of DNA damage in ejaculated human spermatozoa. Rev Reprod *4*, 31-37.

Sakkas, D., Moffatt, O., Manicardi, G., Mariethoz, E., Tarozzi, N., and Bizzaro, D. (2002). Nature of DNA damage in ejaculated human spermatozoa and the possible involvement of apoptosis. Biol Reprod *66*, 1061-1067.

Scherthan, H., Jerratsch, M., Dhar, S., Wang, Y., Goff, S., and Pandita, T. (2000). Meiotic telomere distribution and Sertoli cell nuclear architecture are altered in Atm- and Atm-p53-deficient mice. Mol Cell Biol *20*, 7773-7783.

Schultz, N., Hamra, F.K., and Garbers, D.L. (2003). A multitude of genes expressed solely in meiotic or postmeiotic spermatogenic cells offers a myriad of contraceptive targets. Proceedings of the National Academy of Sciences of the United States of America *100*, 12201-12206.

Setchell, B.P. (1969). Do Sertoli cells secrete fluid into the seminiferous tubules? J Reprod Fertil *19*, 391-392.

Setchell, B.P. (1998). The Parkes Lecture. Heat and the testis. J Reprod Fertil *114*, 179-194.

Shaman, J., Prisztoka, R., and Ward, W. (2006). Topoisomerase IIB and an extracellular nuclease interact to digest sperm DNA in an apoptotic-like manner. Biol Reprod *75*, 741-748.

Shannon, M. (1999). Characterization of the Mouse Xpf DNA Repair Gene and Differential Expression during Spermatogenesis. Genomics *62*, 427-435.

Shrivastav, M., de Haro, L.P., and Nickoloff, J.A. (2008). Regulation of DNA double-strand break repair pathway choice. Cell research *18*, 134-147.

Spano, M., Bonde, J.P., Hjøllund, H.I., Kolstad, H.A., Cordelli, E., and Leter, G. (2000). Sperm chromatin damage impairs human fertility. The Danish First Pregnancy Planner Study Team. Fertility and sterility *73*, 43-50.

Stevanin, G., Giunti, P., David, G., and Belal, S. (1998). De novo expansion of intermediate alleles in spinocerebellar ataxia 7. Human molecular ….

Tanphaichitr, N., Sobhon, P., Taluppeth, N., and Chalermisarachai, P. (1978). Basic nuclear proteins in testicular cells and ejaculated spermatozoa in man. Exp Cell Res *117*, 347-356.

Thomas, N.S., Durkie, M., Van Zyl, B., Sanford, R., Potts, G., Youings, S., Dennis, N., and Jacobs, P. (2006). Parental and chromosomal origin of unbalanced de novo structural chromosome abnormalities in man. Hum Genet *119*, 444-450.

Tóth, G., Gáspári, Z., and Jurka, J. (2000). Microsatellites in different eukaryotic genomes: survey and analysis. Genome research *10*, 967-981.

Turley, H., Comley, M., Houlbrook, S., Nozaki, N., Kikuchi, A., Hickson, I., Gatter, K., and Harris, A. (1997). The distribution and expression of the two isoforms of DNA topoisomerase II in normal and neoplastic human tissues. Br J Cancer *75*, 1340-1346.

van der Heijden, G., Derijck, A., Ramos, L., Giele, M., van der Vlag, J., and de Boer, P. (2006). Transmission of modified nucleosomes from the mouse male germline to the zygote and subsequent remodeling of paternal chromatin. Dev Biol *298*, 458-469.

Venkatesh, S., Kumar, R., Deka, D., Deecaraman, M., and Dada, R. (2011). Analysis of sperm nuclear protein gene polymorphisms and DNA integrity in infertile men. Systems Biology in Reproductive Medicine.

Vogl, A.W., Vaid, K.S., and Guttman, J.A. (2008). The Sertoli cell cytoskeleton. Adv Exp Med Biol *636*, 186-211.

Walter, C., Intano, G., McCarrey, J., McMahan, C., and Walter, R. (1998). Mutation frequency declines during spermatogenesis in young mice but increases in old mice. Proc Natl Acad Sci USA *95*, 10015-10019.

Ward, W.S. (1993). Deoxyribonucleic acid loop domain tertiary structure in mammalian spermatozoa. Biol Reprod *48*, 1193-1201.

Watanabe, S., Tanaka, A., Fujii, S., Mizunuma, H., Fukui, A., Fukuhara, R., Nakamura, R., Yamada, K., Tanaka, I., Awata, S., *et al.* (2011). An investigation of the potential effect of vacuoles in human sperm on DNA damage using a chromosome assay and the TUNEL assay. Human Reproduction.

Weng, S., Taylor, S., Morshedi, M., Schuffner, A., Duran, E., Beebe, S., and Oehninger, S. (2002). Caspase activity and apoptotic markers in ejaculated human sperm. Mol Hum Reprod *8*, 984-991.

West, S.C. (2003). Molecular views of recombination proteins and their control. Nature reviews Molecular cell biology *4*, 435-445.

Wojtczak, A., Popłońska, K., and Kwiatkowska, M. (2008). Phosphorylation of H2AX histone as indirect evidence for double-stranded DNA breaks related to the exchange of nuclear proteins and chromatin remodeling in Chara vulgaris spermiogenesis. Protoplasma *233*, 263-267.

Wold, M.S. (1997). Replication protein A: a heterotrimeric, single-stranded DNA-binding protein required for eukaryotic DNA metabolism. Annual review of biochemistry *66*, 61-92.

Xie, A., Kwok, A., and Scully, R. (2009). Role of mammalian Mre11 in classical and alternative nonhomologous end joining. Nature structural & molecular biology *16*, 814-818.

Yan, W., Ma, L., Burns, K., and Matzuk, M. (2003). HILS1 is a spermatid-specific linker histone H1-like protein implicated in chromatin remodeling during mammalian spermiogenesis. Proc Natl Acad Sci USA *100*, 10546-10551.

Yen, P. (1998). A Long-Range Restriction Map of Deletion Interval 6 of the Human Y Chromosome: A Region Frequently Deleted in Azoospermic Males. Genomics *54*, 5-12.

Zaalishvili, G.T., Tsetskhladze, Z.R., Margiani, D.O., Gabriadze, I.I., and Zaalishvili, T.M. (2005). ADP-ribosylation intensifies cleavage of DNA loops in the nuclear matrix. Mol Biol (Mosk) *39*, 317-320.

Zalenskaya, I.A., Bradbury, E.M., and Zalensky, A.O. (2000). Chromatin structure of telomere domain in human sperm. Biochem Biophys Res Commun *279*, 213-218.

Zini, A. (2011). Are sperm chromatin and DNA defects relevant in the clinic? Systems Biology in Reproductive Medicine *57*, 78-85.

Zini, A., Boman, J.M., Belzile, E., and Ciampi, A. (2008). Sperm DNA damage is associated with an increased risk of pregnancy loss after IVF and ICSI: systematic review and meta-analysis. Human Reproduction *23*, 2663-2668.

Zühlke, C., Rless, O., Bockel, B., Lange, H., and Thies, U. (1993). Mitotic stability and meiotic variability of the (CAG) nrepeat in the Huntington disease gene. Human Molecular Genetics *2*, 2063-2067.

17

BRCA2 Mutations and Consequences for DNA Repair

Erika T. Brown
Medical University of South Carolina
United States

1. Introduction

The *BRCA2* gene was the second gene discovered to be associated with early-onset, familial breast cancer. The BRCA2 protein is expressed in breast, ovarian, prostate, and pancreatic tissues and is associated with cancer predisposition in all four, with breast cancer being the most predominant (Goggins, Schutte et al. 1996). BRCA2 is functionally defined as a tumor suppressor and is most critical in maintenance of genomic integrity and DNA repair fidelity. The importance of BRCA2 in maintaining genomic integrity is based on its function to specifically repair double-strand DNA breaks (DSBs) via the process of homologous recombination (HR). However, BRCA2 resolves genomic lesions in concert with a number of DNA repair proteins, the most significant being RAD51 (Sharan, Morimatsu et al. 1997),(Yuan, Lee et al. 1999). RAD51 is a recombinase that is highly conserved, having homologues in *E. coli* and yeast, as well as in mammals. BRCA2 modulates the activity of RAD51 during DNA repair, and they both are found in nuclear DNA damage-induced foci, which are complexes of DNA repair proteins bound to DNA during the process of repair (Roth, Porter et al. 1985; Roth and Wilson 1986; Derbyshire, Epstein et al. 1994; Jackson and Jeggo 1995; Takata, Sasaki et al. 1998; Johnson and Jasin 2000). The relationship between BRCA2 and RAD51 has been determined to be a fundamental interaction in the repair of DSBs.

The role of BRCA2 as a tumor suppressor has been established by its importance in maintaining genomic integrity. The inability of the cell to repair DSBs can potentially cause small-scale lesions in regions of the DNA that encode single genes and incite large-scale lesions, such as chromosomal anomalies. The consequence of such damage can disrupt the normal expression of gene products that are required to regulate cell growth and arrest and induce apoptosis, thereby establishing a cellular environment that can foster malignant transformation.

Cancer cells that express mutated BRCA2 have been shown to have elevated sensitivity to the anti-cancer therapeutics called PARP (Poly [ADP-ribose] polymerase) inhibitors. PARP inhibitors prevent the binding of PARP to sites of damaged DNA, which serves as a signal to initiate DNA repair (Schreiber, Dantzer et al. 2006); (Ratnam and Low 2007). The effectiveness of PARP inhibitors in BRCA2-mutated cells is based on the premise of synthetic lethality, which is when two pathway defects alone are innocuous, but combined become lethal (Ratnam and Low 2007). The unresolved DSBs of BRCA2-mutated cells combined with the inhibition of PARP activity are effective in promoting DNA damage-induced apoptosis. This finding has established mutated BRCA2 as a potential target in improving present anti-cancer therapeutic regimens.

The information that follows will provide a comprehensive understanding of BRCA2, starting from its functions at the molecular level in maintaining genomic integrity, to describing how deregulation can lead to disease predisposition and development, and concluding with the development of PARP inhibitors that use the DNA repair defects of BRCA2-mutations to improve the sensitivity of anti-cancer treatments towards BRCA2-tumors.

2. The role of BRCA2 in DNA repair

The BRCA2 protein specifically repairs double-strand DNA breaks (DSBs) via the process of homologous recombination (HR), thereby establishing its importance in maintaining genomic integrity. The *BRCA2* gene is found on chromosome 13q12.3 and encodes a protein of 3,418 amino acids, resulting in a molecular weight of approximately 340 kDa. BRCA2 resolves genomic lesions in a complex with several additional DNA repair proteins, the most significant being RAD51 (Sharan, Morimatsu et al. 1997; Yuan, Lee et al. 1999). RAD51 is a highly conserved recombinase, having homologues in *E. coli* and yeast, as well as in mammals. BRCA2 modulates the activity of RAD51 during DNA repair and this relationship is determined to be a fundamental interaction in repair of DSBs.

2.1 The interaction between BRCA2 and the RAD51 recombinase

RAD51 catalyzes the strand exchange of DNA homologues to promote gene conversion and repair DSBs by HR (Ogawa, Yu et al. 1993) (Benson, Stasiak et al. 1994). HR is one of two pathways of repair of DSBs in mammals—the other being nonhomologous end-joining (NHEJ) (Derbyshire, Epstein et al. 1994), (Jackson and Jeggo 1995), (Roth, Porter et al. 1985), (Roth and Wilson 1986), (Takata, Sasaki et al. 1998) and (Johnson and Jasin 2000), (Figure 1). HR requires the damaged DNA molecule to use the undamaged homologue as a template in order to repair the DSB. NHEJ involves ligation of the DNA ends at the breakpoint junction regardless of whether the original genetic information is still present. As a result, HR confers greater accuracy in repair than NHEJ (Derbyshire, Epstein et al. 1994), (Jackson and Jeggo 1995), (Roth, Porter et al. 1985), (Roth and Wilson 1986), (Takata, Sasaki et al. 1998) and (Johnson and Jasin 2000). Studies performed in mice in which the *Rad51* gene was either mutated or completely knocked out have shown its importance in genomic stability and cell viability (Taki, Ohnishi et al. 1996) and (Sonoda, Sasaki et al. 1998). Nonfunctional RAD51 does not repair chromosome breaks and other DNA lesions, thereby leading to an accumulation of DSBs and stalled replication forks (Taki, Ohnishi et al. 1996) and (Sonoda, Sasaki et al. 1998). In addition, inactivation of the *RAD51* gene causes embryonic lethality (Tsuzuki, Fujii et al. 1996).

2.2 The structure of BRCA2

Yeast two-hybrid screening assays were used in the discovery of the interaction between RAD51 and BRCA2 (Mizuta, LaSalle et al. 1997), (Wong, Pero et al. 1997), (Chen, Chen et al. 1998) and (Marmorstein, Ouchi et al. 1998). And, studies examining the interaction between the two proteins have collectively shown that BRCA2 has two regions for RAD51 binding. The first region is in the mid-portion of BRCA2 and consists of eight highly conserved amino acid motifs called BRC repeats (Figure 2). The repeats have different binding affinities for RAD51:

repeats 1–4, 7, and 8 all interact with RAD51, with repeats 3 and 4 having the strongest affinity (Wong, Pero et al. 1997) (Bignell, Micklem et al. 1997). The second RAD51 binding site is located on the CTD (C-terminal domain) of BRCA2. This RAD51 binding site is described as playing a major role in the regulation of RAD51 recombination activity by displacing the single-strand DNA binding protein replication protein A (RPA) from the exonucleolytically processed 3′-single-strand overhangs of the DSBs, thus allowing RAD51 to bind and form nucleoprotein filaments (Yang, Jeffrey et al. 2002). The CTD portion of BRCA2 has been shown to be highly active in HR-mediated repair with RAD51 (Yang, Jeffrey et al. 2002). This region consists of five domains significant in DNA repair. The first is the α-helical domain, which interacts with the DMC1 protein—a meiosis specific paralog of RAD51 that forms nucleoprotein filaments and catalyzes strand exchange, and that BRCA2 requires for meiotic recombination (Thorslund, Esashi et al. 2007); (Jensen, Carreira et al.). The next three domains are the oligonucleotide–oligosaccharide binding domains (OB1, OB2, OB3) that have structural similarities with ssDNA binding proteins such as replication protein A (RPA). And, the fifth domain is the tower domain, which extends from OB2, and has structural similarities with the DNA binding domains of bacterial site-specific recombinases able to bind double-strand DNA (Yang, Jeffrey et al. 2002).

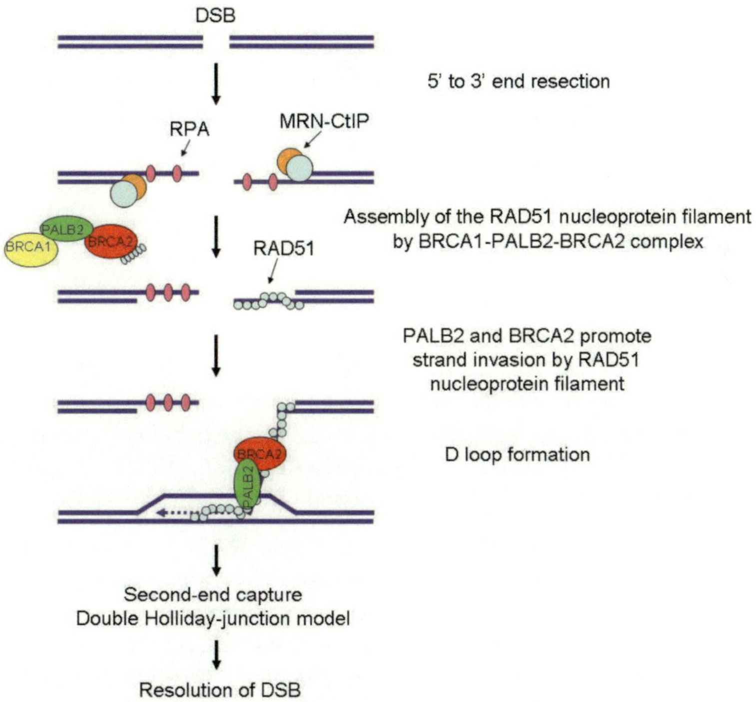

Fig. 1. Model of homologous recombination (HR)-mediated repair. After a DSB has occurred, the MRN-CtIP complex resects the 5′ends of the break. The 3′ssDNA overhangs are coated with replication protein A (RPA), which is displaced by RAD51. The BRCA1-PALB2-BRCA2 complex facilitates binding of RAD51 to form nucleoprotein filaments which invade the homologous strand, resulting in the D loop intermediate. This is followed by formation of the Holliday junction and resolution of the DSB.

Also located on the C-terminus of BRCA2 are its two nuclear localization signals (NLSs) (Spain, Larson et al. 1999) and (Yano, Morotomi et al. 2000). As a result, C-terminal mutations which disrupt, or truncations which remove, the NLSs are extremely detrimental to BRCA2 DNA repair functions, because they prevent nuclear localization. And, cell lines that have nonfunctional or absent BRCA2 NLSs primarily exhibit cytoplasmic localization of RAD51 after induction of DSBs by ionizing radiation (IR) (Spain, Larson et al. 1999). BRCA2 also interacts with RAD51 via a separate motif located at its C-terminus (Esashi, Christ et al. 2005). This interaction is regulated by cell cycle (CDK)-dependent phosphorylation of serine 3291 in exon 27 (and has been referred to, in some instances, as the "TR2" domain) and appears to function as a "switch" controlling recombinational repair activity during the transition from S/G2 to M phase in the cell cycle (Esashi, Christ et al. 2005). This phosphorylation site appears to be crucial in the checkpoint control mechanisms involved in the DNA repair pathway involving BRCA2.

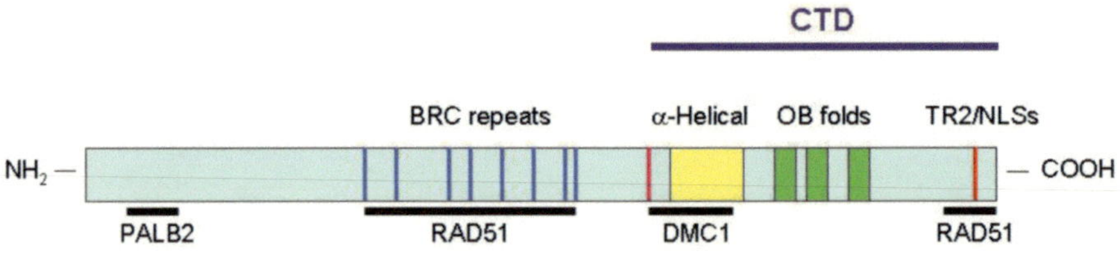

Fig. 2. Schematic of BRCA2. Starting at the N-terminus, the PALB2, the DMC1 and the two RAD51 binding sites on BRCA2 are indicated by black bars. The mid-portion contains eight highly-conserved BRC repeats. The CTD contains the α-helical domain, three OB-folds, the TR2 (location of S3291) domain, and putative nuclear localization signals (NLSs). The tower domain (not shown) extends from the second OB-fold (OB2).

The N-terminal region of BRCA2 does not bind RAD51; however, it does interact with a protein that is equally crucial to maintenance of genomic integrity, which is PALB2 (partner and localizer of BRCA2) (Xia, Sheng et al. 2006); (Rahman, Seal et al. 2007). PALB2 has been observed complexed with DNA damage-induced BRCA1/BRCA2 nuclear foci (Sy, Huen et al. 2009), (Zhang, Fan et al. 2009; Zhang, Ma et al. 2009). Subsequent studies have shown that PALB2 is crucial in the localization of BRCA2 to sites of DNA damage via associations with chromatin structures and in HR-mediated DNA repair ((Sy, Huen et al. 2009), (Zhang, Fan et al. 2009; Zhang, Ma et al. 2009). This indirectly influences the localization of RAD51 to sites of DNA damage, due to its reliance on BRCA2. During the process of HR-mediated repair, PALB2 appears to be crucial in "D-loop" formation, (Buisson, Dion-Cote et al.)2010) (figure 2). This is the step in which the 3′ overhangs of the dsDNA break, resulting from resection of the 5′ ends of the break, are coated with RAD51 protein to form nucleoprotein filaments which invade the homologous template and form a Holliday junction. In the absence of PALB2, cells exhibit genomic instability and treatment with drugs that cause inter-strand crosslinks leads to increased chromosome breakage.

3. Mutations of BRCA2, DNA repair fidelity and disease predisposition

BRCA2 and its predecessor, *BRCA1*, were the first genes to be discovered that were associated with early-onset, familial breast cancer. Furthermore, germline mutations of *BRCA2* are also responsible for hereditary forms of ovarian, prostate and pancreatic cancer; however, the risk of acquiring breast cancer is most prevalent. Moreover, the risk for breast cancer is 50-80%, however, the degree of penetrance has been shown to vary (Tonin, Weber et al. 1996).

3.1 Mutated BRCA2 in familial cancers

Most mutations in BRCA2 are the result of small deletions and insertions. In fact, a *BRCA2* mutation that has been of interest for almost two decades is the 6174delT mutation, in which the thymine at position 6174 is deleted. This mutation disrupts BRC repeats 5 and 6, and introduces a premature stop codon that abruptly truncates the protein (Neuhausen, Gilewski et al. 1996; Oddoux, Struewing et al. 1996; Roa, Boyd et al. 1996; Abeliovich, Kaduri et al. 1997; Levy-Lahad, Catane et al. 1997). The truncated form no longer possesses the CTD region, which comprises the domains required for DNA repair and recombination, the second RAD51 binding site, TR2/S3291, and the putative nuclear localization signals. As a consequence, cells with this mutation exhibit inefficient repair of DSBs, loss of genomic stability, and sensitivity to radiation and DNA crosslinking agents (Goggins, Schutte et al. 1996),(Ozcelik, Schmocker et al. 1997). The 6174delT is a founder mutation in the Ashkenazi Jewish population at a frequency of 1.36% ((Tonin, Weber et al. 1996)). And, it is the only BRCA2 mutation, along with three BRCA1 mutations, that is carried in 78-96% of Ashkenazi Jews with detectable mutations (Oddoux, Guillen-Navarro et al. 1999) (Mangold, Wang et al.)

Another *BRCA2* mutation that was also discovered to have a founder's effect is the 999del5 mutation, which was discovered in an Icelandic population (Thorlacius, Olafsdottir et al. 1996). It is a five base-pair deletion that starts at nucleotide 999, codon 257 in exon 9. The mutation introduces a frame-shift that prematurely truncates the protein, and renders it nonfunctional, similar to the effect of the 6174delT founder mutation in the Ashkenazi Jewish population. Carriers of the mutation exhibit familial forms of male or female breast, prostate or pancreatic cancer. However, there are varying forms of penetrance, in which some carriers have never been diagnosed with cancer. In fact, there is either absolutely no phenotypic expression or diagnosis of varying forms of cancer (Thorlacius, Olafsdottir et al. 1996).

In a study of BRCA1/2 mutations performed in a Serbian population, one family was shown to carry a BRCA2 mutation that was an insertion of two nucleotides, c.4367_4368dupTT (Dobricic, Brankovic-Magic et al.). The mutation causes a frame-shift that alters codons 1381-1387 and introduces a premature stop codon at position 1388, resulting in a loss of > 2,000 amino acids at the C-terminus. The protein product lacks BRC repeats 3-8, as well as the crucial CTD and TR2 domains, rendering BRCA2 completely non-functional in regulating RAD51 activity, as well as in promoting HR-mediated repair of DSBs (Dobricic, Brankovic-Magic et al.)

3.2 Mutated BRCA2 in the development of Fanconi Anemia

Another inheritable condition resulting from mutated BRCA2 is the disorder Fanconi Anemia (FA). The disorder is rare and is characterized by aplastic anemia in childhood, susceptibility to leukemia and cancer, and hypersensitivity of FA cells to interstrand crosslinking agents, such as cisplatin (D'Andrea, 2010). The FA proteins are the products of 13 genes that comprise the following subtypes, FA-A, B, C, D1, D2, E, F, G, I, J, L, M, and N. And, eight of those gene products encoding proteins FANCA-C, FANCE-G, FANCL, and FANCM form a nuclear multi-protein core complex (the FA complex) that functions in the DNA repair pathway. Furthermore, it was discovered that genes underlying the FA-D1 (*FANCD1*) and FA-N (*FANCN*) subtypes were *BRCA2* and *PALB2*, respectively. Ultimately, the multi-protein core complex is responsible for monoubiquitylating FANCD2 on lysine 561 in order to activate the Fanconi Anemia pathway in response to S-phase progression or DNA damage (Zhi, Wilson et al. 2009), (Figure 3).

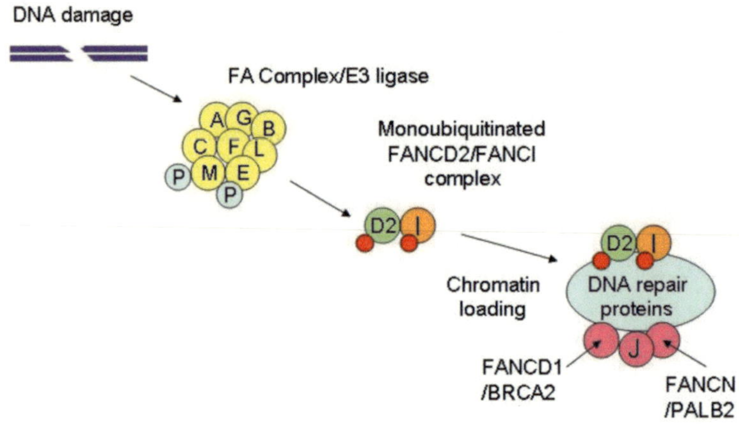

Fig. 3. Schematic of the Fanconi Anemia Pathway. After DNA damage, the ATR kinase phosphorylates and activates the FA core complex, comprised of FANCA, -B, -C, -E, -F, -G, -L, and –M. The complex functions as an E3 ligase and monoubiquitinates the FANCD2/FANCI complex, which then targets chromatin, where it assembles with other DNA repair proteins and FANCD1/BRCA2 and FANCN/PALB2 to repair damaged DNA.

The discovery of the FANCD1 protein being identified as BRCA2 was surprising, yet quite rational given the similarities between FANCD1 and BRCA2 mutated cells. They both exhibit chromosomal instabilities, sensitivity to ionizing radiation and crosslinking agents, and inefficient HR-mediated repair of DSBs. The role of FANCD1/BRCA2 in this protein complex is to act downstream in concert with the FA complex, additional FA members, and DNA repair proteins. However, Fanconi Anemia, subtype D1 is caused by biallelic inactivation of BRCA2; however, risk of breast, ovarian, prostate, and pancreatic cancers are associated with heterozygous BRCA2 mutations (Howlett, Taniguchi et al. 2002).

The FA proteins function in a DNA damage repair pathway, with the multi-protein core complex ultimately being responsible for monoubiquitylating the FANCD2 and FANC1 proteins, in response to DNA damage or entry into S phase of the cell cycle. Activation of the core complex is initiated by phosphorylation of FA proteins by the DNA damage sensing kinases ATM and ATR. After phosphorylation, the core complex assembles to form a nuclear ubiquitin E3 ligase complex. The complex proceeds to monoubiquitylate the FANCD2 and FANC1 proteins thereby causing them to move to chromatin structures and form nuclear foci at sites of DNA damage. The FA complex interacts with FA members, FANCD1/BRCA2, FANCN/PALB2 and FANCJ, along with other DNA repair proteins to promote HR-mediated resolution of DSBs. Given that this pathway is involved in HR-mediated repair, it was not surprising to discover the involvement of RAD51 and BRCA1 downstream in the FA DNA repair pathway. And, because of the involvement of BRCA2, along with BRCA1, this pathway is now referred to as the Fanconi Anemia/BRCA pathway or network (D'Andrea).

3.3 BRCA2 in cell cycle signaling and the DNA damage response

To activate BRCA2, a sequence of cell signaling events is initiated in response to DNA damage, called the DNA damage response (or DDR). When the cell has experienced DSBs, either by exogenous sources such as ionizing radiation or exposure to crosslinking agents such as cisplatin, or endogenous sources such as free radicals and stalled replication forks, the goal is to immediately arrest cell division and repair the damage. When efficient DNA repair does not occur, apoptosis is induced to prevent propagation of genetic mutations. The phosphoinositide 3-kinase related kinases (PIKKs), ataxia-telangiectasia mutated kinase (ATM), and ATM and Rad 3-related kinase (ATR), are crucial in the detection and subsequent resolution of DNA damage. Furthermore, they are also involved in the Fanconi Anemia pathway, as previously described. ATM and ATR "cross-talk" with each other, given that ATM activates ATR in response to ionizing radiation, and ATR activates ATM in response to ultraviolet light. With respect to the DDR pathway that involves BRCA2, resolution of DSBs is initiated by activation of ATR, after phosphorylation by ATM. ATR proceeds to phosphorylate and active Chk1, which then phosphorylates RAD51. Chk1 arrests the cells in S and G2 phases to ensure DNA is repaired before synthesis and cell division. At this point, RAD51 is now able to engage in HR-mediated repair of DSBs under the regulation of BRCA2 (McNeely, Conti et al.), (Connell, Shibata et al.).

BRCA2 appears to play a crucial role during S and G2 phases of the cell cycle. First, during S phase, replication forks can stall and collapse due to exogenous or endogenous sources of damage. A DNA strand break at a replication fork can mimic a DSB as a result of the nascent DNA chain that is being synthesized at the fork. At this point, activated RAD51 is required to repair the break and subsequently stalled fork. It has been proposed that deficient BRCA2, which functions to regulate RAD51 during HR-mediated repair, may be a major cause of diseases resulting from an accumulation of stalled replication forks and consequential DNA breaks that remain unrepaired (Lomonosov, Anand et al. 2003). And, with respect to G2 phase, in a study where the binding of BRCA2 with RAD51 was inhibited in cells expressing the BRC4 repeat, which competed against endogenous full-length BRCA2, there was a failure to initiate radiation-induced G2/M checkpoint arrest. These results implied that the interaction between BRCA2 and RAD51 was imperative for G2/M checkpoint control (Chen, Chen et al. 1999).

The majority of *BRCA2* mutations that are associated with cancer predisposition tend be truncations that remove substantial portions of the CTD, which is where the domains required for DNA repair are located. This region of the protein also appears to be significant in cell cycle changes due to the DNA damage response, via the TR2 domain. The TR2 domain contains a serine at 3291 that is CDK phosphorylated and appears to be one method in which binding between BRCA2 and RAD51 is regulated (Esashi, Christ et al. 2005). There is reduced phosphorylation at this site during S phase, which allows BRCA2 and RAD51 to interact, and engage in HR-mediated repair resulting from replication-induced DNA breaks. In addition, phosphorylation is reduced in response to ionizing radiation. However, phosphorylation of S3291 increases during G2/M to inactivate HR from occurring during mitosis. Further support for this region of the protein being a cancer-related mutation site is evidenced by the association of the P3292L mutation with breast cancer incidence (Esashi, Christ et al. 2005). The TR2 domain also only interacts with multimeric forms of RAD51, both in the presence and absence of DNA (Esashi, Galkin et al. 2007). And, RAD51 monomers bearing mutations that prevent self-association do not interact with the TR2 domain. The impact that this has on BRCA2 function is quite remarkable and has been elegantly summarized (Esashi, Galkin et al. 2007). In the absence of DNA damage, the TR2 domain is phosphorylated at S3291, preventing association of the C-terminus of BRCA2 with RAD51, as well as keeping BRCA2 inactive. However, concurrently, RAD51 is associated with BRCA2 via the BRC repeats in monomeric form. And, it has been noted that the BRC repeats may serve as a negative regulator of RAD51 by preventing it from forming nucleoprotein filaments with ssDNA until after damage has been detected and the DNA has been prepped for HR-mediated repair. After DNA damage has been detected, S3291 is dephosphorylated, now allowing BRCA2 to become activated. The C-terminus can now bind with RAD51 in multimeric form, and the OB folds which possess ssDNA binding activity, deliver RAD51 to sites of DNA damage. This change in BRCA2 function from negatively regulating RAD51 to mobilizing it to sites of damage may be driven by the self-assembly of RAD51 from a monomeric to a multimeric state in response to DNA damage (Esashi, Galkin et al. 2007). This detrimental function of the C-terminus of BRCA2 further substantiates how truncations of this region of the protein, which are commonly seen in BRCA2-cancers, incite genomic instability and subsequent malignant transformation.

The role of the BRC repeat region has been somewhat controversial. It has been described as the region of BRCA2 that is responsible for delivering RAD51 to ssDNA at sites of DNA damage (Carreira, Hilario et al. 2009), (Shivji, Davies et al. 2006) but, conversely, as a negative regulator of RAD51, which was described in the previous section (Nomme, Takizawa et al. 2008), (Davies and Pellegrini 2007). Results of a study investigating cancer-associated mutations of BRC repeats supported their role as a negative regulator that binds and inhibits RAD51 from engaging in HR. But, then releases RAD51 monomers upon detection of DNA damage, thus allowing RAD51 to multimerize and interact with the BRCA2 TR2 region for mobilization to sites of damage. At this point, RAD51 is ready to form nucleoprotein filaments on the 3′ ssDNA overhangs at the breakpoint junction, which will invade the DNA homologue to be used as the template for repair. Considering that the BRC repeats are important for modulating RAD51 activity, several cancer-associated mutations, primarily point mutations, have been identified in this highly conserved region of BRCA2. Cancer-associated mutations have been identified in BRC motifs 1(T1011R), 2(F1219L, S1221P), 4(G1529R), and 7(T1980I) (Esashi, Galkin et al. 2007). The effect of mutations in BRC motifs 2 and 4 on RAD51-mediated HR repair was assessed. The results determined that such mutations prevent binding of monomeric RAD51 to the BRC repeats, which prevents recruitment of RAD51 to DSBs, thereby inhibiting nucleoprotein filament formation and impairing HR-mediated repair (Tal, Arbel-Goren et al. 2009).

A great deal of attention has been focused on the role of the C-terminus and BRC repeat region of BRCA2 in HR-mediated repair. However, mutations of the N-terminus also have detrimental effects on protein function. The N-terminus of BRCA2 binds the protein PALB2 (partner and localizer of BRCA2) (Xia, Sheng et al. 2006); (Rahman, Seal et al. 2007), (Figure 2). PALB2 is also a member of the Fanconi Anemia pathway, denoted as FANCN, in the same manner in which BRCA2/FANCD1 is involved, as well (Figure 3). And, just as biallelic mutations of BRCA2/FANCD1 cause a subtype of Fanconi Anemia, and susceptibility to childhood cancers, biallelic mutations of PALB2/FANCN have a similar phenotype (D'Andrea). With respect to the interaction with BRCA2, PALB2 is responsible for localizing BRCA2 to the sites of DNA damage in order to promote repair (Xia, Sheng et al. 2006). Mutations of the PALB2 binding site on BRCA2 prevent this interaction, causing impaired formation of RAD51 damage-induced foci, and unresolved DSBs (Xia, Sheng et al. 2006). Furthermore, PALB2 is also able to bind DNA and enhance the recombination activity of RAD51 (Dray, Etchin et al.).

4. Therapeutic regimens designed to target BRCA2 defects

Cells that are defective in BRCA1 and BRCA2 retain unresolved DSBs. This attribute, which is detrimental in terms of genomic instability and risk for cancer, is actually a potent target for inhibitors of Poly(ADP-ribose) polymerase, or PARP, in the eradication of transformed cells.

4.1 Efficacy of PARP inhibitors in treating BRCA2-tumors

PARPs are a family of 17 enzymes, with PARP-1 and -2 having been shown to be involved in DNA repair. PARP-1 is a nuclear protein with a zinc-finger DNA binding domain (Amir, Seruga et al.). It is responsible for binding to the sites of single-strand breaks, signaling damage at the site, and the initiating repair. The zinc finger domain binds to ssDNA breaks, cleaves NAD+, and attaches multiple ADP-ribose units to the protein. This results in an extremely negatively charged target which causes unwinding of the damaged DNA, followed by repair by the Base-Excision Repair (BER) pathway (Schreiber, Dantzer et al. 2006); (Ratnam and Low 2007). However, PARP-1 has also been shown to serve as an anti-recombinogenic factor at sites of damage where it has bound, thereby having implications on inhibiting HR-mediated repair (Amir, Seruga et al.), (Sandhu, Yap et al.). BRCA1 and -2 mutant cells are defective in repair of DSBs, and as a consequence, are sensitive to agents that induce DSBs. PARP-1 inhibitors have been shown to be effective in selectively targeting BRCA1 and -2 defective cells by converting SSBs, which have been induced by the use of chemotherapeutic agents, ionizing radiation, or occurring in normal cellular processes, such as stalled replication forks, to DSBs. The SSBs would have normally been identified and resolved by PARP-1 binding and the BER pathway; however, PARP-1 inhibitors prevent such resolution, and during DNA synthesis, the SSBs are converted to DSBs. The DSBs are normally resolved by HR-mediated repair involving BRCA1, and most important BRCA2, with the recombinase RAD51. However, this is deficient in BRCA-mutant cells and the addition of PARP inhibition enhances DNA-damage induced cell cycle arrest and apoptosis. This process eradicates the tumor cells.

4.2 Development of PARP inhibitors

The first PARP-1 inhibitor created was 3-aminobenzamide (3-AB). It causes inhibition of PARP-1 by competing with NAD+ as a substrate. However, 3-AB showed poor specificity and inhibited de-novo purine synthesis (Purnell, Stone et al. 1980); (Drew and Plummer). Approximately, twenty years have passed since the synthesis of 3-AB, and the focus has been to create PARP-1 inhibitors with greater specificity for PARP-1 inhibition, only. In 2003, the PARP-1 inhibitor AG014699 was the first to enter clinical trials (Plummer and Calvert 2007), (Drew and Plummer). Xenograft studies showed significant delay of tumor growth when AG014699 was combined with irinotecan and irradiation and tumor regression when combined with temozolomide (Ratnam and Low 2007). There are presently at least eight PARP inhibitors in clinical trials (Drew and Plummer), (Amir, Seruga et al.), (Table 1). PARP inhibitors are effective at sensitizing tumor cells to other chemotherapeutic agents, and can be used as a combination therapy with platinums, temozolomide, topopisomerase I inhibitors, and γ-/X-radiation (Ratnam and Low 2007), (Curtin, Wang et al. 2004), (Miknyoczki, Jones-Bolin et al. 2003), (Nguewa, Fuertes et al. 2006), (Chalmers, Johnston et al. 2004), (Fernet, Ponette et al. 2000), (Veuger, Curtin et al. 2003). Due to PARP inhibitors effectively promoting cell cycle arrest and subsequent apoptosis, clinical trials are testing their efficacy as single-agents in the treatment of BRCA1- and BRCA2-tumors (Ratnam and Low 2007).

Agent	Single/combination therapy	Disease
Olaparib (AZD2281)	Single agent Combination trials	BRCA-related tumors Solid tumors
BSI-201	Single agent Combination trials (gemcitabine/carboplatin)	Triple negative breast cancer Advanced solid tumors
AG014699	Single agent Combination trials (temozolomide [TMZ]	Solid tumors Melanoma
ABT-888	Single agent	Solid tumors and lymphoid malignancies
INO-1001	Single agent Combination with TMZ	Melanoma Glioblastoma mutiforme
MK4827	Single agent	Solid tumors BRCA ovarian
GPI21016	Combination with TMZ	Solid tumors
CEP-9722	Combination with TMZ	Solid tumors

Table 1. PARP inhibitors presently in clinical trials

4.3 Clinical implications of PARP inhibitor use

In general, there is very high enthusiasm for the use of PARP inhibitors in the treatment of *BRCA2*-cancers. The requirement for specificity is met because the *BRCA1/2*-mutated cells are most sensitive to the inhibitors, due to their DNA repair defects, and the premise of "synthetic lethality", which is when two pathway defects alone are innocuous, but combined become lethal (Ratnam and Low 2007). The combination of impaired HR-mediated repair due to the *BRCA1/2*-mutation and the inhibition of PARP-1 to signal the DNA breaks provides the "synthetic lethality" that is necessary for the efficacy of PARP inhibitors in the treatment of *BRCA*-tumors. Furthermore, the therapeutic benefit of PARP inhibitors appears to greatly outweigh the undesirable side effects; however, there are areas of concern. First and foremost, PARP inhibitors are still in the early stages of clinical testing. Therefore, the optimal dosage and duration of treatment have not been definitively determined. And, although PARP inhibitors are effective against BRCA-tumors, there is the potential for possible toxicity in normal tissues. In the Olaparib phase I study, DSB accumulations were observed in normal tissues (eyebrow hair follicles), (Drew and Plummer). In addition to toxicity, the inhibitors may disrupt DNA repair pathways in normal tissue from DNA damage acquired through sun exposure or other environmental agents (Ratnam and Low 2007). And, the potential for secondary cancers to occur through genomic instability from inhibition of PARP-1 is possible. In an in vivo study of PARP-1 deficiency, female mice developed mammary carcinoma (Tong, Yang et al. 2007); (Drew and Plummer). Furthermore, secondary mutations after PARP inhibitor treatment may lead to drug resistance. Previous reports have observed intragenic secondary mutations/deletions of BRCA2 occurring after treatment with PARP-1, and the anti-cancer agent cisplatin, which restored the open-reading frame and led to the expression of new BRCA2 isoforms. This resulted in reversal of the original BRCA2 mutation and resistance to PARP inhibitors (Edwards, Brough et al. 2008), (Sakai, Swisher et al. 2008), (Drew and Plummer).

5. Conclusion

Overall, the use of PARP inhibitors appears to be very promising in the treatment of BRCA-tumors as a single agent, and as a chemotherapeutic/radiation sensitizer when used in combination with anticancer therapeutics or γ-radiation. The on-going clinical trials will provide more information about the aspects of PARP inhibitor usage that are presently vague, such as proper dosage and duration of treatment, possible effects on DNA repair mechanisms in normal cells, possible induction of secondary mutations, and acquired resistance of tumors over the course of treatment.

6. References

Abeliovich, D., L. Kaduri, et al. (1997). "The founder mutations 185delAG and 5382insC in BRCA1 and 6174delT in BRCA2 appear in 60% of ovarian cancer and 30% of early-onset breast cancer patients among Ashkenazi women." *Am J Hum Genet* 60(3): 505-14.

Amir, E., B. Seruga, et al. "Targeting DNA repair in breast cancer: a clinical and translational update." *Cancer Treat Rev* 36(7): 557-65.

Benson, F. E., A. Stasiak, et al. (1994). "Purification and characterization of the human Rad51 protein, an analogue of E. coli RecA." *Embo J* 13(23): 5764-71.

Bignell, G., G. Micklem, et al. (1997). "The BRC repeats are conserved in mammalian BRCA2 proteins." *Hum Mol Genet* 6(1): 53-8.

Buisson, R., A. M. Dion-Cote, et al. "Cooperation of breast cancer proteins PALB2 and piccolo BRCA2 in stimulating homologous recombination." *Nat Struct Mol Biol* 17(10): 1247-54.

Carreira, A., J. Hilario, et al. (2009). "The BRC repeats of BRCA2 modulate the DNA-binding selectivity of RAD51." *Cell* 136(6): 1032-43.

Chalmers, A., P. Johnston, et al. (2004). "PARP-1, PARP-2, and the cellular response to low doses of ionizing radiation." *Int J Radiat Oncol Biol Phys* 58(2): 410-9.

Chen, C. F., P. L. Chen, et al. (1999). "Expression of BRC repeats in breast cancer cells disrupts the BRCA2-Rad51 complex and leads to radiation hypersensitivity and loss of G(2)/M checkpoint control." *J Biol Chem* 274(46): 32931-5.

Chen, P. L., C. F. Chen, et al. (1998). "The BRC repeats in BRCA2 are critical for RAD51 binding and resistance to methyl methanesulfonate treatment." *Proc Natl Acad Sci* U S A 95(9): 5287-92.

Connell, C. M., A. Shibata, et al. "Genomic DNA damage and ATR-Chk1 signaling determine oncolytic adenoviral efficacy in human ovarian cancer cells." *J Clin Invest* 121(4): 1283-97.

Curtin, N. J., L. Z. Wang, et al. (2004). "Novel poly(ADP-ribose) polymerase-1 inhibitor, AG14361, restores sensitivity to temozolomide in mismatch repair-deficient cells." *Clin Cancer Res* 10(3): 881-9.

D'Andrea, A. D. "Susceptibility pathways in Fanconi's anemia and breast cancer." *N Engl J Med* 362(20): 1909-19.

Davies, O. R. and L. Pellegrini (2007). "Interaction with the BRCA2 C terminus protects RAD51-DNA filaments from disassembly by BRC repeats." *Nat Struct Mol Biol* 14(6): 475-83.

Derbyshire, M. K., L. H. Epstein, et al. (1994). "Nonhomologous recombination in human cells." *Mol Cell Biol* 14(1): 156-69.

Dobricic, J., M. Brankovic-Magic, et al. "Novel BRCA1/2 mutations in Serbian breast and breast-ovarian cancer patients with hereditary predisposition." *Cancer Genet Cytogenet* 202(1): 27-32.

Dray, E., J. Etchin, et al. "Enhancement of RAD51 recombinase activity by the tumor suppressor PALB2." *Nat Struct Mol Biol* 17(10): 1255-9.

Drew, Y. and R. Plummer "The emerging potential of poly(ADP-ribose) polymerase inhibitors in the treatment of breast cancer." *Curr Opin Obstet Gynecol* 22(1): 67-71.

Edwards, S. L., R. Brough, et al. (2008). "Resistance to therapy caused by intragenic deletion in BRCA2." *Nature* 451(7182): 1111-5.

Esashi, F., N. Christ, et al. (2005). "CDK-dependent phosphorylation of BRCA2 as a regulatory mechanism for recombinational repair." *Nature* 434(7033): 598-604.

Esashi, F., V. E. Galkin, et al. (2007). "Stabilization of RAD51 nucleoprotein filaments by the C-terminal region of BRCA2." *Nat Struct Mol Biol* 14(6): 468-74.

Fernet, M., V. Ponette, et al. (2000). "Poly(ADP-ribose) polymerase, a major determinant of early cell response to ionizing radiation." *Int J Radiat Biol* 76(12): 1621-9.

Goggins, M., M. Schutte, et al. (1996). "Germline BRCA2 gene mutations in patients with apparently sporadic pancreatic carcinomas." *Cancer Res* 56(23): 5360-4.

Howlett, N. G., T. Taniguchi, et al. (2002). "Biallelic inactivation of BRCA2 in Fanconi anemia." *Science* 297(5581): 606-9.

Jackson, S. P. and P. A. Jeggo (1995). "DNA double-strand break repair and V(D)J recombination: involvement of DNA-PK." *Trends Biochem Sci* 20(10): 412-5.

Jensen, R. B., A. Carreira, et al. "Purified human BRCA2 stimulates RAD51-mediated recombination." *Nature* 467(7316): 678-83.

Johnson, R. D. and M. Jasin (2000). "Sister chromatid gene conversion is a prominent double-strand break repair pathway in mammalian cells." *Embo J* 19(13): 3398-407.

Levy-Lahad, E., R. Catane, et al. (1997). "Founder BRCA1 and BRCA2 mutations in Ashkenazi Jews in Israel: frequency and differential penetrance in ovarian cancer and in breast-ovarian cancer families." *Am J Hum Genet* 60(5): 1059-67.

Lomonosov, M., S. Anand, et al. (2003). "Stabilization of stalled DNA replication forks by the BRCA2 breast cancer susceptibility protein." *Genes Dev* 17(24): 3017-22.

Mangold, K. A., V. Wang, et al. "Detection of BRCA1 and BRCA2 Ashkenazi Jewish founder mutations in formalin-fixed paraffin-embedded tissues using conventional PCR and heteroduplex/amplicon size differences." *J Mol Diagn* 12(1): 20-6.

Marmorstein, L. Y., T. Ouchi, et al. (1998). "The BRCA2 gene product functionally interacts with p53 and RAD51." *Proc Natl Acad Sci* U S A 95(23): 13869-74.

McNeely, S., C. Conti, et al. "Chk1 inhibition after replicative stress activates a double strand break response mediated by ATM and DNA-dependent protein kinase." *Cell Cycle* 9(5): 995-1004.

Miknyoczki, S. J., S. Jones-Bolin, et al. (2003). "Chemopotentiation of temozolomide, irinotecan, and cisplatin activity by CEP-6800, a poly(ADP-ribose) polymerase inhibitor." *Mol Cancer Ther* 2(4): 371-82.

Mizuta, R., J. M. LaSalle, et al. (1997). "RAB22 and RAB163/mouse BRCA2: proteins that specifically interact with the RAD51 protein." *Proc Natl Acad Sci* U S A 94(13): 6927-32.

Neuhausen, S., T. Gilewski, et al. (1996). "Recurrent BRCA2 6174delT mutations in Ashkenazi Jewish women affected by breast cancer." *Nat Genet* 13(1): 126-8.

Nguewa, P. A., M. A. Fuertes, et al. (2006). "Poly(ADP-ribose) polymerase-1 inhibitor 3-aminobenzamide enhances apoptosis induction by platinum complexes in cisplatin-resistant tumor cells." *Med Chem* 2(1): 47-53.

Nomme, J., Y. Takizawa, et al. (2008). "Inhibition of filament formation of human Rad51 protein by a small peptide derived from the BRC-motif of the BRCA2 protein." *Genes Cells* 13(5): 471-81.

Oddoux, C., E. Guillen-Navarro, et al. (1999). "Mendelian diseases among Roman Jews: implications for the origins of disease alleles." *J Clin Endocrinol Metab* 84(12): 4405-9.

Oddoux, C., J. P. Struewing, et al. (1996). "The carrier frequency of the BRCA2 6174delT mutation among Ashkenazi Jewish individuals is approximately 1%." *Nat Genet* 14(2): 188-90.

Ogawa, T., X. Yu, et al. (1993). "Similarity of the yeast RAD51 filament to the bacterial RecA filament." *Science* 259(5103): 1896-9.

Ozcelik, H., B. Schmocker, et al. (1997). "Germline BRCA2 6174delT mutations in Ashkenazi Jewish pancreatic cancer patients." *Nat Genet* 16(1): 17-8.

Plummer, E. R. and H. Calvert (2007). "Targeting poly(ADP-ribose) polymerase: a two-armed strategy for cancer therapy." *Clin Cancer Res* 13(21): 6252-6.

Purnell, M. R., P. R. Stone, et al. (1980). "ADP-ribosylation of nuclear proteins." *Biochem Soc Trans* 8(2): 215-27.

Rahman, N., S. Seal, et al. (2007). "PALB2, which encodes a BRCA2-interacting protein, is a breast cancer susceptibility gene." *Nat Genet* 39(2): 165-7.

Ratnam, K. and J. A. Low (2007). "Current development of clinical inhibitors of poly(ADP-ribose) polymerase in oncology." *Clin Cancer Res* 13(5): 1383-8.

Roa, B. B., A. A. Boyd, et al. (1996). "Ashkenazi Jewish population frequencies for common mutations in BRCA1 and BRCA2." *Nat Genet* 14(2): 185-7.

Roth, D. B., T. N. Porter, et al. (1985). "Mechanisms of nonhomologous recombination in mammalian cells." *Mol Cell Biol* 5(10): 2599-607.

Roth, D. B. and J. H. Wilson (1986). "Nonhomologous recombination in mammalian cells: role for short sequence homologies in the joining reaction." *Mol Cell Biol* 6(12): 4295-304.

Sakai, W., E. M. Swisher, et al. (2008). "Secondary mutations as a mechanism of cisplatin resistance in BRCA2-mutated cancers." *Nature* 451(7182): 1116-20.

Sandhu, S. K., T. A. Yap, et al. "Poly(ADP-ribose) polymerase inhibitors in cancer treatment: a clinical perspective." *Eur J Cancer* 46(1): 9-20.

Schreiber, V., F. Dantzer, et al. (2006). "Poly(ADP-ribose): novel functions for an old molecule." *Nat Rev Mol Cell Biol* 7(7): 517-28.

Sharan, S. K., M. Morimatsu, et al. (1997). "Embryonic lethality and radiation hypersensitivity mediated by Rad51 in mice lacking Brca2." *Nature* 386(6627): 804-10.

Shivji, M. K., O. R. Davies, et al. (2006). "A region of human BRCA2 containing multiple BRC repeats promotes RAD51-mediated strand exchange." *Nucleic Acids Res* 34(14): 4000-11.

Sonoda, E., M. S. Sasaki, et al. (1998). "Rad51-deficient vertebrate cells accumulate chromosomal breaks prior to cell death." *Embo J* 17(2): 598-608.

Spain, B. H., C. J. Larson, et al. (1999). "Truncated BRCA2 is cytoplasmic: implications for cancer-linked mutations." *Proc Natl Acad Sci* U S A 96(24): 13920-5.

Sy, S. M., M. S. Huen, et al. (2009). "PALB2 is an integral component of the BRCA complex required for homologous recombination repair." *Proc Natl Acad Sci* U S A 106(17): 7155-60.

Takata, M., M. S. Sasaki, et al. (1998). "Homologous recombination and non-homologous end-joining pathways of DNA double-strand break repair have overlapping roles in the maintenance of chromosomal integrity in vertebrate cells." *Embo J* 17(18): 5497-508.

Taki, T., T. Ohnishi, et al. (1996). "Antisense inhibition of the RAD51 enhances radiosensitivity." *Biochem Biophys Res Commun* 223(2): 434-8.

Tal, A., R. Arbel-Goren, et al. (2009). "Cancer-associated mutations in BRC domains of BRCA2 affect homologous recombination induced by Rad51." *J Mol Biol* 393(5): 1007-12.

Thorlacius, S., G. Olafsdottir, et al. (1996). "A single BRCA2 mutation in male and female breast cancer families from Iceland with varied cancer phenotypes." *Nat Genet* 13(1): 117-9.

Thorslund, T., F. Esashi, et al. (2007). "Interactions between human BRCA2 protein and the meiosis-specific recombinase DMC1." *Embo J* 26(12): 2915-22.

Tong, W. M., Y. G. Yang, et al. (2007). "Poly(ADP-ribose) polymerase-1 plays a role in suppressing mammary tumourigenesis in mice." *Oncogene* 26(26): 3857-67.

Tonin, P., B. Weber, et al. (1996). "Frequency of recurrent BRCA1 and BRCA2 mutations in Ashkenazi Jewish breast cancer families." *Nat Med* 2(11): 1179-83.

Tsuzuki, T., Y. Fujii, et al. (1996). "Targeted disruption of the Rad51 gene leads to lethality in embryonic mice." *Proc Natl Acad Sci* U S A 93(13): 6236-40.

Veuger, S. J., N. J. Curtin, et al. (2003). "Radiosensitization and DNA repair inhibition by the combined use of novel inhibitors of DNA-dependent protein kinase and poly(ADP-ribose) polymerase-1." *Cancer Res* 63(18): 6008-15.

Wong, A. K., R. Pero, et al. (1997). "RAD51 interacts with the evolutionarily conserved BRC motifs in the human breast cancer susceptibility gene brca2." *J Biol Chem* 272(51): 31941-4.

Xia, B., Q. Sheng, et al. (2006). "Control of BRCA2 cellular and clinical functions by a nuclear partner, PALB2." *Mol Cell* 22(6): 719-29.

Yang, H., P. D. Jeffrey, et al. (2002). "BRCA2 function in DNA binding and recombination from a BRCA2-DSS1-ssDNA structure." *Science* 297(5588): 1837-48.

Yano, K., K. Morotomi, et al. (2000). "Nuclear localization signals of the BRCA2 protein." *Biochem Biophys Res Commun* 270(1): 171-5.

Yuan, S. S., S. Y. Lee, et al. (1999). "BRCA2 is required for ionizing radiation-induced assembly of Rad51 complex in vivo." *Cancer Res* 59(15): 3547-51.

Zhang, F., Q. Fan, et al. (2009). "PALB2 functionally connects the breast cancer susceptibility proteins BRCA1 and BRCA2." *Mol Cancer Res* 7(7): 1110-8.

Zhang, F., J. Ma, et al. (2009). "PALB2 links BRCA1 and BRCA2 in the DNA-damage response." *Curr Biol* 19(6): 524-9.

Zhi, G., J. B. Wilson, et al. (2009). "Fanconi anemia complementation group FANCD2 protein serine 331 phosphorylation is important for fanconi anemia pathway function and BRCA2 interaction." *Cancer Res* 69(22): 8775-83.

18

Roles of MicroRNA in DNA Damage and Repair

Xinrong Chen and Tao Chen
National Center for Toxicological Research/US Food and Drug Administration
U.S.A.

1. Introduction

DNA damage mainly results from either endogenous metabolic activity, such as oxidative stress, or environmental exposure, such as ionizing irradiation. In human cells, endogenous and exogenous genotoxic agents produce as many as 1 million molecular lesions per cell per day. If the unrepaired lesions occur in certain critical genes, they can cause mutations that can lead to tumors (Lodish H, 2004).

There are several different types of DNA damage, including DNA hydrolysis, DNA adduction, DNA crosslinking, and DNA strand breakage. DNA hydrolysis is the breaking of DNA through the addition of water. Hydrolysis of DNA bases consists of deamination, depurination, and depyrimidination. A DNA adduct is a piece of DNA covalently bonded to a chemical. DNA crosslinks are links formed within a single (intrastrand) or between strands of DNA (interstrand). There are two types of DNA strand breaks, single strand breaks and double strand breaks. DNA double strand breaks are particularly hazardous to the cells because they can lead to genome rearrangements. (Rich et al., 2000).

Cells respond to DNA damage through a variety of different mechanisms, such as apoptosis, senescence, and DNA repair. Excessive DNA damage induces apoptosis, or programmed cell death, that eliminates cells with heavily damaged DNA, thus protecting the organism from the mutations potentially induced by the damage. Unrepaired DNA damage is a driving force for senescence. Senescence serves as a functional alternative to apoptosis in cases where the physical presence of cells is required for spatial reasons. If DNA replication occurs before DNA damage is repaired, mutations can be formed in the cells. To prevent mutation formation, cells have developed DNA repair mechanisms to correct DNA.

There are several different types of DNA repair. They are direct reversal, base excision repair (BER), nucleotide excision repair (NER), mismatch repair (MMR), non-homologous end-joining (NHEJ), and homologous recombination repair (HRR). Direct reversal can remove DNA damage by chemically reversing it. Since the correction only occurs in one of the four bases and not the phosphodiester backbone, this type of repair does not need any DNA template. For example, methylation of guanine bases can be directly reversed by methyl guanine methyl transferase (MGMT) that removes the methyl group. BER amends damage to single nucleotides produced by oxidation, alkylation, or hydrolysis. NER corrects ethylation products, bulky DNA adducts, helix-distorting changes, such as thymine dimers, and single-strand breaks. MMR repairs mismatched bases in double-stranded DNA (e.g., A:C or G:T). HRR is a mechanism for DNA double-strand repair that reconstitutes the original sequence using the sister chromatid as a template. NHEJ is a relatively simple way for DNA double-strand repair and it just rejoins two broken ends without correcting any deletions or rearrangements of DNA.

2. Biogenesis of miRNA

A microRNA gene can be located in an intron of another gene, in either the sense or antisense orientation. miRNA can be coordinately expressed with its host gene, or it can have its own promoter independent of its host gene (Ozsolak et al., 2008). The biogenesis of miRNA is a complex process as shown in Figure 1. miRNA is first transcribed as a long primary miRNA (pri-miRNA) by RNA polymerase II in the nucleus (Lee et al., 2004). Pri-miRNA is structurally similar to mRNA, but contains a stable stem-loop structure (Cai et al., 2004). Recognition of the hairpin and selection of a cleavage site are mediated by DGCR8. Nuclear RNase III (Drosha) then cleaves the pri-miRNA to release the hairpin-shaped precursor miRNA (pre-miRNAs). The pre-miRNA is exported from the nucleus to the cytoplasm by Exportin 5 (Exp5). In the cytoplasm, the pre-miRNA is subsequently cut by cytoplasmic RNase III (Dicer) in complex with Argonaute2 (Ago2) and TRBP, a double-stranded RNA-binding protein. This process cleaves the pre-miRNA hairpins to remove its hairpin loop, resulting in a miRNA duplex with the appropriate length (Gregory et al., 2005; Han et al., 2004; Lee et al., 2003). Normally, one strand of the duplex is then degraded. The mature miRNA are incorporated into an RNA-induced silencing complex (RISC) (Gregory, et al., 2005; Grishok et al., 2001; Hutvagner et al., 2001; Ketting et al., 2001; Maniataki and Mourelatos, 2005). RISC recognizes target mRNAs through full or partial base-pairing interactions between the miRNA and the to "3'-untranslated region (UTR) of the target mRNA. Depending on pairing interactions between miRNAs and their targets, miRNAs suppress their target gene expression by either mRNA cleavage or translational repression. If an mRNA target match perfectly or near-perfectly to the miRNA, the mRNA will be degraded; otherwise, the mRNA will be translationally suppressed (Meister and Tuschl, 2004).

3. Alteration of miRNA biogenesis in response to DNA damage and repair

Because miRNAs are actively involved in regulation of genes that are related to DNA damage and repair, it was not surprising to find that miRNA biogenesis changes in response to DNA damage and repair. Several studies demonstrated that both miRNA transcription and maturation process are altered in response to DNA damage and repair.

Recent studies show that transcription of miRNA can be directly affected by DNA damage. The *P53* gene plays a critical role in this regulation. For example, miR-34a can be up-regulated by the *P53* gene in response to DNA damage (Chang et al., 2007; Corney et al., 2007; He et al., 2007; Raver-Shapira et al., 2007; Welch et al., 2007). Up-regulation of miR-34a results in apoptosis, cell-cycle arrest, and DNA repair. miR-34a is a direct transcriptional target of P53 because the promoter region of miR-34a contains a canonical P53 binding site. When DNA damage activates the *P53* gene, P53 protein binds to the promoter of miR-34a and up-regulates miRNA expression. In *Caenorhabditis elegans*, miR-34a expression was enhanced by irradiation in a P53 independent manner, and knocking down of the *Cep1* gene (homolog of the *P53* gene) had no effect on the miR-34a response to irradiation (Kato et al., 2009). Up-regulation of miR-34a in response to genotoxin exposure is also observed in different biological systems (Chen et al., 2011; Li et al., 2010;

Li et al., 2011; Zenz et al., 2009). miR-34c, another member of miR-34 family, is transcriptionally up-regulated by P53 following DNA damage (Cannell et al., 2010). In addition to miR-34a, P53 can also regulate the expression of miR-192, miR-194, and miR-215. These miRNAs are considered tumor suppressor miRNAs (Braun et al., 2008; Georges et al., 2008).

miRNA biogenesis is globally induced upon DNA damage in an ATM (ataxia telangiectasia mutated) dependent manner (Zhang et al., 2011). The ATM gene encodes a DNA damage-inducible kinase. ATM controls cell grow rate by interacting with other proteins, for example BRCA1, following DNA damage. In response to strand breaks or other type of DNA damage, the ATM protein coordinates DNA repair by activating other proteins. Because of its central role in cell division and DNA repair, the ATM protein is important in carcinogenesis. More than one-fourth of miRNAs were significantly upregulated after DNA damage, while loss of ATM activity abolished their induction. Their results show that DNA damage activates the ATM kinase that directly binds to and phosphorylates KH-type splicing regulatory protein (KSRP), leading to enhanced interaction between KSRP and pri-miRNAs and increased KSRP activity in miRNA processing. The increased activity, in turn, results in more pre-miRNAs from pri-miRNAs, so that more miRNA products are produced to respond to the DNA damage.

Other studies show a different mechanism by which DNA damage signaling is linked to the miRNA maturation processes. Several miRNAs with growth suppressive function, including miR-16-1, miR-143 and miR-145, were regulated at the post transcriptional level through a P53-mediated miRNA maturation process in response to DNA damage (Suzuki et al., 2009; Toledo and Bardot, 2009). The P53 tumor suppressor protein binds to Drosha to facilitate the processing of pri-miRNAs to pre-miRNAs. Mutation in the DNA-binding domain of P53 decreases processing of pri-miRNAs by Drosha, and reduces the expression of the related miRNAs. In silico analyses, all three component of the P53 tumor suppressor, P53, P63, and P73, can regulate the major components of miRNA processing, such as Drosha-DGCR8, Dicer-TRBP2, and Agronaute proteins. Thus, when DNA damage activates the P53 gene, the activated P53 gene can modulate miRNA expression by affecting the miRNA biogenesis processes.

miR-24 regulates the DNA damage response by down-regulation of H2AX, the initial sensor protein for the DNA damage response. miR-100, miR-101 and miR-421 suppress ATM, the chief transducer of the DNA damage response, by targeting the 3'-UTR of ATM. miR-16 can up-regulate ATM activity by suppressing levels of Wip1. DNA repair pathways are regulated by a number of miRNAs involved in different types of DNA damage correction. the NER protein RAD23B was down-regulated by miR-373. MMR protein MSH2 and MSH6 were down regulated by miR-21 and MLH1/MSH2 were suppressed by miR-155. The HRR protein BRCA1 was down-regulated by miR-182 and RAD52 was suppressed by miR-210 and miR-373. The NHEJ protein DNA-PKcs was suppressed by miR-101 (Yan, Ng. 2010).

4. miRNA regulation of signal transduction for DNA damage

miRNAs regulate multiple aspects of the DNA damage response pathway, including regulation of signal transduction of DNA damage, changing expression level of master regulatory proteins such as P53, modulating key protein expression in different types of DNA repair such as MMR, NER, NHEJ and HRR. Figure 2 and Table 1 summarize recently reported miRNAs associated with DNA damage and repair.

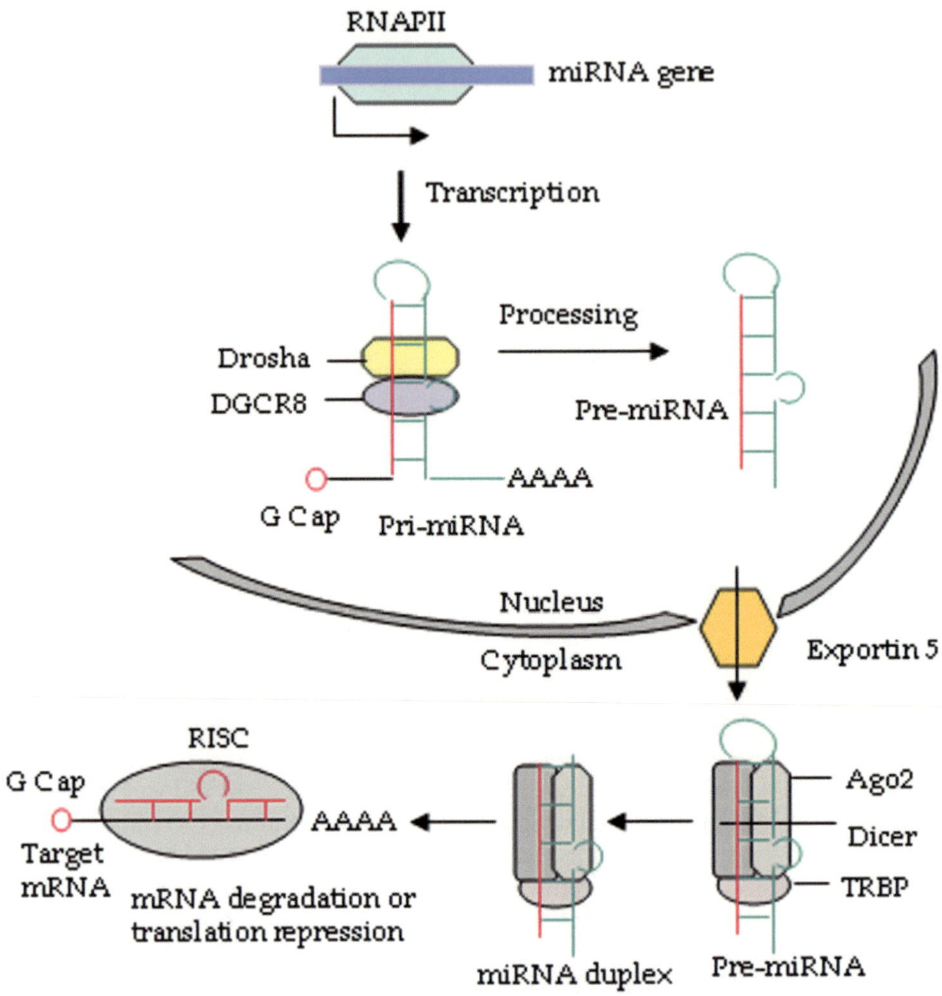

Fig. 1. MicroRNA biogenesis. A microRNA gene is transcribed by RNA polymerase II (RNAPII) to produce a pri-miRNA. The pri-miRNA is formed by RNase III family Drosha, cooperating in a complex with dsRNA-binding proteins DGCR8. The Drosha–DGCR8 complex processes the pri-miRNA into an ~70-nucleotide pre-miRNA, which is exported to the cytoplasm by expotin 5. The cytoplasm pre-miRNA is cleaved by Dicer, assisted by TRBP and AGO2, and yields an ~20-bp miRNA/miRNA* duplex. One strand of the miRNA/miRNA* duplex is preferentially incorporated into a miRNA-induced silencing complex (RISC), whereas the other strand is degraded (not shown). RISC recognizes target mRNAs and lets the miRNA binds to its target mRNA to suppress gene expression, either by mRNA cleavage or translational repression.

DNA damage activates the signal transduction process that leads to cell cycle arrest, which can lead to apoptosis or DNA repair. This DNA-damage response is mainly regulated at the transcriptional and posttranslational levels. Recent evidence suggests that miRNAs offer another degree of regulation at the posttranscriptional level in response to DNA damage. The DNA damage response to UV light was severely attenuated after the key components of

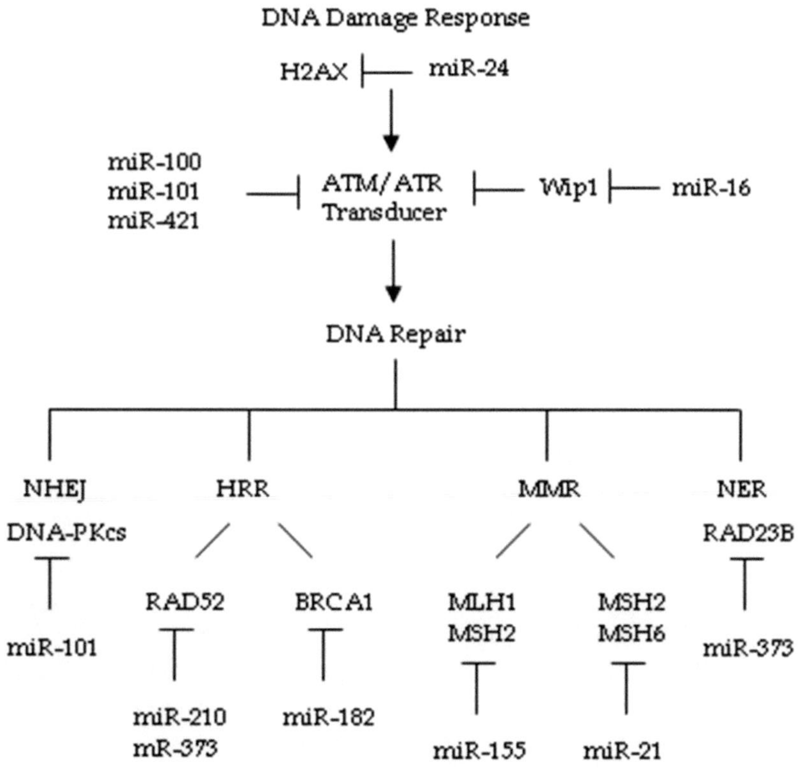

Fig. 2. miRNAs directly regulate DNA repair

the miRNA-processing pathway (Dicer and Ago2) were knocked down. miRNA mediated gene regulation operates earlier than most other transcriptional responses following genotoxic stress (Pothof et al., 2009).

H2AX, a histone variant, is an initial sensor protein for the DNA damage response. The function of H2AX is associated with DNA double strand break repair. miR-24 expression is up-regulated during hematopoietic cell differentiation into multiple lineages. miR-24 regulates H2AX expression through binding to its 3'-UTR. Both H2AX mRNA and protein levels are dramatically reduced by high levels of miR-24 in terminal differentiated human blood cells. miR-24 mediated suppression of H2AX in terminally differentiated blood cells renders them hypersensitive to gamma-irradiation, deficient in DSB repair, and susceptible to chromosomal instability (Lal et al., 2009).

Wild-type p53-induced phosphatase 1 (Wip1) is an oncogene with critical function in the ATM/ATR-p53 DNA damage signaling pathway. Wip1 reverses DNA damage–induced cell cycle checkpoints by dephosphorylating several key DNA damage responsive proteins. Recently, miRNAs are found to play an important role in suppressing Wip1 activity. Knockdown of miR-15a and miR-16 promotes survival, proliferation and invasiveness of untransformed prostate cells, and tumor formation in immunodeficient NOD-SCID mice. Conversely, reconstitution of miR-15a and miR-16 expression results in marked regression of prostate tumor xenografts. The function of miR-15a and miR-16 is considered through their regulation of Wip1 expression. miR-16 can down-regulate the expression level of Wip1 by targeting the 3′ UTR of Wip1. As a result, the Wip1 protein level is significantly deceased, which prevents a premature inactivation of ATM/ATR signaling and allows a functional completion of the early DNA damage response (Zhang et al., 2010).

miRNA	Pathway Involved	Target Protein	Net Effect	Reference
miR-24	DDR	H2AX	-	Lal, Pan. 2009
miR-16	DDR	Wip1	+	Zhang, Wan. 2010
miR-100	DDR	ATM	-	Ng, WL. 2010
miR-101	DDR	ATM	-	Yan, Ng. 2010
miR-421	DDR	ATM	-	Hu, Du. 2010)
miR-373	NER	RAD23B	-	Crosby, Kulshreshtha. 2009
miR-21	MMR	MSH2, MSH6	-	Valeri, Gasparini. 2010)
miR-155	MMR	MLH1, MSH2	-	Volinia, Calin. 2006
miR-182	HRR	BRCA1	-	Moskwa, Buffa. 2011
miR-210	HRR	RAD52	-	Crosby, Kulshreshtha. 2009
miR-373	HRR	RAD52	-	Crosby, Kulshreshtha. 2009
miR-101	NHEJ	DNA-PKcs		Yan, Ng. 2010
miR-29	P53	P85a, CDC42	+	Park, Lee. 2009
miR-34a	P53	SIRT1	+	Yamakuchi, Ferlito. 2008)
miR122	P53	Cyclin G1	+	Fornari, Gramantieri. 2009
miR-125b	P53	P53	-	Le, Teh. 2009
miR-504	P53	P53	-	Hu, Chan. 2010

Table 1. miRNAs involved in DNA repair (notes: - means inhibite and + means stimulate)

ATM is a serine/threonine kinase that transfers the DNA damage signals to down-steam events, such as cell cycle arrest, apoptosis and DNA repair (Lavin, 2008; Shiloh, 2003). ATM plays a critical role in the maintenance of genomic stability by activating cell cycle checkpoints and promoting DNA double-strand breaks repair. M059J is a human malignant glioma cell line with high sensitivity to ionizing radiation due to low-expression of ATM. The low-expression of ATM is related to miR-100 (Ng et al., 2010). Both computational analysis and luciferase reporter gene assay indicate that miR-100 can target the 3'-UTR of ATM. miR-100 was found to be highly-expressed in M059J cells by RNase protection assay and qRT-PCR. Up-regulation of miR-100 in M059K cells reduces ATM expression and renders them hypersensitive to ionizing radiation, while Knock-down of miR-100 promotes ATM expression in M059J cells. These results indicate that the low-expression of ATM in M059J cells is mainly due to the high expression of miR-100.

Another miRNA miR-421 is also involved in ATM regulation. miR-421 suppresses the expression of ATM by targeting the 3′ UTR of ATM. Ectopic expression of miR-421 lead to a deficient cell cycle checkpoint in S-phase and increased sensitivity to ionizing radiation (Hu et al., 2010a). Blocking the interaction between miR-421 and ATM with chemically synthesized oligonucleotides rescued the defective phenotype caused by miR-421 over expression, suggesting that ATM mediates the effect of miR-421 on cell-cycle checkpoints followed by radiation.

5. miRNA regulation of core components of DNA damage response

miRNAs are involved in DNA repair by regulating critical components of the DNA repair pathways, such as P53. As a transcription factor, the tumor suppressor P53 is a powerful regulator of diverse cellular processes including cell-cycle arrest, DNA repair, apoptosis and cellular senescence. P53 and its signaling pathway, play a pivotal role in maintaining genomic stability and tumor suppression (Levine et al., 2004; Levine et al., 2006). Recently, P53 activity was found to be widely regulated by a number of miRNAs. These miRNAs either directly target the 3′ UTR of P53 or indirectly regulate P53 activity by modulating proteins associated with P53 (Figure 3). Among these miRNAs, miR-504 negatively regulate p53 expression through binding to two DNA *cis* element located in the P53 3′ UTR. Ectopic expression of miR-504 reduces the protein level of P53 and impairs P53-mediated apoptosis and cell cycle arrest (Hu et al., 2010b). miR-125b is another negative regulator of P53 in both zebrafish and humans (Le et al., 2009). Knocking down of miR-125b increased the expression level of P53; and over-expression of miR-125b suppressed the expression of P53. Interestingly, miR-125b was down-regulated when the Zebrafish embryo was exposed to gamma irradiation, corresponding to the up-regulation of P53 protein induced by the irradiation exposure.

In addition to the direct binding to P53, several miRNA including miR-34a, miR-29 and miR-122 can indirectly modify P53 activity (Fornari et al., 2009; Park et al., 2009; Yamakuchi et al., 2008). miR-34a is a direct transcriptional target of P53 (Chang, et al., 2007; Corney, et al., 2007; Raver-Shapira, et al., 2007). P53 can up-regulate miR-34a expression by binding to a palindromic sequence located in miR-34a promoter region. miR-34a can positively regulate P53-dependent apoptosis through another intermediate protein, SIRT1 (Yamakuchi, et al., 2008). miR-34 inhibition of SIRT1 leads to an increase in acetylated P53. As a result, miR-34 suppression of SIRT1 ultimately leads to P53 mediated apoptosis in human colon cancer cells. miR-29 family members directly suppress P85a and CDC42, both of which negatively regulate P53. As a result, miR-29 positively up-regulates P53 level and induces apoptosis and DNA repair in a P53-dependent manner (Park, et al., 2009). miR-122 is a liver-specific miRNA accounting for 70% of the total miRNA population. miR-122 can down-regulate the expression of cyclin G1, which has the potential to inhibit P53 activity and promote cancer development. From a therapeutic perspective, miR-122 has potential to become a miRNA based therapy for hepatocellular carcinoma (HCC) patients (Fornari, et al., 2009).

6. Functions of miRNAs in mismatch repair (MMR)

MMR corrects erroneous deletion, insertion, or mis-incorporation of bases resulting from DNA replication, DNA recombination, or DNA damage. Human mutS homolog 2 (hMSH2) and mutL homolog 1 (hMLH1) function as core proteins in MMR. They form heterodimers with protein homologs hMSH3 or hMSH6 (Fishel, 2001). The over-expression of miR-21 is linked to progression of human colorectal cancer (Link et al., 2010; Ng et al., 2009). It was reported recently that miR-21 directly targeted the 3' UTRs of both the hMSH2 and hMSH6 mRNAs (Valeri et al., 2010a). Protein levels of hMSH2 and hMSH6 in the cells transfected with a locked nucleic acid (LNA) against miR-21 were significantly increased over the control cells. In addition, the over-expression of miR-21 was inversely correlated with the down regulation of hMSH2 in colorectal cancer tumors. Because the hMSH2-hMSH6 heterodimer is the key initiation component of MMR, the down regulation of hMSH2 is likely to suppress MMR, and ultimately enhance tumor progression.

miR-155 also plays a critical role in MMR. Over-expression of miR-155 reduced the levels of the human mismatch repair genes MLH1, MSH2 and MSH6 in a colorectal cancer cell line.

In addition, high expression of miR-155 was inversely correlated with the low expression of MLH1 and MSH2 protein in human colorectal cancer. More importantly, human tumors with unexplained MMR inactivation showed miR-155 over expression (Valeri et al., 2010b; Volinia et al., 2006). These results indicate that increased expression of miR-155 down-regulates MMR genes and results in an increase in genomic instability.

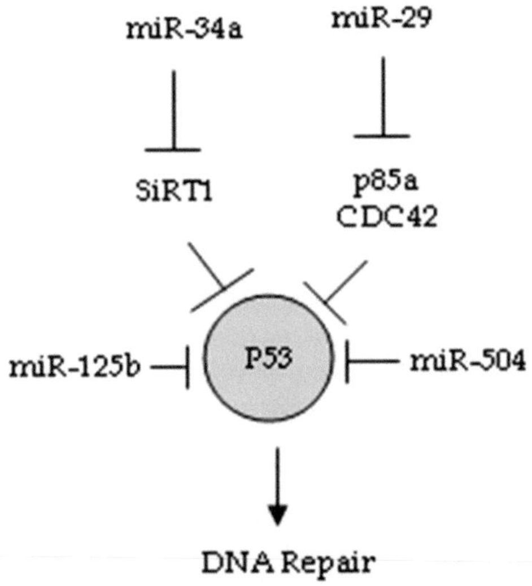

Fig. 3. miRNA indirectly regulates DNA repair through P53

miR-504 and miR-125b directly bind to the P53 3'-UTR and down-regulate P53 activity. miR-34a positively up-regulates P53 through SIRT1 inhibition, a negative regulator of P53. miR-29 down-regulates the P85a regulatory subunit of PI3K, which enhances P53 activity through the negative feedback loop between PI3K-AKT-MDM2 and P53.

7. Functions of miRNAs in nucleotide excision repair (NER)

NER recognizes bulky, helix distorting defects, such as cross-linking thymine dimmers. NER is particularly important for removing the vast majority of UV-induced DNA damage. Currently, only one miRNA is reported to be related with NER (Crosby et al., 2009). miR-373 suppresses the expression of a NER protein called RAD23B. RAD23B is a key component of the XPC/RAD23B complex that mediates damage recognition in the NER pathway (Batty et al., 2000). NER activity is functionally reduced in hypoxic cells (Yuan et al., 2000). A possible mechanism for the hpoxia-induced down-regulation of RAD23B is that hpoxia can up-regulate miR-373 expression, and the up-regulated miR-373 then suppresses RAD23B expression. This mechanism was supported by the fact that pre-treating cells with anti-miR-373 reversed the hypoxia-mediated down-regulation of RAD23B in hypoxic cells (Crosby, et al., 2009).

8. Functions of miRNAs in non-homologous end-joining (NHEJ)

NHEJ is a relatively simple but error prone DNA double strand break repair. It ligates broken ends, without the need for a homologous template. DNA protein kinase (DNA-PK) is a core component of mammalian NHEJ and involves a catalytic subunit (DNA-PKcs) that can act as a regulatory element. DNA-PKcs is a molecular sensor for DNA damage that enhances the signal via phosphorylation of many downstream targets. Therefore, DNA-PKcs is an essential factor for NHEJ. Yan et al. found that miR-101 could efficiently target DNA-PKcs and ATM via binding to their 3'- UTRs. Up-regulating miR-101 efficiently reduced the protein levels of DNA-PKcs and ATM in tumor cells, and most importantly, sensitized the tumor cells to radiation in vitro and in vivo (Yan et al., 2010). Radiotherapy kills tumor-cells by inducing DNA double strand breaks (DSBs). However, the efficient repair of double strand breaks in tumors frequently prevents successful treatment. Therefore, miR-101 could be used to target DNA DSB repair genes, in order to sensitize tumors to radiation and improve tumor radiotherapy.

9. Functions of miRNAs in homologous recombination repair (HRR)

HRR is the most widely used repair mechanism which can accurately repair DNA double strand breaks. HRR reconstitutes the genetic information using the sister chromatid as a template. Several proteins are involved in the HRR process. Rad 52 protein recognizes double-strand breaks and adheres to the free ends of the break while the Rad51 protein, together with tumor-suppressor protein BRCA1, searches the undamaged sister chromatid for homologous pairing (Haber, 2000; Orelli and Bishop, 2001).

Both miR-210 and miR-373 were up-regulated in hypoxic cells. Up-regulation of miR-210 significantly suppressed the expression level of RAD51, while up-regulation of miR-373 inhibited the expression of RAD52. The modulation of miR-210 to RAD51 and miR-373 to RAD52 were verified by microarray analysis and luciferase reporter gene assay. Both of the miRNAs can bind to the binding sites in the 3′ UTRs of their respective target mRNAs (Crosby, et al., 2009). Thus, hypoxia-inducible miR-210 and miR-373 regulate HRR via targeting RAD51 and RAD52.

BRCA1 is a constituent of several different protein complexes and is a key protein for HRR. Expression of BRCA1 is commonly decreased in sporadic breast tumors, and this correlates with poor prognosis of breast cancer patients (Mueller and Roskelley, 2003). It was recently reported that miR-182 down-regulated BRCA1 expression. As a result, the HRR efficiency for DNA double strand break repair was impaired (Moskwa et al., 2011; Yao and Ventura, 2011). Antagonizing miR-182 enhanced BRCA1 protein level, which, in turn, protected cells from irradiation exposure. Over-expressing of miR-182 reduced BRCA1 protein level, which impaired HRR efficiency and rendered cells hypersensitive to irradiation. The impaired HRR phenotype due to miR-182 over-expression was able to be fully rescued by over-expressing of BRCA1. Thus, these data demonstrate miR-182-mediated down-regulation of BRCA1 suppresses HRR.

10. Conclusion

miRNAs appear to be involved in DNA damage and repair in many ways. miRNA biogenesis, including miRNA gene transcription and miRNA maturation processes, is readily altered in response to DNA damage. miRNAs regulate the ATM and P53 that are the regulators of the global induction of miRNA biogenesis upon DNA damage. miRNAs are also involved in signal transduction processes that leads to cell cycle arrest, apoptosis or DNA repair upon DNA damage. miR-100 and miR-421 can regulate expression of ATM, a critical protein in DNA damage signalling. miR-24 suppresses gene expression of H2AX, an initial sensor protein for DNA damage response. miR-16 down-regulates the expression level of Wip1, an inhibitor of ATM/ATR-p53 DNA damage signalling pathway. miRNAs can mediate the activity of P53, a core component of the DNA damage response. miR-504 and miR-125b negatively regulate p53 expression. miR-34a, miR-29 and miR-122 can indirectly modify P53 activity by regulating the P53-related factors. miRNAs play important roles in different types of DNA repair. miR-21 down-regulates MMR proteins, MSH2 and MSH6, while miR-155 reduced the expression of the MMS genes MLH1, MSH2 and MSH6. miR-373 suppresses expression of RAD23B, a key component of the NER. miR-101 down-regulates the protein level of DNA-PKcs, an essential factor for NHEJ. miR-210, miR-373 and miR-182 down-regulate the expression of RAD51, RAD52 and BRCA1, respectively. RAD51, RAD52 and BRCA1 are all key components of HRR. With increased studies of miRNAs' roles in DNA damage and repair, more miRNAs will be discovered to involve in the DNA damage and repair pathways.

11. Acknowledgements

The views presented in this article do not necessarily reflect those of the Food and Drug Administration. We would like to thank Dr. Barbara Parsons and Mr. Jian Yan for their review of this manuscript.

12. References

Batty, D., Rapic'-Otrin, V., Levine, A. S. and Wood, R. D. (2000). Stable binding of human XPC complex to irradiated DNA confers strong discrimination for damaged sites. J Mol Biol 300, 275-90.

Braun, C. J., Zhang, X., Savelyeva, I., Wolff, S., Moll, U. M., Schepeler, T., Orntoft, T. F., Andersen, C. L. and Dobbelstein, M. (2008). p53-Responsive micrornas 192 and 215 are capable of inducing cell cycle arrest. Cancer Res 68, 10094-104.

Cai, X., Hagedorn, C. H. and Cullen, B. R. (2004). Human microRNAs are processed from capped, polyadenylated transcripts that can also function as mRNAs. RNA 10, 1957-66.

Cannell, I. G., Kong, Y. W., Johnston, S. J., Chen, M. L., Collins, H. M., Dobbyn, H. C., Elia, A., Kress, T. R., Dickens, M., Clemens, M. J., Heery, D. M., Gaestel, M., Eilers, M., Willis, A. E. and Bushell, M. (2010). p38 MAPK/MK2-mediated induction of miR-34c following DNA damage prevents Myc-dependent DNA replication. Proc Natl Acad Sci U S A 107, 5375-80.

Chang, T. C., Wentzel, E. A., Kent, O. A., Ramachandran, K., Mullendore, M., Lee, K. H., Feldmann, G., Yamakuchi, M., Ferlito, M., Lowenstein, C. J., Arking, D. E., Beer, M. A., Maitra, A. and Mendell, J. T. (2007). Transactivation of miR-34a by p53 broadly influences gene expression and promotes apoptosis. Mol Cell 26, 745-52.

Chen, D. H., Li, Z. and Chen, T. (2011). Increased Expression of miR-34a in mouse spleen one day after exposure to N-ethyl-N-nitrosourea. Applied Journal of Toxicology.

Corney, D. C., Flesken-Nikitin, A., Godwin, A. K., Wang, W. and Nikitin, A. Y. (2007). MicroRNA-34b and MicroRNA-34c are targets of p53 and cooperate in control of cell proliferation and adhesion-independent growth. Cancer Res 67, 8433-8.

Crosby, M. E., Kulshreshtha, R., Ivan, M. and Glazer, P. M. (2009). MicroRNA regulation of DNA repair gene expression in hypoxic stress. Cancer Res 69, 1221-9.

Fishel, R. (2001). The selection for mismatch repair defects in hereditary nonpolyposis colorectal cancer: revising the mutator hypothesis. Cancer Res 61, 7369-74.

Fornari, F., Gramantieri, L., Giovannini, C., Veronese, A., Ferracin, M., Sabbioni, S., Calin, G. A., Grazi, G. L., Croce, C. M., Tavolari, S., Chieco, P., Negrini, M. and Bolondi, L. (2009). MiR-122/cyclin G1 interaction modulates p53 activity and affects doxorubicin sensitivity of human hepatocarcinoma cells. Cancer Res 69, 5761-7.

Georges, S. A., Biery, M. C., Kim, S. Y., Schelter, J. M., Guo, J., Chang, A. N., Jackson, A. L., Carleton, M. O., Linsley, P. S., Cleary, M. A. and Chau, B. N. (2008). Coordinated regulation of cell cycle transcripts by p53-Inducible microRNAs, miR-192 and miR-215. Cancer Res 68, 10105-12.

Gregory, R. I., Chendrimada, T. P., Cooch, N. and Shiekhattar, R. (2005). Human RISC couples microRNA biogenesis and posttranscriptional gene silencing. Cell 123, 631-40.

Grishok, A., Pasquinelli, A. E., Conte, D., Li, N., Parrish, S., Ha, I., Baillie, D. L., Fire, A., Ruvkun, G. and Mello, C. C. (2001). Genes and mechanisms related to RNA interference regulate expression of the small temporal RNAs that control C. elegans developmental timing. Cell 106, 23-34.

Haber, J. E. (2000). Partners and pathwaysrepairing a double-strand break. Trends Genet 16, 259-64.

Han, J., Lee, Y., Yeom, K. H., Kim, Y. K., Jin, H. and Kim, V. N. (2004). The Drosha-DGCR8 complex in primary microRNA processing. Genes Dev 18, 3016-27.

He, L., He, X., Lim, L. P., de Stanchina, E., Xuan, Z., Liang, Y., Xue, W., Zender, L., Magnus, J., Ridzon, D., Jackson, A. L., Linsley, P. S., Chen, C., Lowe, S. W., Cleary, M. A. and Hannon, G. J. (2007). A microRNA component of the p53 tumour suppressor network. Nature 447, 1130-4.

Hu, H., Du, L., Nagabayashi, G., Seeger, R. C. and Gatti, R. A. (2010a). ATM is down-regulated by N-Myc-regulated microRNA-421. Proc Natl Acad Sci U S A 107, 1506-11.

Hu, W., Chan, C. S., Wu, R., Zhang, C., Sun, Y., Song, J. S., Tang, L. H., Levine, A. J. and Feng, Z. (2010b). Negative regulation of tumor suppressor p53 by microRNA miR-504. Mol Cell 38, 689-99.

Hutvagner, G., McLachlan, J., Pasquinelli, A. E., Balint, E., Tuschl, T. and Zamore, P. D. (2001). A cellular function for the RNA-interference enzyme Dicer in the maturation of the let-7 small temporal RNA. Science 293, 834-8.

Kato, M., Paranjape, T., Muller, R. U., Nallur, S., Gillespie, E., Keane, K., Esquela-Kerscher, A., Weidhaas, J. B. and Slack, F. J. (2009). The mir-34 microRNA is required for the DNA damage response in vivo in C. elegans and in vitro in human breast cancer cells. Oncogene 28, 2419-24.

Ketting, R. F., Fischer, S. E., Bernstein, E., Sijen, T., Hannon, G. J. and Plasterk, R. H. (2001). Dicer functions in RNA interference and in synthesis of small RNA involved in developmental timing in C. elegans. Genes Dev 15, 2654-9.

Lal, A., Pan, Y., Navarro, F., Dykxhoorn, D. M., Moreau, L., Meire, E., Bentwich, Z., Lieberman, J. and Chowdhury, D. (2009). miR-24-mediated downregulation of

H2AX suppresses DNA repair in terminally differentiated blood cells. Nat Struct Mol Biol 16, 492-8.

Lavin, M. F. (2008). Ataxia-telangiectasia: from a rare disorder to a paradigm for cell signalling and cancer. Nat Rev Mol Cell Biol 9, 759-69.

Le, M. T., Teh, C., Shyh-Chang, N., Xie, H., Zhou, B., Korzh, V., Lodish, H. F. and Lim, B. (2009). MicroRNA-125b is a novel negative regulator of p53. Genes Dev 23, 862-76.

Lee, Y., Ahn, C., Han, J., Choi, H., Kim, J., Yim, J., Lee, J., Provost, P., Radmark, O., Kim, S. and Kim, V. N. (2003). The nuclear RNase III Drosha initiates microRNA processing. Nature 425, 415-9.

Lee, Y., Kim, M., Han, J., Yeom, K. H., Lee, S., Baek, S. H. and Kim, V. N. (2004). MicroRNA genes are transcribed by RNA polymerase II. EMBO J 23, 4051-60.

Levine, A. J., Finlay, C. A. and Hinds, P. W. (2004). P53 is a tumor suppressor gene. Cell 116, S67-9, 1 p following S69.

Levine, A. J., Hu, W. and Feng, Z. (2006). The P53 pathway: what questions remain to be explored? Cell Death Differ 13, 1027-36.

Li, Z., Branham, W. S., Dial, S. L., Wang, Y., Guo, L., Shi, L. and Chen, T. (2010). Genomic analysis of microRNA time-course expression in liver of mice treated with genotoxic carcinogen N-ethyl-N-nitrosourea. BMC Genomics 11, 609.

Li, Z., Fuscoe, J. C. and Chen, T. (2011). MicroRNAs and their predicted target messenger RNAs are deregulated by Exposure to a Carcinogenic Dose of Comfrey in Rat Liver. Environ Mol Mutagen.

Link, A., Balaguer, F., Shen, Y., Nagasaka, T., Lozano, J. J., Boland, C. R. and Goel, A. (2010). Fecal MicroRNAs as novel biomarkers for colon cancer screening. Cancer Epidemiol Biomarkers Prev 19, 1766-74.

Lodish H, B. A., Matsudaira P, Kaiser CA, Krieger M, Scott MP, Zipursky SL, Darnell J. (2004). Molecular Biology of the Cell, p963.

Maniataki, E. and Mourelatos, Z. (2005). A human, ATP-independent, RISC assembly machine fueled by pre-miRNA. Genes Dev 19, 2979-90.

Meister, G. and Tuschl, T. (2004). Mechanisms of gene silencing by double-stranded RNA. Nature 431, 343-9.

Moskwa, P., Buffa, F. M., Pan, Y., Panchakshari, R., Gottipati, P., Muschel, R. J., Beech, J., Kulshrestha, R., Abdelmohsen, K., Weinstock, D. M., Gorospe, M., Harris, A. L., Helleday, T. and Chowdhury, D. (2011). miR-182-mediated downregulation of BRCA1 impacts DNA repair and sensitivity to PARP inhibitors. Mol Cell 41, 210-20.

Mueller, C. R. and Roskelley, C. D. (2003). Regulation of BRCA1 expression and its relationship to sporadic breast cancer. Breast Cancer Res 5, 45-52.

Ng, E. K., Chong, W. W., Jin, H., Lam, E. K., Shin, V. Y., Yu, J., Poon, T. C., Ng, S. S. and Sung, J. J. (2009). Differential expression of microRNAs in plasma of patients with colorectal cancer: a potential marker for colorectal cancer screening. Gut 58, 1375-81.

Ng, W. L., Yan, D., Zhang, X., Mo, Y. Y. and Wang, Y. (2010). Over-expression of miR-100 is responsible for the low-expression of ATM in the human glioma cell line: M059J. DNA Repair (Amst) 9, 1170-5.

Orelli, B. J. and Bishop, D. K. (2001). BRCA2 and homologous recombination. Breast Cancer Res 3, 294-8.

Ozsolak, F., Poling, L. L., Wang, Z., Liu, H., Liu, X. S., Roeder, R. G., Zhang, X., Song, J. S. and Fisher, D. E. (2008). Chromatin structure analyses identify miRNA promoters. Genes Dev 22, 3172-83.

Park, S. Y., Lee, J. H., Ha, M., Nam, J. W. and Kim, V. N. (2009). miR-29 miRNAs activate p53 by targeting p85 alpha and CDC42. Nat Struct Mol Biol 16, 23-9.

Pothof, J., Verkaik, N. S., van, I. W., Wiemer, E. A., Ta, V. T., van der Horst, G. T., Jaspers, N. G., van Gent, D. C., Hoeijmakers, J. H. and Persengiev, S. P. (2009). MicroRNA-mediated gene silencing modulates the UV-induced DNA-damage response. EMBO J 28, 2090-9.

Raver-Shapira, N., Marciano, E., Meiri, E., Spector, Y., Rosenfeld, N., Moskovits, N., Bentwich, Z. and Oren, M. (2007). Transcriptional activation of miR-34a contributes to p53-mediated apoptosis. Mol Cell 26, 731-43.

Rich, T., Allen, R. L. and Wyllie, A. H. (2000). Defying death after DNA damage. Nature 407, 777-83.

Shiloh, Y. (2003). ATM and related protein kinases: safeguarding genome integrity. Nat Rev Cancer 3, 155-68.

Suzuki, H. I., Yamagata, K., Sugimoto, K., Iwamoto, T., Kato, S. and Miyazono, K. (2009). Modulation of microRNA processing by p53. Nature 460, 529-33.

Toledo, F. and Bardot, B. (2009). Cancer: Three birds with one stone. Nature 460, 466-7.

Valeri, N., Gasparini, P., Braconi, C., Paone, A., Lovat, F., Fabbri, M., Sumani, K. M., Alder, H., Amadori, D., Patel, T., Nuovo, G. J., Fishel, R. and Croce, C. M. (2010a). MicroRNA-21 induces resistance to 5-fluorouracil by down-regulating human DNA MutS homolog 2 (hMSH2). Proc Natl Acad Sci U S A 107, 21098-103.

Valeri, N., Gasparini, P., Fabbri, M., Braconi, C., Veronese, A., Lovat, F., Adair, B., Vannini, I., Fanini, F., Bottoni, A., Costinean, S., Sandhu, S. K., Nuovo, G. J., Alder, H., Gafa, R., Calore, F., Ferracin, M., Lanza, G., Volinia, S., Negrini, M., McIlhatton, M. A., Amadori, D., Fishel, R. and Croce, C. M. (2010b). Modulation of mismatch repair and genomic stability by miR-155. Proc Natl Acad Sci U S A 107, 6982-7.

Volinia, S., Calin, G. A., Liu, C. G., Ambs, S., Cimmino, A., Petrocca, F., Visone, R., Iorio, M., Roldo, C., Ferracin, M., Prueitt, R. L., Yanaihara, N., Lanza, G., Scarpa, A., Vecchione, A., Negrini, M., Harris, C. C. and Croce, C. M. (2006). A microRNA expression signature of human solid tumors defines cancer gene targets. Proc Natl Acad Sci U S A 103, 2257-61.

Welch, C., Chen, Y. and Stallings, R. L. (2007). MicroRNA-34a functions as a potential tumor suppressor by inducing apoptosis in neuroblastoma cells. Oncogene 26, 5017-22.

Yamakuchi, M., Ferlito, M. and Lowenstein, C. J. (2008). miR-34a repression of SIRT1 regulates apoptosis. Proc Natl Acad Sci U S A 105, 13421-6.

Yan, D., Ng, W. L., Zhang, X., Wang, P., Zhang, Z., Mo, Y. Y., Mao, H., Hao, C., Olson, J. J., Curran, W. J. and Wang, Y. (2010). Targeting DNA-PKcs and ATM with miR-101 sensitizes tumors to radiation. PLoS One 5, e11397.

Yao, E. and Ventura, A. (2011). A new role for miR-182 in DNA repair. Mol Cell 41, 135-7.

Yuan, J., Narayanan, L., Rockwell, S. and Glazer, P. M. (2000). Diminished DNA repair and elevated mutagenesis in mammalian cells exposed to hypoxia and low pH. Cancer Res 60, 4372-6.

Zenz, T., Mohr, J., Eldering, E., Kater, A. P., Buhler, A., Kienle, D., Winkler, D., Durig, J., van Oers, M. H., Mertens, D., Dohner, H. and Stilgenbauer, S. (2009). miR-34a as part of the resistance network in chronic lymphocytic leukemia. Blood 113, 3801-8.

Zhang, X., Wan, G., Mlotshwa, S., Vance, V., Berger, F. G., Chen, H. and Lu, X. (2010). Oncogenic Wip1 phosphatase is inhibited by miR-16 in the DNA damage signaling pathway. Cancer Res 70, 7176-86.

Zhang, X., Wan, G., Berger, F. G., He, X. and Lu, X. (2011). The ATM kinase induces microRNA biogenesis in the DNA damage response. Mol Cell 41, 371-83.

Part 2

Evolution of DNA Repair

19

Meiosis as an Evolutionary Adaptation for DNA Repair

Harris Bernstein[1], Carol Bernstein[1] and Richard E. Michod[2]
[1]*Department of Cellular and Molecular Medicine, University of Arizona*
[2]*Department of Ecology and Evolutionary Biology, University of Arizona*
USA

1. Introduction

The adaptive function of sex remains, today, one of the major unsolved problems in biology. Fundamental to achieving a resolution of this problem is gaining an understanding of the function of meiosis. The sexual cycle in eukaryotes has two key stages, meiosis and syngamy. In meiosis, typically a diploid cell gives rise to haploid cells. In syngamy (fertilization), typically two haploid gametes from different individuals fuse to generate a new diploid individual. A unique feature of meiosis, compared to mitosis, is recombination between non-sister homologous chromosomes. Usually these homologous chromosomes are derived from different individuals. In mitosis, recombination can occur, but it is ordinarily between sister homologs, the two products of a round of chromosome replication. Birdsell & Wills (2003) have reviewed the various hypotheses for the origin and maintenance of sex and meiotic recombination, including the hypothesis that sex is an adaptation for the repair of DNA damage and the masking of deleterious recessive alleles. Recently, we presented evidence that among microbial pathogens, sexual processes promote repair of DNA damage, especially when challenged by the oxidative defenses of their biologic hosts (Michod et al., 2008). Here, we present evidence that meiosis is primarily an evolutionary adaptation for DNA repair. Since our previous review of this topic (Bernstein et al., 1988), there has been a considerable increase in relevant information at the molecular level on the DNA repair functions of meiotic recombination, and this new information is emphasized in the present chapter.

2. Meiosis in protists and simple multicellular eukaryotes is induced in response to stressful conditions that likely cause DNA damage

Eukaryotes appeared in evolution more than 1.5 billion years ago (Javaux et al., 2001). Among extant eukaryotes, meiosis and sexual reproduction are ubiquitous and appear to have been present early in eukaryote evolution. Malik et al. (2008) found that 27 of 29 tested meiotic genes were present in *Trichomonas vaginalis*, and 21 of these 29 genes were also present in *Giardia intestinalis*, indicating that most meiotic genes were present in a common ancestor of these species. Since these lineages are highly divergent among eukaryotes, these authors concluded that each of these meiotic genes were likely present in the common ancestor of all eukaryotes. Dacks and Roger (1999) also proposed that sex has a single evolutionary origin and was present in the last common ancestor of eukaryotes. Recently, this view received further support from a study of amoebae. Although amoebae generally have been assumed to be asexual, Lahr et al. (2011) showed that the majority of amoeboid lineages were likely anciently sexual, and that most asexual groups have probably arisen recently and independently.

Eukaryotes arose in evolution from prokaryotes, and eukaryotic meiosis may have arisen from bacterial transformation, a naturally occurring sexual process in prokaryotes. The fundamental similarities between transformation and meiosis have been explored (H. Bernstein & C. Bernstein, 2010). Bacterial transformation, like meiosis, involves alignment and recombination between non-sister homologous chromosomes (or parts of chromosomes) originating from different parents. Both during transformation and meiosis, homologs of the bacterial *recA* gene play a central role in the strand transfer reactions of recombination, indicating a mechanistic similarity. Also, bacterial transformation is induced by environmental stresses that are similar to those that induce meiosis in protists and simple multicellular eukaryotes, suggesting that there was continuity in the evolutionary transition from prokaryotic sex to eukaryotic sex. Evidence indicates that bacterial transformation is an adaptation for repairing DNA (Michod et al., 1988; Hoelzer & Michod, 1991; Michod & Wojciechowski, 1994; reviewed by Michod et al., 2008). Thus meiosis may have emerged from transformation as an adaptation for repairing DNA.

Among extant protists and simple multicellular eukaryotes sexual reproduction is ordinarily facultative. Meiosis and sex in these organisms is usually induced by stressful conditions. The paramecium tetrahymena can be induced to undergo conjugation leading to meiosis by washing, which causes rapid starvation (Elliott & Hayes, 1953). Depletion of the nitrogen source in the growth medium of the unicellular green alga *Chlamydomonas reinhardi* leads to differentiation of vegetative cells into gametes (Sager & Granick 1954). These gametes can then mate, form zygotes and undergo meiosis. Upon nitrogen starvation or desiccation, the human fungal pathogen *Cryptococcus neoformans* undergoes mating or fruiting, both processes involving meiosis (Lin et al., 2005).

In addition to starvation, oxidative stress is another condition that induces meiosis and sex. The haploid fission yeast *Schizosaccharomyces pombe* is induced to undergo sexual development and mating when the supply of nutrients becomes limiting (Davey et al., 1998). Moreover, treatment of late-exponential-phase *S. pombe* vegetative cells with hydrogen peroxide, which causes oxidative stress, increases the frequency of mating and production of meiotic spores by 4- to 18-fold (C. Bernstein & Johns, 1989). The oomycete *Phytophthora cinnamomi* is induced to undergo sexual reproduction by exposure to the oxidizing agent hydrogen peroxide or mechanical damage to hyphae (Reeves & Jackson, 1974). In the simple multicellular green algae *Volvox carteri,* sex is induced by heat shock (Kirk & Kirk, 1986). This effect can be inhibited by antioxidants, indicating that the induction of sex by heat shock is mediated by oxidative stress (Nedelcu & Michod, 2003). Furthermore, induction of oxidative stress by an inhibitor of the mitochondrial electron transport chain also induced sex in *V. carteri* (Nedelcu et al., 2004). The budding yeast *Saccharomyces cerevisiae* reproduces as mitotically dividing diploid cells when nutrients are plentiful, but undergoes meiosis to form haploid spores when starved (Herskowitz, 1988). When *S. cerevisiae* are starved, oxidative stress is increased and DNA double-strand breaks (DSBs) and apurinic/apyrimidinic sites accumulate (Steinboeck et al., 2010). Perhaps, in *S. cerevisiae,* the induction of sex by starvation is mediated by oxidative stress, analogous to the way induction of sex by heat is mediated by oxidative stress in *V. carteri.*

These observations suggest that meiosis is an adaptation for dealing with stress, particularly oxidative stress. It is well established that oxidative stress induces a variety of DNA damages including DNA DSBs, single-strand breaks and modified bases (Slupphaug et al., 2003). Thus we hypothesize that, in facultative sexual protists and simple multicellular eukaryotes, sex, with the central feature of meiosis, is an adaptive response to DNA damage, particularly oxidative DNA damage.

3. DNA damages induced by exogenous agents cause increased meiotic recombination

If recombination during meiosis is an adaptation for repairing DNA damages, then it would be expected that exposure to DNA damaging treatments would increase the frequency of recombination, as measured by crossovers between allelic markers. Stimulation of allelic recombination was reported in the fruitfly *Drosophila melanogaster* in response to exposure to the DNA damaging agents UV light (Prudhommeau & Proust, 1973), X-rays (Suzuki & Parry, 1964), and mitomycin C (Schewe et al., 1971). X-rays induce recombination in meiotic cells not only of *D. melanogaster* females, but also of males, which normally display no recombination during meiosis (Hannah-Alava, 1964).

Increased meiotic recombination in response to X-irradiation has also been reported in *Caenorhabditis elegans* (Kim & Rose, 1987), and in *S. cerevisiae* (Kelly et al., 1983).

4. During mitosis and meiosis, DNA damages caused by diverse exogenous agents can be repaired by homologous recombination

Molecular recombination (that is homologous physical exchange or informational exchange) during mitosis and meiosis functions as a DNA repair process designated homologous recombinational repair (HRR). Many of the gene products employed in mitotic HRR are also employed in recombination during meiosis. It is this consistent function of recombination across meiosis and mitosis in eukaryotes and transformation in prokaryotes that we seek to understand through the repair hypothesis. Mutants defective in HRR genes in *D. melanogaster* and yeast have reduced ability to repair DNA damages arising from a variety of exogenous sources. These mutants are also defective in recombination during meiosis. In general, loss of HRR capability causes increased sensitivity to killing by agents that harm cells primarily through induction of DNA damage. These agents are listed in Table 1. There have been no reports, that we know of, that HRR defective cells are sensitive to agents that harm cells by mechanisms other than primarily causing DNA damage.

In *D. melanogaster*, mutants defective in genes *mei-41, mei-9, hdm, spnA* and *brca2* have reduced spontaneous allelic recombination (crossing over) during meiosis and increased sensitivity to killing by exposure to numerous DNA damaging agents (Table 1). The Mei-41 protein is a structural and functional homolog of the human Atm (ataxia telangiectasia) protein (Hari et al., 1995), which plays a central role in HRR. The Mei-9 and Hdm proteins are components of a multiprotein complex that resolves meiotic recombination intermediates (Joyce et al., 2009). The SpnA protein is a homolog of yeast Rad51 (Staeva-Vieira et al., 2003), and Rad51 plays a central role in strand-exchange during HRR. The *D. melanogaster* Brca2 protein, a homolog of the human Brca2 protein that protects against breast cancer, regulates the activity of Rad51 protein in HRR. The Brca2 protein is required for HRR of DSBs during meiosis (Klovstad et al., 2008).

In *S. cerevisiae,* numerous mutant genes have been identified that confer sensitivity to radiation and/or genotoxic chemicals (Haynes & Kunz, 1981). Several of these mutant genes are also defective in meiotic recombination. For instance, the *rad52* gene is required for meiotic recombination (Game et al., 1980) as well as for mitotic recombination (Malone & Esposito, 1980). Mutants defective in the *rad52* gene are sensitive to killing by several DNA damaging agents (Table 1). Diploid cells of *S. cerevisiae* are able to repair DNA DSBs introduced by ionizing radiation, and this ability is lost in mutant strains defective in the *rad52* gene (Resnick & Martin, 1976). The Rad52 protein promotes the DNA strand exchange reaction of recombination during meiosis and mitosis (Mortensen et al., 2009).

Taken as a whole, these findings indicate that the products of genes *mei-41, mei-9, hdm, spnA, and brca2* in *D. melanogaster* and the *rad52* gene of yeast are required in meiosis for recombination and in somatic cells for HRR of potentially lethal DNA damages. Since the gene products that function in mitotic HRR are able to repair DNA damages from different sources, it can be reasonably assumed that these genes serve a similar DNA repair function during recombination in meiosis.

In the nematode *C. elegans* gonad, oocyte nuclei in the pachytene stage of meiosis, the stage in which HRR occurs, are hyper-resistant to X-ray irradiation compared to oocytes in the subsequent diakinesis stage of meiosis (Takanami et al., 2000). This hyper-resistance depends on expression of gene *ce-rdh-51*, a homolog of yeast *rad51* and *dmc1* that play a central role in meiotic HRR. Meiotic pachytene nuclei are also more resistant to heavy ion particle irradiation than the subsequent meiotic diplotene or diakinesis stages (Takanami et al., 2003). This resistance also depends on the *ce-rdh-51* gene, as well as on gene *ce-atl-1*. *ce-atl-1* is related to *atm* (ataxia –telangiectasia mutated), a gene necessary for repair of DSBs by HRR.

Coogan & Rosenblum (1988) measured repair of DSBs following γ-irradiation of rat spermatogenic cells during successive stages of germ cell formation. The stages were spermatagonia and preleptotene spermatocytes, pachytene spermatocytes and spermatid spermatocytes. The greatest repair capability was observed in pachytene, the stage of meiosis when HRR occurs. These findings indicate that HRR of γ-ray-induced DSBs occurs during meiosis. Several mammalian germ cell stages, including pachytene spermatocytes, produce levels of reactive oxygen species (ROS) sufficient to cause oxidative stress (Fisher & Aitkin, 1997). This observation suggests that HRR during meiosis may also remove DNA damages caused by natural endogenously produced ROS.

The results reviewed in this section indicate that, in both meiosis and mitosis, DNA damages caused by different exogenous agents are repaired by HRR, suggesting that DNA damages from natural endogenous sources (e.g. ROS) are similarly repaired. In general, DNA damage appears to be a fundamental problem for life. As noted by Haynes (1988), DNA is composed of rather ordinary molecular subunits, which are not endowed with any peculiar kind of quantum mechanical stability. He observed that its very "chemical vulgarity" makes DNA subject to all the "chemical horrors" that might befall any such molecule in a warm aqueous medium. The average amount of oxidative DNA damage occurring per cell per day is estimated to be about 10,000 in humans, and in rat, with a higher metabolic rate, about 100,000 (Ames et al., 1993). Most of these damages affect only one strand of the DNA, but a fraction, about 1-2%, are double-strand damages such as DSBs (Massie et al., 1972). These damages can be repaired accurately by HRR.

Organism	Mutant gene	Meiotic recomb-ination	DNA damaging agent(s)	Sensitivity to killing by agent(s)	Reference
D. melano-gaster	*mei-41*	Reduced	X-rays, UV, methyl methanesulfonate, nitrogen mustard, benzo(s)pyrene, 2-acetyl-aminofluorene	Increased	Baker et al., 1976; Boyd, 1978; Rasmuson, 1984
	mei-9	Reduced	X-rays, UV, methyl methanesulfonate, nitrogen mustard, benzo(s)pyrene, 2-acetyl-aminofluorene	Increased	Baker et al., 1976; Boyd, 1978; Rasmuson, 1984
	hdm	Reduced	methyl methanesulfonate	Increased	Joyce et al., 2009
	spnA	Reduced	X-rays	Increased	Staeva-Vieira et al., 2003
	brca2	HRR of DSBs is reduced	X-rays, methyl methanesulfonate	Increased	Klovstad et al., 2008
S. cerevisiae	*rad52*	Reduced	X-rays, methyl methanesulfonate, crosslinking agent 8-methoxypsoralen plus UV light	Increased	Haynes & Kunz, 1981; Henriques & Moustacchi, 1980; Game et al., 1980

Table 1. Mutants with reduced meiotic recombination and sensitive to killing by specific DNA damaging agents.

5. In humans and rodents, defects in HRR enzymes lead to infertility, as would be expected if removal of DNA damages is an essential function of meiosis

About 15% of all couples in the US are infertile, and an important cause of male infertility appears to be oxidative stress during gametogenesis (Makker et al., 2009). During spermatogenesis in the mouse, DNA repair capability declines after meiosis is complete, allowing accumulation of DNA damage (Marchetti & Wyrobek, 2008). Lewis & Aitken (2005) reviewed evidence that DNA damages in the germ line of men are associated with poor semen quality, low fertilization rates, impaired pre-implantation development, increased abortion, and elevated incidence of disease in the offspring including childhood cancer. They noted that the natural causes of this DNA damage are uncertain, but the major candidate is oxidative stress. On the hypothesis that meiosis is an adaptation for DNA repair, it is expected that loss of ability to repair DNA damages during meiosis would have adverse effects, including infertility. Although the finding of such adverse effects is expected on the hypothesis that meiosis is an adaptation for repairing naturally caused DNA

damages, this finding does not prove the hypothesis. Another possibility is that during meiosis damages are introduced in a programmed fashion, leading to HRR. Such HRR may be necessary for proper pairing and segregation of chromosomes, and this process may be required for fertility (see section 8 below).
Inherited mutations in genes that specify proteins necessary for HRR cause infertility (Table 2) indicating that production of functional gametes depends on HRR. Genes *brca1, atm,* and *mlh1* are expressed in mitosis, but at a higher level in meiosis, and gene *dmc1* is expressed exclusively in meiosis (Table 2).

Gene	Species	Fold-increased expression in testes vs. somatic cells	Infertility in mutant females/males	References
brca1	Mouse	3×	male mice are infertile	Galetzka et al., 2007; Cressman et al., 1999
atm	human, mouse	4×	females and males in both humans and mice are infertile	Galetzka et al., 2007; Barlow et al., 1998
mlh1	Mouse	1.7×	female and male mice are infertile	Galetzka et al., 2007; Wei et al., 2002
dmc1	Mouse	specific for meiotic cells	female and male mice are infertile	Pittman et al., 1998

Table 2. Mutant genes defective in HRR that cause infertility in human and/or mouse

Brca1 functions during both meiotic and mitotic recombination. The inheritance of a mutant *brca1* allele substantially increases a woman's lifetime risk for developing breast or ovarian cancer due to a deficiency in HRR of DNA DSBs in somatic cells. Male *brca1* defective mice are infertile due to meiotic failure during spermatogenesis (Table 2), indicating that HRR is necessary during meiosis.
The Atm protein acts during both meiotic and mitotic recombination in detection and signaling of DSBs, and is necessary for fertility of females and males in both humans and mice (Table 2). Gametogenesis is severely disrupted in Atm-deficient mice as early as the leptonema stage of prophase I, resulting in apoptotic degeneration (Barlow et al., 1998).
Mismatch repair protein Mlh1 (homolog of *E. coli* MutL) is necessary for meiotic recombination (Wei et al., 2002). Mutation in the *mlh1* gene causes blockage at the pachytene stage of meiosis and female and male infertility (Table 2).
Dmc1 is a meiosis specific gene. Dmc1 protein (a homolog of *E. coli* RecA protein) functions during meiotic recombination to promote recognition of homologous DNA and to catalyze strand exchange. *Dmc1* deficient female and male mice are infertile due to arrest of gametes in meiotic prophase (Table 2).
The evidence reviewed in this section indicates that defective HRR of DNA damages during meiosis causes infertility.

6. Non-crossover (NCO) recombination during meiosis is likely an adaptation for DNA repair

Meiotic recombination appears to be a near universal feature of meiosis [although it may be absent in some situations, such as in *Drosophila* males (Chovnick et al., 1970)]. There are two major classes of meiotic recombination. If, during recombination, the chromosome arms on opposite sides of a DSB exchange partners, the recombination event is referred to as a crossover (CO). If the original configuration of chromosome arms is maintained, the recombination event is referred to as a non-crossover (NCO) (see Figure 1). The relative occurrence of NCO or CO recombination events is relevant to evolutionary theories of meiosis which assume producing genetic variation is the function of meiosis. NCO events have little effect on linkage disequilibrium (the statistical association of genes at different loci) and so produce very little genetic variation in terms of new combinations of genes. However, CO and NCO events are equivalent from the point of view of HRR.

Data based on tetrad analysis from several species of fungi indicates that the majority (about 2/3) of recombination events during meiosis are NCOs [see Whitehouse (1982), Tables 19 and 38, for summaries of data from *S. cerevisiae*, *Podospora anserine*, *Sordaria fimicola* and *Sordaria brevicollis*]. More recent work also supports a bias towards NCOs during meiosis. In mouse meiosis there are $\geq$ 10-fold more DSBs than CO recombinants (Moens et al., 2002), suggesting that most DSBs are repaired by NCO recombination. In *D. melanogaster* there is at least a 3:1 ratio of NCOs to COs (Mehrotra & McKim, 2006). These observations indicate that the majority of recombination events are NCOs. These NCOs involve informational exchange between two homologs but not physical exchange, and little genetic variation is created. Thus explanations for the adaptive function of meiosis that focus exclusively on crossing over are inadequate to explain the majority of recombination events.

Andersen & Sekelsky (2010) have argued that a common mechanism called "synthesis dependent strand annealing" (see section 7, below) is employed in both meiotic HRR of the NCO type and mitotic HRR (which is largely of the NCO type), and thus meiotic and mitotic NCOs probably have a similar function. Substantial evidence indicates that HRR during mitosis is an adaptation to repair DNA damages that originate from diverse endogenous and exogenous sources (e.g. endogenous ROS from oxidative metabolism and exogenous X-rays, UV, chemical carcinogens) (see examples in Table 1; also Lisby & Rothstein, 2009). Thus NCO recombination during meiosis, as in mitosis, likely functions to repair of DNA damages from diverse sources.

7. NCO recombination likely occurs by synthesis-dependent strand annealing

Molecular models of meiotic recombination have evolved over the years as relevant evidence accumulated. The model that has been most influential in recent decades has been the Double-Strand Break Repair model (Szostak et al. 1983). By this model, during each recombination event two Holliday Junctions (HJs) are formed and resolved (see Figure 1). Thus the Double-Strand Break Repair model can also be referred to as the Double Holliday Junction (DHJ) model. The DHJ model was considered to provide an explanation for both CO and NCO types of recombination events. However, Allers & Lichten (2001) showed that, although CO recombinants are likely formed by a pathway involving resolution of Holliday junctions, NCO recombinants arise by a different pathway that acts earlier in meiosis. Allers & Lichten (2001), McMahill et al. (2007) and Andersen & Sekelsky (2010) have presented evidence that NCO recombinants are generated during meiosis by an HRR repair process referred to as "Synthesis-Dependent Strand Annealing" or "SDSA" (see Figure 1). During SDSA the invading strand from a chromosome with a DSB is displaced from the D-loop structure of an intact chromosome and its newly synthesized sequence anneals to the other side of the break on the chromosome with the original DSB. This process can accurately repair DNA DSBs by copying the information lost in the damaged homolog from the other intact homolog without the need for physical exchange of DNA. This process contributes little to genetic variation since the arms of the chromosomes flanking the recombination event remain in the parental position.

Youds et al. (2010) presented evidence that the RTEL-1 protein of *C. elegans* physically dissociates strand invasion events, thereby promoting NCO repair by SDSA (Figure 1). HRR events initiated by DSBs consequently divide into two subsets, a larger subset which undergoes SDSA forming NCO recombinants, and a smaller subset which undergo DHJ repair and form CO recombinants. Perhaps SDSA is the preferred mode of HRR for unprogrammed double-strand damages, and DHJ repair is used primarily for programmed DSBs to promote proper chromosome segregation.

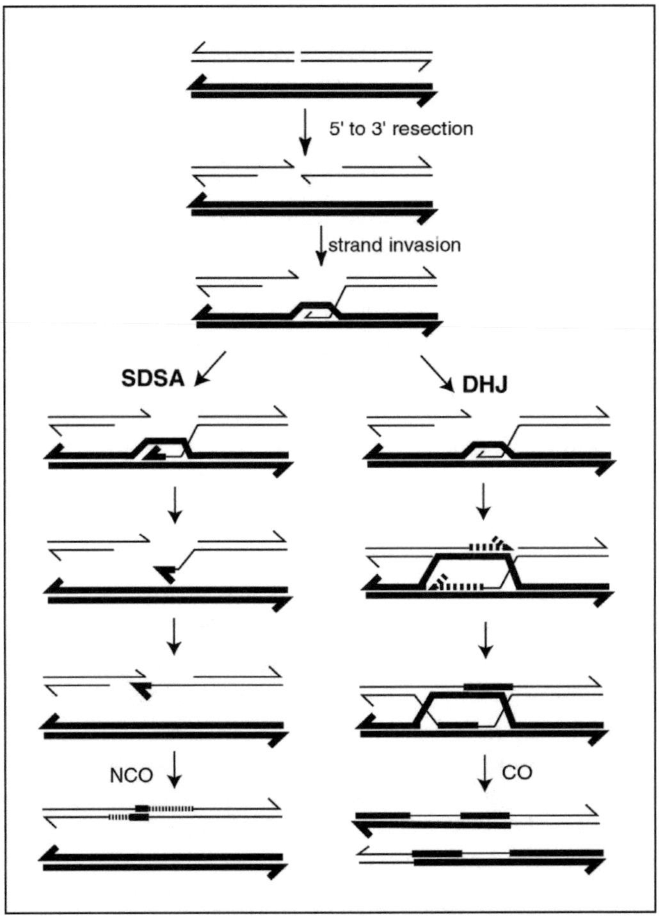

Fig. 1. Current models of meiotic recombination are initiated by a double-strand break or gap, followed by pairing with an homologous chromosome and strand invasion to initiate the recombinational repair process. Repair of the gap can lead to crossover (CO) or non-crossover (NCO) of the flanking regions. CO recombination is thought to occur by the Double Holliday Junction (DHJ) model, illustrated on the right, above. NCO recombinants are thought to occur primarily by the Synthesis Dependent Strand Annealing (SDSA) model, illustrated on the left, above. Most recombination events appear to be the SDSA type.

Although the SDSA model starts with a DSB, it would also be applicable to other types of double-strand damages such as interstrand-crosslinks, or a single-strand damage (e.g. an altered base) opposite a break in the other strand. In principle, both of these types of double-strand damages could be converted by nucleases to a DSB that would then be subject to SDSA.

8. The role of Spo11 in promoting accurate DNA repair can also facilitate proper chromosome segregation

In the budding yeast *S. cerevisiae,* synapsis (pairing of homologous chromosomes) and synaptonemal complex formation depend on Spo11, a nuclease related to type II topoismerases. Spo11 induces DSBs leading to HRR events of the CO type that form the physical association between homologs (chiasmata) needed for synaptonemal complex formation and proper disjunction of non-sister homologs at the first meiotic division. On the basis of these properties of Spo11, it is sometimes assumed that the primary function of meiotic recombination is to promote synapsis. However, as reviewed by Barzel & Kupiec (2008), this theme cannot be generalized, as synapsis occurs independently of Spo11 induced recombination in the nematode worm *C. elegans* and the fruitfly *D. melanogaster*. In *C. elegans,* synapsis between homologs occurs normally in a *spo-11* mutant (Dernburg et al., 1998). The *D. melanogaster* gene *mei-W68* encodes a *spo11* homolog (McKim & Hayashi-Hagihara, 1998). In *D. melanogaster* females, meiotic chromosome synapsis occurs in the absence of *mei-W68* mediated CO recombination (McKim et al., 1998). Electron microscopy of oocytes from females homozygous for *mei-W68* mutations that eliminated meiotic recombination revealed normal synaptonemal complex formation. In *D. melanogaster* females, meiotic recombination does not appear to be necessary for synapsis. Since the role of Spo11 is of substantial interest in current discussions of the adaptive significance of meiotic recombination, we offer a speculation on its possible role consistent with the DNA repair hypothesis. As shown in Figure 1, both the DHJ and SDSA models for HRR start with a DSB. During meiosis in *S. cerevisiae,* DSBs are formed by a process that usually depends on Spo11. In *S. pombe,* Spo11 homolog Rec12 generates meiotic recombinants and meiosis specific DSBs. In *C. elegans,* a Spo11 homolog seems to have a similar role. We propose that DNA damages of various types are converted to DSBs, a "common currency," in order to initiate their recombinational repair (see also H. Bernstein et al., 1988). Spo11 appears to be employed in this process. Our reasoning is based on the precedents of the well-established pathways of nucleotide excision repair and base excision repair. In nucleotide excision repair, the initial steps of the pathway involve recognition of a wide variety of bulky damages followed by their removal to generate a single-strand gap, the "common currency" which is then repaired by a gap filling process. In base excision repair, a variety of altered bases are recognized by a corresponding variety of DNA glycosylases that generate an intermediate apurinic/apyrimidinic site, the "common currency" for further repair. On this reasoning, formation of DSBs by a Spo11-dependent process is part of an overall DNA repair sequence. In those species where the resolution of meiotic HRR by CO recombination is beneficial in promoting proper chromosome segregation at the first meiotic division, we think this benefit arose secondarily to the primary benefit of accurate DNA repair.

The function of recombination as a repair process may have arisen very early in the evolution of life [perhaps in the RNA world (H. Bernstein et al., 1984)], and the function of promoting synapsis during meiosis probably arose later in evolution in some eukaryotic lineages. If, in mammals, a major function of meiotic CO recombination, as distinct from NCO recombination, is to promote synapsis and proper chromosome segregation, then one might expect CO events to be localized to specific hot-spot sequences. Hot-spot determinants may also include specific proteins that bind to hot-spot sequences and facilitate CO recombination such as Prdm9 (Hochwagen and Marals, 2010). It is estimated that, in humans, the average number of endogenous DNA DSBs per somatic cell occurring at each cell generation is about 50 (Vilenchik & Knudson, 2003). This rate of DSB formation likely reflects unprogrammed damages, such as may be caused by ROS, and can be taken as an indication of the level of unprogrammed DSBs present in cells undergoing meiosis as well. In the human genome 25,000 hotspots for meiotic recombination have been identified (Myers et al., 2006). The average number of CO recombination events per hotspot is one CO event per 1,300 meioses. The large number of recombination hotspots is consistent with a wide distribution of sites vulnerable to unprogrammed DNA damage as well as specific sites where recombination would need to be induced to promote synapsis. A challenge for future research is the identification of the types of natural damages and programmed damages, and their frequencies, that are removed by CO recombinational repair during meiosis.

9. During meiosis, CO recombination can repair DNA damages independently of Spo11

In a *spo11* mutant of *S. cerevisiae*, the meiotic defects in recombination and synapsis are alleviated by X-irradiation, indicating that X-ray induced DNA damages can initiate CO recombination leading to synapsis independently of Spo11 (Thorne & Byers, 1993). Also, in *C. elegans*, Spo11 is required for meiotic recombination, but radiation induced-breaks alleviate this dependence (Dernberg et al., 1998). These findings indicate that unprogrammed DNA damages induced by X-rays can be repaired by HRR during meiosis independently of Spo11. In both *S. pombe* and *C. elegans*, mutants deficient for Spo11 undergo meiotic CO recombination when single base lesions of the type dU:dG are produced in their DNA (Pauklin et al., 2009). This recombination does not involve production of large numbers of DSBs, but does require uracil DNA-glycolylase, an enzyme that removes uracil from the DNA backbone and initiates base excision repair. These authors proposed that base excision repair of a uracil base, an abasic site, or a single-strand nick are sufficient to initiate meiotic CO recombination in *S pombe* and *C. elegans*.

In a Rec12 (Spo11 homolog) mutant strain of *S. pombe*, meiotic recombination can be restored to near normal levels by a deletion in *rad2* that encodes an endonuclease involved in Okazaki fragment processing (Farah et al., 2005). Both CO and NCO recombination were increased, but DSBs were undetectable. On the basis of the biochemical properties of Rad 2, these authors proposed that meiotic recombination can be initiated by non-DSB lesions, such as nicks and gaps, which accumulate during premeiotic DNA replication when Okasaki fragment processing is deficient.

In general the findings reviewed in this section indicate that DNA damages arising from a variety of sources can be repaired by meiotic HRR of the CO type, and that this repair may occur independently of Spo11.

10. DNA repair likely provides the strong short-term advantage that maintains meiosis, while genetic variation may provide a long-term advantage

Evolutionary explanations for sex have often assumed that the adaptive advantage of meiosis arises from the genetic variation produced. A variety of models and reviews have been presented in this active area of research (e.g. Barton & Charlesworth, 1998; Otto & Gerstein, 2006; Agrawal, 2006). However, Otto & Gerstein (2006) have also pointed out that in a fairly stable environment, individuals surviving to reproductive age have genomes that function well in their current environment. They raise the question of why such individuals should risk shuffling their genes with those of another individual, as happens during meiotic recombination. This consideration, and others, have led many investigators to question whether production of genetic diversity is the principal adaptive advantage of sex.

Heng (2007) and Gorelick & Heng (2010) reviewed evidence that sex actually decreases most genetic variation. Their view is that sex acts like a coarse filter, weeding out major changes, such as chromosomal rearrangements, but allowing minor variation, such as changes at the nucleotide or gene level (that are often neutral), to flow through the sexual sieve. Thus, they consider that sex acts as a constraint on genomic variation, thereby limiting adaptive evolution.

We consider that the major adaptive advantage of meiosis is enhanced recombinational repair. In contrast to the variation hypothesis, DNA repair provides an appropriate explanation for the adaptive advantage of sex (and meiosis) in the short-term, since its benefits are large enough (removal of DNA damages that would be deleterious/lethal to gametes or progeny) to plausibly balance the large costs of sex. The large costs of sex include the "cost of males" (Maynard Smith, 1978; Williams, 1975), "recombinational load" that arises from the randomization of genetic information during sex and loss of coadapted gene complexes (Shields, 1982), the cost of mating (Bernstein et al., 1985b), and cost of sexually transmitted disease (Michod et al., 2008).

The hypothesis that meiosis is an adaptation for DNA repair can be consistently applied to all organisms that have sex, including the facultative sexual organisms discussed above, as well as species that undergo meiosis but experience little or no outcrossing, as described below. If, in the long-term, the genetic variation produced by sex increases the rate of adaptation, as proposed by a number of authors (Goddard et al., 2005; Colegrave et al., 2002; Kaltz & Bell, 2002; Cooper et al., 2005; de Visser & Elena, 2007; Peters & Otto, 2003), this would be an added benefit. However, in the short-term, we consider it unlikely that the benefit of variation is large enough to maintain sex.

In nature, many organisms that undergo meiosis outcross only rarely or not at all. In these cases, meiosis generates little or no genetic variation. In the budding yeast *S. cerevisiae*, outcrossing sex, in contrast to inbreeding sex, appears to be very infrequent in nature. Ruderfer et al. (2006) estimated that the ancestors of three *S. cerevisiae* strains outcrossed in nature only about once every 50,000 generations. On the other hand, mating between closely related yeast cells is likely to have been much more common in nature. Mating can occur when haploid cells of opposite mating types, MATa and MATα, come into contact. As pointed out by Zeyl & Otto (2007), mating between closely related cells is common for two reasons; (1) the close physical proximity of cells of opposite mating type from the same ascus (the sac that contains the products from a single meiosis), and (2) homothallism, the ability of haploid cells of one mating type to produce daughter cells of the opposite mating type. Thus, in nature, the meiotic events that produce little or no recombinational variation are much more frequent than meiotic events that do produce recombinational variation. This disparity is consistent with the idea that the primary adaptive function of meiosis in *S. cerevisiae* is HRR of DNA damages, since this benefit is realized in meiosis resulting from either inbreeding or outcrossing. If the primary adaptive function of meiosis were to generate genetic variation, it is difficult to understand how the complex process of meiosis could be selectively maintained in *S. cerevisiae* during the many generations in which there is no outcrossing.

Various levels of inbreeding due to consanguineous mating are known in many species. One extreme, but well studied, example among vertebrate species is the Mangrove Killifish, *Kryptolebias marmoratus*, which inhabits brackish water mangrove habitats from Brazil to Florida. These fish produce sperm and eggs by meiosis and reproduce routinely by self-fertilization. Each hermaphroditic individual normally fertilizes itself when a sperm and egg that it has produced by an internal organ unite inside the fish's body (Sakakura et al., 2006; for review see Avise, 2008). In this highly inbred hermaphroditic species meiotic recombination does not produce significant allelic variation, suggesting that meiosis is retained for some other adaptive benefit.

In higher plants, outcrossing sexual reproduction is the most common mode of reproduction, but about 15% of plants undergo meiosis and are principally self-fertilizing (C. Bernstein & H. Bernstein, 1991). We infer from these examples that the generation of genetic variation is not likely to be the adaptive benefit maintaining meiosis in these organisms. However, meiosis may be maintained by the adaptive benefit of HRR of DNA damage, since this benefit does not depend on outcrossing, nor that the participating chromosomes carry different alleles.

The meiotic function of repairing DNA damages primarily acts to preserve the existing genome. The generation of new genomic variants, a consequence of recombinational repair processes, appears to be a secondary effect that may provide a benefit in the long-term.

As discussed above, most HRR events during meiosis are of the NCO type, which generate minimal genetic variation compared to the CO type. This is consistent with the DNA repair hypothesis, since both the CO and NCO types of recombination can repair DNA. On the assumption that the generation of variation is the primary benefit of meiosis, the majority of HRR events, those of the NCO type, provide no significant benefit and hence are wasteful.

Even though, during meiosis, the frequency of CO recombination is ordinarily substantially less than the frequency of NCO recombination, during mitosis the frequency of CO compared to NCO recombination is even lower (e.g. Virgin et al., 2001; Prado et al., 2003). The higher frequency of CO recombinants during meiosis compared to mitosis may reflect the role of CO recombinants in promoting synapsis during meiosis (see section 8, above), a process distinct to meiosis.

11. During meiosis, HRR may remove a class of damages that cannot be accurately repaired during mitosis

HRR during meiosis offers unique advantages compared to HRR during mitosis, based on the opportunity for non-sister homologs to pair and recombine during meiosis, which does not happen during mitosis. In mitosis, HRR involves interaction between the sister-chromosomes formed upon DNA replication. Thus, in mitosis, HRR is limited to the phases of the cell cycle during DNA replication (S phase) and after DNA replication (G2/M). Prior to DNA replication (G1 phase) in mitosis, double-strand DNA damages, such as DSBs, are repaired by an inaccurate process, non-homologous end-joining (NHEJ), which generates mutation. Double strand damages arising after DNA replication, may be repaired during mitosis by HRR between sisters (Tichy et al., 2010). However, meiotic recombination can cope in a non-mutagenic way with double strand damages which arise at any point in the cell cycle.

Meiotic G1 phase cells appear to be more resistant to the lethal effects of X-irradiation than mitotic G1 phase cells (Kelly et al., 1983). This finding suggests that repair of DSBs is more efficient during meiotic than mitotic G1 phase, as DSBs are a common consequence of X-irradiation. We speculate that during meiosis, in contrast to mitosis, double-strand damages occurring prior to DNA replication may be accurately repaired by HRR because pairing occurs between non-sister chromosomes. If this is so, meiotic cells have the advantage, compared to mitotic cells, of being able to accurately and efficiently repair double-strand damages that occur both before and after replication. As a result, germ cells would tend to be protected against the mutagenic effect of inaccurate NHEJ that typically occurs prior to replication in mitotic cells.

Mao et al. (2008) presented evidence that one type of somatic cell, human fibroblasts, utilizes error-prone NHEJ as the major DSB repair pathway at all cell cycle stages. In these cells, HRR is nearly absent prior to replication (G1 phase) and is used, when it occurs, primarily in the S phase. Even after the S phase when two sister-chromosomes are present (the G2/M phase), NHEJ is elevated and HRR is in decline.

The situation is somewhat different in mammalian embryonic stem (ES) cells compared to differentiated somatic cells (Tichy et al., 2010). ES cells give rise to all of the cell types of an organism. Because mutations at this early embryonic stage are passed on to all clonal descendents, they can be seriously detrimental to the organism as a whole. Therefore robust mechanisms are needed in ES cells for reducing DNA damages (or eliminating damaged cells) in order to reduce mutations. Mouse ES cells were found to predominantly use high fidelity HRR to repair DSBs, compared to somatic cells that predominantly used NHEJ (Tichy et al., 2010). Furthermore mouse ES cells lack a G1 checkpoint and do not undergo cell-cycle arrest upon receiving DNA damage prior to DNA replication. Rather, they undergo p53-independent apoptosis in response to DNA damage (Aladjem et al., 1998). Consistent with these findings, mouse ES stem cells have a mutation frequency about 100-fold lower than that of isogenic mouse somatic cells (Cervantes et al., 2002), but, as discussed next, at a likely cost resulting from somatic selection against cells with unrepairable DSBs which arise before DNA replication.

These results imply that a low mutation rate is achievable in mitotic cells by using apoptosis to remove cells with DNA damages that are present prior to replication, and using HRR, rather than NHEJ, to remove double-strand damages present subsequent to DNA replication. The non-sister chromosomes present in every diploid somatic cell during mitosis, in principal, might pair and undergo accurate HRR (as in meiosis), but this does not ordinarily occur, presumably because, in somatic cells, the benefit is outweighed by costs [e.g. loss of heterozygosity and expression of deleterious recessive alleles including those leading to cancer]. Meiosis is therefore unique, in that DNA damages occurring both prior to and after DNA replication can be subject to high fidelity HRR between non-sister homologs. This would avoid the high costs of both deleterious mutation and loss of potential gametes due to apoptosis.

In humans at each cell division, 30,000-50,000 DNA replication origins are activated (Mechali et al., 2010). Thus the chromosome is ordinarily replicated in segments. We postulate that any segment containing a DSB will fail to complete its replication until the DSB is repaired. This limited and temporary blockage of replication may result directly from the break itself, or occur as a response to regulatory events set off by proteins that specifically bind to the broken ends. In any case, HRR can be carried out during the subsequent prophase I stage of meiosis, when the segment containing a DSB pairs with a non-sister homologue. This repair would then allow chromosome replication to be completed.

12. DNA damage during the mitotic divisions of the germ line in multicellular organisms

In multicellular eukaryotes there are typically many mitoses during germ line development, and only a single final meiosis leading to gamete formation. During the mitotic cell divisions in the germ line, DSBs and other double-strand damages occurring after DNA replication are likely repaired by HRR or eliminated from the cell lineage by death and/or apoptosis of the damaged cell. We have argued above (section 11) that because of the lack of pairing of non-sister homologs during mitosis, HRR is unable to accurately repair double-strand damages occurring before replication. Thus when double-strand damages occur prior to replication during the mitotic divisions in the germ line the consequence will be either increased mutation or increased apoptosis. By analogy with the strategy used by somatic stem cells (section 11, above), we think that the preferred strategy during these mitotic divisions is likely to be apoptosis, since this avoids mutations in the germ line that could be passed on to progeny. However, double-strand damages occurring prior to replication during meiosis need not lead to apoptosis (which would likely decrease fecundity), since these can be accurately repaired by HRR between non-sister chromosomes. The consequence will be enhanced gamete viability and fecundity, that is, enhanced fitness. In the mitotic divisions of the germ-line prior to meiosis, loss of cells due to DNA damage-induced apoptosis need not be very costly to organism fitness, since such losses could be made up by extra cell divisions of undamaged cells. However, the loss of sperm or egg cells due to unrepaired DNA damage would likely have substantial costs to fitness due to loss of fertility and progeny, as discussed above in section 5.

13. Why is meiosis frequently associated with outcrossing?

While the focus of this article is on the adaptive benefit of meiosis itself, we briefly consider why meiosis is frequently associated with outcrossing, where the chromosomes involved in recombination come from different unrelated parents in a prior generation. Previously, we discussed examples of meiosis occurring in association with inbreeding and self-fertilization. Meiosis with inbreeding will be favored when the costs of mating are high (e.g. the cost of finding a mate at low population density). These examples of inbred meiosis were presented to illustrate our argument that meiosis provides an adaptive advantage (accurate DNA repair) independent of whether significant recombinational variation is also produced. However, meiosis is often associated with outcrossing, and we now consider why.

A disadvantage of inbreeding, especially of self-fertilization, is expression of deleterious recessive mutations, resulting in inbreeding depression. Analysis of the effects of masking deleterious recessive mutations (genetic complementation) using heuristic modes and arguments indicated that complementation provides benefits sufficient to maintain outcrossing (H. Bernstein et al., 1985a, 1987; Michod, 1995). However, more explicit population genetic models have raised some issues that are in need of further clarification. In population genetics terms, the basic effect of outcrossing is to bring populations to Hardy-Weinberg (HW) equilibrium. Thus, outcrossing can be beneficial if there is another force that pushes the population away from HW equilibrium (generating either an excess or a deficit of heterozygotes) and if it's advantageous to go closer to HW equilibrium. One possible force that generates departure from HW equilibrium is dominance: for example if deleterious alleles tend to be recessive, after selection there will be an excess of heterozygotes (and a deficit of homozygotes). However in this case outcrossing is costly in the short term (because it tends to expose deleterious alleles), but beneficial in the long term (because purging them becomes more efficient). Otto (2003) showed that under this scenario high rates of outcrossing are favored only if deleterious alleles are weakly recessive (dominance close to 0.5). Another potential force pushing away from HW equilibrium considered by Roze and Michod (2010) is gene conversion which creates homozygosity. Gene conversion could result from mitotic HRR between sister chromosomes as discussed above. In this case (and if deleterious alleles tend to be partially recessive) outcrossing is beneficial in the short term (because it masks deleterious alleles) but disadvantageous in the long term (because purging is less efficient). The magnitude of this force may be estimated from rates of loss of heterozygosity during development [discussed in Roze and Michod (2010)]. The few estimates which exist indicate that the loss of heterozygosity is low, and thus this selective force for outcrossing may be weak. Clearly, we need more estimates of this critical parameter to know how large this force for outcrossing may be.

Another consequence of outcrossing is the generation of new genetic variants which may provide an additional long-term advantage.

14. The special case of asexual bdelloid rotifers

Bdelloid rotifers are common invertebrate animals. They are apparently obligate asexuals that reproduce by parthenogenesis. These organisms are extraordinarily resistant to ionizing radiation (Gladyshev and Meselson, 2008). This resistance appears to be a consequence of an evolutionary adaptation to survive desiccation in ephemerally aquatic habitats. Such desiccation causes extensive DNA breakage, which they are able to repair. Bdelloid primary oocytes are in the G1 phase of the cell cycle and thus lack sister chromatids. Welch et al. (2008) proposed a mechanism of repair involving interaction of non-sister co-linear chromosome pairs, which are maintained as templates for repair of DNA DSBs caused by the frequent desiccation and rehydration. Thus although these organisms apparently lack sex and meiosis, an essential feature of meiosis, HRR between non-sister homologs appears to be retained.

15. Conservation among eukaryotes of RecA-like proteins as key components of the HRR machinery acting during meiosis

Sex appears to be universally based on RecA-like proteins. RecA-like proteins play a key role in HRR, and the HRR machinery and its mechanism of action appear to be highly conserved among eukaryotes. The r*ad51* and d*mc1* genes in the eukaryotic yeasts *S. cerevisiae* and *S. pombe* are orthologs of the bacterial *recA* gene. The *dmc1* gene is found in many different eukaryote species, and has been reported, for instance, in the protists *Giardia, Trypanosoma, Leishmania, Entamoeba* and *Plasmodium* (Ramesh et al., 2005). Rad51 and Dmc1 proteins are recombinases that interact with single-stranded DNA to form filamentous intermediates called presynaptic filaments, and these filaments initiate HRR (Sauvageau et al., 2005; San Filippo et al., 2008). Dmc1 recombinase functions only during meiosis, whereas Rad51 recombinase acts in both somatic HRR and in meiosis. When it functions in meiosis, Rad51 mainly uses a sister chromosome for HRR. In contrast, Dmc1 mainly uses the non-sister homologous chromosome. The yeast Rad51 recombinase catalyzes ATP-dependent homologous DNA pairing and strand exchange, as does the bacterial RecA recombinase (Sung, 1994). The tertiary structure of the Dmc1 recombinase has an overall similarity to the bacterial RecA recombinase (Story et al., 1993). These observations suggest that the bacterial RecA that functions in the bacterial sexual process of transformation, and the yeast Rad51 and Dmc1 recombinases that act in meiosis have similar functions, consistent with the idea that meiotic recombination evolved from simpler sexual processes in bacteria

We next consider evidence that RecA orthologs play a key role in meiosis, not only in protists, but also in multicellular eukaryotes. RecA orthologs act in meiosis in a range of animals (e.g. nematodes, chickens, humans and mice) and plants (e.g. *Arabidopsis*, rice and lilies). The *rad51* gene is expressed at a high level in mouse testis and ovary, suggesting that Rad51 protein is involved in meiotic recombination (Shinohara et al., 1993). In mice, mutations in the *dmc1* gene cause sterility, failure to undergo intimate pairing of homologous chromosomes and an inability to complete meiosis (Pittman et al., 1998; Yoshida et al., 1998; see also Table 2). In the nematode *C. elegans*, resistance to DNA damage caused by X-irradiation in the meiotic pachytene nuclei depends on a RecA-like gene (Takanami et al., 2000). *RecA* gene orthologs are also expressed in chicken testis and ovary and in human testis. In humans, Dmc1, the meiosis-specific recombinase, forms nucleoprotein complexes on single-stranded DNA that promote a search for homology and carry out strand exchange, the two necessary steps of genetic recombination (Sehorn et al, 2004; Bugreev et al., 2005).

In lily plants, genes *lim15* and *rad51* are orthologs, respectively, of the *dmc1* and *rad51* genes of yeast. The lily proteins Lim15 and Rad51 colocalize on chromosomes in various stages of meiotic prophase I, and form discrete foci (Terasawa et al., 1995). The proteins of these foci are considered to participate in the search for, and pairing of, homologous sequences of DNA. In another plant, *Arabidopsis thaliana*, meiotic recombination requires Dmc1 (Couteau et al., 1999) and Rad51 (Li et al., 2004). In the rice plant, an ortholog of dmc1 is necessary for meiosis and has a key function in the pairing of homologous chromosomes (Deng and Wang, 2007).

In general, both animals and plants have RecA-like proteins that appear to have a central function in meiotic HRR. Furthermore, bacterial RecA and its animal and plant orthologs have very similar roles in the HRR events during the sexual processes of bacterial transformation and eukaryotic meiosis. In all cases, the RecA protein or RecA-like protein assembles on single-stranded DNA to form a pre-synaptic filament. This filament then attaches to a duplex DNA molecule and searches for homology in its target. When the presynaptic molecule locates an homologous sequence in the duplex molecule, it is able to form a DNA joint [Figure 2]. These joints are then processed further to complete the HRR event.

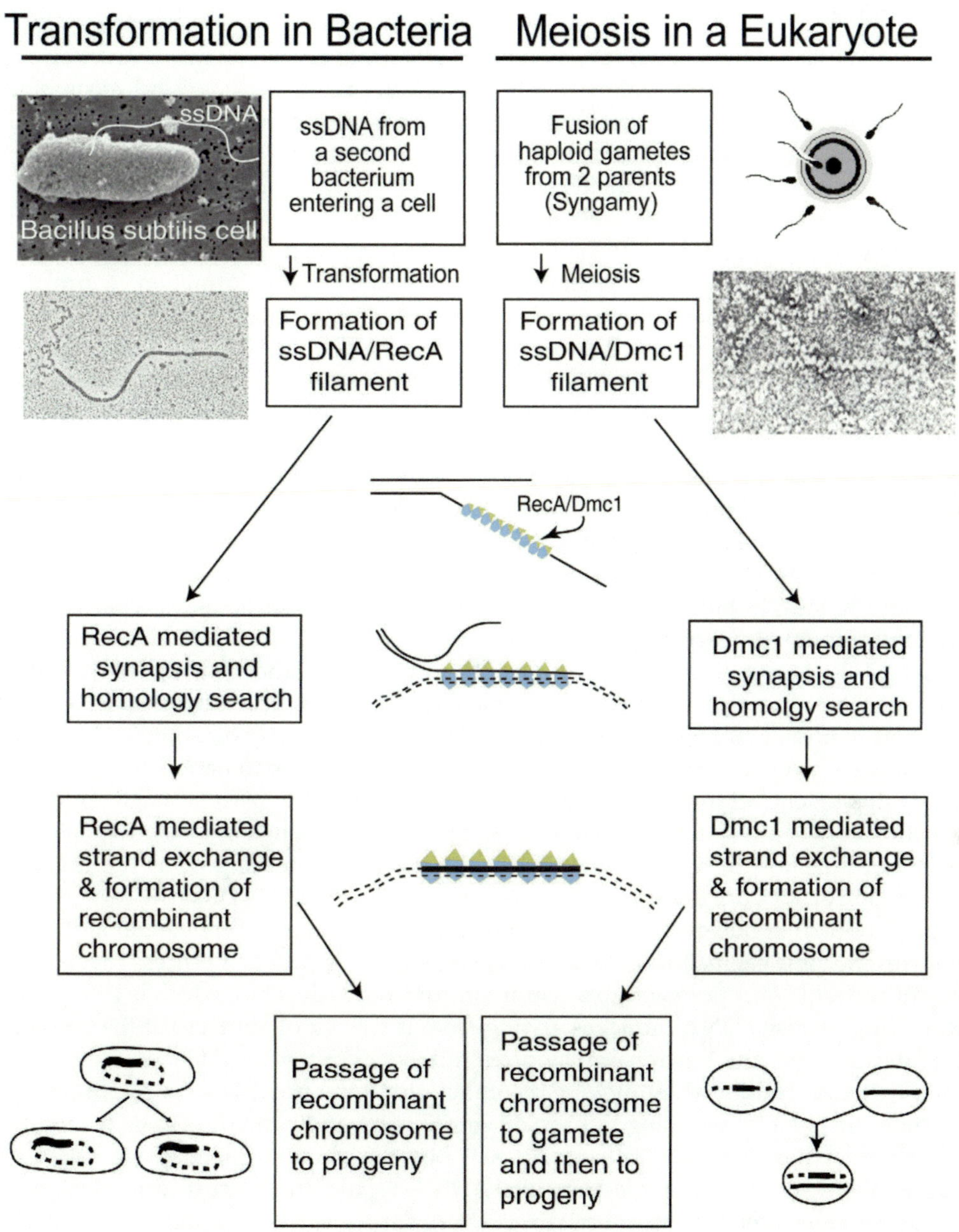

Fig. 2. Conservation of the key components of the HRR machinery during the sexual process of transformation in bacteria and during meiosis in eukaryotes. The bacterial RecA protein or the eukaryotic RecA-like protein, Dmc1, assembles on single-stranded DNA to form a pre-synaptic filament. This filament then attaches to a duplex DNA molecule and searches for homology in its target. When the pre-synaptic molecule locates an homologous sequence in the duplex molecule, it is able to form a DNA joint. These joints are then processed further to complete the HRR event.

16. Summary

Currently there is no general agreement among biologists on the adaptive function of sex. Meiosis, a key stage of the sexual cycle, involves close pairing and physical recombination and information exchange between homologous chromosomes ordinarily derived from two different parents. Fundamental to solving the problem of why sex exists is achieving an understanding of the function of meiosis.

A primitive form of meiosis was likely present early in the evolution of eukaryotes, perhaps in the single-celled ancestor of all eukaryotes that arose from ancestral bacteria over 1.5 billion years ago. Meiosis may be derived from bacterial transformation, a prokaryotic sexual process that promotes homologous recombinational repair of DNA as shown in Figure 2. Among extant single-cell eukaryotes, meiosis and facultative sex are ubiquitous. Entry into the sexual cycle ordinarily occurs in response to stressful conditions, such as oxidative stress, that tend to be associated with DNA damage. Thus meiosis may be an adaptation for dealing with such stresses and the resulting DNA damages. Consistent with this idea, exposure of eukaryotes to various DNA damaging agents increases meiotic recombination. Both in mitosis and meiosis, DNA damages caused by different exogenous agents are repaired by HRR, suggesting that DNA damages from natural sources (e.g. ROS) are also repaired by HRR. The consistent function of recombination in DNA repair across meiosis and mitosis in eukaryotes, and transformation in prokaryotes, is what we seek to understand through the repair hypothesis.

Defective HRR during meiosis causes infertility in humans and rodents, suggesting that removal of DNA damages is an essential function of meiosis. The majority of HRR events during both mitosis and meiosis are of the NCO type. NCO recombination is able to repair DNA damages from diverse sources. Furthermore NCO recombination likely occurs by synthesis-dependent strand annealing, a mechanism that involves a small exchange of information between two chromosomes but not physical exchange of DNA. Explanations of the adaptive function of meiosis that focus exclusively on crossing over, the minority of recombination events, are inadequate to explain the majority, the NCO type.

The Spo11 protein, a nuclease, produces DSBs that can initiate recombination and promote proper chromosome segregation. We speculate that Spo11 is part of a process that converts a variety of types of DNA damages to a "common currency," the DSB, which is then subject to HRR. During meiosis, DNA damages arising from a variety of sources can be repaired by HRR of the CO type, and this repair may occur independently of Spo11.

Genetic variation produced by meiotic recombination may provide a long-term benefit at the population level by reducing linkage disequilibrium and providing gene combinations on which selection can more effectively act, but the short-term adaptive benefit that maintains the machinery of meiosis is likely DNA repair. In contrast to mitosis, meiosis may allow greater accuracy in the repair of DNA damages, since double-strand damages occurring prior to DNA replication can, in principle, be accurately removed by HRR between non-sister homologous chromosomes, a process that is largely unavailable during mitosis.

Among different species, meiosis is frequently associated with outcrossing. This probably reflects the benefit of masking deleterious recessive alleles. However, numerous species that undergo meiosis are largely inbreeding or self-fertilizing. This implies that meiosis provides a benefit (accurate DNA repair) independently of the benefit of outcrossing and masking deleterious recessive alleles.

Animals and plants have RecA-like proteins that have key functions in meiotic recombination involving homology recognition and strand exchange. The function of these eukaryotic proteins is similar to the bacterial RecA protein that acts during the bacterial sexual process of transformation, further suggesting that eukaryotic meiosis may have evolved from simpler sexual processes in bacteria.

17. Conclusion

DNA damages appear to be a ubiquitous and serious problem for all of life. We consider that the heightened ability of meiosis to repair such damages in the DNA to be passed on to the next generation is a capability sufficient to explain its widespread occurrence.

18. Acknowledgment

We thank Deborah Shelton, Denis Roze and Mike Berman for their thoughtful and very helpful comments on drafts of the manuscript. This work was supported in part by Arizona Biomedical Research Commission Grant #0803 and the Department of Veterans Affairs (VA), Veterans Health Administration, Office of Research and Development, VA Merit Review Grant 0142 of the Southern Arizona Veterans Affairs Health Care System. This work was also supported by National Science Foundation grant DEB-0742383 and the College of Science at the University of Arizona.

19. References

Agrawal, A.P. (2006). Evolution of sex: why do organisms shuffle their genotypes? *Current Biology,* Vol.16, pp. R696-R704.

Aladjem, M.I., Spike, B.T., Rodewald, L.W., Hope, T.J., Klemm, M., Jaenishc, R. & Wahl, G.M. (1998). ES cells do not activate p53-dependent stress responses and undergo p53-independent apoptosis in response to DNA damage. *Current Biology,* Vol. 8, pp. 145-155.

Allers, T. & Lichten, M. (2001). Differential timing and control of noncrossover and crossover recombination during meiosis. *Cell,* Vol. 106, pp. 47-57.

Ames, B.N., Shigenaga, M.K. & Hagen, T.M. (1993). Oxidants, antioxidants, and the degenerative diseases of aging. *Proceedings of the National Academy of Sciences USA,* Vol. 90, pp. 7915-7922.

Andersen, S.L. & Sekelsky. J. (2010). Meiotic versus mitotic recombination: two different routes for double-strand break repair. *Bioessays,* Vol. 32, pp. 1058-1066.

Avise, J.C. (2008). Clonality: *The genetics, ecology, and evolution of sexual abstinence in vertebrate animals.* Oxford University Press, New York, NY

Baker, B.S., Boyd, J.B., Carpenter, A.T.C., Green, M.M., Nguyen, T.D., Ripoll, P. & Smith, P.D. (1976). Genetic controls of meiotic recombination and somatic DNA metabolism in *Drosophila melanogaster*. *Proceedings of the National Academy of Sciences USA,* Vol. 73, pp. 4140-4144.

Barlow, C., Liyanage, M., Moens, P.B., Tarsounas, M., Nagashima, K., Brown, K., Rottinghaus, S., Jackson, S.P., Tagle, D., Ried, T. & Wynshaw-Boris, A. (1998). Atm deficiency results in severe meiotic disruption as early as leptonema of prophase I. *Development,* Vol. 125, pp. 4007-4017.

Barton, N.H. & Charlesworth, B. (1998). Why sex and recombination? *Science,* Vol. 281, pp. 1986-1989.

Barzel, A. & Kupiec, M. (2008). Finding a match: how do homologous sequences get together for recombination? *Nature Reviews/Genetics,* Vol. 9, pp. 27-37.

Bernstein, C & Johns, V. (1989). Sexual reproduction as a response to H_2O_2 damage in *Schizosaccharomyces pombe. Journal of Bacteriology,* Vol. 171, pp.1893-1897.

Bernstein, C. & Bernstein, H. (1991). *Aging, Sex and DNA Repair*. Academic Press, San Diego

Bernstein, H., Byerly, H.C., Hopf, F.A. & Michod, R.E. (1984). Origin of sex. *Journal of Theoretical Biology,* Vol. 110, pp. 323-351.

Bernstein, H., Byerly, H.C., Hopf, F.A. & Michod, R.E. (1985a). Genetic damage, mutation and the evolution of sex. *Science,* Vol. 229, pp.1277-1281.

Bernstein, H., Byerly, H.C., Hopf, F.A. & Michod, R.E. (1985b). Sex and the emergence of species. *Journal of Theoretical Biology,* Vol. 117, pp. 665-690.

Bernstein, H., Hopf, F.A. & Michod, R.E. (1987). The molecular basis of the evolution of sex. *Advances in Genetics,* Vol. 24, pp. 323-370.

Bernstein, H., Hopf, F.A. & Michod, R.E. (1988). Is meiotic recombination an adaptation for repairing DNA, producing genetic variation, or both? In *The Evolution of Sex: An Examination of Current Ideas* R.E. Michod. & B.R. Levin (Eds.). pp. 139-160 Sinauer, Sunderland, Mass.

Bernstein, H. & Bernstein, C. (2010). Evolutionary origin of recombination during meiosis. *BioScience,* Vol. 60, No. 7, pp. 498-505.

Birdsell, J.A. & Wills, C. (2003) The evolutionary origin and maintenance of sexual recombination: A review of contemporary models. In: *Evolutionary Biology*. R.G. MacIntyre, M.T. Clegg, (Eds.), pp. 27-138. Kluwer Academic/Plenum Publishers.

Boyd J.B. (1978). DNA repair in *Drosophila*. In *DNA Repair Mechanisms* P.C. Hanawalt, E.C. Friedberg & C.F. Fox. (Eds.) pp. 449-452. Academic Press, New York.

Bugreev, D.V., Golub, E.I., Stasiak, A.Z., Stasiak, A. & Mazin A.V. (2005). Activation of human meiosis-specific recombinase Dmc1 by Ca2+. *Journal of Biological Chemistry,* Vol. 280, pp. 26886-26895.

Cervantes, R.B., Stringer, J.R., Shao, C., Tischfield, J.A. & Stambrook, P.J. (2002) Embryonic stem cells and somatic cells differ in mutation frequency and type. *Proceedings of the National Academy of Sciences USA,* Vol. 99, pp.3586-3590.

Chovnick, A., Ballantyne, G.H., Baillie, D.L., Holm, D.G. (1970). Gene conversion in higher organisms: half-tetrad analysis of recombination within the rosy cistron of *Drosophila melanogaster. Genetics,* Vol. 66, pp 315-329.

Colegrave, N., Kaltz, O. & Bell, G. (2002). The ecology and genetics of fitness in *Chlamydomonas*. VIII. The dynamics of adaptation to novel environments after a single episode of sex. *Evolution,* Vol. 56, pp. 14-21.

Cooper, T.F., Lenski, R.E. & Elena, S.P. (2005). Parasites and mutational load: an experimental test of a pluralistic theory for the evolution of sex. *Proceedings of the Royal Society B,* Vol. 272, pp. 311-317.

Coogan, T.P. & Rosenblum, I.Y. (1988). DNA double-strand damage and repair following gamma-irradiation in isolated spermatogenic cells. *Mutation Research,* Vol. 194, pp. 183-191.

Couteau, F., Belzile, F., Horlow, C., Granjean, O., Vezon, D. & Doutriaux, M.P. (1999). Random chromosome segregation without meiotic arrest in both male and female meiocytes of a Dmc1 mutant of Arabidopsis. *Plant Cell*, Vol. 11, 1623-1634.

Cressman, V.L., Backlund, D.C., Avrutskaya, A.V., Leadon, S.A., Godfrey, V. & Koller, B.H. (1999). Growth retardation, DNA repair defects, and lack of spermatogenesis in BRCA1-deficient mice. *Molecular and Cellular Biology*, Vol. 19, No. 10, pp. 7061-7075.

Dacks, J. & Roger, A.J. (1999). The first sexual lineage and the relevance of facultative sex. *Journal of Molecular Evolution*, Vol. 48, pp. 779-783.

Davey, J. (1998). Fusion of a fission yeast. *Yeast*, Vol. 14, pp. 1529-1566.

Deng, Z.Y. & Wang, T. (2007). OsDMC1 is required for homologous pairing in Oryza sativa. Plant Molecular Biology, Vol. 65, pp. 31-42.

Dernberg, A.F., McDonald, K., Moulder, G., Barstead, R., Dresser, M. & Villeneuve, A.M. (1998). Meiotic recombination in *C. elegans* initiates by a conserved mechanism and is dispensable for homologous chromosome synapsis. *Cell*, Vol. 94, pp. 387-398.

DeVisser, J.A. & Elena, S.F. (2007). The evolution of sex: empirical insights into the roles of epistasis and drift. *Nature Reviews/Genetics*, Vol. 8, pp.139-149.

Elliott, A.M. & Hayes, R.E. (1953). Mating types in tetrahymena. *Biological Bulletin*, Vol., 105, pp. 269-284.

Farah, J.A., Cromie, G., Davis, L., Steiner, W.W. & Smith, G.R. (2005). Activation of an alternative, Rec12 (Spo11)-independent pathway of fission yeast meiotic recombination in the absence of a DNA flap endonuclease. *Genetics*, Vol. 171, pp. 1499-1511.

Fisher, H.M. & Aitken, R.J. (1997) Comparative analysis of the ability of precursor germ cells and epididymal spermatozoa to generate reactive oxygen metabolites. *The Journal of Experimental Zoology*, Vol. 277, pp. 390-400.

Galetzka, D., Weis, E., Kohlschmidt, N., Bitz, O., Stein, R. & Haaf, T. (2007). Expression of somatic DNA repair genes in human testes. *Journal of Cellular Biochemistry*, Vol. 100, pp. 1232-1239.

Game, J.C., Zamb, T.J., Braun, R.J., Resnick, M. & Roth, R.M. (1980). The role of radiation (rad) genes in meiotic recombination in yeast. *Genetics*, Vol. 94, pp. 51-68.

Gladyshev, E. & Meselson, M. (2008). Extreme resistance of bdelloid rotifers to ionizing radiation. *Proceedings of the National Academy of Sciences USA*, Vol. 105, pp. 5139-5144.

Goddard, M.R., Godfray, H.C. & Burt, A. (2005). Sex increases the efficacy of natural selection in experimental yeast populations. *Nature*, Vol. 434, pp. 636-640.

Gorelick, R. & Heng, H.H.Q. (2011). Sex reduces genetic variation: A multidisciplinary review. *Evolution*, Vol. 65, pp. 1088-1098.

Hannah-Alava, A (1964). The brood pattern of X-ray-induced mutational damage in the germ cells of *Drosophila melanogaster* males. *Mutation Research*, Vol. 1, pp. 414-436.

Hari, K.L., Santerre, A., Sekelsky, J.J., McKim, K.S., Boyd, J.B. & Hawley, R.S. (1995). The *mei-41* gene of *D. melanogaster* is a structural and functional homolog of the human ataxia telangiectasia gene. *Cell*, Vol. 82, pp. 815-821.

Haynes, R.H. (1988). Biological context of DNA repair. In: *Mechanisms and Consequences of DNA Damage Processing,* E.C. Friedberg & P.C. Hanawalt (Eds), pp. 577-584. Alan R. Liss, New York

Haynes, R.H. & Kunz, B.A. (1981)/ DNA Repair and mutagenesis in yeast. In: *The Molecular Biology of the Yeast Saccharomyces. Life Cycle and Inheritance,* J. Strathern, E. Jones & J. Broach (Eds.) Cold Spring Harbor Laboratory, Cold Spring Harbor, N.Y.

Heng, H.H.Q. (2007) Elimination of altered karyotypes by sexual reproduction preserves species identity. *Genome,* Vol. 50, pp. 517-524.

Henriques, J.A.P. & Moustacchi, E. (1980). Sensitivity to photoaddition of mono- and bifunctional furocoumarins of X-ray sensitive mutants of *Saccharomyces cerevisiae. Photochemistry and Photobiology,* Vol. 31, pp. 557-561.

Herskowitz, I. (1988). Life cycle of the budding yeast *Saccharomyces cerevisiae. Microbiological Reviews,* Vol. 52, pp. 536-553.

Hochwagen A & Marais G.A.B. (2010). Meiosis: APRDM9 guide to the hotspots of recombination. *Current Biology,* Vol. 20, pp. R271-R274.

Hoelzer, M.A. & Michod, R.E. (1991). DNA repair and the evolution of transformation in *Bacillus subtilis.* III Sex with damaged DNA. *Genetics,* Vol.128, pp. 215-223.

Javaux, E.J., Knoll, A.H. & Walter, M.R. (2001). Morphological and ecological complexity in early eukaryote ecosystems. *Nature,* Vol. 412, pp. 66-69.

Joyce, E.F., Tanneti, S.N. & McKim, K.S. (2009). Drosophila Hold'em is required for a subset of meiotic crossovers and interacts with the DNA repair endonuclease complex subunits MEI-9 and ERCC1. *Genetics,* Vol. 181, pp. 335-340.

Kaltz, O. & Bell, G. (2002). The ecology and genetic of fitness in Chlamydomonas. XII. Repeated sexual episodes increase rates of adaptation to novel environments. *Evolution,* Vol. 56, pp. 1743-1753.

Kelly, S.L., Merrill, C. & Parry, J.M. (1983). Cyclic variations in sensitivity to X-irradiation during meiosis in *Saccharomyces cerevisiae. Molecular and General Genetics,* Vol. 191, pp. 314-318.

Kim, J.S. & Rose, A.M. (1987). The effect of gamma radiation on recombination frequency in *Caenorhabditis elegans. Genome,* Vol. 29, pp. 457-462.

Kirk, D.L. & Kirk, M. (1986). Heat shock elicits production of sexual inducer in *Volvox. Science,* Vol. 231, pp. 51-54.

Klovstad, M., Abdu, U. & Schupbach, T. (2008). Drosophila *brca2* is required for mitotic and meiotic DNA repair and efficient activation of the meiotic recombination checkpoint. *PloS Genetics,* Vol. 4, No. 2: e31.doi:10.1371/journal.pgen.0040031

Lahr, D.J.G., Parfrey, L.W., Mitchell, E.A.D., Katz, L.A. & Lara, E. (2011). The chastity of amoebae: re-evaluating evidence for sex in amoeboid organisms. *Proceedings of the Royal Society B: Biological Sciences.* Published online 23 March 2011. doi: 10.1098/rspb.so11.0289

Lewis, S.E.M. & Aitken, R.J. (2005). DNA damage to spermatozoa has impacts on fertilization and pregnancy. *Cell Tissue Research,* Vol. 322, pp. 33-41.

Li, W., Chen, C., Markmann-Mulisch, U., Timofejeva, I., Schmeizer, E., Ma, H. & Reiss, B. (2004). The Arabidopsis AtRAD51 gene is dispensable for vegetative development but required for meiosis. *Proceedings of the National Academy of Sciences,* Vol. 101, 10596-10601.

Lin, X., Hull, C.M. & Heitman, J. (2005). Sexual reproduction between partners of the same mating type in *Cryptococcus neoformans*. *Nature*, Vol. 434, pp. 1017-1021.

Lisby, M. & Rothstein, R. (2009). Choreography of recombination proteins during DNA damage response. *DNA Repair*, Vol. 8, pp. 1068-1076.

Makker, K., Agarwal, A. & Sharma, R. (2009). Oxidative stress & male infertility. *Indian Journal of Medical Research*, Vol. 129, pp. 357-367.

Malik, S-B., Pightling, A.W., Stefaniak, L.M., Schurko, A.M. & Logsdon, J.M. Jr. (2008). An expanded inventory of conserved meiotic genes provides evidence for sex in *Trichomonas vaginalis*. *PloS ONE*, Vol. 3, No. 8: e2879. doi:10.1371/journal.pone.0002879

Malone, R.E. & Esposito, R.E. (1980). The RAD52 gene is required for homothallic interconversion of mating types and spontaneous mitotic recombination in yeast. *Proceedings of the National Academy of Sciences USA*, Vol. 77, No. 1, pp. 503-507.

Mao, Z., Bozzella, M., Seluanov, A. & Gorbunova, V. (2008). DNA repair by nonhomologous end joining and homologous recombination during cell cycle in human cells. *Cell Cycle*, Vol. 7, pp. 2902-2906.

Marchetti, F. & Wyrobek, A.J. (2008). DNA repair decline during mouse spermiogenesis results in the accumulation of heritable DNA damage. *DNA Repair*, Vol. 7, pp. 572-581.

Massie, H.R., Samis, H.V. & Baird, M.B. (1972) The kinetics of degradation of DNA and RNA by H_2O_2. *Biochimica et Biophysica Acta*, Vol. 272, pp. 539-548.

Maynard Smith, J. (1978). *The Evolution of Sex*, Cambridge University Press, London

McKim, K.S., Green-Marroquin, B.L., Sekelsky. J.J., Chin, G., Steinberg, C., Khodosh, R. & Hawley, R.S. (1998). Meiotic synapsis in the absence of recombination. *Science*, Vol. 279, pp. 876-878.

McKim, K.S. & Hayashi-Hagihara, A. (1998). *mei-W68* in *Drosophila melanogaster* encodes a SPO11 homolog: evidence that the mechanism for initiating meiotic conversations is conserved. *Genes & Development*, Vol. 12, No. 18, pp. 2932-2942.

McMahill, M.S., Sham, C.W. and Bishop, D.K. (2007). Synthesis-dependent strand annealing in meiosis. *PloS Biology*, Vol. 5, No. 11: e299. doi:10.1371/journal.pbio.0050299

Mechali, M. (2010). Eukaryotic DNA replication origins: many choices for appropriate answers. *Nature Reviews: Molecular Cell Biology*, Vol. 11, pp. 728-738.

Mehrotra, S. & McKim, K.S. (2006). Temporal analysis of meiotic DNA double-strand break formation and repair in Drosophila females. *PloS Genetics*, Vol. 2, No.11: e200.doi:10.1371/journal.pgen.0020200

Michod, R.E., Wojciechowski, M.F. & Hoelzer, M.A. (1988). DNA repair and the evolution of transformation in the bacterium *Bacillus subtilis*. *Genetics*, Vol. 118, pp. 31-39.

Michod, R.E. & Wojciechowski, M.F. (1994). DNA repair and evolution of transformation IV. DNA damage increases transformation. *Journal of Evolutionary Biology*, Vol. 7, pp. 147-175.

Michod, R.E. (1995). *Eros and Evolution: A Natural Philosophy of Sex*. Addison-Wesley, Reading, MA.

Michod, R.E., Bernstein, H. & Nedelcu, A.M. (2008). Adaptive value of sex in microbial pathogens. *Infection, Genetics and Evolution*, Vol. 8, pp. 267-285.

Moens, P.B., Kolas, N.K., Tarsounas, M., Marcon, E., Cohen, P.E. & Spyropoulos, B. (2002). The time course and chromosomal localization of recombination-related proteins at meiosis in the mouse are compatible with models that can resolve the early DNA-DNA interactions without reciprocal recombination. *Journal of Cell Science*, Vol. 115, pp.1611-1622.

Mortensen, U.H., Lisby, M. & Rothstein, R. (2009). Rad52. *Current Biology*, Vol. 19, No.16, pp. R676-677.

Myers, S., Spencer, C.C.A., Auton, A., Bottolo, L., Freeman, C., Donnelly, P. & McVean, G. (2006). The distribution and causes of meiotic recombination in the human geneome. *Biochemical Society Transactions*, Vol. 34, No. 4, pp. 526-530.

Nedelcu, A.M. & Michod, R.E. (2003). Sex as a response to oxidative stress: The effect of antioxidants on sexual induction in a facultatively sexual lineage. *Proceedings of the Royal Society B (suppl.)*, Vol. 270, pp. S136-S139.

Nedelcu, A.M., Marcu, O. & Michod, R.E. (2004). Sex as a response to oxidative stress: a two-fold increase in cellular reactive oxygen species activates sex genes. *Proceedings of the Royal Society B*, Vol. 271, 1591-1596.

Otto, S.P. (2003). The advantages of segregation and the evolutionof sex. Genetics, Vol. 164, pp. 1099-1118.

Otto, S.P. & Gerstein, A.C. (2006). Why have sex? The population genetics of sex and recombination. *Biochemical Society Transactions*, Vol. 34, pp. 519-522.

Pauklin, S., Burkert, J.S., Martin, J., Osman, F., Weller, S., Boulton, S.J., Whitby, M.C. & Petersen-Mahrt, S.K. (2009). Alternative induction of meiotic recombination from single-base lesions of DNA deaminases. *Genetics*, Vol. 182, pp. 41-54.

Peters, A.D. & Otto, S.P. (2003). Liberating genetic variance through sex. *BioEssays*, 25: 533-537.

Pittman, D.L., Cobb, J., Schimenti, K.J., Wilson, L.A., Cooper, D.M., Brignull, E., Handel, M.A. & Schimenti, J.C. (1998). Meiotic prophase arrest with failure of chromosome synapsis in mice deficient for *Dmc1*, a germline-specific RecA homolog. *Molecular Cell*, Vol.1, pp. 697-705.

Prado, F., Cortes-Ledesma, F., Huertas, P. & Aguilera, A. (2003). Mitotic recombination in *Saccharomyces cerevisiae*. *Current Genetics*, Vol. 42, pp. 185-198.

Prudhommeau, C. & Proust, J. (1973). UV irradiation of polar cells of *Drosophila melanogaster* embryos. V. A study of the meiotic recombination in females with chromosomes of different structure. *Mutation Research*, Vol. 23, pp. 63-66.

Ramesh, M.A., Malik, S.B. & Logsdon, J.M. Jr. (2005). A phylogenomic inventory of meiotic genes: Evidence for sex in *Giardia intestinalis*. *Science*, Vol. 319, pp. 185-191.

Rasmuson, A. (1984). Effects of DNA-repair-deficient mutants on somatic and germ line mutagenesis in the UZ system of *Drosophila melanogaster*. *Mutation Research*, Vol. 141, pp. 29-33.

Reeves, R.J. & Jackson, R.M. (1974). Stimulation of sexual reproduction in *Phytophthora* by damage. *Journal of General Microbiology*, Vol. 84, pp. 303-310.

Resnick, M.A. & Martin, P. (1976). The repair of double-strand breaks in the nuclear DNA of *Saccharomyces cerevisiae* and its genetic control. *Molecular and General Genetics*, Vol. 143, pp. 119-129.

Roze, D. & Michod, R.E. (2010). Deleterious mutations and selection for sex in finite diploid populations. *Genetics*, Vol. 184, pp. 1095-1112.

Ruderfer, D.M., Pratt, S.C., Seidel, H.S. & Kruglyak, L. (2006). Population genomic analysis of outcrossing and recombination in yeast. *Nature Genetics*, Vol. 38, pp.1077-1081.

Sager, R. & Granick, S. (1954). Nutritional control of sexuality in *Chlamydomonas reinhardi. Journal of General Physiology*, Vol. 37, pp. 729-742.

Sakakura, Y., Soyano, K., Noakes, D.L.G. & Hagiwara, A. (2006). Gonadal morphology in the self-fertilizing mangrove killifish, *Kryptolebias marmoratus. Ichthyological Research*, Vol. 53, pp. 427-430.

San Filippo, J., Sung, P., & Klein H. (2008). Mechanism of eukaryotic homologous recombination. *Annual Review of Biochemistry*, Vol. 77: pp. 229-257.

Sauvageau, S., Stasiak, A.Z., Banville, I, Ploquin, M., Stasiak, A. & Masso, J.Y. (2005). Fission yeast RAD51 and Dmc1, two efficient DNA recombinases forming helical nucleoprotein filaments. *Molecular and Cellular Biology,* Vol. 25, pp. 4377-4387.

Schewe, M.J., Suzuki, D.T. & Erasmus, U. (1971). The genetic effects of mitomycin C in *Drosophila melanogaster*. II. Induced meiotic recombination. *Mutation Research,* Vol. 12, pp. 269-279.

Sehorn, M.G., Sigurdsson, S., Bussen, W., Unger, V.M. & Sung P. (2004). Human meiotic recombinase Dmc1 promotes ATP-dependent homologous DNA strand exchange. *Nature*, Vol. 429, 433-437.

Shields, W.M. (1982). *Philopatry, Inbreeding, and the Evolution of Sex,* State University of NY Press, Albany, NY.

Shinohara, A., Ogawa, H., Matsuda, Y., Ushio,N., Ikeo, K. & Ogawa, T. (1993). Cloning of human, mouse and fission yeast recombination genes homologous to RAD51 and RecA. *Nature Genetics*, Vol. 4, pp.239-243.

Slupphaug, G., Kavli, B. & Krokan, H.E. (2003). The interacting pathways for prevention and repair of oxidative DNA damage. *Mutation Research*, Vol. 531, pp. 231-251.

Staeva-Vieira, E., Yoo, S. & Lehmann, R. (2003). An essential role of DmRad51/SpnA in DNA repair and meiotic check point control. *The EMBO Journal*, Vol. 22, No. 21, pp. 5863-5874.

Steinboeck, F., Hubmann, M., Bogusch, A., Dorninger, P., Lengheimer, T. & Heidenreich, E. (2010). The relevance of oxidative stress and cytotoxic DNA lesions for spontaneous mutagenesis in non-replicating yeast cells. *Mutation Research*, Vol. 688, pp. 47-52.

Story, R.M., Bishop, D.K., Kleckner, N. & Steitz, T.A. (1993). Structural relationship of bacterial RecA proteins to recombination proteins from bacteriophage T4 and yeast. *Science*, Vol. 259, pps. 1892-1896.

Sung, P. (1994). Catalysis of ATP-dependent homologous DNA pairing and strand exchange by yeast RAD51 protein. *Science,* Vol. 265, pp.1241-1243.

Suzuki, D.T. & Parry, D.M. (1964). Crossing over near the centromere of chromosome 3 in *Drosophila melanogaster* females. *Genetics*, Vol. 50, pp.1427-1432.

Szostak, J.W., Orr-Weaver, T.L., Rothstein, R.J. & Stahl, F.W. (1983). The double-strand-break repair model for recombination. *Cell*, Vol. 33, pp. 25-35.

Takanami, T., Mori, A., Takahashi, H. & Higashitani, A. (2000). Hyper-resistance of meiotic cells to radiation due to a strong expression of a single recA-like gene in *Caenorhabditis elegans. Nucleic Acids Research*, Vol. 28, No. 21, pp. 4232-4236.

Takanami, T., Zhang, Y., Aoki, H., Abe, T., Yoshida, S., Takahashi, H., Horiuchi, S. & Higashitani, A. (2003). Efficient repair of DNA damage induced by heavy ion particles in meiotic prophase I nuclei of *Caenorhabditis elegans*. *Journal of Radiation Research*, Vol. 44, pp. 271-276.

Terasawa, M., Shinohara, A., Hotta, Y., Ogawa, H. & Ogawa, T. (1995). Localization of RecA-like recombination protein on chromosomes of the lily at various meiotic stages. *Genes and Development*, Vol. 9, pp. 925-934.

Thorne, L.W. & Byers, B. (1993). Stage-specific effects of X-irradiation on yeast meiosis. *Genetics*, Vol. 134, pp. 29-42.

Tichy, E.D., Pillai, R., Deng, L., Liang, L., Tischfield, J., Schwemberger, S.J., Babcock, G.F. & Stambrook, P.J. (2010). Mouse embryonic stem cells, but not somatic cells, predominantly use homologous recombination to repair double-strand breaks. *Stem Cells and Development*, Vol. 19, No. 11, pp. 1699-1711.

Vilenchik, M.M. & Knudson, A.G. (2003). Endogenous DNA double-stand breaks: Production, fidelity of repair and induction of cancer. *Proceedings of the National Academy of Sciences USA*, Vol. 100, pp. 12871-12876.

Virgin, J.B., Bailey, J.P., Hasteh, F., Neville, J., Cole, A. & Tromp, G. (2001). Crossing over is rarely associated with mitotic intragenic recombination in *Schizosaccharomyces pombe*. *Genetics*, Vol. 157, pp. 63-77.

Wei, K., Kucherlapati, R. & Edelmann, W. (2002). Mouse models for human DNA mismatch-repair gene defects. *TRENDS in Molecular Medicine*, Vol. 8, No. 7, pp. 346-353.

Welch, D.B.M., Welch, J.L.M. & Meselson, M. (2008). Evidence for degenerate tetraploidy in bdelloid rotifers. *Proceedings of the National Academy of Sciences USA* , Vol. 105, pp. 5145-5149.

Whitehouse, H.L.K. (1982). *Genetic Recombination*, Wiley, New York.

Williams, G.C. (1975). *Sex and Evolution*, Princeton University Press, Princeton, NJ

Yoshida, K., Kondoh, G., Matsuda, Y., Habu, T., Nishimune, Y. & Morita, T. (1998). The mouse RecA-like gene Dmc1 is required for homologous chromosome synapsis during meiosis. *Molecular Cell*, Vol. 1, pp. 707-718.

Youds, J.L., Mets, D.G., McIlwraith, M.J., Martin, J.S., Ward, J.D., Oneil, N.J., Rose, A.M., West, S.C., Meyer, B.J. & Boulton, S.J. (2010). RTEL-1 enforces meiotic crossover interference and homeostasis. *Science*, Vol. 327, pp.1254-1258.

Zeyl, C.W. & Otto, S.P. (2007). A short history of recombination in yeast. *Trends in Ecology and Evolution*, Vol. 22, No. 5, pp. 223-225.

20

From Seed to Tree: The Functioning and Evolution of DNA Repair in Plants

Jaana Vuosku[1,2], Marko Suokas[1], Johanna Kestilä[1],
Tytti Sarjala[2] and Hely Häggman[1]
[1]*Department of Biology, University of Oulu, Oulu*
[2]*Finnish Forest Research Institute, Parkano Research Unit, Parkano*
Finland

1. Introduction

In order to alleviate harmful effects of DNA damage and maintain genome integrity, all living organisms have developed a complex network of DNA repair mechanisms. However, the biochemical and genetic studies of DNA repair pathways have hitherto focused mostly on bacterial, yeast and mammalian systems (Sancar et al., 2004; Pan et al., 2006; Goosen & Moolenaar, 2008; Jackson & Bartek, 2009), whereas plants have been somewhat neglected in this respect. In plant cells, DNA damages can be generated "spontaneously" by reactive metabolites and by mistakes that occur during DNA replication and recombination processes or they can arise from exposure to environmental DNA damaging agents (Tuteja et al., 2001 & 2009). Plants are sessile organisms, which are continuously exposed to a wide variety of biotic and abiotic stresses, which can cause DNA damages directly or indirectly via the generation of reactive oxygen species (ROS) (Roldán-Arjona & Ariza, 2009). In plants, mutations, which initially arise in somatic cells, may also be present in gametes because plants lack a reserved germline and produce meiotic cells late in development (Walbot and Evans, 2003). However, the mutation rate in long-lived coniferous forest trees, such as pines, is not unexpectedly high, which indicates that the activities responsible for maintaining genome integrity must be efficient in somatic cells (Willyard et al., 2007).

This chapter gives an overview of the special requirement of DNA repair in plants particularly from the point of view of longevity and the lifestyle of plants. We introduce the sequences of the Scots pine (*Pinus sylvestris* L.) putative *RAD51* and *KU80* genes which are involved in the repair of double-strand breaks (DSBs) by homologous recombination (HR) and non-homologous end-joining (NHEJ), respectively. The novel sequence data is used in the reconstruction of the evolutionary history of the *RAD51* and *KU80* genes in eukaryotes. In addition, the use of the HR and NHEJ pathways is demonstrated during the Scots pine seed development. From its early stages of development in the mother plant onwards, a pine seed is exposed to developmentally programmed as well as environmental stresses which are potentially damaging to the genome. Furthermore, the pine seed represents an interesting inheritance of seed tissues as well as anatomically well-described sequences of embryogenesis. Thus, we consider the pine seed to be a model system for studying the DNA repairing mechanisms, yet not solely within plants, but in wider use – for eukaryotes in general.

2. Searching for a fountain of youth in pines

Organismal ageing is generally connected to deterioration. With the passage of time, organisms accumulate stochastic damage to DNA, proteins and other macromolecules (Rattan, 2008). If damages are left unrepaired, they impair important biological functions and, furthermore, result in age-related physiological changes, an increased susceptibility to diseases and environmental stress, reduced fertility, and finally, to increased mortality (Watson & Riha, 2011). The rate of damage accumulation should be approximately equal in all organisms. However, both the rate of senescence and the length of lifespan vary largely among organisms, which suggests that they are genetically determined (Finch, 2001).

Plants have adopted many survival strategies that are totally different from those of animals, and in relation to plants, even the terms individual, aging and lifespan may sometimes be difficult to define (Thomas, 2002; Munné-Bosch, 2007). Furthermore, vegetative propagation is common in plants, and even entire forests can consist of one tree clone. In quaking aspen (*Populus tremuloides* Michx.), clones are formed by sprouting of stems from the root systems of aspens that originally are derived from a seed (Lanner, 2002). The development of plants differs completely from the development of animals, which must be taken into account in inquiries into age-related changes in plants. In plants, only a fundamental body plan is established during embryogenesis, and practically all structures and organs are formed by the proliferation of meristematic cells throughout adult life (Watson & Riha, 2011). In plants, new organs develop asynchronously during a plant's life and these have shorter lifespans than the plant as a whole (Aphalo, 2010). Concerning plant ageing, it is essential to underline that senescence can also be a highly regulated physiological process, such as a development-related physiological cell death, which is significant when compared to the death of the whole organism. In annual plants, leaf senescence is connected with the death of the whole plant, whereas in perennials, leaf senescence is a regulated physiological process that contributes to nutrient recycling and allows the rest of the plant to benefit from the nutrients which have accumulated in leafs (Lim, 2007). In trees, the biomass may mostly consist of dead cells that form a supporting structure for a thin layer of newly emerged organs (Watson & Riha, 2011).

A walk through a park is enough to show that plants age as well and that the rate of senescence and the length of lifespan are species-specific. Plants can live from a few weeks to as long as millennia (Thomas, 2002; Lanner 2002). Monocarpic plants flower, set seed and die. The monocarpic habit is well exemplified by the model plant *Arabidopsis thaliana* (L.), which may go through its entire life cycle in 8 to 10 weeks, but may nevertheless produce thousands of offspring during that time (Hensel et al., 1993). In association with massive reproductive effort, the leaves, stems and fruits of the adult Arabidopsis plant undergo progressive senescence that ultimately results in the death of the plant (Hensel et al., 1993). Despite the fact that Arabidopsis is considered to be a mere weed, due to its small size, small genome, quick generation time, ease of genetic transformation, and the availability of mutant plants, it has been found to be useful both as a model for plants in general and for the study of a variety of fundamental biological processes (Meyerowitz, 1989; Swarbreck et al., 2008). In contrast to Arabidopsis, trees are examples of long-living organisms. Trees usually remain reproductive into great old age, and hence, the characteristics that prolong life are thought to be naturally selected because they increase fitness by multiplying reproductive opportunities (Lanner, 2002). In fact, the oldest living individual organism known on earth is a tree – a Great Basin bristlecone pine (*Pinus longaeva*), which has attained at least 4862 years (Lanner, 2002). While several Great Basin bristlecone pines have exceeded 4000 years of age, they do not show evident signs of senescence (Lanner & Connor, 2001). The grafting experiments with Scots pine indicated that age-related regulation in the growth is mainly caused by physical factors and not by the age itself (Vanderklein et al., 2007).Thus, the lifetime of trees seems to be mostly limited by external factors such as the activities of pests, the frequency and intensity of fires, and ultimately, by how long it takes for the soil to erode away from their roots (Lanner, 2002).

The two major groups of seed plants, angiosperms and gymnosperms, shared a common ancestor approximately 285 million years ago (Bowe et al. 2000). For several decades, Arabidopsis has provided the leading model for angiosperms (Meyerowitz, 1989), whereas pines, *Pinus* species, have been suggested as a model for gymnosperms and woody plants (Lev-Yadun & Sederoff 2000). The genus *Pinus* has a rich history of phylogenetic analysis, and the relationships between the approximately 120 extant species are well documented (Gernandt et al. 2005), as are the development, reproduction, ecology and genetics of many pine species (Lev-Yadun & Sederoff 2000). Although pines and other gymnosperms are generally considered to be difficult subjects for genetic studies e.g. due to their long generation times, large genome size and outbred mating system, they have one remarkable advantage: the haploid megagametophyte tissue represents a single meiotic product and makes the direct analysis of inheritance of genetic loci possible without the use of controlled crosses (Devey et al. 1995). Five pines were ranked to be the most interesting on the basis of their biological, geographical or economical importance. The economically dominant pines are loblolly pine (*P. taeda*), Monterey pine (*P. radiata*) and Scots pine (Lev-Yadun & Sederoff 2000). Scots pine is the most widely distributed Eurasian conifer and one of the keystone species in the Eurasian boreal forest zone, growing in a range of environments from Spain and Turkey to the subarctic forests of northern Scandinavia and Siberia (Mirov, 1967). Additionally, two bristlecone pines, *P. aristata* and *P. longaeva*, were selected to the top five due to their greatest longevity (Lev-Yadun & Sederoff 2000). Several reports have suggested that the activities responsible for the maintenance of genome integrity must be efficient in pines. Despite the long lifetime, the observed mutation rates in the somatic cells of pines were not unexpectedly high (Willyard et al., 2007). Furthermore, no age-dependent decline was detected in the telomeres of extremely long-lived bristlecone pines, although a positive correlation was found between telomere length and life expectancy in a study in which six tree species were compared (Flanary and Kletetschka, 2005). The results suggested that answers to many intriguing questions about the maintenance of genomic integrity during organismal ageing may be found in pine trees.

3. A future vision: From weed to seed

The seed represents the main vector of plant propagation and thus, in a plant's life, it is a critical stage with many special characteristics (Rajjou & Debeaujon, 2008). According to the practical instructions for plant seed storage (Bonner, 2008), plant seeds can be classified into five types: true orthodox, sub-orthodox, intermediates class between orthodox and recalcitrant (Ellis et al. 1990), temperate recalcitrant, and tropical-recalcitrant. The seeds of most tree species with high economic value (e.g. *Abies, Betula, Pinus, Picea*) at the Northern Temperate Zone as well as many tree species (e.g. *Cauarina, Eucalyptus, Tectona*) at tropics and subtropics are true orthodox. The water content of a seed is determined by seed composition and, in addition, it is in equilibrium with the prevailing relative humidity.

Orthodox seeds are able to withstand the reduction of moisture content to around 5% (Berjak & Pammenter, 2002) and they can be stored for long periods (10 to 50+ years) at subfreezing temperatures (Bonner, 2008). Embryo development, reserve accumulation and maturation / drying are the three typical stages of orthodox seed development, leading from a zygotic embryo to a mature, quiescent seed. The maturation drying causes severe stress, and a wide range of mechanisms such as protection, detoxification and repair are needed for the surviving of a seed during the dry state and to preserve the high germination ability (Buitink & Leprince, 2008; Rajjou & Debeaujon, 2008). The longevity of seeds during storage has a major ecological, agronomical as well as economical importance (Rajjou & Debeaujon, 2008), and seed conservation is one of the useful strategies to conserve plant genetic diversity (Cochrane, 2007). Furthermore, the seeds of particular plant species such as canna (*Canna compacta*), sacred lotus (*Nelumbo nucifera* Gaertn.) and date palm (*Phoenix dactylifera* L.) represent the most impressive examples of organismal longevity (Lerman & Cigliano, 1971; Shen-Miller, 2002; Sallon et al., 2008).

Seeds are subjected to DNA damage during maturation drying, but also during seed storage. Due to the fairly easy detection of chromosome breakage or translocations, DNA lesions during seed ageing has been demonstrated for a long time. As early as in 1969, it was shown that, in the seeds of crop species such as barley (*Hordeum vulgare* L.), broad bean (*Vicia faba* L.) and pea (*Pisum sativum* L.), chromosomal damages appeared as a result of the cumulative effects of temperature, moisture and oxygen during the ageing of seeds (Abdallah & Roberts, 1969). Later, the accumulation of chromosomal aberrations appeared to be a significant factor by its contribution to the loss of seed viability during storage (Cheah & Osborne, 1978). In maize (*Zea mays* L.) seed, the maturation drying / rehydration cycle creates thousands of single strand breaks (SSBs) in the genome of each cell (Dandoy et al., 1987). During germination, a seed recovers physically from maturation drying, resumes a sustained intensity of metabolism, completes essential cellular events to allow the embryo to emerge, and induces subsequent seedling growth (Nonogaki et al., 2010). Quantitative trait loci (QTL) mapping in Arabidopsis (Clerkx et al., 2004) and rice (*Oryza sativa* L.) (Miura et al., 2002) revealed that seed longevity during storage and germination is controlled by several genetic factors. In particular, the maintenance of genetic information during the seed dehydration and rehydration cycle has been found to be essential for plant survival (Osborne et al., 2002). It has been suggested that the capability to restore genetic integrity during rehydration in an embryo whose DNA is damaged is a major factor in the determining of the seed desiccation tolerance (Boubriak et al., 1997).

In seeds, DNA repair mechanisms improve emergence and germination, particularly under stress conditions. Artificially, DNA repair can be facilitated by seed priming, that is, by controlled hydration of seeds (Rajjou & Debeaujon, 2008). Due to incomplete hydration, seeds remain desiccation-tolerant and can be re-dried after treatment (Heydecker et al., 1973). For example, in *Artemisia sphaerocephala* and *Artemisia ordosia*, DNA repair during seed priming improves seed viability under harsh desert conditions (Huang et al., 2008). Although DNA repair has been demonstrated to occur during seed priming, the molecular mechanisms involved in DNA repair in seeds are still poorly known. In Arabidopsis seed, the activities of poly (ADP-ribose) polymerases (PARP enzymes) that are implicated in DNA base-excision repair are important for germination (Hunt et al., 2007). Also, DNA ligase VI (Waterworth et al., 2010) and one of the three *RAD21* gene homologues, *AtRAD21.1* (da Costa-Nunes et al., 2006), play critical roles in the recovery from DNA damage during Arabidopsis seed imbibition, prior to germination.

4. The lifestyle of plants - living hard, repairing smart

Although ageing may involve damage to various cellular constituents, the imperfect maintenance of genetic information has been suggested to be a critical contributor to ageing (Lombard et al., 2005). Thus, the necessity of appropriate and effective responses to potential mutagenic events is emphasized by several features in the plant's lifestyle which expose them to both external and internal sources of DNA damage. As sessile organisms, plants are continuously exposed to a wide variety of abiotic stresses such as infection by various pathogens, the ultraviolet (UV) component of sunlight, ozone, dehydration and wounding which may cause DNA damages directly or indirectly via the generation of reactive oxygen species (ROS) (Roldán-Arjona & Ariza, 2009). Plants and algae are the only photosynthetic eukaryotes able to capture energy from sun light. Thus, ROS are continuously produced within plant cells also as a result of normal oxidative cellular processes such as photosynthesis and mitochondrial respiration, and they may treat the integrity and viability of cells if they are not removed (Mittler et al., 2004). Oxidative stress, a situation in which ROS exceed cellular antioxidant defenses, can cause lipid peroxidation, protein damage as well as several types of DNA lesions (Lombard et al., 2005). Although ROS are toxic molecules, they also control many different processes in plants. Therefore, the level of ROS in plant cells is tightly regulated, and the intensity, duration and localization of different ROS signals are determined by interplay between the ROS production and ROS scavenging pathways (Mittler et al., 2004). Plant cells respond to persistent DNA stress by losing their competence to divide, which may lead to meristem arrest, but normally, meristems proliferate for the entire plant's lifetime which can be even millennia in some long-lived trees. That is, meristematic cells may divide thousands of times, which inevitably results in a replication-dependent loss of telomeres if their maintance is impaired (Watson & Riha, 2011).

Exogenous and endogenous genotoxic agents may produce various kinds of DNA lesions such as altered base, missing base, mismatch base, deletion, insertion, linked pyrimidines, single (SSB) and double strand breaks (DSB) as well as intra- and inter-strands cross-links (Tuteja et al., 2001). Therefore, organisms have developed a complex network of DNA repair mechanisms both to alleviate harmful effects of DNA damage and to maintain genome integrity (Hakem, 2008). In many cases, the same type of DNA lesions can be processed by several repairing mechanisms (Boyko et al., 2006). Depending on the severity and type of the DNA damage, cellular response can either be the activation of DNA repair pathways, but also a cell cycle arrest or a programmed cell death (PCD) (Barzilai et al., 2004), which indicates that DNA repair systems are tightly connected with other fundamental cellular processes. Particularly, DSBs can be extremely deleterious lesions. Even a single unprocessed DSB can cause a cell death (Rich et al., 2000) by inactivating key genes or by leading serious chromosomal aberrations (van Gent et al., 2001). On the other hand, cellular processes such as DNA replication and the repair of other kinds of DNA lesions give rise to DSBs, and thus, the consequences of DSBs are not always solely harmful to the cell (Bleuyard et al., 2006). Diploid cells can use homology-directed repair (HDR) in DSB repair. The most common form of HDR is homologous recombination (HR), which involves extensive sequence homology between the interacting DNA molecules (Lieber, 2010). In non-dividing haploid cells or in diploid cells that are not in S-phase, a homology donor is not nearby, but they can get over DSBs by non-homologous recombination (NHEJ), which acts independently of significant homology and simply rejoins the two ends of the break

(Bleuyard et al., 2006, Lieber, 2010). These two pathways have different repair fidelity: HR has been considered to be a more accurate pathway that ensures the repair of DSB without any loss of genetic information (Bleuyard et al., 2006), whereas NHEJ results in various mutations varying from single nucleotide substitutions to deletions or insertions of several nucleotides (Pelczar et al., 2003, Kovalchuk et al., 2004). However, HR has frequently found to lead to large segmental duplication, gene duplication, gene loss, or gene inactivation (Boyko et al., 2006). Thus both HR and NHEJ may have roles in genome evolution due to genome rearrangements. Especially in plants, genetic change in somatic cells is relevant for evolutionary considerations because mutations in meristematic cells can be transferred to the offspring (Walbot, 1996). Kirik et al. (2000) analyzed the formation of deletions during DSB repair in two dicotyledonous plant species, Arabidopsis and tobacco (*Nicotiana tabacum* L.), which differ over 20-fold in genome size. They found a putative inverse correlation between genome size and the average length of deletions, which suggested that species-differences in DSB repair may influence genome evolution in plants (Kirik et al., 2000). Pelczar et al. (2003) studied genome maintenance strategies of organisms belonging to different kingdoms (animals versus plants) but of similar genome size. They found that in human HeLa cells, 50–55% DSBs were repaired precisely - a high percentage when compared to as little as 15–30% in tobacco cells - and, moreover, the DSB repair in plants resulted in 30–40% longer deletions and significantly shorter insertions. The findings suggested that the strategies for DSB repair and genome maintenance may be different in plants and animals (Pelczar et al., 2003).

The molecular components of HR and NHEJ pathways are highly conserved amongst eukaryotes and both of the pathways are required for the repairing of DSB also in plants (Bray and West, 2005; Bleuyard et al., 2006). One of the central proteins in HR is RAD51, which ensures high fidelity DNA repair by facilitating strand exchange between damaged and undamaged homologous DNA segments (Baumann & West, 1998). In addition, several RAD51-like proteins such as XRCC2 appear to help with this process (Tambini et al., 2010). In the mediation of NHEJ, a DNA dependent protein kinase (DNA-PK) complex which comprises a KU70-KU80 heterodimer and a catalytic subunit (PKcs) plays a central role (Tamura et al., 2002). The key regulatory mechanisms that direct which pathway is used for DSB repair are still poorly known if they exist at all (Boyko et al., 2006). The suggestion that HR and NHEJ compete for available DNA ends at break sites is based at the molecular level on the equilibrium between RAD52 (HR) and KU70-KU80 dimer (NHEJ) in animals (Ray and Langer, 2002). However, Arabidopsis genome contains no *RAD52* homolog (Bleuyard et al., 2006), whereas *RAD51* homolog has been identified (Doutriaux et al., 1998). Thus, the availability of the key proteins, such as RAD51 and KU proteins, at the time of DSB repair may also be one of the regulatory mechanisms. In Arabidopsis, the rate of HR decreased with plant age, whereas the frequency of strand breaks and point mutations increased. These events were parallel by a decrease in the abundance of *RAD51* transcripts as well as increase in the abundance of *KU70* transcripts and KU70 protein (Boyko et al., 2006). These results of Boyko et al. (2006) suggest that the involvement of HR and NHEJ in DSB repair may be developmentally controlled in plants.

5. DNA fragmentation and repair during Scots pine seed development

As an orthodox seed, a developing pine seed goes through maturation drying during which metabolic activity is gradually reduced and the seed enters into a quiescent state. In addition to this, the development of a viable pine seed includes the strictly co-ordinated action of several cell death programs. A characteristic feature of the Scots pine seed development is the presence of more than one embryo in the developing seed (Fig. 1A). In the beginning of the seed development, the fertilization of many egg nuclei results in several embryos of the same ovule (Buchholz 1926). Later, polyzygotic embryos undergo cleavage polyembryony (Sarvas 1962). However, only the dominant embryo survives and completes its development (Fig. 1B), while subordinate embryos, as well as suspensor tissue, are deleted by programmed cell death (PCD) during the progress of seed development (Filonova et al. 2002). Megagametophyte cells in the embryo surrounding region (ESR) die through necrotic-like cell death (Vuosku et al., 2009), and in addition, the maternal cells of the nucellar layers face destruction during early embryogenesis (Hiratsuka et al., 2002; Vuosku et al., 2009).

In a gymnosperm seed, the megagametophyte tissue develops from a haploid megaspore before the actual fertilization of the eggs (Singh 1978). The megagametophyte houses the majority of the storage reserves of a seed (King & Gifford, 1997) and provides nutrition for the developing embryo during seed development as well as for the young seedling during early germination (Fig.1C). We have shown that, in Scots pine seed, the megagametophyte tissue stays alive from the early phases of embryo development until the imbibition phase of early germination of mature seed, except for the cells in the ESR (Vuosku et al., 2009). Positive signals in TUNEL (terminal deoxynucleotidyl transferase-mediated dUTP nick end labelling) assay indicate DNA fragmentation in the nuclei of the megagametophyte cells at the late embryogeny (Fig.1D). However, the megagametophyte cells do not show other morphological signs of cell death, but appear to be viable with the active gene expression. The decreasing expression of the PCD-related metacaspase (*MCA*) and Tat-D nuclease (*TAT-D*) genes during Scots pine seed development confirms that no large-scale PCD or nucleic acid fragmentation occur in the megagametophyte tissue. Instead, the DNA fragmentation may be a consequence of DNA strand breaks caused by maturation drying or by the DNA breaks with free 3′-OH ends that appear during DNA repair. During the seed development, the expression of *RAD51* gene decrease, whereas the expression of the *KU80* and DNA ligase (*LIG*) genes remain constant, which suggests that the proportion of mitotic cells decrease and the DNA breaks are mainly repaired by NHEJ pathway (Vuosku et al., 2009).

Nuclear DNA fragmentation is currently one of the most frequently used sign of PCD. However, in the Scots pine seed, the megagametophyte cells remain metabolically active until the imbibition phase of germination despite DNA fragmentation in the nuclei already during late seed development (Vuosku et al., 2009). In plants, both the tolerance of DNA fragmentation and effective DNA repair mechanisms may be adaptations to the special energy metabolism as well as to a sessile life style which exposes cells to various endogenous and exogenous stresses. Thus, in plants, DNA fragmentation can also be a temporary process and does not always proceed to cell death.

6. Evolution of DNA repair related *recA/RAD51* gene family and *KU80* gene in eukaryotes

Previously, the homologs of both *recA* and *RAD51* genes have been identified from several prokaryotes and eukaryotes (Eisen, 1995; Bishop et al., 1992; Shinohara et al., 1992). In Arabidopsis, nuclear genome codes four recA-like proteins, RECA1, RECA2, REC3 and DRT100 that have been located in mitochondria and chloroplasts (Cao et al., 1997; Pang et al., 1992; Shedge et al., 2007). In addition to RAD51, Arabidopsis genome encodes seven

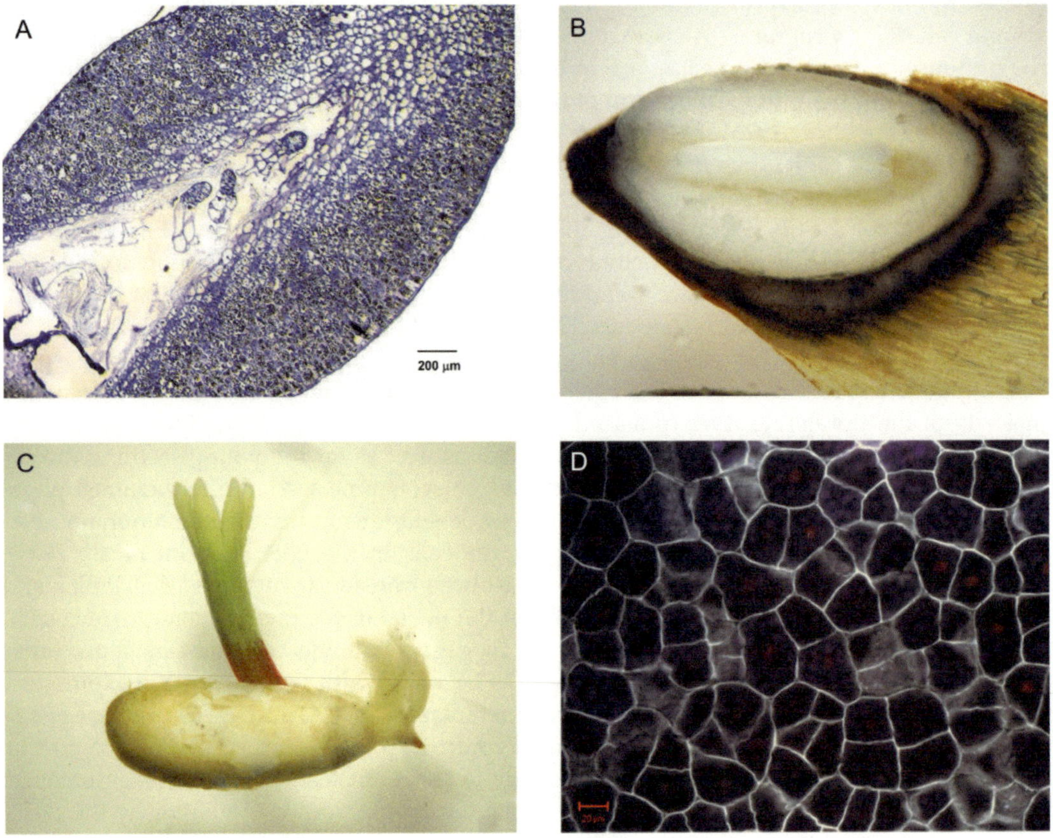

Fig. 1. Scots pine seed development. (A) The dominant embryo and subordinate embryos in the corrosion cavity surrounded by the megagametophyte. (B) A mature Scots pine seed. (C) A young Scots pine seedling. (D) TUNEL positive nuclei in the megagametophyte cells during seed development.

RAD51-like proteins, DMC1, RAD51B, RAD51C, RAD51D, DMC1, XRCC2 and XRCC3 which indicates that Arabidopsis contains the same family of RAD51-like proteins as vertebrates (Klimyuk & Jones, 1997; Doutriaux et al., 1998; Osakabe et al., 2002; Bleuyard et al., 2005). Also, the functions of RAD51 paralogs as well as the different requirements for the RAD51 paralogs in meiosis and DNA repair have been found to be conserved between plants and vertebrates (Bleuyard, et al., 2005). The presence of duplicated intron-free *RAD51* genes in the model moss *Physcomitrella patens* is unique among eukaryotes and may indicate the presence of unusual recombination apparatus in this organism (Markmann-Mulish, 2002). However, NHEJ, rather than HR, has been suggested to be the major pathway for repair DSBs in organisms with complex genomes, including vertebrates and plants (Gorbunova & Levy, 1999). The NHEJ pathway is mediated by KU70-KU80 heterodimer that shows evolutionary conserved functions (Critchlow & Jackson, 1998; Tamura et al., 2002). The KU70 and KU80 proteins of Arabidopsis share about 29% and 23% amino acid sequence identity with human KU70 and KU80 proteins, respectively (Tamura et al., 2002).

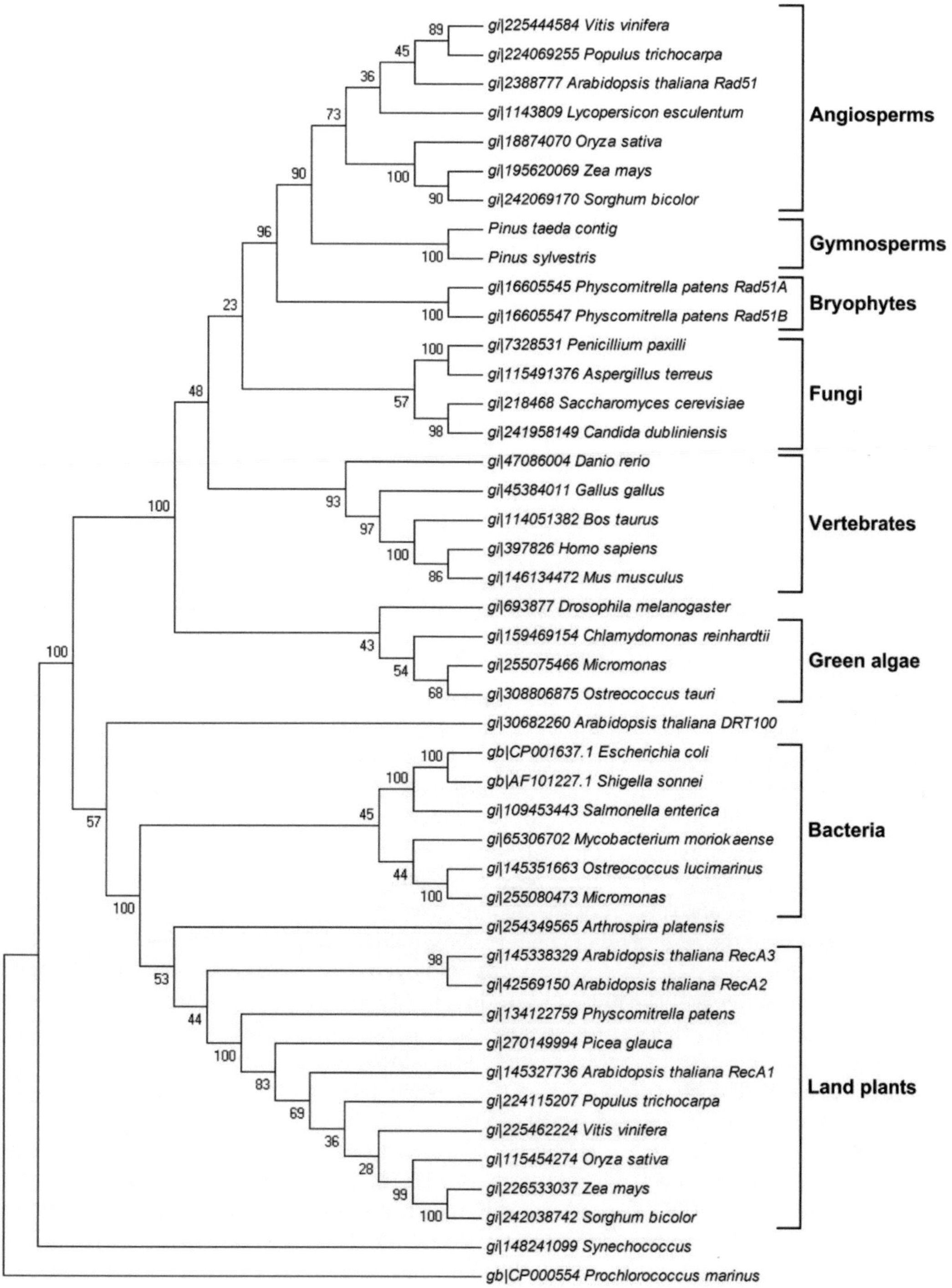

Fig. 2. Phylogenetic analysis of *recA* and *RAD51* sequences.

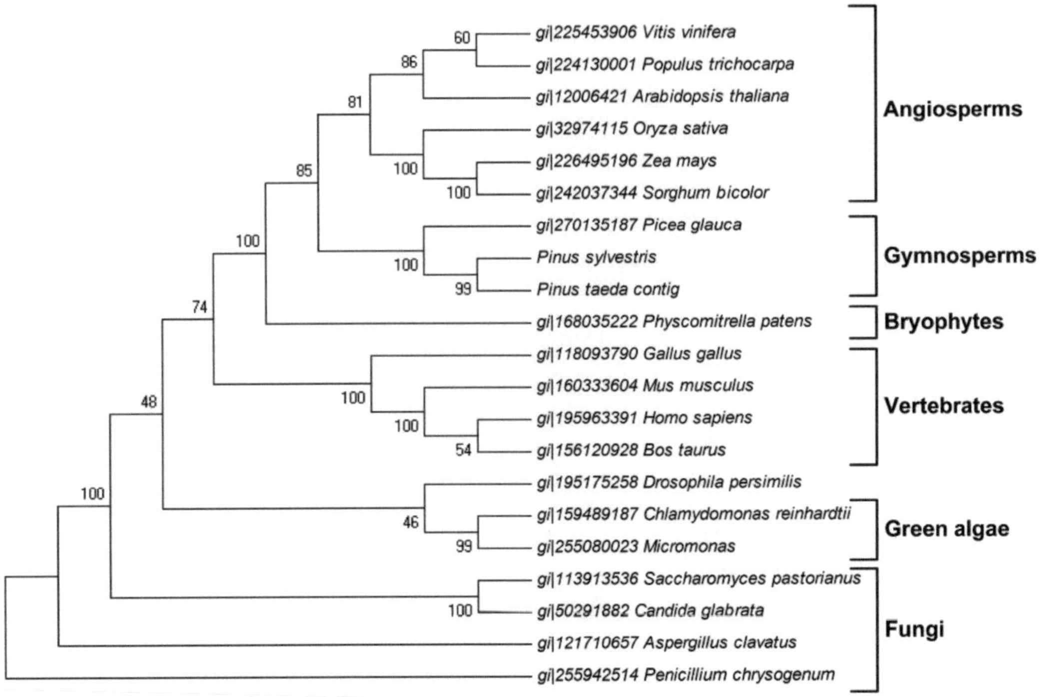

Fig. 3. Phylogenetic analysis of *KU80* sequences.

In the present study, we sequenced the coding regions of the Scots pine putative *RAD51* (GeneBank accession number: JN566226) and *KU80* (GeneBank accession number: JN566225) genes. The predicted amino acid sequences of the Scots pine RAD51 and KU80 proteins showed 77% and 41% identity to the Arabidopsis RAD51 and KU80 proteins, respectively. Blast searches in NCBI databases (http://www.ncbi.nlm.nih.gov) were performed for *recA/RAD51*-like genes as well as for KU80-like genes from various organisms, particularly from the species whose genomes have been completely sequenced. The nucleotide sequences were used for the reconstruction of the evolutionary history of the *recA/RAD51* gene family and *KU80* genes. In the case of other conifers, for which no unigene sequences were available, expressed sequence tag (EST) information was employed to reconstruct a contig containing the complete coding sequence. The nucleotide sequence alignments were performed with ClustalX (Thompson et al. 1997). Phylogenetic analyses were conducted in MEGA4 (Tamura et al. 2007) using the maximum parsimony (MP) method with close-neighbor-interchange algorithm (Nei and Kumar 2000). The bootstrap method (Felsenstein 1985) with 500 replicates was used to evaluate the confidence of the reconstructed trees.

In the phylogenetic tree, *recA* and *RAD51* sequences formed separate branches that were supported by 100% of the bootstraps (Fig. 2). Thus, the result supported the view that eukaryotic *recA* and *RAD51* genes have different evolutionary histories. The phylogenetic analysis suggested a common eukaryotic ancestor for *RAD51* genes, whereas eukaryotes seem to have acquired *recA* genes through horizontal gene transfer from bacteria. Endosymbiotic transfer of *recA* genes may have occurred from mitochondria and chloroplasts to nuclear genomes of ancestral eukaryotes (Lin et al., 2006). Both *RAD51* and *KU80* sequence-based phylogenies (Fig. 2 and 3) were in accordance with the current view of the evolution of green plants (Qiu and Palmer 1999). That is, morphologically simple plants such as *Physcomitrella* are followed by more complex flowering forms with highly developed breeding mechanisms at the top of the plant phylogeny tree. The novel gymnosperm sequences between bryophytes and angiosperms form the link that has been missing until now in the DNA repair genes based phylogenies.

7. Conclusions

Plants are sessile organisms, which are continuously exposed to a wide variety of biotic, abiotic or developmental stresses, which can cause DNA damages directly or indirectly via generation of ROS. In pines, the mechanisms maintaining genomic integrity must be efficient because the observed mutation rates in somatic cells are not high despite the long lifetime of the organisms. In pines, seed development includes developmentally programmed stresses as well as the strictly co-ordinated action of several cell death programs. Furthermore, pine seed represents an interesting inheritance of seed tissues and anatomically well-described sequences of embryogenesis. Thus, the pine seed provides a favorable model for the study of the effects of a variety of endogenous DNA damaging agents as well as developmentally regulated and environmental stresses on genome integrity. Due to the high evolutionary conservation of the DNA repair mechanisms, the pine seed, as a model system, may also shed light on the mechanisms that contribute to longevity and ageing in eukaryotes in general – things of great interest also with regard to the health of human beings.

8. Acknowledgements

We thank the personnel of the Finnish Forest Research Institute at the Punkaharju Research Unit and at the Parkano Research Unit for conducting the collections of the research material. The Research was funded by the Academy of Finland (Project 121994 to TS)

9. References

Abdalla, F.H. & Roberts H (1969) Effects of Temperature, Moisture, and Oxygen on the Induction of Chromosome Damage in Seeds of Barley, Broad Beans, and Peas during Storage. *Annals of Botany*, Vol.32, No.1, pp. 119-136

Aphalo, P.J. (2010) On How to Disentangle the Contribution of Different Organs And Processes to the Growth of Whole Plants. *Journal of Experimental Botany*, Vol.61, No.3, pp. 626-628

Barzilai, A. & Yamamoto, K.I. (2004) DNA Damage Responses to Oxidative Stress. *DNA repair*, Vol.3, No.8-9, pp. 1109-1115

Baumann, P. & West, S. (1998) Role of the Human RAD51 Protein in Homologous Recombination and Double-Stranded-Break Repair. *Trends in Biochemical Sciences*, Vol.23, No.7, pp. 247-251

Berjak, P. & Pammenter, N.M. (2002) Orthodox and Recalcitrant Seeds. In: *Tropical Tree Seed Manual*, J.A. Vozzo, (Ed.), 137-147, USDA Forest Service, Washington DC, USA

Bishop, D.K.; Park, D.; Xu L. & Kleckner, N. (1992) DMC1: A Meiosis-Specific Yeast Homolog of *E. coli recA* Required for Recombination, Synaptonemal Complex Formation, and Cell Cycle Progression. *Cell*, Vol.69, No.3, pp. 439-456

Bleuyard, J-Y.; Gallego, M.E., Savigny, F. & White, S.I (2005) Different Requirements for the Arabidopsis Rad51 Paralogs in Meiosis and DNA Repair. *The Plant Journal*, Vol.41, pp. 533-545

Bleuyard, J-Y.; Gallego, M.E. & White, C.I. (2006) Recent Advances in Understanding of the DNA Double-Strand Break Repair Machinery of Plants. *DNA repair*, Vol.5, pp. 1-12

Bonner, F.T. (2008) Storage of Seeds. In: *The Woody Plant Seed Manual*, F.T. Bonner, R.P. Karrfalt (Ed.), 85-95, USDA FS Agriculture Handbook 727

Bowe, L.M.; Coat, G. & dePamphilis, C.W. (2000) Phylogeny of Seed Plants based on All Three Genomic Compartments: Extant Gymnosperms Are Monophyletic and Gnetales' Closest Relatives Are Conifers. *Proceedings of the National Academy of Sciences of the United States of America*, Vol.97, No.8, pp 4092-4097

Bray, C.M. & West, C.E. (2005) DNA Repair Mechanisms in Plants: Crucial Sensors and Effectors for the Maintenance of Genome Integrity. *New Phytologist*, Vol.168, pp. 511-528

Boubriak, I.; Kargiolaki, H.; Lyne, L. & Osborne, D.J. (1997) The Requirement for DNA Repair in Desiccation Tolerance of Germinating Embryos. *Seed Science Research*, Vol.7, No.2, pp. 97-105

Boyko, A.; Zemp, F.; Filkowski, J. & Kovalchuk, I. (2006) Double-Strand Break Repair in Plants Is Developmentally Regulated. *Plant Physiology*, Vol.141, pp. 488-497

Buchholz, J.T. (1926) Origin of Cleavage Polyembryony in Conifers. *Botanical Gazette*, Vol.81, No.1, pp. 55-71

Buitink, J. & Leprince, O. (2008) Intracellular Glasses and Seed Survival in the Dry State. *Comptes Rendus Biologies*, Vol.331, No.10, pp. 788-795

Cao, J.; Combs, C. & Jagendorf, A.T. (1997) The Chloroplast-Located Homolog of Bacterial DNA Recombinase. *Plant and Cell Physiology*, Vol.38, No.12, pp.1319-1325

Cheah, K.S.E. & Osborne, D.J. (1978) DNA Lesions Occur With Loss of Viability in Embryos of Ageing Rye Seed. *Nature*, Vol.272, pp.593-599

Clerkx, E.J.; El-Lithy, M.E.; Vierling, E.; Ruys, G.J.; Blankestijn-De Vries, H.; Groot, S.P.C.; Vreugdenhil, D & Koornneef, M. (2004) Analysis of Natural Allelic Variation of Arabidopsis Seed Germination and Seed Longevity Traits Between the Accessions Landsberg *erecta* and Shakdara, Using a New Recombinant Inbred Line Population. *Plant Physiology*, Vol.135, pp. 432-443

Cochrane, J.A.; Crawford, A.D. & Monks, L.T. (2007) The Significance of Ex Situ Seed Conservation to Reintroduction of Threatened Plants. *Australian Journal of Botany*, Vol.55, No.3, pp. 356-361

Critchlow, S.E. & Jackson, S.P. (1998) DNA End-Joining: from Yeast to Man. *Trends in Biochemical Sciences*. Vol.23, No.10, pp. 394-398

da Costa-Nunes, J.A.; Bhatt, A.M.; O´Shea, S.; West, C.E.; Bray, C.M.; Grossniklaus, U & Dickinson, H.G. (2006) Characterization of the three *Arabidopsis thaliana* RAD21 cohesins reveals differential responses to ionizing radiation. *Journal of Experimental Botany*, Vol.57, No.4, pp. 971-983

Dandoy, E.; Schyns, R.; Deltour, L. & Verly, W.G. (1987) Appearance and Repair of Apurinic/Apyrimidinic Sites in DNA during Early Germination. *Mutation Research*, Vol.181, No.1, pp. 57-60

Devey, M.E.; Delfinomix, A.; Kinloch, B.B. & Neale, D.B. (1995) Random Amplified Polymorphic DNA Markers Tightly Linked to a Gene for Resistance to White-Pine Blister Rust in Sugar Pine. *The Proceeding of the National Academy of Sciences of the United States of America*, Vol.92, No.6, pp. 2066-2070

Doutriaux, M.; Couteau, F.; Bergounioux, C. & White, C. (1998) Isolation and Characterization of the Rad51 and DMC1 Homologs from *Arabidopsis Thaliana*. *Molecular and General Genetics*, Vol.257, No.3, pp. 283-291

Eisen, J.A. (1995) The RecA Protein as a Model Molecule for Molecular Systematic Studies of Bacteria: Comparison of Trees of RecA and 16S rRNAs from the Same Species. *Journal of Molecular Evolution*, Vol.41, No.6, pp. 1105-1123

Ellis, R.H.; Hong, T.D. & Roberts, E.H. (1990) An Intermediate Category of Seed Storage Behavior? I. Coffee. *Journal of Experimental Botany*, Vol.41, No.9, pp. 1167–1174

Felsenstein, J. (1985) Confidence Limits on Phylogenies: an Approach Using the Bootstrap. *Evolution*, Vol.39, No.4, pp. 783-791

Filonova, L.H; von Arnold, S.; Daniel, G & Bozhkov, P.V. (2002) Programmed Cell Death Eliminates All but One Embryo in a Polyembryonic Plant Seed. *Cell Death and Differentiation*, Vol.9, No.10, pp. 1057-1062

Finch, C.E. & Austad, S.N. (2001) History and Prospects: Symposium on Organisms with Slow Aging. *Experimental Gerontology*, Vol.36, No.4-6, pp. 593-597

Flanary, B.E. & Kletetschka, G. (2005) Analysis of Telomere Length and Telomerase Activity in Tree Species of Various Life-Spans, and with Age in the Bristlecone Pine *Pinus longaeva*. *Biogerontology*, Vol.6, No.2, pp.101-111

Gernandt, D.S.; Lopez, G.G.; Garcia, S.O. & Liston, A. (2005) Phylogeny and Classification of Pinus. *Taxon*, Vol.54, No.1, pp. 29-42

Goosen, N. & Moolenaar G.F. (2008) Repair of UV Damage in Bacteria. *DNA Repair*, Vol.7, pp. 353-379

Gorbunova, V. & Levy, A.A. (1999) How Plants Make Ends Meet: DNA Double Strand Break Repair. *Trends in Plants Sciences*, Vol.4, No.7, pp. 263-269

Hakem, R. (2008) DNA-Damage Repair; the Good, the Bad, and the Ugly. *The EMBO Journal*, Vol.27, pp. 589-605

Hensel, L.L.; Grbić, V.; Baumgarten, D.A. & Bleecker, A.B. (1993) Developmental and Age-Related Processes That Influence the Longevity and Senescence of Photosynthetic Tissues in *Arabidopsis*. *The Plant Cell*, Vol.5, pp.553-564

Heydecker, W.; Higgins, J. & Gulliver, R.L. (1973) Acclerated Germination by Osmotic Seed Treatment. *Nature*, Vol.246, No.2, pp.42-44

Hiratsuka, R.; Yamada, Y. & Terasaka, O. (2002) Programmed Cell Death of *Pinus* Nucellus in Response to Pollen Tube Penetration. *Journal of Plant Research*, Vol.115, No.2, pp. 141-8

Huang, Z.; Boubriak, I.; Osborne, D.J.; Dong, M. & Gutterman, Y. (2008) Possible Role of Pectin-Containing Mucilage and Dew in Repairing Embryo DNA of Seeds Adapted to Desert Conditions. *Annals of Botany*, Vol.101, pp. 277-283

Hunt, L.; Holdsworth, M.J. & Gray, J.E. (2007) Nicotinamidase Activity is Important for Germination. *The Plant Journal*, Vol.51, pp. 341-351

Jackson, S.P. & Bartek, J. (2009) The DNA-Damage Response in Human Biology and Disease. *Nature*, Vol.461, pp.1071-1078

King, J.E. & Gifford, D.J. (1997) Amino Acid Utilization in Seeds of Loblolly Pine during Germination and Early Seedling Growth (I. Arginine and Arginase Activity), *Plant Physiology*, Vol.113, No.4, pp. 1125-1135

Kirik, A.; Salomon S. & Puchta H. (2000) Species-Specific Double-strand Break Repair and Genome Evolution in Plants. *The EMBO Journal*, Vol.19, No.20, pp. 5562-5566

Klimyuk, V.I. & Jones, J.D. (1997) *AtDMC1*, the Arabidopsis Homologue of the Yeast DMC1 Gene: Characterization, Transposon-Induced Allelic Variation and Meiosis-Associated Expression. *Plant Journal*, Vol.11, No.1, pp. 1-14

Kovalchuk, I.; Pelczar, P. & Kovalchuk, O. (2004) High Frequency of Nucleotide Misincorporations upon the Processing of the Double-Strand Breaks. *DNA Repair*, Vol.3, No.3, pp. 217-223

Lanner, R.M. (2002) Why do Trees Live so Long? *Ageing Research Reviews*, Vol.1, No.4, pp. 653-671

Lanner, R.M. & Connor, K.F. (2001) Does Bristlecone Pine Senesce? *Experimental Gerontology*, Vol.36, No.4-6, pp. 675-685

Lerman, J.C. & Cigliano, E.M. (1971) New Carbon-14 Evidence for Six Hundred Years Old *Canna compacta* Seed, *Nature*, Vol.232, pp. 568-570

Lev-Yadun, S. & Sederoff, R. (2000) Pines as Model Gymnosperms to Study Evolution, Wood Formation, and Perennial Growth. *Journal of Plant Growth Regulation*, Vol.19, pp. 290-305

Lieber, M.R. (2010) The Mechanism of Double-Strand DNA Break Repair by the Nonhomologous DNA End Joining Pathway. *Annual Review of Biochemistry*, Vol.79, pp. 181-211

Lim, P.O.; Kim, H.J. & Nam, H.G. (2007) Leaf Senescence. *Annual Review of Plant Biology*, Vol.58, pp. 115-136

Lin, Z.; Kong, H.; Nei, M. & Ma, H. (2006) Origins and Evolution of the *recA/RAD51* Gene Family: Evidence for Ancient Gene Duplication and Endosymbiotic Gene Transfer. *The Proceeding of the National Academy of Sciences of the United States of America*, Vol.103, No.27, pp. 10328-10333

Lombard, D.B.; Chua, K.F.; Mostoslavsky, R.; Franco, S.; Gostissa, M. & Alt, F.W. (2005) DNA Repair, Genome Stability, and Aging, *Cell*, Vol.120, pp. 497-512

Markmann-Mulisch, U.; Hadi, M.Z.; Koepchen, K.; Alonso, J.C.; Russo, V.E.A.; Schell, J. & Reiss, B. (2002) The Organization of *Physcomitrella patens Rad51* Genes is Unique among Eukaryotic Organisms. *The Proceeding of the National Academy of Sciences of the United States of America*, Vol.99, No.5, pp. 2959-2964

Meyerowitz, E.M. (1989) Arabidopsis, a Useful Weed. *Cell*, Vol.56, pp. 263-269

Mittler, R.; Vanderauwera, S.; Gollery, M. & Van Breusegem F. (2004) Reactive Oxygen Gene Network of Plants. *Trends in Plant Sciences*, Vol.9, No.10, pp. 1360-1385

Mirov NT (1967) *The Genus Pinus*, The Ronald Press Company, New York

Miura, K.; Lin, Y.; Yano, M. & Nagamine, T. (2002) Mapping Quantitative Trait Loci Controlling Seed Longevity in Rice (*Oryza sativa* L.). *Theoretical and Applied Genetics*, Vol.104, No.6-7, pp.981-986

Munné-Bosch, S. (2007) Aging in Perennials. *Critical Review in Plant Sciences*, Vol.26, 123-138

Nei, M. & Kumar, S (2000) *Molecular Evolution and Phylogenetics*, Oxford University Press, New York

Nonogaki, H.; Bassel, G.W. & Bewley, J.D. (2010) Germination - Still a Mystery. *Plant Science*, Vol.179, No.6, pp. 574-581

Osakabe, K.; Yoshioka, T.; Ichikawa, H. & Toki, S. (2002) Molecular Cloning and Characterization of RAD51-like Genes from *Arabidopsis thaliana*. *Plant Molecular Biology*, Vol.50, No.1, pp. 71-81

Osborne, D.J.; Boubriak, I.; Leprince, O. (2002) Rehydration of Dried Systems: Membranes and the Nuclear Genome. In: *Desiccation and survival in plants: drying without dying*, M. Black & H.W. Pritchard, (Ed), 343-364, CABI Publishing. Wallingford, Oxon, UK

Pan, X.; Ye, P.; Yuan, D.S.; Wang, X.; Bader, J.S.; Boeke, J.D. (2006) A DNA Integrity Network in the Yeast *Saccharomyces cerevisiae*. *Cell*, Vol.124, No.5, pp.1069-1081

Pang, Q.; Hays, J.B. & Rajagopal, I. (1992) A Plant cDNA that Partially Complements *Escherichia coli recA* Mutations Predicts a Polypeptide not Strongly Homologous to RecA Proteins. *Proceeding of the National Academy of Sciences USA*, Vol.89, No.17, pp. 8073-8077

Pelczar, P.; Kalck, V. & Kovalchuk, I. (2003) Different Genome Maintenance Strategies in Human and Tobacco Cells. *Journal of Molecular Biology*, Vol.331, No.4, pp. 771-779

Qiu, Y-L & Palmer, J.D. (1999) Phylogeny of Early Land Plants: Insights from Genes and Genomes. *Trends in Plant Sciences*, Vol.4, No.1, pp. 26-29

Rajjou, L. & Debeaujon I (2008) Seed Longevity: Survival and Maintenance of High Germination Ability of Dry Seeds. *Comptes Rendus Biologies*, Vol.331, No.10, pp. 796-805

Rattan, S.I.S. (2008) Increased Molecular Damage and Heterogeneity as the Basis of Aging. *Biological Chemistry*, Vol.389, pp. 267-272

Ray, A. & Langer, M. (2002) Homologous Recombination: Ends as the Means. *Trends in Plant Science*, Vol.7, No.10, pp. 435-440

Rich, T; Allen, R.L. & Wyllie, A.H. (2000) Defying Death After DNA Damage. *Nature*, Vol.407, pp. 777-783

Roldán-Arjona, T. & Ariza, R.R. (2009) Repair and Tolerance of Oxidative DNA Damage in Plants. *Mutation Research*, Vol.681, No.2-3, pp. 169-179

Sancar, A; Lindsey-Boltz, L.A.; Ünsal-Kaçmaz, K. & Linn, S. (2004) Molecular Mechanisms of Mammalian DNA Repair and the DNA Damage Checkpoints. *Annual Review of Biochemistry*, Vol.73, pp.39-85

Sallon, S.; Solowey, E.; Cohen, Y.; Korchinsky, R.; Egli, M.; Woodhatch, I.; Simchoni, O. & Kislev, M (2008) Germination, Genetics, And Growth of an Ancient Date Seed. *Science*, Vol.320, No.5882, pp. 1464

Sarvas, R. (1962) Investigations on the Flowering and Seed Crop of *Pinus sylvestris*. *Communicationes Instituti Forestale Fennica*, Vol.53, pp. 1-198

Shedge, V.; Arrieta-Montiel, M., Christensen, A.C. & Mackenzie, S.A. (2007) Plant Mitochondrial Recombination Surveillance Requires Unusual *RecA* and *MutS* Homologs. *The Plant Cell*, Vol.19, No.4, pp. 1251-1264

Shen-Miller, J. (2002) Sacred Lotus, the Long-Living Fruits of China Antique. *Seed Science Research*, Vol.12, No.3, pp. 131-143

Shinohara, A.; Ogawa, H. & Ogawa, T. (1992) Rad51 Protein Involved in Repair and Recombination in *S. cerevisiae* is a RecA-like Protein. *Cell*, Vol.69, No.3, pp. 457-470

Singh H (1978) *Embryology of Gymnosperms*, Borntrager, Berlin

Swarbreck, D.; Wilks, C.; Lamesch, P.; Berardini, T.Z; Garcia-Hernandez, M.; Foerster, H.; Li, D.; Meyer, T.; Muller, R.; Ploetz, L.; Radenbaugh, A.; Singh, S.; Swing, V.; Tissier, C.; Zhang, P. & Huala, E. (2008) The Arabidopsis Information Resource (TAIR): Gene Structure and Function Annotation. *Nucleic Acids Research*, Vol.36, pp. D1009-D1014

Tambini, C.E.; Spink, K.G.; Ross, C.J.; Hill, M.A. & Thacker, J. (2010) The Importance of XRCC2 in RAD51-related DNA Damage Repair. *DNA Repair*, Vol.9, No.5, pp. 517-525

Tamura, K.; Adachi, Y.; Chiba, K.; Oguchi, K. & Takahashi, H. (2002) Identification of *Ku70* and *Ku80* Homologues in *Arabidopsis thaliana*: Evidence for a Role in the Repair of DNA Double-Strand Breaks. *The Plant Journal*, Vol.29, No.6, pp. 771-781

Tamura, K.; Dudley, J.; Nei, M. & Kumar, S. (2007) MEGA4: Molecular Evolutionary Genetics Analysis (MEGA) Software Version 4.0. *Molecular Biology and Evolution*, Vol.24, No.8, pp.1596-1599

Thomas, H. (2002) Ageing in Plants. *Mechanisms of Ageing and Development*. Vol.123, No.7, pp. 747-753

Thompson, J.D.; Gibson, T.J.; Plewniak, F.; Jeanmougin, F. & Higgins, D.G. (1997) The CLUSTAL_X Windows Interface: Flexible Strategies for Multiple Sequence Alignment Aided by Quality Analysis Tools. *Nucleic Acid Research*, Vol.25, No.24, pp. 4876-4882

Tuteja, N.; Ahmad, P.; Panda, B.B. & Tuteja, R. (2009) Genotoxic Stress in Plants: Shedding Light on DNA Damage, Repair and DNA Repair Helicases. *Mutation Research*, Vol.681, No.2-3, pp. 134-149

Tuteja, N.; Singh,M.B.; Misra, M.K.; Bhalla, P.L. & Tuteja, R. (2001) Molecular Mechanisms of DNA Damage and Prepair: Progress in Plants. *Critical Reviews in Biochemistry and Molecular Biology*, Vol.36, No.4, pp. 337-397

van Gent, DC.; Hoeijmakers, J.H.J.& Kanaar, R. (2001) Chromosomal Stability and the DNA Double-Stranded Break Connection. *Nature Review Genetics*, Vol.2, pp. 196-206

Vanderklein, D.; Martínez-Vilalta, J.; Lee, S. & Mencuccini, M. (2007) Plant Size, not Age, Regulates Growth and Gas Exchange in Grafted Scots Pine Trees. *Tree Physiology*, Vol.24, pp. 71-79

Vuosku, J.; Sarjala, T.; Jokela, A.; Sutela, S.; Sääskilahti, M.; Suorsa, M.; Läärä, E. & Häggman, H. (2009) One Tissue, Two Fates: Different Roles of Megagametophyte Cells during Scots Pine Embryogenesis, *Journal of Experimental Botany*, Vol.60, No.4, pp. 1375-86

Walbot, V. (1996) Sources and Consequences of Phenotypic and Genotypic Plasticity in Flowering Plants. *Trends in Plant Science*, Vol.1, No.1, pp. 27-33

Walbot, V. & Evans, M.M. (2003) Unique Features of the Plant Life Cycle and Their Consequences. *Nature Reviews Genetics*, Vol.4, pp. 369-379

Waterworth, W.M.; Masnavi, G.; Bhardwaj, R.M.; Jiang, Q.; Bray, C.M. & West, C.E. (2010) A Plant DNA Ligase is an Important Determinant of Seed Longevity. *The Plant Journal*, Vol.63, No.5, pp. 848-860

Watson, J.M. & Riha, K. (2011) Telomeres, Aging, and Plants: From Weeds to Methuselah – A Mini-Review. *Gerontology*, Vol.57, pp. 129-136

Willyard, A.; Syring, J.; Gernandt, D.S.; Liston, A. & Cronn, R. (2007) Fossil Calibration of Molecular Divergence Infers a Moderate Mutation Rate and Recent Radiations for *Pinus*. *Molecular Biology and Evolution*, Vol.24, No.1, pp. 90-101

Part 3

Mechanisms of DNA Repair

21

The Gratuitous Repair on Undamaged DNA Misfold

Xuefeng Pan[1,2], Peng Xiao[1], Hongqun Li[2], Dongxu Zhao[1] and Fei Duan[2]
[1]*School of Life Science, Beijing Institute of Technology, Beijing*
[2]*Health Science Center, Hebei University, Baoding*
China

A Paradox of Life
B-DNA is needed for maintenance of genetic stability, while it will convert into non-B DNA in replication, repair, transcription or recombination, leading to exposure of bases, single strands, and even introduction of distortions. All these could intrigue gratuitous repair on undamaged DNA using the conventional repair, recombination mechanisms.
Repair or not Repair, turns to be a question?

1. Introduction

In natural genomes, tens of DNA structure analogous to B-DNA conformation have been found to be formed through compiling weak interacting forces, including hydrophobic, Van der Waals and hydrogen-bond accepters and donors and inductions of certain agents (Rao et al., 2010). Of which, hairpins, cruciform junctions, Z-DNA, G-tetrads/quadruplexes, helices, loops and bulges are most studied so far.

Since the late 1950s, the roles of the non-B DNA structures in biological functions have begun to be enlightened (Watson & Crick, 1953; Wilkins et al., 1953a, 1953b; Svozil et al., 2008). Piling up results suggest that non-B conformations, such as cruciforms, triplexes, tetraplexes, can interact with proteins involving DNA metabolism, including replication, gene expression and recombination, or influence nucleosomes and other supramolecular structures formation (Wang & Griffith, 1996; Shimizu et al. 2000). However, non-B DNA secondary structures may also be treated as DNA mis-folds by DNA repair systems. Because of which the non-B DNA secondary structures can serve as end points for several types of genome rearrangements seen in some diseases (Wang & Vasquez, 2006; Wells, 2007; Bacolla & Wells, 2009; Chen et al., 2010).

2. DNA sequences which are susceptible to abnormal folding

The non-B DNA structure forming sequences are found to be rich in genomes from divergent organisms (Table 1) (Cox & Mirkin, 1997; Svozil et al., 2008; Cerz et al., 2011). For example, nearly half of the human genome consists of repetitive sequences, which can be arranged as inverted, direct tandem, and homopurine–homopyrimidine mirror repeats.

These repeat sequences are major contributors to forming non-B DNA structures, although the unusual structures can also be formed by various other sequences that are not repeating tracts (Svozil et al., 2008; Cerz et al., 2011). Repeat DNA sequences may adopt either orthodox right-handed B-DNA or non-B DNA conformations at specific sequence motifs as a function of negative supercoil density, created by transcription, protein binding, and other reasons. For example, inverted repeats can form B conformation in cells, while also forming hairpin structures, slipped structures with looped-out bases, four-stranded G-quartet structures, left-handed Z-DNA and intramolecular triplex DNA structures (H-DNA) depending on the base compositions and the arrangements.

Structural Feature	human	Chimpanzee	Macaque	Dog	Mouse
Cruciform	197910	190736	128334	172032	188532
Slipped Motif	347969	314516	305285	404750	695150
Triplex Motif	179623	105640	140580	303385	565479
Z-DNA Motif	294320	278928	280982	261012	690276
G-Tetraduplex	374545	314171	298142	492535	559280
Direct repeats	871045	787335	765798	968955	1593107
Inverted repeats	1044533	998249	843889	814080	801242
Mirror Repeats	1651723	1485135	1455025	1849897	1651723

Table 1. Non-B DNA motifs in different mammalian genomes (Cer et al., 2011)

2.1 Cruciform motif

DNA sequence that reads the same from 5' to 3' in either strand of a duplex is called as inverted repeat or palindrome DNA sequence. This subset of inverted repeat sequences may fold-back and form intramolecular, antiparallel, double helices stabilized by Watson–Crick hydrogen bonds (van Holde & Zlatanova, 1994; Courey, 1999; Smith, 2008).
As a whole, the interstrand hydrogen bonds in the inverted repeats must be broken, and intrastrand hydrogen bonds form between the complementary bases in each single strand, forming two hairpin-like arms with small (3-4 unpaired bases) loop at their tips. The structure looks similar to a four-way junction, of which the nucleobases in and around the junction are fully involved in base pairing.

2.2 Potential quadruplex sequences

Potential quadruplex sequences are usually G-rich, such as the DNA sequences in eukaryotic telomeres, and in non-telomeric genomic DNA, like the nuclease-hypersensitive promoter regions (Burge et al., 2006; Rawal et al., 2006; Qin & Hurley, 2008; Sannohe & Sugiyama, 2010). To form a quadruplex, the DNA sequences have to form overlapping four G-blocks. Each contains the same number (n) of G bases (n vary from 3 to 7), on each strand, and/ or separated by 1–7 nt (Burge et al., 2006). The potential unimolecular G-quadruplex forming sequences (i.e. intramolecular) can be expressed as follows (Burge et al., 2006):

GaXbGaXcGaXdGa

Where "a" is the number of G residues in each short G-tract, which are usually directly involved in G-tetrad. Xb, Xc and Xd can be any combination of residues, including G, forming the loops.
The potential quadruplex sequences were therefore restricted to:

$$\mathbf{G_{3\text{-}5}NLoop1G_{3\text{-}5}NLoop2G_{3\text{-}5}NLoop3G_{3\text{-}5}}$$

Where NLoop1-3 are loops of unknown length, within the limits 1<NLoop1-3 <7 nt.

2.3 Z-DNA motif

In 1979, DNA sequence of d (CpGpCpGpCpG) was crystallized and found to adopt a left-handed conformation (the Z-DNA conformation) with altered helical parameters relative to right-handed B-form (Rich et al., 1983; Mirkin, 2008). Later, it was realized that DNA sequences with alternating pyrimidines and purines, such as $(CA:TG)_n$ and $(CG:CG)_n$, may wind a double helix into a left-handed zigzag form (Z-DNA). Z-DNA is thinner (18 Å) than B-DNA (20 Å), due to its bases shifting to the outskirts of a double helix. It has only one deep, narrow groove equivalent to the minor groove in B-DNA.
In general, five or more tandem repeats, each comprising an alternating pyrimidine–purine dinucleotide motif, in which the pattern YG is preserved on at least one of the DNA strands can adopt Z-DNA.

2.4 Triplex motif

A subset of mirror repeat sequences comprise only purines (A and G, R) or pyrimidines (C and T, Y) on the same strand of a double stranded DNA, separated by few (0~8) nucleotides. These DNA motifs can adopt various intramolecular three-stranded analogous (triplex, H-DNA) stabilized by Hoogsteen hydrogen bonds (Casey & Glazer, 2001; Mukherjee & Vasquez 2011).
For a sequence requirement in forming triplex DNA is thought to be that only R · Y-containing mirror repeats can yield A: A*T and G: G * C triads. When the hydrogen bonds in the A · T and G · C base pairs are formed in canonical B-form DNA, several hydrogen bond forming groups in the bases can still be free unpaired. Each purine base has two hydrogen bond forming groups on the edges that are posed in the major groove. These unpaired bases can be used to form base triads that are unit blocks of triple-stranded DNA (see the following explanation for detail).
In theory, a homopurine-homopyrimidine duplex can form triplexes of either purine (Pu) motif (purine, antiparallel motif) or pyrimidine (Py) motif (pyrimidine, parallel motif). However, under physiological conditions, cytosine protonation is not favored, and C·G*G becomes therefore the most stable triad in a Pu motif. To form an intermolecular or intramolecular triplex, adjoining homopurine-homopyrimidine tracts of at least 10 base pairs are normally required for a duplex acceptor, since shorter than that the triplexes formed can be unstable under physiological conditions (Fox & Brown, 2011).
A triplex may be mutagenic *in vivo*, as double-strand breaks may occur in or near the triplex site, which if with DNA replication, recombinational repair may produce triplex mediated mutagenesis (Chan et al., 1999; Faruqi et al., 2000).
Triplex can also be formed in RNA transcription, although it is a kinetically unfavored compared to duplex annealing. However triplex RNA and DNA are stable, showing half-lives on the order of days, which may involve the molecular mechanism of Friedreich's ataxia (FRDA) (Pan et al., 2009).

3. The non-B DNA structures and non-B DNA structure-induced genetic instability

3.1 DNA loops/ bulges and slipped DNA

DNA loops and bulges are similar non-B DNA structures sharing common features of unpaired bases of different number (Fig. 1). They can be formed in anywhere by any DNA sequence in natural genome, therefore they may be the most frequent non-B DNA conformations in genomes. For example, $(CA \cdot TG)_n$ DNA sequences are found to exist everywhere in eukaryotic genomes as of 60 base pairs tracts. $(CA \cdot TG)_n$ forms both classical right-handed DNA double helix, and diverse alternative conformations including small DNA loops or bulges (Kladde et al., 1994; Ho, 1994).

Genomic instabilities can also be caused by DNA loops and bulges, which are often seen as slippage instabilities or insertion/deletion (I/ D) instabilities (Pan, 2004). Proteins that bind DNA loops and bulges are also found and mainly known to be mismatch repair proteins (Parker & Marinus, 1992; Carraway & Marinus, 1993; Fang et al., 2003; Kaliyaperumal et al., 2011).

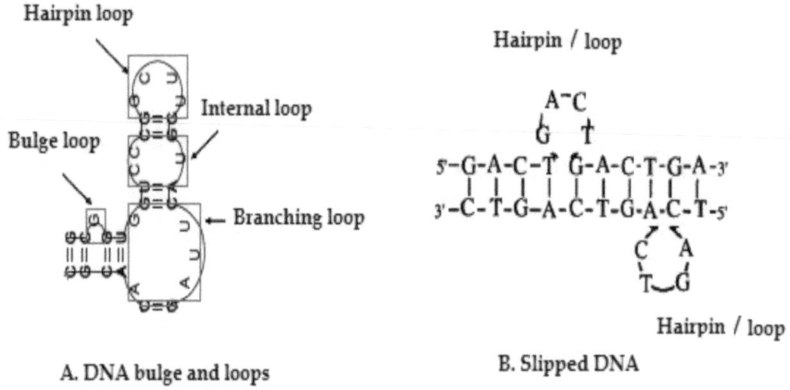

Fig. 1. DNA Loops and bulges

3.2 Branched structures

A branched DNA structure refers to a non-B DNA secondary structure with structured or unstructured "branch". For example, DNA intermediates appeared in homologous recombination as 3- and 4- way junctures are such branched DNA structures with differently oriented double helix arms. Similarly, flapped DNA structures appeared in processing Okazaki fragment in the lagging strand DNA replication also belong to branched DNA. Branched DNA migrates more slowly than their B-DNA conformation having same molecular weight and base composition. Importantly, branched DNA structures can also make genomic instability when in processing.

3.3 Hairpin/ cruciform and genetic instability

A hairpin can be formed at one strand of an inverted repeat, whereas a cruciform consists of two hairpin structures, both in each strand at the same position of the DNA (Fig.2)(Courey, 1999). Similarly some tandem arranged trinucleotide repeats such as CAG, CTG, CCG, CGG,

AAT, ATT etc. can also adopt hairpin structures with mismatched base pairs in the stem (McMurray, 1999; Trotta, et al., 2000).
To form a hairpin/cruciform, DNA duplex needs to be unwound in replication, transcription, and/or DNA repair processing; affording single-stranded repeat sequences the opportunity to base pair with itself in an intramolecular fashion. The term of "cruciform" originates from forming two duplex arms, which adopts either an "open" form, allowing strand migration or a "stacked" (locked) form, where the helices stack on each other (Courey, 1999; Khuu et al., 2006; Lilley, 2010). In both cases, the overall conformation and the intraduplex angles behave like the Holliday junction recombination intermediates (Fig.2A) (Courey, 1999; Khuu et al., 2006;; Lilley, 2010).

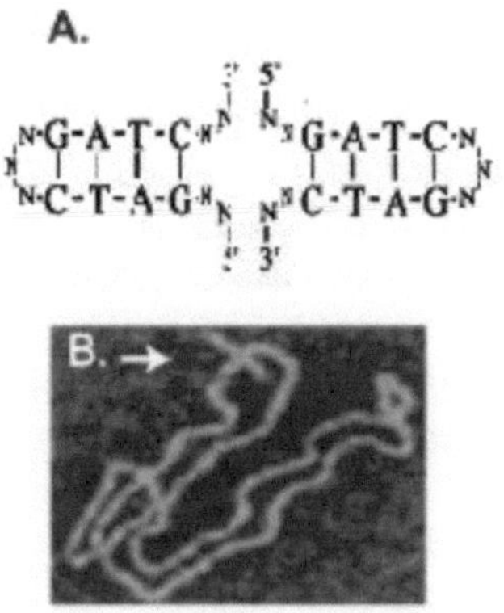

Fig. 2. Hairpin/cruciform of DNA

Both inverted repeats and tandem arranged trinucleotide repeats were found to be mutagenic, causing genomic instability. Inverted repeats were initially found to cause deletions in *E. coli* (Sinden et al., 1991), and then were seen in humans as (8; 22) (q24.13; q11.21), and many types of t (11; 22) translocations. The breakpoints of these translocation mutations were localized at the center of AT-rich palindromic sequences on 11q23 and 22q11, respectively. So far, t (11; 22) is the only known recurrent, non-Robertsonian translocation in humans, in some cases leads to male infertility and recurrent abortion (Kurahashi et al., 2000, 2006, 2010; Kurahashi & Emanuel, 2001). Furthermore, deletions stimulated by a poly (R.Y) sequence from intron 21 of the polycystic kidney disease 1 gene (PKD1) have also been characterized (Bacolla et al., 2001; Patel et al., 2004). And a long $(CCTG\text{-}CAGG)_n$ repeat in *E.coli* was also found to form cruciform (Pluciennik et al., 2002; Dere & Wells, 2006). Interestingly, cruciform-forming inverted repeats have mediated many of the microinversions in evolution that distinguish the human and chimpanzee genomes (Kolb et al., 2009).
In cells, DNA double strand breaks can be derived from cruciform, because hairpin/ cruciform are substrates for several structure-specific nucleases and/ or repair enzymes, such as SbcCD in *E.coli* and Mre11-Rad50 in eukaryotes. The actions of such enzymes make strand breaks, which may result in rearrangements or translocation of chromosomes (Smith, 2008).
In addition, proteins working in nucleotide excisonal repair (NER) can also recognize the helical distortions in hairpin, therefore NER may recognize DNA hairpin to resolve the hairpin in the DNA.

Besides, some other proteins were also found to bind the structural elements in cruciforms. For example, HMG proteins, replication initiation protein RepC, cruciform binding protein CBP, and four-way junction resolvases have all been indentified to bind cruciforms (Pearson et al., 1996; Jin et al., 1997; Novac et al., 2002; Lange et al., 2009; lilley, 2010).

3.4 Z-DNA and genetic instability

Z-DNA can be seen as the high-energy conformers of B-DNA that forms *in vivo* during transcription as a result of torsion strain generated by a moving polymerase (Wang, 1984; Casasnovas & Azorin, 1987; Johnston, 1988; Hebert & Rich, 1996). It has been thoroughly studied since 1957, how a right-handed B-DNA adopting a Z-DNA *in vitro* through "flipping" the base pairs upside down, and rotating every other purine from *anti* to *syn* conformation (Johnston, 1988; Hebert & Rich, 1996). Compared to B-DNA, Z-DNA does not have a major groove, therefore could potentially impact transcription by physically blocking RNA polymerase, or by relaxing negative supercoiling turns, or by acting as an enhancer through recruiting transacting factors.

In Z-DNA, the guanosine nucleotides are in *syn* position where the bases are found over the sugar without protection, thus more accessible to DNA damaging factors, more resistant to processing by DNA repair enzymes. For example, alkylating damage such as N^7-methylguanine, which is typically removed by a DNA glycosylase in B-DNA is not efficiently repaired when present in Z-DNA (Pfohl-Leszkowicz et al., 1983; Boiteux et al., 1985).

Further, DNA sequences with the potential to adopt Z-DNA are associated with recombination hot spots in eukaryotic cells (Wang et al., 2006). A hot spot of 1000 bp in the major histocompatibility complex (MHC) in mice, containing several copies of long GT repeats, may account for up to 2% of the recombination events occurring on the chromosome (Crouau-Roy, 1999). In *E.coli*, the RecA molecules show a much higher binding affinity for Z-DNA than for normal B-DNA and single-stranded DNA, and show a Z-DNA structure-stimulated ATPase activity, implicating a recombination hot spot of Z-DNA in prokaryotes as well. Genetic recombination in Z-DNA can potentially induce deletion instability and/ or produce DNA double-strand breaks. For example, a CG (12) sequence forming Z-DNA induces high levels of genetic instability in both bacterial and mammalian cells (Casasnovas & Azorin, 1987).

Recently, proteins binding Z-DNA are found, including specific proteins, such as Zα domain-containing proteins ADAR1 and ESL, and fairly low specific proteins, such as HMG proteins (Suda et al., 1996; Lange et al., 2009).

3.5 H-DNA and H-DNA induced DSBs and genetic instability

H-DNA, alternatively known as triplex DNA can be classified into either pyrimidine motif or purine motif according to the orientation and composition of the third strand in a triple stranded DNA structure (Fig. 3). The third strand can form either Hoogsteen or reverse-Hoogsteen hydrogen bonds with the purine-rich strand of the duplex DNA. Therefore, the third strand can be both pyrimidine-rich and parallel to the complementary strand (Y* R: Y) or purine-rich and antiparallel to the complementary strand (R* R: Y), producing either pyrimidine motif or purine motif triple stranded DNA (as described previously).

Whereas (R* R: Y) triplexes form under conditions of physiological pH, triplex of the (Y* R: Y) composition form most readily under conditions of acidic pH. At physiological pH, triplex may be stabilized by negative supercoiling, modified with phosphorothioate groups, or polyvalent cations such as spermine and spermidine. For the R* R: Y intramolecular triplexes and T: A* T and C^+: G* C triplets for the Y* R: Y intramolecular triplexes are included since these are considered the most stable triplet combinations.

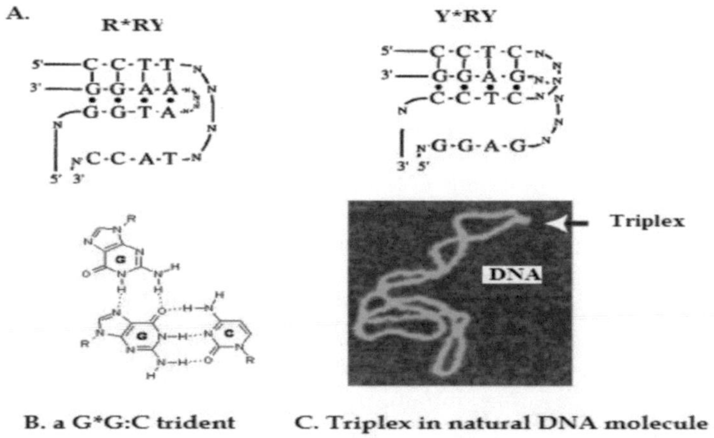

Fig. 3. H-DNA (Star/ Dot marks Hoogsteen hydrogen bonded bases; colon/ line shows Watson–Crick hydrogen bonded bases)

In general, formation of a triplex DNA was a role of sequence, topology (supercoil density), ionic conditions, protein binding, methylation, carcinogen binding, and other factors. Global negative supercoil density acts in concert with local transient waves of topological changes produced by replication or transcription, and both have a critical influence on forming and stabilizing triplex DNA *in vivo*. It has been reported that a higher negative supercoiling destabilized long CTG · CAG, CCG · CGG, and GAA · TTC repeats in *Escherichia coli.* Similarly a 2.5-kb poly (R · Y) tract from the human PKD1 gene lowered the viability of the host cells (Bacolla et al., 2001; Patel et al., 2004).

Several types of DNA damages induced by H-DNA have been reported, including single and/ or double strand breaks. For example, the endogenous H-DNA forming sequences from the human *c-myc* promoter was shown to be intrinsically mutagenic in mammalian cells because of the generation of either single or double strand breaks in the H-DNA, or near the H-DNA locus. Besides, the single-stranded area, or the triplex region is also a target of various nucleases, resulting in single or DSBs formation, and the increased mutagenesis or recombination (Wang & Vasquez, 2006).

Although triplex (H-DNA) DNA occurs mainly at poly (purine·pyrimidine) ($(R \cdot Y)_n$) tracts, it can also be induced to form with the sequence specific DNA recognition and binding of some synthetic triplex-forming oligonucleotides (TFOs) (Casey & Glazer, 2001; Mukherjee & Vasquez, 2011). TFOs bind to the major groove of homopurine-homopyrimidine stretches of double-stranded DNA to induce forming the triplex (Casey & Glazer, 2001; Mukherjee & Vasquez, 2011). During which the duplex DNA may have to undergo helical distortions on TFO binding and the distortions trigger endogenous recombination and repair mechanisms in the cell (Raghavan et al., 2004, 2005).

Indeed it has been reported that formation of TFO-induced triplex can induce sequence-specific DNA damages both in cells and in animals (Chan, et al., 1999; Kalish et al., 2005).

However, mismatch repair proteins are not involved in this TFO-induced mutagenesis. Several reports have now shown that cells that are deficient in the MutS and MutL homologues MSH2, MLH1, MSH3, or MSH6, do not show any change in TFO-induced mutagenesis. In contrasts, NER factors can recognize the intermolecular triplex at least in part. Therefore NER was involved in the triplex-induced mutagenesis and recombination in cells. For example, in *E.coli*, NER proteins, such as UvrB and UvrC, were necessary for H-DNA-induced cell growth retardation and cell lysis, similarly, recombination induced by TFOs depends also on the NER pathway (Faruqi et al., 2000).

3.6 G-tetraduplex and genetic instability

G-quadruplexes are higher-order DNA or RNA structures formed from G-rich DNA or RNA sequences that are built around tetrads of hydrogen-bonded guanine bases (Lipps & Rhodes, 2009; Sannohe & Sugiyama, 2010). Despite the wide prevalence of genomic sequences that have G-rich property and that can potentially fold into tetraplex / quadruplexes structures, a direct demonstration of their existence *in vivo* proved to be a difficult undertaking. Only recently has there evidence started to increase for their presence and role *in vivo* (Lipps & Rhodes, 2009), since most of the tetraplex/ quadruplexes forming sequences are fairly short and quadruplexes are likely to be transiently formed. G-quadruplexes (tetraduplex) may have several isomers which can be formed intramolecularly and intermolecularly (Fig. 4).

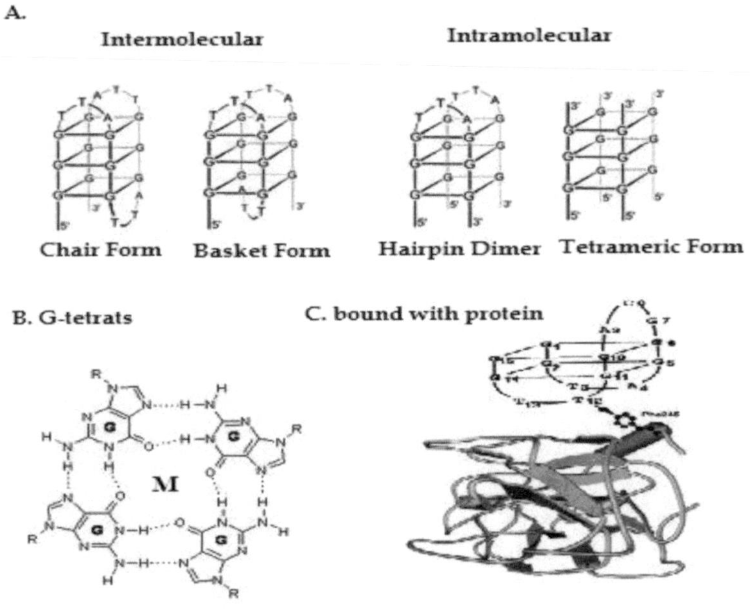

Fig. 4. Tetraplex DNA

Recent progress of the related studies revealed that G-quadruple could provide a nucleic acid based mechanism, such as regulating telomere maintenance, transcription, replication as well as translation. In the same time, various G-quadruplexes binding proteins, such as, a G4 quadruplex and purine Motif triplex nucleic acid-binding protein have also been characterized (Dyke et al.,2004), many others have been summarized in the reference (Fry, 2007).
The existence of cellular proteins that preferentially interact with tetraplex DNA provides a strong argument for the existence of quadruplex formations in genomic DNA.

3.7 Unwound DNA

Unwound DNA is known to be formed by A+T -rich sequences (Fig. 5). Since A · T base pairs contain two hydrogen bonds and C · G base pairs contain three, A · T-rich tracts are less thermally stable than C · G -rich tracts in DNA. In the presence of superhelical energy, A+T -rich regions can unwind and remain unwound under conditions normally found in the cell. Such sites often provide places for DNA replication proteins to enter DNA to begin the chromosome duplication. Unwound DNA can therefore be alternatively called as DNA unwinding elements (DUEs) that have been identified in both prokaryotic and eukaryotic DNA sequences. DUEs are AT-rich sequences about 30-100 bp long. They share little sequence similarity except for being AT-rich. Under torsion stress, unwinding of the double helix occurs first in AT-rich sequences; therefore, DUEs can be maintained as unpaired DNA regions in the presence of negative supercoiling. The single-stranded area of the unwound structure may be target of nuclease activity resulting in single or DSBs, leading to enhanced mutagenesis or recombination.

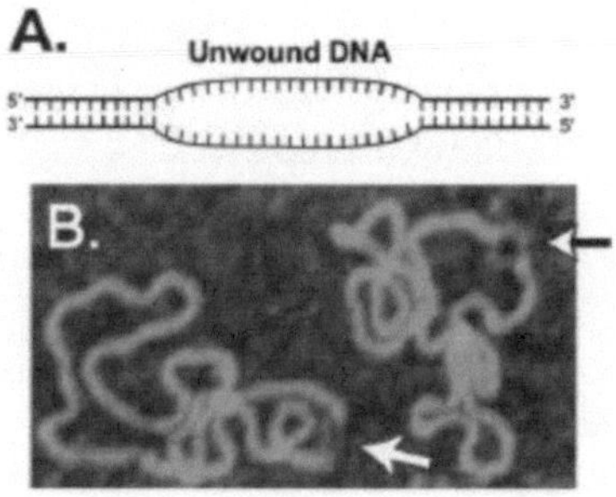

Fig. 5. Unwound DNA

3.8 Curved DNA

Normally, curved DNA is often seen in DNA segment containing runs of three or four bases of A in one strand and a similar run of T in the other and spaced at 10-base pair intervals. Interestingly we have recently found that trinucleotide repeats AAT can also adopt curved DNA in *E.coli*, which can be repressed by H-NS and its stimulated IS1E transposition (Pan et al., 2010)

4. Biological significance of DNA abnormal folding

Apart from the roles in DNA replication, transcription and gene regulation, non-B DNA may also lead to gene instability, including chromosomal translocation, deletion and amplification in cancer and other human diseases (Bacolla & Wells, 2009; Chen et al., 2010). Since non-B DNA abnormal folds have been addressed with generating DNA breaks, including both single and double strand DNA breaks. Non-B DNA structures recruit DNA repair machinery to the breaking sites, which then make gene mutations and chromosomal rearrangements during repair.

4.1 Effects of non-B DNA structures on DNA replication / transcription

Some regions of DNA forming non-B DNA structures in replication or transcription, which may turn to affect the DNA transactions (Van Holde & Zlatanova, 1994; Samadashwily et al., 1997; Krasilnikova et al., 2004; Lin et al., 2006; Mirkin & Mirkin, 2007)

One of the well-studied effects of the non-B structures on replication is a block to polymerases because of template folding, which was shown for cruciforms/ hairpins and H-DNA (Samadashwily et al., 1997; Krasilnikova et al., 2004; Voineaqu et al., 2009).
It has been found that triplex DNA can adversely affect DNA replication and potentially lead to replication fork collapse (Samadashwily et al., 1997; Krasilnikova et al., 2004; Voineaqu et al., 2009). The polypurine strand of a triplex forming duplex may not be a potential template, therefore giving increased chance of being single stranded, and forming intermolecular or intramolecular triplex (Hile & Eckert, 2004; Urban et al.,2010). Besides,a non-B DNA structure itself may also directly slow the progression of replication fork (Samadashwily et al., 1997; Mirkin & Mirkin, 2007; Trinh & Sinden, 1991). Such non-B DNA structures may be an obstacle to fork progression or a target for nucleolytic attack, thus allowing DNA breakage leading to deletion or recombination (Mirkin, 2006; Kim et al., 2006).
In contrast, the single-stranded parts in a cruciform or H-DNA may serve as the recognition elements for replication initiation proteins. For example, cruciform binding proteins (CBP), such as 14-3-3sigma in HeLa cells recruits replication proteins to a cruciform to start replication (Alvarez et al., 2002; Novac et al., 2002). Therefore, it is possible for a hairpin/cruciform DNA sequence behaves like a replication "origin", inducing an origin independent DNA replication. The similar way of DNA replication has been found in *E.coli* and named as stable DNA replication. More interestingly, the origin independent DNA replication has also been proposed as a mechanism for the production of expanded DNA repeats (Pan 2006).
In addition, certain non-B DNA structures can also interfere with RNA transcription and recombination (Van Holde & Zlatanova, 1994; Broxson et al., 2011). Similarly RNA transcription can also promote forming non-B DNA structures, including hairpin, triplexs and G_4DNA (Van Holde & Zlatanova, 1994; Broxson et al., 2011).

4.2 Modulation of supercoiling and promoting transcription

The extent of supercoiling in a DNA segment is known to affect transcription, recombination, and replication such that an ideal DNA topology may be critical for them. It has been found that formation of cruciforms, Z-DNA and H-DNA caused partial relaxation of excessive superhelicity in a topological domain. Specific cases of DNA replication and gene expression have also been described as superhelicity dependent events induced by formation of cruciforms, Z-DNA and H-DNA.

4.3 Accumulation of DNA Damages causing increased mutability within non-B DNA structure forming sequences or their flanking sequences

DNA sequences that are prone to adopting non-B DNA secondary structures are associated with hot spots of genomic instability, where repeat expansions, chromosomal fragility, or gross chromosomal rearrangements can be often seen. For example, long repeating tracts of CTG · CAG, CCTG · CAGG, and GAA · TTC are associated with the etiology of myotonic dystrophy type 1 (DM1), type 2(DM2), and Friedreich's ataxia (FRDA) (Wells, 2007). The repeating sequences involved have potentials to adopt a variety of non-B DNA secondary structures (McMurray, 1999; Pan, 2004, 2006, 2009). Studies in various model systems, including *Escherichia coli* and mammalian cell lines, such as COS-7, CV-1, and HEK-293, have revealed that conditions promoting formation of non-B DNA structures enhanced the repeats instabilities. Such instabilities can occur both within the repeat sequences and in the flanking sequences of up to ~4 kbp (Wojciechowska et al., 2006).

Indeed, it has been found that DNA double-stranded breaks (DSBs) can sometimes be accumulated at or around the repeating sequences, and error-prone repair pathways were also proposed to be involved in forming gross DNA rearrangements (Kurahashi et al., 2006). Moreover, DNA breaks may also happen in the single-stranded area, or the structured region when they serve as targets of nuclease activity, leading to enhanced mutagenesis or recombination. The breakpoints of the disease-causing translocation cluster within a 150-bp genomic region of the *bcl-2* gene were seen potentially form a triplex DNA structure (Adachi & Tsujimoto, 1990; Raghavan et al., 2004, 2005).

It has long been found that, the efficacies of DNA replication in the leading and lagging strand templates were differently performed in *E. coli* chromosome. Replication errors and SOS mutator effects occurred preferentially in the lagging strand, while intermolecular strand switch events during DNA replication occurred preferentially in the leading strand (Iwaki et al., 1995; Trinh & Sinden, 1995; Iwaki et al., 1996; Fijalkowska et al., 1998; Sinden et al., 1999; Maliszewska-Tkaczyk, 2002; Gawel et al., 2002; Hashem & Sinden, 2005). Similarly, unequal fidelities have also been found with deletions between direct repeats in the leading strand template (Hashem & Sinden, 2005). This may attribute to potential of non-B DNA structure formation in the leading and lagging strand template in DNA replication. Similarly, the replication fidelities of various inverted repeats, direct repeats, including trinucleotide repeats can also be compromised if they adopt non-B DNA conformations, such as hairpin, cruciform, triplex, tetra-duplex DNA, leading potentially to mutations or rearrangements (Pan & Leach, 2000; Sinden et al., 2002).

4.4 Nucleosome exclusion

In eukaryotes, chromosomal DNA wrapping around histones in nucleosomes interferes with the protein binding to promoters and origins of replication. Nucleosome formations, on one hand, and formation of cruciform, Z-DNA and triplex DNA, on the other hand, are mutually exclusive. Thus, the alternative structure-forming DNA sequences may expose nucleosome-free DNA, making them accessible to transcription, replication, recombination proteins as well as nucleases, producing fragile sites in chromosome (chwartz et al., 2006; Lukusa & Fryns, 2008).

Fragile sites are specific loci that appear as constrictions, gaps, or breaks on chromosomes from cells exposed to partial inhibition of DNA replication (Schwartz et al., 2006; Lukusa & Fryns, 2008). In chromosomal level, fragile sites always lack nucleosomes, and sometimes can be associated with trinucleotide repeats (TNRs) of CGG · CCG, CAG · CTG, GAA · TTC and GCN · NGC, with specific G-rich tetra- to dodecanucleotide repeats or with long AT-rich repeats, such as the 33 or 42 minisatellites in the FRA16B and FRA10B common fragile sites (Wang & Griffith, 1996). In the same time, fragile sites can be classified as rare or common, depending on their frequency within the population and their specific mode of induction. So far, there are more than 89 common fragile sites listed in GDB (Gene Databases), which are considered to be an intrinsic part of the chromosomal structure presented in all individuals. Six common fragile sites have been cloned and characterized, including FRA3B (Huebner & Croce, 2001; Lettessier et al., 2011), FRA7G, FRA7H, FRA16D (Shah et al., 2010), FRAXB , and FRA6F. Common fragile site instability was attributed to the fact that they contain sequences prone to form secondary structures that may impair replication fork movement, possibly leading to fork collapse and resulting in DNA breaks.

Most rare fragile sites are induced by folate shortage, and others are induced by DNA minor groove binders. So far, seven folate sensitive (FRA10A, FRA11B, FRA12A, FRA16A, FRAXA,

FRAXE and FRAXF) and two nonfolate sensitive (FRA10B and FRA16B) fragile sites have been molecularly characterized. Interestingly, almost all these fragile sites are found to have expanded DNA repeats resulting from mutation involving the normally occurring polymorphic CCG/CGG trinucleotide repeats and AT-rich minisatellite repeats (Balakumaran et al., 2000; Voineagu et al., 2009).

The expanded repeats were also demonstrated to have the potentials, at least under certain circumstances, to form stable secondary non-B DNA structures, including intrastrand hairpins, slipped strand DNA or tetrahelical structures, or to present flexible repeat sequences. Both of which are expected to affect the replication. In addition, these DNA sequences are also found to decrease the efficiency of nucleosome assembly, resulting in decondensation defects seen as fragile sites (Wang & Griffith, 1996; Freudenreich, 2007).

5. Genes and gene products that are involved in abnormal folding

A numerous proteins that interact with non-B DNA secondary structures have been characterized recently. These proteins may also be called as DNA structure-specific proteins, such as Rad1, Rad2, Rad10, Msh2, Msh3, BLM, WRN and Sgs1 (Bhattacharyya & Lahue, 2004; Nag & Cavallo, 2007; Kantelinen et al., 2010; Pichierri et al., 2011). These DNA structure-specific proteins can be further classified by function into several distinct groups, depending on their possible effects on the formation/ stability of non-B DNA structure. Some of the binding proteins may increase the stability of the bound non-B DNA secondary structures; and some may promote forming non-B DNA secondary structures; or destabilize non-B DNA secondary structures. Indeed, the available data implicate various proteins participating in mismatch repair, nucleotide excision repair, base excision repair, homologous recombination, recognize non-B DNA secondary structures in trying to avoid "so called" structure-directed mutagenesis.

As discussed previously, DNA structures can often induce DNA mutations. This DNA structure mediated mutagenesis may be because of the following reasons: the abnormal positioning of the bases and sugar in non-B DNA conformations, which impact the function of some DNA repair proteins on damaged DNA. For example, alkylating damage such as N^7-methylguanine or O^6-methylguanine is not repaired as efficiently in Z-DNA as it is in B-DNA. Alternatively, forming DNA secondary structures near DNA damage sites might influence the damage repair processing, depending on the types of damages, the environments, and the nature of the secondary structures (Pfohl-Leszkowicz et al., 1983; Boiteux et al., 1985).

5.1 MMR proteins

It has long been studied that MMR deficiency is associated with microsatellite sequence instability and human disease. For example, the instability of TNRs and AT-rich minisatellites is associated with their capacity of adopting unusual secondary structures, such as hairpins or DNA triplexes. This feature is common to different types of repeated DNA. Therefore, repeat instability is dependent on MMR in mice and yeast, consistent with the observation that sequences at repetitive DNA sites form short hairpins or small loops that are targets of the Msh2–Msh6 MMR (Modrich, 2006).

MMR proteins bind to non-B DNA secondary structures mainly through its capacity of recognizing mismatched base pairs. It has been found that MMR binds mismatches in a CNG triplet repeats hairpin stem. Although the MSH2–MSH3 complex of MMR also binds perfect hairpin formed by inverted repeats (lacking mismatched regions), affinity is low, suggesting that mismatches are important for the MMR protein binding (Kantelinen et al., 2008). In addition, MutS has also been reported to bind parallel G4 DNA in humans (Fry, 2007).

5.2 NER and HR proteins

NER proteins, such as the UvrB and UvrC in *E.coli*, and the XPA, XPG, XPC in eukaryotes and homologous recombination proteins, such as RecA, HsRad51, were found to be involved in H-DNA mediated repair and recombination (Bacolla et al., 2001). UvrB and UvrC may preferentially recognize the helical distortions, while RecA recognizing single stranded DNA region in an H-DNA.

5.3 Helicases and junction resolvases

Proteins that preferentially catalyze the unwinding of DNA non-B DNA secondary structures are DNA helicases in ATP-hydrolysis dependent manner. Helicases are DNA unwinding enzymes that preferentially melt some of the non-B DNA structures. The selectivity of helicases on non-B DNA secondary structures has been identified in simian virus 40 (SV40), yeast and human cells. The most studied helicases are members of RecQ family, whose roles are found in a broad range of organisms from *E. coli* RecQ to humans WRN, BLM and RecQL4 (Mohaghegh et al., 2001; Bachrati & Hickson, 2003; Cobb & Bjergbaek, 2006; Masai, 2011). All the non-B DNA secondary structure unwinding helicases act catalytically and all require for their hydrolysis of nucleotide triphosphate, normally ATP, and the presence of Mg^{2+} ions. For example, G-quadruplex DNA substrates are unwound by RecQ helicase with a 3'→5' polarity and need the tetraplex to hold a short 3' single-stranded tail that serves as a "loading dock" for these enzymes (Jain et al., 2010). It should be emphasized, however, that none of the described helicases unwinds tetraplex DNA only and all the enzymes are also able to unfold, although at a lower efficiency, other DNA structures such as duplex DNA, Holliday junctions or triplex. Recently, DHX9 helicase from human cells was found to co-immunoprecipitate with triplex DNA, suggesting a role in maintaining genome stability (Jain et al., 2010). DHX9 displaced the third strand from a specific triplex DNA and catalyzed the unwinding with a 3′ to 5′ polarity for the displaced third strand ((Jain et al., 2010).

5.3.1 RecQ helicases BLM, WRN, RECQL4 and Sgs1

RecQ helicases are a group of DNA helicases that are conserved from bacteria to man (Bachrati & Hickson, 2003). *Rec*Q helicase is named after the *rec*Q gene of *Escherichia coli* and has the activity of unwinding DNA in the 3′–5′ direction in relation to the DNA strand in which the enzyme is bound (Mohaghegh et al., 2001). There are at least five homologues in humans, three of which are associated with genetic diseases. The yeast homologue of RecQ is Sgs1, whose function was found to be similar to most of the members in the RecQ family (Bachrati & Hickson, 2003; Cejka & Kowalczykowski, 2010; Masai, 2011).
It has been reported that, without a functional RecQ helicase, DNA replication does not advance normally. In humans, lacking of WRN or BLM protein accumulates aberrant replication intermediates (Harrigan et al., 2003; Cheok et al., 2005), this may allow for certain non-B DNA structure forming (Mohaghegh et al., 2001; Bacolla et al., 2011). Therefore, it is not surprising to see that more and more reports are going to be published

which specify the important roles of RecQ in resolving the non-B DNA structures, including those G4-DNA (Kamath-Loeb et al., 2001; Fry & loeb, 1999). Similarly the large T antigen and Dna2 helicase/ exonuclease have also been found to unwind the G-tetraduplex (Masuda-Sasa et al., 2008).

5.3.2 Junction resolvases

A cruciform is similar in appearance to a recombination intermediate, a four-way Holliday junction. Therefore, Holliday junction resolvases, RuvABC in prokaryotes, or Mus81, Sgs1 and Sgs2 in yeast might also have activity on cruciforms formed at inverted repeats (Cejka & Kowalczykowski, 2010; Lilley, 2010; Ashton et al., 2011; Mankouri et al., 2011),.

5.4 Topoisomerase

Non-B DNA structures can be substrates for DNA topoisomerase I and II (Howard et al., 1993; Froelich-Ammon et al., 1994). It has shown that DNA topoisomerase II binds and cleaves hairpins (e.g., hairpin formed at a negatively supercoiled 52-bp palindromic sequence in the human β-globin gene), but not cruciforms. DNA topoisomerase II cleavage sites near human immunodeficiency virus integration sites in the human genome consist of Z-DNA forming sequences and other repetitive sequence (Howard et al., 1993); in contrast, DNA topoisomerase I promotes forming parallel G4 DNA in humans. Similarly RAP1, Hop1 in yeast, and Thrombin in humans are also found to promote form of G4 DNA.

5.5 Single strand binding protein (SSB/RPA)

RPA–ssDNA serves as intermediate in many DNA repair processes. For example, ssDNA-RPA can be made through nuclease and helicase actions in repair of UV-induced thymine dimers by nucleotide excision repair, and in a replication fork where DNA polymerase is paused but without pausing DNA helicase accompanied. RPA may prevent or destabilize a non-B DNA structure formation. For example, RPA in humans has been found to destabilize a G′4 DNA (Fig. 1). As for a triplex, the polypyrimidine strands are preferred to bind with RPA, which will then form complex with XPA, XPC-hHR23B (Vasquez et al., 2002; Thomas et al., 2005). In mammalian cells, RPA binds 50-fold more strongly to pyrimidines than to purines, therefore, makes the polypyrimidine strand single-stranded in an intramolecular triplex structure at neutral pH. Moreover, persistent RPA binding may lead to RPA hyper-phosphorylation that triggers repair reactions (Thomas et al., 2005). In addition, RPA-ssDNA and an ssDNA–dsDNA junction can also act as initial signals for cells response to DNA damages, which activates the ATR pathway (Ball et al., 2004; Choi et al., 2010) .

5.6 DNA structure-specific nucleases

Proteins consist of nucleases that specifically cleave DNA next to or within a non-B DNA secondary structures have been well studied. The earliest protein having such functions was identified in *Saccharomyces cerevisiae*, the gene *KEM*1 (also called SEP1, DST2, XRN1 and RAR5) (Liu et al., 1994, 1995). *KEM*1 was initially characterized as a telomere binding protein, and later, it was found to cleave DNA that includes a four-stranded G4 domain but show low or no nucleolytic activity toward single- or double-stranded DNA substrates. Other well-known DNA structure specific nucleases are SbcCD (Connelly & Leach, 1992,

1996, 2004; Connelly et al., 1998, 1999) and its eukaryotic homologue of Mre11-Rad50 (Paull & Gellert, 1998, 2000; Sonoda et al., 2006; Carter et al., 2007; Delmas et al., 2009).

5.6.1 SbcCD

It is now known that influences of repetitive DNA sequences on genomic instabilities were often attributable to forming non-B DNA secondary structures *in vivo*. Once a non-B DNA structure is stable, which will interfere with DNA replication, repair and/ or transcription *in vivo*, resulting in unstable genome. These deleterious non-B DNA secondary structures have already been found to form in *E.coli*, such as the large hairpin formed by the long palindrome DNA sequences (Leach, 1994). The stable hairpin can be cleaved by SbcCD, leading to forming DNA double strand breaks, and then be repaired by using homologous recombination (Connelly & Leach, 1996,; Connelly et al., 1992, 1998, 1999).

Long palindrome sequences are significantly more stable in nuclease-deficient (SbcCD) strains of *E. coli* than in wild-type strains. The SbcCD protein complex is a member of the structural maintenance of chromosomes (SMCs) family found in bacteriophage, bacteria, yeast, *Drosophila*, mouse, and human. SbcCD has both 3′–5′ exonuclease activity on double-stranded DNA and endonuclease activity on single-stranded DNA (Connelly et al., 1999). *In vitro*, it can recognize and bind hairpin structures and cleave at the loop, 5′ immediately next to the loop/ stem junction.

Further degradation of the hairpin cleavage products can occur by the ATP-dependent double-stranded DNA exonuclease activity of the SbcCD protein complex. This structure-specific endonuclease activity does not need a 3′ or 5′ terminus (Connelly & Leach, 1992, 1996; Connelly et al., 1998, 1999).

5.6.2 Mre11-Rad50-Nbs1 (MRN) / Mre11-Rad50-Xrs2 (MRX)

Rad50 and Mre11 are the eukaryotic homologues of SbcCD that have not been shown to bind hairpin/cruciform directly. Mre11 and Rad50, forming complex with Nbs1 (in human cells) or Xrs2 (in yeast), show a hairpin structure cleaving activity *in vitro*. And which participate in processing double strand breaks *in vivo* by homologous recombination or non-homologous end-joining (Paull & Gellert, 1998, 2000; Sonoda et al., 2006; Delmas et al., 2009). In hairpin cleavage, MRN/ MRX interacts with BRCA1 which preferentially binds four-way branched DNA, similar to cruciforms. Mre11 shows an incision activity at hairpin/ cruciform, and acts as a selective endonuclease in yeast to bind to G4 DNA or to G'2 quadruplex DNA and cleaves the G4 DNA.

5.6.3 other nucleases

Besides the DNA structure specific nucleases such as SbcCD and its eukaryotic homologue Mre11-Rad50-Nbs1 (Xrs1), many other DNA structure-specific DNA nucleases have also been determined. These nucleases recognize and cleave the non-B DNA structures or even the DNA sequences that have non-B DNA secondary structures adopted, playing important roles in various DNA transactions including DNA replication, repair and recombination. For example, Rad1-Rad10 (XPF or ERCC1) has shown to cleave branched intermediates/ Flapped DNA in repair (Li et al., 2008; Muñoz et al., 2009). And Rad2 family of nucleases, such as human XPG (Class I), FEN1 (Class II), and HEX1/ hEXO1 (Class III), have shown both substrate specific 5' to 3' exonuclease activity and endonuclease activity in repair, recombination, and/ or replication. Among them, Rad2 domain of human exonuclease 1

(HEX1-N2) has high activity on single- and double-stranded DNA substrates as well as a flap structure-specific endonuclease activity but does not have specific endonuclease activity at 10-base pair bubble-like structures, G:T mismatches, or uracil residues (Lee & Wilson, 1999). FEN-1, a structure-specific endonuclease is essential for DNA replication and repair, removes RNA and DNA 5' flaps (Tsutakawa et al., 2011). FEN-1 was thought to be involved in hairpin structure processing, and was found to be involved in CNG triplet repeat stability in the lagging strand template (Spiro et al., 1999; Singh et al., 2007). Similarly, Deletions in PCNA, RPA, and the Bloom protein (BLM), a 3′-5′ helicase can also increase CNG repeat expansion or deletion, which reportedly interacts with FEN-1 in cleaving flaps. Recently NucS from *Pyrococcus abyssi* was found to be the equivalent of FEN-1 that cleaves the flapped DNA in Okazaki frangment processing in the lagging strand DNA replication (Ren et al., 2009; Creze et al., 2011).

SLX1 and SLX4 are other structure-specific endonucleases acting as heteromer that cleave branched DNA substrates, particularly simple-Y, 5'-flap, or replication fork structures. It also cleaves the strand bearing the 5' nonhomologous arm at the branch junction and generates ligatable nicked products from 5'-flap or replication fork substrates (Fricke & Brill, 2003).

RAGs is a complex consisting of RAG1, RAG2, and HMGB1 that cleaves 3′ overhangs in multiple locations at the duplex/ single-stranded transitions (Fugmann, 2001). RAGs complex is able to cleave different non-B DNA structures such as symmetric bubbles, heterologous loops and proposed triplex DNA. For example, RAGs complex cleaves the *bcl-2* Mbr at 3′ overhang and non-B DNA structures under physiological buffer conditions (Adachi & Tsujimoto, 1990; Fugmann, 2001; Raghavan et al., 2004, 2005).

In addition, many single-strand specific nucleases, like S1, P1, and mung bean nucleases, are also efficient at cleaving single stranded DNA in the non-B DNA structures, though at low pH. Since some non-B DNA structures, e.g. H-DNA and G4 DNA disclose an unstructured single-stranded DNA region, which therefore serve as substrates for those single-strand specific nucleases. Recently, a more specific nuclease that cuts single-stranded DNA 5' to a G4 domain was isolated from human cells. This enzyme, initially named G quartet nuclease 1 (GQN1) is thought to be involved in immunoglobulin heavy chain class switch recombination in B cells, does not digest single- or double-stranded DNA, Holliday junctions or tetraplex RNA. It specifically cuts single-stranded DNA located few nucleotides 5' to either G'2 or G4 domains (Sun et al., 2001). However, GQN1 cannot incise tetraplex RNA, showing a significant difference from a mouse cytoplasmic exoribonuclease (mXRN1p) which cleaves G4 RNA (Bashkirov et al., 1997).

6. Gratuitous repair on undamaged DNA misfolds by multiple proteins

DNA damage and repair are always active in living cells regardless of the proliferation status of the cells. And unpaired bases and the helix distortions/ junctions in most of the non-B DNA secondary structures can therefore be targets for the structure specific proteins working in DNA repair, e.g. mismatch repair, nucleotide excision repair etc., launching DNA repairs or activating checkpoints repair (Voineagu et al., 2009).

6.1 Repair by singular pathway of DNA repair

Small DNA loops/ bulges, triplex DNA may be readily corrected by an individual repair, such as a mismatch repair or a nucleotide excision repair. For example, helix distortion and/ or mismatched base pairs in a hairpin, which sometime also occurs with imperfect hairpin structures at CAG repeats, can be recognized by mismatch repair machinery (Yang, 2006). Msh2/ Msh3 complex in eukaryotic cells specifically binds CAG-hairpins, and the ATP-ase activity of the Msh2 / Msh3 complex can be altered by the binding. However, the repair is dependent on the number of loops/ bulges. A few of them may be repaired by MMR, but too many may not because of interfering MMR by multiple MutS binding, suggesting that repair on a particular non-B DNA conformation will be conditional, depending on locations and environments. Further, nucleotide excision repair (NER) proteins can bind intermolecular triplex, which are involved in the triplex mediated mutagenesis and recombination (Wang & Vasquez, 2006). In bacterial cells, NER proteins UvrB and UvrC were responsible for triplex-induced cell growth retardation. Given the likenesses of the intermolecular and intramolecular triplex, it is possible for NER contributing to the H-DNA-induced mutagenesis and recombination.

6.2 Competitions among multiple repair proteins

Apart from initiating an individual pathway of DNA repair, some non-B DNA structures can also be recognized by more than one repair proteins working in different repair pathways, resulting in competitions between proteins on same DNA structures.

Competition of repair proteins on a non-B DNA structure may be needed for a cooperative repair, setting up a cooperative new DNA repair to repair; in contrast, the competition may sometimes be internecine, failing in repair of either pathway. Under this circumstance, the repair on a non-B DNA structure by the compositing actions of the DNA structural recognition proteins would be compromised. For example, a stable hairpin may be needed for starting DNA replication, but such a stable hairpin would also be repaired by SbcCD or Mre11-Rad50, making a DNA break for homologous recombination to repair (Leach, 1994). Similarly, unwound DNA or small DNA loops may also be needed for DNA replication or for transcription. While they may also be recognized and bound by repair proteins, such as DNA mismatch and nucleotide-excision repair proteins, recombination proteins, instead of SSB/ RPA (Kirkpatrick & Petes, 1997).

A good demonstration for the internecine competition between multiple repair proteins was the foldings of TGG and AGG repeats in the lagging strand template in a replication fork (Pan & Leach, 2000; Pan et al., to be published results). TGG, AGG and CGG repeats are a group of NGG repeats which own significant potential of folding into non-B DNA secondary structures (Usdin, 1998; Pan & Leach, 2000). AGG repeats formed triplex (Suda et al., 1996; Mishima et al., 1996, 1997), homoduplex (Suda et al.,1995), tetra-duplex (Yang & Hurley, 2006), and a special G-quadruplex, known as tetrad:heptad:heptad:tetrad ((G:H:H:G) or (T:H:H:T)) (Matsugami et al., 2001a, 2001b, 2002, 2003), while CGG and TGG repeats formed pseudo-hairpin and tetra-duplex, respectively (Darlow & Leach, 1998; Usdin, 1998; Pan & Leach, 2000; Zemánek et al., 2005).

It was shown by Pan and Leach, that replication of TGG repeats in the lagging strand template experiences repeats misfolding, during which both MutS and SbcCD were found to affect the later processing by homologous recombination. Binding MutS to the non-B DNA structure formed by TGG repeats may stabilize the structure, while hindering SbcCD cleaving the structure. Interestingly, the roles of MutS and SbcCD in this case seemed complex, since TGG repeats can replicate either without MutS or SbcCD, suggesting that they also play same role in stabilizing the TGG repeat structure. In contrast, similar sized AGG repeats was found also to fold into non-B DNA structures in a similar lagging strand template of a replication fork.

However, the non-B DNA structure formed by AGG repeats was found to be incapable of binding with MutS protein, and being cleaved by SbcCD. This made consistence with the reports though AGG repeats belong to a same group of NGG trinucleotide repeats with TGG repeats, they form various G-rich DNA secondary structures, including quadruplex, triple helical, homoduplex and tetrad:heptad:heptad:tetrad ((G:H:H:G) or (T:H:H:T)). Obviously, some of these non-B DNA structures folded may not be recognized by MutS protein *in vivo*, making significant differences in DNA structure formation between AGG repeats and TGG repeats (Pan et al., unpublished results).

The examples of a coordinated repair by different repair proteins on the same non-B DNA structures are the repair of DNA loops by MMR and NER proteins (Kirkpatrick & Petes, 1997; Zhao et al., 2009, 2010). It has been found that both MSH2 and XPA proteins are involved in the instabilities of CAG repeats, possibly through some so far unidentified roles (Kirkpatrick & Petes, 1997; Lin & Wilson, 2009; Zhao etal., 2009, 2010). Knocking down both MSH2 and XPA proteins did not further reduce CAG repeat contraction, suggesting a new role for these proteins in the same pathway. Similarly, it has also been reported the MSH2 and XPA are also involved in H-DNA metabolism but once again the DNA structure may not be processed via canonical MMR or NER mechanisms (Zhao et al., 2009, 2010).

6.3 Repair proteins can be defeated by DNA secondary structure

It may be feasible by postulating that more non-B DNA structures might be formed by DNA sequences in the genomes. However the repair machinery in the cells may only be limited to a few types, such as those MMR, NER single / double strand breaks etc. It therefore raises a question as if all non-B DNA structures possibly form could be recognized and processed by those repair proteins? The answer to this question is presently unknown; however some of the known secondary structures cannot easily be repaired, including large DNA loops and the flapped DNA etc.

6.3.1 Large loops

Stable base pairing prevents recognition by repair enzymes of bases or junctions requiring repair. For example, in *E.coli*, small loops (or secondary structure) may allow mispairing of bases that are corrected by MMR enzymes, leading to loss of base interruption (Parker & Marinus, 1992; Carraway & Marinus, 1993). However, DNA loops made up of less than four unpaired bases are efficiently corrected by methyl-directed mismatch repair (MMR), but loops larger than that cannot be repaired effectively (Parker & Marinus, 1992; Carraway & Marinus, 1993; Fang et al., 2003). The reason for this inefficacy was found to be due to the failure in loop recognition using MutS proteins, leaving the large looped DNA unrepaired by MMR.

6.3.2 Flapped DNA

Flap endonuclease (RAD27 in *Saccharomyces cerevesiae*; FEN-1 in humans) can destabilize simple tandem repeat loci. The 5′ to 3′ flap endonuclease FEN-1/ RAD27 is a structure-specific nuclease required for Okazaki fragment processing in the lagging strand DNA replication. FEN-1, a structure-specific endonuclease is also thought to be involved in CNG triplet repeat stability. It has been reported that a stable hairpin formed by CTG or CAG repeats at the flap region can block the activity of FEN-1. Which then join the upstream Okazaki fragment, resulting in repeats expansion during the next cycle of replication, marking the activity of FEN-1 can be defeated by stable DNA structure (Spiro et al., 1999; Singh et al., 2007).

6.4 Cellular response to non-B DNA structures by activating checkpoints

The existence of cellular proteins that interact with non-B DNA structures provides both strong argument for the existence of non-B DNA structure formations in genomic DNA, and suggestion for cell having intrinsic response to the formation of non-B DNA structures. However, it seems that not all non-B DNA secondary structures, unless they make severe troublesome to DNA metabolism such as making DNA double strand breaks, or generating long single stranded region, were recognized as "DNA damage". Even if cruciforms / hairpins, triplexes, slipped conformations, quadruplexes, and left-handed Z-DNA have all been reported to be chromosomal targets for DNA repair, recombination, and aberrant DNA synthesis, leading to repeat expansion or genomic rearrangements associated with neurodegenerative and genomic disorders. Some of them may also raise more severe response by cells (Voineagu et al., 2009).

The situations for a non-B DNA secondary structure intriguing a cellular response may be addressed at the competing recognition and processing by multiple repair proteins, resulting in incomplete / partial / opposing processing of the non-B DNA structure. Such intermediates may be recognized by proteins capable of activating a cellular response. Alternatively non-B DNA structure bears components that can be recognized by proteins capable of activating a cellular response (Voineagu et al., 2009). In support of this idea, DNA structure-specific proteins Rad1, Msh2, Msh3, and Sgs1 were found to play opposite roles in yeast gene targeting, a triple stranded DNA mediated process. During which Rad1, Msh2, and Msh3 facilitated forming triplex DNA, while Sgs1 prevented forming triplex DNA (Langston & Symington, 2005), therefore should a cellular response be intrigued in gene targeting may have to wait for processing the structure-specific proteins.

The ssDNA region in a non-B DNA structure may likely be coated by single-stranded DNA-binding protein (RPA) directly, or RPA coats the ssDNA after the non-B DNA structure is processed. Either way makes a common intermediate of ssDNA-RPA that activates ATR signaling in response to all of the genotoxic lesions (Krejci et al., 2003; Hu et al., 2007). Indeed, the ssDNA-RPA complex has been found to be a common intermediate in the processing of many types of damaged DNA, including DSBs, UV-induced thymidine dimers, intrastrand cross-links, and mismatches in base-pairing (Ball et al., 2005; Choi et al., 2010). The RPA–ssDNA complex will promote the loading of the 9–1–1 and ATR–ATRIP complexes (Dore et al., 2009). The juxtaposition of these complexes allows ATR to phosphorylate Chk1, which then promotes cell cycle arrest, causing a cellular response to non-B DNA structure formation. Alternatively, ssDNA-RPA complex can recruit Cut5, by which ATR (ATR-ATRIP) (Mec1-Ddc2 in yeast), DNA polymerase α, Rad50-Mre11-Nbs1 (MRN) and clamp loader Rad24 (Rad17 in mammals) can all be recruited to the ssDNA-RPA (Cortez et al., 2001; Zou & Elledge, 2003; Robison et al., 2004).

The purpose of activating DNA damage checkpoint in response to the formation of non-B DNA secondary structure is to regulate cell cycle events, for mediating appropriate repair and fork restart processes. While non-B DNA structure forming sequences per se are probably an infrequent trigger of DNA damage checkpoint responses, and, thus, should not be regarded as a real DNA damage by cells. There has extensive evidence suggesting that non-B DNA structure forming sequences can only induce checkpoint-triggering events when stable non-B DNA structures are adopted. The stable DNA structures may affect normal DNA metabolism, making DSBs or causing more severe effects on DNA metabolism, such as replication fork stalling, formation of nucleosome free sites (Chromosomal Fragile Sites) etc.

Consisting with that, mutations in checkpoint genes, such as Mec1, Ddc2, Rad9, Rad17, Rad24, or Rad53, produce repeat instabilities by a $CAG_{\sim70}$, including both expansion and contraction instabilities. These suggested that DNA structure formed by long CAG repeats activated checkpoints in eukaryotes (Lahiri et al., 2004; Sundararajan & Freudenreich, 2011). Similarly, a CAG_{175} repeat on plasmids can also be recognized as "DNA damage" in *E. coli*, as witnessed by inducing SOS response (Majchrzak et al., 2006).

Surprisingly, it was found that even those shorter CAG repeats (containing 13–20 triplets) can also intrigue DNA damage checkpoint. By which repeats expansion can be prevented when the repeats formed non-B structures, suggesting that cells have endowed the checkpoint mechanism of responding to non-B DNA structure formation (Razidlo & Lahue, 2008).

Another example as intriguing cellular response for non-B DNA structure formation by derived structure processing is also found with human PKD1 gene. The 2.5-kb polypurine-polypyrimidine tract in intron 21 in human PKD1 gene potentially forms H-DNA structure, contributing to the high mutation rate of the PKD1 gene (Bacolla et al., 2001; Patel et al., 2004). A plasmid carrying this polypurine–polypyrimidine tract induced a stronge SOS response and severely delayed the host cell growth, resulting in a dramatic decrease in colony formation (Patel et al., 2004). However, the effect was largely reduced without UvrA (100-fold decrease in colony formation), and nearly vanished without UvrB or UvrC. These suggested the polypurine–polypyrimidine repeat sequence or the structure formed by the repeats per se was not involved in the effects, while the NER processing was essential (Bacolla et al., 2001).

6.5 Mre11-Rad50-Nbs1 (MRN)/ Mre11-Rad50-Xrs2 (MRX)

Apart from the nucleolytic activity, MRN / MRX can also play roles in activating the checkpoints as mentioned above (van den Bosch, et al., 2003; Sundararajan & Freudenreich, 2011). It was believed that a single stranded region in a non-B DNA structure forms ssDNA-RPA to the amount of triggering a checkpoint response (normally exceeds 300 bp). One way of Rad50-Mre11-Nbs1 (MRN) contributing to checkpoint response might be through Cut5 recruitment. Rad50-Mre11-Nbs1 (MRN) can be recruited to the single stranded region in the non-B DNA structure, and then participates in ATR checkpoint. Alternatively Rad50-Mre11-Nbs1 (MRN) can also secure DNA replication as implicated by its ortholog SbcCD in *E.coli* (Darmon et al., 2007; Zahra et al., 2007). Indeed, the MRN / MRX complex has been co localized in the replication machinery. In this context, the resection role of MRN / MRX on DSB initiated recombination repair may be no more necessary as long as the checkpoints mechanism prevented the DSB formation by checkpoint proteins (Mimitou & Symington, 2008; Zhu et al., 2008).

Non-B DNA structure forming sequences are potential triggers of DNA damage checkpoint responses mainly by inducing replication fork stalling and chromosomal breaks. Since the non-B DNA structures have specific DNA conformations at the damaged site, which may influence the checkpoint signaling, and the dynamics of checkpoint activation are likely to differ at different types of non-B DNA structure forming sequences.

7. Future perspectives

Many lines of evidence suggest that unusual DNA structures can form *in vivo* and play significant roles in DNA metabolism, while they may also serve as a source for the generation of genomic instability. Strikingly, unusual DNA structures were often found to trigger some kinds of repair actions or avoidance responses that promote their removal of the structures once formed. Under this later circumstance, it becomes obvious that formation of non-B DNA structures *in vivo* was somehow similar to the appearances of some real DNA damages as induced by environmental DNA damaging agents. Certain unusual DNA structures have unpaired bases and regions with helix distortions/junctions etc., which may experience unprovoked repair in cells. Therefore triggering cellular responses of a non-B DNA structure is subject to its morphological/ topological properties, which could attract recognizing repair proteins. In fact, a non-B DNA structure is often recognized by more than one repair proteins, such as the proteins working in MMR, NER and recombination. Questions rose therefore as if individual pathways of DNA repair accounts enough for the repair of the non-B DNA structures? Or does it need multiple proteins working in different repair pathways reconstitute synthesized pathway(s) to repair? Nevertheless, progress in this field seems support an idea that enzymes/ proteins that recognize and/ or process the possible non-B DNA structures may be different because of the non-B DNA structures formed. Proteins that have been found to associate with non-B DNA instability might take part in an unexpected way in processing the non-B DNA structures. Therefore studies in the coming future may have to focus on the identifications of the types of non-B DNA structures that elicit certain kinds of mutations and the enzyme systems involved. It could be expected that more diseases will be recognized as because of mutations at non-B DNA structures. Also, strategies will have to make toward developing therapeutics to appease the devastating effects of the syndromes.

8. References

Adachi, M. & Tsujimoto. Y. (1990). Potential Z-DNA elements surround the breakpoints of chromosome translocation within the 5′ flanking region of *bcl*-2 gene. *Oncogene,* 5:1653–1657.

Alvarez, D., Novac, O., Callejo, M., Ruiz, M. T., Price, G. B. & Zannis-Hadjopoulos, M. (2002).14-3-3sigma is a cruciform DNA binding protein and associates in vivo with origins of DNA replication. *J Cell Biochem.* 87(2):194-207.

Antony, S., Arimondo, P. B., Sun, J-S. & Pommier, Y. (2004). Position- and orientation-specific enhancement of topoisomerase I cleavage complexes by triplex DNA structures. *Nucleic Acids Res.*, 32 (17): 5163-5173.

Arimondo, P. B., Riou, J-F., Mergny, J-L., Tazi, J., Sun, J-S., Garestier, T. & Hélène, C. (2000). Interaction of human DNA topoisomerase I with G-quartet structures. *Nucleic Acids Res.*, 28 (24): 4832-4838.

Ashton, T. M., Mankouri, H. W., Heidenblut, A., McHugh, P. J. & Hickson, I. D. (2011). Pathways for Holliday Junction Processing during Homologous Recombination in *Saccharomyces cerevisiae*. *Mol Cell Biol.*, 31(9):1921-1933.

Bachrati, C. Z. & Hickson, I. D. (2003). RecQ helicases: suppressors of tumorigenesis and premature aging. *Biochem J.*, 374(Pt 3):577-606.

Bacolla, A., Jaworski, A., Connors, T. D. & Wells, R. D. (2001). Pkd1 unusual DNA conformations are recognized by nucleotide excision repair. *J Biol Chem.*, 276:18597–18604.

Bacolla, A. & Wells, R. D. (2009). Non-B DNA conformations as determinants of mutagenesis and human disease. *Mol Carcinog.*, 48:273-285.

Bacolla, A., Wang, G., Jain, A., Chuzhanova, N. A., Cer, R. Z., Collins, J. 1 R., Cooper, D. N., Bohr, V. A. & Vasquez, K. M. (2011). Non-B DNA-forming sequences and WRN deficiency independently increase the frequency of base substitution in human cells. *J Biol Chem.*, 286(12):10017-10026.

Balakumaran, B. S., Freudenreich, C. H. & Zakian, V. A. (2000). CGG / CCG repeats exhibit orientation-dependent instability and orientation-independent fragility in Saccharomyces cerevisiae. *Hum Mol Genet.*, 9(1):93-100.

Ball, H. L, Myers, J. S. & Cortez, D. (2005). ATRIP binding to replication protein A-single-stranded DNA promotes ATR-ATRIP localization but is dispensable for Chk1 phosphorylation. *Mol Biol Cell.*, 16(5):2372-2381.

Bashkirov, V. I., Scherthan, H., Solinger, J. A., Buerstedde, J. M. & Heyer, W. D. (1997). A mouse cytoplasmic exoribonuclease (mXRN1p) with preference for G4 tetraplex substrates. *J Cell Biol.*, 136(4):761-773.

Bhattacharyya, S. & Lahue, R. S. (2004). *Saccharomyces cerevisiae* Srs2 DNA helicase selectively blocks expansions of trinucleotide repeats. *Mol Cell Biol.*, 24(17):7324-7330.

Boiteux, S., Costa de Oliveira, R. & Laval, J. (1985). The *Escherichia coli* O6-methylguanine-DNA methyltransferase does not repair promutagenic O6-methylguanine residues when present in Z-DNA. *J Biol Chem.*, 260(15):8711-8715.

Boiteux, S. & Laval, F. (1985). Repair of O6-methylguanine, by mammalian cell extracts, in alkylated DNA and poly (dG-m5dC)·(polydG-m5dC) in B and Z forms. *Carcinogenesis*, 6:805–807.

Broxson, C., Beckett, J. & Tornaletti, S. (2011). Transcription arrest by a G quadruplex forming-trinucleotide repeat sequence from the human *c-myb* gene. *Biochemistry.*, [Epub ahead of print]

Burge, S., Parkinson, G. N., Hazel, P., Todd, A. K. & Neidle, S. (2006). Quadruplex DNA: sequence, topology and structure. *Nucleic Acids Res.*, 34(19):5402-5415..

Carraway, M. & Marinus, M. G. (1993). Repair of heteroduplex DNA molecules with multibase loops in *Escherichia coli*. *J Bacteriol.*, 175(13):3972-3980.

Casasnovas, J. M. & Azorin, F. (1987). Supercoiled induced transition to the Z-DNA conformation affects the ability of a $d(CG/GC)_{12}$ sequence to be organized into nucleosome-cores. *Nucleic Acids Res.*, 15:8899–8918.

Casey, B. P. & Glazer, P. M. (2001). Gene targeting via triple-helix formation. *Prog Nucleic Acid Res Mol Biol.*, 67:163-192.

Cejka, P. & Kowalczykowski, S. C. (2010). The full-length *Saccharomyces cerevisiae* Sgs1 protein is a vigorous DNA helicase that preferentially unwinds holliday junctions. *J Biol Chem.*, 285(11):8290-82301.

Cer, R. Z., Bruce, K. H., Mudunuri, U. S., Yi, M., Volfovsky, N., Luke, B. T., Bacolla, A., Collins, J. R. & Stephens, R. M. (2011). Non-B DB: a database of predicted non-B DNA-forming motifs in mammalian genomes. *Nucleic Acids Res.*, 39 (Database issue):D383-391.

Chan, P. P., Lin, M., Faruqi, A. F., Powell, J., Seidman, M. M. & Glazer, P. M. (1999). Targeted correction of an episomal gene in mammalian cells by a short DNA fragment tethered to a triplex-forming oligonucleotide. *J Biol Chem.*, 274, 11541-11548.

Chen, J. M., Cooper, D. N., Ferec, C., Kehrer-Sawatzki, H. & Patrinos, G. P. (2010). Genomic rearrangements in inherited disease and cancer. *Semin Cancer Biol.*, 20(4):222-233.

Cheok, C. F., Bachrati, C. Z., Chan, K. L., Ralf, C., Wu, L. & Hickson, I. D. (2005). Roles of the Bloom's syndrome helicase in the maintenance of genome stability. *Biochem Soc Trans.*, 33(Pt 6):1456-1459.

Choi, J. H., Lindsey-Boltz, L. A., Kemp, M., Mason, A. C., Wold, M. S. & Sancar, A. (2010). Reconstitution of RPA-covered single-stranded DNA-activated ATR-Chk1 signaling. *Proc Natl Acad Sci USA.*, 107(31):13660-13665.

Connelly, J., de Leau, E. S. & Leach, D. (1992). DNA cleavage and degradation by the SbcCD complex from *Escherichia coli*. *Nucleic Acid Res.*, 27, 1039-1046

Connelly, J. & Leach, D. (1996). The *sbc*C and *sbc*D genes of *Escherichia coli* encode a nuclease involved in palindromic inviability and genetic recombination. *Genes to Cell.*, 1,285-291.

Connelly, J., Kirkham, L. A. & Leach, D. (1998). The SbcCD nuclease of *Escherichia coli* is a structural maintenance of chromosomes (SMC) family protein that cleaves hairpin DNA. *Proc Natl Acad Sci U S A.*, 95, 7969-7974.

Connelly, J., delau, E.S. & Leach, D. R. F. (1999). DNA cleavage and degradation by the SbcCD complex from *Escherichia coli, Nucleic Acid Res.*, 27:1039–1046.

Courey, A. J. (1999). Analysis of altered DNA structures: cruciform DNA. *Methods Mol Biol.* 94:29-40.

Cox, R. & Mirkin, S. M. (1997). Characteristic enrichment of DNA repeats in different genomes. *Proc Natl Acad Sci USA.*, 94: 5237–5242.

Creze, C., Lestini, R., Kühn, J., Ligabue, A., Becker, H. F., Czjzek, M., Flament, D. & Myllykallio H. (2011). Structure and function of a novel endonuclease acting on branched DNA substrates. *Biochem Soc Trans.*, 39(1):145-9.

Crouau-Roy, B. (1999). Trans-speciation maintenance in the MHC region of a polymorphism which includes a polymorphic dinucleotide locus, and the *de novo* arisal of a polymorphic tetranucleotide microsatellite. *Tissue Antigens.*, 54(6):560-4.

Darmon, E., Lopez-Vernaza, M. A., Helness, A. C., Borking, A., Wilson, E., Thacker, Z., Wardrope, L. & Leach, D. R. F., (2007). SbcCD regulation and localization in *Escherichia coli*. *J Bacteriol.*, 189(18), 6686-6694.

Dere, R. & Wells, R. D. (2006). DM2 CCTG*CAGG repeats are crossover hotspots that are more prone to expansions than the DM1 CTG*CAG repeats in *Escherichia coli*. *J Mol Biol.*, 360(1):21-36.

Dore´, A. S., Kilkenny, M. L., Rzechorzek, N. J. & Pearl, L. H. (2009). Crystal structure of the Rad9-Rad1-Hus1 DNA damage checkpoint complex— implications for clamp loading and regulation. *Mol Cell*, 34, 735–745.

Dyke, M. W. V., Nelson, L. D., Weilbaecher, R. G. & Mehta, D. V. (2004). Stm1p, a G4 Quadruplex and purine motif triplex nucleic acid-binding protein, interacts with ribosomes and subtelomeric Y' DNA in *Saccharomyces cerevisiae*. *J Biol Chem.*, 279, 24323-24333.

Fang, W. H., Wang, B. J., Wang, C. H., Lee, S. J., Chang, Y. T., Chuang, Y. K. & Lee, C. N. (2003). DNA loop repair by *Escherichia coli* cell extracts. *J Biol Chem.*, 278(25):22446-22452.

Faruqi, A. F., Datta, H. J., Carroll, D., Seidman, M. M. & Glazer, P. M. (2000). Triple-helix formation induces recombination in mammalian cells via a nucleotide excision repairdependent pathway. *Mol Cell Biol.*, 20, 990-1000.

Fox, K. R. & Brown, T. (2011). Formation of stable DNA triplexes. *Biochem Soc Trans.*, 39(2):629-34.

Freudenreich, C. H. (2007). Chromosome fragility: molecular mechanisms and cellular consequences. *Front. Biosci.*, 12:4911-24.

Froelich-Ammon, S. J., Gale, K. C. & Osheroff, N. (1994). Site-specific cleavage of a DNA hairpin by topoisomerase II. DNA secondary structure as a determinant of enzyme recognition/cleavage. *J Biol Chem.*, 269:7719–7725.

Fry, M. & Loeb, L. A. (1999). Human werner syndrome DNA helicase unwinds tetrahelical structures of the fragile X syndrome repeat sequence $d(CGG)_n$. *J Biol Chem.*, 274(18):12797-802.

Fry, M. (2007). Tetraplex DNA and its interacting proteins. *Frontiers in Bioscience*, 12, 4336-4351.

Fugmann, S. D. (2001). RAG1 and RAG2 in V (D) J recombination and transposition. *Immunol Res.*, 23(1):23-39.

Gur-Arie, R., Cohen, C. J., Eitan, Y., Shelef, L., Hallerman, E. M. & Kashi, Y. (2000). Simple Sequence Repeats in *Escherichia coli*: Abundance, Distribution, Composition, and Polymorphism. *Genome Res.*, 10: 62-71.

Harrigan, J. A., Opresko, P. L., von Kobbe, C., Kedar, P. S., Prasad, R., Wilson, S. H. & Bohr, V. A. (2003). The Werner syndrome protein stimulates DNA polymerase beta strand displacement synthesis via its helicase activity. *J Biol Chem.*, 278(25):22686-22695.

Hebert, A. & Rich, A. (1996). The Biology of Left-handed Z-DNA. *J Biol Chem.*, 271(20): 11595–11598.

Ho, P. S. (1994). The non-B DNA structure of $d(CA/TG)_n$ does not differ from that of Z-DNA. *Proc Natl Acad Sci U S A.*, 91(20):9549-9553.

Howard, M.T. & Griffith, J. D. (1993). A cluster of strong topoisomerase II cleavage sites is located near an integrated human immunodeficiency virus. *J Mol Biol.*, 232:1060–1068.

Inagaki, H., Ohye, T., Kogo, H., Kato, T., Bolor, H., Taniguchi, M., Shaikh, T. H., Emanuel, B. S. & Kurahashi, H. (2009). Chromosomal instability mediated by non-B DNA:Cruciform conformation and not DNA sequence is responsible for recurrent translocation in humans. *Genome Res.*, 19:191–198.

Jain, A., Bacolla, A., Chakraborty, P., Grosse, F., Vasquez, K. M. (2010). Human DHX9 helicase unwinds triple-helical DNA structures. *Biochemistry.*, 49(33):6992-6999.

Jin, R., Fernandez-Beros, M. E. & Novick, R. P. (1997). Why is the initiation nick site of an AT-rich rolling circle plasmid at the tip of a GC-rich cruciform? *EMBO J.*, 16(14):4456-66.

Johnston, B. H. (1988). Chemical probing of the B-Z transition in negatively supercoiled DNA. *J Biomol Struct Dyn.*, 6(1):153-166.

Kalish, J. M., Seidman, M. M., Weeks, D. L. & Glazer, P. M. (2005). Triplex-induced recombination and repair in the pyrimidine motif. *Nucleic Acids Res.*, 33(11):3492-502.

Kaliyaperumal, S., Patrick, S. M. & Williams, K. J. (2011). Phosphorylated hMSH6: DNA mismatch versus DNA damage recognition. *Mutat Res.*, 706(1-2):36-45.

Kamath-Loeb, A. S., Loeb, L. A., Johansson, E., Burgers, P. M. & Fry, M. (2001). Interactions between the Werner syndrome helicase and DNA polymerase delta specifically facilitate copying of tetraplex and hairpin structures of the $d(CGG)_n$ trinucleotide repeat sequence. *J Biol Chem.*, 276(19):16439-16446.

Kantelinen, J., Kansikas, M., Korhonen, M. K., Ollila, S., Heinimann, K., Kariola, R., Nystrm, M. (2010). MutSbeta exceeds MutSalpha in dinucleotide loop repair. *Br J Cancer.*, 102(6):1068-1073.

Khuu, P. A., Voth, A. R., Hays, F. A. & Ho, P. S. (2006). The stacked-X DNA Holliday junction and protein recognition. *J Mol Recognit.*, 19(3):234-242.

Kirkpatrick, D. T. & Petes T. D. (1997). Repair of DNA loops involves DNA mismatch and nucleotide-excision repair proteins. *Nature*, 387:929–931.

Kladde, M. P., Kohwi, Y., Kohwi-Shigematsu, T. & Gorski J. (1994). The non-B DNA structure of $d(CA/TG)_n$ differs from that of Z-DNA. *Proc Natl Acad Sci U S A.*, 91(5):1898-902.

Kolb. (2009). Cruciform-forming inverted repeats appear to have mediated many of the microinversions that distinguish the human and chimpanzee genomes. *Chromosome Res.*, 17:469–483

Kurahashi, H., Shaikh, T. H., Hu, P., Roe, B. A., Emanuel, B. S. & Budarf, M. L. (2000). Regions of genomic instability on 22q11 and 11q23 as the etiology for the recurrent constitutional t(11;22). *Hum Mol Genet*, 9:1665–1670.

Kurahashi, H. & Emanuel, B. S. (2001). Long AT-rich palindromes and the constitutional t(11;22) breakpoint. *Hum Mol Genet.*, 10(23):2605-17.

Kurahashi, H., Inagaki, H., Ohye, T., Kogo, H., Kato, T. & Emanuel, B. S. (2006). Palindrome-mediated chromosomal translocations in humans. *DNA Repair (Amst).*, 5(9-10):1136-45.

Kurahashi, H., Inagaki, H., Ohye, T., Kogo, H., Tsutsumi, M., Kato, T., Tong, M. & Emanuel, B. S. (2010). The constitutional t(11;22): implications for a novel mechanism responsible for gross chromosomal rearrangements. *Clin Genet.*, 78(4):299-309.

Lahiri, M., Gustafson, T. L., Majors, E. R. & Freudenreich, C. H. (2004). Expanded CAG repeats activate the DNA damage checkpoint pathway. *Mol Cell.*, 15(2):287-93.

Lange, S. S., Reddy, M. C. & Vasquez, K. M. (2009). Human HMGB1 directly facilitates interactions between nucleotide excision repair proteins on triplex-directed psoralen interstrand crosslinks. *DNA Repair (Amst).*, 8(7):865-72.

Langston, L. G. & Symington, L. S. (2005). Opposing roles for DNA structure-specific proteins Rad1, Msh2, Msh3, and Sgs1 in yeast gene targeting. *EMBO J.*, 24, 2214–2223

Lee, B. I. & Wilson, D. M. 3rd. (1999). The RAD2 domain of human exonuclease 1 exhibits 5' to 3' exonuclease and flap structure-specific endonuclease activities. *J Biol Chem.*, 274(53):37763-9.

Letessier, A., Millot, G. A., Koundrioukoff, S., Lachagès, A. M., Vogt, N., Hansen, R. S., Malfoy, B., Brison, O. & Debatisse, M. (2011). Cell-type-specific replication initiation programs set fragility of the FRA3B fragile site. *Nature.*, 470(7332):120-3.

Li, F., Dong, J., Pan, X., Oum, J. H., Boeke, J. D. & Lee, S. E. (2008). Microarray-based genetic screen defines SAW1, a gene required for Rad1 / Rad10-dependent processing of recombination intermediates. *Mol Cell.,* 30(3):325-335.

Lilley, D. M. (2010). The interaction of four-way DNA junctions with resolving enzymes. *Biochem Soc Trans.,* 38(2):399-403.

Lin, Y. & Wilson, J. H. (2009). Diverse effects of individual mismatch repair components on transcription-induced CAG repeat instability in human cells. *DNA Repair (Amst).,* 8(8):878-885.

Lipps, H. J. & Rhodes, D. (2009). G-quadruplex structures: *in vivo* evidence and function. Trends *Cell Biol.* 19(8):414-22.

Liu, Z. & Gilbert, W. (1994). The yeast KEM1 gene encodes a nuclease specific for G4 tetraplex DNA: implication of in vivo functions for this novel DNA structure. *Cell,* 77(7):1083-1092.

Liu, Z., Lee, A. & Gilbert, W. (1995). Gene disruption of a G4-DNA-dependent nuclease in yeast leads to cellular senescence and telomere shortening. *Proc Natl Acad Sci USA.,* 92(13):6002-6002.

Lukusa, T. & Fryns, J. P. (2008). Human chromosome fragility. *Biochim Biophys Acta.,* 1779(1):3-16.

Majchrzak, M., Bowater, R. P., Staczek, P. & Parniewski, P. (2006). SOS repair and DNA supercoiling influence the genetic stability of DNA triplet repeats in *Escherichia coli. J Mol Biol.,* 364(4):612-24.

Mankouri, H. W., Ashton, T. M., Hickson, I. D. (2011). Holliday junction-containing DNA structures persist in cells lacking Sgs1 or Top3 following exposure to DNA damage. *Proc Natl Acad Sci U S A.,* 108(12):4944-4949.

Masai, H. (2011). RecQL4: a helicase linking formation and maintenance of a replication fork. *J Biochem.,* 2011:149(6):629–631.

Masuda-Sasa, T., Polaczek, P., Peng, X. P., Chen, L. & Campbell, J. L. (2008). Processing of G4 DNA by Dna2 helicase / nuclease and replication protein A (RPA) provides insights into the mechanism of Dna2 / RPA substrate recognition. *J Biol Chem.,* 283(36):24359-24373.

Mäueler, W., Bassili, G., Epplen, C., Key, H. G. & Epplen, J. T. (1999). Protein binding to simple repetitive sequences depends on DNA secondary structure(s). *Chromosome Res.,* 7(3):163-166.

McMurray, C. T. (1999). DNA secondary structure: A common and causative factor for expansion in human disease. *Proc Natl Acad Sci U S A.,* 96: 1823–1825.

Mimitou, E. P. & Symington, L. S. (2008). Sae2, Exo1 and Sgs1 collaborate in DNA double-strand break processing. *Nature,* 455(7214):770-774.

Mirkin, S. M. (2008). Discovery of alternative DNA structures: a heroic decade (1979-1989). *Front Biosci.* , 13:1064-1071.

Mishima, Y., Kaizu, H. & Kominami, R. (1997). Pairing of DNA fragments containing (GGA: TCC)$_n$ repeats and promotion by high mobility group protein 1 and histone H1. *J Biol Chem,* 272, 26578–26584

Mukherjee, A. & Vasquez, K. M. (2011). Triplex technology in studies of DNA damage, DNA repair, and mutagenesis. *Biochimie,* 2011:93(8):1197-1208.

Muñoz, I. M., Hain, K., Déclais, A. C., Gardiner, M., Toh, G. W., Sanchez-Pulido, L., Heuckmann, J. M., Toth, R., Macartney, T., Eppink, B., Kanaar, R., Ponting, C. P.,

Lilley, D. M. & Rouse, J. (2009). Coordination of structure-specific nucleases by human SLX4/BTBD12 is required for DNA repair. *Mol Cell,* 35(1):116-127.

Nag, D. K. & Cavallo, S. J. (2007). Effects of mutations in SGS1 and in genes functionally related to SGS1 on inverted repeat-stimulated spontaneous unequal sister-chromatid exchange in yeast. *BMC Mol Biol.,* 8:120.

Novac, O., Alvarez, D., Pearson, C. E., Price, G. B., Zannis-Hadjopoulos, M. (2002). The human cruciform-binding protein, CBP, is involved in DNA replication and associates *in vivo* with mammalian replication origins. *J Biol Chem.,* 277(13):11174-11183.

Novara, F., Beri, S., Bernardo, M. E., Bellazzi, R., Malovini, A., Ciccone, R., Cometa, A. M., Locatelli, F., Giorda, R. And Zuffardi, O. (2009). Different molecular mechanisms causing 9p21 deletions in acute lymphoblastic leukemia of childhood. *Hum Genet.,* 126:511-520.

Pan, X. & Leach, D. (2000). The roles of *mut*S, *sbc*CD and *rec*A in the propagation of TGG repeat in *Escherichia coli. Nucleic Acids Res,* 28: 3178–3184.

Pan, X. (2004). Self-maintenance of gene and occurrence of genetic diseases, *Science Press Beijing,* pp.1–403.

Pan, X. (2006). Mechanism of trinucleotide repeats instabilities: the necessities of repeat non-B secondary structure formation and the roles of cellular trans-acting factors. *J Genet Genomics,* 33: 1–11.

Pan, X., Ding, Y. F. & Shi, L. F. (2009). The roles of SbcCD and RNaseE in the transcription of GAA · TTC repeats in Escherichia coli. *DNA Repair* (Amst) , 8:1321–1327.

Pan, X., Liao, Y., Liu, Y., Chang, P., Liao, L., Yang, L. & Li, H. Q. (2010). Transcription of AAT · ATT Triplet Repeats in *Escherichia coli* Is Silenced by H-NS and IS1E Transposition. *PLoS ONE,* 5(12): e14271.

Pan, X., Chang, P., Long, J., Xiao, P., Li, H. Q. & Duan, F. (2011). The molecular maintenance of trinucleotide repeats AGG in *Escherichia coli* relies on both homologous recombination and UmuDC -catalyzed DNA translesion synthesis. *DNA Res.,* (submitted).

Parker, B. O. & Marinus, M. G. (1992). Repair of DNA heteroduplexes containing small heterologous sequences in *Escherichia coli. Proc Natl Acad Sci U S A.,* 89(5):1730-1734.

Patel, H. P., Lu, L., Blaszak, R. T. & Bissler, J. J. (2004). PKD1 intron 21: triplex DNA formation and effect on replication. *Nucleic Acids Res.,* 32(4):1460-1468.

Pearson, C. E., Zorbas, H., Price, G. B. & Zannis-Hadjopoulos, M. (1996). Inverted repeats, stem-loops, and cruciforms: significance for initiation of DNA replication. *J Cell Biochem.,* 63(1):1-22.

Pfohl-Leszkowicz A, Boiteux S, Laval J, Keith G, Dirheimer G. (1983). Enzymatic methylation of chemically alkylated DNA and poly(dG-dC) X poly(dG-dC) in B and Z forms. *Biochem Biophys Res Commun.,* 116(2):682-688.

Qin, Y. & Hurley, L. H. (2008). Structures, folding patterns, and functions of intramolecular DNA G-quadruplexes found in eukaryotic promoter regions. *Biochimie.,* 90(8):1149-1171.

Qiu, J. F. & Pan, X. (2008). The linkage of DNA replication, recombination and repair, *Prog. Biochem. Biophys.,* 35: 751–756.

Raghavan, S. C., Swanson, P. C., Wu, X., Hsieh, C. L. & Lieber, M. R. (2004). A non-B-DNA structure at the Bcl-2 major breakpoint region is cleaved by the RAG complex. *Nature*, 428, 88-93.

Raghavan, S. C., Chastain, P., Lee, J. S., Hegde, B. G., Houston, S., Langen, R., Hsieh, C. L., Haworth, I. S. & Lieber, M. R.(2005). Evidence for a triplex DNA conformation at the *bcl*-2 major breakpoint region of the t(14;18) translocation. *J Biol Chem.*, 280, 22749-22760.

Rao,S. R., Trivedi, S., Emmanuel, D., Merita, K., & Hynniewta, M. (2010). DNA repetitive sequences-types, distribution and function: A review. *J Cell and Mol Biol.*, 7(2) & 8(1): 1-11.

Rawal, P., Kummarasetti, V. B., Ravindran, J., Kumar, N., Halder, K., Sharma, R., Mukerji, M., Das, S. K. & Chowdhury, S. (2006). Genome-wide prediction of G4 DNA as regulatory motifs: role in *Escherichia coli* global regulation. *Genome Res.*, 16(5):644-55.

Razidlo, D. F. & Lahue, R. S. (2008). Mrc1, Tof1 and Csm3 inhibit CAG·CTG repeat instability by at least two mechanisms. *DNA Repair* (Amst), 7(4):633-640.

Ren, B., Kühn, J., Meslet-Cladiere, L., Briffotaux, J., Norais, C., Lavigne, R., Flament, D., Ladenstein, R. & Myllykallio, H. (2009). Structure and function of a novel endonuclease acting on branched DNA substrates. *EMBO J.*, 28(16):2479-2489.

Rich, A., Nordheim, A. & Azorin, F. (1983). Stabilization and detection of natural left-handed Z-DNA. *J Biomol Struct Dyn.*, 1(1):1-19.

Sannohe, Y. & Sugiyama, H. (2010). Overview of formation of G-quadruplex structures. *Curr Protoc Nucleic Acid Chem.*, Chapter 17:Unit 17.2.1-17.

Schwartz, M., Zlotorynski, E. & Kerem, B. (2006). The molecular basis of common and rare fragile sites. *Cancer Lett.*, 232(1):13-26.

Shah, S. N., Opresko, P. L., Meng, X., Lee, M. Y. & Eckert, K. A. (2010). DNA structure and the Werner protein modulate human DNA polymerase delta-dependent replication dynamics within the common fragile site FRA16D. *Nucleic Acids Res.*, 38(4):1149-1162.

Shimizu, M., Mori, T., Sakuri, T. & Shindo, H. (2000).Destablization of nucleosomes by an unusual DNA conformation adopted by poly(dA)poly(dT) tracts *in vivo*. *EMBO J.*,19(13):3358-3365.

Sinden, R. R., Zheng, G. X., Brankamp R. G. & Allen, K. N. (1991). On the deletion of inverted repeated DNA in *Escherichia coli*: effects of length, thermal stability, and cruciform formation *in vivo*. *Genetics*, 129, 991–1005.

Sinden, R. R., Hashem, V. I. & Rosche, W. A. (1999). DNA-directed mutations. Leading and lagging strand specificity. *Ann N Y Acad Sci.*, 870,173-189

Singh, P., Zheng, L., Chavez, V., Qiu, J. & Shen, B. (2007). Concerted action of exonuclease and Gap-dependent endonuclease activities of FEN-1 contributes to the resolution of triplet repeat sequences $(CTG)_n$- and $(GAA)_n$-derived secondary structures formed during maturation of Okazaki fragments. *J Biol Chem.*, 282(6):3465-3477.

Smith, R. (2008). Meeting DNA palindromes head-to-head. *Genes Dev.*, 22: 2612-2620.

Spiro, C., Pelletier, R., Rolfsmeier, M. L., Dixon, M. J., Lahue, R. S., Gupta, G., Park, M. S., Chen, X, Mariappan, S. V. & McMurray, C. T. (1999). Inhibition of FEN-1 processing by DNA secondary structure at trinucleotide repeats. *Mol Cell*, 4(6):1079-1085.

Stros, M., Muselíková-Polanská, E., Pospísilová, S. & Strauss, F. (2004). High-affinity binding of tumor-suppressor protein p53 and HMGB1 to hemicatenated DNA loops. *Biochemistry.*, 43(22):7215-7225.

Suda,T., Mishma,Y., Takayanagi, K., et al. (1996). A novel activity of HMG domains promotion of the triple-stranded complex formation between DNA containing $(GGA/TCC)_{11}$ and $d(GGA)_{11}$ Oligonucleotides. *Nucleic Acids Res.*, 24, 4733-4740

Sun, H., Yabuki, A. & Maizels, N. (2001). A human nuclease specific for G4 DNA. *Proc Natl Acad Sci U S A.*, 98(22):12444-12449.

Sundararajan, R. & Freudenreich, C. H. (2011). Expanded CAG / CTG Repeat DNA Induces a checkpoint response that impacts cell Proliferation in Saccharomyces cerevisiae. *PLoS Genet.*, 7(3):e1001339.

Svozil, D., Kalina, J., Omelka, M. & Schneider, B. (2008). DNA conformations and their sequence preferences. *Nucleic Acids Res.*, 36(11):3690-3706.

Tsutakawa, S. E., Classen, S., Chapados, B. R., Arvai, A. S., Finger, L. D., Guenther, G., Tomlinson, C. G., Thompson, P., Sarker, A. H., Shen, B., Cooper, P. K., Grasby, J. A. & Tainer, J. A. (2011). Human Flap Endonuclease Structures, DNA Double-Base Flipping, and a Unified Understanding of the FEN1 Superfamily. *Cell.*, 145(2):198-211.

Urban, M., Joubert, N., Purse, B. W., Hocek, M. & Kuchta, R. D. (2010). Mechanisms by which human DNA primase chooses to polymerize a nucleoside triphosphate. *Biochemistry.*, 49(4):727-735.

Van Holde, K. & Zlatanova, J. (1994). Unusual DNA structures, chromatin and transcription. *Bioessays.*, 16(1):59-68.

Vasquez, K. M., Christensen, J., Li, L., Finch, R. A. & Glazer, P. M. (2002). Human XPA and RPA DNA repair proteins participate in specific recognition of triplex-induced helical distortions. *Proc Natl Acad Sci U S A.*, 99(9):5848-5853.

Voineagu, I., Freudenreich, C. H. & Mirkin, S. M. (2009).Checkpoint responses to unusualstructures formed by DNA repeats. *Mol. Carcinogenesis,* 48:309 - 318.

Voineagu, I., Surka, C. F., Shishkin, A. A., Krasilnikova, M. M. & Mirkin, S. M. (2009). Replisome stalling and stabilization at CGG repeats, which are responsible for chromosomal fragility. *Nat Struct Mol Biol.*, 16(2):226-228.

Wang, G. & Vasquez, K. M. (2004). Naturally occurring H-DNA-forming sequences are mutagenic in mammalian cells. *Proc Natl Acad Sci U S A.*, 101(37):13448-13453.

Wang, G. & Vasquez, K. M. (2006). Non-B DNA structure induced genetic instability. *Mutat Res.*, 598, 103-119

Wang, J. C. (1984). DNA supercoiling and its effects on the structure of DNA. *J Cell Sci.* Suppl., 1:21-29.

Wang, Y. W. & Griffith, J. D. (1996). Methylation of expanded CCG triplet repeat DNA from fragile X syndrome patients enhances nucleosome exclusion. *J Biol Chem.*, 271, 22937-22940.

Watanabe, Y. & Maekawa, M. (2010). Spatiotemporal regulation of DNA replication in the human genome and its association with genomic instability and disease. *Curr Med Chem.*, 17:222-233.

Watson, J. D. & Crick, F. H. C. (1953). Structure for deoxyribose nucleic acid, *Nature,* 171:737 - 738.

Weber, J. L. & Wong, C. (1993). Mutation of human short tandem repeats. *Hum Mol Genet.*, 2(8):1123-1128.

Wells, R. D. (2007). Non-B DNA conformations, mutagenesis and disease. *Trends Biochem Sci.*, 32(6): 271-278.

Wilkins, M. H. F., Stokes, A. R. & Wilson, H. R. (1953a). Molecular structure of DNA, *Nature*,171:738-740.

Wilkins, M. H. F., Seeds, W. E., Stokes, A. R. & Wilson, H. R. (1953b). Helical structure of crystalline DNA, *Nature*, 172: 759 - 762.

Wojciechowska, M., Napierala, M., Larson, J. E. & Wells, R. D. (2006). Non-B DNA conformations formed by long repeating tracts of Myotonic Dystrophy Type 1, Myotonic Dystrophy Type 2, and Friedreich's Ataxia genes, not the sequences per se, promote mutagenesis in flanking regions. *J Biol Chem.*, 281(34):24531-24543.

Yang, W. (2006). Poor base stacking at DNA lesions may initiate recognition by many repair proteins. *DNA Repair* (Amst), 5(6):654-666.

Zahra, R., Blackwood, J. K., Sales, J. & Leach, D. R. F. (2007). Proofreading and secondary structure processing determine the orientation dependence of CAG • CTG trinucleotide repeat instability in *Escherichia coli. Genetics.*, 276:27-41.

Zhao, J., Jain, A., Iyer, R. R., Modrich, P. L. & Vasquez, K. M. (2009). Mismatch repair and nucleotide excision repair proteins cooperate in the recognition of DNA interstrand crosslinks. *Nucleic Acids Res.*, 37(13):4420-4429.

Zhao, J., Bacolla, A., Wang, G. & Vasquez, K. M. (2010). Non-B DNA structure-induced genetic instability and evolution. *Cell Mol Life Sci.*, 67:43-62.

22

ATP-Binding Cassette Properties of Recombination Mediator Protein RecF

Sergey Korolev
Saint Louis University School of Medicine
USA

1. Introduction

1.1 Recombinational repair

*H*omologous *r*ecombination (HR) is essential for genetic diversity and genome stability. The conserved RecA-like recombinases promote pairing and consequent exchange of fragments between two homologous DNA molecules during conjugation in bacteria and meiotic recombination in eukaryotes. HR is a main DNA repair pathway particularly important in case of large-scale DNA damages, including chromosome or *d*ouble-*s*tranded (ds) *D*NA *b*reaks (DSBs) and long *s*ingle-*s*tranded (ss) DNA *g*aps (SSGs) (Cox, 1991; Kowalczykowski et al., 1994). The broken chain is paired with the intact DNA, which serves as a template for the synthesis of the damaged DNA. The same recombinases are also involved in the repair and origin-independent restart of stalled DNA replication, a frequently occurring event in every cell (Cox et al., 2000; Kowalczykowski, 2000; Kuzminov, 2001).

HR is initiated by the cooperative binding of RecA recombinase to ssDNA hundreds or thousands nucleotides long forming nucleoprotein filament, a so called presynaptic complex often designated as RecA*. The presynaptic complex can bind homologous dsDNA and exchange a DNA strands. RecA* has multiple activities beyond the strand invasion and exchange (Figure 1). Those include triggering DNA damage SOS response through stimulation of LexA autocleavage (Rehrauer et al., 1996) and activation of UmuD subunit of the error-prone DNA polymerase PolV important for translesion synthesis to bypass small-scale DNA errors (Jiang et al., 2009; Rajagopalan et al., 1992). RecA* was also suggested to stabilize and maintain stalled replication fork during DNA repair (Courcelle et al., 1997). Consequently, RecA binding to DNA is regulated at multiple levels (Cox, 2007).

1.2 Recombination mediator proteins

Transient ssDNA regions generated during replication are protected by ssDNA binding proteins like bacterial *ss*DNA *b*inding (SSB) protein and eukaryotic *r*eplication *p*rotein *A* (RPA), which prevent recombinase binding. Under DNA damage conditions, ubiquitous *r*ecombination *m*ediator *p*roteins (RMPs) overcome inhibitory effect of SSB and initiate presynaptic complex formation (Fig. 1)(Beernink and Morrical, 1999; Symington, 2002). RMPs are not directly involved in the repair of specific DNA damages, but they regulate initiation of multiple DNA repair pathways and damage response signaling cascades (Courcelle, 2005; Kowalczykowski, 2005; Lee and Paull, 2005; Moynahan et al., 2001;

Williams et al., 2007). In addition to presynaptic complex formation, many RMPs also promote DNA annealing (Luisi-DeLuca and Kolodner, 1994; Sugiyama et al., 1998). The importance of RMPs is reflected by the fact that recombination and repair pathways are often named after specific RMPs, e. g. RecF, RecBC, Rad52 pathways. RMPs include phage UvsY (Sweezy and Morrical, 1999), prokaryotic RecBCD and RecFOR proteins (Fujii et al., 2006; Kolodner et al., 1985; Lloyd and Thomas, 1983; Wang and Smith, 1983), and numerous eukaryotic members (Symington, 2002). Mutations of human RMPs are associated with cancer predisposition, mental retardation, UV-sensitivity and premature aging (Ouyang et al., 2008; Powell et al., 2002; Tal et al., 2009; Thompson and Schild, 2002).

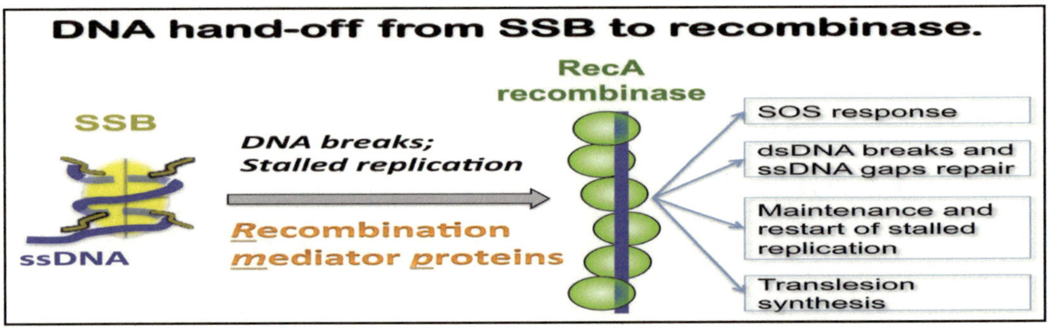

Fig. 1. The ssDNA hand-off from ssDNA binding proteins to RecA-like recombinase triggers multiple DNA damage response pathways important for DNA repair and origin-independent restart of stalled replication. Such DNA transaction is regulated by RMPs.

While ssDNA-binding proteins and RecA-like recombinases are well characterized, the mechanism of RMPs function remains poorly understood. Recent studies revealed a variety of RMPs structural domains. (Koroleva et al., 2007; Lee et al., 2004; Leiros et al., 2005; Makharashvili et al., 2004; Singleton et al., 2002; Yang et al., 2002). The diversity of RMPs structural domains reflects the plethora of different DNA damage response scenarios regulated by these proteins. The focus of this review is prokaryotic RMP RecF. Although a major bacterial recombination repair pathway is named after RecF, the mechanism of RecF activity and even its functional role remains one of the least understood and most controversial issues.

2. RecFOR recombination mediators

2.1 RecF pathway

The RecF was discovered as an alternative to RecBC pathway in genetic screens based on frequency of conjugation recombination in *E. coli*, and was found to be important for postreplication repair of extended SSGs (Horii and Clark, 1973; Lovett and Clark, 1983; Wang and Smith, 1984). Later, it was shown that *recF* mutants are even more hypersensitive to UV radiation than *RecBC,* that RecF pathway plays a major role in replication restart under UV damage conditions, and that RecF is involved in DSBs repair in the absence of RecBC and SbcBC (Clark, 1991; Courcelle, 2005; Courcelle et al., 1997; Ivancic-Bace et al., 2003; Kidane et al., 2004; Kusano et al., 1989; Whitby and Lloyd, 1995; Zahradka et al., 2006). Sequencing of new genomes revealed the ubiquitous nature of RecF pathway proteins found in most bacteria (Rocha et al., 2005), including the radiation resistant bacteria *Deinococcus radiodurans* (Bentchikou et al., 2010; Cox et al., 2010; Chang et al., 2010; Makarova et al.,

2001). RecF forms an epistatic group with RecO and RecR proteins (Asai and Kogoma, 1994; Courcelle et al., 1997; Courcelle and Hanawalt, 2003; Horii and Clark, 1973; Kolodner et al., 1985; Wang and Smith, 1984). All three proteins are equally important for recombinational repair in most genetic screens, although they do not form triple complex in solution. RecF and RecR genes are often located in DNA replication operons on chromosome, with the exception of extremophiles like *T. thermophiles* and *D. radiodurans* (Ream and Clark, 1983; Ream et al., 1980). In *E. coli*, RecF is co-transcribed with major subunits of replication machinery, DnaA and DnaN (Perez-Roger et al., 1991; Villarroya et al., 1998). RecF pathway proteins share either sequence or structural homology or functional similarities with eukaryotic proteins such as WRN, BLM, RAD52, and BRCA2, which are associated with cancer predisposition and premature aging when mutated (Karow et al., 2000; Kowalczykowski, 2005; Mohaghegh and Hickson, 2001; Yang et al., 2005).

Genetic studies demonstrated that RecF regulates several DNA repair and recombination pathways but is not directly involved in repair of specific DNA damage. For example, in *RecF* mutants DNA lesions are removed with the efficiencies comparable to wild-type cells, while the UV resistance is strongly compromised (Courcelle et al., 1999; Rothman and Clark, 1977). RecF-mediated loading of RecA on ssDNA is required for the maintenance of arrested replication forks, fot the protection and processing of DNA ends to permit DNA repair and replication restart at the site of disruption.

The regulatory role of RecF in replication restart is further supported by examples where RecF impairs cell survival, like in thymine starvation experiments (Nakayama et al., 1982). Another example is revealed by genetic studies of DNA helicases UvrD and Rep (Petit and Ehrlich, 2002). Mutants lacking both helicases are not viable and *RecF* mutations suppress the lethality of the E. coli *Rep/UvrD* double mutant. UvrD helicase disassembles RecA* filaments, the reaction opposite to that of RecFOR, while Rep helicase promotes replication through transcription sites (Boubakri et al., 2010; Centore and Sandler, 2007; Heller and Marians, 2005; Lane and Denhardt, 1975; Veaute et al., 2005). The frequent pausing of the replication fork can potentially stimulate RecF-mediated initiation of RecA* filament formation leading to illegitimate recombination in the absence of UvrD (Mahdi et al., 2006).

2.2 Mechanism of RecOR activities

The involvement of all three RecF, -O and -R proteins in HR initiation is well documented by genetic studies. However, the mechanism of their activities in the initiation process remains poorly understood, particularly with respect to RecF. RecO and RecR alone are sufficient to promote formation of the RecA filament on SSB-bound ssDNA (Cox, 2007; Umezu et al., 1993). RecO binds DNA and the C-terminal tail of SSB and these interactions are critical for RecOR function, at least in the absence of RecF (Inoue et al., 2011; Manfredi et al., 2010; Ryzhikov et al., 2011; Sakai and Cox, 2009; Umezu and Kolodner, 1994). In addition, RecO anneals complimentary ssDNA strands protected by cognate SSB (Kantake et al., 2002; Luisi-DeLuca and Kolodner, 1994), resembling the properties of the eukaryotic RMPs, Rad52 and BRCA2 (Grimme et al., 2010; Mazloum et al., 2007; Sugiyama et al., 1998). RecR binds either RecO or RecF (Makharashvili et al., 2009; Umezu and Kolodner, 1994; Webb et al., 1995, 1997). Although *E. coli* RecR does not bind DNA at submillimolar concentrations, it significantly affects DNA binding properties of both RecO and RecF (Kantake et al., 2002; Makharashvili et al., 2009; Webb et al., 1999). RecR inhibits DNA annealing properties of RecO, even though RecOR complex binds both ss- and dsDNA. In addition to initial loading of RecA, RecOR further stimulate homologous recombination by preventing the dissociation of RecA* filament from ssDNA in *E. coli* (Bork et al., 2001). Somewhat different properties were reported for *Bacillus subtilis* RecO, which does not require RecR for initiation of RecA* formation (Manfredi et al., 2008; Manfredi et al., 2010).

Crystal structures of all three proteins and of the RecOR complex from *D. radiodurans* have been reported (Koroleva et al., 2007; Lee et al., 2004; Leiros et al., 2005; Makharashvili et al., 2004; Timmins et al., 2007). RecR structure resembles that of a DNA clamp-like tetramer (Lee et al., 2004). However, the role of a potential DNA clamp in RMPs-mediated reaction is unknown. Moreover, in the crystal structure of RecOR complex RecO occupies large portion of the clamp inner space. Such conformation makes it challenging to predict functionally relevant interaction of the complex with DNA. Another intriguing fact is that the crystal structure of RecO did not resemble any structural features of its functional eukaryotic analog Rad52 (Leiros et al., 2005; Makharashvili et al., 2004; Singleton et al., 2002), which supports two identical reactions.

2.3 Ambiguities of RecF function

In contrast to genetic data, initial biochemical studies did not reveal the function of RecF in recombination initiation (Umezu et al., 1993). RecF binds both ss- and dsDNA in the presence of ATP, and it is a weak DNA-dependent ATPase (Griffin and Kolodner, 1990; Madiraju and Clark, 1991, 1992). It interacts with RecR in the presence of ATP and DNA (Webb et al., 1999). Surprisingly however, RecF was initially shown to play an inhibitory role during RecOR-mediated loading of RecA on SSB-protected ssDNA (Umezu et al., 1993).

The UV-sensitivity of *RecF* mutant can be suppressed by RecOR overexpression, suggesting that RecF plays a regulatory role (Sandler and Clark, 1994). In agreement with this hypothesis, RecF dramatically increases the efficiency of RecOR-mediated RecA loading at ds/ssDNA junctions with a 3′ ssDNA extension under specific conditions (Morimatsu and Kowalczykowski, 2003). RecF was suggested to recognize specific DNA junction structure to direct RecA loading at the boundary of SSGs. While initial experiments demonstrated such a preference (Hegde et al., 1996), later work did not support the binding preference of RecF to DNA junction (Webb et al., 1999). Purified RecF tends to gradually aggregate in solution (Webb et al., 1999). Apparently, nonspecific high molecular weight RecF aggregates interact with DNA resulting in the inhibitory effect of RecF or false positive interactions of RecF with specific DNA substrates (Hegde et al., 1996). In addition, RecFR complex limits the extension of RecA* beyond SSGs, the observation indirectly supporting RecF specificity towards boundaries of SSGs while in complex with other proteins (Webb et al., 1997).

RecF is co-transcribed with the replication initiation protein DnaA and with the β-clamp subunit of DNA polymerase III DnaN. However, its open reading frame is usually shifted by one or two nucleotides relatively to that of DnaN (Villarroya et al., 1998). *E. coli RecF* gene also has multiple rear codons. Thus, expression of RecF is likely to be down regulated at translational level. Consequently, there are only a few copies of RecF in an *E. coli* cell.

How RecF promotes recombination remains an open question. The ability of RecFR complex to limit extension of RecA* filament beyond the SSGs suggests that the RecFR complex may specifically interact with RecA*. However, no direct observation of such interactions has been reported so far. RecF also binds RecX protein (Lusetti et al., 2006). RecX is a negative regulator of presynaptic complex formation, which inhibits filament extension by binding to RecA. RecF scavenges RecX from solution through direct interaction, thus diminishing negative regulatory effect of RecX (Drees et al., 2004; Lusetti et al., 2006). Additional evidence of direct involvement of RecF in the initiation of RecA* filament formation was recently demonstrated in experiments with the SSB mutant lacking conserved C-terminus peptide. This SSB mutant inhibits RecOR-mediated recombination initiation, likely due to lack of interaction of SSB with RecO (Sakai and Cox, 2009). Surprisingly, RecF rescues the RecOR function with this SSB mutant, even on ssDNA plasmids without ds/ssDNA junction.

3. Structural studies of RecF

3.1 RecF is an ABC ATPase

The amino acid sequence of RecF contains three conserved motifs characteristic of ATP-binding cassette (ABC) ATPases: Walker A, Walker B, and a "signature" motif. Walker A, or P-loop, is a nucleotide binding site found in a variety of ATPases (Walker et al., 1982). Walker B motif provides acidic amino acids important for coordination of a water molecule and a metal ion during the hydrolysis of a triphosphate nucleotide bound to the Walker A motif. The signature motif is a unique feature of ABC ATPases, a diverse family of proteins ranging from membrane transporters to DNA-binding proteins (review in (Hopfner and Tainer, 2003). ATP-dependent dimerization is a common feature of this class of proteins. Signature motif residues interact with the nucleotide bound to an opposite monomer (Hopfner et al., 2000). This motif is important for both ATP-dependent dimerization and subsequent ATP hydrolysis. ABC ATPases are not motor proteins and utilize ATP binding and hydrolysis as a switch or sensor mechanism, regulating diverse signaling pathways and reactions.

DNA-binding ABC ATPases include DNA mismatch and nucleotide excision repair enzymes (Ban and Yang, 1998; Junop et al., 2001; Obmolova et al., 2000; Tessmer et al., 2008), structural maintenance of chromosome (SMC) proteins cohesin and condensin (Strunnikov, 1998), and DSBs repair enzyme Rad50 (Hirano et al., 1995). SMCs and Rad50 are characterized by the presence of a long coiled-coil structural domain inserted between N- and C-terminal halves of the globular head domain (Haering et al., 2002). RecF lacks a coiled-coil region, but it does exhibit an ATP-dependent DNA binding and a slow DNA-dependent ATP hydrolysis activity (Hegde et al., 1996; Madiraju and Clark, 1992; Webb et al., 1995). However, the SMC-like properties of RecF and their role in recombinational repair have not been addressed. Previously, only Walker A motif has been shown to be critical for RecF function (Sandler et al., 1992; Webb et al., 1999). All known ABC-type ATPases function as a heterooligomeric complexes in which a sequence of inter- and intra-molecular interactions is triggered by the ATP-dependent dimerization and the dimer-dependent ATP hydrolysis (Deardorff et al., 2007; Dorsett, 2011; Hopfner and Tainer, 2003; Junop et al., 2001; Moncalian et al., 2004; Smith et al., 2002). Thus, RecF may function in recombination initiation through a multistep pathway of protein-protein and DNA-protein interactions regulated by ATP-dependent RecF dimerization.

3.2 Structural similarity of RecF with Rad50 head domain

The diversity of ABC ATPases makes it difficult to predict to which subfamily RecF belongs to based on sequence comparison. RecF is a globular protein lacking long coiled-coil domains of Rad50 and SMC proteins. However, it does not have significant sequence similarity beyond three major motifs with globular DNA binding proteins like MutS. We crystalized and solved a high resolution structure of RecF from *D. radiodurans* (DrRecF) (Fig.

2) (Koroleva et al., 2007). The structure was solved with resolution of 1.6 Å using native and selenomethionine protein derivative crystals. The structure is comprised of two domains. The ATPase domain I is formed by two β-sheets wrapped around central α-helix A and is similar to the corresponding subdomain of the Rad50 head domain (Figure 2, right). Structures of nucleotide-binding domains are similar in all ABC ATPases. In contrast, structure of subdomain containing signature motif (Lobe II in Rad50) is highly diverse among even DNA binding ABC ATPases. However, all structural elements presented in RecF domain II are present in Rad50 Lobe II subdomain and these domains are structurally more similar than ATP-binding domains. The only difference is two long α-helixes of RecF which are connected at the apical part of this "arm-like" domain. In Rad50 analogous α-helixes are extended into an extremely long coiled-coil structure, absent in RecF. High degree of structural similarity unequivocally puts RecF in the same family together with Rad50 and SMC proteins. Therefore, RecF represents the only known globular protein with a structure highly homologous to that of the head domains of Rad50, cohesin and condensin.

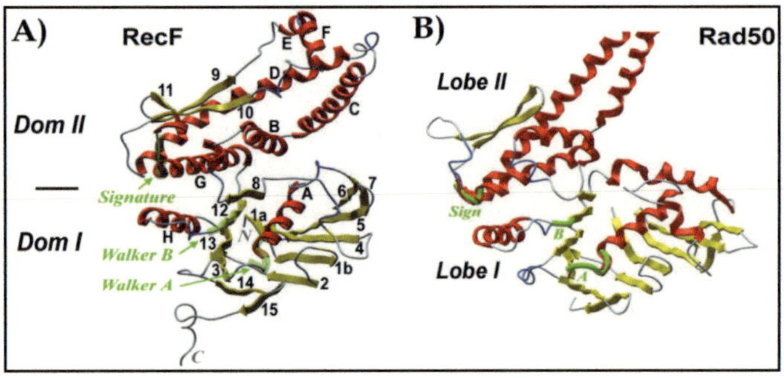

Fig. 2. Cartoon representation of **A**) RecF and **B**) Rad50 head domain structures. α-helixes are shown in red and β-sheets in yellow. In RecF, α-helixes are lettered and β -strands are numbered. Walker A, B, and signature motifs are highlighted in green and labeled. In RecF, ATP-binding domain is designated as Domain I and signature motif domain as Domain II. In Rad50 corresponding domains are referred as Lobe I and Lobe II subdomains.

3.3 The model of ATP-dependent dimer suggests mechanism of DNA binding

RecF was crystallized as a monomer. ATP-dependent dimer was modeled based on known intersubunit interactions conserved in ABC ATPases and, specifically, based on a known structure of Rad50 dimer (Fig. 3)(Hopfner et al., 2000). In all proteins of this family, a conserved serine of the signature motif interacts with a γ-phosphate group of ATP. The ATP bound to Walker A motif was modeled accordingly to its highly conserved conformation in all Walker A and B containing structures. These constrains unambiguously dictate a single conformation of the potential RecF dimer (Fig. 3A). The model suggests a potential DNA binding site located on the top of two nucleotide-binding domains, in a conformation similar to the proposed DNA binding site of Rad50 (Figs. 3B-D). The resulting RecF dimer forms a semi-clamp or a symmetrical crab-claw with two arms extending in the directions similar to those of coiled-coil regions of Rad50 dimer (Hopfner et al, 2001). The claw structure contains sufficient space to accommodate and cradle dsDNA. In this model, the majority of conserved residues map to the dimerization interface and pocket region of the claw, where DNA binding is expected to occur.

The proposed model explains an ATP-dependence of RecF DNA binding. First, it is an acidic protein with mostly negatively charged surface area. In the model of an ATP-dependent dimer, small patches of positively charged surface area are aligned on the top of the dimer, creating the extended basic surface area. Second, the arms of domain II form a deep cleft, sufficient to engulf a DNA helix. The constrains of a signature motif interaction with a γ-phosphate group of ATP does not allow to alter the distance between these arms in the model without significant structural clashes of surface exposed residues of the two monomers. Thus, the ATP-dependent dimerization leads to favorite juxtaposition of the surface charges and to surface complementarity, which stimulate DNA binding.

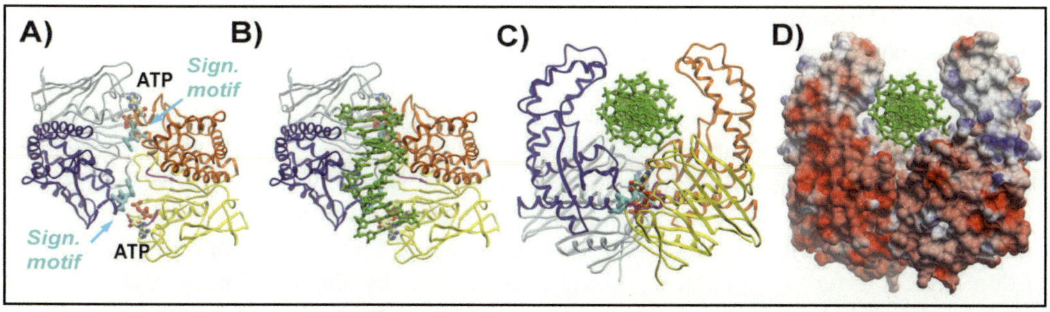

Fig. 3. A model of RecF dimer. **A**) Domains I and II of one RecF monomer are color-coded in yellow and orange, and of the other monomer in grey and blue. Signature motif residues are shown by stick representation in cyan and ATP by stick representation with nitrogen, oxygen, carbon and phosphate atoms are colored in blue, red, yellow and orange, correspondingly. **B**) The same dimer representation with bound dsDNA shown by stick representation in green. **C**) Orthogonal view of the dimer shown in B). **D**) Surface representation of DrRecF dimer in same orientation as in C) color-coded according to the surface electrostatic potential.

Proving ATP-dependent dimerization of RecF in solution was quite challenging due to poor solubility and a tendency of RecF to form nonspecific soluble aggregates (Webb et al., 1999). Initial attempts with size *e*xclusion *c*hromatography (SEC) yielded the monomeric form of E. coli RecF in the presence of ATP (Webb et al., 1999). The caveat of such experiment is in low protein solubility, when only solution with limited protein concentration can be run through column, and in a non-equilibrium nature of SEC, which may lead to dissociation of weak dimers. Later, it was shown that DrRecF nonspecifically interacts with the column resin even in a 1M KCl buffer (Koroleva et al., 2007). Therefore, a combination of SEC with static light scattering was utilized to determine the true molecular weight of eluted fractions. DrRecF does form an ATP-dependent dimer, though relatively unstable, which could dissociate on the column under non-equilibrium conditions at low protein concentration. The dimerization of wild type protein and specific mutants under equilibrium conditions was tested with a *d*ynamic *l*ight *s*cattering (DLS). DrRecF dimerizes only in the presence of ATP but not with ADP. Mutation of signature motif S276R resulted in lack of dimerization, as well as mutation of Walker motif A K39M, which prevents ATP binding. Walker A motif mutant K39R which binds, but does not hydrolyses ATP, forms dimer as well as mutants of Walker B motif D300N. Surprisingly, non-hydrolizable ATP analogs did not support dimerization in initial experiments, suggesting that RecF dimerization is highly sensitive to specific ATP-bound conformation. While DLS method is not suitable for quantitative analysis, it is highly sensitive to the presence of high molecular weight protein aggregates, and it was utilized to optimize RecF solution conditions for other experiments.

4. Functional significance of ABC-type ATPase properties of RecF

4.1 ATP-dependent dimerization is required for DNA binding

The DNA binding properties of RecF and their role in recombination initiation remain poorly understood and controversial. Different publications presented contradicting results of DNA junction recognition by RecF (Hegde et al., 1996; Webb et al., 1999). RecR was shown to stabilize ATP-dependent interaction of RecF with DNA. However, RecR also stimulated ATP hydrolysis, which theoretically should lead to destabilizing of RecF complex with DNA (Webb et al., 1995). Therefore, multiple complimentary equilibrium binding techniques were utilized to comprehensively address the relationship between dimerization, DNA binding and ATP binding and hydrolysis (Makharashvili et al., 2009). Quantitative characterization of RecF dimerization was performed using Föster (or Fluorescence) Resonance Energy Transfer (FRET) technique with a mixture of Cy3- and FAM(fluorescein)-labeled DrRecF (Fig. 4). The cysteine substitutions were introduced either at a topical part of domain II arm or at the C-terminal tail to crosslink DrRecF with fluorophores. The labeling of domain II interfered with DNA-binding (Makharashvili, 2009), indirectly confirming the dimer model presented in Fig. 3, where apical parts of domain II arms are situated close to each other in the dimer and the presence of bulky polar fluorophores may interfere with DNA binding. C-terminally labeled protein (A355C) was fully functional. Apparent dimerization constant of $L_d = 0.15 \pm 0.02$ μM was calculated from the plot of FRET signal versus DrRecF concentration (Fig. 4C). Alternatively, multiple data sets (Fig. 4B) were globally fitted into a two-step reaction model consisting of the ATP-binding and dimerization processes resulting in a dimerization constant of $L_d = 0.13 \pm 0.02$ μM and an ATP-binding constant of $K_d^{ATP} = 13 \pm 2$ μM.

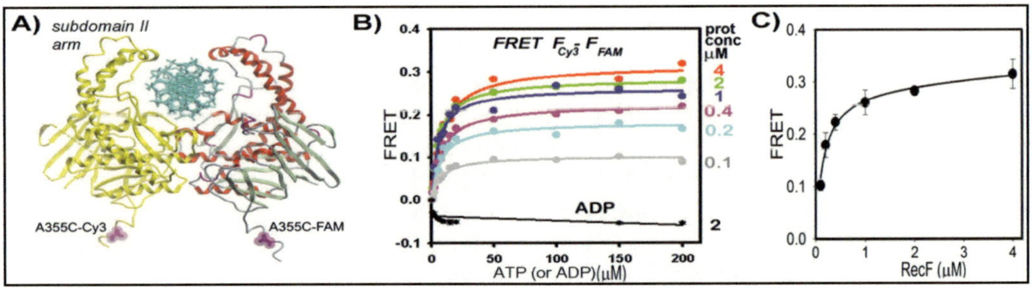

Fig. 4. ATP-dependent dimerization of DrRecF. **A**) Location of cysteines (A355C) are shown by magenta spheres on the model of DrRecF dimer with one monomer is colored in yellow and the other color-coded accordingly to its secondary structure elements with α-helixes in red and β-strands in green. The DNA is shown in cyan. **B**) Titration of labeled DrRecF by ATP. Different isotherms represent different concentration of DrRecF in solution (values are shown on the right). The black isotherm corresponds to titration of 2 μM DrRecF by ADP. **C**) A plot of maximal FRET signal versus DrRecF concentrations.

The DNA binding was first assayed using short FAM-labeled oligonucleotides with the fluorescent polarization anisotropy method (Fig. 5). To address initial DNA binding rate, reactions were performed for a relatively short time (10-15 min) and with the excess of ATP, taking an advantage of RecF being a slow ATPase (Fig. 6C, below). Alternatively, the rate of ATP hydrolysis was measured over 1 or 2 hours time upon titration of RecF by different DNA oligonucleotides (Fig. 6B). The binding of all DNA substrates was relatively weak with the apparent dissociation constants greater than 15 μM (Fig. 5). Neither a wild type DrRecF in the presence of ADP nor a signature motif mutant S279R in the presence of ATP were able to bind DNA (Fig. 5), suggesting that the ATP-dependent dimerization is essential for RecF interaction with all DNA substrates.

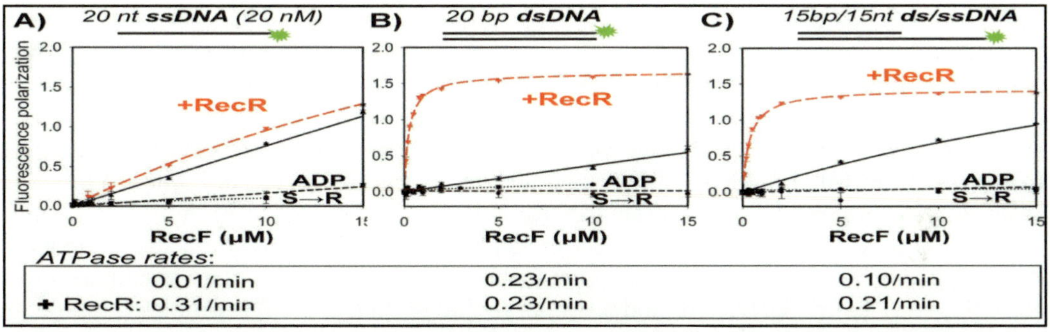

Fig. 5. ATP-dependent binding of DrRecF to different DNA substrates (top) and DNA-dependent ATP hydrolysis rates (bottom). DNA substrates are schematically represented above each plot with **A)** ssDNA, **B)** dsDNA and **C)** ds/ssDNA junction. Solid isotherms correspond to binding in the presence of ATP, dashed black - in the presence of ADP, dotted - to the binding of signature motif mutant S279R in the presence of ATP. Red isotherms correspond to DrRecF binding in the presence of ATP and 50 μM DrRecR. The maximum estimated ATP hydrolysis rates of DrRecF (Fig. 6A) are shown at the bottom with the top lane corresponding to reactions without DrRecR and the bottom - with RecR. DrRecF concentration is 10 μM, DNA- 20 nM, ATP - 2 mM.

4.2 RecR-dependent DNA specificity of RecF

DNA binding of DrRecF is drastically alters in the presence of DrRecR (red isotherms in Fig. 5). DrRecR significantly increases the affinity of DrRecF to dsDNA (Fig. 5B) with the estimated association binding constant at least two orders of magnitude stronger than without DrRecR. DrRecR does not alter DrRecF ssDNA binding according to the DNA binding assay. However, the ATPase assay clearly demonstrated interaction of DrRecR with DrRecF in the presence of ssDNA. ssDNA does not stimulate ATP hydrolysis by DrRecF, while the presence of both DrRecR and ssDNA results in strongest ATPase rate. This suggests that DrRecR stimulates the ATPase rate of DrRecF bound to ssDNA, potentially destabilizing dimerization and ssDNA binding. In case of dsDNA, maximum ATPase rates were similar with and without DrRecR. Therefore, DrRecR stabilizes DrRecF complex with dsDNA without increasing its ATPase rate. Due to this stabilization effect of RecR, we are able to measure DNA binding and dimerization of DrRecF in the presence of ATP analogs (Fig. 6B). Curiously, a weak dimerization is observed at highest DrRecF concentration even in the presence of ADP. Therefore, DrRecR selectively stimulates binding of DrRecF dimer to dsDNA, while potentially destabilizing DrRecF complex with ssDNA. Both dimerization and DNA binding reactions were also measured as a function of time to verify that under these conditions ATP hydrolysis does not significantly alter either interaction within first 10 minutes (Fig. 6C).

DrRecR is characterized by a weak DNA binding affinity in a millimolar range, while binding of *E. coli* RecR to DNA was not detected. DrRecR forms a tetrameric DNA clamp-like structure (Lee et al., 2004). This conformation is likely to be conserved for other RecR homologs since *E. coli* RecR is either a dimer or tetramer in solution (Umezu et al., 1993), and *H. influenzae* RecR also was crystallized in a similar tetrameric conformation (Koroleva, O., Baranova, E., Korolev, S. unpublished data). One way to explain the DNA-dependent interaction of RecR with RecF is through the binding of both proteins to a shared DNA substrate, as beads on a string. Moreover, since dimer to tetramer transition was proposed as a clamp loading mechanism (although not confirmed), the ATP-dependent dimerization of RecF may stimulate such loading of RecR clamp on DNA. To test the hypothesis of shared DNA substrate requirement for RecF interaction with RecR, the RecR-stimulated DNA binding of RecF and the ATPase rate were tested in the presence of different length dsDNA substrates. Surprisingly, 10 bp short oligonucleotide stimulates DrRecF interaction with DrRecR. Structural modeling suggests that RecF dimer can bind 12-15 bp long DNA, while RecR clamp may cover up to 8-12 bp. These results rule out the beads-on-a-string model of RecFR binding to dsDNA. Alternatively, RecR may interact with the domain II arms encircling RecF bound DNA in a model similar to that of Rad50/Mre11 complex (Hopfner et al., 2001; Lammens et al., 2011; Williams et al., 2011).

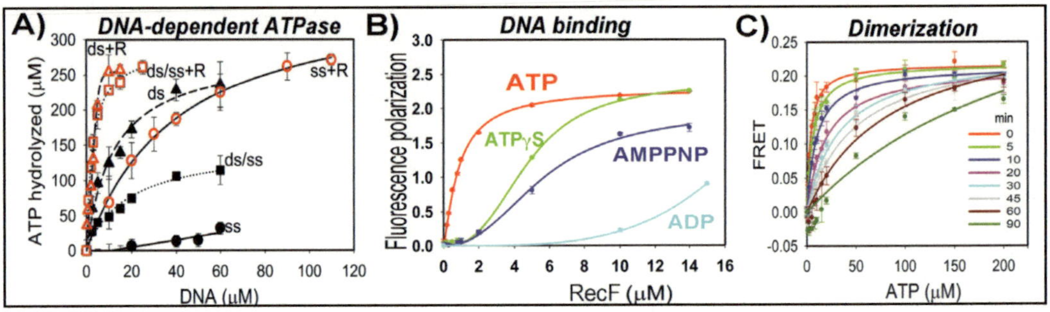

Fig. 6. **A**) ATP hydrolysis by DrRecF over 120 min was measured upon titration by different DNA substrates, with circles corresponding to ssDNA, triangles to dsDNA, and squares to ds/ssDNA. Red symbols correspond to titrations in the presence of 50 μM RecR. Concentration of RecF is 10 μM, and ATP 2 mM. **B**) dsDNA binding by RecFR in the presence of ATP analogs measured with the fluorescence polarization assay performed similarly to that in Fig. 5 with the following nucleotides: ATP (red), ATPγS (green), AMPPNP (blue), and ADP (cyan). **C**) Time dependence of RecF dimerization upon titration with ATP as measured by FRET of labeled RecF. Isotherms of different colors correspond to the FRET value at different time points shown on the right.

4.3 The lack of ss/dsDNA junction specificity

The steps of RecF interaction with DNA and RecR are schematically represented in Fig. 7. ATP binding stimulates RecF dimerization, essential for binding of all DNA substrates. The DNA-bound RecF dimer interacts with RecR, which either stabilizes the complex with dsDNA or destabilizes with ssDNA. Importantly, neither of the performed assays revealed any specificity of RecF and RecFR complex for ss/dsDNA junction. Both DNA binding and

ATPase rates had an average between ss- and dsDNA substrates values. Although all data were obtained with *D. radiodurans* proteins, RecF and RecR are highly homologous proteins. Moreover, *E. coli* RecR stimulates DNA binding of *D. radiodurans* RecF similarly to that of *D. radiodurans* RecR suggesting that DrRecF binds both Dr- and *E. coli* RecR proteins with similar affinities (Makharashvili, 2009). Therefore, the described above properties of *D. radiodurans* proteins are likely to be conserved for *E. coli* homologs. While DNA binding and ATPase assays did not reveal specificity of RecF towards DNA junction, functional studies clearly evidence the role of RecF at ss/dsDNA junction (Chow and Courcelle, 2004; Handa et al., 2009; McInerney and O'Donnell, 2007; Morimatsu and Kowalczykowski, 2003; Webb et al., 1997). The potential specificity of RecF to ds/ssDNA junction is likely to require additional protein partners of recombination initiation reaction including SSB, RecO and RecA. For example, RecR can be recruited to SSB-bound ssDNA while in complex with RecO (Ryzhikov et al., 2011). The increased local concentration of RecR on SSB-coated ssDNA may subsequently stimulate RecF interaction with the adjacent dsDNA region.

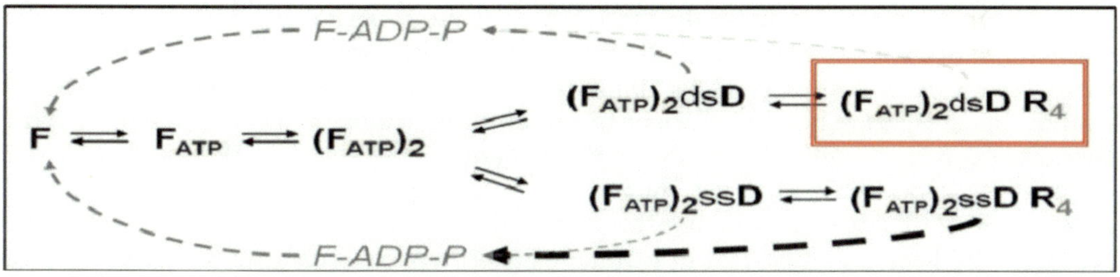

Fig. 7. Schematic representation of RecF interaction with ATP, ATP-dependent dimerization, DNA binding, and the effect of RecR on DNA binding and ATP hydrolysis. The complex formed on dsDNA in the presence of RecR (red box) is the most stable intermediate. In case of *D. radiodurans* homologs, RecF dimer interacts with RecR tetramer.

4.4 In vivo function of RecF conserved motifs

The role of RecF SMC motifs *in vivo* was initially addressed with *E. coli RecF* mutant cells transformed with RecF-containing vector (Koroleva et al., 2007). Only wild type RecF complemented the UV sensitivity of a *recF* cells. Mutations of Walker A, -B and signature motifs did not restore the UV resistance. Since the overexpression of RecF can potentially affect its function, similar mutants of *RecF* were constructed in chromosome (Michel-Marks et al., 2010). Importantly, different steps of RecFOR function were tested with each mutant. Those include the rate of DNA synthesis, degradation of nascent DNA, the presence of DNA intermediates, and cell survival upon UV irradiation. Mutants included Walker A motif K36M, deficient in ATP binding, a Walker A motif K36R and a Walker B D303N, which both retain ATP binding but are deficient in ATP hydrolysis, and two signature motif mutants S270R and Q273A, which prevent an ATP-dependent dimerization.

Following the UV-induced arrest of replication, the nascent DNA is partially degraded at the replication fork by RecQ helicase and RecJ nuclease and RecF limits such degradation (Courcelle and Hanawalt, 1999). The degree of nascent DNA degradation was measured with pulse labeling of growing cell culture with [^{14}C]thymine and [^{3}H]thymidine. Similarly to a null mutant(Courcelle and Hanawalt, 1999), approximately 50% of nascent DNA was degraded with all mutants with the exception of D303N, where degradation was less severe.

Therefore, all steps of the dynamic interactions of RecF with ATP and DNA are important for the very first step of RecFOR function in replication repair. The weak functionality of D303N can be explained by a potential residual ATPase activity of this mutant, as shown for other SMC proteins (Lammens et al., 2004). Experiments with ATP analogs (Fig. 6B) demonstrated that even minor conformational changes significantly affect RecF properties. Therefore, an alternative explanation may be that D303N mutant introduces the least conformational distortion at the ATP-binding site and may retain conformation of a wild type wild type dimer and DNA-binding activities better than K36R mutant.

The rate of DNA synthesis is reduced by approximately 90% immediately after UV irradiation, but is recovered to nearly initial rate within 100 min in wild-type cells. The overall accumulation of DNA is increased at that time approaching the level of unirradiated cells. In *recF* cells the initial reduction of DNA synthesis rate is similar, but there is no recovery. Like in the previous assay, all mutants with exception of D303N were similar to the null mutant. D303N mutant did support slight recovery of DNA replication rate, yet it was significantly weaker than that of a wild type. RecF is associated with appearance of specific replication intermediates during DNA damage, as visualized on two-dimensional agarose gel (Courcelle et al., 2003). In this assay, all mutants were equally deficient in accumulation of such intermediates similarly to the null mutant, although the detection level of this assay may not be sufficient to reveal weak activity of D303N mutant. Finally, the survival rate of cell culture after UV irradiation was assayed. D303N mutant was partially resistant, while all other mutants were as hypersensitive to UV irradiation as deletion of *recF*. These studies demonstrate that all steps of ATP binding, dimerization and hydrolysis by RecF are important to maintain stalled replication and to restart cell growth after DNA damage.

5. Conclusions

RecFOR proteins regulate RecA binding to ssDNA under DNA damage conditions. This reaction initiates a variety of DNA repair pathways including maintenance and restart of stalled replication. Correspondingly, recombinational repair is tightly regulated in cell. While the exact role and mechanism of RecF in these pathways remain controversial, the majority of known data suggest a regulatory function of RecF during initiation and subsequent steps of recombinational DNA repair. Intricate properties of the ATP-dependent interaction of RecF with DNA and of the DNA-dependent ATP hydrolysis as well as the dependence of these interactions on RecR strongly supports this hypothesis.

Regulatory function is further reinforced by the sequence and structural homology with the head domain of Rad50 and SMC proteins. Rad50 is involved in multiple steps of DNA damage response including initial detection of DSBs, triggering of cell signaling cascades, and in resection of dsDNA to create 3′ ssDNA tail for recombinase binding (Nicolette et al., 2010). In bacteria, RecF is likely to be involved in multiple steps of replication restart as well, including initial detection of replication arrest. Neither Rad50 nor RecF specifically recognizes functionally relevant DNA substrates, blunt-end DNA and ss/dsDNA junction, correspondingly (de Jager et al., 2002). Rad50 functions in complex with other DNA binding proteins, including Mre11 nuclease, and protein-protein interactions regulate DNA binding and ATPase activities (Lammens et al., 2011; Lim et al., 2011; Williams et al., 2011). By analogy, we can speculate that ATP binding and hydrolysis may not simply control DNA binding and dissociation of RecF, but also regulate binding of RecF dimer to different protein partners. For example, the ability of short DNA fragments to promote RecR binding suggests that the DNA-dependent conformational changes of RecF are important for protein-protein recognition rather than simple binding to the shared DNA substrate.

It is important to note that RecF does not represent the exact analog of Rad50. It is a much smaller protein without long coiled-coil structures. RecF does not support DNA unwinding or resection, as well as additional adenylate kinase activity of Rad50 and SMC proteins (Bhaskara et al., 2007; Lammens and Hopfner, 2010). Instead, it is involved in the initiation of the presynaptic complex formation, the function performed by BRCA2 or Rad52 in eukaryotes (Moynahan et al., 2001; New et al., 1998; Shinohara and Ogawa, 1998; Sung, 1997; Yang et al., 2005). While Rad52 is rather unique protein (Singleton et al., 2002), structural and functional motifs of BRCA2 resemble that of RecFOR system (Yang et al., 2002). BRCA2 interacts with ssDNA through OB-fold domain, similarly to RecO, and has a putative dsDNA-binding domain. The latter function is likely to be performed by RecF, even with the lack of structural similarity.

RecF regulates RecQJ-dependent resection of nascent DNA at stalled replication fork (Courcelle and Hanawalt, 1999). This step occurs prior to RecA loading and initiation of SOS response. How RecF recognizes stalled replication remains unknown. It is tempting to speculate that RecF is a part of replisome (Kogoma, 1997) based on co-translation of RecF with replication initiation protein DnaA and polymerase subunit DnaN and on its early involvement in detection of replication arrest. However, no interactions of RecF with replication proteins have been identified so far. RecF may represent an alternative to PriA pathway of replication restart in case of arrested replication or postreplication repair (Sandler, 1996). Thus, it is important to find additional RecF-binding proteins. The detection of novel interactions is problematic due to low copy number of RecF in cells and poor solubility of purified RecF. The potential requirement of ATP- and DNA-dependent dimerization for RecF interaction with other proteins further complicates the search for interacting proteins.

The relationship of specific steps of ATP-dependent reactions with the DNA damage recognition and processing by RecF and Rad50 remains elusive. Since RecF is the smallest known DNA-biding ABC ATPase composed of the head domain only, it represents an excellent model system to address the role of allosteric regulations, governing function of this class of proteins. Importantly, both ATP binding and hydrolysis are likely to play an important mechanistic role in most of reactions (Fig. 7). For example, the first step of limiting degradation of nascent lagging DNA by RecQJ and loading of RecA may only require formation of a stable RecF dimer at DNA junction, while ATP hydrolysis and dimer dissociation may be important for the following steps. However, the involvement of all the conserved motifs to prevent degradation of nascent DNA suggests that both ATP binding and hydrolysis are important even for this initial step. Therefore, all steps of RecF function in DNA repair are likely to depend on dynamic interactions of RecF with ATP, DNA and DNA repair proteins. Delineating molecular basis and principles of these interactions is essential for understanding fundamental mechanisms of DNA repair, recombination and replication.

6. Acknowledgment

The research was supported by National Institutes of Health grant GM073837. The author is grateful for help during manuscript preparation to Mikhail Ryzhikov and Ekaterina Los. Significant portion of RecF studies were performed by graduate student Nodar Makharashvili.

7. References

Asai, T., and Kogoma, T. (1994). The RecF pathway of homologous recombination can mediate the initiation of DNA damage-inducible replication of the Escherichia coli chromosome. J Bacteriol *176*, 7113-7114.

Ban, C., and Yang, W. (1998). Crystal structure and ATPase activity of MutL: implications for DNA repair and mutagenesis. Cell *95*, 541-552.

Beernink, H.T., and Morrical, S.W. (1999). RMPs: recombination/replication mediator proteins. Trends Biochem Sci *24*, 385-389.

Bentchikou, E., Servant, P., Coste, G., and Sommer, S. (2010). A major role of the RecFOR pathway in DNA double-strand-break repair through ESDSA in Deinococcus radiodurans. PLoS Genet *6*, e1000774.

Bhaskara, V., Dupre, A., Lengsfeld, B., Hopkins, B.B., Chan, A., Lee, J.H., Zhang, X., Gautier, J., Zakian, V., and Paull, T.T. (2007). Rad50 adenylate kinase activity regulates DNA tethering by Mre11/Rad50 complexes. Mol Cell *25*, 647-661.

Bork, J.M., Cox, M.M., and Inman, R.B. (2001). The RecOR proteins modulate RecA protein function at 5' ends of single- stranded DNA. Embo J *20*, 7313-7322.

Boubakri, H., de Septenville, A.L., Viguera, E., and Michel, B. (2010). The helicases DinG, Rep and UvrD cooperate to promote replication across transcription units in vivo. Embo J *29*, 145-157.

Chang, X., Yang, L., Zhao, Q., Fu, W., Chen, H., Qiu, Z., Chen, J.A., Hu, R., and Shu, W. (2010). Involvement of recF in 254 nm ultraviolet radiation resistance in Deinococcus radiodurans and Escherichia coli. Curr Microbiol *61*, 458-464.

Centore, R.C., and Sandler, S.J. (2007). UvrD limits the number and intensities of RecA-green fluorescent protein structures in Escherichia coli K-12. J Bacteriol *189*, 2915-2920.

Chow, K.H., and Courcelle, J. (2004). RecO acts with RecF and RecR to protect and maintain replication forks blocked by UV-induced DNA damage in Escherichia coli. J Biol Chem *279*, 3492-3496.

Clark, A.J. (1991). rec genes and homologous recombination proteins in Escherichia coli. Biochimie *73*, 523-532.

Courcelle, J. (2005). Recs preventing wrecks. Mutat Res *577*, 217-227.

Courcelle, J., Carswell-Crumpton, C., and Hanawalt, P.C. (1997). recF and recR are required for the resumption of replication at DNA replication forks in Escherichia coli. Proc Natl Acad Sci U S A *94*, 3714-3719.

Courcelle, J., Crowley, D.J., and Hanawalt, P.C. (1999). Recovery of DNA replication in UV-irradiated Escherichia coli requires both excision repair and recF protein function. J Bacteriol *181*, 916-922.

Courcelle, J., Donaldson, J.R., Chow, K.H., and Courcelle, C.T. (2003). DNA damage-induced replication fork regression and processing in Escherichia coli. Science *299*, 1064-1067.

Courcelle, J., and Hanawalt, P.C. (1999). RecQ and RecJ process blocked replication forks prior to the resumption of replication in UV-irradiated Escherichia coli. Mol Gen Genet *262*, 543-551.

Courcelle, J., and Hanawalt, P.C. (2003). RecA-dependent recovery of arrested DNA replication forks. Annu Rev Genet *37*, 611-646.

Cox, M.M. (1991). The RecA protein as a recombinational repair system. Mol Microbiol *5*, 1295-1299.

Cox, M.M. (2007). Regulation of bacterial RecA protein function. Crit Rev Biochem Mol Biol *42*, 41-63.

Cox, M.M., Goodman, M.F., Kreuzer, K.N., Sherratt, D.J., Sandler, S.J., and Marians, K.J. (2000). The importance of repairing stalled replication forks. Nature *404*, 37-41.

Cox, M.M., Keck, J.L., and Battista, J.R. (2010). Rising from the Ashes: DNA Repair in Deinococcus radiodurans. PLoS Genet *6*, e1000815.

de Jager, M., Wyman, C., van Gent, D.C., and Kanaar, R. (2002). DNA end-binding specificity of human Rad50/Mre11 is influenced by ATP. Nucleic Acids Res *30*, 4425-4431.

Deardorff, M.A., Kaur, M., Yaeger, D., Rampuria, A., Korolev, S., Pie, J., Gil-Rodriguez, C., Arnedo, M., Loeys, B., Kline, A.D., *et al.* (2007). Mutations in cohesin complex members SMC3 and SMC1A cause a mild variant of cornelia de Lange syndrome with predominant mental retardation. Am J Hum Genet *80*, 485-494.

Dorsett, D. (2011). Cohesin: genomic insights into controlling gene transcription and development. Curr Opin Genet Dev *21*, 199-206.

Drees, J.C., Lusetti, S.L., and Cox, M.M. (2004). Inhibition of RecA protein by the Escherichia coli RecX protein: modulation by the RecA C terminus and filament functional state. J Biol Chem *279*, 52991-52997.

Fujii, S., Isogawa, A., and Fuchs, R.P. (2006). RecFOR proteins are essential for Pol V-mediated translesion synthesis and mutagenesis. Embo J *25*, 5754-5763.

Griffin, T.J.t., and Kolodner, R.D. (1990). Purification and preliminary characterization of the Escherichia coli K-12 recF protein. J Bacteriol *172*, 6291-6299.

Grimme, J.M., Honda, M., Wright, R., Okuno, Y., Rothenberg, E., Mazin, A.V., Ha, T., and Spies, M. (2010). Human Rad52 binds and wraps single-stranded DNA and mediates annealing via two hRad52-ssDNA complexes. Nucleic Acids Res *38*, 2917-2930.

Haering, C.H., Lowe, J., Hochwagen, A., and Nasmyth, K. (2002). Molecular architecture of SMC proteins and the yeast cohesin complex. Mol Cell *9*, 773-788.

Handa, N., Morimatsu, K., Lovett, S.T., and Kowalczykowski, S.C. (2009). Reconstitution of initial steps of dsDNA break repair by the RecF pathway of E. coli. Genes Dev *23*, 1234-1245.

Hegde, S.P., Rajagopalan, M., and Madiraju, M.V. (1996). Preferential binding of Escherichia coli RecF protein to gapped DNA in the presence of adenosine (gamma-thio) triphosphate. J Bacteriol *178*, 184-190.

Heller, R.C., and Marians, K.J. (2005). Unwinding of the nascent lagging strand by Rep and PriA enables the direct restart of stalled replication forks. J Biol Chem *280*, 34143-34151.

Hirano, T., Mitchison, T.J., and Swedlow, J.R. (1995). The SMC family: from chromosome condensation to dosage compensation. Curr Opin Cell Biol *7*, 329-336.

Hopfner, K.P., Karcher, A., Craig, L., Woo, T.T., Carney, J.P., and Tainer, J.A. (2001). Structural biochemistry and interaction architecture of the DNA double-strand break repair Mre11 nuclease and Rad50-ATPase. Cell *105*, 473-485.

Hopfner, K.P., Karcher, A., Shin, D.S., Craig, L., Arthur, L.M., Carney, J.P., and Tainer, J.A. (2000). Structural biology of Rad50 ATPase: ATP-driven conformational control in DNA double-strand break repair and the ABC-ATPase superfamily. Cell *101*, 789-800.

Hopfner, K.P., and Tainer, J.A. (2003). Rad50/SMC proteins and ABC transporters: unifying concepts from high-resolution structures. Curr Opin Struct Biol *13*, 249-255.

Horii, Z., and Clark, A.J. (1973). Genetic analysis of the recF pathway to genetic recombination in Escherichia coli K12: isolation and characterization of mutants. J Mol Biol *80*, 327-344.

Inoue, J., Nagae, T., Mishima, M., Ito, Y., Shibata, T., and Mikawa, T. (2011). A mechanism for single-stranded DNA-binding protein (SSB) displacement from single-stranded DNA upon SSB-RecO interaction. J Biol Chem *286*, 6720-6732.

Ivancic-Bace, I., Peharec, P., Moslavac, S., Skrobot, N., Salaj-Smic, E., and Brcic-Kostic, K. (2003). RecFOR Function Is Required for DNA Repair and Recombination in a RecA Loading-Deficient recB Mutant of Escherichia coli. Genetics *163*, 485-494.

Jiang, Q., Karata, K., Woodgate, R., Cox, M.M., and Goodman, M.F. (2009). The active form of DNA polymerase V is UmuD'(2)C-RecA-ATP. Nature *460*, 359-363.

Junop, M.S., Obmolova, G., Rausch, K., Hsieh, P., and Yang, W. (2001). Composite active site of an ABC ATPase: MutS uses ATP to verify mismatch recognition and authorize DNA repair. Mol Cell *7*, 1-12.

Kantake, N., Madiraju, M.V., Sugiyama, T., and Kowalczykowski, S.C. (2002). Escherichia coli RecO protein anneals ssDNA complexed with its cognate ssDNA-binding protein: A common step in genetic recombination. Proc Natl Acad Sci U S A *99*, 15327-15332.

Karow, J.K., Wu, L., and Hickson, I.D. (2000). RecQ family helicases: roles in cancer and aging. Curr Opin Genet Dev *10*, 32-38.

Kidane, D., Sanchez, H., Alonso, J.C., and Graumann, P.L. (2004). Visualization of DNA double-strand break repair in live bacteria reveals dynamic recruitment of Bacillus subtilis RecF, RecO and RecN proteins to distinct sites on the nucleoids. Mol Microbiol *52*, 1627-1639.

Kogoma, T. (1997). Is RecF a DNA replication protein? Proc Natl Acad Sci U S A *94*, 3483-3484.

Kolodner, R., Fishel, R.A., and Howard, M. (1985). Genetic recombination of bacterial plasmid DNA: effect of RecF pathway mutations on plasmid recombination in Escherichia coli. J Bacteriol *163*, 1060-1066.

Koroleva, O., Makharashvili, N., Courcelle, C.T., Courcelle, J., and Korolev, S. (2007). Structural conservation of RecF and Rad50: implications for DNA recognition and RecF function. Embo J *26*, 867-877.

Kowalczykowski, S.C. (2000). Initiation of genetic recombination and recombination-dependent replication. Trends Biochem Sci *25*, 156-165.

Kowalczykowski, S.C. (2005). Cancer: catalyst of a catalyst. Nature *433*, 591-592.

Kowalczykowski, S.C., Dixon, D.A., Eggleston, A.K., Lauder, S.D., and Rehrauer, W.M. (1994). Biochemistry of homologous recombination in Escherichia coli. Microbiol Rev *58*, 401-465.

Kusano, K., Nakayama, K., and Nakayama, H. (1989). Plasmid-mediated lethality and plasmid multimer formation in an Escherichia coli recBC sbcBC mutant. Involvement of RecF recombination pathway genes. J Mol Biol *209*, 623-634.

Kuzminov, A. (2001). DNA replication meets genetic exchange: chromosomal damage and its repair by homologous recombination. Proc Natl Acad Sci U S A *98*, 8461-8468.

Lammens, A., and Hopfner, K.P. (2010). Structural basis for adenylate kinase activity in ABC ATPases. J Mol Biol *401*, 265-273.

Lammens, A., Schele, A., and Hopfner, K.P. (2004). Structural biochemistry of ATP-driven dimerization and DNA-stimulated activation of SMC ATPases. Curr Biol *14*, 1778-1782.

Lammens, K., Bemeleit, D.J., Mockel, C., Clausing, E., Schele, A., Hartung, S., Schiller, C.B., Lucas, M., Angermuller, C., Soding, J., *et al.* (2011). The Mre11:Rad50 Structure Shows an ATP-Dependent Molecular Clamp in DNA Double-Strand Break Repair. Cell *145*, 54-66.

Lane, H.E., and Denhardt, D.T. (1975). The rep mutation. IV. Slower movement of replication forks in Escherichia coli rep strains. J Mol Biol *97*, 99-112.

Lee, B.I., Kim, K.H., Park, S.J., Eom, S.H., Song, H.K., and Suh, S.W. (2004). Ring-shaped architecture of RecR: implications for its role in homologous recombinational DNA repair. Embo J *23*, 2029-2038.

Lee, J.H., and Paull, T.T. (2005). ATM activation by DNA double-strand breaks through the Mre11-Rad50-Nbs1 complex. Science *308*, 551-554.

Leiros, I., Timmins, J., Hall, D.R., and McSweeney, S. (2005). Crystal structure and DNA-binding analysis of RecO from Deinococcus radiodurans. Embo J *24*, 906-918.

Lim, H.S., Kim, J.S., Park, Y.B., Gwon, G.H., and Cho, Y. (2011). Crystal structure of the Mre11-Rad50-ATP{gamma}S complex: understanding the interplay between Mre11 and Rad50. Genes Dev. 25, 1091-1104

Lloyd, R.G., and Thomas, A. (1983). On the nature of the RecBC and RecF pathways of conjugal recombination in Escherichia coli. Mol Gen Genet *190*, 156-161.

Lovett, S.T., and Clark, A.J. (1983). Genetic analysis of regulation of the RecF pathway of recombination in Escherichia coli K-12. J Bacteriol *153*, 1471-1478.

Luisi-DeLuca, C., and Kolodner, R. (1994). Purification and characterization of the Escherichia coli RecO protein. Renaturation of complementary single-stranded DNA molecules catalyzed by the RecO protein. J Mol Biol *236*, 124-138.

Lusetti, S.L., Hobbs, M.D., Stohl, E.A., Chitteni-Pattu, S., Inman, R.B., Seifert, H.S., and Cox, M.M. (2006). The RecF protein antagonizes RecX function via direct interaction. Mol Cell *21*, 41-50.

Madiraju, M.V., and Clark, A.J. (1991). Effect of RecF protein on reactions catalyzed by RecA protein. Nucleic Acids Res *19*, 6295-6300.

Madiraju, M.V., and Clark, A.J. (1992). Evidence for ATP binding and double-stranded DNA binding by Escherichia coli RecF protein. J Bacteriol *174*, 7705-7710.

Mahdi, A.A., Buckman, C., Harris, L., and Lloyd, R.G. (2006). Rep and PriA helicase activities prevent RecA from provoking unnecessary recombination during replication fork repair. Genes Dev *20*, 2135-2147.

Makarova, K.S., Aravind, L., Wolf, Y.I., Tatusov, R.L., Minton, K.W., Koonin, E.V., and Daly, M.J. (2001). Genome of the extremely radiation-resistant bacterium Deinococcus radiodurans viewed from the perspective of comparative genomics. Microbiol Mol Biol Rev *65*, 44-79.

Makharashvili, N. (2009). What RecFOR are for: Structure-function studies of recombination mediator proteins. In Biochemistry (Saint Louis, Missouri, USA, Saint Louis University), pp. 152.

Makharashvili, N., Koroleva, O., Bera, S., Grandgenett, D.P., and Korolev, S. (2004). A novel structure of DNA repair protein RecO from Deinococcus radiodurans. Structure (Camb) *12*, 1881-1889.

Makharashvili, N., Mi, T., Koroleva, O., and Korolev, S. (2009). RecR-mediated modulation of RecF dimer specificity for single- and double-stranded DNA. J Biol Chem *284*, 1425-1434.

Manfredi, C., Carrasco, B., Ayora, S., and Alonso, J.C. (2008). Bacillus subtilis RecO nucleates RecA onto SsbA-coated single-stranded DNA. J Biol Chem *283*, 24837-24847.

Manfredi, C., Suzuki, Y., Yadav, T., Takeyasu, K., and Alonso, J.C. (2010). RecO-mediated DNA homology search and annealing is facilitated by SsbA. Nucleic Acids Res *38*, 6920-6929.

Mazloum, N., Zhou, Q., and Holloman, W.K. (2007). DNA binding, annealing, and strand exchange activities of Brh2 protein from Ustilago maydis. Biochemistry *46*, 7163-7173.

McInerney, P., and O'Donnell, M. (2007). Replisome fate upon encountering a leading strand block and clearance from DNA by recombination proteins. J Biol Chem *282*, 25903-25916.

Michel-Marks, E., Courcelle, C.T., Korolev, S., and Courcelle, J. (2010). ATP binding, ATP hydrolysis, and protein dimerization are required for RecF to catalyze an early step in the processing and recovery of replication forks disrupted by DNA damage. J Mol Biol *401*, 579-589.

Mohaghegh, P., and Hickson, I.D. (2001). DNA helicase deficiencies associated with cancer predisposition and premature ageing disorders. Hum Mol Genet *10*, 741-746.

Moncalian, G., Lengsfeld, B., Bhaskara, V., Hopfner, K.P., Karcher, A., Alden, E., Tainer, J.A., and Paull, T.T. (2004). The rad50 signature motif: essential to ATP binding and biological function. J Mol Biol *335*, 937-951.

Morimatsu, K., and Kowalczykowski, S.C. (2003). RecFOR Proteins Load RecA Protein onto Gapped DNA to Accelerate DNA Strand Exchange. A Universal Step of Recombinational Repair. Mol Cell *11*, 1337-1347.

Moynahan, M.E., Pierce, A.J., and Jasin, M. (2001). BRCA2 is required for homology-directed repair of chromosomal breaks. Mol Cell *7*, 263-272.

Nakayama, H., Nakayama, K., Nakayama, R., and Nakayama, Y. (1982). Recombination-deficient mutations and thymineless death in Escherichia coli K12: reciprocal effects of recBC and recF and indifference of recA mutations. Can J Microbiol *28*, 425-430.

New, J.H., Sugiyama, T., Zaitseva, E., and Kowalczykowski, S.C. (1998). Rad52 protein stimulates DNA strand exchange by Rad51 and replication protein A. Nature *391*, 407-410.

Nicolette, M.L., Lee, K., Guo, Z., Rani, M., Chow, J.M., Lee, S.E., and Paull, T.T. (2010). Mre11-Rad50-Xrs2 and Sae2 promote 5' strand resection of DNA double-strand breaks. Nat Struct Mol Biol *17*, 1478-1485.

Obmolova, G., Ban, C., Hsieh, P., and Yang, W. (2000). Crystal structures of mismatch repair protein MutS and its complex with a substrate DNA. Nature *407*, 703-710.

Ouyang, K.J., Woo, L.L., and Ellis, N.A. (2008). Homologous recombination and maintenance of genome integrity: cancer and aging through the prism of human RecQ helicases. Mech Ageing Dev *129*, 425-440.

Perez-Roger, I., Garcia-Sogo, M., Navarro-Avino, J.P., Lopez-Acedo, C., Macian, F., and Armengod, M.E. (1991). Positive and negative regulatory elements in the dnaA-dnaN-recF operon of Escherichia coli. Biochimie *73*, 329-334.

Petit, M.A., and Ehrlich, D. (2002). Essential bacterial helicases that counteract the toxicity of recombination proteins. EMBO J *21*, 3137-3147.

Powell, S.N., Willers, H., and Xia, F. (2002). BRCA2 keeps Rad51 in line. High-fidelity homologous recombination prevents breast and ovarian cancer? Mol Cell *10*, 1262-1263.

Rajagopalan, M., Lu, C., Woodgate, R., O'Donnell, M., Goodman, M.F., and Echols, H. (1992). Activity of the purified mutagenesis proteins UmuC, UmuD', and RecA in replicative bypass of an abasic DNA lesion by DNA polymerase III. Proc Natl Acad Sci U S A *89*, 10777-10781.

Ream, L.W., and Clark, A.J. (1983). Cloning and deletion mapping of the recF dnaN region of the Escherichia coli chromosome. Plasmid *10*, 101-110.

Ream, L.W., Margossian, L., Clark, A.J., Hansen, F.G., and von Meyenburg, K. (1980). Genetic and physical mapping of recF in Escherichia coli K-12. Mol Gen Genet *180*, 115-121.

Rehrauer, W.M., Lavery, P.E., Palmer, E.L., Singh, R.N., and Kowalczykowski, S.C. (1996). Interaction of Escherichia coli RecA protein with LexA repressor. I. LexA repressor cleavage is competitive with binding of a secondary DNA molecule. J Biol Chem *271*, 23865-23873.

Rocha, E.P., Cornet, E., and Michel, B. (2005). Comparative and evolutionary analysis of the bacterial homologous recombination systems. PLoS Genet *1*, e15.

Rothman, R.H., and Clark, A.J. (1977). The dependence of postreplication repair on uvrB in a recF mutant of Escherichia coli K-12. Mol Gen Genet *155*, 279-286.

Ryzhikov, M., Koroleva, O., Postnov, D., Tran, A., and Korolev, S. (2011). Mechanism of RecO recruitment to DNA by single-stranded DNA binding protein. Nucleic Acids Res.

Sakai, A., and Cox, M.M. (2009). RecFOR and RecOR as distinct RecA loading pathways. J Biol Chem *284*, 3264-3272.

Sandler, S.J. (1996). Overlapping functions for recF and priA in cell viability and UV-inducible SOS expression are distinguished by dnaC809 in Escherichia coli K-12. Mol Microbiol *19*, 871-880.

Sandler, S.J., Chackerian, B., Li, J.T., and Clark, A.J. (1992). Sequence and complementation analysis of recF genes from Escherichia coli, Salmonella typhimurium, Pseudomonas putida and Bacillus subtilis: evidence for an essential phosphate binding loop. Nucleic Acids Res *20*, 839-845.

Sandler, S.J., and Clark, A.J. (1994). RecOR suppression of recF mutant phenotypes in Escherichia coli K-12. J Bacteriol *176*, 3661-3672.

Shinohara, A., and Ogawa, T. (1998). Stimulation by Rad52 of yeast Rad51-mediated recombination. Nature *391*, 404-407.

Singleton, M.R., Wentzell, L.M., Liu, Y., West, S.C., and Wigley, D.B. (2002). Structure of the single-strand annealing domain of human RAD52 protein. Proc Natl Acad Sci U S A *99*, 13492-13497.

Smith, P.C., Karpowich, N., Millen, L., Moody, J.E., Rosen, J., Thomas, P.J., and Hunt, J.F. (2002). ATP binding to the motor domain from an ABC transporter drives formation of a nucleotide sandwich dimer. Mol Cell *10*, 139-149.

Strunnikov, A.V. (1998). SMC proteins and chromosome structure. Trends Cell Biol *8*, 454-459.

Sugiyama, T., New, J.H., and Kowalczykowski, S.C. (1998). DNA annealing by RAD52 protein is stimulated by specific interaction with the complex of replication protein A and single-stranded DNA. Proc Natl Acad Sci U S A *95*, 6049-6054.

Sung, P. (1997). Function of yeast Rad52 protein as a mediator between replication protein A and the Rad51 recombinase. J Biol Chem *272*, 28194-28197.

Sweezy, M.A., and Morrical, S.W. (1999). Biochemical interactions within a ternary complex of the bacteriophage T4 recombination proteins uvsY and gp32 bound to single-stranded DNA. Biochemistry *38*, 936-944.

Symington, L.S. (2002). Role of RAD52 epistasis group genes in homologous recombination and double-strand break repair. Microbiol Mol Biol Rev *66*, 630-670, table of contents.

Tal, A., Arbel-Goren, R., and Stavans, J. (2009). Cancer-associated mutations in BRC domains of BRCA2 affect homologous recombination induced by Rad51. J Mol Biol *393*, 1007-1012.

Tessmer, I., Yang, Y., Zhai, J., Du, C., Hsieh, P., Hingorani, M.M., and Erie, D.A. (2008). Mechanism of MutS searching for DNA mismatches and signaling repair. J Biol Chem *283*, 36646-36654.

Thompson, L.H., and Schild, D. (2002). Recombinational DNA repair and human disease. Mutat Res *509*, 49-78.

Timmins, J., Leiros, I., and McSweeney, S. (2007). Crystal structure and mutational study of RecOR provide insight into its mode of DNA binding. Embo J *26*, 3260-3271.

Umezu, K., Chi, N.W., and Kolodner, R.D. (1993). Biochemical interaction of the Escherichia coli RecF, RecO, and RecR proteins with RecA protein and single-stranded DNA binding protein. Proc Natl Acad Sci U S A *90*, 3875-3879.

Umezu, K., and Kolodner, R.D. (1994). Protein interactions in genetic recombination in Escherichia coli. Interactions involving RecO and RecR overcome the inhibition of RecA by single-stranded DNA-binding protein. J Biol Chem *269*, 30005-30013.

Veaute, X., Delmas, S., Selva, M., Jeusset, J., Le Cam, E., Matic, I., Fabre, F., and Petit, M.A. (2005). UvrD helicase, unlike Rep helicase, dismantles RecA nucleoprotein filaments in Escherichia coli. EMBO J *24*, 180-189.

Villarroya, M., Perez-Roger, I., Macian, F., and Armengod, M.E. (1998). Stationary phase induction of dnaN and recF, two genes of Escherichia coli involved in DNA replication and repair. EMBO J *17*, 1829-1837.

Walker, J.E., Saraste, M., Runswick, M.J., and Gay, N.J. (1982). Distantly related sequences in the alpha- and beta-subunits of ATP synthase, myosin, kinases and other ATP-requiring enzymes and a common nucleotide binding fold. Embo J *1*, 945-951.

Wang, T.C., and Smith, K.C. (1983). Mechanisms for recF-dependent and recB-dependent pathways of postreplication repair in UV-irradiated Escherichia coli uvrB. J Bacteriol *156*, 1093-1098.

Wang, T.V., and Smith, K.C. (1984). recF-dependent and recF recB-independent DNA gap-filling repair processes transfer dimer-containing parental strands to daughter strands in Escherichia coli K-12 uvrB. J Bacteriol *158*, 727-729.

Webb, B.L., Cox, M.M., and Inman, R.B. (1995). An interaction between the Escherichia coli RecF and RecR proteins dependent on ATP and double-stranded DNA. J Biol Chem *270*, 31397-31404.

Webb, B.L., Cox, M.M., and Inman, R.B. (1997). Recombinational DNA repair: the RecF and RecR proteins limit the extension of RecA filaments beyond single-strand DNA gaps. Cell *91*, 347-356.

Webb, B.L., Cox, M.M., and Inman, R.B. (1999). ATP hydrolysis and DNA binding by the Escherichia coli RecF protein. J Biol Chem *274*, 15367-15374.

Whitby, M.C., and Lloyd, R.G. (1995). Altered SOS induction associated with mutations in recF, recO and recR. Mol Gen Genet *246*, 174-179.

Williams, G.J., Williams, R.S., Williams, J.S., Moncalian, G., Arvai, A.S., Limbo, O., Guenther, G., Sildas, S., Hammel, M., Russell, P., *et al.* (2011). ABC ATPase signature helices in Rad50 link nucleotide state to Mre11 interface for DNA repair. Nat Struct Mol Biol *18*, 423-431.

Williams, R.S., Williams, J.S., and Tainer, J.A. (2007). Mre11-Rad50-Nbs1 is a keystone complex connecting DNA repair machinery, double-strand break signaling, and the chromatin template. Biochem Cell Biol *85*, 509-520.

Yang, H., Jeffrey, P.D., Miller, J., Kinnucan, E., Sun, Y., Thoma, N.H., Zheng, N., Chen, P.L., Lee, W.H., and Pavletich, N.P. (2002). BRCA2 function in DNA binding and recombination from a BRCA2-DSS1-ssDNA structure. Science *297*, 1837-1848.

Yang, H., Li, Q., Fan, J., Holloman, W.K., and Pavletich, N.P. (2005). The BRCA2 homologue Brh2 nucleates RAD51 filament formation at a dsDNA-ssDNA junction. Nature *433*, 653-657.

Zahradka, K., Simic, S., Buljubasic, M., Petranovic, M., Dermic, D., and Zahradka, D. (2006). sbcB15 And DeltasbcB mutations activate two types of recf recombination pathways in Escherichia coli. J Bacteriol *188*, 7562-7571.

23

DNA Damage Recognition for Mammalian Global Genome Nucleotide Excision Repair

Kaoru Sugasawa
Biosignal Research Center, Organization of Advanced Science and Technology
Kobe University
Japan

1. Introduction

As a blueprint for genetic information, the structural and functional integrity of DNA must be maintained during cell division and gamete formation. However, this fundamental principle is threatened continuously by the vulnerability of DNA itself and/or by assaults from endogenously produced agents, such as reactive oxygen species and other metabolites, as well as various environmental agents including ultraviolet light (UV), ionizing radiation and chemical compounds (Friedberg et al., 2006). Among the DNA components, bases in particular are frequently the targets for such insults. Because DNA replication and transcription rely on the formation of specific base pairs, even a subtle change in the base structures can compromise faithful propagation and the expression of genetic information. For instance, replicative DNA polymerases, which exhibit very high intrinsic fidelity, are often blocked at sites where template bases are modified, which can lead to replication fork collapse and consequent chromosomal aberrations and/or cell death. This problem is overcome, at least partly, by translesion DNA synthesis, which is an error-prone process (Friedberg et al., 2005). To minimize the risk of mutagenesis, it is crucial for growing cells to detect and to remove damaged bases as much as possible before replication forks collide with them.

Nucleotide excision repair (NER) is a major DNA repair pathway that can eliminate an extremely broad spectrum of base damage. The NER substrates include dipyrimidinic UV photolesions, such as cyclobutane pyrimidine dimers (CPDs) and pyrimidine-pyrimidone (6-4) photoproducts (6-4PPs), intrastrand crosslinks caused by bifunctional alkylating agents (e.g., cisplatin), and bulky base adducts induced by numerous chemical carcinogens (Gillet & Schärer, 2006). The common feature shared by all of these insults does not reside in their chemical structure, but rather in the accompanying distortions of the otherwise regular DNA helical structure. Two subpathways are associated with mammalian NER: global genome NER (GG-NER) and transcription-coupled NER (TC-NER). GG-NER is a general pathway that operates throughout the genome. It minimizes the collision of replication forks with damaged bases and, thereby, contributes to the maintenance of genome integrity (Gillet & Schärer, 2006). TC-NER is specialized to remove transcription-blocking lesions from the template DNA strands, which ensures rapid recovery of transcriptional activity and thus averts apoptosis (Hanawalt & Spivak, 2008). In humans, hereditary defects in NER are associated with several autosomal recessive disorders, including xeroderma pigmentosum (XP), Cockayne syndrome (CS) and trichothiodystrophy (TTD) (Bootsma et al., 2001). The clinical hallmarks exhibited by patients with XP, which include marked photosensitivity and a predisposition to skin cancer, explicitly indicate that the impaired repair of UV-induced DNA photolesions promotes mutagenesis and carcinogenesis in the skin. Numerous genetic complementation groups have been identified for the above diseases, including 8 for XP (XP-A through -G, and variant), 2 for CS (CS-A and -B) and 1 for TTD (TTD-A). Cloning of the responsible genes has revealed that all of them encode proteins involved in the NER pathway. The notable exception is the XP variant (*XPV*) gene encoding DNA polymerase η that is involved in translesion DNA synthesis, but not in NER. Another important milestone in elucidating the NER mechanism has been the establishment of the cell-free system, which faithfully recapitulates the NER reaction with human whole cell extracts. Together, genetic and biochemical studies have successfully identified more than 30 polypeptides that are involved in mammalian GG-NER (Fig. 1). A fundamental challenge for GG-NER is that the cells must detect a small number of injured bases among the vast excess of normal bases comprising the huge genome. Although the complete network of mechanisms has not yet been entirely uncovered, recent studies have revealed some of the sophisticated molecular mechanisms that accomplish this difficult task, which involves concerted actions of multiple protein factors. This chapter overviews the latest progress in our understanding of the damage-recognition mechanism for mammalian GG-NER.

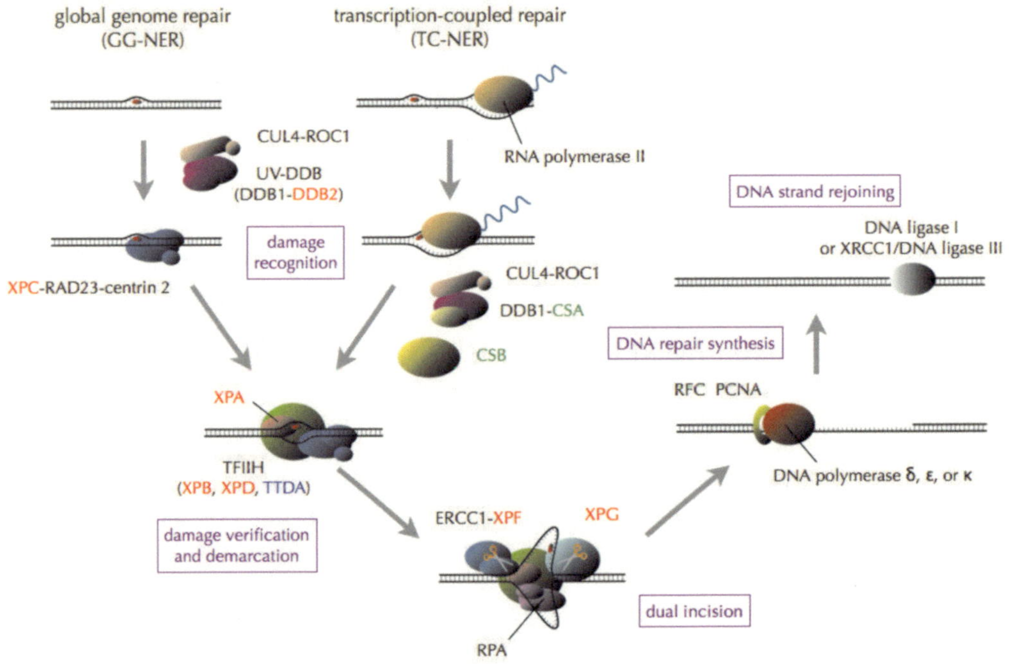

Fig. 1. Model of the mammalian NER mechanism. The 2 subpathways, GG-NER and TC-NER, differ in their strategies for initial damage recognition, but converge into a common process. The disease-related gene products are indicated by letters in different colors: XP, red; CS, green; TTD, blue.

2. Primary damage sensors for the initiation of GG-NER

One of the remarkable characteristics of GG-NER resides in its extremely broad substrate specificity, which encompasses UV-induced photolesions and other bulky base adducts that can be induced by numerous chemical compounds (Gillet & Schärer, 2006). These GG-NER substrates are associated with considerable levels of DNA helical distortion. This situation is in marked contrast to substrates for base excision repair (BER), such as uracils and oxidative base lesions, which are supposed to induce only marginal structural distortions. Initial damage detection for BER is accomplished by a set of DNA glycosylases, each of which exhibits a certain (partially overlapping) range of substrate specificity. In contrast, a virtually infinite spectrum of helix-distorting insults can be handled by the unified molecular machinery in GG-NER. In addition, GG-NER must survey the huge genome continuously and discriminate a small number of injured bases from normal bases with very high efficiency and accuracy. Recent biochemical studies have uncovered some of the sophisticated molecular mechanisms that achieve this difficult task.

2.1 Indirect sensing of DNA damage by XPC

The *XPC* gene was isolated from a cDNA expression library (Legerski & Peterson, 1992) that corrected the UV sensitivity of fibroblasts from patients with XP-C. Cells lacking XPC are incompetent for GG-NER, but TC-NER functions normally (Venema et al., 1990). By using the cell-free NER system, a protein factor that is missing in XP-C cells was purified from HeLa cell extracts (Masutani et al., 1994; Shivji et al., 1994). This biochemical approach revealed that the XPC protein forms a stable complex in vivo with 1 of the 2 human homologues of *Saccharomyces cerevisiae* Rad23p (designated RAD23A and RAD23B). Depletion of RAD23 markedly destabilized the XPC protein, thereby compromising GG-NER function (Ng et al., 2003; Okuda et al., 2004). Another component of the XPC complex, centrin-2 (Araki et al., 2001; Nishi et al., 2005), belongs to the calmodulin superfamily of small calcium-binding proteins containing 4 conserved EF-hand motifs. A subpopulation of centrin-2 localizes to the centrosomes and plays a vital role in cell cycle regulation (Lutz et al., 2001; Salisbury et al., 2002). Centrin-2 also binds to an α-helix near the C-terminus of XPC: this interaction potentiates the DNA-binding activity of the complex (Bunick et al., 2006; Nishi et al., 2005; Popescu et al., 2003; Thompson et al., 2006).
The XPC protein complex has been known to be associated with DNA-binding activity since it was first purified (Masutani et al., 1994; Shivji et al., 1994), although its preference for damaged DNA was discovered sometime later (Batty et al., 2000; Sugasawa et al., 1998). With conventional electrophoretic mobility shift assays (EMSAs) and DNase I footprint analyses with defined DNA substrates, we demonstrated that XPC prefers to associate with sites containing a helix-distorting lesion, such as 6-4PP or *N*-(guanin-8-yl) *N*-acetyl-2-aminofluorene (dG-AAF) adduct (Sugasawa et al., 1998; Sugasawa et al., 2001). However, the addition of an appropriate competitor DNA was necessary to reveal the damage specificity, by preventing XPC from binding to the undamaged part of the DNA. Several physicochemical approaches subsequently were undertaken to assess the affinities of XPC for various DNA structures in more dynamic states (Hey et al., 2002; Roche et al., 2008; Trego & Turchi, 2006).
Involvement of the XPC complex in the very early stages of NER was first proposed on the basis of the results obtained with the cell-free NER system (Sugasawa et al., 1998). In this system, 2 plasmid DNAs containing AAF adducts were preincubated separately with

different sets of NER factors, for which either XP cell extracts or purified recombinant proteins were used. After the 2 mixtures were combined and missing NER factors, if any, were supplemented, the initial repair rates of the 2 damaged DNA substrates were compared directly in one reaction. Damaged DNA preincubated in the presence of XPC was always repaired preferentially compared to DNA preincubated in its absence. Because a similar repair bias was not observed with other NER factors, these findings strongly suggest that XPC initiates in vitro NER, and its binding to damaged DNA is sufficient to recruit the whole repair machinery.

Several subsequent studies have supported this model. Local UV irradiation through micropore membrane filters has been used to visualize the recruitment of NER factors in cultured cells to the sites of DNA damage. Use of this method revealed that XPC accumulates at subnuclear UV-damaged areas, even when any other XP genes were mutated (Volker et al., 2001). Conversely, none of the other NER-related XP proteins (except for DDB2; see below) was recruited to the sites of DNA damage in *XPC*-deficient cells, consistent with the role of XPC as the initiator of GG-NER. Through the use of paramagnetic beads immobilized with a damaged DNA substrate, more refined biochemical studies were undertaken to determine the order of arrival and departure of individual NER proteins at the lesion: these studies also concluded that XPC arrives first (Riedl et al., 2003). It should be noted that only GG-NER is impaired in XP-C (and also XP-E) cells, unlike other NER-deficient XP cells, in which both GG-NER and TC-NER are affected. Considering that TC-NER is supposed to be triggered by RNA polymerase II stumbling at damaged bases on the template DNA strand, it could be assumed that the 2 NER subpathways vary only in their strategies for initial damage recognition and eventually merge into a common process.

Because XPC appeared to bind specifically to various lesions that did not share any common chemical structure, it was of great interest to understand which feature of DNA determined its binding specificity. To examine this, using EMSA, we tested XPC binding with various DNA substrates containing a defined lesion and/or artificial structure (Sugasawa et al., 2001; Sugasawa et al., 2002). XPC was able to recognize and to bind DNA duplexes containing a partially single-stranded region, such as bubble and loop structures, even though these substrates contained only base mismatches, but no chemical modifications. Further analyses using various oligonucleotides as competitors revealed that XPC was targeted preferentially to a branched DNA structure containing a double-stranded region attached to a single-stranded 3'-overhang. On the basis of these results, it might be better to refer to XPC as a *structure-specific DNA-binding factor*, rather than as a damage recognition factor.

The binding of XPC to sites of DNA damage seems to depend solely on the extent of local unwinding of the DNA duplex caused by a given lesion: typically, XPC showed very little affinity for sites of CPD, because of the subtle DNA helical distortion associated with this lesion. In contrast, the presence of 1 or 2 mismatched bases opposite the photodimer significantly enhanced binding by XPC (Sugasawa et al., 2001). Accordingly, this biochemical feature of XPC may provide an important molecular basis for the substrate specificity of GG-NER, including an infinite range of helix-distorting lesions, but not a number of nonbulky lesions, such as oxidized and deaminated bases.

More recently, a structural study corroborated this DNA-binding mode of XPC (Min & Pavletich, 2007). The *S. cerevisiae* NER protein Rad4p is presumed to be the counterpart of mammalian XPC: both proteins share several conserved structural domains in their C-terminal regions, including the transglutaminase-homology domain (TGD) and 3 consecutive β-hairpin domains (designated BHD1, BHD2, and BHD3). The X-ray crystal structure was solved with the C-terminal region of Rad4p bound to a short DNA duplex containing a CPD (which was placed within 3-base mismatches to enhance recognition by Rad4p). Consistent with the results of our footprint analyses with XPC, the results showed that Rad4p binds asymmetrically to the damaged DNA: it interacts with an 11-base pair segment of DNA duplex on the 3' side of CPD, mainly through TGD and BHD1, leaving the other double-stranded part on the 5' side of the lesion completely free. In the closer vicinity of the lesion, BHD3 is inserted into the major groove, such that BHD2 and BHD3 appear to pinch the phosphate-sugar backbone of the undamaged strand. As a result, 2 "normal" bases on the undamaged DNA strand are flipped out and held by BHD2-BHD3, while the CPD is also flipped out structurally disordered, and devoid of any contact with the protein (Fig. 2). The Rad4p binding results in a ~42° bend of DNA, as observed by our scanning force microscopy with the XPC-DNA complex (Janićijević et al., 2003). In conclusion, XPC/Rad4p appears to function as a versatile damage-recognition factor that senses the presence of oscillating normal bases within the DNA duplex.

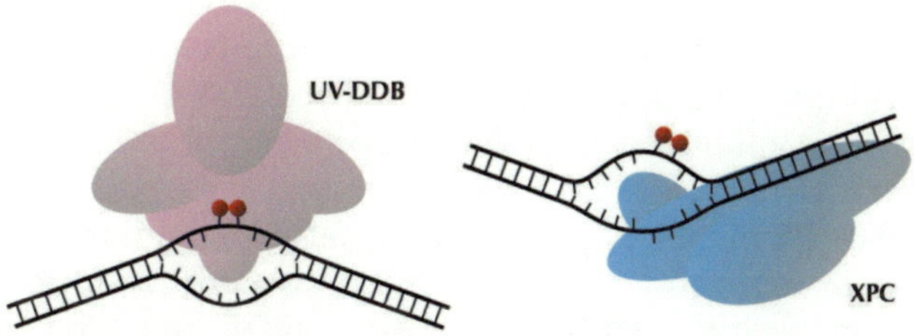

Fig. 2. Different binding modes of UV-DDB and XPC to damaged DNA sites. The β-hairpin of UV-DDB on the DDB2 β-propeller is inserted between the two strands of the DNA, so that DDB2 interacts directly with the damaged nucleotides flipped out of the DNA duplex. In contrast, XPC interacts with normal bases on the undamaged DNA strand without any contact with the damaged bases.

2.2 UV-DDB facilitates detection of UV-induced photolesions

In accordance with the proposed function of XPC as the initiator of GG-NER, most of the DNA lesions that are subject to GG-NER in vivo are recognized by XPC in vitro. However, CPD serves as a noticeable exception. Like other GG-NER substrates, CPDs are not removed from the global genome in *XPC*-deficient cells, although XPC by itself cannot find this type of insult (as described above). From this apparent discrepancy, it can be assumed that a certain factor (other than XPC) is responsible for the initial detection of CPDs, whereas XPC must be involved in later steps.

UV-damaged DNA-binding protein complex (UV-DDB) was first discovered as a factor that bound UV-damaged DNA with high affinity and specificity. The factor responsible for this binding activity was purified and revealed as a complex consisting of 2 subunits, designated DDB1 and DDB2, respectively (for a review, see Tang & Chu, 2002). It was later demonstrated that mutations in the *DDB2* gene constitute the XP genetic complementation group E (Rapić-Otrin et al., 2003). Recent studies have redefined DDB1 as an adaptor protein that mediates interactions between the CUL4-ROC1 ubiquitin ligase complex and a member of the substrate-recruiting subunit family, called DDB1-CUL4 associating factor (DCAF)

(Angers et al., 2006; Lee & Zhou, 2007). The DNA-binding specificity of purified UV-DDB has been characterized extensively (Fujiwara et al., 1999; Payne & Chu, 1994; Reardon et al., 1993; Treiber et al., 1992; Wittschieben et al., 2005). Concerning UV-induced photolesions, UV-DDB exhibits extraordinarily high affinity and specificity for 6-4PPs, although it also binds CPDs moderately. Although binding to chemical-induced base adducts seems not to be pronounced, abasic sites are relatively good substrates for UV-DDB.

Despite the above biochemical characteristics that explicitly point to roles in UV-damage recognition, the impact of defects in UV-DDB on NER has remained enigmatic. Cells from patients with XP-E have defects in GG-NER, but not in TC-NER. However, in contrast to XP-C, cells from patients with XP-E are proficient in removal of 6-4PPs from the global genome, while repair of CPDs seems to be affected profoundly (Hwang et al., 1999; Tang et al., 2000). As a result, among the NER-deficient XP groups, XP-E cells show the highest levels of residual UV-induced unscheduled DNA synthesis (>50% of normal cells) and resistance to killing by UV (Tang & Chu, 2002).

Unlike other XP-related gene products, DDB2 reportedly accumulates to local UV-damaged areas within the nucleus, even in the absence of XPC (Wakasugi et al., 2002), although XPC can relocate to sites containing UV-induced DNA damage in a DDB2-independent manner (Moser et al., 2005). Although UV-DDB and XPC appear to be recruited independently, UV irradiation always induces a mixture of various sorts of DNA injuries, including 6-4PPs, CPDs, and other less frequent insults. To solve this problem, elegant experiments have been undertaken, in which 6-4PPs were erased soon after local UV irradiation with the aid of an ectopically expressed 6-4PP photolyase (Fitch et al., 2003). Under these conditions where the remaining photolesions were mostly CPDs, DDB2-dependent recruitment of XPC became evident. These results clearly indicate that differential pathways are used for the deployment of XPC to sites of UV damage, depending on the type of lesions.

Considering the role for UV-DDB in CPD repair and its much stronger binding to 6-4PPs, one could assume that UV-DDB plays a role in the detection and repair of 6-4PPs. However, 6-4PPs are rapidly removed from the global genome even in the absence of DDB2 (most likely through direct recognition by XPC), so that stimulation by UV-DDB, if any, cannot be clearly discerned. Additionally, DDB2 undergoes degradation by the proteasome in response to UV irradiation (see below) (Fitch et al., 2003; Rapić-Otrin et al., 2002). Since this degradation is quite fast - particularly at relatively high UV doses - this situation further overshadows possible effects of UV-DDB on the repair of 6-4PPs.

Recently, the local UV irradiation technique has been applied to the quantification of 6-4PPs, which appear as fluorescent spots developed by an antibody specific for the photolesion (Moser et al., 2005). With this method, the total number of generated photolesions per cell was reduced substantially, and retardation of 6-4PP repair in the absence of UV-DDB became discernable. Similar conclusions were drawn from our experiments using fluorescence recovery after photobleaching (FRAP) (Nishi et al., 2009), which is a widely used method to assess the in vivo mobility of fluorescence-labeled proteins. With cells expressing NER factors fused to green fluorescent protein (GFP), global UV irradiation before photobleaching resulted in the significant retardation of fluorescence recovery within the bleached subnuclear region. This result indicated that the proteins concerned are sequestered at the sites of UV photolesions and engaged in NER (Houtsmuller et al., 1999).

The reduction in the mobility of GFP-XPC showed a unique biphasic relationship with the pre-UV dose. The immobilization of GFP-XPC was saturated at relatively low UV doses (5~10 J/m^2): higher UV doses resulted in further dose-dependent retardation of fluorescence recovery, which eventually became saturated again at extremely high doses (around 80~100 J/m^2). Notably, the reduction in XPC mobility seemed to depend on the remaining 6-4PPs rather than on CPDs. Overexpression and siRNA knockdown of DDB2 revealed that the first immobilization of GFP-XPC (observed with low UV doses) was due to entrapment by UV-DDB bound to 6-4PPs (Nishi et al., 2009). These results indicate that UV-DDB likely contributes to the efficient detection of both of the major photolesions, particularly when the density of the induced lesions is low enough (in terms of physiologically relevant levels), and thereby recruits XPC and other NER factors.

Although the precise molecular mechanism underlying XPC recruitment by UV-DDB remains unclear, we have shown the presence of a direct physical interaction between these 2 damage-recognition factors by coimmunoprecipitation experiments (Sugasawa et al., 2005). Among the components of each complex, XPC and DDB2 appeared to be responsible for the interaction. More recently, researchers have solved the crystal structure for UV-DDB bound to a DNA duplex containing a 6-4PP (Scrima et al., 2008). DDB1 shows a unique structure containing 3 β-propeller domains (designated BPA, BPB, and BPC), whereas DDB2 has a β-propeller that is exclusively involved in its interaction with DNA. The N-terminal extension of DDB2 contains a helix-loop-helix motif, which mediates its interaction with DDB1. In this structure, UV-DDB approaches the lesion and inserts its evolutionarily conserved β-hairpin on the surface of the DDB2 β-propeller into the minor groove of the DNA, thereby causing a ~40° kink in the DNA. This β-hairpin seems to push the 2 affected bases out of the DNA duplex: these bases interact extensively with the amino acids that form a binding pocket on the surface of DDB2 (Fig. 2). The size of the binding pocket seems fit to accommodate 2 nucleotides, which suggests that DDB2 has evolved to recognize dinucleotide lesions, such as UV-induced photodimers. Considering that XPC interacts with the undamaged strand, XPC may gain access to the lesion from the side opposite to UV-DDB, sandwiching the DNA in between. However, the formation of such a ternary complex has not been demonstrated by EMSA or other methods.

2.3 Roles of ubiquitylation in GG-NER damage recognition

As mentioned above, UV-DDB is thought to be part of the ubiquitin ligase complex. Expression of the epitope-tagged DDB2 in cells and isolation of the protein complexes under relatively mild conditions have revealed that DDB2 associates in vivo with not only DDB1, but also with CUL4A-ROC1 and the COP9 signalosome (CSN) (Groisman et al., 2003). CSN, which is an 8-subunit complex possessing deneddylation and deubiquitylation activities, is believed to function as a negative regulator of the cullin-based ubiquitin ligase family (Lyapina et al., 2001; Yang et al., 2002). Upon UV irradiation of cells, UV-DDB relocates onto chromatin, where the associating ubiquitin ligase seems to be activated, judging from dissociation of CSN and neddylation of CUL4A (Groisman et al., 2003).

We have demonstrated that XPC is one of the substrates for this ubiquitin ligase (Sugasawa et al., 2005). After UV irradiation, slowly migrating, ubiquitylated forms of XPC became apparent. The appearance of these forms peaked around 1 h postirradiation, at which time the repair of 6-4PPs was rapidly ongoing. This transient ubiquitylation of XPC was detected even in NER-deficient XP and CS cells, with the only exception being XP-E cells. Notably, treatment of cells with a protein synthesis inhibitor, cycloheximide, revealed that ubiquitylated XPC had mostly reverted to its unmodified form, instead of being degraded. Subsequently, the recombinant DDB1-DDB2-CUL4A-ROC1 ubiquitin ligase complex was purified and successfully used for in vitro reconstitution of the XPC ubiquitylation. In this reaction, not only XPC but also DDB2 and CUL4A were found to be polyubiquitylated. It was previously reported that DDB2 undergoes degradation by the proteasome in response to UV irradiation (Fitch et al., 2003; Rapić-Otrin et al., 2002). These results suggest that the fates of the modified XPC and DDB2 are different, even though they seem to be ubiquitylated by the same ligase.

To elucidate the roles of ubiquitylation in the mechanism of GG-NER, we performed DNA-binding assays using paramagnetic beads immobilized with DNA containing the UV photolesions, CPD or 6-4PP (Sugasawa et al., 2005). In vitro ubiquitylation reactions in the presence of these DNA beads revealed that polyubiquitylation of DDB2 completely abolished the strong damaged DNA-binding activity of UV-DDB. In contrast, polyubiquitylated XPC in the same reaction continued to bind to DNA, with a slightly higher affinity than the unmodified form. Considering the remarkable difference in their affinities for UV-damaged DNA, it is conceivable that XPC cannot simply displace UV-DDB that is already bound to the site containing a photolesion.

When UV-DDB was added to cell-free NER reactions involving 6-4PP as a defined DNA substrate, only inhibition (and not stimulation) of dual incision was observed (Sugasawa et al., 2005). This finding suggested that UV-DDB tightly bound to the lesion may adversely block access to XPC and other NER factors, at least in vitro. Since this inhibition was partially alleviated by the addition of all of the components required for ubiquitylation, we proposed that damage handover from UV-DDB (strong binder) to XPC (weak binder) may be promoted by polyubiquitylation (Sugasawa et al., 2005; Sugasawa, 2006). Apart from these insights into the damage-recognition mechanism, the precise biological meanings of the UV-induced proteasomal degradation of DDB2 and the reversible polyubiquitylation of XPC remain to be understood.

Ddb2-deficient mice are characterized by a defect in UV-induced cellular apoptosis, in addition to a predisposition to skin cancer that was predicted from the phenotypes of human patients with XP-E (Itoh et al., 2004; Yoon et al., 2005). Although there have been some contradictory reports (Stubbert et al., 2007; Stubbert et al., 2009), the disappearance of DDB2 and/or the modification of XPC may be involved in a signal transduction pathway that regulates cellular responses to UV (Stoyanova et al., 2009). Among the known NER proteins, the expression of DDB2 and XPC is under the control of the p53 tumor suppressor (Adimoolam & Ford, 2002; Amundson et al., 2002; Hwang et al., 1999), whereas DDB2 conversely regulates p53 expression, thereby forming a regulatory circuit (Itoh et al., 2003).

Structural studies have suggested that the N-terminus of the rod-shaped CUL4 molecule anchors to the BPB domain of DDB1 (Angers et al., 2006; Scrima et al., 2008). In contrast to DDB2 and the other 2 β-propellers of DDB1 that seem to be fixed on the lesion, the BPB domain is supposed to exhibit considerable conformational flexibility. As a result, the ubiquitin ligase catalytic center assembled on the other tip of CUL4 is expected to move around within a certain spatial range (like a crane arm), and potentially ubiquitylate various targets around the lesion. Other substrates for the UV-DDB ubiquitin ligase include histones H2A (Kapetanaki et al., 2006), H3, and H4 (Wang et al., 2006). H3 and H4 ubiquitylation by the ligase reportedly leads to the dissociation of histone octamers from DNA. In this regard, it should be noted that the nucleosome assembly of DNA containing 6-4PPs interferes in vitro with lesion access to XPC, as well as the subsequent dual incision (Hara et al., 2000; Yasuda et al., 2005). On the other hand, owing to the substantial nonspecific DNA-binding activity of XPC, its specific binding to 6-4PP (observed with EMSAs) was easily competed out by the addition of undamaged DNA: this inhibition was dramatically attenuated by the organization of the competitor DNA into nucleosomes. Taken together, these studies indicate that nucleosome assembly may contribute to the masking of the undamaged part of the genomic DNA from useless surveillance by XPC, so that specific remodeling of the chromatin structures at relevant lesion sites can enhance damage discrimination tremendously.

In addition to ubiquitin ligase, the histone acetyltransferases CBP/p300 reportedly interact with UV-DDB (Datta et al., 2001; Rapić-Otrin et al., 2002), which suggests that multiple histone modifications may be involved in the reorganization of chromatin environments to allow the initiation of GG-NER. In the reconstituted cell-free system, UV-DDB is dispensable for and could even inhibit the repair of 6-4PPs, as described above. Moreover, its influence on CPD repair has been somewhat elusive, despite the obvious stimulatory effect observed in vivo. In some studies, significant stimulation of dual incision was obtained with the CPD substrate (Aboussekhra et al., 1995; Wakasugi et al., 2001; Wakasugi et al., 2002). However, other systems (including ours) showed no or only a minimal effect of UV-DDB on CPD repair, even in the presence of the components required for ubiquitylation (Reardon & Sancar, 2003; Sugasawa et al., 2005). As suggested by others, the involvement of chromatin structures may be important to reproduce the role for UV-DDB in the efficient recognition and repair of CPDs (Rapić Otrin et al., 1998).

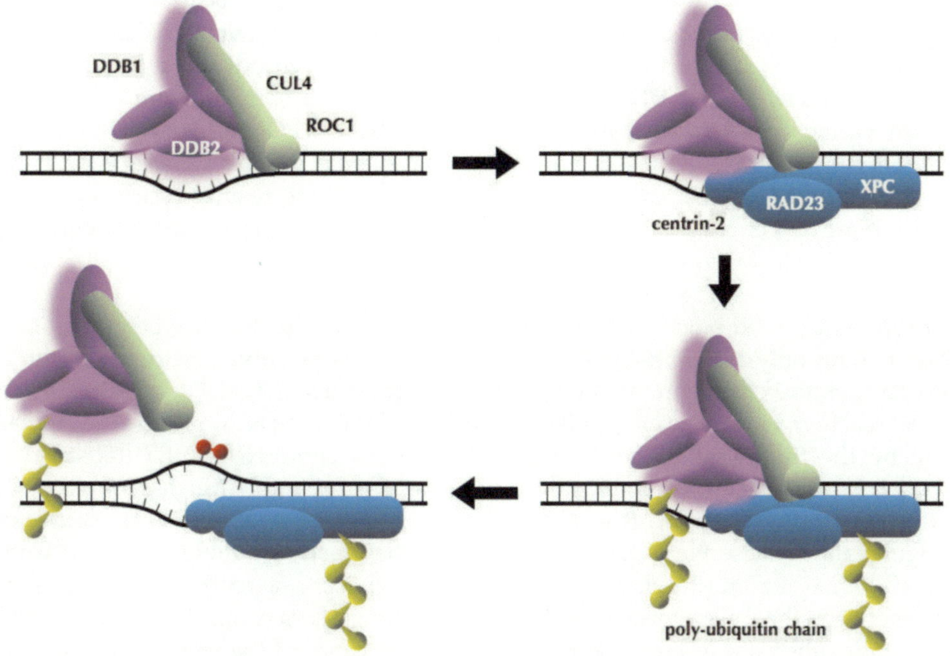

Fig. 3. Ubiquitylation-mediated damage handover model. Once UV-DDB binds to a UV photolesion, it recruits the XPC complex. The associating CUL4-ROC1 ubiquitin ligase is subsequently activated, thereby polyubiquitylating both XPC and DDB2. With the polyubiquitylation of DDB2, UV-DDB loses its affinity for damaged DNA, which results in the successful transfer of the lesion from UV-DDB to XPC.

3. The contribution of damage verification to the accuracy of GG-NER

As discussed in the previous section, there are at least 2 branches of damage-recognition pathways in GG-NER: sensing by XPC of unpaired bases associated with a wide variety of highly distorting lesions, and UV-DDB-dependent deployment of XPC that works specifically for UV-induced photolesions. However, particularly in the former pathway, XPC may bind to sites devoid of damage (e.g., bubble-like structures). The reason for this binding is that XPC can detect certain secondary structure of DNA, but not any feature of DNA chemistry. To avoid incision by NER at damage-free sites that could adversely challenge genomic stability, the verification of damage after XPC binding is fundamental.

3.1 Bipartite substrate discrimination model

Important clues to understand the structural determinants of NER substrate specificity were obtained from a series of biochemical studies. Among the key substrates were artificial DNA backbone lesions at the C4' position of the deoxyribose moiety (Buschta-Hedayat et al., 1999; Hess et al., 1997). Although these lesions were associated with little helix distortion and, thus, were hardly excised in human cell-free extracts, they were excised efficiently when combined with a small bubble structure. On the other hand, bubble structures devoid of lesions were never incised by NER. Based on these findings, the *bipartite substrate discrimination theory* was proposed, which states that efficient NER substrates must simultaneously contain 2 structural elements: disruption of canonical Watson-Crick base pairing (i.e., the presence of unpaired bases), and some aberrant modification of DNA chemistry. It should be noted that XPC senses the former, but not the latter, as described above. We later tested other DNA substrates containing a bubble structure and a dG-AAF adduct in various combinations (Sugasawa et al., 2001). XPC could bind to the bubble regardless of the presence or absence of the lesion, whereas in vitro NER incision occurred only when the AAF adduct existed at the bubble site. These results clearly indicate that DNA binding by XPC does not lead to dual incision in a straightforward manner. Instead, the presence of an alteration of DNA chemistry must be verified thereafter: in the case of no lesion, the repair process is aborted at a certain step.

One of difficulties with biochemical studies of the NER mechanism has been that its early process includes only assembly/disassembly of protein factors and unwinding of the DNA duplex: no chemical change in DNA occurs before dual incision, which is quite a late step in the repair reaction. However, mechanistic dissection of the early NER process was advanced recently by the finding that the 2 structural elements comprising NER substrates (i.e., unpaired base and chemical modification) are spatially separable (Sugasawa et al., 2009). With the C4' backbone lesions, it was already shown that those abnormal structures could be recognized and incised by NER in vitro, even if they resided a few bases apart from the end of a bubbled region (Buschta-Hedayat et al., 1999). Very recently, we showed that the distance between the 2 elements can be much longer (Sugasawa et al., 2009). Although CPDs are very poor substrates in our in vitro NER system because of the small helical distortion, enormous stimulation of dual incision was observed when a 3-base bubble was inserted about 60 bases on the 5' side of the lesion. Footprint analyses revealed that XPC was targeted to the bubble site, rather than to the CPD. This result indicated that the NER machinery was capable of searching around the XPC-bound site and finding the lesion at a distal position. More intriguingly, this stimulatory effect upon CPD recognition was abolished when the bubble was moved to the 3' side of the lesion.

The observed position specificity provided crucial insights into the molecular mechanism underlying the damage search. This mechanism was difficult to explain, if we assumed that the NER factors assembled at the XPC-bound site interacted in trans with the distal CPD. Instead, it seemed more likely that the damage search was accomplished by scanning the DNA strand in the 5' to 3' direction. This scanning mechanism was further supported by the observation that the stimulation of CPD removal was attenuated reciprocally by increasing the distance between the bubble and CPD. The damage search seemed to reach at least 160 bases from the bubble, but the efficiency declined if the distance was 400 bases or more.

3.2 Roles for TFIIH helicases in damage verification

Given the existence of a 5' to 3' scanning mechanism in damage verification, the transcription factor IIH (TFIIH) is thought to be the most likely candidate for performing the scan. TFIIH was originally identified as a basal transcription factor that is essential for the initiation of transcription by RNA polymerase II. TFIIH consists of 10 subunits, including 3 disease-related gene products, XPB, XPD, and TTDA (Giglia-Mari et al., 2004). Electron microscopic analyses of the purified TFIIH complex have revealed a ring-shaped structure, in which the spatial arrangement of individual subunits has been proposed (Chang & Kornberg, 2000; Schultz et al., 2000). Notably, the XPB and XPD subunits possess DNA-dependent ATPase and helicase activities: the XPD helicase translocates on a DNA strand in the 5' to 3' direction (Schaeffer et al., 1994; Sung et al., 1993), whereas the contribution of XPB helicase activity with the opposite (3' to 5') polarity seems only marginal (Coin et al., 1998; Schaeffer et al., 1994). These activities have been implicated in the local unwinding of the DNA duplex at promoter sites (for transcriptional initiation) (Holstege et al., 1996) and at sites containing DNA damage (for NER) (Evans et al., 1997; Mu et al., 1997).

The XPB ATPase activity is necessary for both transcription and NER (Hwang et al., 1996; Tirode et al., 1999). In contrast, ATP-hydrolysis by XPD seems dispensable for transcription, but not for NER (Winkler et al., 2000). TTDA (also known as p8) is a very small protein that recently was identified as a subunit of TFIIH (Giglia-Mari et al., 2004). TTDA stimulates the ATPase activity of XPB in the NER reaction, but it is not directly involved in transcription, which suggests that it performs NER-dedicated roles (Coin et al., 2006). However, TTDA appears to affect the stability of the gross TFIIH complex, because cells from patients with TTD-A show substantially reduced levels of TFIIH and transcriptional activity (Giglia-Mari et al., 2004).

The observed polarity of the XPD helicase coincides with the 5' to 3' scanning model of damage verification. In this regards, there have been notable reports that the helicase activity of Rad3p, the *S. cerevisiae* XPD homolog, is inhibited in the presence of DNA damage (Naegeli et al., 1992). This finding evokes the notion that damage verification may depend on obstruction of the TFIIH helicase translocation at sites where the DNA structure is chemically altered (Dip et al., 2004; Gillet & Schärer, 2006; Wood, 1999). Similar results were obtained recently with an archaeal XPD homologue (Mathieu et al., 2010), although some contradictory data have been also documented (Rudolf et al., 2010), which might be explained by differences in the DNA substrates used. Using paramagnetic beads immobilized with DNA containing a CPD and a 5'-loop, we showed that a certain NER protein complex assembled at the loop site indeed moves to the CPD in an ATP-dependent manner (Sugasawa et al., 2009). In addition to XPC, both XPB and XPD ATPase activities as well as XPA seemed to be involved in this process. Considering that XPB, another TFIIH-related helicase, exhibits the opposite (3' to 5') polarity, it has been proposed that XPB and XPD may be loaded onto different DNA strands and may move toward the same direction (Dip et al., 2004). This process would enable the simultaneous inspection of both strands, so that discrimination between damaged and undamaged strands can be made depending on which helicase is blocked. However, our results strongly suggest that only 1 strand is subjected to scanning, such that lesions on the other strand, if any, are ignored. Recent mutational analyses have revealed that the ATPase, but not the helicase, activity of XPB is required for NER (Coin et al., 2007): this finding implies that XPB may not mediate the opening of the DNA duplex or movement along a DNA strand.

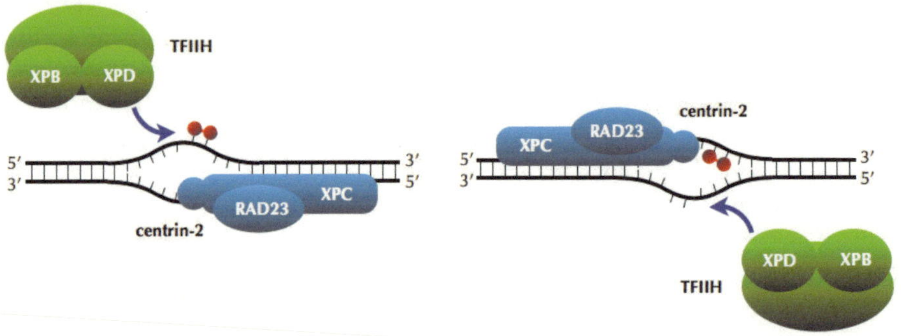

Fig. 4. Polarity of the XPC binding regulates which DNA strand is scanned by the XPD helicase. For successful loading of XPD onto the damaged strand, XPC must interact with the undamaged strand.

Another point made by this study was the importance of the XPC binding polarity. As demonstrated by the aforementioned biochemical and structural studies (Min & Pavletich, 2007; Sugasawa et al., 2002), XPC binds to a site containing unpaired bases in an asymmetric fashion. This binding polarity can be controlled intentionally by using a loop structure, in which only 1 DNA strand has unpaired bases. When a loop with either polarity was substituted for a bubble positioned on the 5' side of the CPD, incision at the lesion site was stimulated only by a looped-out sequence in the "undamaged" (CPD-free) DNA strand. In the case where both the loop and CPD were present in the same strand, incision was completely blocked (Sugasawa et al., 2009). These findings strongly suggest that, after XPC interacts with unpaired bases in 1 DNA strand, the XPD helicase in subsequently recruited TFIIH may be loaded onto the other strand and may start scanning in the 5' to 3' direction. According to this model, XPD would be forced to bind the undamaged strand erroneously, if the damage-containing strand is looped out.

Although this model was deduced from the results of in vitro experiments using rather artificial DNA substrates, it might also apply to normal NER reactions, in which unpaired bases and chemical modifications coexist in close proximity. To induce productive NER, XPC must interact with unpaired bases opposite the lesion, so that the XPD helicase can be loaded successfully onto the damaged strand immediately on the 5' side of the lesion. Intriguingly, with DNA containing a bulky lesion (such as the dG-AAF adduct), XPC exhibits a propensity to bind in a correct orientation in the absence of other factors, most likely because of steric effects preventing interactions between XPC and the modified base (Sugasawa et al., 2009). On the other hand, footprints of XPC on a 6-4PP appear rather symmetric (Sugasawa et al., 1998), which suggests that a substantial fraction of 6-4PP repair events that are initiated directly by XPC may be abortive. In the UV-DDB-mediated damage recognition pathway, however, XPC may be properly guided to interact with the undamaged strand, because the UV photolesions are already occupied by UV-DDB.

3.3 Possible roles for XPA and RPA

XPA, which was the first cloned XP gene (Tanaka et al., 1990), complemented UV sensitivity of fibroblasts from patients with XP-A. Cultured cells lacking expression of functional *XPA* are defective in both GG-NER and TC-NER, and show extreme sensitivity to killing by UV. The *XPA* gene product is a relatively small protein that is essential for in vitro NER. It shows a DNA-binding activity with a significant preference for various types of damaged DNA (Asahina et al., 1994; Jones & Wood, 1993).

Replication protein A (RPA) is a heterotrimeric protein complex exhibiting remarkable single-stranded DNA-binding activity. RPA is supposed to promote the unwinding of the DNA duplex, stabilize the single-stranded conformation, and stimulate various enzymatic activities, such as DNA polymerases. As the eukaryotic counterpart of bacterial SSB, RPA has been implicated in various DNA metabolisms, including replication, repair, and recombination (Wold, 1997). Its involvement in NER was demonstrated by fractionation and reconstitution of human cell-free extracts used for in vitro NER (Coverley et al., 1991). RPA also binds damaged DNA with significant specificity (Burns et al., 1996; Clugston et al., 1992; He et al., 1995), and the reported interaction between XPA and RPA seems to enhance their damage-specific DNA-binding activities (Buschta-Hedayat et al., 1999; He et al., 1995; Li et al., 1995; Wakasugi & Sancar, 1999).

Although the above findings suggest that the XPA-RPA complex could be responsible for initial damage recognition, the observed specificity and affinity of this complex for damaged DNA seem less pronounced than those of XPC or UV-DDB. In addition, accumulating evidence from biochemical and cell biological studies has supported the conclusion that these factors are more likely to be involved in later stages of the NER process. Both XPA and RPA are essential for the assembly of the NER preincision intermediate complex that contains the fully opened DNA duplex. RPA likely stabilizes the single-stranded conformation of DNA and protects the undamaged strand specifically, while XPA binds around the end of the unwound region on the 5' side of the lesion (Krasikova et al., 2010). Considering the reported physical interactions with a number of NER factors, one of the roles for these factors may be orchestrating the assembly of the preincision complex and correctly arranging other factors, including the 2 incision endonucleases, ERCC1-XPF and XPG.

The XPA protein possesses a zinc-finger domain, which NMR studies revealed is involved in the interaction with RPA. In contrast, its DNA-binding functionality was assigned to a different domain in the protein (Buchko et al., 1998; Buchko et al., 1999; Ikegami et al., 1998). Intriguingly, the DNA-binding domain in XPA shows structural resemblance to DNA binding β-hairpins (particularly BHD2) in XPC/Rad4p (Min & Pavletich, 2007), which suggests their evolutionary and functional relationship.

So far, the precise roles for the (rather weak) damage-specific DNA-binding activity of XPA remain unclear. XPA reportedly exhibits remarkable binding affinities for DNA containing highly kinked conformations, such as 3-way junctions and the Holliday junction-like structure (Camenisch et al., 2006; Missura et al., 2001). From mutational analyses, it has been proposed that XPA may be suitable for sensing abnormal electrostatic potentials of DNA, which could be caused by certain distorted DNA conformations in the damage-containing DNA duplex that are unwound by the helicase activities of TFIIH (Camenisch et al., 2007). In addition to such "proofreading" functions, our recent DNA-binding assays have raised the possibility that XPA may be required for launching the DNA scanning complex from the XPC-bound sites (Sugasawa et al., 2009). We also have shown that XPA may stimulate the TFIIH helicase activity under certain conditions, presumably through their reported physical interaction (Li et al., 1998; Park et al., 1995). Based on these findings, it is conceivable that a ternary complex involving XPC, XPA, and TFIIH scans DNA strands to search for damage: this model is reminiscent of the damage-recognition mechanism in the bacterial NER system. As for *E. coli*, 2 damage recognition pathways have been proposed (Van Houten et al., 2005): the UvrA homodimer directly recognizes and binds to distorted sites and then recruits UvrB, or preassembled complexes involving 2 UvrA and 1 or 2 UvrB molecules bind DNA in a nonspecific manner and then search for damage by scanning the DNA strands. In this analogy, UvrB seems to correspond to TFIIH as the driving subunit with ATPase/helicase activities, whereas UvrA may have evolved into XPC and/or XPA. Although little amino acid sequence homology exists between these bacterial and mammalian counterparts, the fundamental principles underlying NER damage recognition may have been conserved throughout evolution.

3.4 Implications in the damage surveillance mechanism

Although the specific DNA binding of UV-DDB and XPC has been observed in vitro, it still remains to be understood how these factors survey DNA and eventually reach relevant sites. For many DNA-binding proteins with sequence- and/or structure-specificity, it has been supposed that the proteins first bind DNA in a nonspecific manner and then "slide" or "hop" to search for their target sites (Gorman & Greene, 2008). A recent report has suggested that BHD1 and BHD2 in XPC may serve as dynamic damage sensors by binding to DNA and rapidly scanning for the integrity of base pairing (Camenisch et al., 2009). Once it encounters a distorted site, BHD3 may be inserted into the duplex to form a stabilized damage-recognition complex.

Apart from these models, our findings that the NER protein complex driven by the XPD helicase can scan DNA strands provides interesting insights into the molecular mechanism underlying in vivo damage surveillance: for instance, the association of XPC even with inappropriate (damage-free) sites could help the NER machinery to survey the local genomic region and find damage at rather distal positions. Possible candidates for such XPC anchoring sites include base mismatches (caused by errors of replication/repair and deamination of bases), thermodynamic "breathing" of the DNA duplex, and other sequences that are intrinsically prone to melting (e.g., transcriptional promoters and replication origins), especially in the presence of topological stresses imposed by chromatin structure. In addition, some endogenous DNA damage, such as abasic sites and single-strand breaks, also may target XPC and thereby launch the "patrolling" system. It would be of great interest to examine how the timing and efficiency of GG-NER are regulated at different genomic loci.

4. Conclusion

Multiple protein factors are involved in the detection and verification of DNA damage, which, in conjunction with the GG-NER system, determine whether to incise DNA or not.

These factors sample all different structural aspects of DNA damage. XPC senses the presence of oscillating unpaired bases, which allows GG-NER to target an extremely broad spectrum of DNA insults. UV-DDB seems more customized for the detection and repair of UV-induced photolesions through direct interaction with the affected bases. As for CPDs (which are refractory to detection by XPC), UV-DDB further extends the substrate specificity of GG-NER. The XPD helicase in TFIIH scans DNA strands as a fine sensor of chemical changes in DNA structure. By integrating these different strategies, GG-NER as a whole can work as a highly versatile, efficient, and accurate system. Numerous biochemical and cell biological studies have confirmed that checks for different structural abnormalities in DNA are conducted in a sequential manner. Additionally, possible stochastic mathematical models have been also discussed (Kesseler et al., 2007; Luijsterburg et al., 2010; Politi et al., 2005). Considering the in vivo situations, decondensation and some remodeling of the chromatin structure would also be expected to precede damage recognition by UV-DDB and XPC, although the underlying mechanism involved in this process remains unclear. These key issues need to be addressed at the molecular level in the near future.

5. Acknowledgement

This work was supported by Grants-in-Aid from the Ministry of Education, Culture, Sports, Science and Technology of Japan, by a Health and Labour Sciences Research Grant (Research on Intractable Diseases) from the Ministry of Health, Labour and Welfare of Japan, and by the Takeda Science Foundation.

6. References

Aboussekhra, A., Biggerstaff, M., Shivji, M.K., Vilpo, J.A., Moncollin, V., Podust, V.N., Protić, M., Hübscher, U., Egly, J.M., & Wood, R.D. (1995). Mammalian DNA nucleotide excision repair reconstituted with purified protein components. *Cell,* Vol.80, No.6, pp. 859-868, ISSN 0092-8674.

Adimoolam, S. & Ford, J.M. (2002). p53 and DNA damage-inducible expression of the xeroderma pigmentosum group C gene. *Proceedings of the National Academy of Sciences of the United States of America,* Vol.99, No.20, pp. 12985-12990, ISSN 0027-8424.

Amundson, S.A., Patterson, A., Do, K.T., & Fornace, A.J. (2002). A nucleotide excision repair master-switch: p53 regulated coordinate induction of global genomic repair genes. *Cancer Biology & Therapy,* Vol.1, No.2, pp. 145-149, ISSN 1538-4047.

Angers, S., Li, T., Yi, X., MacCoss, M.J., Moon, R.T., & Zheng, N. (2006). Molecular architecture and assembly of the DDB1-CUL4A ubiquitin ligase machinery. *Nature,* Vol.443, No.7111, pp. 590-593, ISSN 1476-4687.

Araki, M., Masutani, C., Takemura, M., Uchida, A., Sugasawa, K., Kondoh, J., Ohkuma, Y., & Hanaoka, F. (2001). Centrosome protein centrin 2/caltractin 1 is part of the xeroderma pigmentosum group C complex that initiates global genome nucleotide excision repair. *The Journal of Biological Chemistry,* Vol.276, No.22, pp. 18665-18672, ISSN 0021-9258.

Asahina, H., Kuraoka, I., Shirakawa, M., Morita, E.H., Miura, N., Miyamoto, I., Ohtsuka, E., Okada, Y., & Tanaka, K. (1994). The XPA protein is a zinc metalloprotein with an ability to recognize various kinds of DNA damage. *Mutation Research,* Vol.315, No.3, pp. 229-237, ISSN 0027-5107.

Batty, D., Rapic'-Otrin, V., Levine, A.S., & Wood, R.D. (2000). Stable binding of human XPC complex to irradiated DNA confers strong discrimination for damaged sites. *Journal of Molecular Biology,* Vol.300, No.2, pp. 275-290, ISSN 0022-2836.

Bootsma, D., Kraemer, K.H., Cleaver, J.E., & Hoeijmakers, J.H. (2001). Nucleotide excision repair syndromes: xeroderma pigmentosum, Cockayne syndrome, and trichothiodystrophy, In: *Metabolic and Molecular Bases of Inherited Disease,* Scriver, C. et al. (Eds.) Chap. 28, McGraw-Hill, New York.

Buchko, G.W., Daughdrill, G.W., de Lorimier, R., Rao B, K., Isern, N.G., Lingbeck, J.M., Taylor, J.S., Wold, M.S., Gochin, M., Spicer, L.D., Lowry, D.F., & Kennedy, M.A. (1999). Interactions of human nucleotide excision repair protein XPA with DNA and RPA70 Delta C327: chemical shift mapping and 15N NMR relaxation studies. *Biochemistry,* Vol.38, No.46, pp. 15116-15128, ISSN 0006-2960.

Buchko, G.W., Ni, S., Thrall, B.D., & Kennedy, M.A. (1998). Structural features of the minimal DNA binding domain (M98-F219) of human nucleotide excision repair protein XPA. *Nucleic Acids Research,* Vol.26, No.11, pp. 2779-2788, ISSN 0305-1048.

Bunick, C.G., Miller, M.R., Fuller, B.E., Fanning, E., & Chazin, W.J. (2006). Biochemical and structural domain analysis of xeroderma pigmentosum complementation group C protein. *Biochemistry,* Vol.45, No.50, pp. 14965-14979, ISSN 0006-2960.

Burns, J.L., Guzder, S.N., Sung, P., Prakash, S., & Prakash, L. (1996). An affinity of human replication protein A for ultraviolet-damaged DNA. *The Journal of Biological Chemistry,* Vol.271, No.20, pp. 11607-11610, ISSN 0021-9258.

Buschta-Hedayat, N., Buterin, T., Hess, M.T., Missura, M., & Naegeli, H. (1999). Recognition of nonhybridizing base pairs during nucleotide excision repair of DNA. *Proceedings of the National Academy of Sciences of the United States of America,* Vol.96, No.11, pp. 6090-6095, ISSN 0027-8424.

Camenisch, U., Dip, R., Schumacher, S.B., Schuler, B., & Naegeli, H. (2006). Recognition of helical kinks by xeroderma pigmentosum group A protein triggers DNA excision repair. *Nature Structural & Molecular Biology,* Vol.13, No.3, pp. 278-284, ISSN 1545-9993.

Camenisch, U., Dip, R., Vitanescu, M., & Naegeli, H. (2007). Xeroderma pigmentosum complementation group A protein is driven to nucleotide excision repair sites by the electrostatic potential of distorted DNA. *DNA Repair,* Vol.6, No.12, pp. 1819-1828, ISSN 1568-7864.

Camenisch, U., Träutlein, D., Clement, F.C., Fei, J., Leitenstorfer, A., Ferrando-May, E., & Naegeli, H. (2009). Two-stage dynamic DNA quality check by xeroderma pigmentosum group C protein. *The EMBO Journal,* Vol.28, No.16, pp. 2387-2399, ISSN 1460-2075.

Chang, W.H. & Kornberg, R.D. (2000). Electron crystal structure of the transcription factor and DNA repair complex, core TFIIH. *Cell,* Vol.102, No.5, pp. 609-613, ISSN 0092-8674.

Clugston, C.K., McLaughlin, K., Kenny, M.K., & Brown, R. (1992). Binding of human single-stranded DNA binding protein to DNA damaged by the anticancer drug cis-diamminedichloroplatinum (II). *Cancer Research,* Vol.52, No.22, pp. 6375-6379, ISSN 0008-5472.

Coin, F., Marinoni, J.C., Rodolfo, C., Fribourg, S., Pedrini, A.M., & Egly, J.M. (1998). Mutations in the XPD helicase gene result in XP and TTD phenotypes, preventing interaction between XPD and the p44 subunit of TFIIH. *Nature Genetics,* Vol.20, No.2, pp. 184-188, ISSN 1061-4036.

Coin, F., Oksenych, V., & Egly, J.M. (2007). Distinct roles for the XPB/p52 and XPD/p44 subcomplexes of TFIIH in damaged DNA opening during nucleotide excision repair. *Molecular Cell,* Vol.26, No.2, pp. 245-256, ISSN 1097-2765.

Coin, F., Proietti De Santis, L., Nardo, T., Zlobinskaya, O., Stefanini, M., & Egly, J.M. (2006). p8/TTD-A as a repair-specific TFIIH subunit. *Molecular Cell,* Vol.21, No.2, pp. 215-226, ISSN 1097-2765.

Coverley, D., Kenny, M.K., Munn, M., Rupp, W.D., Lane, D.P., & Wood, R.D. (1991). Requirement for the replication protein SSB in human DNA excision repair. *Nature,* Vol.349, No.6309, pp. 538-541, ISSN 0028-0836.

Datta, A., Bagchi, S., Nag, A., Shiyanov, P., Adami, G.R., Yoon, T., & Raychaudhuri, P. (2001). The p48 subunit of the damaged-DNA binding protein DDB associates with the CBP/p300 family of histone acetyltransferase. *Mutation Research,* Vol.486, No.2, pp. 89-97, ISSN 0027-5107.

Dip, R., Camenisch, U., & Naegeli, H. (2004). Mechanisms of DNA damage recognition and strand discrimination in human nucleotide excision repair. *DNA Repair,* Vol.3, No.11, pp. 1409-1423, ISSN 1568-7864.

Evans, E., Moggs, J.G., Hwang, J.R., Egly, J.M., & Wood, R.D. (1997). Mechanism of open complex and dual incision formation by human nucleotide excision repair factors. *The EMBO Journal,* Vol.16, No.21, pp. 6559-6573, ISSN 0261-4189.

Fitch, M.E., Cross, I.V., Turner, S.J., Adimoolam, S., Lin, C.X., Williams, K.G., & Ford, J.M. (2003). The DDB2 nucleotide excision repair gene product p48 enhances global genomic repair in p53 deficient human fibroblasts. *DNA Repair,* Vol.2, No.7, pp. 819-826, ISSN 1568-7864.

Fitch, M.E., Nakajima, S., Yasui, A., & Ford, J.M. (2003). In vivo recruitment of XPC to UV-induced cyclobutane pyrimidine dimers by the DDB2 gene product. *The Journal of Biological Chemistry,* Vol.278, No.47, pp. 46906-46910, ISSN 0021-9258.

Friedberg, E.C., Lehmann, A.R., & Fuchs, R.P. (2005). Trading places: how do DNA polymerases switch during translesion DNA synthesis? *Molecular Cell,* Vol.18, No.5, pp. 499-505, ISSN 1097-2765.

Friedberg, E.C., Walker, G.C., Siede, W., Wood, R.D., Schultz, R.A., & Ellenberger, T. (Eds.) (2006). *DNA Repair and Mutagenesis, Second Edition,* ASM Press, ISBN 1-55581-319-4, Washington, DC.

Fujiwara, Y., Masutani, C., Mizukoshi, T., Kondo, J., Hanaoka, F., & Iwai, S. (1999). Characterization of DNA recognition by the human UV-damaged DNA-binding protein. *The Journal of Biological Chemistry,* Vol.274, No.28, pp. 20027-20033, ISSN 0021-9258.

Giglia-Mari, G., Coin, F., Ranish, J.A., Hoogstraten, D., Theil, A., Wijgers, N., Jaspers, N.G., Raams, A., Argentini, M., van der Spek, P.J., Botta, E., Stefanini, M., Egly, J.M., Aebersold, R., Hoeijmakers, J.H., & Vermeulen, W. (2004). A new, tenth subunit of TFIIH is responsible for the DNA repair syndrome trichothiodystrophy group A. *Nature Genetics,* Vol.36, No.7, pp. 714-719, ISSN 1061-4036.

Gillet, L.C. & Schärer, O.D. (2006). Molecular mechanisms of mammalian global genome nucleotide excision repair. *Chemical Reviews*, Vol.106, No.2, pp. 253-276, ISSN 0009-2665.

Gorman, J. & Greene, E.C. (2008). Visualizing one-dimensional diffusion of proteins along DNA. *Nature Structural & Molecular Biology*, Vol.15, No.8, pp. 768-774, ISSN 1545-9985.

Groisman, R., Polanowska, J., Kuraoka, I., Sawada, J., Saijo, M., Drapkin, R., Kisselev, A.F., Tanaka, K., & Nakatani, Y. (2003). The ubiquitin ligase activity in the DDB2 and CSA complexes is differentially regulated by the COP9 signalosome in response to DNA damage. *Cell*, Vol.113, No.3, pp. 357-367, ISSN 0092-8674.

Hanawalt, P.C. & Spivak, G. (2008). Transcription-coupled DNA repair: two decades of progress and surprises. *Nature Reviews. Molecular Cell Biology*, Vol.9, No.12, pp. 958-970, ISSN 1471-0080.

Hara, R., Mo, J., & Sancar, A. (2000). DNA damage in the nucleosome core is refractory to repair by human excision nuclease. *Molecular and Cellular Biology*, Vol.20, No.24, pp. 9173-9181, ISSN 0270-7306.

He, Z., Henricksen, L.A., Wold, M.S., & Ingles, C.J. (1995). RPA involvement in the damage-recognition and incision steps of nucleotide excision repair. *Nature*, Vol.374, No.6522, pp. 566-569, ISSN 0028-0836.

Hess, M.T., Schwitter, U., Petretta, M., Giese, B., & Naegeli, H. (1997). Bipartite substrate discrimination by human nucleotide excision repair. *Proceedings of the National Academy of Sciences of the United States of America*, Vol.94, No.13, pp. 6664-6669, ISSN 0027-8424.

Hey, T., Lipps, G., Sugasawa, K., Iwai, S., Hanaoka, F., & Krauss, G. (2002). The XPC-HR23B complex displays high affinity and specificity for damaged DNA in a true-equilibrium fluorescence assay. *Biochemistry*, Vol.41, No.21, pp. 6583-6587, ISSN 0006-2960.

Holstege, F.C., van der Vliet, P.C., & Timmers, H.T. (1996). Opening of an RNA polymerase II promoter occurs in two distinct steps and requires the basal transcription factors IIE and IIH. *The EMBO Journal*, Vol.15, No.7, pp. 1666-1677, ISSN 0261-4189.

Houtsmuller, A.B., Rademakers, S., Nigg, A.L., Hoogstraten, D., Hoeijmakers, J.H., & Vermeulen, W. (1999). Action of DNA repair endonuclease ERCC1/XPF in living cells. *Science*, Vol.284, No.5416, pp. 958-961, ISSN 0036-8075.

Hwang, B.J., Ford, J.M., Hanawalt, P.C., & Chu, G. (1999). Expression of the p48 xeroderma pigmentosum gene is p53-dependent and is involved in global genomic repair. *Proceedings of the National Academy of Sciences of the United States of America*, Vol.96, No.2, pp. 424-428, ISSN 0027-8424.

Hwang, J.R., Moncollin, V., Vermeulen, W., Seroz, T., van Vuuren, H., Hoeijmakers, J.H., & Egly, J.M. (1996). A 3' --> 5' XPB helicase defect in repair/transcription factor TFIIH of xeroderma pigmentosum group B affects both DNA repair and transcription. *The Journal of Biological Chemistry*, Vol.271, No.27, pp. 15898-15904, ISSN 0021-9258.

Ikegami, T., Kuraoka, I., Saijo, M., Kodo, N., Kyogoku, Y., Morikawa, K., Tanaka, K., & Shirakawa, M. (1998). Solution structure of the DNA- and RPA-binding domain of the human repair factor XPA. *Nature Structural Biology*, Vol.5, No.8, pp. 701-706, ISSN 1072-8368.

Itoh, T., Cado, D., Kamide, R., & Linn, S. (2004). DDB2 gene disruption leads to skin tumors and resistance to apoptosis after exposure to ultraviolet light but not a chemical carcinogen. *Proceedings of the National Academy of Sciences of the United States of America,* Vol.101, No.7, pp. 2052-2057, ISSN 0027-8424.

Itoh, T., O'Shea, C., & Linn, S. (2003). Impaired regulation of tumor suppressor p53 caused by mutations in the xeroderma pigmentosum DDB2 gene: mutual regulatory interactions between p48(DDB2) and p53. *Molecular and Cellular Biology,* Vol.23, No.21, pp. 7540-7553, ISSN 0270-7306.

Janićijević, A., Sugasawa, K., Shimizu, Y., Hanaoka, F., Wijgers, N., Djurica, M., Hoeijmakers, J.H., & Wyman, C. (2003). DNA bending by the human damage recognition complex XPC-HR23B. *DNA Repair,* Vol.2, No.3, pp. 325-336, ISSN 1568-7864.

Jones, C.J. & Wood, R.D. (1993). Preferential binding of the xeroderma pigmentosum group A complementing protein to damaged DNA. *Biochemistry,* Vol.32, No.45, pp. 12096-12104, ISSN 0006-2960.

Kapetanaki, M.G., Guerrero-Santoro, J., Bisi, D.C., Hsieh, C.L., Rapić-Otrin, V., & Levine, A.S. (2006). The DDB1-CUL4ADDB2 ubiquitin ligase is deficient in xeroderma pigmentosum group E and targets histone H2A at UV-damaged DNA sites. *Proceedings of the National Academy of Sciences of the United States of America,* Vol.103, No.8, pp. 2588-2593, ISSN 0027-8424.

Kesseler, K.J., Kaufmann, W.K., Reardon, J.T., Elston, T.C., & Sancar, A. (2007). A mathematical model for human nucleotide excision repair: damage recognition by random order assembly and kinetic proofreading. *Journal of Theoretical Biology,* Vol.249, No.2, pp. 361-375, ISSN 0022-5193.

Krasikova, Y.S., Rechkunova, N.I., Maltseva, E.A., Petruseva, I.O., & Lavrik, O.I. (2010). Localization of xeroderma pigmentosum group A protein and replication protein A on damaged DNA in nucleotide excision repair. *Nucleic Acids Research,* Vol.38, No.22, pp. 8083-8094, ISSN 1362-4962.

Lee, J. & Zhou, P. (2007). DCAFs, the missing link of the CUL4-DDB1 ubiquitin ligase. *Molecular Cell,* Vol.26, No.6, pp. 775-780, ISSN 1097-2765.

Legerski, R. & Peterson, C. (1992). Expression cloning of a human DNA repair gene involved in xeroderma pigmentosum group C. *Nature,* Vol.359, No.6390, pp. 70-73, ISSN 0028-0836.

Li, L., Lu, X., Peterson, C.A., & Legerski, R.J. (1995). An interaction between the DNA repair factor XPA and replication protein A appears essential for nucleotide excision repair. *Molecular and Cellular Biology,* Vol.15, No.10, pp. 5396-5402, ISSN 0270-7306.

Li, R.Y., Calsou, P., Jones, C.J., & Salles, B. (1998). Interactions of the transcription/DNA repair factor TFIIH and XP repair proteins with DNA lesions in a cell-free repair assay. *Journal of Molecular Biology,* Vol.281, No.2, pp. 211-218, ISSN 0022-2836.

Luijsterburg, M.S., von Bornstaedt, G., Gourdin, A.M., Politi, A.Z., Moné, M.J., Warmerdam, D.O., Goedhart, J., Vermeulen, W., van Driel, R., & Höfer, T. (2010). Stochastic and reversible assembly of a multiprotein DNA repair complex ensures accurate target site recognition and efficient repair. *The Journal of Cell Biology,* Vol.189, No.3, pp. 445-463, ISSN 1540-8140.

Lutz, W., Lingle, W.L., McCormick, D., Greenwood, T.M., & Salisbury, J.L. (2001). Phosphorylation of centrin during the cell cycle and its role in centriole separation preceding centrosome duplication. *The Journal of Biological Chemistry,* Vol.276, No.23, pp. 20774-20780, ISSN 0021-9258.

Lyapina, S., Cope, G., Shevchenko, A., Serino, G., Tsuge, T., Zhou, C., Wolf, D.A., Wei, N., Shevchenko, A., & Deshaies, R.J. (2001). Promotion of NEDD-CUL1 conjugate cleavage by COP9 signalosome. *Science,* Vol.292, No.5520, pp. 1382-1385, ISSN 0036-8075.

Masutani, C., Sugasawa, K., Yanagisawa, J., Sonoyama, T., Ui, M., Enomoto, T., Takio, K., Tanaka, K., van der Spek, P.J., Bootsma, D., Hoeijmakers, J.H.J., & Hanaoka, F. (1994). Purification and cloning of a nucleotide excision repair complex involving the xeroderma pigmentosum group C protein and a human homologue of yeast RAD23. *The EMBO Journal,* Vol.13, No.8, pp. 1831-1843, ISSN 0261-4189.

Mathieu, N., Kaczmarek, N., & Naegeli, H. (2010). Strand- and site-specific DNA lesion demarcation by the xeroderma pigmentosum group D helicase. *Proceedings of the National Academy of Sciences of the United States of America,* Vol.107, No.41, pp. 17545-17550, ISSN 1091-6490.

Min, J.H. & Pavletich, N.P. (2007). Recognition of DNA damage by the Rad4 nucleotide excision repair protein. *Nature,* Vol.449, No.7162, pp. 570-575, ISSN 1476-4687.

Missura, M., Buterin, T., Hindges, R., Hübscher, U., Kaspárková, J., Brabec, V., & Naegeli, H. (2001). Double-check probing of DNA bending and unwinding by XPA-RPA: an architectural function in DNA repair. *The EMBO Journal,* Vol.20, No.13, pp. 3554-3564, ISSN 0261-4189.

Moser, J., Volker, M., Kool, H., Alekseev, S., Vrieling, H., Yasui, A., van Zeeland, A.A., & Mullenders, L.H. (2005). The UV-damaged DNA binding protein mediates efficient targeting of the nucleotide excision repair complex to UV-induced photo lesions. *DNA Repair,* Vol.4, No.5, pp. 571-582, ISSN 1568-7864.

Mu, D., Wakasugi, M., Hsu, D.S., & Sancar, A. (1997). Characterization of reaction intermediates of human excision repair nuclease. *The Journal of Biological Chemistry,* Vol.272, No.46, pp. 28971-28979, ISSN 0021-9258.

Naegeli, H., Bardwell, L., & Friedberg, E.C. (1992). The DNA helicase and adenosine triphosphatase activities of yeast Rad3 protein are inhibited by DNA damage. A potential mechanism for damage-specific recognition. *The Journal of Biological Chemistry,* Vol.267, No.1, pp. 392-398, ISSN 0021-9258.

Ng, J.M., Vermeulen, W., van der Horst, G.T., Bergink, S., Sugasawa, K., Vrieling, H., & Hoeijmakers, J.H. (2003). A novel regulation mechanism of DNA repair by damage-induced and RAD23-dependent stabilization of xeroderma pigmentosum group C protein. *Genes & Development,* Vol.17, No.13, pp. 1630-1645, ISSN 0890-9369.

Nishi, R., Alekseev, S., Dinant, C., Hoogstraten, D., Houtsmuller, A.B., Hoeijmakers, J.H., Vermeulen, W., Hanaoka, F., & Sugasawa, K. (2009). UV-DDB-dependent regulation of nucleotide excision repair kinetics in living cells. *DNA Repair,* Vol.8, No.6, pp. 767-776, ISSN 1568-7864.

Nishi, R., Okuda, Y., Watanabe, E., Mori, T., Iwai, S., Masutani, C., Sugasawa, K., & Hanaoka, F. (2005). Centrin 2 stimulates nucleotide excision repair by interacting with xeroderma pigmentosum group C protein. *Molecular and Cellular Biology,* Vol.25, No.13, pp. 5664-5674, ISSN 0270-7306.

Okuda, Y., Nishi, R., Ng, J.M., Vermeulen, W., van der Horst, G.T., Mori, T., Hoeijmakers, J.H., Hanaoka, F., & Sugasawa, K. (2004). Relative levels of the two mammalian

Rad23 homologs determine composition and stability of the xeroderma pigmentosum group C protein complex. *DNA Repair,* Vol.3, No.10, pp. 1285-1295, ISSN 1568-7864.

Park, C.H., Mu, D., Reardon, J.T., & Sancar, A. (1995). The general transcription-repair factor TFIIH is recruited to the excision repair complex by the XPA protein independent of the TFIIE transcription factor. *The Journal of Biological Chemistry,* Vol.270, No.9, pp. 4896-4902, ISSN 0021-9258.

Payne, A. & Chu, G. (1994). Xeroderma pigmentosum group E binding factor recognizes a broad spectrum of DNA damage. *Mutation Research,* Vol.310, No.1, pp. 89-102, ISSN 0027-5107.

Politi, A., Moné, M.J., Houtsmuller, A.B., Hoogstraten, D., Vermeulen, W., Heinrich, R., & van Driel, R. (2005). Mathematical modeling of nucleotide excision repair reveals efficiency of sequential assembly strategies. *Molecular Cell,* Vol.19, No.5, pp. 679-690, ISSN 1097-2765.

Popescu, A., Miron, S., Blouquit, Y., Duchambon, P., Christova, P., & Craescu, C.T. (2003). Xeroderma pigmentosum group C protein possesses a high affinity binding site to human centrin 2 and calmodulin. *The Journal of Biological Chemistry,* Vol.278, No.41, pp. 40252-40261, ISSN 0021-9258.

Rapić Otrin, V., Kuraoka, I., Nardo, T., McLenigan, M., Eker, A.P., Stefanini, M., Levine, A.S., & Wood, R.D. (1998). Relationship of the xeroderma pigmentosum group E DNA repair defect to the chromatin and DNA binding proteins UV-DDB and replication protein A. *Molecular and Cellular Biology,* Vol.18, No.6, pp. 3182-3190, ISSN 0270-7306.

Rapić-Otrin, V., McLenigan, M.P., Bisi, D.C., Gonzalez, M., & Levine, A.S. (2002). Sequential binding of UV DNA damage binding factor and degradation of the p48 subunit as early events after UV irradiation. *Nucleic Acids Research,* Vol.30, No.11, pp. 2588-2598, ISSN 1362-4962.

Rapić-Otrin, V., Navazza, V., Nardo, T., Botta, E., McLenigan, M., Bisi, D.C., Levine, A.S., & Stefanini, M. (2003). True XP group E patients have a defective UV-damaged DNA binding protein complex and mutations in DDB2 which reveal the functional domains of its p48 product. *Human Molecular Genetics,* Vol.12, No.13, pp. 1507-1522, ISSN 0964-6906.

Reardon, J.T. & Sancar, A. (2003). Recognition and repair of the cyclobutane thymine dimer, a major cause of skin cancers, by the human excision nuclease. *Genes & Development,* Vol.17, No.20, pp. 2539-2551, ISSN 0890-9369.

Reardon, J.T., Nichols, A.F., Keeney, S., Smith, C.A., Taylor, J.S., Linn, S., & Sancar, A. (1993). Comparative analysis of binding of human damaged DNA-binding protein (XPE) and Escherichia coli damage recognition protein (UvrA) to the major ultraviolet photoproducts: T[c,s]T, T[t,s]T, T[6-4]T, and T[Dewar]T. *The Journal of Biological Chemistry,* Vol.268, No.28, pp. 21301-21308, ISSN 0021-9258.

Riedl, T., Hanaoka, F., & Egly, J.M. (2003). The comings and goings of nucleotide excision repair factors on damaged DNA. *The EMBO Journal,* Vol.22, No.19, pp. 5293-5303, ISSN 0261-4189.

Roche, Y., Zhang, D., Segers-Nolten, G.M., Vermeulen, W., Wyman, C., Sugasawa, K., Hoeijmakers, J., & Otto, C. (2008). Fluorescence correlation spectroscopy of the binding of nucleotide excision repair protein XPC-hHr23B with DNA substrates. *Journal of Fluorescence,* Vol.18, No.5, pp. 987-995, ISSN 1053-0509.

Rudolf, J., Rouillon, C., Schwarz-Linek, U., & White, M.F. (2010). The helicase XPD unwinds bubble structures and is not stalled by DNA lesions removed by the nucleotide excision repair pathway. *Nucleic Acids Research,* Vol.38, No.3, pp. 931-941, ISSN 1362-4962.

Salisbury, J.L., Suino, K.M., Busby, R., & Springett, M. (2002). Centrin-2 is required for centriole duplication in mammalian cells. *Current Biology : CB,* Vol.12, No.15, pp. 1287-1292, ISSN 0960-9822.

Schaeffer, L., Moncollin, V., Roy, R., Staub, A., Mezzina, M., Sarasin, A., Weeda, G., Hoeijmakers, J.H., & Egly, J.M. (1994). The ERCC2/DNA repair protein is associated with the class II BTF2/TFIIH transcription factor. *The EMBO Journal,* Vol.13, No.10, pp. 2388-2392, ISSN 0261-4189.

Schultz, P., Fribourg, S., Poterszman, A., Mallouh, V., Moras, D., & Egly, J.M. (2000). Molecular structure of human TFIIH. *Cell,* Vol.102, No.5, pp. 599-607, ISSN 0092-8674.

Scrima, A., Konícková, R., Czyzewski, B.K., Kawasaki, Y., Jeffrey, P.D., Groisman, R., Nakatani, Y., Iwai, S., Pavletich, N.P., & Thomä, N.H. (2008). Structural basis of UV DNA-damage recognition by the DDB1-DDB2 complex. *Cell,* Vol.135, No.7, pp. 1213-1223, ISSN 1097-4172.

Shivji, M.K., Eker, A.P., & Wood, R.D. (1994). DNA repair defect in xeroderma pigmentosum group C and complementing factor from HeLa cells. *The Journal of Biological Chemistry,* Vol.269, No.36, pp. 22749-22757, ISSN 0021-9258.

Stoyanova, T., Roy, N., Kopanja, D., Raychaudhuri, P., & Bagchi, S. (2009). DDB2 (damaged-DNA binding protein 2) in nucleotide excision repair and DNA damage response. *Cell Cycle (Georgetown, Tex.),* Vol.8, No.24, pp. 4067-4071, ISSN 1551-4005.

Stubbert, L.J., Hamill, J.D., Spronck, J.C., Smith, J.M., Becerril, C., & McKay, B.C. (2007). DDB2-independent role for p53 in the recovery from ultraviolet light-induced replication arrest. *Cell Cycle (Georgetown, Tex.),* Vol.6, No.14, pp. 1730-1740, ISSN 1551-4005.

Stubbert, L.J., Smith, J.M., Hamill, J.D., Arcand, T.L., & McKay, B.C. (2009). The anti-apoptotic role for p53 following exposure to ultraviolet light does not involve DDB2. *Mutation Research,* Vol.663, No.1-2, pp. 69-76, ISSN 0027-5107.

Sugasawa, K. (2006). UV-induced ubiquitylation of XPC complex, the UV-DDB-ubiquitin ligase complex, and DNA repair. *Journal of Molecular Histology,* Vol.37, No.5-7, pp. 189-202, ISSN 1567-2379.

Sugasawa, K., Akagi, J., Nishi, R., Iwai, S., & Hanaoka, F. (2009). Two-step recognition of DNA damage for mammalian nucleotide excision repair: Directional binding of the XPC complex and DNA strand scanning. *Molecular Cell,* Vol.36, No.4, pp. 642-653, ISSN 1097-4164.

Sugasawa, K., Ng, J.M., Masutani, C., Iwai, S., van der Spek, P.J., Eker, A.P., Hanaoka, F., Bootsma, D., & Hoeijmakers, J.H. (1998). Xeroderma pigmentosum group C protein complex is the initiator of global genome nucleotide excision repair. *Molecular Cell,* Vol.2, No.2, pp. 223-232, ISSN 1097-2765.

Sugasawa, K., Okamoto, T., Shimizu, Y., Masutani, C., Iwai, S., & Hanaoka, F. (2001). A multistep damage recognition mechanism for global genomic nucleotide excision repair. *Genes & Development,* Vol.15, No.5, pp. 507-521, ISSN 0890-9369.

Sugasawa, K., Okuda, Y., Saijo, M., Nishi, R., Matsuda, N., Chu, G., Mori, T., Iwai, S., Tanaka, K., Tanaka, K., & Hanaoka, F. (2005). UV-induced ubiquitylation of XPC protein mediated by UV-DDB-ubiquitin ligase complex. *Cell,* Vol.121, No.3, pp. 387-400, ISSN 0092-8674.

Sugasawa, K., Shimizu, Y., Iwai, S., & Hanaoka, F. (2002). A molecular mechanism for DNA damage recognition by the xeroderma pigmentosum group C protein complex. *DNA Repair,* Vol.1, No.1, pp. 95-107, ISSN 1568-7864.

Sung, P., Bailly, V., Weber, C., Thompson, L.H., Prakash, L., & Prakash, S. (1993). Human xeroderma pigmentosum group D gene encodes a DNA helicase. *Nature,* Vol.365, No.6449, pp. 852-855, ISSN 0028-0836.

Tanaka, K., Miura, N., Satokata, I., Miyamoto, I., Yoshida, M.C., Satoh, Y., Kondo, S., Yasui, A., Okayama, H., & Okada, Y. (1990). Analysis of a human DNA excision repair gene involved in group A xeroderma pigmentosum and containing a zinc-finger domain. *Nature,* Vol.348, No.6296, pp. 73-76, ISSN 0028-0836.

Tang, J. & Chu, G. (2002). Xeroderma pigmentosum complementation group E and UV-damaged DNA-binding protein. *DNA Repair,* Vol.1, No.8, pp. 601-616, ISSN 1568-7864.

Tang, J.Y., Hwang, B.J., Ford, J.M., Hanawalt, P.C., & Chu, G. (2000). Xeroderma pigmentosum p48 gene enhances global genomic repair and suppresses UV-induced mutagenesis. *Molecular Cell,* Vol.5, No.4, pp. 737-744, ISSN 1097-2765.

Thompson, J.R., Ryan, Z.C., Salisbury, J.L., & Kumar, R. (2006). The structure of the human centrin 2-xeroderma pigmentosum group C protein complex. *The Journal of Biological Chemistry,* Vol.281, No.27, pp. 18746-18752, ISSN 0021-9258.

Tirode, F., Busso, D., Coin, F., & Egly, J.M. (1999). Reconstitution of the transcription factor TFIIH: assignment of functions for the three enzymatic subunits, XPB, XPD, and cdk7. *Molecular Cell,* Vol.3, No.1, pp. 87-95, ISSN 1097-2765.

Trego, K.S. & Turchi, J.J. (2006). Pre-steady-state binding of damaged DNA by XPC-hHR23B reveals a kinetic mechanism for damage discrimination. *Biochemistry,* Vol.45, No.6, pp. 1961-1969, ISSN 0006-2960.

Treiber, D.K., Chen, Z., & Essigmann, J.M. (1992). An ultraviolet light-damaged DNA recognition protein absent in xeroderma pigmentosum group E cells binds selectively to pyrimidine (6-4) pyrimidone photoproducts. *Nucleic Acids Research,* Vol.20, No.21, pp. 5805-5810, ISSN 0305-1048.

Van Houten, B., Croteau, D.L., DellaVecchia, M.J., Wang, H., & Kisker, C. (2005). 'Close-fitting sleeves': DNA damage recognition by the UvrABC nuclease system. *Mutation Research,* Vol.577, No.1-2, pp. 92-117, ISSN 0027-5107.

Venema, J., van Hoffen, A., Natarajan, A.T., van Zeeland, A.A., & Mullenders, L.H. (1990). The residual repair capacity of xeroderma pigmentosum complementation group C fibroblasts is highly specific for transcriptionally active DNA. *Nucleic Acids Research,* Vol.18, No.3, pp. 443-448, ISSN 0305-1048.

Volker, M., Moné, M.J., Karmakar, P., van Hoffen, A., Schul, W., Vermeulen, W., Hoeijmakers, J.H., van Driel, R., van Zeeland, A.A., & Mullenders, L.H. (2001).

Sequential assembly of the nucleotide excision repair factors in vivo. *Molecular Cell,* Vol.8, No.1, pp. 213-224, ISSN 1097-2765.

Wakasugi, M. & Sancar, A. (1999). Order of assembly of human DNA repair excision nuclease. *The Journal of Biological Chemistry,* Vol.274, No.26, pp. 18759-18768, ISSN 0021-9258.

Wakasugi, M., Kawashima, A., Morioka, H., Linn, S., Sancar, A., Mori, T., Nikaido, O., & Matsunaga, T. (2002). DDB accumulates at DNA damage sites immediately after UV irradiation and directly stimulates nucleotide excision repair. *The Journal of Biological Chemistry,* Vol.277, No.3, pp. 1637-1640, ISSN 0021-9258.

Wakasugi, M., Shimizu, M., Morioka, H., Linn, S., Nikaido, O., & Matsunaga, T. (2001). Damaged DNA-binding protein DDB stimulates the excision of cyclobutane pyrimidine dimers in vitro in concert with XPA and replication protein A. *The Journal of Biological Chemistry,* Vol.276, No.18, pp. 15434-15440, ISSN 0021-9258.

Wang, H., Zhai, L., Xu, J., Joo, H.Y., Jackson, S., Erdjument-Bromage, H., Tempst, P., Xiong, Y., & Zhang, Y. (2006). Histone H3 and H4 ubiquitylation by the CUL4-DDB-ROC1 ubiquitin ligase facilitates cellular response to DNA damage. *Molecular Cell,* Vol.22, No.3, pp. 383-394, ISSN 1097-2765.

Winkler, G.S., Araújo, S.J., Fiedler, U., Vermeulen, W., Coin, F., Egly, J.M., Hoeijmakers, J.H., Wood, R.D., Timmers, H.T., & Weeda, G. (2000). TFIIH with inactive XPD helicase functions in transcription initiation but is defective in DNA repair. *The Journal of Biological Chemistry,* Vol.275, No.6, pp. 4258-4266, ISSN 0021-9258.

Wittschieben, B.Ø., Iwai, S., & Wood, R.D. (2005). DDB1-DDB2 (xeroderma pigmentosum group E) protein complex recognizes a cyclobutane pyrimidine dimer, mismatches, apurinic/apyrimidinic sites, and compound lesions in DNA. *The Journal of Biological Chemistry,* Vol.280, No.48, pp. 39982-39989, ISSN 0021-9258.

Wold, M.S. (1997). Replication protein A: a heterotrimeric, single-stranded DNA-binding protein required for eukaryotic DNA metabolism. *Annual Review of Biochemistry,* Vol.66, pp. 61-92, ISSN 0066-4154.

Wood, R.D. (1999). DNA damage recognition during nucleotide excision repair in mammalian cells. *Biochimie,* Vol.81, No.1-2, pp. 39-44, ISSN 0300-9084.

Yang, X., Menon, S., Lykke-Andersen, K., Tsuge, T., Di Xiao, Wang, X., Rodriguez-Suarez, R.J., Zhang, H., & Wei, N. (2002). The COP9 signalosome inhibits p27(kip1) degradation and impedes G1-S phase progression via deneddylation of SCF Cul1. *Current Biology : CB,* Vol.12, No.8, pp. 667-672, ISSN 0960-9822.

Yasuda, T., Sugasawa, K., Shimizu, Y., Iwai, S., Shiomi, T., & Hanaoka, F. (2005). Nucleosomal structure of undamaged DNA regions suppresses the non-specific DNA binding of the XPC complex. *DNA Repair,* Vol.4, No.3, pp. 389-395, ISSN 1568-7864.

Yoon, T., Chakrabortty, A., Franks, R., Valli, T., Kiyokawa, H., & Raychaudhuri, P. (2005). Tumor-prone phenotype of the DDB2-deficient mice. *Oncogene,* Vol.24, No.3, pp. 469-478, ISSN 0950-9232.

24

DNA Double-Strand Break Repair Through Non-Homologous End-Joining: Recruitment and Assembly of the Players

Radhika Pankaj Kamdar[1,2] and Yoshihisa Matsumoto[1]
[1]*Research Laboratory for Nuclear Reactors, Tokyo Institute of Technology, Tokyo*
[2]*Department of Human Genetics, Emory University, Atlanta, Georgia*
[1]*Japan*
[2]*USA*

1. Introduction

DNA, this vitally important genetic macromolecule, is under constant assault via endogenous and exogenous agents which cause damage to DNA and thus to cells leading to genomic instability. The primary endogenous cause of DNA damage is caused during continuous replication of DNA at the S phase of the cell cycle effecting spontaneous mutations. Other endogenous DNA damaging agents are reactive oxygen species (ROS) produced as metabolic byproducts. Additionally, breaks are introduced to DNA in the process of recombination, *e.g.*, V(D)J recombination in immune systems and meiotic recombination in reproductive organs. The exogenous DNA damaging agents are ionizing radiations and chemical compounds, which are intercalated into major or minor grooves of DNA strand or form chemical bond with bases.

DNA damages include base elimination, modification, cross-linking and strand break. Strand break includes single-strand break (SSB) and double-strand break (DSB). Among these various types of DNA damages, DSB is considered most fatal. Hence healing DSB is vital to circumvent genomic instability encompassing chromosomal aberrations, translocations and tumorigenesis. Eukaryotes have evolved two major pathways to repair DSBs, *i.e.*, homologous recombination (HR) and non-homologous end-joining (NHEJ). This chapter will review the mechanisms of the latter, especially how the players are recruited to the sites of DSBs and are assembled into multi-protein repair machinery.

2. DNA double-strand break repair through non-homologous end-joining pathway

2.1 Homologous Recombination and Non-Homologous End-Joining

HR is a reaction wherein the genetic material is exchanged between two similar or identical strands of DNA. In the repair of DSB through HR, undamaged DNA serves as a template to reconsitute the original sequence across the break. On the other hand, NHEJ is the direct rejoining of the broken DNA ends without much regard for homology at these ends.

Therefore, NHEJ may sometimes incur nucleotide deletions or insertions at the junction or joining with incorrect partner, leading to chromosomal abberations like duplications, inversions or translocations. Hence it is considered that NHEJ is less accurate than HR but, nevertheless, important especially in vertebrates.

In HR, the template should be found in homologous chromosome or in sister chromatid. Organisms like budding yeast can avail homologous chromosome as the template. However, vertebrate can utilize only sister chromatid, but not homologous chromosome, as the template for HR and, therefore, the repair of DSB through HR is limited to late S and G2 phases. The majolity of the cells reside in G0 or G1 phases in vertebrate body, where only NHEJ can operate.

Additionally, only small portions of the genome in vertebrate are encoding protein or functional RNA and other portions are intervening or repetitive sequences. These regions may have important roles in the structural maintenance of the genome, proper replication/segregation of the genome or spatiotemporal regulation of the genen expression. Nevertheless, small deletion or insertion of nucleotides might be tolerated in most portion of the vertebrate genome.

Finally, whereas HR is utilized in meiotic recombination in reproductive organs, NHEJ is utilized in V(D)J recombination in immune system to establish diversity of immunogloblins and T cell recepters. Thus, genetic defect in either one of NHEJ components results not only in elevated sensitivity toward radiation and radiomimetic agents but also in immunodeficiency.

2.2 Processes of NHEJ

NHEJ process may be divided into three steps, i.e., (i) detection, (ii) processing and (iii) ligation of DSB ends (Fig.1). The detection and ligation steps comprises the core reaction while the processing step is required only when the ends are not readily ligatable. In the detection step, Ku protein, heterodimer consisting of Ku70 and Ku86 (also known as Ku80), first binds to the ends of double-stranded DNA and then recruits DNA-PK catalytic subunit (DNA-PKcs). The complex consisting of Ku70, Ku86 and DNA-PKcs is termed DNA-dependent protein kinase (DNA-PK). Upon binding of DNA-PKcs to DNA ends, it exerts kinase catalytic activity to phosphorylate substrate proteins. Thus, DNA-PK is considered the molecular sensor of DSB, triggering the signalling cascade. At the final ligation step, DNA ligase IV in a tight association with XRCC4 catalyzes the reaction to join the two DNA ends. XRCC4-like factor, XLF, which is also known as Cernunnos, is also essential at this step, especially when two ends are not compatible. Thus, six polypeptides, i.e., Ku70, Ku86, DNA-PKcs, DNA ligase IV, XRCC4 and XLF are core components of NHEJ. Processing step might involve a number of enzymes depending on the shape of each DNA end and compatibility of two ends to be ligated. Presumed processing enzymes contain Artemis, DNA polymerase μ/λ, polynucleotide kinase/phosphatase (PNKP), Aprataxin (APTX) and Aprataxin and PNKP-like factor (APLF, also known as PALF, C2orf13 or Xip1).

2.3 Components of NHEJ

2.3.1 Ku

Ku protein was initially found as the antigen of autoantibody in a patient of polymyositis-scleroderma overlap syndrome (Mimori et al., 1981). Biochemical approach, including immunoprecipitation of [^{32}P]orthophosphate or [^{35}S]methionine-labeled cell extract and

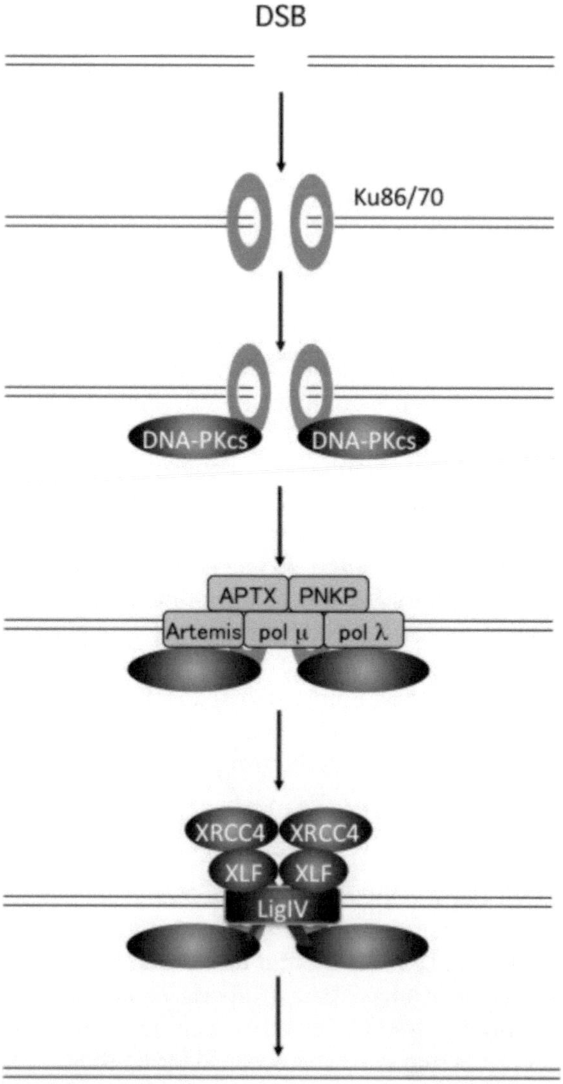

Fig. 1. Repair of DSB through NHEJ.

immunoaffinity purification, lead to identify Ku as a DNA-binding protein made up of two subunits of 70,000Da and 80,000Da, respectively, which are now known as Ku70 and Ku80 (or Ku86) (Mimori et al., 1986). It is also estimated that Ku is an abundant protein, existing as 400,000 copies in logarithmically growing HeLa cells. Protein-DNA interaction studies, including footprint analysis, led to the finding that Ku binds to the ends of double-stranded DNA without requirement for specific sequence (Mimori & Hardin, 1986). Because of this striking property, possible role of Ku in DNA repair or in transposition was suspected. In early 1990s, Ku was found to be an essential component of DNA-PK (Dvir et al., 1992, 1993; Gottlieb and Jackson, 1993). It was also found that Ku80 is equivalent to XRCC5 (X-ray repair cross complementing) gene product, which is missing in X-ray sensitive rodent cell lines including *xrs*-5, -6, XR-V9B and XR-V15B (Taccioli et al., 1994; Smider et al., 1994).

These cell lines also exhibit defect in V(D)J recombination, indicating the role of Ku in this process. Ku80 knockout mice showed immunodeficiency and radiosensitivity, like *scid* mice (below) and also exhibited growth defect; body weight was 40-60% of age-matched control (Nussenzweig et al., 1996; Zhu et al., 1996). Ku70 knockout mice also showed immunodeficiency, radiosensitivity and growth defect. However, immunological defect in Ku70 knockout mice was less severe than in Ku80 knockout mice, as it shows partial production and differentiation of T cells (Gu et al., 1997; Ouyang et al., 1997). Ku is also implied to play critical roles in telomere capping in mammalian cells (Hsu et al., 2000).

Homologues of Ku proteins were identified not only in mammals but also in other eukaryota including budding yeast, where it is referred to as HDF1 and HDF2 (high- affinity DNA binding factor), or Yku70 and Yku80, respectively (Feldmann & Winnacker, 1993; Milne et al., 1996; Feldmann et al., 1996; Boulton & Jackson, 1996). Yeast Ku is shown to play important roles in NHEJ, telomere maintenance and silencing (Boulton & Jackson, 1996, 1998; Porter et al., 1996).

Ku70 and Ku80 show low but significant sequence similarity, indicating common evolutional origin, and share a similar structural configuration (Dynan & Yoo, 1998; Gell & Jackson, 1999). Expectedly, "single" Ku orthologue was identified in bacteria and in bacteriophage (Weller et al., 2002; d'Adda di Fagagna et al., 2003). As revealed by X-ray crystallography, Ku 70 and Ku80 fold to form an asymmetric ring shaped structure forming an aperture large enough to let DNA thread through it; thus playing a crucial role in DSB recognition (Walker et al., 2001). The core of Ku required to form dimer and aperture is conserved among all Ku orthologues. Both of Ku70 and Ku80 bear von Willebrant factor A domain, which may be essential for heterodimer formation. The C-termial of Ku70 bears SAP domain, which may mediate DNA binding, and the C-terminal of Ku80 bears a conserved motif to interact with DNA-PKcs (Gell & Jackson, 1999; Falck et al.., 2005).

Ku translocates along DNA in an ATP-independent manner, allowing several dimers to bind on a single DNA molecule (Zhang and Yaneva, 1992; Bliss and Lane, 1997). Ku was identified also as a ssDNA dependent ATPase stimulating the DNA polymerase α primase activity (Vishwanatha and Baril, 1990; Cao et al., 1994) and as an ATP dependent DNA helicase II (HDH II) (Tuteja et al., 1994). Recent study demonstrated that Ku has 5'-RP/AP lyase activity, nicking 3'-side of abasic site (Roberts et al., 2010). Thus, Ku might exert multiple functions, not only binding to DSBs but also activating damage signal via DNA-PKcs and processing DSB ends removing the obstacle for ligation.

2.3.2 DNA-PKcs

DNA-PK activity was first found as an activity to phosphorylate Hsp90 in the presence of double-stranded DNA in the extracts of HeLa cell, rabbit reticulocyte, Xenopus egg and sea urchin egg (Walker et al., 1985). DNA-PK was purified from Hela cell nuclei as a 300-350 kDa protein, which is now called DNA-PKcs for DNA-PK catalytic subunit (Carter et al., 1990; Lees-Miller et al., 1990). Later it was found that Ku is an essential component of DNA-PK and that DNA-PK requires binding to DNA ends to be activated (Dvir et al., 1992, 1993; Gottlieb and Jackson, 1993). Following the finding that XRCC5 is equivalent to Ku80, DNA-PKcs is found to correspond to XRCC7, which is deficient in *scid* (severe combined immunodeficiency) mouse (Kirchgessner et al., 1995; Blunt et al., 1995; Peterson et al., 1995), lacking mature B and T cells due to a defect in V(D)J recombination (Bosma et al., 1983; Lieber et al., 1988; Fulop & Phillips, 1990; Biederman et al., 1991). Scid due to defect in DNA-

PKcs is also found in horse (Wiler et al., 1995; Shin and Meek, 1997) and in dog (Meek et al., 2001). M059J, a human glioma cell line, defective in DNA-PKcs, also showed radiosensitivity with defective DSB repair (Lees-Miller et al., 1995). Recently, DNA-PKcs missense mutation was identified in human radiosensitive T- B- severe combined immunodeficiency (TB-SCID) (van der Burg et al., 2009). Cells from the patient exhibit normal DNA-PK activity but may have defect in Artemis activation (below).

Cloning of gene revealed that DNA-PKcs is a 4,127 amino acid polypeptide, one of the largest molecules in the cell (Hartley et al., 1995). The carboxy-terminal between amino acid residues 3719 - 4127 compose the catalytic domain that is categolized into phosphatidylinositol-3 kinase and like kinase (PIKK) family (Hartley et al., 1995; Poltoratsky et al., 1995). PIKK family include ataxia-telangiectasia mutated (ATM) (Savitsky et al., 1995) and ATM- and Rad3-related (ATR) (Cimprich et al., 1996), both of which are protein kinases with roles in DNA repair and cell cycle checkpoint as sensors of DNA damages. Although orthologues of ATM and ATR can be found in fruit fly, nematoda, plants and yeast, DNA-PKcs has been found only in vertebrate, some arthropods (Dore et al., 2004) and dictyostelium (Hudson et al., 2005).

In vitro studies had revealed that DNA-PK can phosphorylate a number of nuclear, DNA binding proteins with supposed functions in transcription, replication, recombination and repair (Lees-Miller et al., 1992). The sites phosphorylated by DNA-PK were identified as serine and threonine that are immediately followed by a glutamine on the linear sequence; SQ/TQ (Lees-Miller et al., 1992), although there are a considerable number of exceptions reported. The protein phosphorylation by DNA-PK should be essential for NHEJ, as catalytically inactive form of DNA-PKcs can restore at most partial NHEJ activity to DNA-PKcs deficient cells (Kurimasa et al., 1999). However, it is presently unclear what is/are the *in vivo* phosphorylation target(s) essential for DNA repair.

Recent studies have shed light on the phosphorylation of DNA-PKcs itself. At least 16 sites of autophosphorylation have been identified (Chan et al., 2002; Douglas et al., 2002; Ding et al., 2003). Most of them are clustered within 2023 - 2056 (PQR cluster), 2609 - 2647 (ABCDE cluster) and 2671 - 2677. Some of them may be phosphorylated by ATM or ATR *in cellulo* (Chen et al., 2007; Yajima et al., 2006) It has been demonstrated that, *in vitro*, autophosphorylation of DNA-PK leads to loss of kinase activity and dissociation from Ku (Chan et al., 1996). It should be also noted that substitution of serines and threonines within ABCDE cluster with alanine results in greater radiation sensitivity than DNA-PKcs null cells and also in reduced rates of HR. Thus, autophosphorylation, especially within ABCDE cluster might regulate DNA-PK activity negatively or switch repair pathway from NHEJ to HR.

2.3.3 XRCC4-DNA ligase IV

XRCC4 was isolated and cloned from a human cDNA sequence whose expression in the XR-1 cells, derived from Chinese Hamster ovary and phenotypically similar to *scid* and *xrs*, conferred normal V(D)J recombination ability and also DSB repair activity (Li et al., 1995). Biochemical studies lead to finding that it is associated with DNA ligase IV (Critchlow et al., 1997; Grawunder et al., 1997). Mutations in DNA ligase IV gene have been identified in radiosensitive leukemia patient (Badie et al, 1995; Riballo et al., 1999) and in patients exhibiting developmental delay and immunodeficiency, which is called ligase IV syndrome (O'Driscoll et al., 2001). Although mutation in XRCC4 gene has not been found in humans, there are some polymorphisms associated with colorectal cancer and childfood leukemia (Bau et al., 2010; Wu et al., 2010). Disruption of either XRCC4 or DNA Ligase IV gene in mice leads to embryonic lethality with a primary defect in neurogenesis and severe neuronal apoptosis (Barnes et al., 1998; Frank et al., 1998; Gao et al., 1998). Mutants of *DNL4* and *LIF1* genes, the yeast orthologue of human DNA Ligase IV and XRCC4, respectively, exhibited a phenotype similar to that of HDF1 and 2 mutants, indicating its role in recombination and repair (Wilson et al., 1997; Teo and Jackson, 1997, 2000).

XRCC4-DNA Ligase IV is a critical complex formed *in vivo* (Critchlow et al., 1997; Grawunder et al., 1997) for the ligation of the broken DNA ends via NHEJ pathway. The presence of XRCC4 stabilize and activates DNA Ligase IV (Grawunder et al., 1997; Bryans et al., 1999) by stimulating its adenylation which is the first chemical step in ligation (Modesti et al., 1999). XRCC4 forms a homodimer and associates with a polypeptide at the C-terminus of DNA Ligase IV (Critchlow et al., 1997; Junop et al., 2000; Sibanda et al., 2001). This interaction is mapped to the central coiled coil domain of XRCC4 and the inter BRCT linker region at the C-terminus of DNA Ligase IV. This region within DNA Ligase IV, termed as the XRCC4-interacting region (XIR) was deemed necessary and sufficient for XRCC4-Ligase IV interaction (Grawunder et al., 1998). Recently a high resolution crystal structure of human XRCC4 bound to the C-terminal tandem BRCT repeat of DNA Ligase IV was reported. It revealed an extensive binding interface formed by helix-loop-helix structure within the inter-BRCT linker region of Ligase IV, as well as significant interactions involving the second BRCT domain that induces a kink in the tail region of XRCC4 (Wu et al., 2009). This interaction was demonstrated as essential to stabilize the interaction between the XIR of DNA Ligase IV and XRCC4, while the first BRCT domain was considerably dispensable.

2.3.4 XLF/ cernunnos

Although above five factors had been identified by 1998, there were indications of the existence of additional factor essential for mammalian NHEJ. First, 2BN cell line, which is derived from radiosensitive and immunodeficient patient, showed defective NHEJ but all the known NHEJ components were normal. Second, in 2001, NEJ1/LIF2 was identified as a new essential factor of NHEJ in budding yeast (Kegel et al., 2001; Valencia et al., 2001; Ooi et al., 2001; Frank-Vaillant & Marcand, 2001).

XLF was identified in the yeast two hybrid screen for XRCC4 inteacting protein (Ahnesorg et al., 2006) and named XRCC4-like factor, as it was predicted to have 3D structure similar to that of XRCC4. It is also identified as Cernunnos missing in patients with growth retardation, microcephaly, immunodeficiency, increased cellular sensitivity to ionizing radiation and a defective V(D)J recombination (Buck et al, 2006). It is a 33kDa protein with 299 amino acid residues. NHEJ deficient 2BN cells lacked XLF due to a frameshift mutation (Ahnesorg, 2006). XLF was found to be a genuine homologue of Nej1p from budding yeast (Callebaut et al., 2006). XLF was also shown to be conserved across evolution (Hentges et al., 2006) and to be a paralogue of XRCC4 (Callebaut et al., 2006).

Chromatographic analyses established XLF existing as dimer and crystallographic studies demonstrated its interaction through globular head-to-head domain with that of XRCC4 (Andres et al., 2007; Li et al., 2008). Three-dimensional X-ray scattering characterized a tetramer formation of XRCC4, while the XRCC4-XLF interaction was still mediated through glogular head domains which rendered it suitable for DNA alignment and Ligase IV function (Hammel et al., 2010). XLF possesses DNA binding activity dependent on the length of DNA (Lu et al., 2007a) and ability to ligate mismatched and non-cohesive ends (Tsai et al., 2007).

2.3.5 Processing enzymes

Pathologic and physiologic breaks create incompatible DNA ends which are not as easy to rejoin as those created *in vitro* by restriction enzyme digestion. It requires removal of excess DNA and fill-in of gaps and overhangs in order to make them compatible for the DNA ligase activity.

Artemis was identified as the causative gene for human RS-SCID (Moshous et al., 2001). Artemis forms a complex with DNA-PKcs and expresses 5′ to 3′ exonuclease activity and endonuclease and endonuclease activity at the junction of single-stranded and double-stranded DNA (Ma et al., 2002). Although, the signal joint formation during V(D)J recombination does not require Artemis or DNA-PKcs for joining, all of the components of NHEJ including Artemis are required for coding ends. Artemis in association with DNA-PKcs is deemed necessary for the opening of hairpin structures (Lu et al., 2007b). Artemis is phosphorylated both by DNA-PKcs and ATM (Poinsignon et al., 2004; Zhang et al., 2004).

Polymerases μ and λ belong to pol X family and might fill gaps and 5′overhangs (Ramadan et al., 2003). Polynucleotide kinase/phosphatase (PNKP) adds phosphate group to 5'-hydroxyl end and also removes phosphate group from 3′-phosphorylated end (Koch et al., 2004; Clements et al., 2004;Whitehouse et al., 2001). Aprataxin (APTX) is initially identified as the product of the gene defective in genetic disorder early-onset ataxia with oculomoter apraxia (Date et al., 2001) and later shown to remove AMP from abortive intermediates of ligation (Ahel et al., 2009). PNK- and APTX-like FHA protein (PALF, also known as APLF, C2orf13 or Xip1) has AP endonuclease activity (Kanno et al., 2007; Iles et al., 2007). Recent study showed that APLF also has histone chaperone activity (Mehrotra et al., 2011) and that it co-operates with PARP-3, which is newly found as a DSB sensor (Rulten et al., 2011). It might be noted that all of these factors bears BRCT or FHA domain as module to bind phosphorylated proteins. Polymerases μ and λ possess BRCT domain. PNKP, APTX and PALF possess FHA domain, which is structurally similar to each other and known to interact with CKII-phosphorylated XRCC1 or XRCC4 (see below).

2.4 Alternative NHEJ pathways

Apart from the classical NHEJ model, there are also studies by several groups highlighting NHEJ as a more sophisticated and complex mechanism involving a cross–talk between pathways including proteins other than DNA-PKcs, Ku, XRCC4-DNA Ligase IV.

2.4.1 ATM dependent pathway

Human genetic disorder, Ataxia Telangiectasia (AT) is caused by mutation in the ATM (Ataxia Telangiectasia mutated) gene and is characterized by chromosomal instability, immunodeficiency, radiosensitivity, defective cell cycle checkpoint activation and predisposition to cancer indicating its responsibility in genome surveillance (Jorgensen and Shiloh, 1996). ATM deficiency causes early embryonic lethality in Ku or DNA-PKcs deficient mice, thus providing NHEJ an independent role for the DNA-PK holoenzyme (Sekiguchi et al., 2001). ATM and Artemis, together with NBS1, Mre11 and 53BP1 function in a sub-pathway that repairs approximately 10% of DSBs, probably requiring end-processing (Riballo et al., 2004). Another study suggested three parallel, but mutually crosstalking, pathways of NHEJ, *i.e.*, core pathway mediated by DNA-PKcs and Ku, ATM-Artemis pathway and 53BP1 pathway, all of which finally converge on XRCC4-DNA Ligase IV (Iwabuchi et al., 2006).

2.4.2 Back-up NHEJ pathway

Repair in IR-induced DSBs in higher eukaryotes is mainly dominated by NHEJ which is faster as compared to other mechanisms. However, it is severely compromised in case of defects in DNA-PKcs, Ku and DNA Ligase IV (DiBiase et al., 2000; Wang et al., 2001). An array of biochemical and genetic studies have shown that despite the prevalence of DNA-PK dependent pathway, cells deficient in either of its components are still able to rejoin a majority of DSBs, operating with slower kinetics, using an alternative pathway (Nevaldine et al., 1997; Wang et al., 2003). Chicken DT40 cells defective in HR rejoin IR induced DSBs with kinetics similar to those of other cells with much lower levels of HR. Nevertheless, rejoining of DSBs with slow kinetics is associated with incorrect DNA end-joining which is incompatible with the mechanism of HR (Löbrich et al., 1995). These observations led to the model that DNA DSBs are rejoined by two pathways, one of which is DNA-PK dependent (D-NHEJ) and an alternative pathway termed as Back-up (B-NHEJ) pathway (Wang et al., 2003) possibly prone to erroneous re-joining and utilization of microhomologies (Roth DB, 1986). Further investigations ascertained the role of DNA-PK in the functional co-ordination of D-NHEJ and B-NHEJ, suggesting that the binding of inactive DNA-PK to DNA ends not only blocks the D-NHEJ but also interferes with the function of B-NHEJ (Perrault et al., 2004). The DNA-PK and Ku complex is believed to recruit other repair proteins like XRCC4-DNA Ligase IV complex and stimulate the ligation of DNA ends (Ramsden and Gellert, 1998) in D-NHEJ pathway.

DNA Ligase IV deficient mouse embryonic fibroblasts retained significant DNA end-joining activity which was reduced upto 80% by knocking down DNA Ligase III. Thus DNA Ligase III was identified as a vital component of B-NHEJ (Wang et al., 2005). PARP-1 was initially pointed to bind to DSBs with a higher efficacy than to SSBs (Weinfeld et al., 1997) and with a greater affinity than that of DNA-PKcs (D'Silva et al., 1999). It has also been shown to interact with both the subunits of DNA-PK (Galande and Kohwi-Shigematsu, 1999; Ariumi et al., 1999) catalyzing their poly(ADP-ribosyl)ation (Li et al., 2004; Ruscetti et al., 1998). Using chemically potent producer of DSBs, calicheamicin $\gamma 1$, a new mechanism was identified operating independently but complementing the classical NHEJ pathway. Proteins such as, PARP-1, XRCC1 and DNA Ligase III, which were believed to be otherwise involved in Base Excision Repair (Caldecott, 2003) and SSB repair (Caldecott, 2001) surmised a new mechanism encompassing synapsis and end-joining activity.

Above mentioned studies evidently illustrate alternative DNA end-joining pathways to contribute in the repair of DSBs in order to maintain the genomic integrity when D-NHEJ is compromised. However, due to their low fidelity, they are directly implicated in genomic instability (Ferguson et al., 2000), aberrant coding and signal joint formation during V(D)J recombination (Taccioli et al., 1993;Bogue et al., 1997) as well as formation of soft tissue sarcomas (Sharpless et al., 2001) that potentially leads to cancer.

3. Recruitment and assembly of NHEJ factors at DSB

The key players of NHEJ are named, but the mechanism of their recruitment and hierarchy of assembly on the DNA DSB is not yet well clarified. Many proteins in the HR pathway, *e.g.*, Nbs1-Mre11-Rad50, BRCA1 and Rad51, exhibit local accumulation after DSB induction, forming microscopically visible structures, termed ionizing radiation-induced foci (IRIF) (Maser et al., 1997). Such change in the localization of HR proteins has been observed also in partial volume irradiation (Nelms et al., 1998) and laser micro-irradiation experiments (Kim et al., 2002). As the distribution of these proteins after irradiation, at least partially, overlapped with irradiated area or DSBs, visualized by DNA end labeling or immunofluorescence analysis of γ-H2AX, these phenomena are believed to reflect the accumulation of these proteins around DSB sites. In the case of NHEJ proteins, however, IRIF has been observed only for autophosphorylated form of DNA-PKcs (Chan et al., 2002). Recently, there are increasing number of studies using laser micro-irradiation demonstrating the accumulation of NHEJ molecules in irradiated area. Another approach to examine the association of DNA repair proteins with damaged DNA is sequential extraction with increasing concentration of detergent or salt.

3.1 Recruitment of XRCC4 to chromatin DNA in response to ionizing radiation

We employed sequential extraction with detergent-containing buffer to examine the binding of XRCC4 to DSB (Kamdar and Matsumoto, 2010). The retention of XRCC4 to subcellular fraction consisting of chromatin DNA and other nuclear matrix structures increased in response to irradiation. Micrococcal nuclease enzyme which specifically cleaves the chromatin DNA into smaller nucleosomal fragments revealed that XRCC4 is tethered to chromatin DNA after irradiation.

Through quantitative analyses, it was estimated that only one or few XRCC4 molecules might be recruited to each DNA end at the DSB site. This can be speculated based on the stoichiometric results depicting a complex consisting of two XRCC4 molecules forming a dimer and one Ligase IV molecule (Junop et al., 2000). The accumulation of XRCC4 on the damaged chromatin is very rapid and sensitive as the response after radiation is observed in $\leq$ 0.1hr and is stable until at least 4 hrs. This phenomenon is in parallel to the appearance of phosphorylation of H2AX which is observed as foci until the DSBs are repaired and then their disappearance from the resealed DNA (Svetlova et al., 2010). XRCC4 could be retained on the damaged chromatin as long as the repair complex carries out the rejoining of the DNA ends which pivotally includes ligation by XRCC4-DNA Ligase IV. In addition, the residence of XRCC4 on chromatin might be very transient, particularly after the irradiation with small and conventional doses. These observations can reasonably explain why it has been difficult to capture the movement of NHEJ enzymes to DSB sites.

Using a similar approach, the movement of NHEJ molecules in response to DSB induction by neocarzinostatin or bleomycin was reported (Drouet et al., 2005). Conversely, there are several differences between the results of the two studies. First, they observed that DNase I treatment released DNA-PKcs and Ku but not XRCC4 and DNA Ligase IV, leading to the idea that XRCC4 and DNA Ligase IV were bound to nuclear matrix or other structures rather than chromatin itself. In the present study, XRCC4 retained after buffer extraction could be released by micrococcal nuclease treatment, indicating its binding to chromatin DNA. Second, they mentioned that the movement of NHEJ molecules could be observed only after high doses of irradiation in their study. The present study has demonstrated small but significant increase in the chromatin binding of XRCC4 even after physiologically relevant dose, *i.e.*, 2Gy, of irradiation.

3.2 Phosphorylation of XRCC4

Several studies have shown that DNA-PK can phosphorylate XRCC4 *in vitro*, decreasing its interaction with DNA, although the significance of this phenomenon is presently unclear (Critchlow et al., 1997; Leber et al., 1998; Modesti et al., 1999). Moreover, our research group demonstrated XRCC4 phosphorylation in living cells, which was induced by ionizing radiation in a manner dependent on DNA-PKcs (Matsumoto et al., 2000), indicating that XRCC4 is an *in vivo* and not merely an *in vitro*, substrate of DNA-PK. However, the presence of DNA-PK did not seem as a pre-requisite for XRCC4 recruitment to chromatin as demonstrated by siRNA and specific kinase inhibitors against DNA-PKcs.

DNA-PK is autophosphorylated and leads to the phosphorylation events on the target proteins. An earlier study also detected XRCC4 on DNA ends in a phosphorylated form dependent on DNA-PK. However, phosphorylation was deemed dispensable for XRCC4-DNA Ligase IV loading at DNA ends since stable complexes involving DNA-PK and the ligation complex were recovered in the presence of wortmannin which is a PIKK inhibitor (Calsou et.al 2003). A recent study using laser irradiation demonstrated XRCC4 accumulation in irradiated area, which also did not require DNA-PKcs (Mari et al., 2006; Yano et al., 2008). All these observations in aggregate thus lead to the unanswered question as to what mechanism is involved in XRCC4 recruitment to damaged chromatin DNA.

Then, what is the importance of the phosphorylation of XRCC4, if any? It has been awaited to find the biological consequence of XRCC4 phosphorylation by DNA-PK through the identification and elimination of the phosphorylation site(s). Several groups, employing mass spectrometry, identified Ser260 and Ser318 as the major phosphorylation sites in XRCC4 by DNA-PK *in vitro* (Lee et al., 2002; Yu et al., 2003; Lee et al., 2003; Wang et al., 2004). However, it is presently unclear whether these sites are phosphorylated in living cells, especially, in response to DNA damage. Furthermore, the mutants lacking these phosphorylation sites appeared fully competent in the restoration of radioresistance and V(D)J recombination in CHO-derived XRCC4-deficient XR-1 cells and also exhibited normal activity in DNA joining reaction in cell-free system, leading to the conclusion that XRCC4 phosphorylation by DNA-PK was unnecessary for these functions (Lee et.al 2003; Yu et.al 2003). However, our group recently identified four additional phosphorylation sites in XRCC4 by DNA-PK and found that at least three of them would be important for DSB repair, because disruption of these sites resulted in elevated radiosensitivity (Sharma, Matsumoto et al., unpublished results).

3.3 Recruitment dynamics of NHEJ complex on damaged chromatin

XRCC4 associates in a tight complex with DNA Ligase IV. XRCC4 is essential for the stability of ligase IV in mammalian cells (Bryans et.al 1999). It also initiates the chemical reaction of ligation reaction by bringing about the adenylation on Ligase IV to rejoin the DNA. Radiation induced modification, i.e phosphorylation of XRCC4 is also observed in the cells harboring the ligase IV gene. Although, it is evident from the above reports that phosphorylation is not a necessary phenomenon required for XRCC4 recruitment to chromatin, it occurs as a modification induced in response to radiation. These observations lead to two possible hierarchies; (a) ionizing radiation induces phosphorylation on DNA-PKcs which then in turn phosphorylates XRCC4 and the phosphorylated form is recruited to DSBs or (b) ionizing radiation stimulates XRCC4 recruitment to DSBs, chaperoned by other factors like ligase IV, and also recruitment of DNA-PKcs independently and then the kinase would bring about the phosphorylation events. However, since current evidences render phosphorylation dispensable for recruitment of XRCC4, the second mechanism may seem more plausible.

Moreover, movement of DNA-PKcs to chromatin DNA is also diminished in the absence of DNA Ligase IV and Ku. In addition, structural and crystallographic studies have displayed that the interaction between XRCC4 dimer and DNA Ligase IV is via the linker region on ligase IV between the tandem BRCT domains (Grawunder et al., 1998). A recent high resolution crystallographic study has revealed an extensive DNA Ligase IV binding interface for XRCC4 forming a helix-loop-helix structure forming a clamp within the inter-BRCT linker region. This loop buries and packs against a large hydrophobic surface of XRCC4, thus inducing a kink in the tail region of XRCC4, thereby involving numerous interactions between the BRCT2 domain of ligase IV and XRCC4 which are expected to play a major role in the interactions between the two proteins (Wu et.al., 2009). Mutational analysis in several of these hydrophobic residues would give a better insight in the mode of interaction alterating the conformation of both the molecules for recruitment on DNA ends.

XLF or Cernnunos is also considered a vital component of the ligation complex to reseal the DNA ends. XLF has been demonstrated to interact with XRCC4 via the globular head domains at the amino-terminal region of both the proteins forming a heterodimeric structure (Andres et al., 2007). The response to ionizing radiation could thus be expected to be similar to that evoked in XRCC4. Conversely, the protein was not found to be tethered to chromatin even after extraction with a high detergent concentration. Contrasting to that observed in case of XRCC4, XLF accumulation was neither rapid or transient nor sensitive to be observed at conventional radiation dose. This leads to the possibility that XLF association to XRCC4 is highly unstable and does not directly adhere to chromatin structures. A parallel observation was drawn by another study wherein they demonstrated that XRCC4 was dispensable for XLF recruitment to DSBs, although it could act as a stabilizing factor and cause a dynamic exchange between the free and bound protein once XLF is recruited on the DNA free ends (Yano et.al., 2008). Very recent study indicated that 10 amino acid region at the C-terminal of XLF is essential for interaction with Ku and for recruitment to DSB (Yano et al., 2011).

Intriguingly, transgenetically expressed XLF protein demonstrated a similar trend, except that the retention was observed in the subcellular nucleosolic fraction, alleged as tethered to chromatin. This disparity in the observation can be attributed to the difference in behaviour between endogenous and exogenously expressed molecules.

Owing to the recruitment of XRCC4 during the inhibition of phosphorylation by the kinases, a possible speculation leads to the idea that either or both of ligase IV and XLF molecules could play a role as a chaperone responsible for the recruitment of XRCC4 to damaged chromatin.

Live cell imaging studies have demonstrated that Ku recruits XLF and is also likely to mediate the XLF-DNA interaction (Yano et al., 2008). Therefore, the vital component of NHEJ, Ku might be mediating the interaction between XRCC4 and DSB via DNA Ligase IV or also between Ligase IV and DSB via XRCC4, though ligase IV possess a DNA-binding region at the N-terminus.

Another very intriguing analysis has exhibited that PARP-3, whose function was previously unknown, accumulates APLF (Aprataxin-like factor) to the site of DSBs which in turn supports the retention of XRCC4-DNA Ligase IV on the chromatin (Rulten et al., 2011).

Another possibility is that XRCC4 moves to a DSB site autonomously due to its intrinsic DNA end-binding activity (Modesti et al., 1999). Furthermore, XRCC4 was shown to interact with polynucleotide kinase (PNK) (Koch et al., 2004) or aprataxin (APTX) (Clements et al., 2004), depending on the phosphorylation by casein kinase II. Unexpectedly, unphosphorylated XRCC4 interacts with PNKP, although with a lower affinity, but CKII mediated XRCC4 phosphorylation inhibited the PNKP activity (Mani et al., 2010). In addition, XRCC4 has been shown to undergo monoubiquitination (Foster et al., 2006) and SUMOylation (Yurchenko et al., 2006), the former of which was shown to be DNA damage-inducible. The role of such posttranslational modifications on the chromatin-recruitment of XRCC4 is of another interest.

Additionally, studies by several groups have suggested that NHEJ is more sophisticated than thought initially and involves many proteins other than DNA-PKcs, Ku, XRCC4-DNA ligase IV, XLF/Cernunnos. In order to investigate into the entirety of the complex compounding several molecules from NHEJ and particularly from other repair or physiological pathways: XRCC4 associated complex bound to chromatin, supposedly at the last step of resealing the DNA nicks and gaps, can be isolated and analysed.

One of the other speculations is that the unwinding may be carried out by Ku since it possesses helicase activity in an ATP dependent manner (Blier et al., 1993) and is supposedly the earliest protein in repair hierarchy. Certain studies have shown a functional interaction between the Ku heterodimer and WRN (Karmakar et al., 2002) emphasizing its significance in DNA repair and metabolism pathways. The exonuclease but not the helicase activity of WRN is stimulated by physical interaction with XRCC4-ligase IV (Kusumoto et al., 2008).

ATM and Artemis, together with Nbs1, Mre11 and 53BP1, function in a subpathway of NHEJ that repairs approximately 10% of DSBs, probably those require DNA end processing (Riballo et. al, 2004). Another study suggested three parallel, but mutually crosstalking, pathways of NHEJ, *i.e.,* core pathway mediated by DNA-PKcs and Ku, ATM-Artemis pathway and 53BP1 pathway, all of which finally converge on XRCC4-DNA ligase IV (Iwabuchi et al., 2006). Recent studies indicated the requirement of chromatin remodeling factors, like ALC1 and ACF1, for the recruitment of NHEJ molecules to DSB (Ahel et al., 2009; Lan et al., 2010).

It will be of interest to investigate whether all of the above mentioned proteins play some role in the recruitment of XRCC4-DNA Ligase IV to DSB sites or, conversely, are recruited to DSB sites through interaction with XRCC4. This entire conglomerate of proteins has yet to reveal complex mechanisms and cross-talk between other repair and cellular pathways.

These questions may be addressed by examining the chromatin-recruitment of deletion or point mutants of XRCC4 and by applying siRNA or inhibitors of the above listed molecules in experimental systems. They could then be optimized for use as adjuvants in radiotherapy.

Proteomic analysis is one of the vital instruments to examine any kinase network involving *in vivo* substrates. Such modern technologies have helped to understand that the DNA damage repair response is much sophisticated and complicated than anticipated earlier. It connects NHEJ with chromatin remodelling as well as transcription processes which are also pivotal to cellular functions; thereby aspiring to investigate the cross-talks involved in the repair mechanics.

3.4 Future perspectives

There have been several studies including ours, demonstrating various mechanisms for the dynamics and assembly of the repair machinery on the damaged DNA site in response to various forms of endogenous and exogenous stress. A certain study also suggests that the DNA damage response does not require the DNA damage but the stable association of the repair factors for a prolonged period of time with chromatin which is likely a critical step in triggering, amplifying and maintaining the DNA damage response signal (Soutoglou and Misteli, 2008). It will thus be interesting to investigate the capricious questions as to what are the exact signalling mechanisms to trigger the DSB repair response or the role of several macromolecules involved in different cellular processes. Thus, the assembly of non-homologous end joining protein complex at DSB was not as simple as thought in classical models and further studies are warranted to fully elucidate the processes. Another important aspect, not clarified, is to understand the hierarchy and mechanism of the disassembly of the repair machinery, involved in NHEJ or from cross-talk pathways, from the site of refurbished DNA. Finally, understanding the mechanisms of DNA repair at molecular levels might bring us a new approach to be applied in cancer radiotherapy or chemotherapy.

4. Conclusions

DSB repair through NHEJ has been considered rather simple reaction, basically comprised of six core factors, Ku70, Ku80, DNA-PKcs, XRCC4, DNA Ligase IV and XLF. However, the mechanism how these molecules are recruited to DSBs and assembled into repair machinery is not fully understood. It has been difficult even to observe the recruitement of NHEJ molecules by immunofluorescence or simple labeling with fluorescent proteins. However, laser microirradiation technique combined with fluorescent protein and biochemical fractionation enabled us to capture the binding of NHEJ factors to DSBs. NHEJ would involve a number of processing enzymes, whose function or regulation is largely unclear. Additionally, most recent study shed light on the importance of chromatin remodeling prior to the binding of Ku. Obviously, further studies are warranted to elucidate this complexity.

5. Acknowledgements

Our work was supported in part by Grant-in-Aid for Scientific Research from the Ministry of Education, Culture, Sport, Science and Technology of Japan to Y.M. Y.M. also received supports from Foundation for Promotion of Cancer Research, Sato Memorial Foundation for Cancer Research, Public Trust Haraguchi Memorial Cancer Research Fund and Osaka Cancer Research Foundation. A part of the work is the result of "Initiating Events in the Recognition and Repair of DNA Double-Strand Breaks" carried out under the Strategic Promotion Program for Basic Nuclear Research, the Ministry of Education, Culture, Sport, Science and Technology, Japan.

6. References

Ahel, D., Horejsi, Z., Wiechens, N., Polo, S.E., Garcia-Wilson, E., Ahel, I., Flynn, H., Skehel, M., West, S.C., Jackson, S.P., Owen-Hughes, T. & Boulton, S.J. (2009) Poly(ADP-ribose)-dependent regulation of DNA repair by the chromatin remodeling enzye ALC1. *Science*, Vol. 325, pp. 1240-1243.

Ahel, I., Rass, U., El-Khamisy, S., Katyal, S., Clements, P., McKinnon, P., Caldecott, K. & West, S. (2006) The neurodegenerative disease protein aprataxin resolves abortive DNA ligation intermediates. *Nature,* Vol. 443, pp.713-716.

Ahnesorg, P., Smith, P. & Jackson, S. (2006) XLF interacts with the XRCC4-DNA ligase IV complex to promote DNA nonhomologous end-joining. *Cell,* Vol. 124, pp. 301-313.

Andegeko, Y., Moyal, L., Mittelman, L., Tsarfaty, I., Shiloh, Y. & Rotman, G. (2001) Nuclear retention of ATM at sites of DNA double strand breaks. *Journal of Biological Chemistry*, Vol. 276, pp. 38224-38230.

Anderson, C.W. & Lees-Miller, S.P. (1992) The nuclear serine/threonine protein kinase DNA-PK. *Critical Reviews on Eukaryotic Gene Expression,* Vol. 2., No.4, pp. 283-314.

Andres, S.N.; Modesti, M.; Tsai, C.J.; Chu, G. & Junop, M.S. (2007) Crystal structure of human XLF: a twist in nonhomologous DNA end-joining. *Molecular Cell,* Vol. 28, pp. 1093-1101.

Ariumi, Y.; Masutani, M.; Copeland, T.D.; Mimori, T.; Sugimura,T.; Shimotohno, K.; Ueda, K.; Hatanaka, M.; and Noda, M. (1999) Suppression of the poly(ADP-ribose) polymerase activity by DNA-dependent protein kinase in vitro. *Oncogene,* Vol. 18, pp. 4616-4625.

Badie, C.; Iliakis, G.; Foray, N.; Alsbeih, G.; Pantellias, G.E.; Okayasu, R.; Cheong, N.; Russell, N.S.; Begg, A.C.; Arlett, C.F. & Malaise, E.P. (1995) Defective repair of DNA double-strand breaks and chromosome damage in fibroblast from a radiosensitive leukemia patient. Cancer Research, Vol. 55, pp. 1232-1234.

Barnes, D., Stamp, G., Rosewell, I., Denzel, A. & Lindahl, T. (1998) Targeted disruption of the gene encoding DNA ligase IV leads to lethality in embryonic mice. *Current Biology,* Vol. 8, pp. 1395-1398.

Bau, D., Yang, M., Tsou, Y., Lin, S., Wu, C., Hsieh, H., Wang, R., Tsai, C., Chang, W., Hsieh, H., Sun, S. & Tsai, R. (2010) Colorectal cancer and genetic polymorphism of DNA double-strand break repair gene XRCC4 in Taiwan. *Anticancer Research,* Vol. 30, pp. 2727-2730.

Biederman, K.A.; Sun, J.; Giaccia, A.J.; Tosto, L.M. & Brown, J.M. (1991) scid mutation in mice confers hypersensitivity to ionizing radiation and a deficiency in DNA double-strand break repair. *Proceeding of National Academy of Science United States of America,* Vol. 88, pp. 1394-1397.

Blier, P.R.; Griffith, A.J.; Craft, J.; and Hardin, J.A. (1993) Binding of Ku protein to DNA. Measurement of affinity for ends and demonstration of binding to nicks. *J Biol. Chem.,* Vol. 268, pp. 7594-7601.

Bliss, T. & Lane, D. (1997) Ku selectively transfers between DNA molecules with homologous ends. *Journal of Biological Chemistry,* Vol. 272, pp. 5765-5773.

Blunt, T.; Finnie,N.; Taccioli, G.; Smith, G.; Demengeot, J.; Gottlieb, T.; Mizuta, R.; Varghese, A.; Alt, F.; Jeggo, P. & Jackson, S.P. (1995) Defective DNA-dependent protein kinase activity is linked to V(D)J recombination and DNA repair defects associated with the murine scid mutation. *Cell,* Vol. 80, pp. 813-823.

Bogue, M.A.; Wang, C.; Zhu, C. and Roth, D.B. (1997). V(D)J recombination in Ku86-deficient mice: distinct effects on coding, signal, and hybrid joint formation. *Immunity,* Vol. 7, pp. 37-47.

Bosma, G.; Custer, R. & Bosma, M. (1983) A severe combined immunodeficiency mutation in the mouse. *Nature*, Vol. 301, pp. 527-530.

Boulton, S.J. & Jackson, S.P. (1996) Identification of a *Saccharomyces cerevisiae* Ku80 homologue: roles in DNA double strand break rejoining and in telomeric maintenance. *Nucleic Acids Research*, Vol. 24, pp. 4639-4648.

Boulton, S.J. & Jackson, S.P. (1998) Components of the Ku-dependent non-homologous end-joining pathway are involved in telomeric length maintenance and teleomeric silencing. EMBO Journal, Vol. 17, pp. 1819-1828.

Bryans, M., Valenzano, M. & Stamato, T. (1999). Absence of DNA ligase IV protein in XR-1 cells: evidence for stabilization by XRCC4. *Mutation Research*, Vol. 433, pp. 53-58.

Buck, D., Malivert, L., de Chasseval, R., Barraud, A., Fondanèche, M., Sanal, O., Plebani, A., Stéphan, J., Hufnagel, M., le Deist, F., Fischer, A., Durandy, A., de Villartay, J. & Revy, P. (2006) Cernunnos, a novel nonhomologous end-joining factor, is mutated in human immunodeficiency with microcephaly. *Cell*, Vol. 124, pp. 287-299.

Caldecott, K.W. (2001) Mammalian DNA single-strand break repair: an X-ra(y)ted affair. *Bioessays*, Vol. 23, pp. 447-455.

Caldecott, K.W. (2003) XRCC1 and DNA strand break repair. *DNA Repair (Amst)*, Vol. 2, pp. 955-969.

Callebaut, I., Malivert, L., Fischer, A., Mornon, J., Revy, P. & de Villartay, J. (2006) Cernunnos interacts with the XRCC4 x DNA-ligase IV complex and is homologous to the yeast nonhomologous end-joining factor Nej1. *Journal of Biological Chemistry*, Vol. 281, pp. 13857-13860.

Calsou, P., Delteil, C., Frit, P., Drouet, J. & Salles,B. (2003) Coordinated assembly of Ku and p460 subunits of the DNA-dependent protein kinase on DNA ends is necessary for XRCC4-ligase IV recruitment. *Journal of Molecular Biology*, Vol.326, pp.93-103.

Cao, Q., Pitt, S., Leszyk, J. & Baril, E. (1994) DNA-dependent ATPase from HeLa cells is related to human Ku autoantigen. *Biochemistry*, Vol. 33, pp. 8548-8557.

Carter, T.; Vancurova, I.; Sun, I.; Lou, W. & DeLeon, S. (1990) A DNA-activated protein kinase from HeLa cell nuclei. *Molecular and Cellular Biology*, Vol. 10, pp. 6460-6471.

Chan, D.W. & Lees-Miller, S.P. (1996) The DNA-dependent protein kinase is inactivated by autophosphorylation of the catalytic subunit. *Journal of Biological Chemistry*, Vol. 271, pp. 8936-8941.

Chan, D.W., Chen, B.P., Prithivirajsingh, S., Kurimasa, A., Story, M.D., Qin, J. & Chen, D.J. (2002) Autophosphorylation of the DNA-dependent protein kinase catalytic subunit is required for rejoining of DNA double-strand breaks. *Genes & Development*, Vol. 16, pp. 2333-2338.

Chen, B.P.-C.; Uematsu, N.; Kobayashi, J.; Lerenthal, Y.; Krempler, A.; Yajima, H.; Lobrich, M.; Shiloh, Y. & Chenk D.J. (2007) ATM is essential for DNA-PKcs phosphorylation at T2609 cluster upon DNA double-strand break. *Journal of Biological Chemistry*, Vol. 282, pp. 6582-6587.

Chen, L., Trujillo, K., Sung, P. & Tomkinson, A. (2000). Interactions of the DNA ligase IV-XRCC4 complex with DNA ends and the DNA-dependent protein kinase. *Journal of Biological Chemistry*, Vol. 275, pp. 26196-26205.

Clements, P., Breslin, C., Deeks, E., Byrd, P., .Ju, L., Bieganowski, P., Brenner, C., Moreira, M., Taylor, A. & Caldecott, K. (2004). The ataxia-oculomotor apraxia 1 gene product has a role distinct from ATM and interacts with the DNA strand break repair proteins XRCC1 and XRCC4. *DNA Repair (Amst.)*, Vol. 3, pp. 1493-1502.

Cimprich,K.A.; Shin, T.B.; Keith, C.T. & Schreiber,S.L. (1996) cDNA cloning and gene mapping of a candicated human cell cycle checkpoint protein. *Proceeding of National Academy of Science United States of America*, Vol. 93, pp. 2850-2855.

Critchlow, S.; Bowater, R. & Jackson, S. (1997) Mammalian DNA double-strand break repair protein XRCC4 interacts with DNA ligase IV. *Current Biology*, Vol. 7, pp. 588-598.

d'Adda di Fagagna, F.; Weller, G.R.; Doherty, A.J. & Jackson, S.P. (2003) The Gam protein of bacteriophage Mu is an orthologue of eukaryotic Ku. *EMBO Reports*, Vol. 4, pp. 47-52.

Dai, Y., Kysela, B., Hanakahi, K., Manolis, K., Riballo, E., Stumm, M., Harville, T. O., West, S., C., Oettinger, M. A., and Jeggo, P. A. (2003) Nonhomologous end joining and V(D)J recombination require an additional factor. *Proceeding of National Academy of Science United States of America*, Vol. 100, pp. 2462-2467.

Date,H., Onodera,O., Tanaka,H., Iwabuchi,K., Uekawa,K., Igarashi,S., Koike,R., Hiroi,T., Yuasa,T., Awaya, Y., Sakai, T., Takahashi, T., Nagatomo, H., Sekijima, Y., Kawachi, I., Takiyama, Y., Nishizawa, M., Fukuhara, N., Saito, K., Sugano, S. & Tsuji, S. (2001) Early-onset ataxia with ocular motor apraxia and hypoalbuminemia is caused by mutations in a new HIT superfamily gene. *Nature Genetics*, Vol. 29, pp. 184–188.

DiBiase, S.J.; Zeng, Z.C.; Chen, R.; Hyslop, T.; Curran, Jr., W.J. and Iliakis, G. (2000). DNA-dependent protein kinase stimulates an independently active, nonhomologous, end-joining apparatus. *Cancer Res.*, Vol. 60, pp. 1245-1253.

Ding, Q.; Reddy, Y.; Wang, W.; Woods, T.; Douglas, P.; Ramsden, D.; Lees-Miller, S.P. & Meek, K. (2003) Autophosphorylation of the catalytic subunit of the DNA-dependent protein kinase is required for efficient end processing during DNA double-strand break repair. *Molecular and Cellular Biology*, Vol. 23, pp. 5836-5848.

D'Silva, I.; Pelletier, J.D.; Lagueux, J.; D'Amours, D.; Chaudhry, M.A.; Weinfeld, M.; Lees-Miller, S.P. and Poirier, G. G. (1999) Relative affinities of poly(ADP-ribose) polymerase and DNA-dependent protein kinase for DNA strand interruptions. *Biochim. Biophys. Acta.*, Vol. 1430, pp. 119-126.

Dvir, A.; Peterson, S.R.; Knuth, M.W.; Lu, H. & Dynan,W.S. (1992) Ku autoantigen is the regulatory component of a template-associated protein kinase that phosphorylates RNA polymerase II. *Proceeding of National Academy of Science United States of America*, Vol. 89, pp. 11920-11924.

Dvir, A.; Stein, L.Y.; Calore, B.L. & Dynan,W.S. (1993) Purification and characterization of a template-associated protein kinase that phosphorylates RNA polymerase II. *Journal of Biological Chemistry*, Vol. 268, pp.10440-10447.

Dore, A.S.; Drake, A.C., Brewerton, S.C. & Blundell, T.L. Identification of DNA-PK in the arthropods. Evidence for the ancient ancestry of vertebrate non-homologous end-joining. DNA Repair, Vol. 3., pp. 33-41.

Douglas, P., Sapkota, G., Morrice, N., Yu, Y., Goodarzi, A., Merkle, D., Meek, K., Alessi, D. & Lees-Miller, S. (2002) Identification of in vitro and in vivo phosphorylation sites in the catalytic subunit of the DNA-dependent protein kinase. *Biochemical Journal*, Vol. 368, pp.243-251.

Drouet, J., Delteil, C., Lefrancois, J., Concannon, P., Salles, B. & Calsou, P. (2005) DNA-dependent protein kinase and XRCC4-DNA ligase IV mobilization in the cell in response to DNA double strand breaks. *Journal of Biological Chemistry*, Vol. 280 pp. 7060-7069.

Dynan, W.S. & Yoo, S. (1998) Interaction of Ku protein and DNA-dependent protein kinase catalytic subunit with nucleic acids. *Nucleic Acids Research*, Vol. 26, pp. 1551-1559.

Falck, J.; Coates, J. & Jackson, S.P. (2005) Conserved modes of recruitment of ATM, ATR and DNA-PKcs to sites of DNA damage. *Nature*, Vol. 434, pp. 605-611.

Feldmann, H.; Driller, L.; Meier, B.; Mages, G.; Kellermann, J. & Winnacker,E.L. (1996) HDF2, the second subunit of the Ku homologue from *Saccharomyces cerevisiae*. *Journal of Biological Chemistry*, Vol. 271, pp. 27765-27769.

Feldmann, H. & Winnacker, E.L. (1993) A putative homologue of the human autoantigen Ku from Saccharomyces cerevisiae. *Journal of Biological Chemistry*, Vol. 268, pp. 12895-12900.

Ferguson, D.O.; Sekiguchi, J.M.; Chang, S.; Frank, K.M.; Gao, Y.; DePinho, R.A. and Alt, F.W. (2000) The nonhomologous end-joining pathway of DNA repair is required for genomic stability and the suppression of translocations. *Proc. Natl. Acad. Sci. U. S. A*, Vol. 97, pp. 6630-6633.

Foster, R., Nnakwe, C., Woo, L. & Frank, K. (2006) Monoubiquitination of the nonhomologous end joining protein XRCC4. *Biochemical & Biophysical Research Communications*, Vol. 341, pp. 175-183.

Frank, K., Sekiguchi, J., Seidl, K., Swat, W., Rathbun, G., Cheng, H., Davidson, L., Kangaloo, L. & Alt, F. (1998) Late embryonic lethality and impaired V(D)J recombination in mice lacking DNA ligase IV. *Nature*, Vol. 396, pp. 173-177.

Frank-Vaillant, M. & Marcand, S. (2001) NHEJ regulation by mating type is exercised through a novel protein, Lif2p, essential to the Ligase IV pathway. *Genes & Development*, Vol. 15, pp. 3005-3012.

Fulop, G.M. & Phillips, R.A. (1990). The scid mutation in mice causes a general defect in DNA repair. *Nature*, Vol. 347, pp. 479-482.

Gao, Y., Sun, Y., Frank, K., Dikkes, P., Fujiwara, Y., Seidl, K., Sekiguchi, J., Rathbun, G., Swat, W., Wang, J. *et al.* (1998) A critical role for DNA end-joining proteins in both lymphogenesis and neurogenesis. *Cell*, Vol. 95, pp. 891-902.

Galande, S. and Kohwi-Shigematsu, T. (1999) Poly(ADP-ribose) polymerase and Ku autoantigen form a complex and synergistically bind to matrix attachment sequences. *J Biol. Chem.*, Vol. 274, pp. 20521-20528.

Gell, D. & Jackson, S.P. (1999) Mapping of protein-protein interactions within the DNA-dependent protein kinase complex. *Nucleic Acids Research*, Vol. 27, pp.3494-3502.

Gottlieb, T.M. & Jackson,S.P. (1993) The DNA-dependent protein kinase: requirement for DNA ends and association with Ku antigen. *Cell*, Vol. 72, pp.131-142.

Grawunder, U., Wilm, M., Wu, X., Kulesza, P., Wilson, T., Mann, M. & Lieber, M. (1997) Activity of DNA ligase IV stimulated by complex formation with XRCC4 protein in mammalian cells. *Nature*, Vol. 388, pp. 492-495

Grawunder, U., Zimmer, D. & Leiber, M. (1998) DNA ligase IV binds to XRCC4 via a motif located between rather than within its BRCT domains. *Current Biology*, Vol. 8, pp. 873-876.

Gu, Y., Seidl, K., Rathbun, G., Zhu, C., Manis, J., der Van, S., Davidson, L., Cheng, H., Sekiguchi, J., Frank, K., Stanhope-Baker, P., Schlissel, M., Roth, D. & Alt, F. (1997) Growth retardation and leaky SCID phenotype of Ku70-deficient mice. *Immunity*, Vol. 7, pp. 653-665.

Hammel, M., Yu, Y., Fang, S., Lees-Miller, S. & Tainer, J. (2010) XLF regulates filament architecture of the XRCC4·ligase IV complex. *Structure*, Vol. 18, pp. 1431-1442. Hartley, K.; Gell, D.; Smith, C.; Zhang, H.; Divecha, N.; Connelly, M.; Admon, A.; Lees-Miller, S.; Anderson, C. & Jackson, S. (1995) DNA-dependent protein kinase catalytic subunit: a relative of phosphatidylinositol 3-kinase and the ataxia telangiectasia gene product. *Cell*, Vol. 82, pp. 849-856.

Hartley, K.O.; Gell, D.; Smith, G.C.; Zhang, H.; Divecha, N.; Connelly, M.A.; Admon, A.; Lees-Miller, S.P.; Anderson, C.W. and Jackson, S.P. (1995). DNA-dependent protein kinase catalytic subunit: a relative of phosphatidylinositol 3-kinase and the ataxia telangiectasia gene product. *Cell*, Vol. 82, pp. 849-856.

Hentges, P., Ahnesorg, P., Pitcher, R., Bruce, C., Kysela, B., Green, A., Bianchi, J., Wilson, T., Jackson, S. & Doherty, A. (2006). Evolutionary and functional conservation of the DNA non-homologous end-joining protein, XLF/Cernunnos. *Journal of Biological Chemistry*, Vol. 281, pp. 37517-37526.

Herrmann, G.; Lindahl, T. & Schar, P. (1998) Saccharomyces cerevisiae LIF1: a function involved in DNA double-strand break repair related to mammalian XRCC4. EMBO Journal, Vol. 17, pp. 4188-4198.

Hsu, H., Gilley, D., Galande, S., Hande, M., Allen, B., Kim, S., Li, G., Campisi, J., Kohwi-Shigematsu,T. & Chen, D. (2000) Ku acts in a unique way at the mammalian telomere to prevent end joining. *Genes & Development*, Vol. 14, pp. 2807-2812.

Hudson, J.J.; Hsu, D.W.; Guo, K.; Zhukovskaya, N.; Liu, P.H.; Williams, J.G.; Pears, C.J. & Lakin, N.D. (2005) DNA-PKcs-dependent signaling of DNA damage in Dyctyostelium discodeum. *Current Biology*, Vol. 15, pp. 1880-1885.

Iles, N.; Rulten, S.; El-Khamisy, S.F. & Caldecott, K.W. (2007) APLF (C2orf13) is a novel human protein involved in the cellular response to chromosomal DNA strand breaks. *Molecular and Cellular Biology*, Vol. 27, pp. 3793-3803.

Iwabuchi, K., Hashimoto, M., Matsui, T., Kurihara, T., Shimizu, H., Adachi, N., Ishiai, M., Yamamoto, K.-i., Tauchi, H., Takata, M., Koyama, H. and Date, T. (2006) 53BP1 contributes to survival of cells irradiated with X-ray during G1 without Ku70 or Artemis. *Genes to Cells*, Vol. 11, pp. 935-948.

Jorgensen, T.J. and Shiloh, Y. (1996) The ATM gene and the radiobiology of ataxia-telangiectasia. *Int. J Radiat. Biol.*,Vol. 69, pp. 527-537.

Junop, M., Modesti, M., Guarne, A., Ghirlando, R., Gellert, M. & Yang, W. (2000) Crystal structure of the Xrcc4 DNA repair protein and implications for end joining. *EMBO Journal,* Vol. 19, pp. 5962-5970.

Kamdar, R. & Matsumoto, Y. (2010) Radiation-induced XRCC4 association with chromatin DNA analyzed by biochemical fractionation. *Journal of Radiation Research,* Vol. 51, pp. 303-313.

Kanno, S.; Kuzuoka, H.; Sasao, S.; Hong, Z.; Lan, L.; Nakajima, S. & Yasui, A. (2007) A novel human AP endonuclease with conserved zinc-finger-like motifs involved in DNA strand break responses. EMBO Journal, Vol. 26, pp. 2094-2103.

Karmakar, P., Snowden, C.M.; Ramsden, D.A. and Bohr, V.A. (2002) Ku heterodimer binds to both ends of the Werner protein and functional interaction occurs at the Werner N-terminus. *Nucleic Acids Res.,* Vol. 30, pp. 3583-3591.

Kegel, A.; Sjostrand, J.O.O. & Astrom, S.U. (2001) Nej1p, a cell type-specific regulator of nonhomologous end joining in yeast. *Current Biology,* Vol. 11, pp. 1611-1617.

Kienker, L.J.; Shin, E.K. & Meek, K. (2000) Both V(D)J recombination and radioresistance require DNA-PK kinase activity, though minimal levels suffice for V(D)J recombination. *Nucleic Acids Research,* Vol. 28, pp. 2752-2761.

Kim, J. S., Krasieva, T. B., LaMorte, V., Taylor, A. M. R. and Yokomori, K. (2002) Specific recruitment of human cohesin to laser-induce DNA damage. *Journal of Biological Chemistry,* Vol. 277, pp. 45149-45153.

Kirchgessner, C.; Patil, C.; Evans, J.; Cuomo, C.; Fried, L.; Carter, T.; Oettinger, M. & Brown, M. (1995) DNA-dependent kinase (p350) as a candidate gene for the murine SCID defect. *Science,* Vol. 267, pp. 1178-1183.

Koch, C., Agyei, R., Galicia, S., Metalnikov, P., O'Donnell, P., Starostine, A., Weinfeld, M. & Durocher, D. (2004). Xrcc4 physically links DNA end processing by polynucleotide kinase to DNA ligation by DNA ligase IV. *EMBO Journal,* Vol. 23, pp.3874-3885.

Kurimasa, A.; Kumano, S.; Boubnov, N.; Story, M.; Tung, C.; Peterson, S. & Chen, D. (1999) Requirement for the kinase activity of human DNA-dependent protein kinase catalytic subunit in DNA strand break rejoining. *Molecular and Cellular Biology,* Vol. 19, pp. 3877-3884.

Kusumoto, R., Dawut, L., Marchetti, C., Wan, L., Vindigni, A., Ramsden, D. & Bohr, V. (2008) Werner protein cooperates with the XRCC4-DNA ligase IV complex in end-processing. *Biochemistry,* Vol. 47, pp. 7548-7556.

Lan, L.; Ui, A.; Nakajima, S.; Hatakeyama, K.; Hoshi, M.; Watanabe, R.; Janicki, S.M.; Ogiwara, H.; Kohno, T.; Kannno, S. & Yasui, A. (2010) The ACF1 complex is required for DNA double-strand break repair in human cells. *Molecular Cell,* Vol. 40, pp. 976-987.

Leber, R.;.Wise, T.W.; Mizuta, R. and Meek,K.(1998) The XRCC4 gene product is a target for and interacts with the DNA-dependent protein kinase. *J Biol. Chem.,* Vol. 273, pp. 1794-1801.

Lee, K.-J., Dong, X., Wang, J., Takeda, Y., & Dynan, W.S. (2002) Identification of human autoantibodies to the DNA ligase IV/XRCC4 and mapping of an autoimmune epitope to a potential regulatory region. *Journal of Immunology,* Vol. 169, pp. 3413-3421.

Lee, K.-J., Jovanovic, M., Udayakumar, D., Bladen, C.L., & Dynan, W.S. (2003) Identification of DNA-PKcs phosphorylation sites in XRCC4 and effects of mutation at these sites on DNA end joining in a cell-free system. *DNA Repair,* Vol. 3, pp. 267-276.

Lees-Miller, S.P.; Chen,Y.-R. & Anderson,C.W. (1990) Human cells contain a DNA-activated protein kinase that phosphorylates simian virus 40 T antigen, mouse p53, and the human Ku autoantigen. *Molecular and Cellular Biology,* Vol. 10, pp. 6472-6481.

Lees-Miller, S., Sakaguchi, K., Ullrich, S., Appella, E. & Anderson, C. (1992) Human DNA-activated protein kinase phosphorylates serines 15 and 37 in the amino-terminal transactivation domain of human p53. *Molecular and Cellular Biology,* Vol. 12, pp. 5041-5049.

Lees-Miller, S.; Godbout, R.; Chan, D.; Weinfeld, M.; Day III, R.; Barron, G. and Allalunis-Turner, J. (1995). Absence of p350 subunit of DNA-activated protein kinase from a radiosensitive human cell line. *Science*, Vol. 267, pp. 1183-1185.

Li, B.; Navarro, S.; Kasahara, N. and Comai, L. (2004) Identification and biochemical characterization of a Werner's syndrome protein complex with Ku70/80 and poly(ADP-ribose) polymerase-1. *J Biol. Chem.*, Vol. 279, pp. 13659-13667.

Li, Y., Chirgadze, D., Bolanos-Garcia, V., Sibanda, B., Davies, O., Ahnesorg, P., Jackson, S. and Blundell, T. (2008) Crystal structure of human XLF/Cernunnos reveals unexpected differences from XRCC4 with implications for NHEJ. *EMBO Journal*, Vol. 27, pp. 290-300.

Li, Z.; Otevrel, T.; Gao, Y.; Cheng, H.; Seed, B.; Stamato, T.; Taccioli, G. & Alt, F. (1995) The XRCC4 gene encodes a novel protein involved in DNA double-strand break repair and V(D)J recombination. *Cell*, Vol., 83, pp. 1079-1089.

Lieber,M.R.; Hesse, J.E.; Lewis, S.; Bosma, G.C.; Rosenberg, N.; Mizuuchi, K.; Bosma, M.J. & Gellert,M. (1988). The defect in murine severe combined immune deficiency: joining of signal sequences but not coding segments in V(D)J recombination. *Cell*, Vol. 55, pp. 7-16.

Löbrich, M.; Rydberg, B. and Cooper, P.K. (1995) Repair of x-ray-induced DNA double-strand breaks in specific Not I restriction fragments in human fibroblasts: joining of correct and incorrect ends. *Proc. Natl. Acad. Sci. U. S. A.*, Vol. 92, pp.12050-12054.

Lu, H., Pannicke, U., Schwarz, K. & Lieber, M. (2007a) Length-dependent binding of human XLF to DNA and stimulation of XRCC4.DNA ligase IV activity. *Journal of Biological Chemistry*, Vol. 282, pp. 11155-11162.

Lu, H., Schwarz, K. & Lieber, M. (2007b) Extent to which hairpin opening by the Artemis:DNA-PKcs complex can contribute to junctional diversity in V(D)J recombination. *Nucleic Acids Research.*, Vol. 35, pp. 6917-6923.

Ma, Y.; Pannicke, U.; Schwarz, K. & Lieber, M.R. (2002) Hairpin opening and overhang processing by an Artemis/DNA-dependent protein kinase complex in nonhomologous end joining and V(D)J recombination. *Cell*, Vol. 108, pp. 781-794.

Mani, R., Yu, Y., Fang, S., Lu, M., Fanta, M., Zolner, A., Tahbaz, N., Ramsden, D., Litchfield, D., Lees-Miller, S., & Weinfeld, M. (2010) Dual modes of interaction between XRCC4 and polynucleotide kinase/phosphatase: implications for nonhomologous end joining. *J.Biol.Chem.*, Vol. 26, pp. 37619-37629.

Mari, P., Florea, B., Persengiev, S., Verkaik, N., Bruggenwirth, H., Modesti, M., Giglia-Mari, G., Bezstarosti, K., Demmers, J., Luider, T. & van Gent, D.C. (2006) Dynamic assembly of end-joining complexes requires interaction between Ku70/80 and XRCC4. *Proceeding of National Academy of Science United States of America*, Vol. 103, pp. 18597-18602.

Maser, R.S.; Monsen, K.J.; Nelms, B.E. & Petrini, J.H.J. (1997) hMre11 and hRad50 nuclear foci are induced during normal cellular response to DNA double-strand breaks. *Molecular and Cellular Biology*, Vol. 17, pp. 6087-6096.

Matsumoto, Y.; Suzuki, N.; Namba, N.; Umeda, N.; Ma, X.-J.; Morita, A.; Tomita, M.; Enomoto, A.; Serizawa, S.; Hirano, K.; Sakai, K.; Yasuda, H. & Hosoi, Y. (2000) Cleavage and phosphorylation of XRCC4 protein induced by X-irradiation. *FEBS Letters*, Vol. 478, pp. 67-71.

Matsuoka, S., Ballif, B., Smogorzewska, A., McDonald III, E., Hurov, K., Luo, J., Bakalarski, C., Zhao, Z., Solimini, N., Lerenthal, Y., Shiloh, Y., Gygi, S.P. & Elledge, S.J. (2007) ATM and ATR substrate analysis reveals extensive protein networks responsive to DNA damage. *Science,* Vol. 316, pp. 1160-1166.

McElhinny, N., Snowden, C., McCarville, J. & Ramsden, D. (2000). Ku recruits the XRCC4-ligase IV complex to DNA ends. *Molecular and Cellular Biology,* Vol. 20, pp.2996-3003.

Meek, K.; Kienker, L.; Dallas, C.; Wang, W.; Dark, M.J.; Venta, P.J.; Huie, M.L.; Hirschhorn, R. & Bell, T. (2000) SCID in Jack Russell terriers: a new animal model of DNA-PKcs deficiency. *Journal of Immunology,* Vol. 167, pp. 2142-2150.

Mehrotra, P.V.; Ahel, D.; Ryan, D.P.; Weston, R.; Wiechens, N.; Kraehenbuehl, R.; Owen-Hughes, T. & Ahel, I. (2011) DNA repair factor APLF is a histone chaperone. Molecular Cell, Vol. 41, pp. 46-55.

Milne, G.T.; Jin, S.; Shannon, K.B. & Weaver,D.T. (1996) Mutations in two Ku homologs define a DNA end-joining repair pathway in *Saccharomyces cerevisiae. Molecular and Cellular Biology,* Vol. 16, pp. 4189-4198.

Mimori, T.; Akizuki, M.; Yamagata, H.; Inada, S.; Yoshida, S. & Homma, M. (1981) Characterization of a high molecular weight acidic nuclear protein recognized by autoantibodies in sera from patients with polymyositis-scleroderma overlap. *Journal of Clinical Investigations,* Vol. 68, pp. 611-620.

Mimori, T.; Hardin, J.A. & Steitz, J.A. (1986) Characterization of the DNA-binding protein antigen Ku recognized by autoantibodies from patients with rheumatic disorders. *Journal of Biological Chemistry,* Vol. 261, pp.2274-2278.

Mimori, T. & Hardin, J.A. (1986) Mechanism of interaction between Ku protein and DNA. *Journal of Biological Chemistry,* Vol. 261, pp.10375-10379.

Modesti, M., Hesse, J. & Gellert, M. (1999). DNA binding of Xrcc4 protein is associated with V(D)J recombination but not with stimulation of DNA ligase IV activity. *EMBO Journal,* Vol. 18, pp. 2008-2018.

Moshous, D, Callebaut, I., de Chasseval, R., Corneo, B., Cavazzana-Calvo, M., le Deist, F., Tezcan, I., Sanal, O., Bertrand, Y., Philippe, N., Fischer, A. & de Villartay, J.P. (2001) Artemis, a novel DNA double-strand break repair/V(D)J recombination protein, is mutated in human severe combined immune deficiency. *Cell,* Vol. 105, pp.177-186.

Nelms, B.E.; Maser, R.S.; MacKay, J.F.; Lagally, M.G. & Petrini, J.H.J. (1998) In situ visualization of DNA double-strand break repair in human fibroblasts. *Science,* Vol. 280, pp. 590-592.

Nevaldine, B.; Longo, J.A. and Hahn, P.J. (1997). The scid defect results in much slower repair of DNA double-strand breaks but not high levels of residual breaks. *Radiat. Res.,* Vol. 147, pp. 535-540.

Nussenzweig, A.; Chen, C.; de Costa Soares, V.; Sanchez, M.; Sokol, K.; Nussenzweig, M.C. & Li, G.C. (1996) Requirement for Ku80 in growth and immunoglobulin V(D)J recombination. *Nature,* Vol. 382, pp. 551-555.

O'Driscoll, M.; Cerosaletti, K.M.; Girard, P.M.; Dai, Y.; Stumm, M.; Kysela, B.; Hirsch, B.; Gennery, A.; Palmer, S.E.; Seidel, J.; Gatti, R.A.; Varon, R.; Oettinger, M.A.; Neitzel, H.; Jeggo, P.A. & Concannon, P. (2001) DNA ligase IV mutations identified in patients exhibiting developmental delay and immunodeficiency. *Molecular Cell,* Vol. 8, No.6, (December 2001), pp. 1175-1185.

Ooi, S.L.; Shoemaker, D.D. & Boeke, J.D. (2001) A DNA microarray-based genetic screen for nonhomologous end-joining mutants in *Saccharomyces cerevisiae*. *Science*, Vol. 294, pp. 2552-2556.

Ouyang, H., Nussenzweig, A., Kurimasa, A., Soares, V., Li, X., Cordon-Cardo, C., Li, W., Cheong, N., Nussenzweig, M., Iliakis, G., Chen, D. & Li, G. (1997). Ku70 is required for DNA repair but not for T cell antigen receptor gene recombination In vivo. *Journal of Experimental Medicine*, Vol. 186, pp. 921-929.

Perrault, R., Wang, H., Wang, M., Rosidi, B. & Iliakis, G. (2004) Backup pathways of NHEJ are suppressed by DNA-PK. *Journal of Cellular Biochemistry*, Vol. 92, pp. 781-794.

Peterson, S., Kurimasa, A., Oshimura, M., Dynan, W., Bradbury, E. & Chen, D. (1995) Loss of the catalytic subunit of the DNA-dependent protein kinase in DNA double-strand-break-repair mutant mammalian cells. *Proceeding of National Academy of Science United States of America*, Vol. 92, pp. 3171-3174.

Poinsignon, C.; De, C.R.; Soubeyrand, S.; Moshous, D.; Fischer, A.; Hache, R.J.and de Villartay, J.P. (2004). Phosphorylation of Artemis following irradiation-induced DNA damage. *Eur. J Immunol.*, Vol. 34, pp. 3146-3155.

Porter, S.; Greenwell, P.; Ritchie, K. & Petes, T. (1996) The DNA-binding protein Hdf1p (a putative Ku homologue) is required for maintaining normal telomere length in Saccharomyces cerevisiae. *Nucleic Acids Research*, Vol. 24, pp. 582-585.

Poltoratsky,V.; Shi,X.; York, J.; Lieber, M. & Carter, T. (1995) Human DNA-activated protein kinase (DNA-PK) is homologous to phosphatidylinositol kinases. *Journal of Immunology*, Vol. 155, pp. 4529-4533.

Ramadan, K.; Maga, G.; Shevelev, I.V.; Villani, G.; Blanco, L. and Hubscher, U. (2003). Human DNA polymerase lambda possesses terminal deoxyribonucleotidyl transferase activity and can elongate RNA primers: implications for novel functions. *J Mol. Biol.*, Vol. 328, pp. 63-72.

Ramsden, D. & Gellert, M. (1998) Ku protein stimulates DNA end joining by mammalian DNA ligases: a direct role for Ku in repair of DNA double-strand breaks. *EMBO Journal*, Vol. 17, pp. 609-614.

Riballo, E., Kuhne, M., Rief, N., Doherty, A., Smith, G., Recio, M., Reis, C., Dahm, K., Fricke, A., Krempler, A., Parker, A., Jackson, S., Gennery, A., Jeggo, P. & Lobrich, M. (2004). A pathway of double-strand break rejoining dependent upon ATM, Artemis, and proteins locating to gamma-H2AX foci. *Molecular Cell*, Vol. 16, pp. 715-724.

Riballo, E.; Critchlow, S.E.; Teo, S.H.; Doherty, A.J.; Priestley, A.; Broughton, B.; Kysela, B.; Beamish, H.; Plowman N.; Arlett, C.F.; Lehmann, A.R.; Jackson, S.P. & Jeggo, P.A. (1999) Identification of a defect inDNA ligase IV in a radiosensitive leukemia patient. *Current Biology*, Vol. 9, pp. 699-702.

Roberts, S.A.; Strande, N.; Burkhalter, M.D.; Strom, C.; Havener, J.M.; Hasty, P. & Ramsden, D.A. (2008) Ku is a 5′-dRP/AP lyase that excises nucleotide damage near broken ends. *Nature*, Vol. 464, pp. 1214-1217.

Roth, D.B. and Wilson, J.H. (1986) Nonhomologous recombination in mammalian cells: role for short sequence homologies in the joining reaction. *Mol. Cell Biol.*, Vol. 6, pp. 4295-4304.

Rulten, S., Fisher, A., Robert, I., Zuma, M., Rouleau, M., Ju, L., Poirier, G., Reina-San-Martin, B. & Caldecott, K. (2011) PARP-3 and APLF function together to accelerate nonhomologous end-joining. *Molecular Cell,* Vol. 41, pp. 33-45.

Ruscetti, T.; Lehnert, B.E.; Halbrook, J.; Le, T.H.; Hoekstra, M.F.; Chen, D.J.and Peterson, S.R. (1998). Stimulation of the DNA-dependent protein kinase by poly(ADP-ribose) polymerase. *J Biol. Chem.,* Vol. 273, pp. 14461-14467.

Savitsky, K.; Bar-Shira, A.; Gilad, S.; Rotman, G.; Ziv, Y.; Vanagaite, L.; Tagle, D.A.; Smith, S.; Uziel, T.; Sfez, S.; Ashkenazi, M.; Pecker, I.; Frydman, M.; Harnik, R.; Patanjali, S.R.; Simmons, A.; Clines, G.A.; Sartiel, A.; Jaspers, N.G.J.; Taylor, A.M.R.; Arlett, C.F.; Miki, T.; Weissmn, S.M.; Lovett, M.; Collins, F.S. & Shiloh,Y. (1995) A single ataxia telangiectasia gene with a product similar to PI-3 kinase. *Science,* Vol. 268, pp. 1749-1753.

Sekiguchi, J., Ferguson, D., Chen, H., Yang, E., Earle, J., Frank, K., Whitlow, S., Gu, Y., Xu, Y., Nussenzweig, A. & Alt, F.W. (2001) Genetic interactions between ATM and the nonhomologous end-joining factors in genomic stability and development. *Proceeding of National Academy of Science United States of America,* Vol. 98, 3243-3248.

Sharpless, N.E.; Ferguson, D.O.; O'Hagan, R.C.; Castrillon, D.H.; Lee, C.; Farazi, P.A.; Alson, S.; Fleming, J.; Morton, C.C.; Frank, K.; Chin, L.; Alt, F.W and DePinho, R.A. (2001) Impaired nonhomologous end-joining provokes soft tissue sarcomas harboring chromosomal translocations, amplifications, and deletions. *Mol. Cell,* Vol. 8, pp. 1187-1196.

Shin, E., Perryman, L. & Meek, K. (1997). A kinase negative mutation of DNAPKcs in equine SCID results in defective coding and signal joint formation. *Journal of Immunology,* Vol. 158, pp. 565-3589.

Sibanda, B., Critchlow, S., Begun, J., Pei, X., Jackson, S., Blundell, T. & Pellegrini, L. (2001) Crystal structure of an Xrcc4-DNA ligase IV complex. *Nature Structural Bioloty,* Vol. 8, pp. 1015-1019.

Smider, V.; Rathmell, W.K.; Lieber,M.R. & Chu,G. (1994) Restoration of X-ray resistance and V(D)J recombination in mutant cells by Ku cDNA. *Science,* Vol. 266, pp.288-291.

Soutoglou, E. & Misteli, T. (2008) Activation of the cellular DNA damage response in the absence of DNA lesions. *Science,* Vol. 320, pp. 1507-1510.

Svetlova, M.; Solovjeva, L. & Tomilin, N. (2010) Mechanism of elimination of phosphorylated histone H2AX from chromatin after repair of DNA double-strand breaks. *Mutation Research,* Vol. 685, 54-60.

Taccioli, G.E.; Rathbun, G.; Oltz, E.; Stamato, T.; Jeggo, P.A. and Alt, F.W. (1993). Impairment of V(D)J recombination in double-strand break repair mutants. *Science,* Vol. 260, pp. 207-210.

Taccioli, G.E.; Gottlieb, T.M.; Blunt, T.; Priestley, A.; Demengeot, J.; Mizuta, R.; Lehmann, A.R.; Alt, F.W.; Jackson, S.P. & Jeggo, P.A. (1994) Ku80: product of the *XRCC5* gene and its role in DNA repair and V(D)J recombination. *Science,* Vol. 265, pp. 1442-1445.

Teo, S. & Jackson, S. (1997). Identification of Saccharomyces cerevisiae DNA ligase IV: involvement in DNA double-strand break repair. *EMBO Journal,* Vol. 16, pp. 4788-4795.

Teo, S. & Jackson, S. (2000). Lif1p targets the DNA ligase Lig4p to sites of DNA double-strand breaks. *Current Biology,* Vol. 10, pp. 165-168.

Tsai,C., Kim, S. & Chu, G. (2007). Cernunnos/XLF promotes the ligation of mismatched and noncohesive DNA ends. *Proceeding of National Academy of Science United States of America*, Vol. 104, pp. 7851-7856.

Tuteja, N.; Tuteja, R.; Ochem, A.; Taneja, P.; Huang, N.W.; Simoncsits, A.; Susic, S.; Rahman, K.; Marusic, L.; Chen, J.; Zhang, J.; Wang, S; Pongor, S. & Falaschi, A. (1994) Human DNA helicase II: a novel DNA unwinding enzyme identified as the Ku autoantigen. EMBO Journal, Vol .13, pp.4991-5001.

Valencia, M.; Bentele, M.; Vaze, M.B.; Herrmann, G.; Kraus, E.; Lee, S.E.; Schar, P. & Haber, J.E. (2001) NEJ1 controls non-homologous end joining in *Saccharomyces cerevisiae*. *Nature*, Vol. 414, pp. 666-669.

van der Burg, M.; IJspeert, H.; Verkaik, N.S.; Turul, T.; Wiegant, W.W.; Morotomi-Yano, K.; Mari, P.-O.; Tezcan, I.; Chen, D.J.; Zdzienicka, M.Z.; van Dongen, J.J.M.; van Gent, D.C. (2009) A DNA-PK mutation in a radiosensitive T-B- SCID patients inhibits Artemis activation and nonhomologous end-joining. *Journal of Clinical Investigations*, Vol. 119, pp.91-98.

Vishwanatha, J. & Baril, E. (1990). Single-stranded-DNA-dependent ATPase from HeLa cells that stimulates DNA polymerase alpha-primase activity: purification and characterization of the ATPase. *Biochemistry*, Vol. 29, pp. 8753-8759.

Walker, A.I.; Hunt, T.; Jackson, R.J. & Anderson, C.W. (1985) Double-stranded DNA induces the phosphorylation of several proteins including the 90 000 mol. wt. heat-shock protein in animal cell extracts. *EMBO Journal*, Vol. 4., pp. 139-145.

Walker, J.R.; Corpina, R.A. & Goldberg, J. (2001) Structure of the Ku heterodimer bound to DNA and its implication for double-strand break repair. *Nature*, Vol. 412, pp. 607-614.

Wang, H., Zeng, Z., Perrault, A., Cheng, X., Qin, W. & Iliakis, G. (2001). Genetic evidence for the involvement of DNA ligase IV in the DNA-PK-dependent pathway of non-homologous end joining in mammalian cells. *Nucleic Acids Research*, Vol. 29, pp. 1653-1660.

Wang, H., Perrault, R., Takeda, Y., Qin, W., Wang, H. & Iliakis,G. (2003). Biochemical evidence for Ku-independent backup pathways of NHEJ. *Nucleic Acids Research*, Vol. 31, pp. 5377-5388.

Wang, Y., Nnakwe, C., Lane, W., Modesti, M. & Frank, K. (2004). Phosphorylation and regulation of DNA ligase IV stability by DNA-dependent protein kinase. *Journal of Biological Chemistry*, Vol. 279, pp. 37282-37290.

Wang, H., Rosidi, B., Perrault, R., Wang, M., Zhang, L., Windhofer, F. & Iliakis, G. (2005). DNA ligase III as a candidate component of backup pathways of nonhomologous end joining. *Cancer Research*, Vol. 65, pp. 4020-4030.

Weinfeld, M., Chaudhry, M, D'Amours, D., Pelletier, J., Poirier, G., Povirk, L. & Lees-Miller, S. (1997) Interaction of DNA-dependent protein kinase and poly(ADP-ribose) polymerase with radiation-induced DNA strand breaks. *Radiation Research*, Vol. 148, pp. 22-28.

Weller, G.R.; Kysela, B.; Roy, R.; Tonkin, L.M.; Scanlan, E.; Della, M.; Devine, S.K.; Day, J.P.; Wilkinson, A.; d'Adda di Fagagna, F.; Devine, K.M.; Bowarter, R.P.; Jeggo, P.A.; Jackson, S.P. & Doherty, A.J. (2002) Identification of a DNA nonhomologous end-joining complex in bacteria. *Science*, Vol. 297, pp. 1686-1689.

Whitehouse, C.J.; Taylor, R.M.; Thistlethwaite, A.; Zhang, H.; Karimi-Busheri, F.; Lasko, D.D.; Weinfeld, M.and Caldecott, K.W.(2001) XRCC1 stimulates human polynucleotide kinase activity at damaged DNA termini and accelerates DNA single-strand break repair. *Cell,* Vol. 104, pp. 107-117.

Wiler, R.; Leber, R.; Moore, B.B.; VanDyk, L.F.; Perryman, L.E. & Meek, K. (1995) Equine severe combined immunodeficiency: a defect in V(D)J recombination and DNA-dependent protein kinase activity. *Proceeding of National Academy of Science United States of America,* Vol. 92, pp. 11485-11489.

Wilson, T.; Grawunder, U. & Lieber, M. (1997) Yeast DNA ligase IV mediates non-homologous DNA end joining. *Nature,* Vol. 388, pp. 495-498.

Wu, K., Wang, C., Yang, Y., Peng, C., Lin, W., Tsai, F., Lin, D. & Bau D. (2010). Significant association of XRCC4 single nucleotide polymorphisms with childhood leukemia in Taiwan. *Anticancer Research,* Vol. 30, pp. 529-533.

Wu, P., Frit, P., Malivert, L., Revy, P., Biard, D., Salles, B. & Calsou, P. (2007) Interplay between Cernunnos-XLF and nonhomologous end-joining proteins at DNA ends in the cell. *Journal of Biological Chemistry,* Vol. 282, pp. 31937-31943.

Wu, P., Frit, P., Meesala, S., Dauvillier, S., Modesti, M., Andres, S., Huang, Y., Sekiguchi, J. Calsou, P., Salles, B. & Junop, M. (2009) Structural and functional interaction between the human DNA repair proteins DNA ligase IV and XRCC4. *Molecular and Cellular Biology,* Vol. 29, pp. 3163-3172.

Yajima, H.; Lee, K.J. & Chen, B.P. (2006) ATR-dependent phosphorylation of DNA-dependent protein kinase catalytic subunit in response to UV-induced replication stress. *Molecular & Cellular Biology,* Vol. 26, pp. 7520-7528.

Yaneva, M., Wen, J., Ayala, A. & Cook, R. (1989). cDNA-derived amino acid sequence of the 86-kDa subunit of the Ku antigen. *Journal of Biological Chemistry,* Vol. 264, pp. 13407-13411.

Yano, K., Morotomi-Yano, K., Wang, S., Uematsu, N., Lee, K., Asaithamby, A., Weterings, E. & Chen, D. (2008). Ku recruits XLF to DNA double-strand breaks. *EMBO Reports,* Vol. 9, pp. 91-96.

Yano, K.; Morotomi-Yano, K.; Lee, K.J. & Chen, D.J. (2011) Functional significance of the interaction with Ku in DNA double-strand recognition of XLF. FEBS Letters, Vol. 585, pp. 841-846.

Yu, Y., Wang, W., Ding, Q., Ye R., Chen, D., Merkle, D., Schriemer, D., Meek, K. & Lees-Miller, S.P. (2003) DNA-PK phosphorylation sites in XRCC4 are not required for survival after radiation or for V(D)J recombination. *DNA Repair,* Vol. 2, pp. 1239-1252.

Yurchenko, V., Xue, Z., & Sadofsky, M. (2006) SUMO modification of human XRCC4 regulates its localization and function in DNA double-strand break repair. *Molecular & Cellular Biology,* Vol. 26, pp. 1786-1794.

Zhang, W.W. and Yaneva, M. (1992). On the mechanisms of Ku protein binding to DNA. *Biochem. Biophys. Res. Commun.,* Vol. 186, pp. 574-579.

Zhang, X., Succi, J., Feng, Z., Prithivirajsingh, S., Story, M. & R.J.Legerski. (2004) Artemis is a phosphorylation target of ATM and ATR and is involved in the G2/M DNA damage checkpoint response. *Molecular & Cellular Biology,* Vol. 24, pp. 9207-9220.

Zhu, C.; Bogue, M.A.; Lim, D.-S.; Hasty, P. & Roth, D.B. (1996) Ku86-deficient mice exhibit severe combined immunodeficiency and defective processing of V(D)J recombination intermediates. *Cell*, Vol. 86, pp. 379-389.

Part 4

Polymorphism of DNA Repair Genes

25

DNA Repair Capacity-Related to Genetic Polymorphisms of DNA Repair Genes and Aflatoxin B1-Related Hepatocellular Carcinoma Among Chinese Population

Xi-Dai Long[1,2] et al.*
[1]Department of Pathology, Youjiang Medical College for Nationalities
[2]Department of Pathology, Shanghai Jiao Tong University School of Medicine
China

1. Introduction

Primary liver cancer (PLC) is the sixth most commonly occurring cancer and the third most common cause of cancer deaths in the world (1). This tumor has two main pathological types: hepatocellular carcinoma (HCC) and cholangiocellular carcinoma. HCC, the most common pathological form of PLC, occurs more often in specific regions which include eastern and southeastern Asia, Melanesia, and sub-Saharan Africa (1, 2). Once diagnosed, survival rates for HCC are poor: 75% of patients die within 1 year, and 5-year survival rate is only 3 - 5% (3, 4). Therefore, insight into the tumorigenesis mechanisms of HCC will broaden and deepen implications in understanding and preventing occurrence of the cancer.

It has been known that chronic infection with hepatitis virus [including hepatitis virus B (HBV) and hepatitis virus C (HCV)] is the most common cause of HCC worldwide (3). In sub-Saharan Africa and Southern China, chronic exposure of aflatoxin B1 (AFB1) may present a special environmental hazard, especially in individuals chronically infected with HBV (1, 2, 5-8). However, increasing epidemiological evidence has exhibited that although many people are exposed to these risk factors, only a relatively small proportion of chronic infectors or exposure person develop HCC (3, 9, 10). This indicates an individual susceptibility related to genetic factors such as DNA repair capacity might be associated with HCC carcinogenesis (3, 11). In recent years, evidence has been accumulated to support the hypothesis that common genetic polymorphisms in genes involved in long process of

---

* Jin-Guang Yao[3], Zhi Zeng[2], Cen-Han Huang[3], Pinhu Liao[3], Zan-Song Huang[3], Yong-Zhi Huang[1], Fu-Zhi Ban[4], Xiao-Yin Huang[1], Li-Min Yao[5], Lu-Dan Fan[6], and Guo-Hui Fu[2]
[3]*Department of Medicine, Youjiang Medical College for Nationalities, China.*
[4]*Department of Medicine, the Southwestern Affiliated Hospital of Youjiang Medical College for Nationalities, China.*
[5]*Department of Imaging Medicine (Grade 2008), Youjiang Medical College for Nationalities, China.*
[6]*Department of Clinic Medicine (Grade 2009), Youjiang Medical College for Nationalities, China.*

carcinogenesis may be of importance in determining individual susceptibility to HCC (3, 9, 12). Therefore, the existence of low penetrate genetic polymorphisms may explain the reason why only a small portion of individuals, even in high-risk areas, develop HCC in their life span. This study reviews recent efforts in identifying genetic variants which may have impact on risk of HCC.

2. Epidemiology of AFB1-related HCC in China

In China, HCC is the third or fourth most common malignant tumors and accounts for about 55% of the world's HCC cases, more than 340,000 each year (1, 13). This tumor occurs more often in eastern and southeastern China, including Jiangsu, Shanghai, Zhejiang, Fujiang, Guangdong, and Guangxi, mainly because of high AFB1 exposure and/or chronic infection of HBV and HCV (13). In the high AFB1-exposure areas such as Guangxi Zhuang Autonomous Region, this tumor is the most common occuring cancer (13, 14). Moreover, the incidence rate gradually increases with age increasing in above-mentioned AFB1-exposure areas (15). Males are always more frequently affected than females but high male to female ratios of > 3 in the high AFB1-exposure areas (15). Although the incidence rates of this tumor in low AFB1-exposure areas in China have markedly decreased (because of the control of hepatitis virus infection), they have changed little in high AFB1-exposure areas (13, 15). For example, during May 2007 to April 2008, incidence rates were 117.8/100,000 and 103.1/100,000 for Xiangzhou and Fusui (two main high AFB1-exposure areas of China), respectively (13, 16). This was similar to the results before ten years (17).

Because of the very poor prognosis, HCC is the second most common cause of death from cancer in China (18). In the past thirty years, total mortality rate of HCC gradually increased from 12.5/100,000 to 26.26/100,000 (Fig 1A), regardless of countryside areas or urban areas (Fig 1B). This trend was more noticeable in male population than female population (Fig 1C), possibly because male individuals featured more high AFB1 exposure. Supporting aforementioned hypothesis, a recent study from high AFB1-exposure areas has demonstrated these having longer exposure years or higher exposure levels of AFB1 would face lower 5-years survival rate (4).

3. AFB1 exposure and DNA damage and repair

AFB1 is an important mycotoxin produced by the moulds Aspergillus parasiticus and Aspergillus flavus (19). This toxic agent has been found as contaminants of human and animal food, particularly ground nuts (peanuts) and core, in tropical areas such as the Southeastern China as a result of fungal contamination during growth and after harvest which under hot and humid conditions (8, 14, 19, 20). Epidemiological evidence has shown dietary ingestion of high levels of AFB1 presents a significant environmental hazard of HCC (16, 17, 21). Experimental animal models have also shown that AFB1 can induce HCC; whereas DNA damage should play an important role during hepatocellular carcinogenesis (19, 22, 23). Therefore, AFB1 has been classified as a category I known human carcinogen by the International Agency for Research on Cancer (24).

AFB1 is metabolized by cytochrome P450 enzymes to its reactive form, AFB1-8,9-epoxide (AFB1-epoxide), which covalently binds to DNA and induces DNA damage (19, 25-28). DNA damage induced by AFB1 includes AFB1-DNA adducts, oxidative DNA damage,

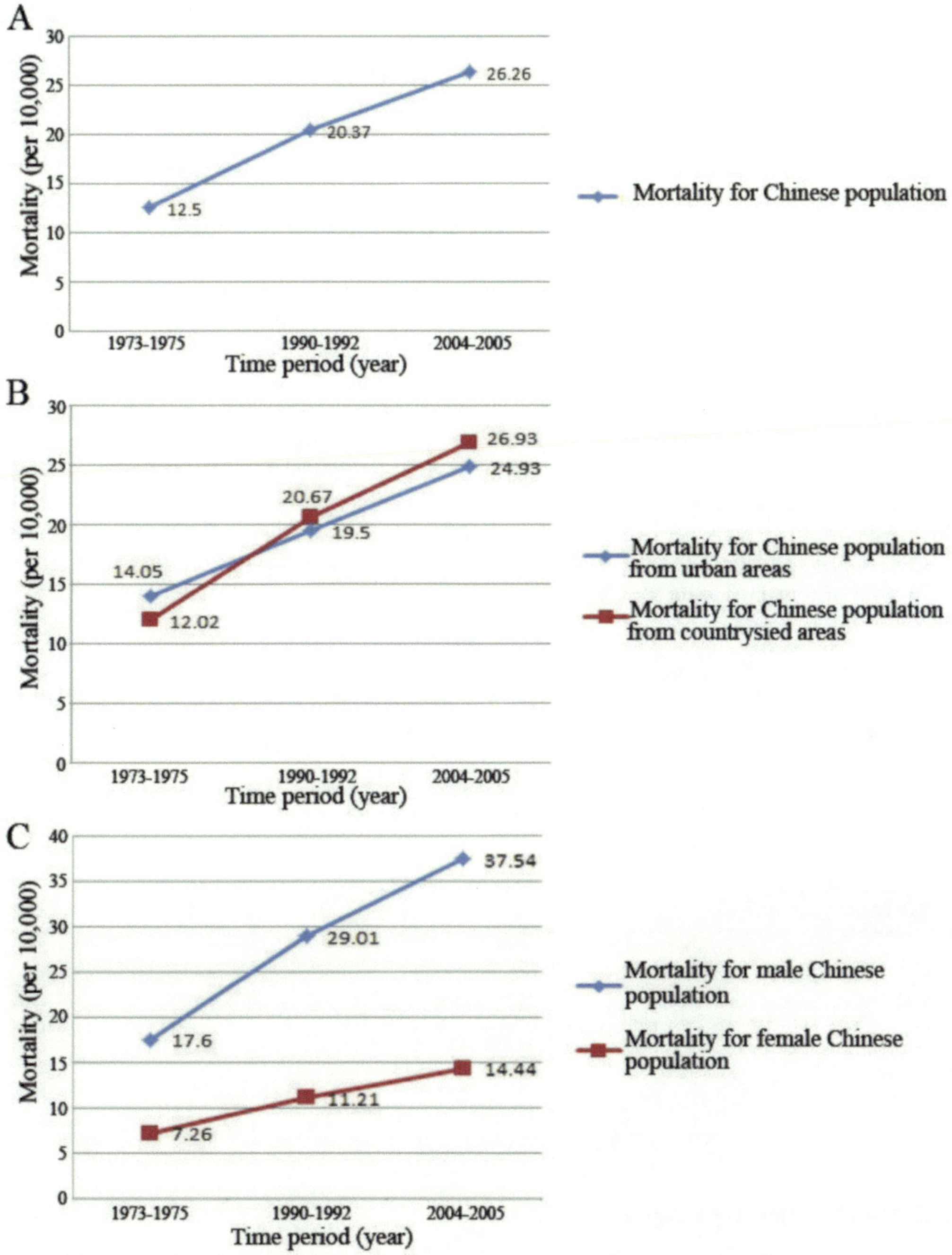

Fig. 1. The mortality rates of HCC in China during 1973 and 2005. Total mortality rates (A), regardless of in urban areas or countryside areas (B), were significantly increasing from during 1973 and 1975 to during 1990 and 1992 or to during 2004 and 2005. This increasing mortality rates were more remarkable among male population (C).

and gene mutation (Fig. 2). Among these AFB1-DNA adducts, 8,9-di-hydro-8-(N^7-guanyl)-9-hydroxy–AFB1 (AFB1-N^7-Gua) adduct is the most common type identified and confirmed in vivo researches (19, 25-27, 29, 30). The formation of this adduct proceeds by a precovalent intercalation complex between double-stranded DNA and the highly electrophilic, unstable AFB1-epoxide isomer (31, 32). After that, the induction of a positive charge on the imidazole portion of the formed AFB1-N^7-Gua adduct gives rise to another important a DNA adduct, a ring-opened formamidopyridine AFB1 (AFB1-FAPy) adduct (33, 34). Accumulation of AFB1-FAPy adduct is characterized by time-dependence, non-enzyme, and may be of biological basis of genes mutation because of its apparent persistence in DNA (19, 33, 34). Furthermore, above adducts are capable of forming subsequent repair-resistant adducts, depurination, or lead to error-prone DNA repair resulting in single-strand breaks (SSBs), double-strand breaks (DSBs), base pair substitution, or frame shift mutations (35, 36). Additionally, AFB1 exposure also induces the formation of such oxidation DNA damage as 8-oxodeoxyguanosine (8-$_{oxod}$G), a common endogenous DNA adduct (36-38). Although these DNA adducts are mainly produced in liver cells, they are also found in the peripheral blood white cells (39, 40). Recent studies have shown that the levels of AFB1-DNA adduct of the peripheral blood white cells are positively and lineally correlated with that of liver cells, implying analysis of AFB1-DNA adducts in the peripheral blood white cells may substitute for the elucidation of tissular levels of adducts (39, 41).

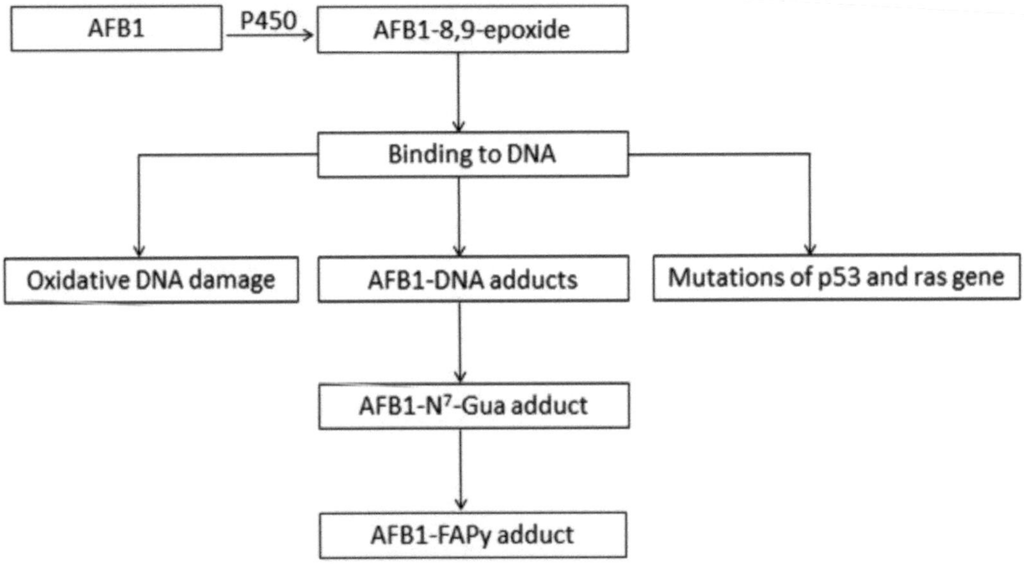

Fig. 2. The DNA damage induced by AFB1.

For genes mutations induced by AFB1 exposure, the experimental and theoretical researches are briefly on the p53 gene (42-49). Reaction with DNA at the N^7 position of guanine preferentially causes a G:C > T:A mutation in codon 249 of this gene, leading to an amino acid substitution of arginine to serine (44-50). In high AFB1-exposure areas, this mutation is present in more than 40% of HCC and can be detected in serum DNA of patients with preneoplastic lesions and HCC (41). While codon 249 transversion mutations are either very rare or absent in low or no AFB1-exposure areas (49, 51, 52). Using the human p53 gene in an in vitro assay, codon 249 has been exhibited to be a preferential site for formation of AFB1-N^7-Gua adducts, evidence consistent with a role for AFB1 in the mutations observed in HCC (50, 53). Therefore, the codon 249 mutation of p53 gene has been defined as the hot-spot mutation of p53 gene resulting from AFB1 and has become the molecular symbol of HCC induced by AFB1 exposure (54-56).

A wide diversity of DNA damage produced by AFB1 exposure, if not repaired, may cause chromosomal aberrations, micronuclei, sister chromatid exchange, unscheduled DNA synthesis, and chromosomal strand breaks, and can be converted into gene mutations and genomic instability, which in turn results in cellular malignant transformation (19). Nevertheless, human cells have evolved surveillance mechanisms that monitor the integrity of genome to minimize the consequences of detrimental mutations (54). AFB1-induced DNA damage can be repaired through the following pathways: nucleotide excision repair (NER), base excision repair (BER), single-strand break repair (SSBR), and double-strand break repair (DSBR) (12, 28, 57). During the process of damage removed by aforementioned repair pathways, DNA repair genes play a central role, because their function determines DNA repair capacity (12). It has been shown that reduction in DNA repair capacity related to DNA repair genes is associated with increased risk of cancers (4, 39-41, 58-62). Thus, genetic polymorphisms in DNA repair genes which contribute to the variation in DNA repair capacity may be correlated with risk of developing cancers, including AFB1-related HCC.

4. Genetic polymorphisms in genes involved in NER pathway and risk of HCC

NER pathway, a major DNA repair pathways in human cells featuring genomic DNA damage, can remove structurally such diverse lesions as pyrimidine dimers, irradiative damage, and bulky chemical adducts, and DNA damage from carcinogens and some chemotherapeutic drugs (63, 64). To date, the mechanism of this pathway is well understood and has been reconstituted in vitro. It consists of several sequential steps: lesion sensing, opening of a denaturation bubble, incision of the damaged strand, displacement of the lesion-containing oligonucleotide, gap filling, and ligation (63, 64). In the fibroblast cells with the deficiency of xeroderma pigmentosum A (XPA) gene, conversion of the initial AFB1-N^7-Gua adduct to the AFB1-FAPy adduct has been found to be more extensive (53). This suggests that NER should be a major mechanism for enzymatic repair of AFB1 adducts (12). It's defects lead to severe diseases related AFB1 exposure, including liver injury and HCC. Accumulating evidence has implied that genetic polymorphisms in NER genes are associated with DNA repair capacity and modulate the risk of cancers (65-69). Molecular epidemiology studies of AFB1-related HCC in China have investigated the associations with several genes involved in NER pathway such as xeroderma pigmentosum C (XPC) and xeroderma pigmentosum D (XPD)(4, 39, 70, 71).

XPC. XPC gene spans 33kb on chromosome 3p25 and contains 16 exons and 15 introns (Genbank accession no. AC090645). This gene encodes a 940-amino acid protein, an important DNA damage recognition molecule which plays an important role in NER pathway (72). It binds tightly with HR23B to form a stable XPC-HR23B complex, the first protein component that recognizes and binds to the DNA damage sites. XPC-HR23B complex can recognize a variety of DNA adducts formed by exogenous carcinogens such as AFB1 and binds to the DNA damage sites (72). Thus, it may play a role in the pathogenesis of HCC-related AFB1. Some recent studies have showed that defects in XPC have been related to many types of malignant tumors (73-82). Transgenic mice studies also revealed predisposition to many types of tumors in XPC gene knockout mice (83). Furthermore, pathological and cellular researches have exhibited that the abnormal expression of this gene is related to hepatocarcinogenesis (84). These studies suggests the polymorphisms localizing at conserved sites of XPC gene might modify the risk of HCC induced by AFB1 exposure. Recently, four studies from high AFB1-exposure areas of China have approved aforementioned hypothesis (4, 70, 71, 85).

The first study conducted by Cai *et al.*(85) is from Shunde area, Guangdong Province. In this 1-1 case-control study (including 78 HCC cases and 78 age- and sex-matching controls), researchers analyzed between two common polymorphisms—Ala499Val and Lys939Gln—of XPC gene and risk of HCC and found these two polymorphisms modified HCC risk [adjusted odds ratios (ORs) were 3.77 with 95% confidence interval (CI)1.34-12.89 for Ala499Lys and 6.78 with 95% CI 2.03-22.69], especially under HBV and HCV infection condition. Although they evaluated the effects of XPC-hepatitis viruses interaction on HCC risk, they did not elucidate the possible interaction of AFB1 exposure.

The other three studies are from Guangxi Zhuang Autonomous Region (4, 70). Li *et al.*(71), Wu *et al.* (70), and Long *et al.* (4) investigated the modifying effects of genetic polymorphisms XPC on HCC based hospitals. The results showed XPC codon 939 Gln alleles increased about 2-times risk of HCC. Furthermore, Wu, *et al.*(70), and Long, *et al.* (4) quantitatively elucidated AFB1 exposure years and levels and their interactive effects with XPC Lys939Gln polymorphism. They found some evidence of AFB1 exposure-risk genotypes of XPC codon 939 on HCC risk (22.33 > 1.88 × 8.69 for the interaction of AFB1-exposure years and XPC risk genotypes and 18.38 > 1.11 × 4.62 for the interaction of AFB1-exposure levels and XPC risk genotypes). Additionally, Gln alleles at codon 939 of XPC gene are observed to be correlated with the decrease of XPC expression levels in cancerous tissues (r = - 0.369, $P < 0.001$) and with the overall survival of HCC patients (the median survival times are 30, 25, and 19 months for patients with XPC gene codon 939 Lys/Lys, Lys/Gln, and Gln/Gln respectively). This decreasing 5-years survival rates would be noticeable under high AFB1 exposure conditions (the median survival times are 15 months for the joint of XPC gene codon 939 Gln/Gln and long-term AFB1-exposure years and 17 month for the joint of XPC gene codon 939 Gln/Gln and high AFB1-exposure level) (4).

These results demonstrate that polymorphism at codon 939 of XPC gene is not only a genetic determinant in the development of HCC induced by AFB1 exposure in Chinese population, but also is an independent prognostic factor influencing the survival of HCC, like AFB1 exposure. However, Li *et al.* (71) reported that the proportional distribution of the Val/Val genotype at codon 499 of XPC gene did not differ between cases with HCC and controls in Guangxi Zhuang Autonomous Region, China ($P > 0.05$), dissimilar to the data from another area of China, Guangdong Province (85). Possible explanations for these inconsistent finding may be either due to unknown confounders or due to small sample size.

XPD. XPD gene-encoding protein, a DNA-dependent ATPase/helicase, is associated with the TFIIH transcription-factor complex and plays a role in NER pathway (86, 87). During NER, XPD participates in the opening of the DNA helix to allow the excision of the DNA fragment containing the damaged base. There are two described polymorphisms that induce amino acid changes in the protein: at codons 312 (Asp to Asn) and 751 (Lys to Gln) (87-89). To date, these two polymorphisms have been extensively studied (87, 88, 90-95).

Several groups have done genotype-phenotype analyses with these two polymorphisms and have shown that the variant allele genotypes are associated with low DNA repair ability (96, 97). Recent studies have showed the polymorphisms at codon 312 and 751 of XPD are correlated with DNA-adducts levels, p53 gene mutation, and cancers risk (88, 94, 98-100).

In a hospital-based case-control study in Guangxi (39), we found that the variant XPD codon 751 genotypes (namely Lys/Gln and Gln/Gln) detected by TaqMan-MGB PCR was significantly different between controls (26.3% and 8.6% for Lys/Gln and Gln/Gln, respectively) and HCC cases (35.9% and 20.1% for Lys/Gln and Gln/Gln, respectively, $P <$ 0.001). Individuals with variant alleles had about 1.5- to 2.5-fold risk of developing the cancer (adjusted OR 1.75 and 95% CI 1.30-2.37 for Lys/Gln; adjusted OR 2.47 and 95% CI 1.62-3.76 for Gln/Gln). Based on relative sample size (including 618 HCC cases and 712 controls), we stratified genotypes of XPD codon 751 according to matching factors and observed some evidence of interaction between XPD codon 751 Gln alleles and sex. These female having Gln alleles, compared to those without these alleles, featured increased HCC risk. Furthermore, the interactive effects of between variant genotypes of XPD gene codon 751 environment variant AFB1 or another NER gene XPC on HCC risk were also found, with interactive value 0.85, 1.04, and 1.71 for AFB1-exposure years, AFB1-exposure levels, and XPC gene codon 939 risk genotypes ($P_{interaction} < 0.05$). Therefore, the XPD gene codon 751 polymorphism may have potential effect on AFB1-related HCC susceptibility among Chinese population. However, the study from AFB1-exposure areas don't exhibit polymorphism at codon 312 of XPD gene significantly associates with the risk of HCC induced by AFB1.

5. Genetic polymorphisms in genes involved in SSBR pathway and risk of HCC

SSB is a common type of DNA damage produced by AFB1 exposure (36). If not repaired, it can disrupt transcription and replication and can be converted into potentially clastogenic and/or lethal DSBs. This DNA damage is repaired via SSBR pathway (101, 102). SSBR pathway includes four basic steps: *a.* SSB detection and signaling, through poly (ADP-ribose) polymerase (PARP); *b.* DNA break end processing, through the role of polynucleotide kinase (PNK), AP endonuclease-1 (APE1), DNA polymerase β (Pol β), tyrosyl phosphodiesterase 1 (TDP1), and flap endonuclease-1 (FEN-1); *c.* gap filling, involving in multiple DNA polymerases; *d.* DNA ligation, involving in multiple DNA ligases. Of the later three steps of SSBR pathway, x-ray repair cross complementary 1 (XRCC1) is indispensible, because it not only acts as the scaffolding protein of SSBR, but also stimulates the activity of PNK (103).

XRCC1 gene encoding protein (633 amino acids), consists of three functional domains — N-terminal domain (NTD), central breast cancer susceptibility protein-1 homology C-terminal (BRCT I), and C-terminal breast cancer susceptibility protein-1 homology C-terminal (BRCT II) (103-106). This protein is directly associated with Pol β, DNA ligase III, and PARP, via their three functional domains and is implicated in the core processes in SSBR and BER pathway (103). Mutant hamster ovary cell lines that lack XRCC1 genes are hypersensitive to DNA damage agents such as ionizing radiation, hydrogen peroxide, and alkylating agents (103). Furthermore, this kind of cells usually face increasing frequency of spontaneous chromosome aberrations and deletions. Three single nucleotide polymorphisms in the coding region of XRCC1 gene that lead to amino acid substitution have been described and investigated (12). Of these polymorphisms, the codon 399 polymorphism is of special concern, because this polymorphism resides in functionally significant regions (BECT II) and may be related to decreasing DNA repair capacity, increasing genes mutation, and running-up risk of cancers (12, 107-114).

In AFB1-exposure areas from China, a total of six molecular epidemiological studies were found in PubMed database, Wangfang Database, and Weipu database (61, 62, 115-118). However, associations between XRCC1 gene codon 399 polymorphism and individual susceptibility to HCC have been reported in these case-control studies with the results being contradictory. We analyzed the possible causes of contradictory using meta-analysis method (Comprehensive Meta Analysis Version 2, http://www.meta-analysis.com/). Fig. 3 showed the meta-analysis results of the modifying effects of XRCC1 gene codon 399 polymorphism on HCC risk. We found these subjects with Gln alleles had increasing risk of HCC (total crude adjusted OR = 1.34, $P < 0.01$), moreover, there were larger relative weight to assign to those studies with OR-value more than 1. Actually, although Yang *et al.* (116) and Ren *et al.* (118) did not observed significantly risk of XRCC1 gene codon 399 polymorphism in crude logistic regression, they found Gln alleles would increase HCC risk in stratified analysis with susceptive environment variants. A individually matching case-controls demonstrated that subjects having Gln alleles might feature remarkably increasing risk of HCC under longer-term AFB1-exposure years or higher AFB1-exposure levels conditions (adjusted OR > 10) (61). This suggests that the genotypes with codon 399 Gln alleles of XRCC1 should be a risk biomarker of Chinese HCC related to AFB1 exposure.

6. Genetic polymorphisms in genes involved in BER pathway and risk of HCC

Of the oxidative DNA damage resulting from AFB1 exposure, the formation of 8-$_{oxod}$G is thought to be important due to being abundant and highly mutagenic and hepatocarcinogenesis (21, 36-38). The 8-$_{oxod}$G lesions are repaired primarily through the BER pathway (119). The BER pathway facilitates DNA repair through two general pathways: *a.* the short-patch BER pathway, leading to a repair tract of a single nucleotide; *b.* the long-patch BER pathway, producing a repair tract of at least two nucleotides (120). In these two repair sub-pathways, DNA glycosylases play a central role because they can recognize and catalyze the removal of damaged bases (120). This suggests that the defect of DNA glycosylases should be related to the decreasing capacity of the BER pathway and might increase the risk of such cancers as HCC.

Human oxoguanine glycosylase 1(hOGG1) is a specific DNA glycosylase that catalyzes the release of 8-$_{oxod}$G and the cleavage of DNA at the AP site (121, 122). Genetic structure study has revealed the presence of several polymorphisms within hOGG1 locus (123). Among them, the polymorphism at position 1245 in exon 7 causes an amino acid substitution (Ser to Cys) at codon 326, suggesting this polymorphism may glycosylase function (123). A functional complementation activity assay showed that hOGG1 protein encoded by the 326 Cys allele had substantially lower DNA repair activity than that encoded by the 326 Ser allele (124). Similar results were observed in human cells in vivo (122, 125). Therefore, low capacity of 8-$_{oxod}$G repair resulting from hOGG1 326Cys polymorphism might contribute to

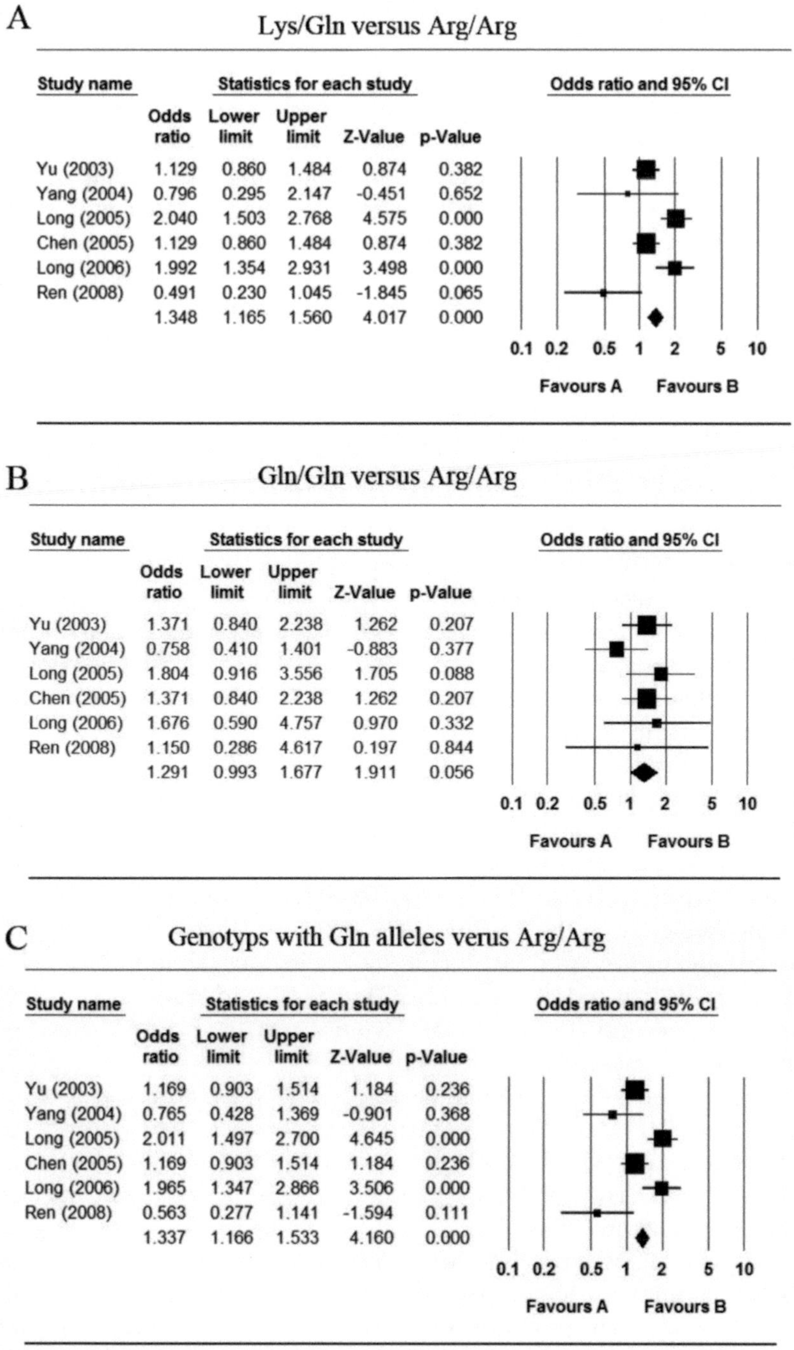

Fig. 3. The meta-analysis of the relationship between XRCC1 codon Lys399Gln polymorphism and HCC risk among China population. Compared with Arg/Arg genotype, Arg/Gln (A) and Gln/Gln (B) genotypes increased HCC risk. This risk effect was also observed in the binding of Arg/Gln and Gln/Gln genotypes (C).

the persistence of 8-$_{oxod}$G in genomic DNA in vivo, which, in turn, could be associated with increased cancer risk (125, 126).

In 2003, Peng *et al.* (126) investigated the correlation among 8-$_{oxod}$G levels, hOGG1 expression, and hOGG1 Cys326Ser polymorphism in Guangxi Autonomous Region. They found that individuals with genotypes with hOGG1 codon 326 Cys alleles faced lower level of hOGG1 expression and higher 8-$_{oxod}$G levels. Supporting their results, Cheng *et al.* (21) reported that hOGG1 expression was significantly linear correlated with HCC. Recently, using the molecular epidemiological methods, Zhang *et al.*(127) found that the distribution of Cys alleles at codon 326 of hOGG1 in HCC cases (43.0%) significantly differed from in controls (33.1%). Logistic regression analysis showed that the genotypes with Cys alleles, compared to without this alleles, increased HCC risk of Chinese population, with adjusted OR-value (95% CI) 1.5 (0.79-2.93) for Cys/Ser and 1.9 (0.83-4.55) for Cys/Cys. These findings suggested pathogenic role of hOGG1 Cys326Ser polymorphism in the hepatocarcinogenesis.

7. Genetic polymorphisms in genes involved in DSBR pathway and risk of HCC

DSBs, although only make up a very small proportion of AFB1-induced DNA damage, are critical lesions that can result in cell death or a wide variety of genetic alterations including large- or small-scale deletions, loss of heterozygosity, translocations, and chromosome loss (19, 128, 129). This type damage is repaired DSBR consisting of non-homologous end-joining (NHEJ) and homologous recombination (HR) (130-133). There are several decades DNA repair genes involves in DSBR pathway and the defects in these genes cause genome instability and promote tumorigenesis (128, 134, 135). In published molecular epidemiological studies, only XRCC3 gene codon Thr241Met polymorphism effects the risk of AFB1-related HCC risk among Chinese population (58, 60).

The product of the XRCC3 gene is one of identified paralogs of the strand-exchange protein RAD51 in human beings (136). This protein correlates directly with DNA breaks and facilitates of the formation of the RAD51 nucleoprotein filament, which is crucial both for homologous recombination and HRR (136-138). Previous studies have shown that a common polymorphism at codon 241 of XRCC3 gene (Thr to Met) modifies the function of this gene ad increases cancers risk (139-143). Two reports from high AFB1-exposure areas of China supported above-mentioned conclusions (58, 60).

In the first frequent case-control study in Guangxiese (58), we observed that the genotypes with XRCC3 codon 241 Met alleles (namely Thr/Met and Met/Met) was significantly different between controls (33.01%) and HCC cases (61.48%, $P < 0.001$). Met alleles increases about 2- to 10-fold risk of HCC and this running-up risk is modulated by the number of Met alleles (adjusted OR 2.48 and 10.06 for one and two this alleles). Considering small sample size in this study, we recruited, in another independent frequent case-control study (60), a relatively larger sample size to compare the results. Subjects included in this study, 491 HCC cases and 862 age-, sex, race, hepatitis virus infection information-matching controls, were permanent residents of Guangxi areas. Similar to the results of the first report, the distribution of XRCC3 codon 241 Met allele frequency was found to be significantly different between cases (59.7%) and controls (32.1%). Individuals having the Thr/Met or Met/Met were at a 2.22-fold or 7.19 fold increased risk of developing HCC cancer. Above two studies showed this allele multiplicatively interacted with AFB1 exposure in the process of hepato-tumorigenesis. These results exhibits that the polymorphism at codon 241 of XRCC3 gene is a genetic determinant in the development of HCC induced by AFB1 exposure among Chinese population.

8. Summary

Like most other human malignant tumors, HCC is a complex disease attributed to environment variation and genetic susceptive factors. In high incidence areas of HCC in China, AFB1 is an important environment variation as well as chronic HBV and HCV infection. This toxic variation is characterized by: *a.* the attraction of specific organs, especially liver; *b.* genotoxicity, mainly inducing the formation of AFB1-DNA adducts and the hot-spot mutation of p53 gene; and *c.* carcinogenicity, primarily causing HCC. In the process of AFB1 hepatocarcinogenesis, AFB1-DNA adducts play a central role because of their genotoxicity and interactions with genetic susceptive factors. Numerous studies reviewed in this paper have demonstrated that the hereditary variations in DNA repair genes are associated with susceptibility to AFB1-related HCC among Chinese population. These molecular epidemiological studies have significantly contributed to our knowledge of the importance of genetic polymorphisms in DNA repair genes in the etiology of HCC related to AFB1 exposure. It would be expected that genetic susceptibility factors involved in DNA repair genes for HCC could serve as useful biomarkers for identifying at-risk individuals and, therefore, targeting prevention of this malignant tumor.

However, there are several issues to be noted. Firstly, the conclusions should be drawn carefully, because of conflicting data existing in the same ethnic population in view of between some genotypes of DNA repair genes and the risk of HCC. Secondly, caution should be taken particularly in extrapolating these data to other ethnic populations, because of the difference of population frequencies corresponding to genetic polymorphisms that depends on ethnicity. Thirdly, when risk of a specific polymorphism is considered, AFB1 exposure should be stressed because AFB1 exposure may differ from areas to areas and from individuals to individuals. Lastly, because of the fact that AFB1-related hepatocarcinogenesis is polygenic, no single genetic marker may sufficiently predict HCC risk. Therefore, a panel of susceptive biomarkers is warranted to define individuals at high-risk for this cancer.

9. Acknowledgments

We are grateful to Yuan-Feng Zhou for the collection and management of data. This study is supported by the Youth Science Foundation of Guangxi (NO. 0832097), the Science Foundation of Youjiang Medical College for Nationalities (NO. 2005 and 2008), and Guangxi Key Construction Project of Laboratory Room (NO. 2009).

10. Abbreviations

AFB1, Aflatoxin B1; AFB1-epoxide, AFB1-8,9-epoxide; AFB1-N^7-Gua, 8,9-di-hydro-8-(N^7-guanyl)-9-hydroxy–AFB1; AFB1-FAPy, ring-opened formamidopyridine AFB1; APE1, AP endonuclease-1; BER, base excision repair; CI, confidence interval; DSB, double-strand break; DSBR, double-strand break repair; HBV, hepatitis virus B; HCV, hepatitis virus C; HCC, hepatocellular carcinoma; hOGG1, Human oxoguanine glycosylase 1; NER, nucleotide excision repair; OR, odds ratio; 8-$_{oxod}$G, 8-oxodeoxyguanosine; PARP, poly (ADP-ribose) polymerase; PLC, Primary liver cancer; PNK, polynucleotide kinase; Pol β, DNA polymerase β; SSB, single-strand break; SSBR, single-strand break repair; XPA, xeroderma pigmentosum A; XPC, xeroderma pigmentosum C; XPD, xeroderma pigmentosum D; XRCC1, x-ray repair cross complementary 1; XRCC3, x-ray repair cross complementary 3; XRCC4, x-ray repair cross complementary 4.

11. References

[1] Parkin DM, Bray F, Ferlay J, Pisani P. Global cancer statistics, 2002. CA Cancer J Clin. 2005;55:74-108.

[2] Henry SH, Bosch FX, Troxell TC, Bolger PM. Reducing Liver Cancer--Global Control of Aflatoxin. Science. 1999;286:2453-4.

[3] Dominguez-Malagon H, Gaytan-Graham S. Hepatocellular carcinoma: an update. Ultrastruct Pathol. 2001;25:497-516.

[4] Long XD, Ma Y, Zhou YF, Ma AM, Fu GH. Polymorphism in xeroderma pigmentosum complementation group C codon 939 and aflatoxin B1-related hepatocellular carcinoma in the Guangxi population. Hepatology. 2010;52:1301-9.

[5] de Oliveira CA, Germano PM. [Aflatoxins: current concepts on mechanisms of toxicity and their involvement in the etiology of hepatocellular carcinoma]. Rev Saude Publica. 1997;31:417-24.

[6] Makarananda K, Pengpan U, Srisakulthong M, Yoovathaworn K, Sriwatanakul K. Monitoring of aflatoxin exposure by biomarkers. J Toxicol Sci. 1998;23 Suppl 2:155-9.

[7] Sell S. Mouse models to study the interaction of risk factors for human liver cancer. Cancer research. 2003;63:7553-62.

[8] Wang JS, Huang T, Su J, Liang F, Wei Z, Liang Y, et al. Hepatocellular carcinoma and aflatoxin exposure in Zhuqing Village, Fusui County, People's Republic of China. Cancer Epidemiol Biomarkers Prev. 2001;10:143-6.

[9] Clifford RJ, Zhang J, Meerzaman DM, Lyu MS, Hu Y, Cultraro CM, et al. Genetic variations at loci involved in the immune response are risk factors for hepatocellular carcinoma. Hepatology. 2010;52:2034-43.

[10] Pang RW, Joh JW, Johnson PJ, Monden M, Pawlik TM, Poon RT. Biology of hepatocellular carcinoma. Annals of surgical oncology. 2008;15:962-71.

[11] Wilson DM, 3rd, Thompson LH. Life without DNA repair. Proceedings of the National Academy of Sciences of the United States of America. 1997;94:12754-7.

[12] Long XD, Tang YH, Qu DY, Ma Y. The toxicity and role of aflatoxin B1 and DNA repair (corresponding DNA repair enzymes) Youjiang Medical College for Nationalities Xue Bao. 2006;28:278-80.

[13] J.G. C, sONG XM. An evaluation on incidence cases of liver cancer in China. Zhongguo Zhongliu. 2005;14:28-31.

[14] Wang YW, Lan LZ, Ye BF, Xu YC, Liu YY, Li WG. The association among geographic distribution, climate, and aflatoxin B1 exposure in China. Zhonggou Kexue. 1983;B:431-7.

[15] Zhang WS, Chen WQ, Kong LZ, Li GL, Zhao P. An Annual Repor t: Cancer Incidence in 35 Cancer Registr ies in China, 2003. Zhongguo Zhongliu. 2007;16:497-507.

[16] Ma AM, Luo YX, Wan JL, Long XD, Huang YZ. An investigative analysis of incidence, prevention, and treatment of hepatocellular carcinoma in Xiangzhou, Baise, Guangxi Autonomous Region, China. Youjiang Minzu Yixueyuan Bao. 2010;32:165-6.

[17] Youjiang Medical College for Nationalities and Public Health Bureau of Tiandong. General investigation of hepatocellular carcinoma in Tiandong, China. 1994—2008 China Academic Journal electronic Publishing Househttp://wwwenkinet.

[18] the Ministry of Health of People's Republic of China. Annals of health statistics in China in 2010. ttp://www.moh.gov.cn/publicfiles/business/htmlfiles/zwgkzt/ptjnj/year2010/index2010.html.

[19] Wang JS, Groopman JD. DNA damage by mycotoxins. Mutation research. 1999;424:167-81.

[20] Yeh FS, Mo CC, Yen RC. Risk factors for hepatocellular carcinoma in Guangxi, People's Republic of China. National Cancer Institute monograph. 1985;69:47-8.

[21] Cheng B, Jungst C, Lin J, Caselmann WH. [Potential role of human DNA-repair enzymes hMTH1, hOGG1 and hMYHalpha in the hepatocarcinogenesis]. Journal of Huazhong University of Science and Technology Medical sciences. 2002;22:206-11, 15.

[22] Scholl PF, McCoy L, Kensler TW, Groopman JD. Quantitative analysis and chronic dosimetry of the aflatoxin B1 plasma albumin adduct Lys-AFB1 in rats by isotope dilution mass spectrometry. Chem Res Toxicol. 2006;19:44-9.

[23] Sudhakar P, Latha P, Sreenivasulu Y, Reddy BV, Hemalatha TM, Balakrishna M, et al. Inhibition of Aspergillus flavus colonization and aflatoxin (AfB1) in peanut by methyleugenol. Indian J Exp Biol. 2009;47:63-7.

[24] International Agency for Research on Cancer, Some naturally occurring substances: food items and constituents, heterocyclic aromatic amines and mycotoxins, IARC Monogr. Eval Carcinog Risks Hum 1993;56:245-540.

[25] Ben Rejeb I, Arduini F, Arvinte A, Amine A, Gargouri M, Micheli L, et al. Development of a bio-electrochemical assay for AFB1 detection in olive oil. Biosens Bioelectron. 2009;24:1962-8.

[26] Giri I, Stone MP. Wobble dC.dA pairing 5' to the cationic guanine N7 8,9-dihydro-8-(N7-guanyl)-9-hydroxyaflatoxin B1 adduct: implications for nontargeted AFB1 mutagenesis. Biochemistry. 2003;42:7023-34.

[27] Habib SL, Said B, Awad AT, Mostafa MH, Shank RC. Novel adenine adducts, N7-guanine-AFB1 adducts, and p53 mutations in patients with schistosomiasis and aflatoxin exposure. Cancer Detect Prev. 2006;30:491-8.

[28] Guengerich FP, Johnson WW, Shimada T, Ueng YF, Yamazaki H, Langouet S. Activation and detoxication of aflatoxin B1. Mutation research. 1998;402:121-8.

[29] Essigmann JM, Croy RG, Nadzan AM, Busby WF, Jr., Reinhold VN, Buchi G, et al. Structural identification of the major DNA adduct formed by aflatoxin B1 in vitro. Proceedings of the National Academy of Sciences of the United States of America. 1977;74:1870-4.

[30] Croy RG, Essigmann JM, Reinhold VN, Wogan GN. Identification of the principal aflatoxin B1-DNA adduct formed in vivo in rat liver. Proceedings of the National Academy of Sciences of the United States of America. 1978;75:1745-9.

[31] Gopalakrishnan S, Harris TM, Stone MP. Intercalation of aflatoxin B1 in two oligodeoxynucleotide adducts: comparative 1H NMR analysis of d(ATCAFBGAT).d(ATCGAT) and d(ATAFBGCAT)2. Biochemistry. 1990;29:10438-48.

[32] Johnson WW, Guengerich FP. Reaction of aflatoxin B1 exo-8,9-epoxide with DNA: kinetic analysis of covalent binding and DNA-induced hydrolysis. Proceedings of the National Academy of Sciences of the United States of America. 1997;94:6121-5.

[33] Croy RG, Wogan GN. Temporal patterns of covalent DNA adducts in rat liver after single and multiple doses of aflatoxin B1. Cancer research. 1981;41:197-203.

[34] Groopman JD, Croy RG, Wogan GN. In vitro reactions of aflatoxin B1-adducted DNA. Proceedings of the National Academy of Sciences of the United States of America. 1981;78:5445-9.

[35] Chen JD, Liu CJ, Lee PH, Chen PJ, Lai MY, Kao JH, et al. Hepatitis B genotypes correlate with tumor recurrence after curative resection of hepatocellular carcinoma. Clin Gastroenterol Hepatol. 2004;2:64-71.

[36] Gradelet S, Le Bon AM, Berges R, Suschetet M, Astorg P. Dietary carotenoids inhibit aflatoxin B1-induced liver preneoplastic foci and DNA damage in the rat: role of the modulation of aflatoxin B1 metabolism. Carcinogenesis. 1998;19:403-11.

[37] Farombi EO, Adepoju BF, Ola-Davies OE, Emerole GO. Chemoprevention of aflatoxin B1-induced genotoxicity and hepatic oxidative damage in rats by kolaviron, a natural bioflavonoid of Garcinia kola seeds. European journal of cancer prevention : the official journal of the European Cancer Prevention Organisation. 2005;14:207-14.

[38] Liu J, Yang CF, Lee BL, Shen HM, Ang SG, Ong CN. Effect of Salvia miltiorrhiza on aflatoxin B1-induced oxidative stress in cultured rat hepatocytes. Free radical research. 1999;31:559-68.

[39] Long XD, Ma Y, Zhou YF, Yao JG, Ban FZ, Huang YZ, et al. XPD Codon 312 and 751 Polymorphisms, and AFB1 Exposure, and Hepatocellular Carcinoma Risk. BMC cancer. 2009;9:400.

[40] Long XD, Ma Y, Deng ZL. GSTM1 and XRCC3 polymorphisms: Effects on levels of aflatoxin B1-DNA adducts. Chinese J Cancer Res. 2009;21:177-84.

[41] Long XD, Ma Y, Huang HD, Yao JG, Qu de Y, Lu YL. Polymorphism of XRCC1 and the frequency of mutation in codon 249 of the p53 gene in hepatocellular carcinoma among Guangxi population, China. Mol Carcinog. 2008;47:295-300.

[42] Wild CP, Montesano R. A model of interaction: aflatoxins and hepatitis viruses in liver cancer aetiology and prevention. Cancer letters. 2009;286:22-8.

[43] Shen HM, Ong CN. Mutations of the p53 tumor suppressor gene and ras oncogenes in aflatoxin hepatocarcinogenesis. Mutation research. 1996;366:23-44.

[44] Golli-Bennour EE, Kouidhi B, Bouslimi A, Abid-Essefi S, Hassen W, Bacha H. Cytotoxicity and genotoxicity induced by aflatoxin B1, ochratoxin A, and their combination in cultured Vero cells. J Biochem Mol Toxicol. 2010;24:42-50.

[45] Paget V, Sichel F, Garon D, Lechevrel M. Aflatoxin B1-induced TP53 mutational pattern in normal human cells using the FASAY (Functional Analysis of Separated Alleles in Yeast). Mutation research. 2008;656:55-61.

[46] Van Vleet TR, Watterson TL, Klein PJ, Coulombe RA, Jr. Aflatoxin B1 alters the expression of p53 in cytochrome P450-expressing human lung cells. Toxicol Sci. 2006;89:399-407.

[47] Vahakangas K. TP53 mutations in workers exposed to occupational carcinogens. Hum Mutat. 2003;21:240-51.

[48] Staib F, Hussain SP, Hofseth LJ, Wang XW, Harris CC. TP53 and liver carcinogenesis. Hum Mutat. 2003;21:201-16.

[49] Chan KT, Hsieh DP, Lung ML. In vitro aflatoxin B1-induced p53 mutations. Cancer letters. 2003;199:1-7.

[50] Bressac B, Kew M, Wands J, Ozturk M. Selective G to T mutations of p53 gene in hepatocellular carcinoma from southern Africa. Nature. 1991;350:429-31.

[51] Li D, Cao Y, He L, Wang NJ, Gu JR. Aberrations of p53 gene in human hepatocellular carcinoma from China. Carcinogenesis. 1993;14:169-73.

[52] Kirk GD, Camus-Randon AM, Mendy M, Goedert JJ, Merle P, Trepo C, et al. Ser-249 p53 mutations in plasma DNA of patients with hepatocellular carcinoma from The Gambia. Journal of the National Cancer Institute. 2000;92:148-53.

[53] Loechler, E.L. Mechanisms by which aflatoxins and other bulky carcinogens induce mutations, in: D.L. Eaton, J.D. Groopman (Eds.), The Toxicology of Aflatoxins: Human Health, Veterinary, and Agricultural Significance, Academic Press, San Diego, 1994, pp. 149–178.

[54] Aguilar F, Hussain SP, Cerutti P. Aflatoxin B1 induces the transversion of G-->T in codon 249 of the p53 tumor suppressor gene in human hepatocytes. Proceedings of the National Academy of Sciences of the United States of America. 1993;90:8586-90.

[55] Denissenko MF, Koudriakova TB, Smith L, O'Connor TR, Riggs AD, Pfeifer GP. The p53 codon 249 mutational hotspot in hepatocellular carcinoma is not related to selective formation or persistence of aflatoxin B1 adducts. Oncogene. 1998;17:3007-14.

[56] Duflot A, Hollstein M, Mehrotra R, Trepo C, Montesano R, Cova L. Absence of p53 mutation at codon 249 in duck hepatocellular carcinomas from the high incidence area of Qidong (China). Carcinogenesis. 1994;15:1353-7.

[57] Waters R, Jones CJ, Martin EA, Yang AL, Jones NJ. The repair of large DNA adducts in mammalian cells. Mutation research. 1992;273:145-55.

[58] Long XD, Ma Y, Deng ZL, Huang YZ, Wei NB. [Association of the Thr241Met polymorphism of DNA repair gene XRCC3 with genetic susceptibility to AFB1-related hepatocellular carcinoma in Guangxi population]. Zhonghua yi xue yi chuan xue za zhi = Zhonghua yixue yichuanxue zazhi = Chinese journal of medical genetics. 2008;25:268-71.

[59] Long XD, Ma Y, Huang YZ, Yi Y, Liang QX, Ma AM, et al. Genetic polymorphisms in DNA repair genes XPC, XPD, and XRCC4, and susceptibility to Helicobacter pylori infection-related gastric antrum adenocarcinoma in Guangxi population, China. Mol Carcinog. 2010;49:611-8.

[60] Long XD, Ma Y, Qu de Y, Liu YG, Huang ZQ, Huang YZ, et al. The polymorphism of XRCC3 codon 241 and AFB1-related hepatocellular carcinoma in Guangxi population, China. Ann Epidemiol. 2008;18:572-8.

[61] Long XD, Ma Y, Wei YP, Deng ZL. The polymorphisms of GSTM1, GSTT1, HYL1*2, and XRCC1, and aflatoxin B1-related hepatocellular carcinoma in Guangxi population, China. Hepatol Res. 2006;36:48-55.

[62] Long XD, Ma Y, Wei YP, Deng ZL. X-ray repair cross-complementing group 1 (XRCC1) Arg 399 Gln polymorphism and aflatoxin B1 (AFB1)-related hepatocellular carcinoma (HCC) in Guangxi population. Chinese J Cancer Res. 2005;17:17-21.

[63] Nouspikel T. DNA repair in mammalian cells : Nucleotide excision repair: variations on versatility. Cellular and molecular life sciences : CMLS. 2009;66:994-1009.

[64] Rechkunova NI, Lavrik OI. Nucleotide excision repair in higher eukaryotes: mechanism of primary damage recognition in global genome repair. Sub-cellular biochemistry. 2010;50:251-77.

[65] Rajaraman P, Hutchinson A, Wichner S, Black PM, Fine HA, Loeffler JS, et al. DNA repair gene polymorphisms and risk of adult meningioma, glioma, and acoustic neuroma. Neuro Oncol. 2010;12:37-48.

[66] Matakidou A, Eisen T, Fleischmann C, Bridle H, Houlston RS. Evaluation of xeroderma pigmentosum XPA, XPC, XPD, XPF, XPB, XPG and DDB2 genes in familial early-onset lung cancer predisposition. International journal of cancer. 2006;119:964-7.

[67] Wang M, Yuan L, Wu D, Zhang Z, Yin C, Fu G, et al. A novel XPF -357A>C polymorphism predicts risk and recurrence of bladder cancer. Oncogene. 2010;29:1920-8.

[68] Dogru-Abbasoglu S, Inceoglu M, Parildar-Karpuzoglu H, Hanagasi HA, Karadag B, Gurvit H, et al. Polymorphisms in the DNA repair genes XPD (ERCC2) and XPF (ERCC4) are not associated with sporadic late-onset Alzheimer's disease. Neurosci Lett. 2006;404:258-61.

[69] Romanowicz-Makowska H, Smolarz B, Kulig A. [Polymorphisms in XRCC1 and ERCC4/XPF DNA repair genes and associations with breast cancer risk in women]. Pol Merkur Lekarski. 2007;22:200-3.

[70] X.M. W, Ma Y, Deng ZL, Long XD. The polymorphism at codon 939 of xeroderma pigmentosum C gene and hepatocellular carcinoma among Guangxi population. Zhonghua Xiaohua Zazhi. 2010;30:846-8.

[71] Li LM, Zeng XY, Ji L, Fan XJ, Li YQ, Hu XH, et al. [Association of XPC and XPG polymorphisms with the risk of hepatocellular carcinoma]. Zhonghua gan zang bing za zhi = Zhonghua ganzangbing zazhi = Chinese journal of hepatology. 2010;18:271-5.

[72] Sugasawa K. XPC: its product and biological roles. Advances in experimental medicine and biology. 2008;637:47-56.

[73] Strom SS, Estey E, Outschoorn UM, Garcia-Manero G. Acute myeloid leukemia outcome: role of nucleotide excision repair polymorphisms in intermediate risk patients. Leuk Lymphoma. 2010;51:598-605.

[74] Sakano S, Matsumoto H, Yamamoto Y, Kawai Y, Eguchi S, Ohmi C, et al. Association between DNA repair gene polymorphisms and p53 alterations in Japanese patients with muscle-invasive bladder cancer. Pathobiology. 2006;73:295-303.

[75] Qiu L, Wang Z, Shi X, Wang Z. Associations between XPC polymorphisms and risk of cancers: A meta-analysis. Eur J Cancer. 2008;44:2241-53.

[76] Zhou RM, Li Y, Wang N, Zhang XJ, Dong XJ, Guo W. [Correlation of XPC Ala499Val and Lys939Gln polymorphisms to risks of esophageal squamous cell carcinoma and gastric cardiac adenocarcinoma]. Ai zheng = Aizheng = Chinese journal of cancer. 2006;25:1113-9.

[77] Zhang D, Chen C, Fu X, Gu S, Mao Y, Xie Y, et al. A meta-analysis of DNA repair gene XPC polymorphisms and cancer risk. Journal of human genetics. 2008;53:18-33.

[78] Shore RE, Zeleniuch-Jacquotte A, Currie D, Mohrenweiser H, Afanasyeva Y, Koenig KL, et al. Polymorphisms in XPC and ERCC2 genes, smoking and breast cancer risk. International journal of cancer. 2008;122:2101-5.

[79] Hansen RD, Sorensen M, Tjonneland A, Overvad K, Wallin H, Raaschou-Nielsen O, et al. XPA A23G, XPC Lys939Gln, XPD Lys751Gln and XPD Asp312Asn polymorphisms, interactions with smoking, alcohol and dietary factors, and risk of colorectal cancer. Mutation research. 2007;619:68-80.

[80] Liang J, Gu A, Xia Y, Wu B, Lu N, Wang W, et al. XPC gene polymorphisms and risk of idiopathic azoospermia or oligozoospermia in a Chinese population. International journal of andrology. 2009;32:235-41.

[81] Gangwar R, Mandhani A, Mittal RD. XPC gene variants: a risk factor for recurrence of urothelial bladder carcinoma in patients on BCG immunotherapy. Journal of cancer research and clinical oncology. 2010;136:779-86.

[82] Francisco G, Menezes PR, Eluf-Neto J, Chammas R. XPC polymorphisms play a role in tissue-specific carcinogenesis: a meta-analysis. Eur J Hum Genet. 2008;16:724-34.

[83] Cheo DL, Burns DK, Meira LB, Houle JF, Friedberg EC. Mutational inactivation of the xeroderma pigmentosum group C gene confers predisposition to 2-acetylaminofluorene-induced liver and lung cancer and to spontaneous testicular cancer in Trp53-/- mice. Cancer research. 1999;59:771-5.

[84] Fautrel A, Andrieux L, Musso O, Boudjema K, Guillouzo A, Langouet S. Overexpression of the two nucleotide excision repair genes ERCC1 and XPC in human hepatocellular carcinoma. J Hepatol. 2005;43:288-93.

[85] Cai XL, Gao YH, Yu ZW, Wu ZQ, Zhou WP, Yang Y, et al. [A 1:1 matched case-control study on the interaction between HBV, HCV infection and DNA repair gene XPC Ala499Val, Lys939Gln for primary hepatocellular carcinoma]. Zhonghua liu xing bing xue za zhi = Zhonghua liuxingbingxue zazhi. 2009;30:942-5.

[86] Aloyz R, Xu ZY, Bello V, Bergeron J, Han FY, Yan Y, et al. Regulation of cisplatin resistance and homologous recombinational repair by the TFIIH subunit XPD. Cancer research. 2002;62:5457-62.

[87] Manuguerra M, Saletta F, Karagas MR, Berwick M, Veglia F, Vineis P, et al. XRCC3 and XPD/ERCC2 single nucleotide polymorphisms and the risk of cancer: a HuGE review. American journal of epidemiology. 2006;164:297-302.

[88] Benhamou S, Sarasin A. ERCC2/XPD gene polymorphisms and cancer risk. Mutagenesis. 2002;17:463-9.

[89] Shen MR, Jones IM, Mohrenweiser H. Nonconservative amino acid substitution variants exist at polymorphic frequency in DNA repair genes in healthy humans. Cancer research. 1998;58:604-8.

[90] Sturgis EM, Dahlstrom KR, Spitz MR, Wei Q. DNA repair gene ERCC1 and ERCC2/XPD polymorphisms and risk of squamous cell carcinoma of the head and neck. Arch Otolaryngol Head Neck Surg. 2002;128:1084-8.

[91] Chen S, Tang D, Xue K, Xu L, Ma G, Hsu Y, et al. DNA repair gene XRCC1 and XPD polymorphisms and risk of lung cancer in a Chinese population. Carcinogenesis. 2002;23:1321-5.

[92] Park JY, Lee SY, Jeon HS, Park SH, Bae NC, Lee EB, et al. Lys751Gln polymorphism in the DNA repair gene XPD and risk of primary lung cancer. Lung cancer (Amsterdam, Netherlands). 2002;36:15-6.

[93] Xing D, Qi J, Miao X, Lu W, Tan W, Lin D. Polymorphisms of DNA repair genes XRCC1 and XPD and their associations with risk of esophageal squamous cell carcinoma in a Chinese population. International journal of cancer. 2002;100:600-5.

[94] Stern MC, Johnson LR, Bell DA, Taylor JA. XPD codon 751 polymorphism, metabolism genes, smoking, and bladder cancer risk. Cancer Epidemiol Biomarkers Prev. 2002;11:1004-11.
[95] Sturgis EM, Castillo EJ, Li L, Eicher SA, Strom SS, Spitz MR, et al. XPD/ERCC2 EXON 8 Polymorphisms: rarity and lack of significance in risk of squamous cell carcinoma of the head and neck. Oral Oncol. 2002;38:475-7.
[96] Spitz MR, Wu X, Wang Y, Wang LE, Shete S, Amos CI, et al. Modulation of nucleotide excision repair capacity by XPD polymorphisms in lung cancer patients. Cancer research. 2001;61:1354-7.
[97] Rzeszowska-Wolny J, Polanska J, Pietrowska M, Palyvoda O, Jaworska J, Butkiewicz D, et al. Influence of polymorphisms in DNA repair genes XPD, XRCC1 and MGMT on DNA damage induced by gamma radiation and its repair in lymphocytes in vitro. Radiation research. 2005;164:132-40.
[98] Tang D, Cho S, Rundle A, Chen S, Phillips D, Zhou J, et al. Polymorphisms in the DNA repair enzyme XPD are associated with increased levels of PAH-DNA adducts in a case-control study of breast cancer. Breast cancer research and treatment. 2002;75:159-66.
[99] Terry MB, Gammon MD, Zhang FF, Eng SM, Sagiv SK, Paykin AB, et al. Polymorphism in the DNA repair gene XPD, polycyclic aromatic hydrocarbon-DNA adducts, cigarette smoking, and breast cancer risk. Cancer epidemiology, biomarkers & prevention : a publication of the American Association for Cancer Research, cosponsored by the American Society of Preventive Oncology. 2004;13:2053-8.
[100] Mechanic LE, Marrogi AJ, Welsh JA, Bowman ED, Khan MA, Enewold L, et al. Polymorphisms in XPD and TP53 and mutation in human lung cancer. Carcinogenesis. 2005;26:597-604.
[101] Caldecott KW. Mammalian single-strand break repair: mechanisms and links with chromatin. DNA repair. 2007;6:443-53.
[102] Fortini P, Dogliotti E. Base damage and single-strand break repair: mechanisms and functional significance of short- and long-patch repair subpathways. DNA repair. 2007;6:398-409.
[103] Thompson LH, West MG. XRCC1 keeps DNA from getting stranded. Mutation research. 2000;459:1-18.
[104] Yamane K, Katayama E, Tsuruo T. The BRCT regions of tumor suppressor BRCA1 and of XRCC1 show DNA end binding activity with a multimerizing feature. Biochem Biophys Res Commun. 2000;279:678-84.
[105] Bhattacharyya N, Banerjee S. A novel role of XRCC1 in the functions of a DNA polymerase beta variant. Biochemistry. 2001;40:9005-13.
[106] Dulic A, Bates PA, Zhang X, Martin SR, Freemont PS, Lindahl T, et al. BRCT domain interactions in the heterodimeric DNA repair protein XRCC1-DNA ligase III. Biochemistry. 2001;40:5906-13.
[107] Divine KK, Gilliland FD, Crowell RE, Stidley CA, Bocklage TJ, Cook DL, et al. The XRCC1 399 glutamine allele is a risk factor for adenocarcinoma of the lung. Mutation research. 2001;461:273-8.
[108] Lee JM, Lee YC, Yang SY, Yang PW, Luh SP, Lee CJ, et al. Genetic polymorphisms of XRCC1 and risk of the esophageal cancer. International journal of cancer. 2001;95:240-6.

[109] Ratnasinghe D, Yao SX, Tangrea JA, Qiao YL, Andersen MR, Barrett MJ, et al. Polymorphisms of the DNA repair gene XRCC1 and lung cancer risk. Cancer Epidemiol Biomarkers Prev. 2001;10:119-23.

[110] Kim SU, Park SK, Yoo KY, Yoon KS, Choi JY, Seo JS, et al. XRCC1 genetic polymorphism and breast cancer risk. Pharmacogenetics. 2002;12:335-8.

[111] Schneider J, Classen V, Helmig S. XRCC1 polymorphism and lung cancer risk. Expert Rev Mol Diagn. 2008;8:761-80.

[112] Kiran M, Saxena R, Chawla YK, Kaur J. Polymorphism of DNA repair gene XRCC1 and hepatitis-related hepatocellular carcinoma risk in Indian population. Mol Cell Biochem. 2009;327:7-13.

[113] Li Y, Long C, Lin G, Marion MJ, Freyer G, Santella RM, et al. Effect of the XRCC1 codon 399 polymorphism on the repair of vinyl chloride metabolite-induced DNA damage. J Carcinog. 2009;8:14.

[114] Saadat M, Ansari-Lari M. Polymorphism of XRCC1 (at codon 399) and susceptibility to breast cancer, a meta-analysis of the literatures. Breast cancer research and treatment. 2009;115:137-44.

[115] Yu MW, Yang SY, Pan IJ, Lin CL, Liu CJ, Liaw YF, et al. Polymorphisms in XRCC1 and glutathione S-transferase genes and hepatitis B-related hepatocellular carcinoma. Journal of the National Cancer Institute. 2003;95:1485-8.

[116] Yang JL, Han YN, Zheng SG. Influence of human XRCC1-399 single nucleotide polymorphism on primary hepatocytic carcinoma. Zhongliu. 2004;24:322-4.

[117] Chen CC, Yang SY, Liu CJ, Lin CL, Liaw YF, Lin SM, et al. Association of cytokine and DNA repair gene polymorphisms with hepatitis B-related hepatocellular carcinoma. International journal of epidemiology. 2005;34:1310-8.

[118] Ren y, Wang DS, Li Z, Xin YM, Yin JM, Zahgn B, et al. Study on the Relationship between Gene XRCC1 Codon 399 Single Nucleotide Polymorphisms and Primary Hepatic Carcinoma in Han Nationality. Linchuang Gandang Bing Zazhi. 2008;24:361-4.

[119] Donigan KA, Sweasy JB. Sequence context-specific mutagenesis and base excision repair. Mol Carcinogen. 2009;48:362-8.

[120] Robertson AB, Klungland A, Rognes T, Leiros I. DNA repair in mammalian cells: Base excision repair: the long and short of it. Cellular and molecular life sciences : CMLS. 2009;66:981-93.

[121] Boiteux S, Radicella JP. The human OGG1 gene: structure, functions, and its implication in the process of carcinogenesis. Archives of biochemistry and biophysics. 2000;377:1-8.

[122] Nishimura S. Involvement of mammalian OGG1(MMH) in excision of the 8-hydroxyguanine residue in DNA. Free radical biology & medicine. 2002;32:813-21.

[123] Weiss JM, Goode EL, Ladiges WC, Ulrich CM. Polymorphic variation in hOGG1 and risk of cancer: a review of the functional and epidemiologic literature. Mol Carcinogen. 2005;42:127-41.

[124] Kohno T, Shinmura K, Tosaka M, Tani M, Kim SR, Sugimura H, et al. Genetic polymorphisms and alternative splicing of the hOGG1 gene, that is involved in the repair of 8-hydroxyguanine in damaged DNA. Oncogene. 1998;16:3219-25.

[125] Sakamoto T, Higaki Y, Hara M, Ichiba M, Horita M, Mizuta T, et al. hOGG1 Ser326Cys polymorphism and risk of hepatocellular carcinoma among Japanese. Journal of epidemiology / Japan Epidemiological Association. 2006;16:233-9.

[126] Peng T, Shen HM, Liu ZM, Yan LN, Peng MH, Li LQ, et al. Oxidative DNA damage in peripheral leukocytes and its association with expression and polymorphisms of hOGG1: a study of adolescents in a high risk region for hepatocellular carcinoma in China. World J Gastroenterol. 2003;9:2186-93.
[127] Zhang H, He BC, He FC. [Impact of DNA repair gene hOGG1 Ser326Cys polymorphism on the risk of hepatocellular carcinoma]. Shijie Huaren xiaohua zazhi. 2006;14:2311-4.
[128] Mills KD, Ferguson DO, Alt FW. The role of DNA breaks in genomic instability and tumorigenesis. Immunol Rev. 2003;194:77-95.
[129] Morgan WF, Corcoran J, Hartmann A, Kaplan MI, Limoli CL, Ponnaiya B. DNA double-strand breaks, chromosomal rearrangements, and genomic instability. Mutation research. 1998;404:125-8.
[130] Kanaar R, Hoeijmakers JH, van Gent DC. Molecular mechanisms of DNA double strand break repair. Trends Cell Biol. 1998;8:483-9.
[131] Pardo B, Gomez-Gonzalez B, Aguilera A. DNA repair in mammalian cells: DNA double-strand break repair: how to fix a broken relationship. Cell Mol Life Sci. 2009;66:1039-56.
[132] Shrivastav M, De Haro LP, Nickoloff JA. Regulation of DNA double-strand break repair pathway choice. Cell Res. 2008;18:134-47.
[133] Sonoda E, Hochegger H, Saberi A, Taniguchi Y, Takeda S. Differential usage of non-homologous end-joining and homologous recombination in double strand break repair. DNA repair. 2006;5:1021-9.
[134] Cahill D, Connor B, Carney JP. Mechanisms of eukaryotic DNA double strand break repair. Front Biosci. 2006;11:1958-76.
[135] Valerie K, Povirk LF. Regulation and mechanisms of mammalian double-strand break repair. Oncogene. 2003;22:5792-812.
[136] Bishop DK, Ear U, Bhattacharyya A, Calderone C, Beckett M, Weichselbaum RR, et al. Xrcc3 is required for assembly of Rad51 complexes in vivo. J Biol Chem. 1998;273:21482-8.
[137] Brenneman MA, Wagener BM, Miller CA, Allen C, Nickoloff JA. XRCC3 controls the fidelity of homologous recombination: roles for XRCC3 in late stages of recombination. Mol Cell. 2002;10:387-95.
[138] Brenneman MA, Weiss AE, Nickoloff JA, Chen DJ. XRCC3 is required for efficient repair of chromosome breaks by homologous recombination. Mutation research. 2000;459:89-97.
[139] Sun H, Qiao Y, Zhang X, Xu L, Jia X, Sun D, et al. XRCC3 Thr241Met polymorphism with lung cancer and bladder cancer: a meta-analysis. Cancer science. 2010;101:1777-82.
[140] Jiang Z, Li C, Xu Y, Cai S. A meta-analysis on XRCC1 and XRCC3 polymorphisms and colorectal cancer risk. International journal of colorectal disease. 2010;25:169-80.
[141] Fang F, Wang J, Yao L, Yu XJ, Yu L. Relationship between XRCC3 T241M polymorphism and gastric cancer risk: a meta-analysis. Med Oncol. 2010.
[142] Economopoulos KP, Sergentanis TN. XRCC3 Thr241Met polymorphism and breast cancer risk: a meta-analysis. Breast cancer research and treatment. 2010;121:439-43.
[143] Zhou K, Liu Y, Zhang H, Liu H, Fan W, Zhong Y, et al. XRCC3 haplotypes and risk of gliomas in a Chinese population: a hospital-based case-control study. International journal of cancer. 2009;124:2948-53.

26

Low Penetrance Genetic Variations in DNA Repair Genes and Cancer Susceptibility

Ravindran Ankathil
Human Genome Center, School of Medical Sciences
University Sains Malaysia, Health Campus
Kubang Kerian, Kelantan
Malaysia

1. Introduction

The genetic material, DNA, which encodes genes needed for the production of essential proteins, is vulnerable to damage in a number of ways. Human DNA is assaulted on a daily basis by a variety of exogenous factors including UV light, cigarette smoke, dietary factors, and other carcinogens all of which can cause varying degrees of DNA damage and can lead to mutations. Similarly, endogenous factors such as undue DNA replication which can cause mismatches, hydrolysis leading to spontaneous DNA depurination, replication form collapse which can result in strand breaks, loss of bases because of spontaneous disintegration of chemical bonds, and DNA damage secondary to endogenous reactants such as alkyl groups, metal cations, and reactive oxygen species (ROS) which can induce base oxidation and DNA breaks also contribute to DNA damage (Branzei & Foiani, 2008; Capella et al., 2008)

When DNA is damaged, an intertwined network of surveillance mechanisms will act including

- Sensing and recognizing DNA damage by activation of cell cycle checkpoints, pause that permit assessment and complete of DNA processing , either DNA damage repair or processing of DNA intermediates
- Up regulation a large number of genes
- Programmed cell death or apoptosis when the cell is unable to repair the damage sustained and
- Elicitation of multiple distinct DNA repair responses

DNA damages are repaired by enzymes coded by one or more DNA repair pathways according to their structure, or their location in the cellular genome. DNA repair enzymes can be characterized as cellular proteins acting directly on damaged DNA in an attempt to restore the correct DNA sequence and structure. These relatively specialized enzymes appear to undertake the initial stages of recognition and repair of specific forms of DNA damage. Since there are various kinds of DNA damage, a variety of repair mechanisms are essential. Cells integrate DNA repair process with transcription and apoptosis through a network known as the DNA damage response (DDR) which is orchestrated by the checkpoint proteins.

2. DNA repair pathways

Damages in DNA are repaired by various DNA repair genes belonging to distinct pathways. Each pathway is recognized for efficient repair of specific types of DNA damage. To date, more than 150 human DNA repair genes have been identified, which can be categorized into at least 5 distinct pathways: Base Excision Repair (BER), Nucleotide Excision Repair (NER), Mismatch Repair (MMR), Double Strand Break Repair (DSBR), and Transcription Coupled Repair (TCR) (Wood et al., 2005). The Base Excision Repair Pathway operates on small lesions such as oxidized or reduced bases, fragmented or nonbulky adduct, and adducts produced by methylating agents. The Nucleotide Excision repair (NER) pathway repairs bulky lesions such as pyramidine dimmers, other products of phytochemical reactions, large chemical adducts and DNA crosslinks. For Double Strand Break Repair (DSBR), at least two pathways exist: homologous recombination and non homologous end joining. Replication errors such as base-base or insert-deletion mismatches caused by the DNA polymerase are repaired by Mismatch Repair (MMR) pathway genes. Finally, the suicide enzyme methyl-guanine-DNA, methyl transferase, is an additional category of DNA repair pathway that directly removes the alkylated bases.

The repair gene products operate in a co-ordinated fashion to form repair pathways that control restitution of specific types of DNA damage. Repair pathways are further co-ordinated with other metabolic processes, such as cell cycle control, to optimize the prospects of successful repair. During the cell cycle, checkpoint mechanisms ensure that a cell's DNA is intact before permitting DNA replication and cell division to occur. Failures in these checkpoints can lead to an accumulation of damage, which in turn leads to mutations.

Repair of damaged DNA is of paramount importance and is essential to prevent loss of or in correct transmission of genetic information, to prevent genetic damage from propagating and accumulating, to maintain genome integrity and stability of cells, and also to prevent mutations The failure of the cell to adequately repair the acquired damage and to undergo apoptosis may lead to further errors which can cause developmental abnormalities and neoplastic transformation of the cell and finally to carcinogenesis.

3. Genetic susceptibility to cancer - High and low penetrance DNA repair genes

Genetic susceptibility to cancer result from variations in the genetic code that alter either protein expression, function or localization. Susceptibility to cancer is determined by two types of genes – high penetrance genes and low penetrance genes. High penetrance genes are genes with allelic variants that confer a high degree of risk to the individual. Relatively few individuals in the population carry risk –increasing genotypes at these loci. The proportion of cancer in the population that may be explained by these genotypes will be low. Therefore the population attributable risk also will be low. But high penetrance genes have a large magnitude of effects on cancer risk and usually follow a mendelian autosomal domiant pattern of inheritance and involve multiple cancer sites that form a cancer syndrome. High penetrance genes with an attendant high likelihood of causing cancer, account for only a small proportion of cancer cases. In humans, high penetrance DNA repair genes that cause family or hereditary cancer syndromes can have substantial impact in affected families (eg: BRCA1 and BRCA2 genes in hereditary breast cancer, DNA Mismatch Repair (MMR) genes in Hereditary Non Polyposis Colorectal Cancer (HNPCC), p53 in

LiFraumeni Syndrome). But these genes affect only a small portion of cancer cases and a small percent age of the population.

Loss of function mutations in a significant number of DNA damage response genes predispose to a variety of familial cancers (Spry et al., 2007). There are several examples such as mutations in BRCA1 and BRCA2 belonging to homologous recombination pathways predispose to breast and ovarian cancer (Bertwistle & Ashworth, 2000). So also, mutations in other double strand break repair genes such as ATM predispose to the familial tumorigenic condition ataxia telangiectasia (Lavin & Shiloh 1996) and breast cancer (Renwick et al., 2006). Mutations in NBSI have been reported to predispose to Nijwegen breakage syndrome (Matsuura et al., 2004). Somatic mutations in another DSB repair gebe, ATR, correlate with sporadic microsatellite (MSI) positive stomach cancer (Menoyo et al., 2001). PALB2 gene, which encodes a BRCA2 indicating protein, has also been identified as a breast cancer susceptibility gene (Rahman et al., 2007). Mutations in a group of DNA mismatch repair (MMR) gene predispose to hereditary non-poplyposis colorectal cancer and other cancers in the extra colonic sites in Lynch syndrome (Jacob & Praz, 2002). Biallelic germline mutations of the base excision repair gene MUTYH have been identified in patients with autosomal recessive form of hereditary multiple colorectal adenoma and carcinoma (Jones et al., 2002). Defect in the nucleotide excision repair pathway genes predispose to xeroderma pimentosum (XP), Cockayne syndrome (CS) and Trichothiodystrophy (TTD), which are all autosomal recessive syndromes (Leibeling et al., 2006).

In contrast, in the remaining major portion of sporadic cases, genetic variations in the form of low to moderate penetrance alleles may predispose individuals to cancer in combination with environmental factors and thus affect a large segment of the population. Low penetrance genes, also referred to as modifier genes, are genes in which subtle sequence variants may be associated with a small to moderate increased relative risk for sporadic cancers.

4. Single Nucleotide Polymorohisms (SNPs) in low penetrance genes

Genetic variations seen in human genome includes insertion/deletion of one or more nucleotides (indels) the copy number variations (CNNs) that can involve DNA sequences of a few kilobases up to millions of bases and single nucleotide polymorphisms (SNPs) which are the substitution of a single nucleotide along the DNA. With an estimated number of more than 10 million to be present in the human genome, SNPs are the most common form of genetic variation (Miller et al., 2005).

Variations in several classes of low penetrance genes known as Single nucleotide polymorphism (SNPs) are very common in the population. SNPs are DNA sequence variations that occur when a single nucleotide (A, T, C, or G) in the genome sequence is altered. For a variation to be considered as SNP, it must be present in at least 1% of the population. SNPs are relatively common in the population and as such may be associated with a much higher attributable risk in the population as a whole than the rare high penetrance genes. Therefore, variants in low penetrance genes could explain a greater proportion of sporadic cancers than the high penetrance genes. SNPs acting together with environmental factors are well documented candidates for cancer susceptibility. Even though, SNPs in these low penetrance genes have only small effect when considered singly, they may produce a high risk profile when acting together with other shared genetic variants and environmental factors (Gary et al., 1999). On the basis of biological plausibility,

SNPs in low penetrance genes whose protein products would affect a pathway involved in carcinogenesis have been documented as cancer predisposition or susceptibility risk factors. Low penetrance candidates are found in a wide variety of pathways ranging from metabolism and detoxification or environmental carcinogens to DNA damage repair.

The recognition that carcinogens can also be mutagens that change the DNA sequence gave impetus to the relevance of DNA damage and repair to carcinogenesis. All the effects of exogenous factors and endogenous factors on tumor production could be accounted for by the DNA damage that they cause and by the errors introduced into DNA during the cell's efforts to repair this damage. According to the mutator phenotype hypothesis, cancer phenotypes result from mutations in genes that maintain genetic stability in normal cells. Mutations in genetic stability genes can cause mutations in other genes that govern genetic stability, initiating a cascade of mutations throughout the genome. So, the prompt response of the cells to repair genetic injury and its ability to maintain genomic stability by means of a variety of DNA repair mechanisms are therefore essential in preventing tumor initiation and progression.

Genetic variants or mutations in high penetrance genes are disease causing whereas genetic variations in low penetrance genes are insufficient to cause cancer, but may influence cancer risk. So genetic variants in low penetrance genes are disease risk associated. Individual low penetrance risk alleles are insufficient to cause cancer, but influence cancer risk. Low penetrance genes, with an attendant increased risk of causing cancer, albeit, less likely than high penetrance genes (Ponder, 2001; Shields & Harris, 2000) predispose individuals to cancer upon interacting with environmental factors.

5. SNPs in DNA damage repair genes

DNA repair mechanisms are controlled by specific set of genes encoding the enzymes that catalyze cellular response to DNA damage. It is well documented that loss of repair function, or alteration of the control of repair process, can have very serious consequences for cells and individuals and can lead to development of cancer. Several genes involved in DNA repair pathways are considered to be low penetrance genes. A link between failure of DNA repair and carcinogens was suggested when individuals with chromosome breakage syndrome such as Xeroderma Pigmentosum, Fanconi Anemia, Bloom Syndrome, Ataxia telangiectasia who have inherited genetic defects in certain DNA repair systems were recognized to be at an increased susceptibility to development of certain cancers.

Because DNA damage is associated with cancer development, it was hypothesized that genes involved in DNA damage repair may influence cancer susceptibility. Polymorphisms in DNA repair genes may be associated with differences in the DRC of DNA damage and may influence an individual's risk for cancer, because the variant genotype in those polymorphisms might destroy or alter repair function. A large number of SNPs have been determined among individuals in DNA repair genes. It has been documented that genetic variations in DNA damage repair genes could result in variations in efficacy and accuracy of DNA repair enzymes and could have effect on the sensitivity of the organism to environmental genotoxins.

Genetic variation in DNA repair genes in each of the five DNA repair pathways has been implicated in cancer susceptibility (Berwick & Vineis 2000; Goode et al., 2002). Genetic variations such as SNPs in DNA repair genes are associated with reduced function of their encoded proteins, rather than absence of function and may alter an individual's capability to repair damaged DNA. This may result in gene product (protein) not being formed, or that the protein is less active, or that it is formed in an uncontrolled fashion, may be at the wrong time, or in the wrong amount. Some minor genetic alterations may not affect protein activity, or interactions, whereas others may significantly disrupt cellular function. It is also possible that since certain proteins work in a number of different processes or complexes, the loss or impairment of one type of protein can affect several different functions of the cell and organism. Deficiency or impairment in DNA repair genes which results in alteration of the key gene expression may have an influence on DNA repairs functions and could lead to altered cancer risk. The importance of these mechanisms in cancer prevention is evident from the increased cancer risk associated with disruption of these pathways (Digweed, 2003). So studies on DNA repair as a susceptibility factor for cancer are increasing exponentially. Majority of cancer susceptibility studies have focused on the identification of low-penetrance disease susceptibility alleles applying candidate gene pathway studies and genome wide association studies. Genetic association studies and genome wide association scans have identified a number of polymorphisms in several low penetrance genes and their role in etiology of several cancers, through risk modification (Tomlinson et al., 2008).

DNA double strand breaks (DSBs) which can result from a variety of factors including ionizing radiation, free radicals, replication errors, telomere dysfunction are one of the most severe types of DNA damage (Khanna & Jackson, 2001). Unpaired or misrepaired DSBs can lead to cell death, genomic instability and oncogenic transformation (Jeggo & Jackson, 2001). Homologous recombination (HR) and nonhomologous enjoining (NHEJ) are the two major DSB repair pathways in mammalian cells. Reports are available suggesting that several Single Nucleotide Polymorphisms in the NHEJ genes may be relevant to modify the risk of multiple myloma (Roddam et al., 2002), glioma (Liu et al., 2008) and, breast cancer (Garcia-Closas et al., 2006). Another study by (Tseng et al., 2009), showed significant association between the XRCC4 and LIGH genotypes with non-small cell lung cancer (NSCLC) risk in an analysis of individual polymorphism associations, and the risk of NSCLC increased further in a combined analysis of multiple polymorphisms.

6. XRCC3

The X-ray repair cross-complementing group 3 (XRCC3), the DNA repair gene which codes for a protein participating in homologous recombination repair (HRR) of double strand breaks (DSB), has been of considerable interest as a candidate gene for cancer susceptibility. The variant allele of the Thr241Met had been reported to have relatively high DNA adduct levels in lymphocyte DNA and hence with relatively low DNA repair capacity (Matullo et al., 2001). Several molecular epidemiologic studies have been performed to evaluate the role of XRCC3 polymorphisms such as XRCC3 4541 A>G, XRCC3 17893 A>G, XRCC3 Thr 241 Met on various neoplasms, such as cancer of breast, lung, bladder, colorectal, head and neck, skin etc (Han et al., 2004; Shen et al., 2004; Ritchey et al., 2005; Jin et al., 2005; Matullo et al.,2005; Garcia-Closas et al., 2006; Zienoldding et al., 2006; Yi et al., 2006). But rather than conclusive, the results from these studies remain fairly conflicting. Ahmd Aizat (2011) reported lack of association of XRCC3 Thr 241 Met with sporadic colorectal cancer susceptibility in Malaysian population. (Han et al., 2006) performed a meta -analysis on XRCC3 polymorphism and cancer risk involving 48 case-control studies including 24,975 cancer patients and 34,209 controls. From the analysis results, (Han et al., 2006) reported that individuals carrying the XRCC3 Met/Met genotype showed a. small cancer risk under a recessive genetic model. Specifically, the XRCC3 Met/Met genotype showed significantly increased risk of breast cancer, but not significant risk of cancer for head and neck, bladder, and non-melanoma skin cancer. This meta analysis results support that the XRCC3 might represent a low penetrance susceptible gene especially for cancer of breast, bladder, head and neck, and non-melanoma skin cancer.

7. XRCC1

The X-Ray Cross Complementing group I XRCC1 gene belongs to The Base Excision Repair IBER) pathway. The XRCC1 gene product plays an important role in the BER pathway by acting as a scolfold for the other DNA repair proteins, such as DNA polymerase B (Kubota et al., 1996), and DNA ligase III (Caldecott, 2003). Few common single nucleotide polymoprhisms of the XRCC1 gene have been identified at codon 194 (G>T substitution at position 26304, exon 6, Arg to Trp), codon 280 (G>A substitution at position 27466, exon 9, Arg to His) and 399 (G>A substitution at position 28152, exon 10, Arg to Gln). The individuals carrying XRCC1 399 variants have been shown to have higher levels of DNA adduct (Lunn et al., 2000) and to be at greater risk for tobacco related DNA damage (Lei et al., 2002). Few studies reported XRCC1 399AA genotype to be significantly associated with lung cancer risk in Caucasian population (Divine et al., 2001; Zhou et al., 2003), Korean population (Park et al., 2002), and Indian population (Sreeja et al., 2008).

8. XPD (ERCC2)

Xeroderma Pigmentosum group D (XPD) also known as ERCC2 (Excision Repair Cross Completing group 2) gene encodes a helicase, a major DNA repair protein, which is involved in transcription-coupled NER and in the removal of a variety of structurally unrelatedas DNA lesions (Lehmann, 2001) including those induced by tobacco carcinogens (Leadon & Cooper, 1993), (Tang et al., 2002). The normal functioning XPD protein plays an essential role in NER and participates in the unwinding of DNA at the site of deleterious DNA lesions (Hoeijmakers et al., 1996). Several studies have reported association between A751C variant of XPD and increased risk of lung cancer (Hou et al., 2002; Spitz et al 2003; Ramachandran et al., 2006). Hou et al., 2003 reported a marginally increased risk for those carrying heterozygous A>C transversions, compared to those with wildtype homozygous, indicating that heterozygosity also carry the risk. In a Northeastern Chinese population, XPD 751 AC heterozygous genotype carriers were at 2.7 fold higher risk of lung cancer than carrier of AA genotype (Yin et al., 2006). A significant association of XPD variants in modulating NSCLC risk was reported by Zienolddiny et al (2006) in Norwegian lung cancer population. So also, in an Indian population, Sreeja et al., (2008) also reported significant association of XPD heterozygous variants in modulating Non small cell lung cancer risk. SNPs in genes involved in nucleotide excision repair (ERCC1, XPD, XPC, XPA, XPF and XPG) and mismatch repair genes (MLH1 and MSH2) in 577 colorectal cancer cases and 307 case-affected sibling controls were examined by Joshi et al., (2009). Their results showed that consumption of red meat, heavily brown on the outside or inside, increased colorectal cancer risk only among subjects with XPD codon 751 Lys/Lys or XPD codon 312 Asp/Asp genotypes.

9. P53

The P53 gene plays a critical role in cell cycle control, the initiation of apoptosis, and maintenance of genomic stability and in DNA repair (Levine, 1997). TP53 is highly polymorphic in coding and non coding regions and some of these polymorphisms have been shown to increase cancer susceptibility and modify cancer phenotypes in TP53 mutation carriers (Whibley et al., 2009). Over 80 TP53 polymorphisms have been identified and validated in human populations. (IARC TP53 Database, R13). Nearly 90% are located in introns, outside splice sites, or in non coding exons. Among the P53 polymorphism, the codon 72 polymorphism (Arg72 Pro) in exon 4 of TP53 is the most extensively studied, both in experimental and population studies. Codon 72 is located within a proline rich region and Arg72 has been reported to be more effective in inducing apoptosis than Pro72. The Arg/Pro polymorphism at codon 72 of the P53 gene alters the ability of the P53 protein to induce apoptosis, influences the behaviour of mutant P53, decreases the DNA repair capacity and has been linked to with an increased risk of cancer, especially lung cancer. Several studies have examined the associations between P53 codon 72 (Arg72Pro) polymorphism and risk of different cancers, but with in consistent results. Few studies reported higher risk for lung cancer in individuals with the Arg/Pro or Pro/Pro genotype and especially Pro/Pro genotype with smoking induced lung cancer (Weston et al., 1992; Jin et al., 1995 ; Fan et al., 2000; Zhou et al., 2001). In a Chilean population, Fan et al., (2000) investigated the influence of polymorphic genotype TP53 on lung cancer susceptibility and the Pro/Pro genotype of TP53 was found to contribute significantly to lung cancer susceptibility risk [OR 3.88 (95% CI 1.16 - 13.39)]. The study by Alexandrov et al (2002) were consistent with the hypothesis that Benzo(a)pyrene (Polycyclic aromatic hydrocarbon, PAH) induce G : C to T : A transverse mutations in the hotspot codons of TP53 and are hence involved in the malignant transformation of the lung tissue of smokers. In an Indian case - control study involving 211 lung cancer cases and 211 controls, Sreeja et al (2007) reported an OR of 2.5 (95% CI 1.470 4.302 , p= 0.001) for the TP53 Pro/Pro variant genotype for lung cancer susceptibility and the risk tended to be higher for women [OR =2.4 , p=0.003] . Recently, Ahmd Aizat (2011) reported a significant association of Pro/Pro homozygous variant of p53 with sporadic colorectal cancer susceptibility (OR = 1.886, CI: 1,046 - 3.399 , p= 0,035) and suggested that p53 Pro72Pro genotype carriers might be having a higher risk for Colorectal cancer susceptibility in Malaysian population (personal communication, unpublished data) However, meta-analysis on the risk association of TP53 Arg72Pro polymorphism with lung cancer (Matakidou et al., 2003) and breast cancer (Schmidt et al., 2007) do not support a significant role for this polymorphism in susceptibility.

10. MMR genes

In the maintenance of genomic stability, the DNA mismatch repair (MMR) systems comprising of various MMR genes play a key role. MMR genes mediate DNA repair through removal of mismatched nucleotide pairs and insertion/ deletion heterologies generated during DNA replication. Germ line mutations as well as hypermethylation in MMR genes have been reported in familial/hereditary forms of colorectal cancer. So, it was hypothesized that common variants in relevant genes encoding DNA MMR enzymes might impact the risk of sporadic form of CRC and studies have been carried out to explore this possibility. Even though the functional relevance of majority of polymorphisms in the genes involved in MMR is not known, recent studies suggest an influence of SNPs or biochemical interaction between components of the MMR pathways or on epigenetic mediated functional regulation (Chen et al., 2007).

Several common polymorphisms in DNA repair genes representing different repair pathways have been reported. Many studies have been carried out to elucidate the association between DNA repair gene polymorphisms and cancer susceptibility. But studies have shown inconsistent associations. The impact of many these polymorphisms on repair phenotype and cancer susceptibility remain uncertain (Berwick & Vineis, 2000; Au et al., 2004). In a study on 5 DNA repair genes (XRCC1 Arg194Trp and Arg399gln, PARP Val762Ala and Lys940Arg, XPD Asp312Asn and Lys751Gln, OGG1 Ser326Cys MGMT Leu84Phe) in Singaporean Chinese population, Stern et al., (2007) provided support to the hypothesis that selected variants in DNA repair genes may contribute to colorectal cancer risk and may modify the effects of relevant life style risk factors that have been inconsistently associated with the disease. This study which reported the overall effects of PARP on colorectal cancer risk and XRCC1 SNPs as modifiers of the effects of smoking and alcohol on colorectal cancer risk, also highlighted the role of the base excision repair pathway in colorectal carcinogenesis. Vinies et al (2009) conducted meta-analyses of 241 associations between variants in DNA repair genes and cancer and had found sparse association signals with strong epidemiological credibility. Using 1087 datasets and publicly available data from genome wide association platforms, meta-analysis using dominant and recessive models were performed on 241 associations between individual variants and specific cancer types that had been tested in two or more independent studies. Thirty one nominally statistically significant ($P<0.05$ without adjustment for multiple comparisons) associations were recorded for 16 genes in dominant and/or recessive model analyses (BRCA2, CCND1, ERCC1, ERCC2, ERCC4, ERCC5, MGMT, NBN, PARP1, POL1, TP53, XPA, XRCC1, XRCC2, XRCC3 and XRCC4). XRCC1, XRCC2, TP53, and ERCC2 variants were each nominally associated with several types of cancer. Three associations were graded as having "strong" credibility, another four had "modest" credibility and 24 had "weak" credibility based on Vinies criteria. Requiring more stringent P values to account for multiplicity of comparisons, only the associations of ERCC2 codon 751 (recessive model) and of XRCC1-77 T>C (dominant-model) with lung cancer had $P\leq 0.0001$ and retained $P\leq 0.001$ even when the first published studies on the respective associations were excluded. The analyses suggested that the vast majority of postulated associations between DNA repair alleles and cancer risk have not been replicated sufficiently to give them strong credibility. This meta-analysis implies that larger scale studies would be necessary to establish specific associations of genetic variants in DNA repair and cancer and that the added risk conferred by single variants in DNA repair genes may be small. In another recent meta analysis, (Kiyohara et al.) found XPA G23A, OGG1 Ser326Cys and XPD Lys751Gln polymorphisms were associated with lung cancer risk .

11. Limitations and future prospectives

In SNP association studies, the most important critical point is associated with often too small size of cohort of cases and controls, resulting in a low statistical power and false, by chance, positive or negative outcomes. Another important aspect concerns inclusion of different ethnic groups. Different results may be expected due to intrinsic difference in genetic background among Caucasians, Asians, Afro Americans and other ethnic groups.

There is wide population variability in repair capability phenotype on account of the variation in the polymorphic allele frequencies of DNA repair genes between different ethnic groups. Even through majority of SNPs are common to at least three historic human populations (Caucasians, Africans, Asians), some SNPs are specific to different ethnicities. These differences among human populations has highlighted the need to consider ethnic genetic differences while conducting genetic association studies evaluating disease risk, treatment response and outcome studies. This could also be accounting for a several fold variation in cancer risk and significant heterogeneity across all included studies. So susceptibility factor in one population may not be a factor in another population. Thus, different study designs, differences in the prevalence of genetic polymorphisms and linkage disequilibrium in different ethnic populations are possible explanations for the varying results obtained in different studies across the world. Effect modification by environmental or other genetic risk factors that differ between study populations are also alternative causes. This warrants the need to undertake large studies on homogeneous populations to avoid such influences. .

It is hoped that in future, advances in genotyping utilizing high throughput genotyping methods could facilitate the analysis of multiple polymorphisms within DNA repair genes and also the analysis of multiple genes within DNA repair pathways. Data generated from multiple polymorphisms within a gene can be combined to create haplotypes , the set of multiple alleles on a single chromosome. Because of higher heterozygosity and tighter linkage disequilibrium within disease causing mutations, haplotype analysis can increase the power to detect disease associations. Haplotype analysis also allows for the possibility of an ungenotyped functional variant to be in linkage disequilibrium with the genotyped polymorphisms. Investigations on gene-gene interactions or pathway analysis also would provide more comprehensive insight into the role of low penetrance genetic variants of DNA repair genes in cancer susceptibility. The identification of common, moderate or low penetrance genes for cancer will potentially be of great benefit , because it allows screening to be targeted to those at greatest risk which in turn will help in implementing cancer prevention strategies.

12. Acknowledgements

The author would like to express his sincere thanks and gratitude to Mr. Ahmad Aizat and Mr. Au Zian Liang, postgraduate students in Human Genome Center, University Sains Malaysia, Malaysia for their valuable help in word processing and reference collection related to this work.

13. References

Ahmad Aizat AA, Siti Nurfatimah MS, Aminudin MB, Biswa BM, Venkatesh RN, Zaidi Z, Ahmad Shanwani MS, Ankathil R. Polymorphism Thr241Met of the XRCC3 Gene and Lack of Association with Colorectal Cancer Susceptibility Risk among Malaysian Population -A Preliminary Report (Accepted to publish in International Medical Journal in next issue)

Ahmad Aizat AA , Siti Nurfatimah MS, Aminudin MM, Zaidi Z , Ahmad Shanwani MS , Muhammad Radzi AH , Ankathil R . Increased risk of sporadic Colorectal Cancer in Pro/Pro 72 genotype carriers of TP53 Arg72Pro polymorphism- A Malaysian case control study (In press)

Alexandrov, K. Cascorbi, I. Rojas, M. Bouvier, G. Kriek, E. & Bartsch, H. (2002). CYP1A1 and GSTM1 genotypes affect benzo[a]pyrene DNA adducts in smokers' lung: comparison with aromatic/hydrophobic adduct formation. Carcinogenesis. 23(12): 1969-1977.

Au, W. W., Navasumrit, P. & Ruchirawat, M. (2004) Use of biomarkers to characterize functions of polymorphic DNA repair genotypes. *Int J Hyg Environ Health,* 207, 301-13.

Bertwistle, D. & Ashworth, A. (2000) BRCA1 and BRCA2. *Curr Biol,* 10, R582.

Berwick, M. & Vineis, P. (2000) Markers of DNA repair and susceptibility to cancer in humans: an epidemiologic review. *J Natl Cancer Inst,* 92, 874-97.

Branzei, D. & Foiani, M. (2008) Regulation of DNA repair throughout the cell cycle. *Nat Rev Mol Cell Biol,* 9, 297-308.

Caldecott, K. W. (2003) XRCC1 and DNA strand break repair. *DNA Repair (Amst),* 2, 955-69.

Chen, H., Taylor, N. P., Sotamaa, K. M., Mutch, D. G., Powell, M. A., Schmidt, A. P., Feng, S., Hampel, H. L., De La Chapelle, A. & Goodfellow, P. J. (2007) Evidence for heritable predisposition to epigenetic silencing of MLH1. *Int J Cancer,* 120, 1684-8.

Digweed, M. (2003) Response to environmental carcinogens in DNA-repair-deficient disorders. *Toxicology,* 193, 111-24.

Divine, K. K., Gilliland, F. D., Crowell, R. E., Stidley, C. A., Bocklage, T. J., Cook, D. L. & Belinsky, S. A. (2001) The XRCC1 399 glutamine allele is a risk factor for adenocarcinoma of the lung. *Mutat Res,* 461, 273-8.

Fan, R., Wu, M. T., Miller, D., Wain, J. C., Kelsey, K. T., Wiencke, J. K. & Christiani, D. C. (2000) The p53 codon 72 polymorphism and lung cancer risk. *Cancer Epidemiol Biomarkers Prev,* 9, 1037-42.

Garcia-Closas, M., Egan, K. M., Newcomb, P. A., Brinton, L. A., Titus-Ernstoff, L., Chanock, S., Welch, R., Lissowska, J., Peplonska, B., Szeszenia-Dabrowska, N., Zatonski, W., Bardin-Mikolajczak, A. & Struewing, J. P. (2006) Polymorphisms in DNA double-strand break repair genes and risk of breast cancer: two population-based studies in USA and Poland, and meta-analyses. *Hum Genet,* 119, 376-88.

Gary, R., Park, M. S., Nolan, J. P., Cornelius, H. L., Kozyreva, O. G., Tran, H. T., Lobachev, K. S., Resnick, M. A. & Gordenin, D. A. (1999) A novel role in DNA metabolism for the binding of Fen1/Rad27 to PCNA and implications for genetic risk. *Mol Cell Biol,* 19, 5373-82.

Gilad, S., Bar-Shira, A., Harnik, R., Shkedy, D., Ziv, Y., Khosravi, R., Brown, K., Vanagaite, L., Xu, G., Frydman, M., Lavin, M. F., Hill, D., Tagle, D. A. & Shiloh, Y. (1996) Ataxia-telangiectasia: founder effect among north African Jews. *Hum Mol Genet,* 5, 2033-7.

Goode, E. L., Ulrich, C. M. & Potter, J. D. (2002) Polymorphisms in DNA repair genes and associations with cancer risk. *Cancer Epidemiol Biomarkers Prev,* 11, 1513-30.

Han, J., Colditz, G. A., Samson, L. D. & Hunter, D. J. (2004) Polymorphisms in DNA double-strand break repair genes and skin cancer risk. *Cancer Res,* 64, 3009-13.

Han, S., Zhang, H. T., Wang, Z., Xie, Y., Tang, R., Mao, Y. & Li, Y. (2006) DNA repair gene XRCC3 polymorphisms and cancer risk: a meta-analysis of 48 case-control studies. *Eur J Hum Genet,* 14, 1136-44.

Hoeijmakers, J. H., Egly, J. M. & Vermeulen, W. (1996) TFIIH: a key component in multiple DNA transactions. *Curr Opin Genet Dev,* 6, 26-33.

Hou, S. M., Falt, S., Angelini, S., Yang, K., Nyberg, F., Lambert, B. & Hemminki, K. (2002) The XPD variant alleles are associated with increased aromatic DNA adduct level and lung cancer risk. *Carcinogenesis,* 23, 599-603.

Hou, S. M., Ryk, C., Kannio, A., Angelini, S., Falt, S., Nyberg, F. & Husgafvel-Pursiainen, K. (2003) Influence of common XPD and XRCC1 variant alleles on p53 mutations in lung tumors. *Environ Mol Mutagen,* 41, 37-42.

Jacob, S. & Praz, F. (2002) DNA mismatch repair defects: role in colorectal carcinogenesis. *Biochimie,* 84, 27-47.

Jeggo, P. A. & Lobrich, M. (2006) Contribution of DNA repair and cell cycle checkpoint arrest to the maintenance of genomic stability. *DNA Repair (Amst),* 5, 1192-8.

Jin, X., Wu, X., Roth, J. A., Amos, C. I., King, T. M., Branch, C., Honn, S. E. & Spitz, M. R. (1995) Higher lung cancer risk for younger African-Americans with the Pro/Pro p53 genotype. *Carcinogenesis,* 16, 2205-8.

Jones, S., Emmerson, P., Maynard, J., Best, J. M., Jordan, S., Williams, G. T., Sampson, J. R. & Cheadle, J. P. (2002) Biallelic germline mutations in MYH predispose to multiple colorectal adenoma and somatic G:C-->T:A mutations. *Hum Mol Genet,* 11, 2961-7.

Joshi, A. D., Corral, R., Siegmund, K. D., Haile, R. W., Le Marchand, L., Martinez, M. E., Ahnen, D. J., Sandler, R. S., Lance, P. & Stern, M. C. (2009) Red meat and poultry intake, polymorphisms in the nucleotide excision repair and mismatch repair pathways and colorectal cancer risk. *Carcinogenesis,* 30, 472-9.

Khanna, K. K. & Jackson, S. P. (2001) DNA double-strand breaks: signaling, repair and the cancer connection. *Nat Genet,* 27, 247-54.

Kiyohara, C., Takayama, K. & Nakanishi, Y. (2010) Lung cancer risk and genetic polymorphisms in DNA repair pathways: a meta-analysis. *J Nucleic Acids,* , 701-760.

Kubota, Y., Nash, R. A., Klungland, A., Schar, P., Barnes, D. E. & Lindahl, T. (1996) Reconstitution of DNA base excision-repair with purified human proteins: interaction between DNA polymerase beta and the XRCC1 protein. *EMBO J,* 15, 6662-70.

Lavin, M. F. & Shiloh, Y. (1996). Ataxia telangiectasia: a multifaceted genetic disorder associated with defective signal transduction. Curr Opin immunol. 8: 459-464.

Leadon, S. A. & Cooper, P. K. (1993) Preferential repair of ionizing radiation-induced damage in the transcribed strand of an active human gene is defective in Cockayne syndrome. *Proc Natl Acad Sci U S A,* 90, 10499-503.

Lehmann, A. R. (2001) The xeroderma pigmentosum group D (XPD) gene: one gene, two functions, three diseases. *Genes Dev,* 15, 15-23.

Lei, Y. C., Hwang, S. J., Chang, C. C., Kuo, H. W., Luo, J. C., Chang, M. J. & Cheng, T. J. (2002) Effects on sister chromatid exchange frequency of polymorphisms in DNA repair gene XRCC1 in smokers. *Mutat Res,* 519, 93-101.

Leibeling, D., Laspe, P. & Emmert, S. (2006) Nucleotide excision repair and cancer. *J Mol Histol,* 37, 225-38.

Levine, A. J. (1997) p53, the cellular gatekeeper for growth and division. *Cell,* 88, 323-31.

Liu, Y., Zhou, K., Zhang, H., Shugart, Y. Y., Chen, L., Xu, Z., Zhong, Y., Liu, H., Jin, L., Wei, Q., Huang, F., Lu, D. & Zhou, L. (2008) Polymorphisms of LIG4 and XRCC4 involved in the NHEJ pathway interact to modify risk of glioma. *Hum Mutat,* 29, 381-9.

Lunn, R. M., Helzlsouer, K. J., Parshad, R., Umbach, D. M., Harris, E. L., Sanford, K. K. & Bell, D. A. (2000) XPD polymorphisms: effects on DNA repair proficiency. *Carcinogenesis,* 21, 551-5.

Matakidou, A., Eisen, T. & Houlston, R. S. (2003) TP53 polymorphisms and lung cancer risk: a systematic review and meta-analysis. *Mutagenesis,* 18, 377-85.

Matsuura, S., Kobayashi, J., Tauchi, H. & Komatsu, K. (2004) Nijmegen breakage syndrome and DNA double strand break repair by NBS1 complex. *Adv Biophys,* 38, 65-80.

Matullo, G., Palli, D., Peluso, M., Guarrera, S., Carturan, S., Celentano, E., Krogh, V., Munnia, A., Tumino, R., Polidoro, S., Piazza, A. & Vineis, P. (2001) XRCC1, XRCC3, XPD gene polymorphisms, smoking and (32)P-DNA adducts in a sample of healthy subjects. *Carcinogenesis,* 22, 1437-45.

Menoyo, A., Alazzouzi, H., Espin, E., Armengol, M., Yamamoto, H. & Schwartz, S., Jr. (2001) Somatic mutations in the DNA damage-response genes ATR and CHK1 in sporadic stomach tumors with microsatellite instability. *Cancer Res,* 61, 7727-30.

Miller, R. D., Phillips, M. S., Jo, I., Donaldson, M. A., Studebaker, J. F., Addleman, N., Alfisi, S. V., Ankener, W. M., Bhatti, H. A., Callahan, C. E., Carey, B. J., Conley, C. L., Cyr, J. M., Derohannessian, V., Donaldson, R. A., Elosua, C., Ford, S. E., Forman, A. M., Gelfand, C. A., Grecco, N. M., Gutendorf, S. M., Hock, C. R., Hozza, M. J., Hur, S., In, S. M., Jackson, D. L., Jo, S. A., Jung, S. C., Kim, S., Kimm, K., Kloss, E. F., Koboldt, D. C., Kuebler, J. M., Kuo, F. S., Lathrop, J. A., Lee, J. K., Leis, K. L., Livingston, S. A., Lovins, E. G., Lundy, M. L., Maggan, S., Minton, M., Mockler, M. A., Morris, D. W., Nachtman, E. P., Oh, B., Park, C., Park, C. W., Pavelka, N., Perkins, A. B., Restine, S. L., Sachidanandam, R., Reinhart, A. J., Scott, K. E., Shah, G. J., Tate, J. M., Varde, S. A., Walters, A., White, J. R., Yoo, Y. K., Lee, J. E., Boyce-Jacino, M. T. & Kwok, P. Y. (2005) High-density single-nucleotide polymorphism maps of the human genome. *Genomics,* 86, 117-26.

Park, J. Y., Lee, S. Y., Jeon, H. S., Bae, N. C., Chae, S. C., Joo, S., Kim, C. H., Park, J. H., Kam, S., Kim, I. S. & Jung, T. H. (2002) Polymorphism of the DNA repair gene XRCC1 and risk of primary lung cancer. *Cancer Epidemiol Biomarkers Prev,* 11, 23-7.

Ponder, B. A. (2001) Cancer genetics. *Nature,* 411, 336-41.

Rahman, N., Seal, S., Thompson, D., Kelly, P., Renwick, A., Elliott, A., Reid, S., Spanova, K., Barfoot, R., Chagtai, T., Jayatilake, H., Mcguffog, L., Hanks, S., Evans, D. G., Eccles, D., Easton, D. F. & Stratton, M. R. (2007) PALB2, which encodes a BRCA2-interacting protein, is a breast cancer susceptibility gene. *Nat Genet,* 39, 165-7.

Ramachandran, S., Ramadas, K., Hariharan, R., Rejnish Kumar, R. & Radhakrishna Pillai, M. (2006) Single nucleotide polymorphisms of DNA repair genes XRCC1 and XPD and its molecular mapping in Indian oral cancer. *Oral Oncol,* 42, 350-62.

Renwick, A., Thompson, D., Seal, S., Kelly, P., Chagtai, T., Ahmed, M., North, B., Jayatilake, H., Barfoot, R., Spanova, K., Mcguffog, L., Evans, D. G., Eccles, D., Easton, D. F., Stratton, M. R. & Rahman, N. (2006) ATM mutations that cause ataxia-telangiectasia are breast cancer susceptibility alleles. *Nat Genet,* 38, 873-5.

Ritchey, J. D., Huang, W. Y., Chokkalingam, A. P., Gao, Y. T., Deng, J., Levine, P., Stanczyk, F. Z. & Hsing, A. W. (2005) Genetic variants of DNA repair genes and prostate cancer: a population-based study. *Cancer Epidemiol Biomarkers Prev,* 14, 1703-9.

Roddam, P. L., Rollinson, S., O'driscoll, M., Jeggo, P. A., Jack, A. & Morgan, G. J. (2002) Genetic variants of NHEJ DNA ligase IV can affect the risk of developing multiple myeloma, a tumour characterised by aberrant class switch recombination. *J Med Genet,* 39, 900-5.

Schmidt, M. K., Reincke, S., Broeks, A., Braaf, L. M., Hogervorst, F. B., Tollenaar, R. A., Johnson, N., Fletcher, O., Peto, J., Tommiska, J., Blomqvist, C., Nevanlinna, H. A., Healey, C. S., Dunning, A. M., Pharoah, P. D., Easton, D. F., Dork, T. & Van't Veer, L. J. (2007) Do MDM2 SNP309 and TP53 R72P interact in breast cancer susceptibility? A large pooled series from the breast cancer association consortium. *Cancer Res,* 67, 9584-90.

Shen, H., Wang, X., Hu, Z., Zhang, Z., Xu, Y., Hu, X., Guo, J. & Wei, Q. (2004) Polymorphisms of DNA repair gene XRCC3 Thr241Met and risk of gastric cancer in a Chinese population. *Cancer Lett,* 206, 51-8.

Shields, P. G. & Harris, C. C. (2000) Cancer risk and low-penetrance susceptibility genes in gene-environment interactions. *J Clin Oncol,* 18, 2309-15.

Spry, M., Scott, T., Pierce, H. & D'orazio, J. A. (2007) DNA repair pathways and hereditary cancer susceptibility syndromes. *Front Biosci,* 12, 4191-207.

Sreeja L, Syamala V, Raveendran PB, Santhi S, Madhavan J, Ankathil R., (2008). P53 Arg72Pro polymorphism Predicts Survival Outcome in Lung Cancer Patients in Indian Population. *Cancer Investigation,* 26:41-46.

Sreeja, L., Syamala, V. S., Syamala, V., Hariharan, S., Raveendran, P. B., Vijayalekshmi, R. V., Madhavan, J. & Ankathil, R. (2007) Prognostic importance of DNA repair gene polymorphisms of XRCC1 Arg399Gln and XPD Lys751Gln in lung cancer patients from India. *J Cancer Res Clin Oncol,* 134, 645-52.

Stern, M. C., Conti, D. V., Siegmund, K. D., Corral, R., Yuan, J. M., Koh, W. P. & Yu, M. C. (2007) DNA repair single-nucleotide polymorphisms in colorectal cancer and their role as modifiers of the effect of cigarette smoking and alcohol in the Singapore Chinese Health Study. *Cancer Epidemiol Biomarkers Prev,* 16, 2363-72.

Tang, D., Cho, S., Rundle, A., Chen, S., Phillips, D., Zhou, J., Hsu, Y., SCHNABEL, F., ESTABROOK, A. & PERERA, F. P. (2002) Polymorphisms in the DNA repair enzyme XPD are associated with increased levels of PAH-DNA adducts in a case-control study of breast cancer. *Breast Cancer Res Treat,* 75, 159-66.

Tomlinson, I. P., Webb, E., Carvajal-Carmona, L., Broderick, P., Howarth, K., Pittman, A. M., Spain, S., Lubbe, S., Walther, A., Sullivan, K., Jaeger, E., Fielding, S., Rowan, A., Vijayakrishnan, J., Domingo, E., Chandler, I., Kemp, Z., Qureshi, M., Farrington, S. M., Tenesa, A., Prendergast, J. G., Barnetson, R. A., Penegar, S., Barclay, E., Wood, W., Martin, L., Gorman, M., Thomas, H., Peto, J., Bishop, D. T., Gray, R., Maher, E. R., Lucassen, A., Kerr, D., Evans, D. G., Schafmayer, C., Buch, S., Volzke, H., Hampe, J., Schreiber, S., John, U., Koessler, T., Pharoah, P., Van Wezel, T., Morreau, H., Wijnen, J. T., Hopper, J. L., Southey, M. C., Giles, G. G., Severi, G., Castellvi-Bel, S., Ruiz-Ponte, C., Carracedo, A., Castells, A., Forsti, A., Hemminki, K., Vodicka, P., Naccarati, A., Lipton, L., Ho, J. W., Cheng, K. K., Sham, P. C., Luk, J., Agundez, J. A., Ladero, J. M., De La Hoya, M., Caldes, T., Niittymaki, I., Tuupanen, S., Karhu, A., Aaltonen, L., Cazier, J. B., Campbell, H., Dunlop, M. G. & Houlston, R. S. (2008) A genome-wide association study identifies colorectal cancer susceptibility loci on chromosomes 10p14 and 8q23.3. *Nat Genet,* 40, 623-30.

Tseng, R. C., Hsieh, F. J., Shih, C. M., Hsu, H. S., Chen, C. Y. & Wang, Y. C. (2009) Lung cancer susceptibility and prognosis associated with polymorphisms in the nonhomologous end-joining pathway genes: a multiple genotype-phenotype study. *Cancer,* 115, 2939-48.

Weston, A., Perrin, L. S., Forrester, K., Hoover, R. N., Trump, B. F., Harris, C. C. & Caporaso, N. E. (1992) Allelic frequency of a p53 polymorphism in human lung cancer. *Cancer Epidemiol Biomarkers Prev,* 1, 481-3.

Whibley, C., Pharoah, P. D. & Hollstein, M. (2009) p53 polymorphisms: cancer implications. *Nat Rev Cancer,* 9, 95-107.

Wood, R. D., Mitchell, M. & Lindahl, T. (2005) Human DNA repair genes. *Mutat Res,* 577, 275-83.

Yin, J., Vogel, U., Ma, Y., Guo, L., Wang, H. & Qi, R. (2006) Polymorphism of the DNA repair gene ERCC2 Lys751Gln and risk of lung cancer in a northeastern Chinese population. *Cancer Genet Cytogenet,* 169, 27-32.

Zhou, G., Zhang, X., Lui, S., Lin, D., Liang, C. & Yang, X. (2001) [Pilot study on mutations of p53 gene in laryngeal carcinoma]. *Hua Xi Yi Ke Da Xue Xue Bao,* 32, 359-60, 434.

Zhou, W., Liu, G., Miller, D. P., Thurston, S. W., Xu, L. L., Wain, J. C., Lynch, T. J., Su, L. & Christiani, D. C. (2003) Polymorphisms in the DNA repair genes XRCC1 and ERCC2, smoking, and lung cancer risk. *Cancer Epidemiol Biomarkers Prev,* 12, 359-65.

Zienolddiny, S., Campa, D., Lind, H., Ryberg, D., Skaug, V., Stangeland, L., Phillips, D. H., Canzian, F. & Haugen, A. (2006) Polymorphisms of DNA repair genes and risk of non-small cell lung cancer. *Carcinogenesis,* 27, 560-7.

27

Polymorphisms in Nucleotide Excision Repair Genes and Risk of Colorectal Cancer: A Systematic Review

Rikke Dalgaard Hansen and Ulla Vogel
Danish Cancer Society & National Research Centre for the Working Environment
Denmark

1. Introduction

Various DNA alterations can be caused by exposure to environmental and endogenous carcinogens through direct binding of metabolites (adduct formation). If not repaired the DNA lesions may lead to genetic instability, mutagenesis and oncogenesis. Thus, DNA repair constitutes a first line of defence against cancer.

Environmental factors are likely to cause damage to DNA through direct binding of metabolites (adduct formation). The nucleotide excision repair (NER) pathway is the primary mechanism for removal of large and bulky adducts from DNA.

1.1 Single nucleotide polymorphisms

Common occurring single nucleotide polymorphisms (SNPs) in genes involved in DNA repair may possibly contribute to the variation in the capacity of repair of bulky DNA adducts. Hence, these SNPs may be important biomarkers of susceptibility to cancer.

The present book chapter includes a systematic review of the available scientific literature on associations between SNPs in genes involved in NER and risk of colorectal adenomas and colorectal cancer. The present review of colorectal cancer studies includes 19 studies on 22 different SNPs. The review is focused on SNPs in four genes: *XPD*, *XPC*, *XPA* and *ERCC1* encoding the essential components of NER: xeroderma pigmentosum complementation group A, C, and D and excision repair cross complementary group 1 and risk of colorectal adenomas and colorectal cancer, and on interaction between the polymorphisms and various life style factors in relation to colorectal cancer risk.

The NER polymorphisms studied in the work underlying this book chapter include the polymorphisms: *XPD* Lys751Gln, *XPD* Asp312Asn, *XPA* G23A, *XPC* Lys939Gln, and *ERCC1* Asn118Asn.

1.2 Colorectal cancer

Colorectal cancer is the third most common cancer and the leading cause of cancer deaths in Western industrialised countries. Thus, every year nearly one million people worldwide develop colorectal cancer. Lifetime risk of colorectal cancer may reach 6% of the population in the Western industrialised countries (Jemal et al., 2006). The age-specific incidence of colorectal cancer increases sharply after 35 years of age, with approximately 90% of cancers occurring in persons older than 50 years (Schottenfeld & Winawer, 1996) . The mean age at time for diagnosis in Danish colorectal cancer patients is approximately 70 years for men and 72 years for women (Iversen et al., 2005) . The disease develops either sporadically, as a part of a hereditary cancer syndrome, or induced by inflammatory bowel disease. Ten to fifteen percent of colorectal cancer cases are caused by hereditary syndromes (Schottenfeld & Winawer, 1996) .

Migrant studies and large international variation in incidence rates indicate that life style factors, including dietary, are associated with risk of colorectal cancer, but traditional epidemiological studies based on life style questionnaires and outcome have mostly failed in identifying the exact risk and beneficial factors. Our current knowledge of colorectal carcinogenesis indicates a multi-factorial and multi-step process that involves various genetic alterations and several biological pathways. An understanding of differences in individual susceptibility and better exposure assessment may be crucial in identifying life style risk factors and possible interactions between susceptibility and exposures in relation to risk of colorectal cancer.

2. DNA adducts

Several life style factors and dietary components are suggested to be associated with risk of colorectal cancer, listed in Table 1. The associations may possibly be caused by increased formation of DNA adducts.

2.1 NOC, HCA and PAH

N-nitroso compounds (NOCs) are present in tobacco smoke and in nitrate- or nitrite-treated meats (Hotchkiss, 1989; Hecht & Hoffmann, 1988). NOCs are alkylating agents able to react with DNA and form adducts. More than 85% of 300 NOCs tested for carcinogenicity in experimental animals were observed to be carcinogenic (Mirvish, 1995), but epidemiologic studies have been inconclusive in finding association between the exposure of NOCs and risk of various cancer forms in humans (Burch et al., 1987; Preston-Martin & Mack, 1991; Carozza et al., 1995), although an increased endogenous production of NOCs, suggested primarily by bacterial catalysis, are proposed associated to the etiology of colorectal cancer (Bingham et al., 1996).

Polycyclic aromatic hydrocarbons (PAHs) and heterocyclic aromatic amines (HCAs) constitute a major class of chemical carcinogens present in the environment. When metabolically activated, these compounds act as mutagens and carcinogens in animal models (Culp et al., 1998; Moller et al., 2002; Dingley et al., 2003) and are able to form bulky DNA adducts in humans (Hecht, 2003), (Phillips, 2002) . Many PAHs and HCAs are found to be tumourigenic in humans or experimental animals (International Agency for Research on Cancer (IARC), 1983). Cooking meat at high temperatures and certain preservation and processing procedures leads to the formation of PAHs and HCAs (Sinha et al., 2005; Guillen et al., 1997) . PAHs are ubiquitous environmental contaminants formed by incomplete combustion of organic matter. They are one of several classes of carcinogenic chemicals present in tobacco smoke (Benhamou et al., 2003; Melikian et al., 1999). PAH compounds may not only be formed by high cooking temperatures but are also found in uncooked food, like sea food and plants, due to contamination of the aquatic environment (Meador et al., 1995) or via atmospheric exposure (Guillen et al., 1997).

2.2 Life style factors and DNA adduct formation

Air pollution is not an established risk factor for colorectal cancer in humans, although several studies have shown higher risk among workers exposed to diesel exhaust (Goldberg et al., 2001). Some studies have found an association between ambient air pollution and DNA adduct levels (Poirier et al., 1998; Hemminki et al., 1990b; Binkova et al., 1995; Palli et al., 2001; Nielsen et al., 1996a; Nielsen et al., 1996c), whereas others failed to find such an association (Kyrtopoulos et al., 2001; Peluso et al., 1998). DNA adduct levels are increased following occupational exposure among foundry and coke oven workers and among workers exposed to diesel exhaust (Hemminki et al., 1997; Hemminki et al., 1990a; Hemminki et al., 1994; Perera et al., 1988; Perera et al., 1994; Lewtas et al., 1997; Nielsen et al., 1996a; Nielsen et al., 1996b), while among fire-fighters (Rothman et al., 1993), traffic exposed policemen (Peluso et al., 1998) and aluminium workers (Yang et al., 1998), no associations between occupational exposures and DNA adducts have been found.

Tobacco smoking is an established risk factor for development of adenomas (Ji et al., 2006), and recently an association between tobacco smoking and risk of colorectal cancer has been recognized by IARC. Following tobacco smoking, adducts formed by metabolites of NOCs and PAHs are not only located in airway tissue, but are also found in bladder and cervical tissue from smokers (Benhamou et al., 2003; Melikian et al., 1999).

Life style factor	*Risk of CRC*	*DNA adduct formation*
Air pollution	↑	PAH
Tobacco smoking	↑	PAH, NOC
Alcohol	↑	Acetaldehyde
Red meat	↑	PAH, NOC, HCA
Processed meat	↑	PAH, NOC, HCA
Vegetables	↓	-
Fruit	↓	-

Table 1. Possible environmental risk and beneficial factors of colorectal cancer and their association with DNA adduct formation. Arrows indicate adverse (↑) or preventive (↓) association with risk of colorectal cancer.

A growing body of evidence supports that avoidance of alcohol is recommended to prevent colorectal cancer (Correa Lima & Gomes-da-Silva, 2005). Acetaldehyde is the primary oxidative metabolite of ethanol. Acetaldehyde and malondialdehyde, the end-product of lipid peroxidation by reactive oxygen species, can combine to form the malondialdehyde-acetaldehyde adduct, which is very reactive and avidly binds to DNA (Brooks & Theruvathu, 2005). The level of acetaldehyde DNA adducts in white blood cell DNA in alcohol abusers have been measured up to 13-fold higher than in subjects from the non-drinking control group (Fang & Vaca, 1997).

There is some evidence for adverse associations between intake of red and processed meat and risk of colorectal cancer (Johnson & Lund, 2007; Doyle, 2007; Norat et al., 2005). The elevated risk may be due to an increased endogenous production of NOC, which may enhance the colonic formation of the DNA adduct O6-carboxymethyl guanine (Bingham et al., 1996; Lewin et al., 2006). Cooking meat at high temperatures leads to the formation of polycyclic aromatic hydrocarbons (PAHs) and heterocyclic amines (HCAs) (Sinha et al., 2005). Additionally, intake of charbroiled or smoked meat may be associated with increased levels of DNA adducts (Rothman et al., 1990; van Maanen et al., 1994; Georgiadis et al., 2001; Rothman et al., 1993), due to HCAs and PAHs (Bruemmer et al., 1996; Balbi et al., 2001; Peters et al., 2004; Skog et al., 1995). The levels of some HCAs and PAHs are comparable for red meat, fish and poultry smoked or cooked at high temperatures (Sinha et al., 1995; Gomaa et al., 1993). Intake of red meat, but not of fish and poultry, increases the luminal contents of N-nitrosocompounds (NOCs) in colon (Bingham et al., 1996; Lewin et al., 2006). The increase in endogenous *N*-nitrosation can be attributed to heme iron (Cross et al., 2003), which is 10-fold higher in red meat than in white meat (Pierre et al., 2003).

There is limited evidence for a preventive effect of intake of fruit and vegetables for cancer in colon and rectum (International Agency for Research on Cancer (IARC), 2003). Intake of fruit, vegetables or antioxidant vitamins have been shown to be negatively associated with DNA adduct levels (Palli et al., 2000; Mooney et al., 1997; Palli et al., 2003; Palli et al., 2004), although some studies found no effect (Georgiadis et al., 2001; Nielsen et al., 1996b) and one study found an effect of increased vitamin intake only in females (Mooney et al., 2005).

3. Nucleotide excision repair

The nucleotide excision repair (NER) pathway is the primary mechanism for removal of helix-distorting damages from DNA, including bulky adducts and UV-induced photolesions. The mechanism of NER includes five steps: 1. Damage recognition, 2. Assembly of the repair factors at the site of damage, 3. Dual incisions and excision of the damage-containing oligomers, 4. Resynthesis to fill in the gap, and 5. Ligation of the strands. All these steps involve more than 20 proteins, like recognition factors, replication protein, transcription factor, helicases, endonucleases and polymerases. Steps 1 and 2 are illustrated in Figure 1.

3.1 The NER pathway

There are two sub-pathways of NER, termed the global genome NER (GG-NER), which corrects lesions in the entire genome including the non-transcribed strands of active genes, and transcription-coupled NER (TC-NER), that only repairs lesions in transcribed strands in active genes. The major differences of the two pathways are the damage recognition step: In GG-NER the proteins Xeroderma Pigmentosum complementation group A and C (XPA/XPC) make the recognition complex (Hanawalt, 2002; Reardon & Sancar, 2002; You et al., 2003; Volker et al., 2001), while in TC-NER a stalled RNA polymerase II (blocked by a lesion) and Cockayne syndrome proteins have this function to act as a signal to recruit NER proteins (Kobayashi et al., 2005; Hanawalt, 2002).

In global genomic NER the XPA and XPC enzymes are involved in the damage recognition-complex of NER. Several studies have shown the XPC-hHR23B complex to function at a very early stage of DNA damage recognition (Reardon & Sancar, 2002; You et al., 2003;

Hanawalt, 2002; Volker et al., 2001). The hHR23B (also called Rad23) NER factor co-purifies with XPC (Masutani et al., 1994) and is essential for high XPC activity in NER (Batty et al., 2000; Guzder et al., 1998). XPC-hHR23B complex exhibit a very strong affinity for damaged DNA (Reardon et al., 1996; Batty et al., 2000; Sugasawa et al., 1998), why it is thought to be the initiator in GG-NER. By interaction with the XPC complex XPA and the transcription factor II H (TFIIH) may be recruited to the damaged DNA site (You et al., 2003; Volker et al., 2001). TFIIH is a nine sub-unit protein complex required for opening the DNA helix at the vicinity of the lesion (Schaeffer et al., 1993; Feaver et al., 1993; Drapkin et al., 1994). Biochemical studies have generated conflicting results with regard to association between the XPC-hHR23B complex, XPA and TFIIH. Some have found recruitment of TFIIH to the site of DNA damage to be dependent on XPC (Volker et al., 2001; Yokoi et al., 2000), while others have found XPA to be interacting with TFIIH (Park et al., 1995). Undoubtedly, both XPC and XPA are vital factors in the very early steps of GG-NER, but exactly when

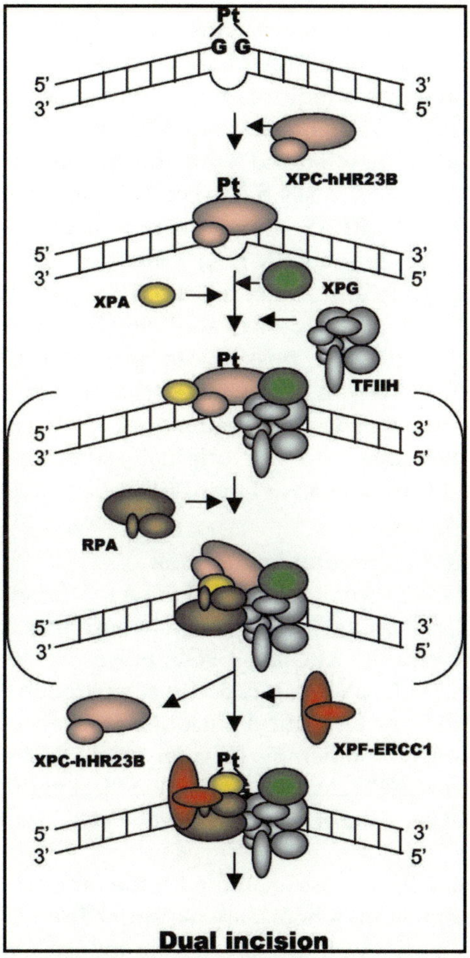

Fig. 1. A proposed molecular mechanism of damage recognition process in the early stage of global genome nucleotide excision repair. Transient steps are indicated with brackets. Adapted from (You et al., 2003) .

XPA enters the site of damage is not clear. XPA physically interacts with replication factor A (RPA) and is essential to efficient NER (Stigger et al., 1998) by stabilizing the interaction between XPA and the damaged DNA. XPA is capable of binding to the XPF-ERCC1 complex with very high affinity (Park & Sancar, 1994). The XPF-ERCC1 is a specific 5´ endonuclease complex, and thus must be located near the site of 5´ incision (Niedernhofer et al., 2001). XPG, a 3´ endonuclease, seems to be the next factor recruited to the site, and is probably positioned at the 3´ incision site (Reardon & Sancar, 2002). Previous studies have observed XPG to co-purify with TFIIH, like XPC, and that XPG exclude XPC when binding to TFIIH (Wakasugi & Sancar, 1999; Wakasugi & Sancar, 1998), which may suggest that the binding of XPG to the NER complex displaces XPC. Hence, XPA is thought to be crucial to the subsequent positioning of the involved NER enzymes by binding to XPF-ERCC1 complex and possibly recruit XPG to the site of DNA damage. XPD and XPB are helicases and parts of the large TFIIH complex. They participate in the unwinding of helix in opposite directions of the region of damaged DNA (Reardon & Sancar, 2002; Schaeffer et al., 1993). When the DNA around the DNA lesion is unwound, the endonucleases XPG and XPF-ERCC1 complex excises an oligonucleotide of 24-32 bases including the damaged site (Mu et al., 1996). The two endonucleases require an opening of approximately 5-8 bases (Evans et al., 1997; de Laat et al., 1998). The final steps of NER are re-synthesis of the strand to fill in the gap and ligation of the new strand with the remaining strand. In mammals the synthesis requires the DNA polymerases δ and/or ε (Hunting et al., 1991; Coverley et al., 1992), the replication protein A (RPA) and replication factor C (RFC) (Shivji et al., 1995) and proliferating cell nuclear antigen (PCNA) (Shivji et al., 1992). The XPF-ERCC1 5´ incision leaves a hydroxyl-group at the 3´ terminus of the gap. This terminus may act as a DNA primer for DNA polymerases (Sijbers et al., 1996). RPA is required for the gap-filling DNA synthesis (Shivji et al., 1995), possibly to protect the template strand against nucleases, and RFC and PCNA as a complex that facilitates the assembly of the polymerases (Shivji et al., 1992). The new fragment of DNA is synthesized and the final step is ligation of the new patch to the original sequence, which possibly may be performed by DNA ligase I (Tomkinson & Levin, 1997).

3.2 SNPs in NER genes and colorectal cancer risk

The variant alleles of *XPA* G23A (Wu et al., 2003), *XPD* Asp312Asn and *XPD* Lys751Gln (Spitz et al., 2001; Qiao et al., 2002) polymorphisms and a polymorphism in *XPC* (Qiao et al., 2002), in full linkage disequilibrium with the *XPC* Lys939Gln polymorphism (Khan et al., 2000), have been associated with a lowered DNA repair capacity compared to the wild type allele. *ERCC1* gene polymorphism is a predictor for clinical outcome in advanced colorectal cancer patients treated with platinum-based chemotherapy (Viguier et al., 2005). Furthermore, the variant alleles of the polymorphisms *XPD* Asp312Asn and *XPD* Lys751Gln have been associated with higher DNA adduct levels (Hou et al., 2002; Matullo et al., 2001; Palli et al., 2001) than the wild type alleles.

Mutations in the NER gene *XPD* are associated with the rare, autosomal-recessive inherited disorder Xeroderma Pigmentosum, where patients suffer from severe photosensitivity and actinic changes leading to early onset of skin cancers induced by sunlight (Cleaver, 2005). Recently the first case of human inherited ERCC1 deficiency was reported (Jaspers et al., 2007). Cells from the patient showed moderate hypersensitivity to ultraviolet rays, but the clinical features were very severe and compatible with a diagnosis of cerebro-oculo-facio-skeletal syndrome. This discovery represents a novel complementation group of patients with defective NER and suggests novel functions for ERCC1.

Overall, the above mentioned studies of the polymorphisms in the genes involved in NER, *XPD* Lys751Gln, *XPD* Asp312Asn, *XPA* G23A, *XPC* Lys939Gln, and *ERCC1* Asn118Asn, indicate that the polymorphisms may modulate DNA repair capacity and may thereby possibly be associated with development of cancer.

There are limited numbers of studies of NER genes in relation to risk of colorectal cancer. A search on the PubMed database of NCBI on January 26th 2011 on the MeSH terms "polymorphism, single nucleotide AND colorectal neoplasms" resulted in 148 hits of which seven studies included polymorphisms in *XPD, XPA, XPC,* and *ERCC1.* In combination with a new search on the PubMed database of NCBI by using different combinations of the words: "XPD XPA XPC ERCC1 polymorphism colorectal colon rectum cancer" 19 studies of SNPs in the four genes in relation to risk of colorectal cancer or prestages to colorectal cancer were identified. The studies are listed in Table 2.

3.2.1 *XPD* Lys751Gln and *XPD* Asp312Asn

The *XPD* Lys751Gln polymorphism is the most frequently studied of the NER polymorphisms in association with risk of cancer. In our Danish prospective study on the Diet, Cancer and Health cohort, we observed no association of the *XPD* Lys751Gln and *XPD* Asp312Asn polymorphisms with risk of colorectal cancer (Hansen et al., 2007). Previously, several studies had similar findings of no association between the *XPD* Lys751Gln (Moreno et al., 2006; Huang et al., 2006; Berndt et al., 2006; Mort et al., 2003; Starinsky et al., 2005; Skjelbred et al., 2006b; Engin et al., 2010; Stern et al., 2009; Stern et al., 2007; Yeh et al., 2005; Joshi et al., 2009; Wang et al., 2010) and the *XPD* Asp312Asn (Moreno et al., 2006; Huang et al., 2006; Berndt et al., 2006; Goodman et al., 2006; Stern et al., 2009; Stern et al., 2007; Joshi et al., 2009) polymorphisms and risk of colorectal cancer. Additionally, Bigler and colleagues found no association of the two polymorphisms with development of adenomas (Bigler et al., 2005). However, they detected a higher risk of colorectal adenomas among individuals with at least two variant alleles of the *XPD* polymorphisms, with an OR of 1.57 (CI: 1.04-2.38). When stratifying by age the association of the two polymorphisms with risk of adenomatous polyps was restricted to the individuals younger than 60 years when diagnosed (OR=3.77, CI: 1.94-7.35). The risk of adenomatous polyps was higher among smokers carrying the homozygous *XPD* variant alleles (OR=3.93, OR: 1.68-9.21) compared with non-smokers carrying the homozygous wild type. A similar finding could not be detected on risk of hyper-plastic polyps. In our Danish study (Hansen et al., 2007) and in a Singapore Chinese study (Stern et al., 2007) did neither of the two XPD polymorphisms, *XPD* Lys751Gln or *XPD* Asp312Asn, modify the effect of smoking on risk of colorectal cancer.

Goodman *et al.,* did not detect any SNP-SNP interaction between the *XPD* Asp312Asn polymorphism and other NER polymorphisms (Goodman et al., 2006). Skjelbred and colleagues detected an association between the *XPD* Lys751Gln polymorphism and development of colorectal adenomas, with an OR of 1.40 (CI: 1.08-1.81), among carriers of the variant allele compared to carriers of the homozygous wild type allele (Skjelbred et al., 2006b). The statistical significance was limited to the low-risk adenoma group (OR: 1.46, CI: 1.11-1.90). The results were contradicted by a large study by Stern *et al.,* including 740 cases with adenomas and 789 controls, where a lower risk of adenomas was observed (OR=0.7, CI:

0.4-1.0) among homozygous carriers of the *XPD* 751Gln allele (Stern et al., 2006). The result was not stratified for ethnicity (Caucasian, African-American, Latinos, Asian-Pacific Islander). When excluding the 1 case and the 17 controls of Latinos, the OR increased to 0.9 (confidence intervals were not reported). An interaction between the *XPD* Lys751Gln polymorphism and alcohol consumption was observed (P=0.04), with higher risk of adenomas among ever-drinkers carrying the *XPD* 751 Gln/Gln genotype (OR=2.5, CI: 1.2-5.2) compared with never-drinkers carrying the same genotype. There was no interaction between the polymorphisms *XPD* Lys751Gln or *XPD* Asp312Asn, respectively, and alcohol consumption on risk of colorectal cancer in our Danish study (Hansen et al., 2007) and in the Singapore Chinese study (Stern et al., 2007).

In a family-based case-control study using a case-only design, an interaction was observed between the two polymorphisms, *XPD* Lys751Gln and *XPD* Asp312Asn, and intake of heavily browned red meat on colorectal cancer risk (Joshi et al., 2009). Intake of red meat heavily brown on the outside or inside increased the risk for colorectal cancer only among carriers of the *XPD* codon 751 Lys/Lys genotype or the *XPD* codon 312 Asp/Asp genotype (case-only interaction P <0.006). There was no association between the meat intake and colorectal cancer risk when the individuals carried at least one copy of the Asn^{321} or Gln^{751} alleles. The results remained statistically significant after accounting for multiple testing. No interaction was observed in our Danish study between the two *XPD* polymorphisms and intake of red meat on risk of colorectal cancer (Hansen et al., 2007).

A higher risk of colorectal cancer has been observed among Ashkenazi Jews below 50 years of age when diagnosed (Starinsky et al., 2005). The risk was higher among carriers of the *XPD* 751Gln allele, but it may be a chance finding due to low number of cases (only 15 cases were diagnosed before their 50 years birthday). Furthermore, the Ashkenazi population is known to have particular genetic characteristics, why the result may not be generalized to other populations.

A large study from Taiwan observed a non-significant tendency for higher risk of colorectal cancer among men carrying the *XPD* 751Gln allele (OR=1.5, CI: 0.9-2.3), while no association was observed for women (OR=0.9, CI: 0.6-1.5) (Yeh et al., 2007). A similar tendency for a gender specific effect of the *XPD* Lys751Gln polymorphism was observed in our Danish study, with lower risk of colorectal cancer among women carrying the variant allele of *XPD* Lys751Gln with an IRR less than 0.62 among carriers of the *XPD* 751Gln allele, compared to women carrying the wild type allele (Hansen et al., 2007) . No association was found among men. The gender differences could hypothetically be caused by a hormonal interaction. However, we observed no interaction between the use of hormone replacement therapy among women and the polymorphism. Thus, we did not find the hypothesis plausible and conclude that our result in the Danish study may be a chance finding.

3.2.2 *XPC* Lys939Gln

In our Danish study and in a Turkish study by Engin *et al.* (Engin et al., 2010) , the *XPC* Lys939Gln polymorphism was not associated with risk of colorectal cancer (Hansen et al., 2007). However, we did observe an interaction between the polymorphism and intake of red meat, with an IRR of 3.70 (CI: 1.70-8.04) for colorectal cancer per 100g red meat intake per day among homozygous carriers of the *XPC* Lys939Gln variant allele (Hansen et al., 2007) . In the light of the sample size and the multiple comparisons being made, this result may be a chance finding. The association was not statistically significant after a Bonferroni correction.

In a large American study by Huang three polymorphisms in *XPC* was studied, including the *XPC* Lys939Gln polymorphism. No association was found between the *XPC* Lys939Gln polymorphism and risk of adenomas (Huang et al., 2006). However, higher risk for development of adenomas was observed among current or recent smokers carrying the *XPC* 939Gln allele (OR=2.0, CI: 1.3-3.0) or a *XPC* haplotype encompassing three linked SNPs in *XPC* (Arg492His, Ala499Val, Lys939Gln) compared with never-smokers carrying the homozygous wild type allele. A study by Joshi *et al.* observed no association between the *XPC* intron 11 polymorphism and risk of colorectal cancer (Joshi et al., 2009) .

In a small study by Berndt *et al.* a tendency for higher risk of proximal colon cancer was observed among homozygous carriers of the variant *XPC* Lys939Gln allele, with an OR of 1.74 (CI: 0.98-3.08) (Berndt et al., 2006). The result may possibly be a chance finding due to sample size and multiple testing. Three other SNPs in the *XPC* gene, see Table 2, were not associated with colorectal cancer risk.

3.2.3 *XPA* G23A

To our knowledge, only three studies have been published on the association of polymorphisms in the *XPA* gene with risk of colorectal cancer: The studies by Berndt *et al.*, Joshi *et al.*, and our study. For a polymorphism positioned in the *XPA* 5´ UTR region, a lower risk for colon cancer cancer was observed among carriers of the T-allele (OR=0.4, 95% CI: 0.2-0.8) compared with homozygous carriers of the C-allele (Joshi et al., 2009) . There was no association for risk of rectal cancer. No association was observed of the *XPA* G23A polymorphism (Hansen et al., 2007) or a polymorphism in the 3´ un-translated region of *XPA* (Berndt et al., 2006) with risk of colorectal cancer.

3.2.4 *ERCC1* Asn118Asn

The results from studies by Skjelbred *et al.* (Skjelbred et al., 2006a) , Joshi *et al.* (Joshi et al., 2009) , and our Danish study (Hansen et al., 2008) on the *ERCC1* Asn118Asn polymorphism suggest no association with risk of colorectal cancer.

Moreno *et al.* examined five polymorphisms in the *ERCC1* gene. A haplotype containing the minor allele of three of the *ERCC1* polymorphisms was associated with a higher risk of colorectal cancer (OR=2.3, 95% CI: 1.0-5.3) compared with carriers of the most frequent haplotype (Moreno et al., 2006). Two other SNPs in the *ERCC1* gene were not associated with risk of colorectal cancer (Mort et al., 2003; Berndt et al., 2006).

3.3 SNPs in NER and risk of other types of cancer than colorectal cancer

Numerous association studies of polymorphisms in genes involved in NER are reported on various types of cancer, with the majority of studies focused on the *XPD* Lys751Gln and *XPD* Asp312Asn polymorphisms. A meta-analysis of lung cancer by Kiyohara *et al.* (with 1913 cases and 1882 controls of different ethnicities) (Kiyohara & Yoshimasu, 2007) suggested among other studies (Xing et al., 2002; Hu et al., 2004; Yin et al., 2006), that carriers of the variant alleles of either of the two *XPD* polymorphisms were found to be at higher risk of lung cancer, while a number of other studies did not observe any association of the two polymorphisms with lung cancer risk (De et al., 2007; Vogel et al., 2005b; Popanda et al., 2004; Hu et al., 2006).

Reference	Polymorphism	Endpoint	Study design	Cases	Controls	Ethnicity	DNA source	Associations (main results)	Interactions
Yeh *et al.*, 2007	*XPD* Lys751Gln	Colorectal cancer	Case-control	727 with carcinomas	736 negative colonoscopy screening	Asian (Taiwan)	Blood samples	Tendency of XPD 751Gln ↑ risk of CRC among men (69 cases/55 controls)	↑risk for colorectal cancer with XPD variant in combinations with several genotypes
Yeh *et al.*, 2005	*XPD* Lys751Gln	Colorectal cancer	Case-control	727 with carcinomas	736 negative colonoscopy screening	Asian (Taiwan)	Blood samples	No association of single SNP	-
Wang *et al.*, 2010	*XPD* Lys751Gln	Colorectal cancer	Case-control	302 with primary colorectal carcinoma	291 free of cancer	Caucasian (India)	Blood samples	No association of single SNP	No GE-interactions with smoking or alcohol consumption
Hansen *et al.*, 2007	*XPD* Lys751Gln *XPD* Asp312Asn *XPA* A23G *XPC* Lys939Gln	Colorectal cancer	Prospective case-cohort	397 with primary colorectal cancer	800 randomly selected from the cohort (10 with colorectal cancer)	Caucasian (Denmark)	Blood samples	No association of single SNPs	GE-interaction between *XPC* polymorphism and intake of red meat No GE-interactions with smoking, alcohol consumption, intake of processed meat, fruit and vegetables
Skjelbred *et al.*, 2006	*XPD* Lys751Gln	Carcinomas and adenomas (high and low-risk)	Case-control	157 with carcinomas, 983 with adenomas (227 high-risk/ 756 low-risk)	399 negative flexible sigmoidoscopy screening	Caucasian (Norway)	Blood samples	↑ risk for low-risk adenomas among carriers of the XPD 751Gln allele compared to homozygous carriers of the wild type allele	No GE-interactions with cigarette smoking
Mort *et al.*, 2003	*XPD* exon 6 *XPD* exon 22 *XPD* exon 23 *ERCC1* exon 4	Colorectal cancer	Case-control	45 with carcinomas	71 hospitalized, not cancer	Caucasian? (England)	Carcinomas/blood samples	No association of single SNPs	-
Engin *et al.*, 2010	*XPD* Lys751Gln *XPD* Asp312Asn	Colorectal cancer	Case-control	110 with carcinomas	116 free of cancer	Caucasian (Turkey)	Blood samples	No association of single SNPs	-
Stern *et al.*, 2009	*XPD* Lys751Gln *XPD* Asp312Asn	Colorectal cancer	Case-control	311 with colorectal cancer	1181 free of cancer	Chinese (Singapore)	Blood/buccal cell samples	No association of single SNPs	-
Stern *et al.*, 2007	*XPD* Lys751Gln *XPD* Asp312Asn	Colorectal cancer	Case-control	310 with colorectal cancer	1176 free of cancer	Chinese (Singapore)	Blood/buccal cell samples	No association of single SNPs	No interaction between XPD polymorphisms and smoking or alcohol consumption, respectively, on colorectal cancer risk
Goodman *et al.*, 2006	*XPD* Asp312Asn	Colon cancer	Case-control	216 men with carcinomas	255 hospitalized men, not cancer, HBV, HIV or HCV	Caucasian, African American (USA)	Primarily blood samples, otherwise colon tissue (some cases)	No association of SNP	No SNP-SNP interaction between the *XPD* polymorphism and other NER polymorphisms
Bigler *et al.*, 2005	*XPD* Lys751Gln *XPD* Asp312Asn	Adenomatous and hyperplastic polyps	Case-control	694 with polyps (384 adenomatous/191 hyperplastic/119 both types)	621 negative colonoscopy screening	Caucasian and Afroamerican (USA)	Blood samples	No association of single SNPs. ↑risk of adenomas for individuals with two *XPD* variant alleles	↑risk of adenomatous polyps among heavy smokers carrying homozygous *XPD* variant compared with nonsmokers who were homozygous wild type. No GE-interactions with consumption of alcohol or meat intake
Stern *et al.*, 2006	*XPD* Lys751Gln	Adenomas	Case-control	740 with adenomas	789 hospitalized, no current or past polyps	Caucasian, African American, Latinos, Asian-Pacific Islander (USA)	Blood samples	↓risk of adenomas among homozygous carriers of the variant allele compared with carriers of the wild type allele	GE-interaction between XPD polymorphism and alcohol consumption No GE-interaction with smoking
Starinsky *et al.*, 2005	*XPD* Lys751Gln	Colorectal cancer	Case-control	456 diagnosed or treated for colorectal cancer	87 hospitalized, not cancer	Jewish (64% Ashkenazi among cases) (Israel)	Blood samples	No association of SNP	↑ risk of colorectal cancer among Ashkenazi Jews age below 50 years when diagnosed, carrying

									the variant allele
Moreno *et al.*, 2006	*XPD* Lys751Gln *XPD* Asp312Asn *ERCC1* 19716 G→C *ERCC1* 19007 T→C *ERCC1* 17677 A→C *ERCC1* 15310 G→C *ERCC1* 8092 C→A	Colorectal adeno-carcinoma	Case-control	377 with carcinomas	329 hospitalized, not cancer	Caucasian (Spain)	Not mentioned	↑ risk of colorectal cancer among carriers of an ERCC1 haplotype (19716C, 19007C, 17677C) No association of single SNPs	No interactions with age
Huang *et al.*, 2006	*XPD* Lys751Gln *XPD* Asp312Asn *XPC* Arg492His *XPC* Ala499Val *XPC* Lys939Gln	Adenomas	Case-control	772 with advanced adenomas in the distal colon	777 negative colonoscopy screening, no family history of CRC	Mixed (USA)	Blood samples	No association of single SNPs	↑ risk of advanced adenomas among current or recent smokers carrying XPC haplotype (492Arg, 499Ala, 939Gln) No interactions with age, gender or ethnicity
Joshi *et al.*, 2009	*XPD* Lys751Gln *XPD* Asp312Asn *XPC* intron 11 *XPA* 5'UTR *ERCC1* 3'UTR	Colorectal cancer	Case-control (case-only analyses)	307 with colorectal cancer	307 unaffected , siblings to the cancer cases	Not mentioned (USA)	Blood samples	No association of SNPs in *XPD*, *XPC* and *ERCC1*. ↑ risk of CRC among homozygous carriers of the variant *XPA* 5'UTR allele (C/C) compared to carriers of the wild type allele.	↑ risk of colorectal cancer from intake of red meat heavily browned on the outside or inside among carriers of the *XPD* codon 751 Lys/Lys or *XPD* codon 312 Asp/Asp genotypes only No GE- interactions with total red meat intake or total intake of red meat cooked by high-temperature methods
Berndt *et al.*, 2006	*XPD* Lys751Gln *XPD* Asp312Asn *XPD* IVS19-70 G→A *XPC* Arg492His *XPC* Ala499Val *XPC* Arg687Arg *XPC* Lys939Gln *XPA* 3'UTR 327 C→G *ERCC1* IVS74 G→C	Colorectal cancer	Case-cohort	250 with carcinomas	2224 (no colorectal cancer diagnosis)	Mixed (98% caucasian among subcohort and full cohort) (USA)	Blood samples	Borderline significant ↑ risk of proximal colon cancer among homozygous carriers of the variant XPC Lys939Gln allele compared to carriers of the wild type allele ↑ risk of colorectal cancer among carriers of 2 or more risk alleles for *XPC* Arg492His and *ERCC6* R1213G (a NER gene)	No interactions with age, gender, smoking, or intake of red meat
Skjelbred *et al.*, 2006	*ERCC1* Asn118Asn	Carcinomas and adenomas (high and low-risk)	Case-control	156 with carcinomas, 981 with adenomas (227 high-risk/ 754 low-risk)	399 negative flexible sigmoidoscopy screening	Caucasian (Norway)	Blood samples	No association of single SNP	No interactions with smoking or alcohol consumption
Hansen *et al.*, 2007	*ERCC1* Asn118Asn	Colorectal cancer	Prospective case-cohort	394 with colorectal cancer	791 randomly selected from the cohort (10 with colorectal cancer)	Caucasian (Denmark)	Blood samples	No association of single SNP	No interactions with smoking or alcohol consumption

Table 2. Studies of possible associations between polymorphisms in *XPD*, *XPA*, *XPC*, and *ERCC1* and risk of colorectal adenomas or colorectal cancer and gene-environment (G E) interaction on risk of colorectal adenomas or colorectal cancer. The results reviewed and included are solely on polymorphisms in the four genes and the environmental factors that are the topic of the present book chapter.

Two large meta-analyses (with 3725 cases and 4152 controls) included identical nine case-control studies but made two dissimilar conclusions: The *XPD* Lys751Gln and *XPD* Asp312Asn polymorphisms are associated with risk of lung cancer (Hu et al., 2004) or no clear association was found (Benhamou & Sarasin, 2005). Some studies suggest an interaction between the two *XPD* polymorphisms and smoking in relation to risk of lung cancer (De et al., 2007; Hu et al., 2006; Xing et al., 2002).

Combinations of the *XPD*, *XPC* and *XPA* genotypes, variant alleles, is suggested to be associated with higher risk of lung cancer (Vogel et al., 2005b). This may be plausible but in the light of multiple testing and the low number of cases this may be a chance finding. The largest breast cancer studies by the number of individuals, 1053 cases/1102 controls (Terry et al., 2004) and 1830 cases/1262 controls (Debniak et al., 2006) observed modest associations of the *XPD* polymorphisms with breast cancer risk. Carriers of the variant *XPD* Lys751Gln allele was associated with a 20% higher risk (OR=1.21, CI: 1.01-1.44) compared with homozygous carriers of the wild type allele. The risk seemed limited to those with a PAH-DNA adduct level above the median, with an OR of 1.61 (CI: 0.99-2.63) among homozygous carriers of the *XPD* 751Gln allele (Terry et al., 2004). Several other studies observed no association of the *XPD* Lys751Gln polymorphism (Debniak et al., 2006; Dufloth et al., 2005; Brewster et al., 2006; Costa et al., 2007; Mechanic et al., 2006; Jorgensen et al., 2007) or the *XPD* Asp312Asn polymorphism (Mechanic et al., 2006; Forsti et al., 2004)to risk of breast cancer. However, higher risk has been detected among ever smoking women carrying the *XPD* 751Gln allele (OR=2.52, CI: 1.27-5.03) compared to ever smoking women carrying the homozygous wild type allele (Metsola et al., 2005). Association with breast cancer risk has been detected when the homozygous variant *XPD* Lys751Gln allele and the homozygous variant *XPD* Asp312Asn allele segregated together, with OR=1.5 ($p<0.05$) and OR=3.69 (CI: 1.76-7.74), respectively (Debniak et al., 2006; Justenhoven et al., 2004). A large study including 2485 cases with single primary melanoma and 1238 cases with second or higher order primary melanomas detected higher melanoma risk among homozygous carriers of the variant *XPD* Lys751Gln allele (OR=1.4, CI: 1.1-1.7) or the variant *XPD* Asp312Asn allele (OR=1.5, CI: 1.2-1.9), respectively (Millikan et al., 2006). Similar results were obtained in a study by Li *et al.* (Li et al., 2006b), while another study observed the inverse association for both polymorphisms (Han et al., 2005). When stratifying by age Baccarelli *et al.* observed an association of the two *XPD* polymorphisms to risk of melanoma only among the individuals older than 50 years when diagnosed (Baccarelli et al., 2004). The *XPD* Lys751Gln (Andrew et al., 2006) and the *XPD* Asp312Asn polymorphism (Wu et al., 2006) have been associated with risk of bladder cancer. An interaction is suggested between the *XPD* Lys751Gln polymorphism and smoking in relation to bladder cancer risk (Andrew et al., 2006; Stern et al., 2002; Schabath et al., 2005). Individuals carrying both the variant *XPD* alleles were more susceptible to development of bladder cancer (Wu et al., 2006; Andrew et al., 2006) than carriers of wild type alleles. The *XPD* Lys751Gln and *XPD* Asp312Asn polymorphisms have not been associated to risk of basal cell carcinoma (Vogel et al., 2005a; Festa et al., 2005; Han et al., 2005; Lovatt et al., 2005), endometrial cancer (Weiss et al., 2006) prostate cancer (Ritchey et al., 2005) or gastric cancer (Huang et al., 2005).

A small study suggest that the variant allele of the polymorphism XPC Lys939Gln is associated with higher risk of bladder cancer (OR=1.49, CI:1.16-1.92) (Sanyal et al., 2004). No association is observed between the polymorphism and risk of lung cancer (Vogel et al., 2005b; Lee et al., 2005; Hu et al., 2006) but a haplotype encompassing more polymorphisms in *XPC* may contribute to a higher risk of lung cancer (Vogel et al., 2005b; Lee et al., 2005;

Hu et al., 2006): Individuals with both putative genotypes of *XPC* Lys939Gln and *XPC* Ala499Val polymorphisms are observed with a 2.4-fold (OR=2.37, CI: 1.33-4.21) higher risk of lung cancer compared with individuals with both wild type genotypes (Vogel et al., 2005b; Lee et al., 2005; Hu et al., 2006), with the higest risk observed among smokers. Polymorphisms in *XPC* have not been associated to risk of basal cell carcinoma (Festa et al., 2005; Nelson et al., 2005), cutaneous melanoma (Blankenburg et al., 2005; Li et al., 2006a) or breast cancer (Mechanic et al., 2006; Jorgensen et al., 2007; Forsti et al., 2004). A lower risk of endometrial cancer may be associated with carriage of at least one variant allele for both *XPC* Lys939Gln and *XPC* Ala499Val polymorphisms (Weiss et al., 2005).

In a Korean population carriers of the wild type allele (G/G or A/G) in the *XPA* G23A polymorphism were reported to have a lower risk of lung cancer compared to carriers of the A/A genotype, with an OR of 0.56 (CI:0.35-0.90) (Park et al., 2002). Similar results were obtained in studies on lung cancer risk in Caucasians and Mexican-Americans (Vogel et al., 2005b; Wu et al., 2003) (Popanda et al., 2004), while a Norwegian study observed the inverse effect with a 1.6-fold higher risk (OR=1.59, CI:1.12-2.27) of lung cancer among carriers of the G/G genotype compared with carriers of the A-allele (Zienolddiny et al., 2006). When stratifying by smoking status the protective effect for lung cancer was only observed among ever smokers (Wu et al., 2003) or current smokers (Park et al., 2002) carrying at least one G-allele or the G/G genotype, respectively. A tendency for lower risk of basal cell carcinoma has been observed among carriers of the variant G-allele, with an OR of 0.82 (CI: 0.66-1.01) and an OR of 0.74 (CI: 0.53-1.03) for homozygous and heterozygous carriers, respectively (Miller et al., 2006). The same tendency was observed for risk of squamous cell carcinoma (Miller et al., 2006). Carriage of at least one A-allele for *XPA* G23A was associated with decreased risk of endometrial cancer, OR=0.47 (CI:0.25-0.82) compared with carriers of the G/G genotype, but only among women with a history of using oral contraceptives (Weiss et al., 2006).

The *ERCC1* Asn118Asn polymorphism is not associated with testicular cancer (Laska et al., 2005). Furthermore, no association has been observed for the *ERCC1* Asn118Asn polymorphism to risk of endometrial cancer (Jo et al., 2007; Weiss et al., 2006), ovarian cancer (Jo et al., 2007) and adult glioma (Wrensch et al., 2005).

All in all the studies suggest that the two *XPD* polymorphisms at amino acid position 312 or 751, the *XPD* Lys751Gln in particular, are associated with risk of cancer in the lung, breast and bladder and seems to modify the effect of smoking on risk of the three cancer forms. The *XPC* Lys939Gln polymorphism may possibly be associated with risk of bladder cancer, and the *XPA* G23A polymorphism may be associated with risk of skin cancer (basal cell carcinoma), endometrial cancer and lung cancer. However, the studies are few and the results are inconsistent.

4. Discussion

In summary, this review, limited by the bias against publication of null findings, highlights the complexities inherent in epidemiological research and, particularly, in molecular epidemiological research on colorectal cancer. Studies on possible associations between SNPs in genes involved in defence of oxidative DNA damages and in nucleotide excision repair and risk of colorectal cancer have not obtained consistent results, why the issue of whether the SNPs are possible biomarkers of susceptibility for colorectal cancer is not satisfactorily clarified at present.

Sample size coupled with allele frequency may have influenced the validity of the results. Differences in the study design, like distribution of gender, age, topology, ethnicity and criteria for recruitment of comparison individuals may have contributed to the dissimilar findings. The application of large, well-designed association studies of the polymorphisms will make it statistically reasonable to make stratified analyses for obtaining information on risk factors in sub-groups and will generally decrease the risk of chance findings. Furthermore, studies including both cases with pre-stages of colorectal cancer and cancer cases will contribute with valuable information of the processes during colorectal carcinogenesis.

Most of the studies analyze individual polymorphisms in genes with modest effect in relation to risk of cancer. Cancer is a complex multigenic and multistage disease involving the interplay of many genetic and environmental factors. Hence, it is unlikely that a single genetic polymorphism in low-penetrance genes would have a dramatic effect on cancer risk. More information may be obtained from haplotyping multiple polymorphisms within genes or from combining multiple polymorphisms within pathways. The continued advances in SNP maps and in high-throughput genotyping methods will facilitate these analyses. Defining haplotypes and whole genome association studies may yield information on unexplored regions of the genome that has impact on colorectal cancer risk and development.

Colorectal cancer is probably caused by a complex interaction between many genetic and environmental factors over time. More and large studies with information on life style factors are required to assess these very possible gene-environment interactions. Identification of gene-environment interactions in cohorts with large relevant exposures has proven to be a useful approach.

Most environmental carcinogens require metabolic activation before they are able to form DNA damages. These activated forms may be detoxified or induce DNA repair or apoptosis. Thus, genetically determined susceptibility to colorectal cancer may depend on the balance among enzymes involved in metabolism and detoxification of carcinogens and on the balance between induction of DNA repair or apoptosis. Further investigations of the combined effects of polymorphisms between genes involved in these four mechanisms may help to clarify the influence of genetic variation in the carcinogenic process and may shed light on the complexities of the many pathways involved in colorectal cancer development, providing hypotheses for future functional studies.

5. Conclusion

In general, the studies suggest that the *XPD* Lys751Gln and *XPD* Asp312Asn polymorphisms may be associated with risk of colorectal adenomas with the possibility of interaction with smoking and alcohol consumption. The reported studies of polymorphisms in *XPC* and *XPA* in relation to risk of colorectal cancer are few, but the results are relatively consistent: In general, no association of the polymorphisms in the genes involved in NER (*XPD, XPC, XPA* and *ERCC1*) was observed with risk of colorectal cancer. A possible interpretation of the results may be that the polymorphisms in the genes *XPD, XPC, XPA* and *ERCC1* are not of major importance in colorectal cancer carcinogenesis, which points towards that lowered repair capacity of the NER pathway may not be a risk factor for development of colorectal cancer.

The results were generally inconsistent or too few to compare to highlight any trend and no strong associations were observed for risk of colorectal adenomas or colorectal cancer.

Overall, the role of genetic variants as SNPs in genes involved in NER is not satisfactorily clarified at present. It is possible that some of the SNPs may contribute to development of adenomas or colorectal cancer only in concomitance with certain dietary and life style factors. Furthermore, it may be only the joint effect of multiple polymorphisms that will provide us with information about genetic susceptibility for colorectal cancer. Larger carefully designed studies with stratified/adjusted analyses of gene-gene and gene-environment interactions may be required in the future to achieve convincing statistically significant results on factors involved in colorectal carcinogenesis.

6. Acknowledgement

Our special thanks go to Anne Tjønneland and Kim Overvad for giving us the opportunity to study the polymorphisms in the Danish prospective cohort Diet, Cancer and Health. We thank Anne-Karin Jensen and Lourdes M. Pedersen for excellent technical assistance for the genotyping in our studies on the Danish cohort. And a thank goes to our co-authors of the manuscripts on the Danish studies for the valuable feedback when writing the manuscripts. The work of the present book chapter was supported by a research grant from the Danish Cancer Society (Grant number R2-A84-09-S2).

7. References

Andrew, A.S., Nelson, H.H., Kelsey, K.T., Moore, J.H., Meng, A.C., Casella, D.P., Tosteson, T.D., Schned, A.R. & Karagas, M.R. (2006). Concordance of multiple analytical approaches demonstrates a complex relationship between DNA repair gene SNPs, smoking and bladder cancer susceptibility. *Carcinogenesis,* Vol. 27, No. 5, pp. (1030-1037)

Baccarelli, A., Calista, D., Minghetti, P., Marinelli, B., Albetti, B., Tseng, T., Hedayati, M., Grossman, L., Landi, G., Struewing, J.P. & Landi, M.T. (2004). XPD gene polymorphism and host characteristics in the association with cutaneous malignant melanoma risk. *Br.J.Cancer,* Vol. 90, No. 2, pp. (497-502)

Balbi, J.C., Larrinaga, M.T., De Stefani, E., Mendilaharsu, M., Ronco, A.L., Boffetta, P. & Brennan, P. (2001). Foods and risk of bladder cancer: a case-control study in Uruguay. *Eur J Cancer Prev,* Vol. 10, No. 5, pp. (453-458)

Batty, D., Rapic'-Otrin, V., Levine, A.S. & Wood, R.D. (2000). Stable binding of human XPC complex to irradiated DNA confers strong discrimination for damaged sites. *J.Mol.Biol.,* Vol. 300, No. 2, pp. (275-290)

Benhamou, S., Laplanche, A., Guillonneau, B., Mejean, A., Desgrandchamps, F., Schrameck, C., Degieux, V. & Perin, F. (2003). DNA adducts in normal bladder tissue and bladder cancer risk. *Mutagenesis,* Vol. 18, No. 5, pp. (445-448)

Benhamou, S. & Sarasin, A. (2005). ERCC2 /XPD gene polymorphisms and lung cancer: a HuGE review. *Am.J.Epidemiol.,* Vol. 161, No. 1, pp. (1-14)

Berndt, S.I., Platz, E.A., Fallin, M.D., Thuita, L.W., Hoffman, S.C. & Helzlsouer, K.J. (2006). Genetic variation in the nucleotide excision repair pathway and colorectal cancer risk. *Cancer Epidemiol.Biomarkers Prev.,* Vol. 15, No. 11, pp. (2263-2269)

Bigler, J., Ulrich, C.M., Kawashima, T., Whitton, J. & Potter, J.D. (2005). DNA repair polymorphisms and risk of colorectal adenomatous or hyperplastic polyps. *Cancer Epidemiol.Biomarkers Prev.,* Vol. 14, No. 11 Pt 1, pp. (2501-2508)

Bingham, S.A., Pignatelli, B., Pollock, J.R., Ellul, A., Malaveille, C., Gross, G., Runswick, S., Cummings, J.H. & O'Neill, I.K. (1996). Does increased endogenous formation of N-nitroso compounds in the human colon explain the association between red meat and colon cancer? *Carcinogenesis,* Vol. 17, No. 3, pp. (515-523)

Binkova, B., Lewtas, J., Miskova, I., Lenicek, J. & Sram, R. (1995). DNA adducts and personal air monitoring of carcinogenic polycyclic aromatic hydrocarbons in an environmentally exposed population. *Carcinogenesis,* Vol. 16, No. 5, pp. (1037-1046)

Blankenburg, S., Konig, I.R., Moessner, R., Laspe, P., Thoms, K.M., Krueger, U., Khan, S.G., Westphal, G., Berking, C., Volkenandt, M., Reich, K., Neumann, C., Ziegler, A., Kraemer, K.H. & Emmert, S. (2005). Assessment of 3 xeroderma pigmentosum group C gene polymorphisms and risk of cutaneous melanoma: a case-control study. *Carcinogenesis,* Vol. 26, No. 6, pp. (1085-1090)

Brewster, A.M., Jorgensen, T.J., Ruczinski, I., Huang, H.Y., Hoffman, S., Thuita, L., Newschaffer, C., Lunn, R.M., Bell, D. & Helzlsouer, K.J. (2006). Polymorphisms of the DNA repair genes XPD (Lys751Gln) and XRCC1 (Arg399Gln and Arg194Trp): relationship to breast cancer risk and familial predisposition to breast cancer. *Breast Cancer Res.Treat.,* Vol. 95, No. 1, pp. (73-80)

Brooks, P.J. & Theruvathu, J.A. (2005). DNA adducts from acetaldehyde: implications for alcohol-related carcinogenesis. *Alcohol,* Vol. 35, No. 3, pp. (187-193)

Bruemmer, B., White, E., Vaughan, T.L. & Cheney, C.L. (1996). Nutrient intake in relation to bladder cancer among middle-aged men and women. *Am J Epidemiol,* Vol. 144, No. 5, pp. (485-495)

Burch, J.D., Craib, K.J., Choi, B.C., Miller, A.B., Risch, H.A. & Howe, G.R. (1987). An exploratory case-control study of brain tumors in adults. *J.Natl.Cancer Inst.,* Vol. 78, No. 4, pp. (601-609)

Carozza, S.E., Olshan, A.F., Faustman, E.M., Gula, M.J., Kolonel, L.N., Austin, D.F., West, E.D., Weiss, N.S., Swanson, G.M., Lyon, J.L. & . (1995). Maternal exposure to N-nitrosatable drugs as a risk factor for childhood brain tumours. *Int.J.Epidemiol.,* Vol. 24, No. 2, pp. (308-312)

Cleaver, J.E. (2005). Cancer in xeroderma pigmentosum and related disorders of DNA repair. *Nat.Rev.Cancer,* Vol. 5, No. 7, pp. (564-573)

Correa Lima, M.P. & Gomes-da-Silva, M.H. (2005). Colorectal cancer: lifestyle and dietary factors. *Nutr.Hosp.,* Vol. 20, No. 4, pp. (235-241)

Costa, S., Pinto, D., Pereira, D., Rodrigues, H., Cameselle-Teijeiro, J., Medeiros, R. & Schmitt, F. (2007). DNA repair polymorphisms might contribute differentially on familial and sporadic breast cancer susceptibility: a study on a Portuguese population. *Breast Cancer Res.Treat.,* Vol. 103, No. 2, pp. (209-217)

Coverley, D., Kenny, M.K., Lane, D.P. & Wood, R.D. (1992). A role for the human single-stranded DNA binding protein HSSB/RPA in an early stage of nucleotide excision repair. *Nucleic Acids Res.,* Vol. 20, No. 15, pp. (3873-3880)

Cross, A.J., Pollock, J.R. & Bingham, S.A. (2003). Haem, not protein or inorganic iron, is responsible for endogenous intestinal N-nitrosation arising from red meat. *Cancer Res.,* Vol. 63, No. 10, pp. (2358-2360)

Culp, S.J., Gaylor, D.W., Sheldon, W.G., Goldstein, L.S. & Beland, F.A. (1998). A comparison of the tumors induced by coal tar and benzo[a]pyrene in a 2-year bioassay. *Carcinogenesis,* Vol. 19, No. 1, pp. (117-124) de Laat, W.L., Sijbers, A.M., Odijk, H., Jaspers, N.G. & Hoeijmakers, J.H. (1998). Mapping of interaction domains between human repair proteins ERCC1 and XPF. *Nucleic Acids Res.*, Vol. 26, No. 18, pp. (4146-4152)

De, R.K., Szaumkessel, M., De, R., I, Dehoorne, A., Vral, A., Claes, K., Velghe, A., Van, M.J. & Thierens, H. (2007). Polymorphisms in base-excision repair and nucleotide-excision repair genes in relation to lung cancer risk. *Mutat.Res.*, Vol. 631, No. 2, pp. (101-110)

Debniak, T., Scott, R.J., Huzarski, T., Byrski, T., Masojc, B., van de, W.T., Serrano-Fernandez, P., Gorski, B., Cybulski, C., Gronwald, J., Debniak, B., Maleszka, R., Kladny, J., Bieniek, A., Nagay, L., Haus, O., Grzybowska, E., Wandzel, P., Niepsuj, S., Narod, S.A. & Lubinski, J. (2006). XPD common variants and their association with melanoma and breast cancer risk. *Breast Cancer Res.Treat.*, Vol. 98, No. 2, pp. (209-215)

Dingley, K.H., Ubick, E.A., Chiarappa-Zucca, M.L., Nowell, S., Abel, S., Ebeler, S.E., Mitchell, A.E., Burns, S.A., Steinberg, F.M. & Clifford, A.J. (2003). Effect of dietary constituents with chemopreventive potential on adduct formation of a low dose of the heterocyclic amines PhIP and IQ and phase II hepatic enzymes. *Nutr.Cancer*, Vol. 46, No. 2, pp. (212-221)

Doyle, V.C. (2007). Nutrition and colorectal cancer risk: a literature review. *Gastroenterol.Nurs.*, Vol. 30, No. 3, pp. (178-182)

Drapkin, R., Reardon, J.T., Ansari, A., Huang, J.C., Zawel, L., Ahn, K., Sancar, A. & Reinberg, D. (1994). Dual role of TFIIH in DNA excision repair and in transcription by RNA polymerase II. *Nature*, Vol. 368, No. 6473, pp. (769-772)

Dufloth, R.M., Costa, S., Schmitt, F. & Zeferino, L.C. (2005). DNA repair gene polymorphisms and susceptibility to familial breast cancer in a group of patients from Campinas, Brazil. *Genet.Mol.Res.*, Vol. 4, No. 4, pp. (771-782)

Engin, A.B., Karahalil, B., Engin, A. & Karakaya, A.E. (2010). Oxidative stress, Helicobacter pylori, and OGG1 Ser326Cys, XPC Lys939Gln, and XPD Lys751Gln polymorphisms in a Turkish population with colorectal carcinoma. *Genet.Test.Mol.Biomarkers*, Vol. 14, No. 4, pp. (559-564)

Evans, E., Fellows, J., Coffer, A. & Wood, R.D. (1997). Open complex formation around a lesion during nucleotide excision repair provides a structure for cleavage by human XPG protein. *EMBO J.*, Vol. 16, No. 3, pp. (625-638)

Fang, J.L. & Vaca, C.E. (1997). Detection of DNA adducts of acetaldehyde in peripheral white blood cells of alcohol abusers. *Carcinogenesis*, Vol. 18, No. 4, pp. (627-632)

Feaver, W.J., Svejstrup, J.Q., Bardwell, L., Bardwell, A.J., Buratowski, S., Gulyas, K.D., Donahue, T.F., Friedberg, E.C. & Kornberg, R.D. (1993). Dual roles of a multiprotein complex from S. cerevisiae in transcription and DNA repair. *Cell*, Vol. 75, No. 7, pp. (1379-1387)

Festa, F., Kumar, R., Sanyal, S., Unden, B., Nordfors, L., Lindholm, B., Snellman, E., Schalling, M., Forsti, A. & Hemminki, K. (2005). Basal cell carcinoma and variants in genes coding for immune response, DNA repair, folate and iron metabolism. *Mutat.Res.*, Vol. 574, No. 1-2, pp. (105-111)

Forsti, A., Angelini, S., Festa, F., Sanyal, S., Zhang, Z., Grzybowska, E., Pamula, J., Pekala, W., Zientek, H., Hemminki, K. & Kumar, R. (2004). Single nucleotide polymorphisms in breast cancer. *Oncol.Rep.*, Vol. 11, No. 4, pp. (917-922)

Georgiadis, P., Topinka, J., Stoikidou, M., Kaila, S., Gioka, M., Katsouyanni, K., Sram, R., Autrup, H. & Kyrtopoulos, S.A. (2001). Biomarkers of genotoxicity of air pollution (the AULIS project): bulky DNA adducts in subjects with moderate to low exposures to airborne polycyclic aromatic hydrocarbons and their relationship to environmental tobacco smoke and other parameters. *Carcinogenesis,* Vol. 22, No. 9, pp. (1447-1457)

Goldberg, M.S., Parent, M.E., Siemiatycki, J., Desy, M., Nadon, L., Richardson, L., Lakhani, R., Latreille, B. & Valois, M.F. (2001). A case-control study of the relationship between the risk of colon cancer in men and exposures to occupational agents. *Am J Ind Med,* Vol. 39, No. 6, pp. (531-546)

Gomaa, E.A., Gray, J.I., Rabie, S., Lopez-Bote, C. & Booren, A.M. (1993). Polycyclic aromatic hydrocarbons in smoked food products and commercial liquid smoke flavourings. *Food Addit.Contam,* Vol. 10, No. 5, pp. (503-521)

Goodman, J.E., Mechanic, L.E., Luke, B.T., Ambs, S., Chanock, S. & Harris, C.C. (2006). Exploring SNP-SNP interactions and colon cancer risk using polymorphism interaction analysis. *Int.J.Cancer,* Vol. 118, No. 7, pp. (1790-1797)

Guillen, M.D., Sopelana, P. & Partearroyo, M.A. (1997). Food as a source of polycyclic aromatic carcinogens. *Rev.Environ.Health,* Vol. 12, No. 3, pp. (133-146)

Guzder, S.N., Sung, P., Prakash, L. & Prakash, S. (1998). Affinity of yeast nucleotide excision repair factor 2, consisting of the Rad4 and Rad23 proteins, for ultraviolet damaged DNA. *J.Biol.Chem.,* Vol. 273, No. 47, pp. (31541-31546)

Han, J., Colditz, G.A., Liu, J.S. & Hunter, D.J. (2005). Genetic variation in XPD, sun exposure, and risk of skin cancer. *Cancer Epidemiol.Biomarkers Prev.,* Vol. 14, No. 6, pp. (1539-1544)

Hanawalt, P.C. (2002). Subpathways of nucleotide excision repair and their regulation. *Oncogene,* Vol. 21, No. 58, pp. (8949-8956)

Hansen, R.D., Sorensen, M., Tjonneland, A., Overvad, K., Wallin, H., Raaschou-Nielsen, O. & Vogel, U. (2007). XPA A23G, XPC Lys939Gln, XPD Lys751Gln and XPD Asp312Asn polymorphisms, interactions with smoking, alcohol and dietary factors, and risk of colorectal cancer. *Mutat.Res.,* Vol. 619, No. 1-2, pp. (68-80)

Hansen, R.D., Sorensen, M., Tjonneland, A., Overvad, K., Wallin, H., Raaschou-Nielsen, O. & Vogel, U. (2008). A haplotype of polymorphisms in ASE-1, RAI and ERCC1 and the effects of tobacco smoking and alcohol consumption on risk of colorectal cancer: a Danish prospective case-cohort study. *BMC.Cancer,* Vol. 8, pp. (54)

Hecht, S.S. (2003). Tobacco carcinogens, their biomarkers and tobacco-induced cancer. *Nat.Rev.Cancer,* Vol. 3, No. 10, pp. (733-744)

Hecht, S.S. & Hoffmann, D. (1988). Tobacco-specific nitrosamines, an important group of carcinogens in tobacco and tobacco smoke. *Carcinogenesis,* Vol. 9, No. 6, pp. (875-884)

Hemminki, K., Dickey, C., Karlsson, S., Bell, D., Hsu, Y., Tsai, W.Y., Mooney, L.A., Savela, K. & Perera, F.P. (1997). Aromatic DNA adducts in foundry workers in relation to exposure, life style and CYP1A1 and glutathione transferase M1 genotype. *Carcinogenesis,* Vol. 18, No. 2, pp. (345-350)

Hemminki, K., Grzybowska, E., Chorazy, M., Twardowska-Saucha, K., Sroczynski, J.W., Putman, K.L., Randerath, K., Phillips, D.H., Hewer, A., Santella, R.M. & . (1990a).

DNA adducts in human environmentally exposed to aromatic compounds in an industrial area of Poland. *Carcinogenesis,* Vol. 11, No. 7, pp. (1229-1231)

Hemminki, K., Randerath, K., Reddy, M.V., Putman, K.L., Santella, R.M., Perera, F.P., Young, T.L., Phillips, D.H., Hewer, A. & Savela, K. (1990b). Postlabeling and immunoassay analysis of polycyclic aromatic hydrocarbons--adducts of deoxyribonucleic acid in white blood cells of foundry workers. *Scand J Work Environ Health,* Vol. 16, No. 3, pp. (158-162)

Hemminki, K., Soderling, J., Ericson, P., Norbeck, H.E. & Segerback, D. (1994). DNA adducts among personnel servicing and loading diesel vehicles. *Carcinogenesis,* Vol. 15, No. 4, pp. (767-769)

Hotchkiss, J.H. (1989). Preformed N-nitroso compounds in foods and beverages. *Cancer Surv.,* Vol. 8, No. 2, pp. (295-321)

Hou, S.M., Falt, S., Angelini, S., Yang, K., Nyberg, F., Lambert, B. & Hemminki, K. (2002). The XPD variant alleles are associated with increased aromatic DNA adduct level and lung cancer risk. *Carcinogenesis,* Vol. 23, No. 4, pp. (599-603)

Hu, Z., Wei, Q., Wang, X. & Shen, H. (2004). DNA repair gene XPD polymorphism and lung cancer risk: a meta-analysis. *Lung Cancer,* Vol. 46, No. 1, pp. (1-10)

Hu, Z., Xu, L., Shao, M., Yuan, J., Wang, Y., Wang, F., Yuan, W., Qian, J., Ma, H., Wang, Y., Liu, H., Chen, W., Yang, L., Jing, G., Huo, X., Chen, F., Jin, L., Wei, Q., Wu, T., Lu, D., Huang, W. & Shen, H. (2006). Polymorphisms in the two helicases ERCC2/XPD and ERCC3/XPB of the transcription factor IIH complex and risk of lung cancer: a case-control analysis in a Chinese population. *Cancer Epidemiol.Biomarkers Prev.,* Vol. 15, No. 7, pp. (1336-1340)

Huang, W.Y., Berndt, S.I., Kang, D., Chatterjee, N., Chanock, S.J., Yeager, M., Welch, R., Bresalier, R.S., Weissfeld, J.L. & Hayes, R.B. (2006). Nucleotide excision repair gene polymorphisms and risk of advanced colorectal adenoma: XPC polymorphisms modify smoking-related risk. *Cancer Epidemiol.Biomarkers Prev.,* Vol. 15, No. 2, pp. (306-311)

Huang, W.Y., Chow, W.H., Rothman, N., Lissowska, J., Llaca, V., Yeager, M., Zatonski, W. & Hayes, R.B. (2005). Selected DNA repair polymorphisms and gastric cancer in Poland. *Carcinogenesis,* Vol. 26, No. 8, pp. (1354-1359)

Hunting, D.J., Gowans, B.J. & Dresler, S.L. (1991). DNA polymerase delta mediates excision repair in growing cells damaged with ultraviolet radiation. *Biochem.Cell Biol.,* Vol. 69, No. 4, pp. (303-308)

International Agency for Research on Cancer (IARC). Polynuclear aromatic compounds. Part I: Chemical, environmental and experimental data. IARC monograph on the evaluation of carcinogenic risk of chemical to man. (32). 1983. Lyon, France, IARC.

International Agency for Research on Cancer (IARC) (2003). *Fruit and vegetables* IARC Press, Lyon

Iversen, L.H., Pedersen, L., Riis, A., Friis, S., Laurberg, S. & Sorensen, H.T. (2005). Population-based study of short- and long-term survival from colorectal cancer in Denmark, 1977-1999. *Br.J.Surg.,* Vol. 92, No. 7, pp. (873-880)

Jaspers, N.G., Raams, A., Silengo, M.C., Wijgers, N., Niedernhofer, L.J., Robinson, A.R., Giglia-Mari, G., Hoogstraten, D., Kleijer, W.J., Hoeijmakers, J.H. & Vermeulen, W. (2007). First reported patient with human ERCC1 deficiency has cerebro-oculo-facio-skeletal syndrome with a mild defect in nucleotide excision repair and severe developmental failure. *Am.J.Hum.Genet.*, Vol. 80, No. 3, pp. (457-466)

Jemal, A., Siegel, R., Ward, E., Murray, T., Xu, J., Smigal, C. & Thun, M.J. (2006). Cancer statistics, 2006. *CA Cancer J.Clin.*, Vol. 56, No. 2, pp. (106-130)

Ji, B.T., Weissfeld, J.L., Chow, W.H., Huang, W.Y., Schoen, R.E. & Hayes, R.B. (2006). Tobacco smoking and colorectal hyperplastic and adenomatous polyps. *Cancer Epidemiol.Biomarkers Prev.*, Vol. 15, No. 5, pp. (897-901)

Jo, H., Kang, S., Kim, S.I., Kim, J.W., Park, N.H., Song, Y.S., Park, S.Y., Kang, S.B. & Lee, H.P. (2007). The C19007T Polymorphism of ERCC1 and Its Correlation with the Risk of Epithelial Ovarian and Endometrial Cancer in Korean Women. A Case Control Study. *Gynecol.Obstet.Invest*, Vol. 64, No. 2, pp. (84-88)

Johnson, I.T. & Lund, E.K. (2007). Review article: nutrition, obesity and colorectal cancer. *Aliment.Pharmacol.Ther.*, Vol. 26, No. 2, pp. (161-181)

Jorgensen, T.J., Visvanathan, K., Ruczinski, I., Thuita, L., Hoffman, S. & Helzlsouer, K.J. (2007). Breast cancer risk is not associated with polymorphic forms of xeroderma pigmentosum genes in a cohort of women from Washington County, Maryland. *Breast Cancer Res.Treat.*, Vol. 101, No. 1, pp. (65-71)

Joshi, A.D., Corral, R., Siegmund, K.D., Haile, R.W., Le, M.L., Martinez, M.E., Ahnen, D.J., Sandler, R.S., Lance, P. & Stern, M.C. (2009). Red meat and poultry intake, polymorphisms in the nucleotide excision repair and mismatch repair pathways and colorectal cancer risk. *Carcinogenesis*, Vol. 30, No. 3, pp. (472-479)

Justenhoven, C., Hamann, U., Pesch, B., Harth, V., Rabstein, S., Baisch, C., Vollmert, C., Illig, T., Ko, Y.D., Bruning, T. & Brauch, H. (2004). ERCC2 genotypes and a corresponding haplotype are linked with breast cancer risk in a German population. *Cancer Epidemiol.Biomarkers Prev.*, Vol. 13, No. 12, pp. (2059-2064)

Khan, S.G., Metter, E.J., Tarone, R.E., Bohr, V.A., Grossman, L., Hedayati, M., Bale, S.J., Emmert, S. & Kraemer, K.H. (2000). A new xeroderma pigmentosum group C poly(AT) insertion/deletion polymorphism. *Carcinogenesis*, Vol. 21, No. 10, pp. (1821-1825)

Kiyohara, C. & Yoshimasu, K. (2007). Genetic polymorphisms in the nucleotide excision repair pathway and lung cancer risk: a meta-analysis. *Int.J.Med.Sci.*, Vol. 4, No. 2, pp. (59-71)

Kobayashi, K., Karran, P., Oda, S. & Yanaga, K. (2005). Involvement of mismatch repair in transcription-coupled nucleotide excision repair. *Hum.Cell*, Vol. 18, No. 3, pp. (103-115)

Kyrtopoulos, S.A., Georgiadis, P., Autrup, H., Demopoulos, N.A., Farmer, P., Haugen, A., Katsouyanni, K., Lambert, B., Ovrebo, S., Sram, R., Stephanou, G. & Topinka, J. (2001). Biomarkers of genotoxicity of urban air pollution. Overview and descriptive data from a molecular epidemiology study on populations exposed to moderate-to-low levels of polycyclic aromatic hydrocarbons: the AULIS project. *Mutat Res*, Vol. 496, No. 1-2, pp. (207-228)

Laska, M.J., Nexo, B.A., Vistisen, K., Poulsen, H.E., Loft, S. & Vogel, U. (2005). Polymorphisms in RAI and in genes of nucleotide and base excision repair are not associated with risk of testicular cancer. *Cancer Lett.*, Vol. 225, No. 2, pp. (245-251)

Lee, K.M., Choi, J.Y., Kang, C., Kang, C.P., Park, S.K., Cho, H., Cho, D.Y., Yoo, K.Y., Noh, D.Y., Ahn, S.H., Park, C.G., Wei, Q. & Kang, D. (2005). Genetic polymorphisms of selected DNA repair genes, estrogen and progesterone receptor status, and breast cancer risk. *Clin.Cancer Res.*, Vol. 11, No. 12, pp. (4620-4626)

Lewin, M.H., Bailey, N., Bandaletova, T., Bowman, R., Cross, A.J., Pollock, J., Shuker, D.E. & Bingham, S.A. (2006). Red meat enhances the colonic formation of the DNA adduct O6-carboxymethyl guanine: implications for colorectal cancer risk. *Cancer Res.*, Vol. 66, No. 3, pp. (1859-1865)

Lewtas, J., Walsh, D., Williams, R. & Dobias, L. (1997). Air pollution exposure-DNA adduct dosimetry in humans and rodents: evidence for non-linearity at high doses. *Mutat Res*, Vol. 378, No. 1-2, pp. (51-63)

Li, C., Hu, Z., Liu, Z., Wang, L.E., Strom, S.S., Gershenwald, J.E., Lee, J.E., Ross, M.I., Mansfield, P.F., Cormier, J.N., Prieto, V.G., Duvic, M., Grimm, E.A. & Wei, Q. (2006a). Polymorphisms in the DNA repair genes XPC, XPD, and XPG and risk of cutaneous melanoma: a case-control analysis. *Cancer Epidemiol.Biomarkers Prev.*, Vol. 15, No. 12, pp. (2526-2532)

Li, H., Yao, L., Ouyang, T., Li, J., Wang, T., Fan, Z., Fan, T., Dong, B., Lin, B., Li, J. & Xie, Y. (2006b). Association of p73 G4C14-to-A4T14 (GC/AT) polymorphism with breast cancer survival. *Carcinogenesis*,

Lovatt, T., Alldersea, J., Lear, J.T., Hoban, P.R., Ramachandran, S., Fryer, A.A., Smith, A.G. & Strange, R.C. (2005). Polymorphism in the nuclear excision repair gene ERCC2/XPD: association between an exon 6-exon 10 haplotype and susceptibility to cutaneous basal cell carcinoma. *Hum.Mutat.*, Vol. 25, No. 4, pp. (353-359)

Masutani, C., Sugasawa, K., Yanagisawa, J., Sonoyama, T., Ui, M., Enomoto, T., Takio, K., Tanaka, K., van der Spek, P.J., Bootsma, D. & . (1994). Purification and cloning of a nucleotide excision repair complex involving the xeroderma pigmentosum group C protein and a human homologue of yeast RAD23. *EMBO J.*, Vol. 13, No. 8, pp. (1831-1843)

Matullo, G., Palli, D., Peluso, M., Guarrera, S., Carturan, S., Celentano, E., Krogh, V., Munnia, A., Tumino, R., Polidoro, S., Piazza, A. & Vineis, P. (2001). XRCC1, XRCC3, XPD gene polymorphisms, smoking and (32)P-DNA adducts in a sample of healthy subjects. *Carcinogenesis*, Vol. 22, No. 9, pp. (1437-1445)

Meador, J.P., Stein, J.E., Reichert, W.L. & Varanasi, U. (1995). Bioaccumulation of polycyclic aromatic hydrocarbons by marine organisms. *Rev.Environ.Contam Toxicol.*, Vol. 143, pp. (79-165)

Mechanic, L.E., Millikan, R.C., Player, J., de Cotret, A.R., Winkel, S., Worley, K., Heard, K., Heard, K., Tse, C.K. & Keku, T. (2006). Polymorphisms in nucleotide excision repair genes, smoking and breast cancer in African Americans and whites: a population-based case-control study. *Carcinogenesis*, Vol. 27, No. 7, pp. (1377-1385)

Melikian, A.A., Sun, P., Prokopczyk, B., El-Bayoumy, K., Hoffmann, D., Wang, X. & Waggoner, S. (1999). Identification of benzo[a]pyrene metabolites in cervical mucus and DNA adducts in cervical tissues in humans by gas chromatography-mass spectrometry. *Cancer Lett*, Vol. 146, pp. (127-134)

Metsola, K., Kataja, V., Sillanpaa, P., Siivola, P., Heikinheimo, L., Eskelinen, M., Kosma, V.M., Uusitupa, M. & Hirvonen, A. (2005). XRCC1 and XPD genetic polymorphisms, smoking and breast cancer risk in a Finnish case-control study. *Breast Cancer Res.*, Vol. 7, No. 6, pp. (R987-R997)

Miller, K.L., Karagas, M.R., Kraft, P., Hunter, D.J., Catalano, P.J., Byler, S.H. & Nelson, H.H. (2006). XPA, haplotypes, and risk of basal and squamous cell carcinoma. *Carcinogenesis,* Vol. 27, No. 8, pp. (1670-1675)

Millikan, R.C., Hummer, A., Begg, C., Player, J., de Cotret, A.R., Winkel, S., Mohrenweiser, H., Thomas, N., Armstrong, B., Kricker, A., Marrett, L.D., Gruber, S.B., Culver, H.A., Zanetti, R., Gallagher, R.P., Dwyer, T., Rebbeck, T.R., Busam, K., From, L., Mujumdar, U. & Berwick, M. (2006). Polymorphisms in nucleotide excision repair genes and risk of multiple primary melanoma: the Genes Environment and Melanoma Study. *Carcinogenesis,* Vol. 27, No. 3, pp. (610-618)

Mirvish, S.S. (1995). Role of N-nitroso compounds (NOC) and N-nitrosation in etiology of gastric, esophageal, nasopharyngeal and bladder cancer and contribution to cancer of known exposures to NOC. *Cancer Lett.,* Vol. 93, No. 1, pp. (17-48)

Moller, P., Wallin, H., Vogel, U., Autrup, H., Risom, L., Hald, M.T., Daneshvar, B., Dragsted, L.O., Poulsen, H.E. & Loft, S. (2002). Mutagenicity of 2-amino-3-methylimidazo[4,5-f]quinoline in colon and liver of Big Blue rats: role of DNA adducts, strand breaks, DNA repair and oxidative stress. *Carcinogenesis,* Vol. 23, No. 8, pp. (1379-1385)

Mooney, L.A., Bell, D.A., Santella, R.M., Van Bennekum, A.M., Ottman, R., Paik, M., Blaner, W.S., Lucier, G.W., Covey, L., Young, T.L., Cooper, T.B., Glassman, A.H. & Perera, F.P. (1997). Contribution of genetic and nutritional factors to DNA damage in heavy smokers. *Carcinogenesis,* Vol. 18, No. 3, pp. (503-509)

Mooney, L.A., Madsen, A.M., Tang, D., Orjuela, M.A., Tsai, W.Y., Garduno, E.R. & Perera, F.P. (2005). Antioxidant vitamin supplementation reduces benzo(a)pyrene-DNA adducts and potential cancer risk in female smokers. *Cancer Epidemiol Biomarkers Prev,* Vol. 14, No. 1, pp. (237-242)

Moreno, V., Gemignani, F., Landi, S., Gioia-Patricola, L., Chabrier, A., Blanco, I., Gonzalez, S., Guino, E., Capella, G. & Canzian, F. (2006). Polymorphisms in genes of nucleotide and base excision repair: risk and prognosis of colorectal cancer. *Clin.Cancer Res.,* Vol. 12, No. 7 Pt 1, pp. (2101-2108)

Mort, R., Mo, L., McEwan, C. & Melton, D.W. (2003). Lack of involvement of nucleotide excision repair gene polymorphisms in colorectal cancer. *Br J Cancer,* Vol. 89, No. 2, pp. (333-337)

Mu, D., Hsu, D.S. & Sancar, A. (1996). Reaction mechanism of human DNA repair excision nuclease. *J.Biol.Chem.,* Vol. 271, No. 14, pp. (8285-8294)

Nelson, H.H., Christensen, B. & Karagas, M.R. (2005). The XPC poly-AT polymorphism in non-melanoma skin cancer. *Cancer Lett.,* Vol. 222, No. 2, pp. (205-209)

Niedernhofer, L.J., Essers, J., Weeda, G., Beverloo, B., de, W.J., Muijtjens, M., Odijk, H., Hoeijmakers, J.H. & Kanaar, R. (2001). The structure-specific endonuclease Ercc1-Xpf is required for targeted gene replacement in embryonic stem cells. *EMBO J.,* Vol. 20, No. 22, pp. (6540-6549)

Nielsen, P.S., Andreassen, A., Farmer, P.B., Ovrebo, S. & Autrup, H. (1996a). Biomonitoring of diesel exhaust-exposed workers. DNA and hemoglobin adducts and urinary 1-hydroxypyrene as markers of exposure. *Toxicol Lett,* Vol. 86, No. 1, pp. (27-37)

Nielsen, P.S., de Pater, N., Okkels, H. & Autrup, H. (1996b). Environmental air pollution and DNA adducts in Copenhagen bus drivers--effect of GSTM1 and NAT2 genotypes on adduct levels. *Carcinogenesis,* Vol. 17, No. 5, pp. (1021-1027)

Nielsen, P.S., Okkels, H., Sigsgaard, T., Kyrtopoulos, S. & Autrup, H. (1996c). Exposure to urban and rural air pollution: DNA and protein adducts and effect of glutathione-S-transferase genotype on adduct levels. *Int Arch Occup Environ Health,* Vol. 68, No. 3, pp. (170-176)

Norat, T., Bingham, S., Ferrari, P., Slimani, N., Jenab, M., Mazuir, M., Overvad, K., Olsen, A., Tjonneland, A., Clavel, F., Boutron-Ruault, M.C., Kesse, E., Boeing, H., Bergmann, M.M., Nieters, A., Linseisen, J., Trichopoulou, A., Trichopoulos, D., Tountas, Y., Berrino, F., Palli, D., Panico, S., Tumino, R., Vineis, P., Bueno-de-Mesquita, H.B., Peeters, P.H., Engeset, D., Lund, E., Skeie, G., Ardanaz, E., Gonzalez, C., Navarro, C., Quiros, J.R., Sanchez, M.J., Berglund, G., Mattisson, I., Hallmans, G., Palmqvist, R., Day, N.E., Khaw, K.T., Key, T.J., San Joaquin, M., Hemon, B., Saracci, R., Kaaks, R. & Riboli, E. (2005). Meat, fish, and colorectal cancer risk: the European Prospective Investigation into cancer and nutrition. *J.Natl.Cancer Inst.,* Vol. 97, No. 12, pp. (906-916)

Palli, D., Masala, G., Peluso, M., Gaspari, L., Krogh, V., Munnia, A., Panico, S., Saieva, C., Tumino, R., Vineis, P. & Garte, S. (2004). The effects of diet on DNA bulky adduct levels are strongly modified by GSTM1 genotype: a study on 634 subjects. *Carcinogenesis,* Vol. 25, No. 4, pp. (577-584)

Palli, D., Masala, G., Vineis, P., Garte, S., Saieva, C., Krogh, V., Panico, S., Tumino, R., Munnia, A., Riboli, E. & Peluso, M. (2003). Biomarkers of dietary intake of micronutrients modulate DNA adduct levels in healthy adults. *Carcinogenesis,* Vol. 24, No. 4, pp. (739-746)

Palli, D., Russo, A., Masala, G., Saieva, C., Guarrera, S., Carturan, S., Munnia, A., Matullo, G. & Peluso, M. (2001). DNA adduct levels and DNA repair polymorphisms in traffic-exposed workers and a general population sample. *Int J Cancer,* Vol. 94, No. 1, pp. (121-127)

Palli, D., Vineis, P., Russo, A., Berrino, F., Krogh, V., Masala, G., Munnia, A., Panico, S., Taioli, E., Tumino, R., Garte, S. & Peluso, M. (2000). Diet, metabolic polymorphisms and dna adducts: the EPIC-Italy cross-sectional study. *Int J Cancer,* Vol. 87, No. 3, pp. (444-451)

Park, C.H., Mu, D., Reardon, J.T. & Sancar, A. (1995). The general transcription-repair factor TFIIH is recruited to the excision repair complex by the XPA protein independent of the TFIIE transcription factor. *J.Biol.Chem.,* Vol. 270, No. 9, pp. (4896-4902)

Park, C.H. & Sancar, A. (1994). Formation of a ternary complex by human XPA, ERCC1, and ERCC4(XPF) excision repair proteins. *Proc.Natl.Acad.Sci.U.S.A,* Vol. 91, No. 11, pp. (5017-5021)

Park, J.Y., Park, S.H., Choi, J.E., Lee, S.Y., Jeon, H.S., Cha, S.I., Kim, C.H., Park, J.H., Kam, S., Park, R.W., Kim, I.S. & Jung, T.H. (2002). Polymorphisms of the DNA repair gene xeroderma pigmentosum group A and risk of primary lung cancer. *Cancer Epidemiol.Biomarkers Prev.,* Vol. 11, No. 10 Pt 1, pp. (993-997)

Peluso, M., Merlo, F., Munnia, A., Valerio, F., Perrotta, A., Puntoni, R. & Parodi, S. (1998). 32P-postlabeling detection of aromatic adducts in the white blood cell DNA of nonsmoking police officers. *Cancer Epidemiol Biomarkers Prev,* Vol. 7, No. 1, pp. (3-11)

Perera, F.P., Dickey, C., Santella, R., O'Neill, J.P., Albertini, R.J., Ottman, R., Tsai, W.Y., Mooney, L.A., Savela, K. & Hemminki, K. (1994). Carcinogen-DNA adducts and gene mutation in foundry workers with low-level exposure to polycyclic aromatic hydrocarbons. *Carcinogenesis,* Vol. 15, No. 12, pp. (2905-2910)

Perera, F.P., Hemminki, K., Young, T.L., Brenner, D., Kelly, G. & Santella, R.M. (1988). Detection of polycyclic aromatic hydrocarbon-DNA adducts in white blood cells of foundry workers. *Cancer Res,* Vol. 48, No. 8, pp. (2288-2291)

Peters, U., Sinha, R., Bell, D.A., Rothman, N., Grant, D.J., Watson, M.A., Kulldorff, M., Brooks, L.R., Warren, S.H. & DeMarini, D.M. (2004). Urinary mutagenesis and fried red meat intake: influence of cooking temperature, phenotype, and genotype of metabolizing enzymes in a controlled feeding study. *Environ Mol Mutagen,* Vol. 43, No. 1, pp. (53-74)

Phillips, D.H. (2002). Smoking-related DNA and protein adducts in human tissues. *Carcinogenesis,* Vol. 23, No. 12, pp. (1979-2004)

Pierre, F., Tache, S., Petit, C.R., Van der, M.R. & Corpet, D.E. (2003). Meat and cancer: haemoglobin and haemin in a low-calcium diet promote colorectal carcinogenesis at the aberrant crypt stage in rats. *Carcinogenesis,* Vol. 24, No. 10, pp. (1683-1690)

Poirier, M.C., Weston, A., Schoket, B., Shamkhani, H., Pan, C.F., McDiarmid, M.A., Scott, B.G., Deeter, D.P., Heller, J.M., Jacobson-Kram, D. & Rothman, N. (1998). Biomonitoring of United States Army soldiers serving in Kuwait in 1991. *Cancer Epidemiol Biomarkers Prev,* Vol. 7, No. 6, pp. (545-551)

Popanda, O., Schattenberg, T., Phong, C.T., Butkiewicz, D., Risch, A., Edler, L., Kayser, K., Dienemann, H., Schulz, V., Drings, P., Bartsch, H. & Schmezer, P. (2004). Specific combinations of DNA repair gene variants and increased risk for non-small cell lung cancer. *Carcinogenesis,* Vol. 25, No. 12, pp. (2433-2441)

Preston-Martin, S. & Mack, W. (1991). Gliomas and meningiomas in men in Los Angeles County: investigation of exposures to N-nitroso compounds. *IARC Sci.Publ.,* No. 105, pp. (197-203)

Qiao, Y., Spitz, M.R., Shen, H., Guo, Z., Shete, S., Hedayati, M., Grossman, L., Mohrenweiser, H. & Wei, Q. (2002). Modulation of repair of ultraviolet damage in the host-cell reactivation assay by polymorphic XPC and XPD/ERCC2 genotypes. *Carcinogenesis,* Vol. 23, No. 2, pp. (295-299)

Reardon, J.T., Mu, D. & Sancar, A. (1996). Overproduction, purification, and characterization of the XPC subunit of the human DNA repair excision nuclease. *J.Biol.Chem.,* Vol. 271, No. 32, pp. (19451-19456)

Reardon, J.T. & Sancar, A. (2002). Molecular anatomy of the human excision nuclease assembled at sites of DNA damage. *Mol.Cell Biol.,* Vol. 22, No. 16, pp. (5938-5945)

Ritchey, J.D., Huang, W.Y., Chokkalingam, A.P., Gao, Y.T., Deng, J., Levine, P., Stanczyk, F.Z. & Hsing, A.W. (2005). Genetic variants of DNA repair genes and prostate cancer: a population-based study. *Cancer Epidemiol.Biomarkers Prev.,* Vol. 14, No. 7, pp. (1703-1709)

Rothman, N., Correa-Villasenor, A., Ford, D.P., Poirier, M.C., Haas, R., Hansen, J.A., O'Toole, T. & Strickland, P.T. (1993). Contribution of occupation and diet to white blood cell polycyclic aromatic hydrocarbon-DNA adducts in wildland firefighters. *Cancer Epidemiol Biomarkers Prev,* Vol. 2, No. 4, pp. (341-347)

Rothman, N., Poirier, M.C., Baser, M.E., Hansen, J.A., Gentile, C., Bowman, E.D. & Strickland, P.T. (1990). Formation of polycyclic aromatic hydrocarbon-DNA adducts in peripheral white blood cells during consumption of charcoal-broiled beef. *Carcinogenesis,* Vol. 11, No. 7, pp. (1241-1243)

Sanyal, S., Festa, F., Sakano, S., Zhang, Z., Steineck, G., Norming, U., Wijkstrom, H., Larsson, P., Kumar, R. & Hemminki, K. (2004). Polymorphisms in DNA repair and metabolic genes in bladder cancer. *Carcinogenesis,* Vol. 25, No. 5, pp. (729-734)

Schabath, M.B., Delclos, G.L., Grossman, H.B., Wang, Y., Lerner, S.P., Chamberlain, R.M., Spitz, M.R. & Wu, X. (2005). Polymorphisms in XPD exons 10 and 23 and bladder cancer risk. *Cancer Epidemiol.Biomarkers Prev.,* Vol. 14, No. 4, pp. (878-884)

Schaeffer, L., Roy, R., Humbert, S., Moncollin, V., Vermeulen, W., Hoeijmakers, J.H., Chambon, P. & Egly, J.M. (1993). DNA repair helicase: a component of BTF2 (TFIIH) basic transcription factor. *Science,* Vol. 260, No. 5104, pp. (58-63)

Schottenfeld, D. & Winawer, S.J. (1996). Cancers of the large intestine, In: *Cancer Epidemiology and Prevention,* Schottenfeld, D. & Fraumeni J.F.Jr., pp. (813-840), Oxford University Press, New York

Shivji, K.K., Kenny, M.K. & Wood, R.D. (1992). Proliferating cell nuclear antigen is required for DNA excision repair. *Cell,* Vol. 69, No. 2, pp. (367-374)

Shivji, M.K., Podust, V.N., Hubscher, U. & Wood, R.D. (1995). Nucleotide excision repair DNA synthesis by DNA polymerase epsilon in the presence of PCNA, RFC, and RPA. *Biochemistry,* Vol. 34, No. 15, pp. (5011-5017)

Sijbers, A.M., de Laat, W.L., Ariza, R.R., Biggerstaff, M., Wei, Y.F., Moggs, J.G., Carter, K.C., Shell, B.K., Evans, E., de Jong, M.C., Rademakers, S., de, R.J., Jaspers, N.G., Hoeijmakers, J.H. & Wood, R.D. (1996). Xeroderma pigmentosum group F caused by a defect in a structure-specific DNA repair endonuclease. *Cell,* Vol. 86, No. 5, pp. (811-822)

Sinha, R., Peters, U., Cross, A.J., Kulldorff, M., Weissfeld, J.L., Pinsky, P.F., Rothman, N. & Hayes, R.B. (2005). Meat, meat cooking methods and preservation, and risk for colorectal adenoma. *Cancer Res.,* Vol. 65, No. 17, pp. (8034-8041)

Sinha, R., Rothman, N., Brown, E.D., Salmon, C.P., Knize, M.G., Swanson, C.A., Rossi, S.C., Mark, S.D., Levander, O.A. & Felton, J.S. (1995). High concentrations of the carcinogen 2-amino-1-methyl-6-phenylimidazo- [4,5-b]pyridine (PhIP) occur in chicken but are dependent on the cooking method. *Cancer Res.,* Vol. 55, No. 20, pp. (4516-4519)

Skjelbred, C.F., Sabo, M., Nexo, B.A., Wallin, H., Hansteen, I.L., Vogel, U. & Kure, E.H. (2006a). Effects of polymorphisms in ERCC1, ASE-1 and RAI on the risk of colorectal carcinomas and adenomas: A case control study. *BMC.Cancer,* Vol. 6, No. 1, pp. (175)

Skjelbred, C.F., Saebo, M., Wallin, H., Nexo, B.A., Hagen, P.C., Lothe, I.M., Aase, S., Johnson, E., Hansteen, I.L., Vogel, U. & Kure, E.H. (2006b). Polymorphisms of the XRCC1, XRCC3 and XPD genes and risk of colorectal adenoma and carcinoma, in a Norwegian cohort: a case control study. *BMC.Cancer,* Vol. 6, pp. (67)

Skog, K., Steineck, G., Augustsson, K. & Jagerstad, M. (1995). Effect of cooking temperature on the formation of heterocyclic amines in fried meat products and pan residues. *Carcinogenesis,* Vol. 16, No. 4, pp. (861-867)

Spitz, M.R., Wu, X., Wang, Y., Wang, L.E., Shete, S., Amos, C.I., Guo, Z., Lei, L., Mohrenweiser, H. & Wei, Q. (2001). Modulation of nucleotide excision repair capacity by XPD polymorphisms in lung cancer patients. *Cancer Res.,* Vol. 61, No. 4, pp. (1354-1357)

Starinsky, S., Figer, A., Ben Asher, E., Geva, R., Flex, D., Fidder, H.H., Zidan, J., Lancet, D. & Friedman, E. (2005). Genotype phenotype correlations in Israeli colorectal cancer patients. *International Journal of Cancer,* Vol. 114, No. 1, pp. (58-73), 0020-7136

Stern, M.C., Butler, L.M., Corral, R., Joshi, A.D., Yuan, J.M., Koh, W.P. & Yu, M.C. (2009). Polyunsaturated fatty acids, DNA repair single nucleotide polymorphisms and colorectal cancer in the Singapore Chinese Health Study. *J.Nutrigenet.Nutrigenomics.,* Vol. 2, No. 6, pp. (273-279)

Stern, M.C., Conti, D.V., Siegmund, K.D., Corral, R., Yuan, J.M., Koh, W.P. & Yu, M.C (2007). DNA repair single-nucleotide polymorphisms in colorectal cancer and their role as modifiers of the effect of cigarette smoking and alcohol in the Singapore Chinese Health Study. *Cancer Epidemiol.Biomarkers Prev.,* Vol. 16, No. 11, pp. (2363-2372)

Stern, M.C., Johnson, L.R., Bell, D.A. & Taylor, J.A. (2002). XPD codon 751 polymorphism, metabolism genes, smoking, and bladder cancer risk. *Cancer Epidemiol.Biomarkers Prev.,* Vol. 11, No. 10 Pt 1, pp. (1004-1011)

Stern, M.C., Siegmund, K.D., Conti, D.V., Corral, R. & Haile, R.W. (2006). XRCC1, XRCC3, and XPD polymorphisms as modifiers of the effect of smoking and alcohol on colorectal adenoma risk. *Cancer Epidemiol.Biomarkers Prev.,* Vol. 15, No. 12, pp. (2384-2390)

Stigger, E., Drissi, R. & Lee, S.H. (1998). Functional analysis of human replication protein A in nucleotide excision repair. *J.Biol.Chem.,* Vol. 273, No. 15, pp. (9337-9343)

Sugasawa, K., Ng, J.M., Masutani, C., Iwai, S., van der Spek, P.J., Eker, A.P., Hanaoka, F., Bootsma, D. & Hoeijmakers, J.H. (1998). Xeroderma pigmentosum group C protein complex is the initiator of global genome nucleotide excision repair. *Mol.Cell,* Vol. 2, No. 2, pp. (223-232)

Terry, M.B., Gammon, M.D., Zhang, F.F., Eng, S.M., Sagiv, S.K., Paykin, A.B., Wang, Q., Hayes, S., Teitelbaum, S.L., Neugut, A.I. & Santella, R.M. (2004). Polymorphism in the DNA repair gene XPD, polycyclic aromatic hydrocarbon-DNA adducts, cigarette smoking, and breast cancer risk. *Cancer Epidemiol.Biomarkers Prev.,* Vol. 13, No. 12, pp. (2053-2058)

Tomkinson, A.E. & Levin, D.S. (1997). Mammalian DNA ligases. *Bioessays,* Vol. 19, No. 10, pp. (893-901)

van Maanen, J.M., Moonen, E.J., Maas, L.M., Kleinjans, J.C. & Van Schooten, F.J. (1994). Formation of aromatic DNA adducts in white blood cells in relation to urinary excretion of 1-hydroxypyrene during consumption of grilled meat. *Carcinogenesis,* Vol. 15, No. 10, pp. (2263-2268)

Viguier, J., Boige, V., Miquel, C., Pocard, M., Giraudeau, B., Sabourin, J.C., Ducreux, M., Sarasin & A., Praz, F. (2005). ERCC1 codon 118 polymorphism is a predictive factor for the tumor response to oxaliplatin/5-fluorouracil combination chemotherapy in patients with advanced colorectal cancer. *Clin.Cancer.Res.,* Vol. 11, pp. (6212-6217)

Vogel, U., Olsen, A., Wallin, H., Overvad, K., Tjonneland, A. & Nexo, B.A. (2005a). Effect of polymorphisms in XPD, RAI, ASE-1 and ERCC1 on the risk of basal cell carcinoma among Caucasians after age 50. *Cancer Detect.Prev.,* Vol. 29, No. 3, pp. (209-214)

Vogel, U., Overvad, K., Wallin, H., Tjonneland, A., Nexo, B.A. & Raaschou-Nielsen, O. (2005b). Combinations of polymorphisms in XPD, XPC and XPA in relation to risk of lung cancer. *Cancer Lett.*, Vol. 222, No. 1, pp. (67-74)

Volker, M., Mone, M.J., Karmakar, P., van, H.A., Schul, W., Vermeulen, W., Hoeijmakers, J.H., van, D.R., Van Zeeland, A.A. & Mullenders, L.H. (2001). Sequential assembly of the nucleotide excision repair factors in vivo. *Mol.Cell*, Vol. 8, No. 1, pp. (213-224)

Wakasugi, M. & Sancar, A. (1998). Assembly, subunit composition, and footprint of human DNA repair excision nuclease. *Proc.Natl.Acad.Sci.U.S.A*, Vol. 95, No. 12, pp. (6669-6674)

Wakasugi, M. & Sancar, A. (1999). Order of assembly of human DNA repair excision nuclease. *J.Biol.Chem.*, Vol. 274, No. 26, pp. (18759-18768)

Wang, J., Zhao, Y., Jiang, J., Gajalakshmi, V., Kuriki, K., Nakamura, S., Akasaka, S., Ishikawa, H., Suzuki, S., Nagaya, T. & Tokudome, S. (2010). Polymorphisms in DNA repair genes XRCC1, XRCC3 and XPD, and colorectal cancer risk: a case-control study in an Indian population. *J.Cancer Res.Clin.Oncol.*, Vol. 136, No. 10, pp. (1517-1525)

Weiss, J.M., Weiss, N.S., Ulrich, C.M., Doherty, J.A. & Chen, C. (2006). Nucleotide excision repair genotype and the incidence of endometrial cancer: effect of other risk factors on the association. *Gynecol.Oncol.*, Vol. 103, No. 3, pp. (891-896)

Weiss, J.M., Weiss, N.S., Ulrich, C.M., Doherty, J.A., Voigt, L.F. & Chen, C. (2005). Interindividual variation in nucleotide excision repair genes and risk of endometrial cancer. *Cancer Epidemiol.Biomarkers Prev.*, Vol. 14, No. 11 Pt 1, pp. (2524-2530)

Wrensch, M., Kelsey, K.T., Liu, M., Miike, R., Moghadassi, M., Sison, J.D., Aldape, K., McMillan, A., Wiemels, J. & Wiencke, J.K. (2005). ERCC1 and ERCC2 polymorphisms and adult glioma. *Neuro.Oncol.*, Vol. 7, No. 4, pp. (495-507)

Wu, X., Gu, J., Grossman, H.B., Amos, C.I., Etzel, C., Huang, M., Zhang, Q., Millikan, R.E., Lerner, S., Dinney, C.P. & Spitz, M.R. (2006). Bladder cancer predisposition: a multigenic approach to DNA-repair and cell-cycle-control genes. *Am.J.Hum.Genet.*, Vol. 78, No. 3, pp. (464-479)

Wu, X., Zhao, H., Wei, Q., Amos, C.I., Zhang, K., Guo, Z., Qiao, Y., Hong, W.K. & Spitz, M.R. (2003). XPA polymorphism associated with reduced lung cancer risk and a modulating effect on nucleotide excision repair capacity. *Carcinogenesis*, Vol. 24, No. 3, pp. (505-509)

Xing, D., Tan, W., Wei, Q. & Lin, D. (2002). Polymorphisms of the DNA repair gene XPD and risk of lung cancer in a Chinese population. *Lung Cancer*, Vol. 38, No. 2, pp. (123-129)

Yang, K., Fang, J.L. & Hemminki, K. (1998). Abundant lipophilic DNA adducts in human tissues. *Mutat Res*, Vol. 422, No. 2, pp. (285-295)

Yeh, C.C., Sung, F.C., Tang, R., Chang-Chieh, C.R. & Hsieh, L.L. (2005). Polymorphisms of the XRCC1, XRCC3, & XPD genes, and colorectal cancer risk: a case-control study in Taiwan. *BMC.Cancer*, Vol. 5, pp. (12)

Yeh, C.C., Sung, F.C., Tang, R., Chang-Chieh, C.R. & Hsieh, L.L. (2007). Association between polymorphisms of biotransformation and DNA-repair genes and risk of colorectal cancer in Taiwan. *J.Biomed.Sci.*, Vol. 14, No. 2, pp. (183-193)

Yin, J., Vogel, U., Ma, Y., Guo, L., Wang, H. & Qi, R. (2006). Polymorphism of the DNA repair gene ERCC2 Lys751Gln and risk of lung cancer in a northeastern Chinese population. *Cancer Genet.Cytogenet.*, Vol. 169, No. 1, pp. (27-32)

Yokoi, M., Masutani, C., Maekawa, T., Sugasawa, K., Ohkuma, Y. & Hanaoka, F. (2000). The xeroderma pigmentosum group C protein complex XPC-HR23B plays an important role in the recruitment of transcription factor IIH to damaged DNA. *J.Biol.Chem.*, Vol. 275, No. 13, pp. (9870-9875)

You, J.S., Wang, M. & Lee, S.H. (2003). Biochemical analysis of the damage recognition process in nucleotide excision repair. *J.Biol.Chem.*, Vol. 278, No. 9, pp. (7476-7485)

Zienolddiny, S., Campa, D., Lind, H., Ryberg, D., Skaug, V., Stangeland, L., Phillips, D.H., Canzian, F. & Haugen, A. (2006). Polymorphisms of DNA repair genes and risk of non-small cell lung cancer. *Carcinogenesis*, Vol. 27, No. 3, pp. (560-567)

28

Variants and Polymorphisms of DNA Repair Genes and Neurodegenerative Diseases

Fabio Coppedè
Contract Professor at Faculty of Medicine, University of Pisa
Italy

1. Introduction

Oxidative DNA damage is one of the earliest detectable events in several neurodegenerative diseases, often preceding the onset of the clinical symptoms. Moreover, neurons in the adult human brain can re-enter the cell division cycle, likely allowing DNA repair. Impairments of DNA repair pathways are reported in neurons of patients suffering from one of several neurodegenative diseases and might result in the accumulation of mutations critical for neurodegeneration. Current investigation aims at understanding the causes of such impairment (Coppedè & Migliore, 2010). One of the most robust set of data that demonstrates association between DNA repair and neurodegenerative diseases comes from studies on early onset ataxia with ocular motor apraxia and hypoalbuminemia/ataxia with oculomotor apraxia type 1 (EAOH/AOA1), an autosomal recessive form of cerebellar ataxia caused by mutations in the aprataxin (*APTX*) gene. It was shown that aprataxin participates in DNA repair suggesting that genes involved in DNA repair pathways might have a role in neurodegeneration (Hirano et al., 2007; Takahashi et al., 2007). Also parkin, encoded by one of the causative genes of Parkinson's disease (PD), seems to contribute to DNA repair (Kao, 2009). Variants and polymorphisms of DNA repair genes, particularly DNA base excision repair (BER) genes, have been investigated as possible risk factors for Alzheimer's disease (AD), Parkinson's disease, amyotrophic lateral sclerosis (ALS), and other neurodegenerative diseases (Coppedè & Migliore, 2010). There is also evidence that BER could contribute to CAG repeat expansion in Huntington's disease (HD) (Kovtun et al., 2007). Most of the genetic association studies have been performed in the last few years and gave often conflicting or inconclusive results, their power was limited by the sample size of case-control groups, gene-gene interactions were missing, and only common polymorphisms have been included with little or no attention paid to rare gene variants (Coppedè, 2011). In this chapter I discuss the current knowledge on DNA repair gene variants and polymorphisms and major neurodegenerative disorders.

2. DNA repair pathways

A brief overview of the major DNA repair pathways in mammals is shown in Table 1. It is estimated that our cells are subjected to a daily average of about one million lesions that, if not properly repaired, can drive mutagenesis, disrupt normal gene expression or create aberrant protein products. Cells have therefore developed several repair systems that can be generally divided into single stand break (SSB) and double strand break (DSB) repair pathways (Table 1).

Pathway	Type of repair	Type of damage
Base excision repair (BER)	SSB	Modifications of DNA bases due to oxidation, alkylation, and deamination
Nucleotide excision repair (NER)	SSB	Repair of UV photoproducts, DNA crosslinks, and bulky lesions.
Mismatch repair (MMR)	SSB	Repair of mismatches and small insertions or deletions during replication.
Homologous recombination (HR)	DSB	Repair of DNA DSBs, such as those caused by ionizing radiations, through recombination with regions of homology (usually a sister chromatid) during late S or G2 phases of the cell cycle
Non homologous end joining (NHEJ)	DSB	Repair of DNA DSBs, such as those induced by radiations, without recombination with regions of homology; it occurs during G0, G1, and early S phases of the cell cycle

Table 1. Major DNA repair pathways in mammalian cells

2.1 Base excision repair (BER)

The DNA base excision repair pathway deserves a detailed description since it is believed to be the major pathway for repairing DNA base modifications caused by oxidation, deamination and alkylation. DNA glycosylases catalyze the first step in the BER process by cleaving the N-glycosylic bond between a damaged base and the sugar moiety; after the cleavage the damaged base is released resulting in the formation of an abasic site which is then cleaved by an AP lyase activity or by the major mammalian apurinic/apyrimidinic endonuclease (APEX1). Repair can then proceed through short or long-patch BER. In short-patch BER, which is the most common sub-pathway, a single nucleotide is incorporated into the gap by DNA polymerase β (Pol β) and ligated by the DNA ligase III/ X-ray repair cross-complementing group 1 (XRCC1) complex. In long-patch BER several nucleotides (two to seven-eight) are incorporated, followed by cleavage of the resulting 5′ flap structure and ligation. It has been suggested that after Pol β adds the first nucleotide into the gap, it is substituted by Pol δ/ε which continues long-patch BER. DNA ligase I completes the long-patch pathway. Several other proteins, including the proliferating cell nuclear antigen (PCNA), the RPA protein, and the 5′-flap endonuclease (FEN-1) participate in long-patch BER. Recent evidence suggests that XRCC1 acts as a scaffold protein in short-patch BER, regulating and coordinating the whole process. XRCC1 recruits DNA Pol β and DNA ligase III required for filling and sealing the damaged strand. Moreover, it also interacts with DNA glycosylases and APEX1, mediating their exchange at the damaged site. XRCC1 also interacts with PARP-1, which is one of the cellular sensors of DNA SSBs and DSBs. BER takes places either in nuclei and mitochondria, and mitochondria have independent BER machinery encoded by nuclear genes. Indeed, several BER enzymes have been identified which have both nuclear and mitochondrial forms. The gaps generated by the action of AP endonucleases/lyases are filled in by Pol γ in the mitochondria, and ligation is mediate by ligase III. To date, there is no evidence of long-patch BER in mitochondria (Weissman et al., 2007).

2.2 Nucleotide excision repair (NER)

The nucleotide excision repair pathway (NER) is required for the removal of a wide variety of forms of DNA damage, including UV induced photoproducts, DNA crosslinks, and other bulky lesions. NER involves at least 20-30 proteins or complexes of proteins, and is divided into global genome repair (GGR) and transcription coupled repair (TCR). The two pathways mainly differ in the initial steps that recognize the DNA lesion, and different initial recognition factors are involved. NER senses the presence of a lesion through the distortion it causes to the DNA structure. In GGR DNA damage recognition requires the xeroderma pigmentosum (XP) complementing protein XPC-HR23B-centrin complex. The DNA damage is verified by opening of the DNA strands surrounding the lesion by the transcription factor TFIIH. This is followed by recruitment of XPA and other components of the transcription factor TFIIH to the lesion site. In TCR the recognition step is initiated when a RNA polymerase stalls at a lesion site and requires the Cockayne's syndrome proteins CSA and CSB. After a correct assembly of the NER complex, a fragment of 24-32 nucleotides is incised and removed from the damaged strand by the simultaneous action of the DNA excision repair cross complementing (ERCC) proteins ERCC5 (XPG; 3′ endonuclease) and ERCC4 (XPF; 5′ endonuclease) complexed with ERCC1. Repair is completed by new DNA synthesis mediated by DNA Pol δ/ε, DNA Pol κ, and ligation (DNA ligase I, DNA ligase III) of the nascent DNA to the parental strands using the undamaged strand as a template. The GGR pathway removes damages overall in the genome irrespective of genome location and point in the cell cycle, whereas TCR is required for the specific repair of bulky lesions in the transcribed strand of active genes. Mitochondria have been shown to lack NER, which operates in the nucleus removing the majority of DNA lesions (Fleck & Nielsen, 2004; Subba Rao, 2007).

2.3 Mismatch repair (MMR)

Mismatch repair (MMR) corrects mismatches and small insertions or deletions during DNA replication, thus eliminating potentially pre-mutagenic bases. Repair involves recognition of the mismatch by MutSα (MSH2 and MSH6 proteins), or by MutSβ (MSH2 and MSH3 proteins) in the case of small insertions/deletions (1-10 nucleotides). MutLα (a heterodimer of MLH1 and PMS2 proteins) is then recruited and serves to coordinate the process that involves, among others, the PCNA protein for strand discrimination and exonuclease 1, DNA Pol δ and a DNA ligase, for DNA repair (Kunkel & Erie, 2005).

2.4 Homologous recombination (HR) and non homologous end joining (NHEJ)

Non homologous end joining (NHEJ) is the major pathway for the repair of DSBs because it can function throughout the cell cycle and does not require a homologous chromosome. Rather, NHEJ involves rejoining of what remains of the two DNA ends, tolerating nucleotide loss or addition at the rejoining site. When a DSB occurs during G0, G1, and early

S phase, the Ku heterodimer (Ku70/Ku80) recognizes DSB ends, aligns them, protects them from excessive degradation, and ultimately prepares them for ligation. The Ku heterodimer is capable of interacting with the nuclease (Artemis-DNA-PKcs) complex, the polymerases (μ and λ), and the ligase (XLF-XRCC4-DNA ligase IV) complex. If complementary ends are not present at the break, the Artemis-DNA-PKcs complex resects some of the overhangs to create single-strand overhangs with short stretches of micro-homology. When necessary, polymerization of missing nucleotides is performed by DNA polymerases. Then, the XLF-XRCC4-LigaseIV complex seals the DSB. When homologous recombination (HR) is used for repair, it is promoted by the recombinase RAD51, the human homolog of the *E. coli* RecA protein, which binds to 3'-tailed single strands at the end of DSBs in a helical fashion and promotes pairing with homologous DNA sequences (usually the sister chromatid) as a prelude to strand invasion and repair of the DSBs. Strand invasion is the invasion of the 3' end of the single-stranded DNA overhang into the region of complementarity in the intact sister chromatid. The process is directed by RAD51 which forms a nucleoprotein filament that directs homology search, strand pairing, and invasion of the homologous chromosome. Rad51 is assisted in this process by several RAD family members (RAD51B, RAD51C, RAD51D, XRCC2, XRCC3, RAD54, and RAD52). During strand invasion, RAD51 creates a four-stranded Holliday junction intermediate. Then, the invading strand is extended by DNA polymerase η and the Holliday junction is resolved by a RAD51C and XRCC3 directed mechanism. Several nucleases and helicases, such as the RecQ family members, also participate in resolving Holliday junctions. Since eukaryotic genomes contain dispersed repeated DNA, repair of DSBs by HR can occur not only through an interaction with the sister chromatid or the homolog chromosome, but also with repeats on non-homolog chromosomes. Numerous factors affect the decision to repair a DSB via these pathways, and accumulating evidence suggests these major repair pathways both cooperate and compete with each other at double-strand break sites to facilitate efficient repair and promote genomic integrity (Kass & Jasin, 2010).

3. Polymorphisms of DNA repair genes and Alzheimer's disease

Alzheimer's disease is a complex multi-factorial neurodegenerative disorder and represents the most common form of dementia in the elderly. In 2006, the worldwide prevalence of AD was 26.6 million. It has been estimated that following the global aging of the world's population this number will quadruple by 2050, suggesting that 1 in 85 persons worldwide will be living with the disease, which is clinically characterized by a progressive neurodegeneration in selected brain regions, including the temporal and parietal lobes and restricted regions within the frontal cortex and the cingulate gyrus, resulting in gross atrophy of the affected regions and leading to memory loss accompanied by changes of behaviour and personality severe enough to affect work, lifelong hobbies or social life (Brookmeyer et al., 2007). Increasing evidence reports oxidative DNA damage in affected brain regions of AD patients, paralleled by a decrease in DNA repair activities, particularly concerning the BER pathway (Lovell et al., 2000; Weissman et al., 2007). This has driven current research to focus on common polymorphisms of BER genes as candidate AD risk factors. Studied genes are those encoding for 8-oxoguanine DNA glycosylase (OGG1), APEX1 and XRCC1. Particularly, we screened 178 Italian late onset AD patients and 146 matched controls for the presence of the *OGG1* Ser326Cys gene polymorphism (rs1052133), observing no difference in allele and genotype frequencies between patients and controls (Coppedè et al., 2007a). Subsequently, 91 sporadic Turkish AD patients and 93 matched controls have been genotyped for the presence of *OGG1* Ser326Cys, *APEX1* Asp148Glu (rs1130409), *XRCC1* Arg280His (rs25489) and *XRCC1* Arg399Gln (rs25487) polymorphisms, but none of them was associated with increased AD risk (Parildar-Karpuzoğlu et al. 2008). Also a small case-control study performed in Poland with 41 AD patients and 51 controls failed to find significant differences in *OGG1* Ser326Cys allele frequencies between groups (Dorszewska et al., 2009). A borderline association with AD risk (*P* =0.06) was observed for the *XRCC1* Arg194Trp (rs1799782) polymorphism in a group of 98 Turkish AD patients and 95 healthy subjects (Doğru-Abbasoğlu et al., 2007), but a recent study failed to replicate this association in a larger case-control group of over 200 Chinese AD patients (Quian et al., 2010). Overall, five common functional polymorphisms of BER genes have been investigated as possible AD risk factors, but none of them resulted significantly associated with increased AD risk (Table 2). Also polymorphisms of NER genes have been evaluated as candidate AD risk factors. Particularly, two common polymorphisms of the *XPD (ERCC2)* gene (namely, rs238406 and rs13181), and a silent mutation in exon 11 (T>C at codon 824) of the *XPF (XRCC4)* gene have been investigated in 97 Turkish AD patients and in 101 matched controls, but none of them resulted to be associated with AD risk (Doğru-Abbasoğlu et al., 2006). Poly-ADP-ribose polymerase-1 (PARP-1) is a zinc-finger DNA binding protein that is activated by DNA SSBs or DSBs. The primary function of PARP-1 is in DNA repair processes through the detection of DNA damage and the prevention of chromatide exchanges. PARP-1 poly-ADP-ribosylates several proteins involved in DNA repair including histones, thus inducing local relaxation of the chromatin structure and facilitating the access of repair proteins to damaged DNA. There is evidence for widespread DNA SSBs and DSBs in AD brains, as well as increased PARP-1 activity (Love et al., 1999). Two independent groups evaluated *PARP-1* gene polymorphisms as putative AD risk factors. Infante and coworkers screened 263 Spanish AD patients and 293 matched controls for the presence of two *PARP-1* promoter polymorphisms (-410 and -1672). If evaluated independently, nor *PARP-1* -410 neither *PARP-1* -1672 resulted associated with increased AD risk (Table 2). However, *PARP-1* -410 and *PARP-1* -1672 polymorphisms resulted in linkage disequilibrium and some haplotypes were associated with increased AD risk. Particularly, haplotypes 2-1 and 1-2 were significantly overrepresented in AD individuals and associated with an increased risk for the disease with an adjusted OR of 1.42 and 5.38, respectively (Infante et al., 2007). More recently two *PARP-1* exonic polymorphisms, 414C>T (rs1805404) and 2456T>C (rs1136410), have been evaluated in 120 Chinese AD patients and 111 matched controls (Liu et al., 2010). Again, none of the polymorphisms resulted independently associated with increased AD risk (Table 2). However, authors found that the distributions of haplotype 3-TT and haplotype 4-CC were significantly associated with an increased risk of AD, whereas the haplotype 1-TC showed a protective effect, with OR of 12.2 and 0.52, respectively (Liu et al., 2010). Overall, both studies support the hypothesis that *PARP1* haplotypes might affect AD risk.

3.1 Searching for BER gene variants in DNA extracted from post-mortem AD brain

Mao and colleagues extracted nuclear DNA from post-mortem brain specimens of 14 late stage AD patients and 10 neurologically healthy controls. They identified and characterized novel *OGG1* mutations (a single base deletion C796del, and two base substitutions leading

Reference	Polymorphism	Number of subjects AD/Controls	Variant allele frequency AD/Controls	Odds Ratio (95% CI)
Coppedè et al., 2007a	OGG1 Ser326Cys	178/146	0.19/0.18	1.04 (0.70-1.55)
Parildar-Karpuzoğlu et al. 2008	OGG1 Ser326Cys	91/93	0.29/0.23	1.32 (0.83-2.11)
Dorszewska et al., 2009	OGG1 Ser326Cys	41/51	0.29/0.21	1.60 (0.81-3.14)
Parildar-Karpuzoğlu et al. 2008	APEX1 Asp148Glu	91/93	0.33/0.31	1.08 (0.70-1.68)
Parildar-Karpuzoğlu et al. 2008	XRCC1 Arg280His	91/93	0.06/0.10	0.53 (0.24-1.14)
Parildar-Karpuzoğlu et al. 2008	XRCC1 Arg399Gln	91/93	034/0.33	1.05 (0.68-1.63)
Doğru-Abbasoğlu et al., 2007	XRCC1 Arg194Trp	98/95	0.11/0.06	2.06 (0.97-4.37)
Quian et al., 2010	XRCC1 Arg194Trp	212/203	0.31/0.31	1.04 (0.70-1.52)
Doğru-Abbasoğlu et al., 2006	ERCC2 rs238406 (XPD exon 6)	97/101	0.40/0.42	0.94 (0.63-1.41)
Doğru-Abbasoğlu et al., 2006	ERCC2 rs13181 (XPD exon 23)	97/101	0.41/0.36	1.24 (0.83-1.86)
Doğru-Abbasoğlu et al., 2006	ERCC4 (XPF exon 11)	97/101	0.37/0.35	1.09 (0.72-1.64)
Infante et al., 2007a	PARP-1 (-410)	263/293	0.35/0.33	1.08 (0.84-1.38)
Infante et al., 2007a	PARP-1 (-1672)	263/293	0.17/0.18	0.94 (0.69-1.27)
Liu et al., 2010	PARP-1 (rs1805404)	120/111	0.53/0.59	0.76 (0.53-1.11)
Liu et al., 2010	PARP-1 (rs1136410)	120/111	0.52/0.59	0.75 (0.52-1.09)

Table 2. DNA repair gene polymorphisms and risk of Alzheimer's disease

to Ala53Thr or Ala288Val amino acidic changes, respectively) in 4 of 14 AD subjects. Particularly, two AD patients carried the C796 deletion, one patient had the Ala53Thr substitution, and another patient carried the Ala288Val substitution. No mutations were found in any of 10 studied age-matched controls (Mao et al., 2007). This study is not an association study for risk assessment but a genetic screening performed on brain DNA specimens searching for novel *OGG1* variants. The authors created the mutant proteins by site-directed mutagenesis observing that the C796del mutant OGG1 lacks glycosylase activity, whereas both Ala53Thr and Ala288Val substitutions result in 40–50% reduced activity (Mao et al., 2007). Therefore, we cannot exclude that the activity of the OGG1 protein might be partially impaired by rare gene variants in some AD subjects. However, given the limited sample-size of the studied case-control group, further studies are required to confirm this hypothesis.

4. Polymorphisms of DNA repair genes and amyotrophic lateral sclerosis

Amyotrophic lateral sclerosis (ALS), also known as motor neuron disease (MND), is one of the major neurodegenerative diseases alongside AD and PD. It is a progressive disorder characterized by the degeneration of motor neurons of the motor cortex, brainstem and spinal cord. The incidence of the disease is similar worldwide and ranges from 1 to 3 cases per 100,000 individuals per year, with the exception of some high-risk areas around the Pacific Rim. Several studies report increased oxidative DNA damage and a compromised DNA repair activity, particularly BER activity, in spinal cords and other tissues of ALS patients (Bogdanov et al., 2000; Ferrante et al., 1997; Kikuchi et al., 2002; Kisby et al., 1997). Missense mutations in the gene encoding *APEX1* were found in DNA obtained from 8 of 11 ALS patients, including the common *APEX1* Asp148Glu polymorphism (Hayward et al., 1999), that was subsequently associated with increased ALS risk in a Scottish cohort of 117 ALS patients and 58 controls, and in an Irish group of 105 ALS individuals and 82 controls (Greenway et al., 2004). The analysis of 88 English ALS patients and 88 matched controls still revealed an increased frequency of the variant allele in the ALS cohort, even if not statistically significant (Tomkins et al. 2000). We have recently performed the largest case-control study aimed at clarifying the role of *APEX1* Asp148Glu in sporadic ALS pathogenesis. No difference in *APEX1* Asp148Glu allele and genotype frequencies was found between 134 ALS patients and 129 controls of Italian origin, nor was the polymorphism associated with disease age or site of onset, or duration of the disease, suggesting that it might not play a major role in ALS pathogenesis in the Italian population (Coppedè et al., 2010a). The ALSGene database (www.alsgene.org) is a public database containing all the ALS genetic association studies, genome-wide association studies and updated meta-analyses of the literature. A meta-analysis of the four studies described above revealed a significant increased frequency of the variant 148Glu allele in ALS cases with respect to controls, suggesting a protective role for the wild type 148Asp variant with an OR = 0.78 (95%CI=0.62-0.97) (www.alsgene.org). Our analysis of the *OGG1* Ser326Cys polymorphism in 136 ALS patients and 129 matched controls of Italian origin revealed a significant association of the variant allele with increased ALS risk (Coppedè et al., 2007b) (Table 3). At best of our knowledge this study is the first in the literature addressing this issue, still pending replication in other populations. More recently, we screened over 400 individuals, including 206 ALS patients and 203 matched controls of Italian origin for the presence of *XRCC1* Arg194Trp, Arg280His and Arg399Gln polymorphisms, observing a significant increased frequency of the 399Gln variant allele and a borderline significant decreased frequency of the 194Trp allele in ALS patients with respect to controls (Coppedè et al., 2010b). Interestingly, others have evaluated the same *XRCC1* polymorphisms and two additional ones (rs939461 and rs915927) in 108 ALS patients and 39 controls from New-England, observing that rs939461 was associated with reduced ALS risk, and Arg399Gln with a borderline significant reduced risk (Fang et al., 2010) (Table 3). Overall, even if still inconclusive, the results of both studies suggest that additional investigation is required to clarify the role of *XRCC1* polymorphisms and haplotypes in ALS pathogenesis.

4.1 Less frequent BER gene variants and polymorphisms

Alongside with common BER gene polymorphisms, less frequent gene variants or polymorphisms have been observed in the DNA of both ALS subjects and matched controls, but with very low allele frequencies and no significant difference between groups. Some examples are *APEX1* 1835C/A (Intron3), *APEX1* 2712A/T (3'UTR), *APEX1* 459C/T (Exon1), and *APEX1* rs1048945 (Q51H) (Hayward et al., 1999; Tomkins et al., 2000).

Reference	Polymorphism	Number of subjects ALS/Controls	Variant allele frequency ALS/Controls	Odds Ratio (95% CI)
Coppedè et al., 2007b	OGG1 Ser326Cys	136/129	0.26/0.18	1.62 (1.07-2.45)
Hayward et al. 1999	APEX1 Asp148Glu	117/58	0.62/0.49	1.66 (1.06-2.60)
Tomkins et al. 2000	APEX1 Asp148Glu	88/88	0.51/0.45	1.28 (0.85-1.95)
Greenway et al. 2004	APEX1 Asp148Glu	105/82	0.60/0.51	1.46 (0.97-2.21)
Coppedè et al. 2010a	APEX1 Asp148Glu	134/129	0.44/0.45	0.99 (0.70-1.40)
Coppedè et al. 2010b	XRCC1 Arg194Trp	206/195	0.05/0.08	0.58 (0.32-1.05)
Coppedè et al. 2010b	XRCC1 Arg280His	205/203	0.09/0.08	1.25 (0.76-2.04)
Coppedè et al. 2010b	XRCC1 Arg399Gln	197/194	0.39/0.28	1.39 (1.05-1.85)
Fang et al. 2010	XRCC1 Arg194Trp	108/39	0.06/0.03	2.4 (0.5-2.2)[a]
Fang et al. 2010	XRCC1 Arg280His	108/39	0.05/0.03	2.0 (0.4-2.0)[a]
Fang et al. 2010	XRCC1 Arg399Gln	108/39	0.35/0.47	0.4 (0.2-1.0)[a]
Fang et al. 2010	XRCC1 rs915927	108/39	0.45/0.33	2.4 (0.5-2.2)[a]
Fang et al. 2010	XRCC1 rs939461	108/39	0.06/0.15	0.4 (0.1-0.9)[a]

Table 3. DNA repair gene polymorphisms and risk of Amyotrophic Lateral sclerosis[a] OR are derived from the original paper and referred to (heterozygous+minor homozygous) vs major homozygous.

5. Polymorphisms of DNA repair genes and Parkinson's disease

Parkinson's disease is the second most common neurodegenerative disorder after AD, affecting 1–2% of the population over the age of 50 years, and is characterized by progressive and profound loss of neuromelanin containing dopaminergic neurons in the *substantia nigra* (SN) resulting in resting tremor, rigidity, bradykinesia, and postural instability. The majority of PD cases are sporadic idiopathic forms, resulting from three interactive events: an individual's inherited genetic susceptibility, subsequent exposure to environmental risk factors, and aging (Bekris et al., 2010). However, in a minority of the cases PD is inherited as a Mendelian trait. Parkin is an E3 ubiquitin ligase that acts on a variety of substrates, resulting in polyubiquitination and degradation by the proteasome or monoubiquitination and regulation of biological activity. Mutation of *parkin* is one of the most prevalent causes of autosomal recessive familial PD and a recent study has shown that parkin is essential for optimal repair of DNA damage. Particularly, DNA damage induces nuclear translocation of parkin leading to interactions with PCNA and possibly other nuclear proteins involved in DNA repair (Kao, 2009). Moreover, parkin protects mitochondrial genome integrity and supports mitochondrial DNA (mtDNA) repair (Rothfuss et al., 2009). DNA polymerase gamma (POLG1) participates in mtDNA replication and repair, thus playing a fundamental role in mtDNA maintenance. Missense mutations in *POLG1* co-segregate with a phenotype that includes progressive external ophthalmoplegia and parkinsonism (Hudson et al., 2007). Moreover, missense mutations in *POLG1* have been reported in case studies, in which parkinsonism was part of the clinical symptoms (Davidzon et al., 2006; Remes et al., 2008). *POLG1* mutations and polymorphisms have been also investigated in sporadic idiopathic PD, among them a polyglutamine (poly-Q) located in the *N*-terminal of POLG1, encoded by a CAG repeat in exon 2. The poly-Q tract normally consists of 10Q (frequency >80%), followed by 11Q (frequency > 6-12%), whereas non-10Q/11Q alleles are considered as less frequent alleles. Several authors investigated whether or not non-10Q alleles are more frequent in PD cases than in matched controls (Hudson et al., 2009; Luoma et al., 2007; Taanman & Shapira, 2005; Tiangyou et al., 2006). Eerola and coworkers recently screened 641 PD patients and 292 controls from USA and performed a pooled analysis of their data with those available in the literature (Hudson et al., 2009; Luoma et al., 2007; Taanman & Shapira, 2005; Tiangyou et al., 2006) for a total of 1163 sporadic PD patients and 1214 controls observing that variant alleles defined as non-10Q were significantly increased in PD patients than in controls (16.3%vs.13.4%, $p = 0.005$) (Eerola et al., 2010). A few months later Anvret and coworkers screened 243 PD patients and 279 matched controls from Sweden, observing that non10Q/11Q alleles were more frequent in PD cases than in controls with an OR of 2.0 (1.3-3.1, 95%CI) strengthening the evidence that non frequent *POLG1* alleles might be more frequent in sporadic PD patients than in controls, thus representing a PD risk factor (Anvret et al., 2010) (Table 4). We screened 139 sporadic PD patients and 211 healthy matched controls for the presence of the *OGG1* Ser326Cys polymorphism. The Cys326 allele frequency was similar between the groups (0.20 in PD patients and 0.19 in controls), and no difference in genotype frequencies was observed. Moreover, the *OGG1* Ser326Cys polymorphism was not associated with PD age at onset (Coppedè et al., 2010c). In human cells the oxidized purine nucleoside triphosphatase MTH1 efficiently hydrolyzes oxidized purines such as 8-oxo-guanine in the nucleotide pools, thus avoiding their incorporation into DNA or RNA. A Val83Met polymorphism of the *MTH1* gene was studied in 73

Japanese patients with sporadic PD and 151 age-matched controls but was not associated with sporadic PD risk (Satoh & Kuroda, 2000). Another *MTH1* polymorphism (Ile45Thr) was investigated in 106 PD patients and 135 unrelated controls from China. The variant allele frequency resulted borderline increased in PD males (Jiang et al., 2008). This finding is pending replication in other populations. *PARP1* promoter polymorphisms (-410C/T, -1672G/A, and a (CA)n microsatellite) have been investigated in 146 Spanish PD cases and 161 matched controls. A protective effect against PD was found for heterozygosity at -410 (OR = 0.44) and (CA)n microsatellite (OR = 0.53) polymorphisms, and heterozygosity at -1672 polymorphism delayed by 4 years on the onset age of PD (Infante et al., 2007). Also these findings are original and waiting for replication in additional case-control groups (Table 4).

Reference	**Polymorphism**	**Number of subjects PD/Controls**	**Variant allele frequency PD/Controls**	**Odds Ratio (95% CI)**
Eerola et al., 2010	POLG1 Poly-Q tract	641/292	0.17/0.12	OR = n.a. *P* = 0.004
Eerola et al., 2010	POLG1 Poly-Q tract	1163/1214[a]	0.16/0.13	OR = n.a. *P* = 0.005
Anvret et al., 2010	POLG1 Poly-Q tract	243/279	0.11/0.06	2.0 (1.3-3.1)
Coppedè et al., 2010c	OGG1 Ser326Cys	139/211	0.20/0.19	1.05 (0.72-1.53)
Satoh & Kuroda, 2000	MTH1 Val83Met	73/151	0.07/0.11	OR = n.a. *P* = 0.219
Jiang et al., 2008	MTH1 Ile45Thr	106/135	0.05/0.02	OR = n.a. *P* = 0.08[b]
Infante et al., 2007b	PARP-1 (-410)	146/161	0.35/0.53[c]	0.44 (0.26-0.75)
Infante et al., 2007b	PARP-1 (-1672)[d]	146/161	0.29/0.27[c]	0.87 (0.50-1.52)
Infante et al., 2007b	PARP-1 (CA)n	146/161	0.36/0.50[c]	0.53 (0.31-0.90)

Table 4. DNA repair gene polymorphisms and risk of Parkinson's disease. [a] = pooled-analysis of (Eerola et al., 2010, Hudson et al., 2009; Luoma et al., 2007; Taanman & Shapira, 2005; Tiangyou et al., 2006). [b] = Allele frequency difference (PD/Controls) approached significance in the male subgroup (0.07/0.02, *P* = 0.05). [c] = Heterozygous genotype frequency. [d] = Associated with PD age at onset

5.1 Other mutations and polymorphisms

As previously observed, several *POLG1* mutations have been observed to co-segregate in families with parkinsonism. For a detailed description I suggest a recent review by Orsucci and coworkers (Orsucci et al., 2010).

6. Other neurodegenerative diseases

6.1 Spinocerebellar ataxias

Hereditary ataxias are a heterogeneous group of diseases with different patterns of inheritance. Some of them are caused by recessive mutations in genes involved in DNA repair pathways that likely predispose the affected individuals to neurodegeneration. Spinocerebellar ataxia with axonal neuropathy 1 (SCAN1) is caused by autosomal recessive mutations in the gene encoding tyrosyl-DNA phosphodiesterase 1 (TDP1), a protein required for the repair of DNA SSBs that arise independent of DNA replication from abortive topoisomerase 1 activity or oxidative stress. Ataxia-telangiectasia (AT), ataxia-telangiectasia-like disorder (ATLD), ataxia oculomotor apraxia type 1 (AOA1) and ataxia oculomotor apraxia type 2A (AOA2) are a subgroup of the autosomal recessive spinocerebellar ataxias characterized by cerebellar atrophy and oculomotor apraxia. The progressive neurodegeneration described in AT and ATLD is due to mutations in genes encoding for ATM and Mre11, respectively. ATM recognizes and signals DNA DSBs to the cell cycle checkpoints and the DNA repair machinery. The Mre11 DNA repair complex, composed of Rad50, Mre11 and Nbs1 proteins, is involved in DNA damage recognition, DNA repair, and initiating cell cycle checkpoints. ATM and the Mre11 complex combine to recognize and signal DNA DSBs. AOA1 is caused by mutations in the gene encoding aprataxin (APTX), a nuclear protein that interacts with several DNA repair proteins, including XRCC1, Polβ, DNA ligase III, PARP-1, and p53. It functions in the endprocessing of DNA SSBs removing 3′-phosphate, 5′-phosphate, and 3′-phosphoglycolate ends. AOA2 is caused by autosomal recessive mutations in the gene encoding senataxin (SETX). SETX is a member of the superfamily I DNA/RNA helicases, likely involved in oxidative DNA damage response. *SETX* mutations have been also linked to juvenile ALS. Overall, spinocerebellar ataxias deficient in DNA damage responses represent the most robust set of data linking mutations in DNA repair genes to neurodegeneration (Gueven et al., 2007; Martin, 2008).

6.2 Huntington's disease

Huntington's disease (HD) is a progressive neurodegenerative disorder resulting in cognitive impairment, choreiform movements and death which usually occurs 15–20 years after the onset of the symptoms. The disease is also characterized by psychiatric and behavioural disturbances. HD is an autosomal dominant disorder caused by a CAG repeat expansion within exon 1 of the gene encoding for huntingtin (*IT15*) on chromosome 4. In the normal population the number of CAG repeats is maintained below 35, while in individuals affected by HD it ranges from 35 to more than 100, resulting in an expanded polyglutamine segment in the protein. Age at onset of the disease is inversely correlated with the CAG repeat length; moreover the length of the expanded polyglutamine segment seems to be related to the rate of clinical progression of neurological symptoms and to the progression of motor impairment, but not to psychiatric symptoms. Somatic CAG repeat expansion in the gene encoding for huntingtin has been observed in several HD tissues, including the striatum which is the region most affected by the disease and the OGG1 protein has been involved in somatic CAG repeat expansion in HD, suggesting that it might contribute to disease age at onset (Kovtun et al. 2007). We recently observed a weak borderline association between the *OGG1* Ser326Cys polymorphism and HD age at onset in a small group of 91 HD subjects (Coppedè et al. 2010d). However, replication of the study in a cohort of more than 400 HD individuals failed to confirm the association between *OGG1* Ser326Cys and HD age at onset (Taherzadeh-Fard et al., 2010).

6.3 Multiple sclerosis

Multiple sclerosis (MS) has been classically regarded as an inflammatory demyelinating disease of the central nervous system. In recent years, it is also becoming increasingly apparent that there is a significant neurodegenerative component in the disease (Moore, 2010). MS is a complex autoimmune disease with a prominent genetic component. The primary genetic risk factor is the human leukocyte antigen *(HLA)-DRB1*1501* allele; however, much of the remaining genetic contribution to MS remains to be elucidated. Briggs and collaborators screened 1,343 MS cases and 1,379 healthy controls of European ancestry for a total of 485 single nucleotide polymorphisms within 72 genes related to DNA repair pathways. Only a single nucleotide polymorphism (rs1264307) within the general transcription factor IIH polypeptide 4 gene (*GTF2H4*), a nucleotide excision repair gene, was significantly associated with MS risk (OR = 0.7) after correcting for multiple testing. However, using a nonparametric approach comprising the Random Forests and CART algorithms, authors observed evidence for a predictive relation for MS based on 9 variants in nucleotide excision repair (rs4134860, rs2974754, rs7783714, rs4134813, rs2957873 and rs4150454), homologous recombination (rs9562605), and nonhomologous end-joining genes (rs9293329 and rs1231201). Specifically, variants within nucleotide excision repair genes were most prominent among predictors of MS (Briggs et al., 2010). Variants of DNA repair genes, particularly *BRCA2* (rs1801406) and *XRCC5* (rs207906), might also increase the risk for the development of secondary acute promyelocytic leukemia in MS patients (Hasan et al., 2011).

6.4 Diseases caused by mutations of NER genes

Xeroderma pigmentosum (XP), Cockayne's syndrome (CS) and trichothiodystropy (TTD) represent a clinically heterogeneous group of progeroid syndromes characterized by defects in NER proteins. A subset of these patients exhibits neurological dysfunction and neurodegeneration, and many XP patients have high cancer predisposition, thus linking DNA repair defects to premature aging, cancer and neurodegeneration. Several studies performed in mice, as well as in cell cultures, suggest that neurodegeneration in XP and CS patients might arise as a consequence of impaired repair of oxidative DNA lesions caused by mutations of NER genes. Details are provided in our recent updated review (Coppedè & Migliore, 2010)

7. Conclusions

The present chapter describes the current knowledge concerning DNA repair genes and neurodegeneration. Studies in ataxias (section 6.1) have undoubtedly linked genes involved in DNA repair to neurodegeneration. These observations, alongside with evidence of increased DNA damage in affected brain regions, have driven researchers to search for variant and polymorphisms of DNA repair genes in major neurodegenerative diseases such as AD, ALS and PD. Studies in sporadic late onset AD patients (Section 3) suggest that common polymorphisms of BER genes, namely *OGG1* Ser326Cys, *APEX1* Asp148Glu, and *XRCC1* (Arg194Trp, Arg280His and Arg399Gln) are unlikely to represent major AD risk factors. However, further studies are required to replicate and clarify the associations observed between *PARP-1* haplotypes and disease risk. Moreover, the power of these studies was limited by the sample size of case-control groups (Table 2), gene-gene interactions were missing, and only common polymorphisms have been included with little or no attention paid to rare gene variants. Concerning ALS, although results are still inconclusive, some studies performed in northern Europe suggest a possible association between the *APEX1* Asp148Glu polymorphism and disease risk, the *OGG1* Ser326Cys polymorphism was associated with increased ALS risk in Italy, and *XRCC1* variants gave conflicting results in different populations (Table 3). Overall, these studies (Section 4) suggest the need of further investigation aimed at addressing the contribution of haplotypes, gene-gene and gene-environment interactions. There is evidence for a contribution of *POLG1* mutations in PD, and parkin seems to be involved in mtDNA repair, thus strengthening the contribution of mtDNA mutations to disease pathogenesis (Section 5). Increasing evidence suggests that BER proteins might be involved in CAG repeat expansion in somatic cells of HD individuals (Section 6.2), however studies aimed at addressing the possible contribution of variant of BER genes to disease age at onset are still in their beginnings. Recent evidence also suggests a possible contribution of NER genes in MS (Section 6.3), and the impaired ability to repair oxidative DNA damage might cause neurodegeneration observed in progeroid syndromes caused by mutations of NER genes (Section 6.4). In summary, increasing evidence supports a role for DNA repair genes in neurodegeneration, making this field a promising area for further investigation.

8. References

Anvret, A., Westerlund, M., Sydow, O., Willows, T., Lind, C., Galter, D. & Belin, A.C. (2010) Variations of the CAG trinucleotide repeat in DNA polymerase gamma (POLG1) is associated with Parkinson's disease in Sweden. *Neurosci Lett.* 485(2): 117-20.

Bekris, L.M., Mata, I.F. & Zabetian, C.P. (2010) The genetics of Parkinson disease. *J Geriatr Psychiatry Neurol.* 23(4): 228-42.

Bogdanov, M., Brown, R.H., Matson, W., Smart, R., Hayden, D., O'Donnell, H., Beal, F.M. & Cudkowicz, M. (2000) Increased oxidative damage to DNA in ALS patients. *Free Radic Biol Med.* 29(7): 652-8.

Briggs, F.B., Goldstein, B.A., McCauley, J.L., Zuvich, R.L., De Jager, P.L., Rioux, J.D., Ivinson, A.J., Compston, A., Hafler, D.A., Hauser, S.L., Oksenberg, J.R., Sawcer, S.J., Pericak-Vance, M.A., Haines, J.L., Barcellos, L.F. & International Multiple Sclerosis Genetics Consortium (2010) Variation within DNA repair pathway genes and risk of multiple sclerosis. *Am J Epidemiol.* 172(2): 217-24.

Brookmeyer, R., Johnson, E., Ziegler-Graham, K. & Arrighi, H.M. (2007) Forecasting the global burden of Alzheimer's disease. *Alzheimers Dement.* 3(3): 186-191.

Coppedè, F., Mancuso, M., Lo Gerfo, A., Manca, M.L., Petrozzi, L., Migliore, L., Siciliano, G., & Murri, L. (2007a) A Ser326Cys polymorphism in the DNA repair gene hOGG1 is not associated with sporadic Alzheimer's disease. *Neurosci Lett.* 414(3): 282-5.

Coppedè, F., Mancuso, M., Lo Gerfo, A., Carlesi, C., Piazza, S., Rocchi, A., Petrozzi, L., Nesti, C., Micheli, D., Bacci, A., Migliore, L., Murri, L. & Siciliano, G. (2007b) Association of the hOGG1 Ser326Cys polymorphism with sporadic amyotrophic lateral sclerosis. *Neurosci Lett.* 420(2): 163-8.

Coppedè, F. & Migliore, L. (2010) DNA repair in premature aging disorders and neurodegeneration. *Curr Aging Sci* 3 (1): 3-19.

Coppedè, F., Lo Gerfo, A., Carlesi, C., Piazza, S., Mancuso, M., Pasquali, L., Murri, L., Migliore, L. & Siciliano, G. (2010a) Lack of association between the APEX1 Asp148Glu polymorphism and sporadic amyotrophic lateral sclerosis. *Neurobiol Aging.* 31(2): 353-5.

Coppedè, F., Migheli, F., Lo Gerfo, A., Fabbrizi, M.R., Carlesi, C., Mancuso, M., Corti, S., Mezzina, N., del Bo, R., Comi, G.P., Siciliano, G. & Migliore, L. (2010b) Association study between XRCC1 gene polymorphisms and sporadic amyotrophic lateral sclerosis. *Amyotroph Lateral Scler.* 11(1-2): 122-4.

Coppedè, F., Ceravolo, R., Migheli, F., Fanucchi, F., Frosini, D., Siciliano, G., Bonuccelli, U. & Migliore, L. (2010c) The hOGG1 Ser326Cys polymorphism is not associated with sporadic Parkinson's disease. *Neurosci Lett.* 473(3): 248-51.

Coppedè, F., Migheli, F., Ceravolo, R., Bregant, E., Rocchi, A., Petrozzi, L., Unti, E., Lonigro, R., Siciliano, G. & Migliore, L. (2010d) The hOGG1 Ser326Cys polymorphism and Huntington's disease. Toxicology 278(2):199-203.

Coppedè, F. (2011) Variants and polymorphisms of DNA base excision repair genes and Alzheimer's disease. *J Neurol Sci.* 300(1-2): 200-1.

Davidzon, G., Greene, P., Mancuso, M., Klos, K.J., Ahlskog, J.E., Hirano, M. & DiMauro, S. (2006) Early-onset familial parkinsonism due to POLG mutations. *Ann Neurol.* 59(5): 859-62

Dogru-Abbasoglu, S., Inceoglu, M., Parildar-Karpuzoglu, H., Hanagasi, H.A., Karadag, B., Gurvit, H., Emre, M., Aykac-Toker, G. & Uysal, M. (2006) Polymorphisms in the DNA repair genes XPD (ERCC2) and XPF (ERCC4) are not associated with sporadic late-onset Alzheimer's disease. *Neurosci Lett.* 404(3):258-61.

Doğru-Abbasoğlu, S., Aykaç-Toker, G., Hanagasi, H.A., Gürvit, H., Emre, M. & Uysal, M. (2007) The Arg194Trp polymorphism in DNA repair gene XRCC1 and the risk for sporadic late-onset Alzheimer's disease. *Neurol Sci.* 28(1):31-4.

Dorszewska, J., Kempisty, B., Jaroszewska-Kolecka, J., Rózycka, A., Florczak, J., Lianeri, M., Jagodziński, P.P. & Kozubski, W. (2009) Expression and polymorphisms of gene 8-oxoguanine glycosylase 1 and the level of oxidative DNA damage in peripheral blood lymphocytes of patients with Alzheimer's disease. *DNA Cell Biol.* 28(11): 579-88.

Eerola, J., Luoma, P.T., Peuralinna, T., Scholz, S., Paisan-Ruiz, C., Suomalainen, A., Singleton ,A.B. & Tienari, P.J. (2010) POLG1 polyglutamine tract variants associated with Parkinson's disease. *Neurosci Lett.* 477(1): 1-5.

Fang, F., Umbach, D.M., Xu, Z., Ye, W., Sandler, D.P., Taylor, J.A. & Kamel, F. (2010) No association between DNA repair gene XRCC1 and amyotrophic lateral sclerosis. *Neurobiol Aging.* Epub Aug 16.

Ferrante, R.J., Browne, S.E., Shinobu, L.A., Bowling, A.C., Baik, M.J., MacGarvey, U., Kowall, N.W., Brown, R.H. Jr. & Beal, M.F. Evidence of increased oxidative damage in both sporadic and familial amyotrophic lateral sclerosis. *J Neurochem.* 69(5): 2064-74.

Fleck, O & Nielsen, O. (2004) DNA repair. *J Cell Sci* 117(Pt4): 515-7.

Greenway, M.J., Alexander, M.D., Ennis, S., Traynor, B.J., Corr, B., Frost, E., Green, A. & Hardiman, O. (2004) A novel candidate region for ALS on chromosome 14q11.2. *Neurology.* 63(10): 1936-8.

Gueven, N., Chen, P., Nakamura, J., Becherel, O.J., Kijas, A.W., Grattan-Smith, P. & Lavin, M.F. (2007) A subgroup of spinocerebellar ataxias defective in DNA damage responses. *Neuroscience.* 145(4): 1418-25.

Hasan, S.K., Buttari, F., Ottone, T., Voso, M.T., Hohaus, S., Marasco, E., Mantovani, V., Garagnani, P., Sanz, M.A., Cicconi, L., Bernardi ,G., Centonze, D. & Lo-Coco, F. (2011) Risk of acute promyelocytic leukemia in multiple sclerosis: Coding variants of DNA repair genes. *Neurology.* 76(12): 1059-65.

Hayward, C., Colville, S., Swingler, R.J. & Brock, D.J. (1999) Molecular genetic analysis of the APEX nuclease gene in amyotrophic lateral sclerosis. *Neurology.* 52(9): 1899-901.

Hirano, M., Yamamoto, A., Mori, T., Lan, L., Iwamoto, T.A., Aoki, M., Shimada, K., Furiya, Y., Kariya, S., Asai, H., Yasui, A., Nishiwaki, T., Imoto, K., Kobayashi, N., Kiriyama, T., Nagata, T., Konishi, N., Itoyama, Y. & Ueno S. (2007) DNA single-strand break repair is impaired in aprataxin-related ataxia. *Ann Neurol* 61(2): 162-74.

Hudson, G., Schaefer, A.M., Taylor, R.W., Tiangyou, W., Gibson, A., Venables, G., Griffiths, P., Burn, D.J., Turnbull, D.M. & Chinnery, P.F. (2007) Mutation of the linker region of the polymerase gamma-1 (POLG1) gene associated with progressive external ophthalmoplegia and Parkinsonism. *Arch Neurol.* 64(4): 553-7.

Hudson, G., Tiangyou, W., Stutt, A., Eccles, M., Robinson, L., Burn, D.J. & Chinnery, P.F. (2009) No association between common POLG1 variants and sporadic idiopathic Parkinson's disease. *Mov Disord.* 24(7): 1092-4.

Infante, J., Llorca, J., Mateo, I., Rodríguez-Rodríguez, E., Sánchez-Quintana, C., Sánchez-Juan, P., Fernández-Viadero, C., Peña, N., Berciano, J. & Combarros, O. (2007) Interaction between poly(ADP-ribose) polymerase 1 and interleukin 1A genes is associated with Alzheimer's disease risk. *Dement Geriatr Cogn Disord.* 23(4): 215-8.

Infante, J., Sánchez-Juan, P., Mateo, I., Rodríguez-Rodríguez, E., Sánchez-Quintana, C., Llorca, J., Fontalba, A., Terrazas, J., Oterino, A., Berciano, J. & Combarros O. (2007) Poly (ADP-ribose) polymerase-1 (PARP-1) genetic variants are protective against Parkinson's disease. *J Neurol Sci.* 256(1-2): 68-70.

Jiang, G., Xu, L., Wang, L., Song, S. & Zhu, C. (2007) Association study of human MTH1 Ile45Thr polymorphism with sporadic Parkinson's disease. *Eur Neurol.* 59(1-2): 15-7.

Kao, S.Y. (2009) Regulation of DNA repair by parkin. *Biochem Biophys Res Commun* 382(2): 321-5.

Kass, E.M. & Jasin, M. (2010) Collaboration and competition between DNA double-strand break repair pathways. *FEBS Lett.* 584(17): 3703-8.

Kikuchi, H., Furuta, A., Nishioka, K., Suzuki, S.O., Nakabeppu, Y. & Iwaki, T. (2002) Impairment of mitochondrial DNA repair enzymes against accumulation of 8-oxo-guanine in the spinal motor neurons of amyotrophic lateral sclerosis. *Acta Neuropathol.* 103(4): 408-14.

Kisby, G.E., Milne, J. & Sweatt, C. (1997) Evidence of reduced DNA repair in amyotrophic lateral sclerosis brain tissue. *Neuroreport.* 8(6): 1337-40.

Kovtun, I.V., Liu, Y., Bjoras, M., Klungland, A., Wilson, S.H. & McMurray, C.T. (2007) OGG1 initiates age-dependent CAG trinucleotide expansion in somatic cells. *Nature* 447 (7143): 447-52.

Kunkel, T.A. & Erie, D.A. (2005) DNA mismatch repair. *Annu Rev Biochem* 74: 681-710.

Liu, H.P., Lin, W.Y., Wu, B.T., Liu, S.H., Wang, W.F., Tsai, C.H., Lee, C.C. & Tsai, F.J. (2010) Evaluation of the poly(ADP-ribose) polymerase-1 gene variants in Alzheimer's disease. *J Clin Lab Anal.* 24(3): 182-6.

Love, S., Barber, R. & Wilcock, G.K. (1999) Increased poly(ADP-ribosyl)ation of nuclear proteins in Alzheimer's disease. *Brain.* 122(Pt 2): 247-53

Lovell, M.A., Xie, C. & Markesbery, W.R. (2000) Decreased base excision repair and increased helicase activity in Alzheimer's disease brain. *Brain Res* 855(1): 116-23 .

Luoma, P.T., Eerola, J., Ahola, S., Hakonen, A.H., Hellström, O., Kivistö, K.T., Tienari, P.J. & Suomalainen, A. (2007) Mitochondrial DNA polymerase gamma variants in idiopathic sporadic Parkinson disease. *Neurology.* 69(11): 1152-9.

Mao, G., Pan, X., Zhu, B.B., Zhang, Y., Yuan, F., Huang, J., Lovell, M.A., Lee, M.P., Markesbery, W.R., Li, G.M. & Gu, L. (2007) Identification and characterization of OGG1 mutations in patients with Alzheimer's disease. *Nucleic Acids Res.* 35(8): 2759-66.

Martin, L.J. (2008) DNA damage and repair: relevance to mechanisms of neurodegeneration. *J Neuropathol Exp Neurol.* 67(5): 377-87.

Moore, G.R. (2010) Current concepts in the neuropathology and pathogenesis of multiple sclerosis. *Can J Neurol Sci.* 37 (Suppl 2) :S5-15.

Orsucci, D., Caldarazzo Ienco, E., Mancuso, M. & Siciliano, G. (2011) POLG1-Related and other "Mitochondrial Parkinsonisms": an Overview. *J Mol Neurosci.* Epub Jan 8.

Parildar-Karpuzoğlu, H., Doğru-Abbasoğlu, S., Hanagasi, H.A., Karadağ, B., Gürvit, H., Emre, M. & Uysal, M. (2008) Single nucleotide polymorphisms in base-excision repair genes hOGG1, APE1 and XRCC1 do not alter risk of Alzheimer's disease. *Neurosci Lett.* 442(3): 287-91.

Qian, Y., Chen, W., Wu, J., Tao, T., Bi, L., Xu, W., Qi, H., Wang, Y. & Guo L. (2010) Association of polymorphism of DNA repair gene XRCC1 with sporadic late-onset Alzheimer's disease and age of onset in elderly Han Chinese. *J Neurol Sci.* 295(1-2): 62-5.

Remes, A.M., Hinttala, R., Kärppä, M., Soini, H., Takalo, R., Uusimaa, J. & Majamaa, K. (2008) Parkinsonism associated with the homozygous W748S mutation in the POLG1 gene. *Parkinsonism Relat Disord.* 14(8): 652-4.

Rothfuss, O., Fischer, H., Hasegawa, T., Maisel, M., Leitner, P., Miesel, F., Sharma, M., Bornemann, A., Berg, D., Gasser, T. & Patenge N. (2009) Parkin protects mitochondrial genome integrity and supports mitochondrial DNA repair. *Hum Mol Genet.* 18(20): 3832-50.

Satoh, J. & Kuroda, Y. (2000) A valine to methionine polymorphism at codon 83 in the 8-oxo-dGTPase gene MTH1 is not associated with sporadic Parkinson's disease. *Eur J Neurol.* 7(6): 673-7.

Subba Rao, K. (2007) Mechanisms of disease: DNA repair defects and neurological disease. *Nat Clin Pract Neurol* 3(3): 162-72.

Taanman, J.W. & Schapira, A.H. (2005) Analysis of the trinucleotide CAG repeat from the DNA polymerase gamma gene (POLG) in patients with Parkinson's disease. *Neurosci Lett.* 376(1): 56-9.

Taherzadeh-Fard, E., Saft, C., Wieczorek, S., Epplen, J.T. & Arning, L. (2010) Age at onset in Huntington's disease: replication study on the associations of ADORA2A, HAP1 and OGG1. *Neurogenetics.* 11(4): 435-9.

Takahashi, T., Tada, M., Igarashi, S., Koyama, A., Date, H., Yokoseki, A., Shiga, A., Yoshida, Y., Tsuji, S., Nishizawa, M. & Onodera O. (2007) Aprataxin, causative gene product for EAOH/AOA1, repairs DNA single-strand breaks with damaged 3'-phosphate and 3'-phosphoglycolate ends. *Nucleic Acids Res* 35(11): 3797-809.

Tiangyou, W., Hudson, G., Ghezzi, D., Ferrari, G., Zeviani, M., Burn, D.J. & Chinnery, P.F. (2006) POLG1 in idiopathic Parkinson disease. Neurology. 67(9):1698-700.

Tomkins, J., Dempster, S., Banner, S.J., Cookson, M.R. & Shaw, P.J. (2000) Screening of AP endonuclease as a candidate gene for amyotrophic lateral sclerosis (ALS). *Neuroreport.* 11(8): 1695-7.

Weissman, L., de Souza-Pinto, N.C., Stevnsner, T. & Bohr, V.A. (2007) DNA repair, mitochondria, and neurodegeneration. *Neuroscience* 145 (12): 1318-29.

Weissman, L., Jo, D.G., Sørensen, M.M., de Souza-Pinto, N.C., Markesbery, W.R., Mattson, M.P. & Bohr V.A. (2007b) Defective DNA base excision repair in brain from individuals with Alzheimer's disease and amnestic mild cognitive impairment. *Nucleic Acids Res* 35(16): 5545-55.

Part 5

Telomeres and DNA Repair

29

Characterization of 5'-Flanking Regions of Various Human Telomere Maintenance Factor-Encoding Genes

Fumiaki Uchiumi[1,4], Takahiro Oyama[1], Kensuke Ozaki[1] and Sei-ichi Tanuma[2,3,4]
[1]*Department of Gene Regulation, Faculty of Pharmaceutical Sciences*
[2]*Department of Biochemistry, Faculty of Pharmaceutical Sciences*
[3]*Genome and Drug Research Center*
[4]*Research Center for RNA Science, RIST, Tokyo University of Science*
Japan

1. Introduction

Telomeres are the unique nucleoprotein complex structures located at the end of linear eukaryotic chromosomes (Blackburn, 2000; de Lange, 2006). They are composed of TTAGGG repeats that are typically 10 kb at birth and gradually shorten with cell divisions (de Lange, 2006). Telomerase is composed of the protein subunit TERT and the RNA subunit TERC (TR). It elongates the telomere by adding telomeric repeats (Greider & Blackburn, 1987). The 50 to 300 nucleotides from the terminal end of the telomeres are single stranded 3'-protluded G-overhang structures which make the t-loop configuration (de Lange, 2006; Griffith et al., 1999). Mammalian telomeres are included in heterochoromatin and attached to the nuclear matrix (Oberdoerffer & Sinclair, 2007; Gonzalez-Suarez & Gonzalo, 2008). Telomere shortening causes instability of the ends of chromosomes to lead to replicative senescence (O'Sullivan & Karlseder, 2010; Lundblad & Szostak, 1989). Therefore, the ends of telomeres should be protected from damaging or cellular activities. The t-loop structures are regulated by shelterin protein factors, TRF1, TRF2, Rap1, TIN2, TPP1, POT1 (Gilson & Geli, 2007; O'Sullivan & Karlseder, 2010), and Rec Q DNA helicases, WRN and BLM (Chu & Hickson, 2009). TRF1 and TRF2, which bind to duplex telomeric DNA and retain shelterin on the telomere repeats, were shown to interact with various functional proteins (Giannone et al., 2010). Molecular structural analysis of Rap1 revealed that its mechanism of action involves interaction with TRF2 and Taz1 proteins (Chen et al., 2011). A recent study showed that depletion of TPP1 and its partner TIN2 causes a loss of telomerase recruitment to telomeres (Abreu et al., 2010). POT1 is an important regulator of telomerase length, in stimulating the RecQ helicases WRN and BLM (Opresko et al., 2005). Tankyrase-1 (TANK1), which is classified as a poly(ADP-ribose) polymerase family protein, is also known to regulate telomere homeostasis by modifying TRF1 (Smith et al., 1998; Schreiber et al., 2006). Dyskerin, which is encoded by the *DKC1* gene, is a key auxiliary protein that is contained in a Cajal body with TERT (Cohen et al., 2007). Defects in the shelterin components and telomerase are thought to down-regulate telomere structure and length (O'Sullivan & Karlseder, 2010). The shelterin proteins also play important roles in protecting chromosomal ends from being recognized by DNA damage response (DDR) machinery (O'Sullivan & Karlseder, 2010). Although the biological significance of the shelterin complex proteins has been studied, the molecular mechanisms that regulate expression of those genes encoding telomere associated proteins is less well-characterized. We hypothesized that expressions of those telomere-associated protein-encoding genes are regulated by a similar mechanism. In order to analyze these promoter activities promptly, we isolated 200 to 300-bp of the 5'-upstream regions of these telomere regulatory protein-encoding genes and applied them to a multiple transfection assay system (Uchiumi et al., 2010a). Previously, we have observed that *WRN* and *TERT* promoter activities were up-regulated by 2-deoxy-D-glucose (2DG) and *trans*-resveratrol (Rsv) in accordance with the activation of telomerase (Zhou et al., 2009; Uchiumi et al., 2011). A potent inhibitor of glucose metabolism, 2DG is thought to mimic glucose deprivation *in vivo* such that it is mimetic of caloric restriction (CR) (Roth et al., 2001). Resveratrol (Rsv), which is a polyphenol contained in grape skins and red wine, activates sirtuin-mediated deacetylation (Stefani et al., 2007; Knutson & Leeuwenburgh, 2008). We report here that most of the promoters of the shelterin protein-encoding genes positively responded to the CR mimetic agents, 2DG and Rsv. These results suggest that telomerase and telomere maintenance factors are simultaneously regulated at the initiation of the transcription.

2. Materials and methods

2.1 Chemicals

The reagents 2-deoxy-D-glucose (2DG) and *trans*-resveratrol (Rsv) were purchased from Wako Chemicals (Tokyo, Japan) and Cayman Chemicals (Ann Arbor, MI), respectively.

2.2 Cells and cell culture

HeLa-S3 cells (Zhou et al., 2009) were cultured in Dulbecco's modified eagle (DME) medium supplemented with heat-inactivated 10% fetal calf serum (FCS) (Sanko-Pure Chemical, Tokyo, Japan), 2 mM L-glutamine (Invitrogen, CA, USA), penicillin (100 IU/mL) (MEIJI SEIKA, Tokyo, Japan), and streptomycin (100 µg/mL) (MEIJI SEIKA).

2.3 Construction of Luc-reporter plasmids

Luc reporter plasmids carrying promoter regions for the human *TERT* and *TERC* genes have been constructed and designated as pGL4-TERT, and pGL4-TERC, respectively (Zhou et al., 2009; Uchiumi et al., 2010a). Extraction of DNA from HeLa-S3 cells, and subsequent PCR for the promoter regions of interest were performed as described previously (Uchiumi et al., 2010a; Zhou et al., 2009). Primer-sets were designed against human genomic sequences from the Cross-Ref NCBI-data base (http://www.ncbi.nlm.nih.gov/sites/gquery/) for the 5'-flanking regions of the genes of interest (Table. 1). PrimeStar Taq polymerase (Takara, Kyoto, Japan) was used for all amplifications.

Amplification conditions consisted of: 30 cycles of 98°C for 10 sec, 55°C for 5 sec, and 72°C for 30 sec. PCR products were digested with *Kpn*I and *Xho*I and then separated on 0.9% agarose gels.

After electrophoresis, DNA bands of the correct length were recovered from the gel with Wizard SV Gel and PCR Clean-Up System (Promega, Madison, WI, USA) and subcloned into the *Kpn*I-*Xho*I site of the pGL4-basic vector (pGL4[luc 2.10]) (Promega). The resultant cloned plasmids were designated pGL4-DKC1, pGL4-POT1, pGL4-RAP1, pGL4-TANK1, pGL4-TANK2, pGL4-TIN2, pGL4-TPP1, pGL4-TRF1, and pGL4-TRF2. Clone sequences were confirmed using a DNA Sequencing System (Applied Biosystems, Foster City, CA) with Rv (5'-TAGCAAAATAGGCTGTCCCC-3' and GL (5'-CTTTATGTTTTTGGCGTCTT-CC-3') primers purchased from Operon Biotechnologies (Tokyo, Japan).

Name	Sequence
hDysk-7065	5'-TCGGTACCGTGAGCCCAGGCGCAGGCGC-3'
AhDysk-7414	5'-ATCTCGAGGGAACGACCGCAGACTCCC-3'
hPOT-1509	5'-TCGGTACCTGAGAACTGAATATTGCTGTG-3'
AhPOT-1164	5'-ATCTCGAGAATATCATCTTACCAAAGAC-3'
hRAP1-5667	5'-TCGGTACCTCGCGGCGCTTCCCAGCCC-3'
AhRAP1-5970	5'-ATCTCGAGCTGTCACCGCAGACGCCTC-3'
hTANK1-8541	5'-TCGGTACCGACTGAAAGTGAGAAATGC-3'
AhTANK1-8860	5'-ATCTCGAGAGCGACGCGACGCCGCCATC-3'
hTANK2-4227	5'-TCGGTACCAGGAGAAAGGGATGTGGAAG-3'
AhTANK2-4519	5'-ATCTCGAGGCGGCGCGAAGGGTTTGTGG-3'
hTIN2-8835	5'-TCGGTACCGCAGGCTCCGCGAAGAAAGC-3'
AhTIN2-8508	5'-ATCTCGAGTGGAGAAGCTGACCGTCTC-3'
hTPP1-8283	5'-TCGGTACCTCGACGATGCTATCGGGAC-3'
AhTPP1-7995	5'-ATCTCGAGCGTGATGACGCAAGAGCGGA-3'
hTRF1-1070	5'-TCGGTACCTCCTCCTATCCTAATCTCGC-3'
AhTRF1-1371	5'-ATCTCGAGGAAACATCCTCCGCCATGTT-3'
hTRF2-9454	5'-TCGGTACCGATCCCGGCCTGTTTTTCAG-3'
AhTRF2-9170	5'-ATCTCGAGCGGGGCCCGCCGTCCCGGC-3'

Table 1. Primers used for amplifying 5'-upstream region of various human telomere-associated genes

2.4 Transient transfection assay

Transient transfection of Luc-reporter plasmids was performed using multi-well culture plates that had been prepared and treated with DNA/DEAE-dextran (Uchiumi et al., 2010a). After 4 h of transfection, 2DG or Rsv was added to the culture medium (Zhou et al., 2009; Uchiumi et al., 2011). After a further incubation (19 to 24 h), cells were collected and lysed with 40 µL of 1 x Cell culture lysis reagent, mixed, and stored at -80°C. Luc assays were performed according to the manufacturer's instructions (Promega). In brief, Luc assay reagent (40 µL) was added to 10 µL of protein sample and mixed briefly. Immediately after mixing, chemiluminescence was measured for 7.5 sec with a Minilumat LB9506 luminometer (Berthold, Bad Wildbad, Germany). Protein assays were performed with the Luc sample (2.5 µL) and Protein Assay Reagent (Bio-Rad Lab., Hercules, CA, USA).

3. Results

3.1 Isolation of 5'-flanking regions of human telomere-associated protein-encoding genes

Previously, we isolated and characterized 5′-flanking regions of the human *TERT* and *TERC* genes (Zhou et al., 2009; Uchiumi et al., 2010a). In this study, those of different human telomere-associated protein-encoding genes were obtained by PCR and inserted into the MCS of the pGL4-basic (pGL4[luc 2.10]) vector. Putative transcription-factor binding elements were found by TF-SEARCH analysis. As summarized in Fig. 1, c-Ets/Elk1, Sp1/GC-box, CREB, OCT, p300, SRY, GATA, E2F, NF-κB/c-Rel, CCAAT-box, and other motifs are located within 300-bp from the 5′-upstream region of the cDNAs. Although all of these telomere-associated protein factors are commonly involved in the maintenance of telomeres, a rigid rule in the order of the *cis*-elements could not be found in their core promoter regions. However, one or more Sp1/GC-box elements are located in 5′-upstream regions of the *DKC1, RAP1, TANK1, TIN2, TPP1, TRF1, TRF2, TERT,* and *TERC* genes, but not in the *POT1* and *TANK2* genes. Similar to the 5′-flanking region of the *WRN* gene, all of the isolated DNA fragments have no obvious TATA-box like sequences except the 5′-flanking region of the *TERC* gene (Uchiumi et al., 2010a).

3.2 Effect of Rsv on the promoter activities of 5'-flanking regions of the shelterin-encoding genes

The natural compound Rsv is known to have life-span promoting properties in yeast and metazoans by affecting the insulin-signaling cascade (Fröjdö et al., 2008). In order to examine the effect of Rsv on the isolated 5′-upstream regions of the shelterin encoding genes, Luc assays were performed. Luc expression plasmids which contained 5′-flanking regions of various telomere maintenance factor-encoding genes were transfected into HeLa-S3 cells by the DEAE-dextran based multiple transfection method (Uchiumi et al., 2010a). Luc activities of reporter plasmid-transfected cells were normalized to that of the pGL4-PIF1 transfected cells, because PIF1 has been suggested to have a negative effect on telomere elongation in yeast cells (Schulz & Zakian, 1994), and it has been shown that the change in the PIF1 promoter activity is largely unaffected after treatment with Rsv (Uchiumi et al., 2011). As shown in Table 2, treatment with Rsv (10 μM) for 24 h augmented Luc activities from the cells transfected with Luc reporter plasmids. Apparent positive responses to the Rsv treatment of the 5′-flanking regions of the *TERT* and *TERC* genes were observed, consistent with the activation of telomerase by Rsv in HeLa-S3 cells (Uchiumi et al., 2011). Although no obvious GC-box like elements are found in the 300-bp 5′-upstream regions of the *POT1* and *TANK2* genes (Fig. 1), Luc activities of these plasmid-transfected cells increased 2.53- and 1.69-fold, respectively, by Rsv treatment.

3.3 Effect of 2DG on the promoter activities of 5'-flanking regions of the shelterin-encoding genes

2DG is known to affect life span by its CR mimetic effect on various species (Roth et al., 2001). We previously observed that treatment with 2DG induces telomerase activity along with transcriptional activation of the *TERT* and *WRN* genes in HeLa-S3 cells (Zhou et al., 2009). Therefore, we examined the effect of 2DG on the promoter activities of shelterin-encoding genes. Although most of the Luc activities of cells transfected with shelterin promoter-Luc expression constructs were diminished by 2DG, the treatment induced

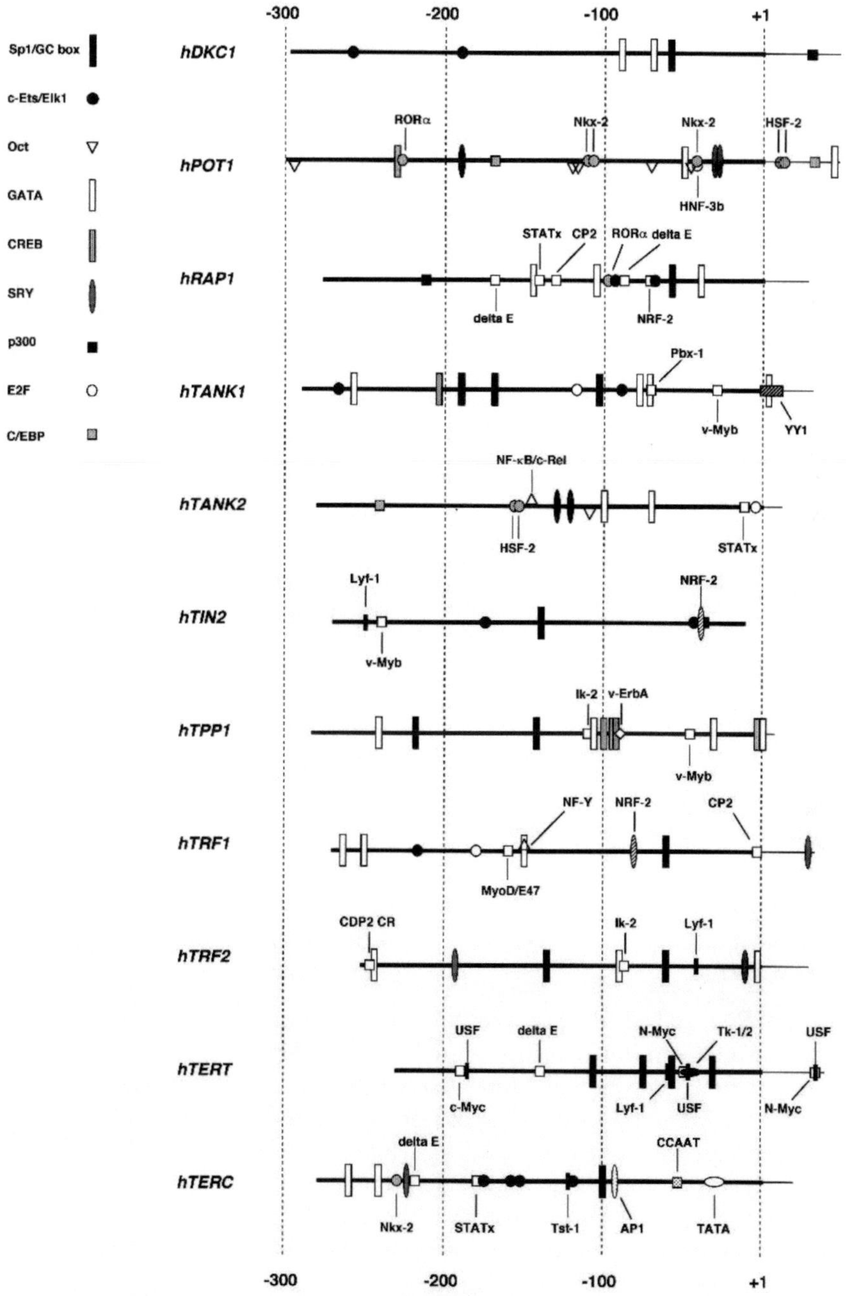

Fig. 1. Promoter regions of the human genes encoding telomere-associated proteins or shelterin protein factors. PCR-amplified 5′-flanking regions of these genes, which were inserted upstream of the *Luciferase* gene of the pGL4-basic vector (pGL4[luc 2.10]), are shown. Transcription start sites (or 5′-end of cDNAs) are designated +1. The TF-SEARCH program (http://www.cbrc.jp/research/db/TFSEARCH.html) was performed and putative transcription-factor binding-elements (score > 85) are shown schematically.

Reporter	Rsv (10 μM)	Relative Luc activity	Fold
pGL4-PIF1	-	1.000 ± 0.033	1.00
pGL4-PIF1	+	1.000 ± 0.088	
pGL4-RTEL	-	2.170 ± 0.119	1.23
pGL4-RTEL	+	2.667 ± 0.326	
pGL4-DKC1	-	1.271 ± 0.117	1.88
pGL4-DKC1	+	2.390 ± 0.325**	
pGL4-POT1	-	0.018 ± 0.003	2.53
pGL4-POT1	+	0.045 ± 0.008**	
pGL4-RAP1	-	0.746 ± 0.023	1.84
pGL4-RAP1	+	1.372 ± 0.164*	
pGL4-TANK1	-	0.069 ± 0.023	1.54
pGL4-TANK1	+	0.107 ± 0.014	
pGL4-TANK2	-	0.0059 ± 0.00155	1.69
pGL4-TANK2	+	0.0099 ± 0.00230	
pGL4-TIN2	-	0.128 ± 0.022	1.48
pGL4-TIN2	+	0.190 ± 0.013	
pGL4-TPP1	-	0.463 ± 0.032	1.54
pGL4-TPP1	+	0.714 ± 0.115*	
pGL4-TRF1	-	0.648 ± 0.078	1.83
pGL4-TRF1	+	1.189 ± 0.104***	
pGL4-TRF2	-	0.139 ± 0.005	1.61
pGL4-TRF2	+	0.224 ± 0.013***	
pGL4-TERT	-	0.794 ± 0.042	1.93
pGL4-TERT	+	1.532 ± 0.081***	
pGL4-TERC	-	0.557 ± 0.142	1.97
pGL4-TERC	+	1.096 ± 0.067*	

Table 2. Effect of Resveratrol (Rsv) on promoter activities of telomere-associated genes in HeLa-S3 cells Various reporter plasmids were introduced into HeLa-S3 cells by multiple DEAE-dextran method transfections. After 4 h of transfection, the culture medium was discarded and changed to Rsv-containing or non-containing medium. Cells were harvested after 24 h of treatment, then Luc assays were performed. Relative values represent Luc activities compared with that of the pGL4-PIF1 transfected cells. Results show means ± S.D. from three independent samples (N=3). Significance of differences between control and Rsv treated cells were analyzed by Student's *t*-test (*$p<0.05$, **$p<0.01$, ***$p<0.005$).

relatively positive values compared to that of the pGL4-PIF1-transfected cells (Table 3). Similar to the response to Rsv (Table 2), the *TERT* and *TERC* promoters were activated by the 2DG treatment. The increase in relative promoter activity (compared with that of the pGL4-PIF1-transfected cells) after 2DG (8 mM) treatment was significant for the *RTEL, DKC1, POT1, RAP1, TANK1, TIN2, TPP1,* and *TRF1* promoters (Table 3). These results suggest that the CR mimetic compound 2DG affects the balance of gene expression to protect telomeres.

Reporter		Relative Luc activity	
	2DG (mM)	4	8
pGL4-PIF1	-	1.000 ± 0.206	1.000 ± 0.141
pGL4-PIF1	+	1.000 ± 0.230	1.000 ± 0.148
pGL4-RTEL	-	1.800 ± 0.802	2.550 ± 0.648
pGL4-RTEL	+	4.011 ± 0.917	6.651 ± 1.958*
pGL4-DKC1	-	1.136 ± 0.111	2.560 ± 0.265
pGL4-DKC1	+	8.767 ± 4.556	6.698 ± 0.921***
pGL4-POT1	-	0.030 ± 0.008	0.027 ± 0.010
pGL4-POT1	+	0.139 ± 0.065	0.102 ± 0.015***
pGL4-RAP1	-	0.993 ± 0.247	2.201 ± 0.236
pGL4-RAP1	+	5.456 ± 1.411*	4.977 ± 0.749***
pGL4-TANK1	-	0.047 ± 0.012	0.106 ± 0.012
pGL4-TANK1	+	0.272 ± 0.110	0.567 ± 0.150*
pGL4-TANK2	-	0.012 ± 0.003	0.006 ± 0.002
pGL4-TANK2	+	0.066 ± 0.011***	0.033 ± 0.032
pGL4-TIN2	-	0.130 ± 0.038	0.213 ± 0.023
pGL4-TIN2	+	0.686 ± 0.273	0.474 ± 0.093**
pGL4-TPP1	-	0.604 ± 0.151	0.751 ± 0.099
pGL4-TPP1	+	3.211 ± 0.237***	5.721 ± 1.302*
pGL4-TRF1	-	0.853 ± 0.131	1.355 ± 0.279
pGL4-TRF1	+	2.178 ± 0.408**	3.442 ± 0.567**
pGL4-TRF2	-	0.173 ± 0.073	0.232 ± 0.022
pGL4-TRF2	+	0.378 ± 0.036*	0.693 ± 0.244
pGL4-TERT	-	0.586 ± 0.094	1.707 ± 0.316
pGL4-TERT	+	1.844 ± 0.498*	3.456 ± 0.963*
pGL4-TERC	-	0.651 ± 0.120	0.897 ± 0.119
pGL4-TERC	+	1.878 ± 0.426**	2.516 ± 0.507**

Table 3. Effect of 2-deoxy-D-glucose (2DG) on promoter activities of telomere-associated genes in HeLa-S3 cells Various reporter plasmids were introduced into HeLa-S3 cells by multiple DEAE-dextran method transfections. After 4 h of transfection, the culture medium was discarded and changed to 2DG-containing (4 and 8 mM) or non-containing medium. Cells were harvested after 24 h (4 mM) or 19 h (8 mM) of the 2DG treatment, then Luc assays were performed. Relative values represent Luc activities compared with that of the pGL4-PIF1 transfected cells. Results show means ± S.D. from three independent samples (N=3). Significance of differences between control and 2DG treated cells were analyzed by Student's *t*-test (*p<0.05, **p<0.01, ***p<0.005).

4. Discussion

4.1 The promoter regions of the shelterin-encoding genes coordinately respond to CR mimetic drugs

In the present study, 5'-flanking regions of different human telomere-associated protein factor-encoding genes were isolated, and these Luc reporter plasmids were used for transient transfection assays. The shelterin- or telomere-associated protein-encoding genes, including *TERT, TERC, DKC1,* and double-stranded break repair protein-encoding genes, such as *ATM* and *ATR*, are conserved among human, mouse and yeast (Stern & Bryan, 2008). Given that these telomere-associated proteins are localized to the telomere t-loop to protect the specific structure, and appear to act in co-operation with each other (O'Sullivan & Karlseder, 2010), their gene expression should be regulated synchronously when the telomeric region needs to be protected. Aging or cellular senescence are thought to be controlled by a genomic maintenance regulatory system (Vieg, 2007). Our hypothesis is that aging or longevity affecting reagents might have an effect on the expression of the telomere-associating protein-encoding genes. The results (Tables 2 and 3) indicate that promoter activities of the shelterin-encoding genes are simultaneously up-regulated by Rsv and 2DG in HeLa-S3 cells when they are compared with *PIF1* promoter activity. Previously, we have reported that multiple GC-boxes are commonly located in the human *TERT* and *WRN* promoter regions and that might play a role in the positive response to Rsv and 2DG in HeLa-S3 cells (Uchiumi et al., 2010c). Although there are no canonical roles of transcription factor binding elements or their order in these promoter regions, Sp1 binding elements or GC-boxes are found in all of them except 5'-upstream of the *POT1* and *TANK2* genes (Fig. 1). Therefore, GC-box binding factors may up-regulate this telomere-associated gene expression. However, there are no GC-box like motifs in the 300-bp up-stream regions of the *POT1* and *TANK2* genes, which are relatively AT-rich and contain Oct-1 binding sites. This observation suggests that POU family proteins might also be involved in the positive regulation of these genes. Apparent up-regulation of promoter activities by Rsv and 2DG treatment was observed in the cells transfected with the Luc reporter plasmids containing 200-bp 5'-upstream regions of the *TERT* and *TERC* genes (Tables 2 and 3). It is noteworthy that the duplicated GGAA-motifs are found in both promoter regions (Uchiumi et al., 2010a, Uchiumi et al., 2011b), suggesting that the GGAA-motif binding factors, including Ets family proteins, might be involved in the positive response to the aging or longevity affecting signals.

Previously, we observed elevation of the human *WRN* promoter activity in accordance with activation of telomerase after Rsv and 2DG treatment of HeLa-S3 cells (Uchiumi et al., 2011; Zhou et al., 2009). 2DG suppresses glucose metabolism to establish a limit for the usage or uptake of glucose into cells (Roth et al., 2001). On the other hand, Rsv is known to activate sirtuin family protein deacetylases (Kaeberlein, 2010). It is thought that both Rsv and 2DG are CR mimetic drugs (Stefani et al., 2007; Roth et al., 2001), and that CR can extend the mean and maximum life spans of numerous organisms (Carvallini et al., 2008; Roth et al., 2001). The present study suggests that induction of telomerase activity in concert with up-regulation of the telomere-associated protein- or shelterin-encoding gene expression may play a role in regulating the aging process through the telomere maintainance system.

4.2 A possible role for telomere maintenance system in aging/senescence regulation

Aging or senescence is a complicated biological process involving various regulatory factors (Campisi & d'Adda di Fagagna, 2007; Kuningas et al., 2008; Sanz & Stefanatos, 2008). Aging could be explained by a mitochondrial free radical theory (Benz & Yau, 2008). On the other hand, cellular senescence could be caused by DNA damage or the associated signals on chromosomes (Vieg, 2007). It is well known that cellular senescence is correlated with the cell growth arrest (Campisi & d'Adda di Fagagna, 2007). DNA damage signals activate ATM or ATR, and then phosphrylate p53 to induce transcription of the *CDKN1A* gene that encodes cyclin-dependent kinase inhibitor 1A (p21). These sequentially occurring events arrest the cell cycle at G1-phase (Meek, 2009). Repair of DNA damage will occur at this stage, unless the cell has initiated apoptosis. Thus, aging is thought to be controlled through both reactive oxygen species (ROS) generated by mitochondria and damages to DNA including telomeric regions of the chromosomes (Sahin & DePinho, 2010). Recently, it was shown that telomere dysfunction causes activation of p53 which directly represses PGC-1α and PGC-1β, leading to mitochondrial compromise (Sahin et al., 2011). Moreover, an experiment to reactivate telomerase in telomerase-deficient mice ameliorated DNA damage signaling and reversed neurodegeneration (Jaskelioff et al., 2011). These lines of evidence suggest that telomeres exert signals to affect mitochondria along with DNA repair systems. The concept that telomere length-associated signaling stimulates mitochondrial function might have combined the mitochondrial free radical theory with the molecular mechanism of chromosomal maintenance system against DNA damaging stresses. Rsv has been shown to have effect activation of PGC-1α to improve mitochondrial function in mouse brown adipose tissue and muscle (Lagouge et al., 2006). The present study indicates that shelterin protein-encoding gene promoters are simultaneously activated by Rsv treatment. Thereby, accumulation of shelterin proteins might lead to stabilization of telomeric regions of the chromosome and activation of PGC-1α.

4.3 Hormesis, the beneficial effects from low doses of toxic stresses, might be a determinant of longevity

The deficiencies in RecQ DNA helicases, including WRN and BLM, are known to cause premature aging (Chu & Hickson, 2009). In the present study, we have observed that CR mimetic drug treatment activates promoters of the shelterin protein-encoding genes, suggesting that CR evokes functions of the telomere maintenance machinery. Hormesis is a phenomenon that generally refers to the beneficial effects from low level toxic or other harmful damage, such as irradiation, heat shock, or food restriction (Schumacher, 2009). High doses of 2DG and Rsv have harmful or toxic effects on cells, leading to cell death or apoptosis (Lin et al., 2003; Cosan, et al., 2010). In contrast, relatively low doses of these CR mimetic reagents, as used in the present study, have effects similar to hormesis. Therefore, resistance to stresses eventually provoked by prolonged low doses of CR mimetic reagents could promote the longevity of organisms. Thus, the results obtained in the present study are consistent with the concept of hormesis.

4.4 Molecules that are involved in the regulation of the aging process

From studies of life spans of the *C. elegans*, it has been suggested that the insulin/IGF-1 pathway influences aging (Kenyon, 2010). In this signaling system, DAF-16 (FoxO transcription factor) plays a role in activating genes that act to extend life span (van der Horst & Burgering, 2007). AMP-activated protein kinase (AMPK), which is known to extend the life span of nematodes (Apfeld et al., 2004), phosphorylates FoxO, PGC-1α, and CREB to induce various genes encoding mitochondrial and oxidative metabolism regulating factors (Cantó & Auwerx, 2010). The other biologically important function of AMPK is that it blocks the mTOR (mammalian target of rapamycin) pathway (Cantó & Auwerx, 2010). A recent study suggested that mTOR is a prime target in the genetic control of aging to determine life span and aging in yeast, worms, flies, and mice (Zoncu et al., 2011). The mTOR pathway accelerates growth by regulating signals downstream of insulin/IGF-1 receptors (Zoncu et al., 2011). Activation of mTOR is thought to speed up aging in adulthood, and reduced mTOR signaling would have the opposite effect, acting downstream of dietary restriction. Thus the anti-aging effect could be expected by mTOR inhibition, such as dietary restriction, rapamycin, introduction of the AMPK expression vector, and genetic inactivation of mTOR by techniques such as RNA interference.

5. Conclusions and future perspectives

It would be advantageous for cells to estimate the state of chromosomes just by monitoring telomeric regions. Monitoring the somatic genes, including promoter, exon, intron or other regions that harbors genetic information, would not work for that purpose, because single or multiple mutations might be lethal to the cell. Thus, microsatellite regions, including telomeres, would be suitable for a DNA damage monitoring system. Recently, it was shown that telomere length regulates mitochondrial function by activating PGC-1α (Sahin et al., 2011). This effect is the same as Rsv treatment (Lagouge et al., 2006). The CR mimetic drugs may have a common role in strengthening telomere maintenance. In the present study, we performed a multiple transfection experiment, which showed that shelterin protein-encoding gene promoters simultaneously respond to CR mimetic drugs in HeLa-S3 cells. Given that anti-aging drugs induce or activate the DNA repair system, especially by maintenance of telomeres, this multiple transfection system has demonstrable potential to contribute to the evaluation and development of such drugs.

6. Acknowledgments

The authors are grateful to Ryosuke Akiyama for outstanding technical assistance. This work was supported in part by a Research Fellowship from the Research Center for RNA Science, RIST, Tokyo University of Science, Tokyo, Japan.

7. References

Abreu, E., Aritonovska, E., Reichenbach, P., Cristofari, G., Culp, B., Terns, R.M., Lingner, J. & Terns, M.P. (2010). TIN2-tethered TPP1 recruits human telomerase to telomeres *in vivo*, *Molecular and Cellular. Biology* 30.(12): 2971–2982.

Blackburn, E.H. (2000). The end of the (DNA) line, *Nature Structural Biology* 7.(10): 847–850.

Campisi, J. & d'Adda di Fagagna, F. (2007). Cellular senescence: when bad things happen to good cells, *Nature Reviews. Molecular Cell Biology* 8.(9): 729–740.

Cantó, C., Auwerx, J. (2010). AMP-activated protein kinase and its downstream transcriptional pathways, *Cellular and Molecular Life Sciences* 67.(20): 3407–3423.

Cavallini, G., Donati, A., Gori, Z. & Bergamini, E. (2008). Towards an understanding of the anti-aging mechanism of caloric restriction, *Current Aging Science* 1.(1): 4–9.

Chen, Y., Rai, R., Zhou, Z.R., Kanoh, J., Ribeyre, C., Yang, Y., Zheng, H., Damay, P., Wang, F., Tsuji, H., Hiraoka, Y., Shore, D., Hu, H.Y., Chang, S. & Lei, M. (2011). A conserved motif within RAP1 has diversified roles in telomere protection and regulation in different organisms, *Nature Structural & Molecular Biology* 18.(2): 213–221.

Chu, W.K. & Hickson, I.D. (2009). RecQ helicases: multifunctional genome caretakers, *Nature Reviews. Cancer* 9.(9): 644–654.

Cohen, S.B., Graham, M.E., Lovrecz, G.O., Bache, N., Robinson, P.J. & Reddel, R.R. (2007). Protein composition of catalytically active human telomerase from immortal cells, *Science* 315.(5820): 1850–1853.

de Lange, T. (2006). Mammalian telomeres, *in* de Lange, T., Lundblad, V. & Blackburn, E. (ed.), *Telomeres (second ed.)*, Cold Spring Harbor Laboratory Press, New York, pp. 387-431.

Fröjdö, S., Durand, C. & Pirola L. (2008). Metabolic effects of resveratrol in mammals--a link between improved insulin action and aging, *Current Aging Science* 1.(3): 145–151.

Giannone, R.J., McDonald, H.W., Hurst, G.B., Shen, R.F., Wang, Y. & Liu, Y. (2010). The protein network surrounding the human telomere repeat binding factors TRF1, TRF2, and POT1, *PLoS One* 5.(8): e12407.

Gilson, E. & Géli, V. (2007). How telomeres are replicated, *Nature Reviews. Molecular Cell Biology* 8.(10): 825–838.

Gonzalez-Suarez, I. & Gonzalo, S. (2008). Crosstalk between chromatin structure, nuclear compartmentalization, and telomere biology, *Cytogenetic and Genome Research* 122.: 202–210.

Greider, C.W. & Blackburn, E.H. (1987). The telomere terminal transferase of *Tetrahymena* is a ribonucleoprotein enzyme with two kinds of primer specificity, *Cell* 51.(6): 887–898.

Griffith, J.D., Comeau, L., Rosenfield, S., Stansel, R.M., Bianchi, A., Moss, H. & de Lange, T. (1999). Mammalian telomeres end in a large duplex loop, *Cell* 97.(4): 503–514.

Jaskelioff, M., Muller, F.L., Paik, J.H., Thomas, E., Jiang, S., Adams, A.C., Sahin, E., Kost-Alimova, M., Protopopov, A., Cadiñanos, J., Horner, J.W., Maratos-Flier, E. & Depinho, R.A. (2011). Telomerase reactivation reverses tissue degeneration in aged telomerase-deficient mice, *Nature* 469.(7328): 102–106.

Kaeberlein, M. (2010). Resveratrol and rapamycin: are they anti-aging drugs? *Bioessays* 32.(2): 96–99.

Kenyon CJ. (2010). The genetics of aging, *Nature* 464. (7288): 504–512.

Knutson, M.D., & Leeuwenburgh, C. (2008). Resveratrol and novel potent activators of SIRT1: effects on aging and age-related diseases, *Nutrition Reviews* 66.(10): 591–596.

Kuningas, M., Mooijaart, S.P., van Heemst, D., Zwaan, B.J., Slagboom, P.E. & Westendorp, R.G. (2008). Genes encoding longevity: from model organisms to humans, *Aging Cell* 7.(2): 270–280.

Lagouge, M., Argmann, C., Gehart-Hines, Z., Meziane, H., Lerin, C., Daussin, F., Messadeq, N., Milne, J., Lambert, P., Elliott, P., Geny, B., Laakso, M., Puigserver, P. & Auwerx, J. (2006). Resveratrol improves mitochondrial function and protects against metabolic disease by activating SIRT1 and PGC-1alpha, *Cell* 127.(6): 1109–1122.

Lin, X., Zhang, F., Bradbury, C.M., Kaushal, A., Li, L., Spitz, D.R., Aft, R.L. & Gius, D. (2003). 2-Deoxy-D-glucose-induced cytotoxicity and radiosensitization in tumor cells is mediated via disruptions in thiol metabolism, *Cancer Research* 63.(12): 3413–3417.

Lundblad, V. & Szostak, J.W. (1989). A mutant with a defect in telomere elongation leads to senescence in yeast, *Cell* 57.(4): 633–643.

Meek, D.W. (2009). Tumor suppression by p53: a role for the DNA damage response? *Nature Reviews. Cancer* 9.(10): 714–723.

Oberdoerffer, P. & Sinclair, D.A. (2007). The role of nuclear architecture in genomic instability and aging, *Nature Reviews. Molecular Cell Biology* 8.(9): 692–702.

Opresko, P.L., Mason, P.A., Podell, E.R., Lei, M., Hickson, I.D., Cech, T.R. & Bohr, V.A. (2005). POT1 stimulates RecQ helicases WRN and BLM to unwind telomeric DNA substrates, *Journal of Biological Chemistry* 280.(37): 32069–32080.

O'Sullivan, R.J. & Karlseder, J. (2010). Telomeres: protecting chromosomes against genome instability, *Nature Reviews. Molecular Cell Biology* 11.(3): 171–181.

Roth, G.S., Ingram, D.K. & Lane, M.A. (2001). Caloric restriction in primates and relevance to humans, *Annals of the New York Academy of Sciences* 928.: 305–315.

Sahin, E. & Depinho, R.A. (2010). Linking functional decline of telomeres, mitochondria and stem cells during aging, *Nature* 464.(7288): 520–528.

Sahin, E., Colla, S., Liesa, M., Moslehi, J., Müller, F.L., Guo, M., Cooper, M., Kotton, D., Fabian, A.J., Walkey, C., Maser, R.S., Tonon, G., Foerster, F., Xiong, R., Wang, Y.A., Shukla, S.A., Jaskelioff, M., Martin, E.S., Heffernan, T.P., Protopopov, A., Ivanova, E., Mahoney, J.E., Kost-Alimova, M., Perry, S.R., Bronson, R., Liao, R., Mulligan, R., Shirihai, O.S., Chin, L. & DePinho, R.A. (2011). Telomere dysfunction induces metabolic and mitochondrial compromise, *Nature* 470.(7334): 359–365.

Sanz, A. & Stefanatos, R.K. (2008). The mitochondrial free radical theory of aging: A critical view, *Current Aging Science* 1.(1): 10–21.

Schumacher, B. (2009). Transcription-blocking DNA damage in aging: a mechanism for hormesis, *Bioessays* 31.(12): 1347–1356.

Schreiber, V., Dantzer, F., Ame, J.-C. & de Murcia, G. (2006). Poly(ADP-ribose): novel functions for an old molecule, *Nature Reviews. Molecular Cell Biology* 7.(7): 517–528.

Schulz, V.P. & Zakian, V.A. (1994). The saccharomyces PIF1 DNA helicase inhibits telomere elongation and de novo telomere formation, *Cell* 76.(1): 145–155.

Smith, S., Giriat, I., Schmitt, A. & de Lange, T. (1998). Tankyrase, a poly(ADP-ribose) polymerase at human telomeres, *Science* 282.(5393): 1484–1487.

Stefani, M., Markus, M.A., Lin, R.C., Pinese, M., Dawes, I.W. & Morris, B.J. (2007). The effect of resveratrol on a cell model of human aging, *Annals of the New York Academy of Sciences* 1114.: 407–418.

Stern, J.L. & Bryan, T.M. (2008). Telomerase recruitment to telomeres, *Cytogenetic and Genome Research* 122.: 243–254.

Cosan, D.T., Soyocak, A., Basaran, A., Degirmenci, I., Gunes, H.V. & Sahin, F.M. (2011). Effects of various agents on DNA fragmentation and telomerase enzyme activities in adenocarcinoma cell lines, *Molecular Biology Reports* 38.(4): 2463-2469.

Uchiumi, F., Sakakibara, G., Sato, J. & Tanuma, S. (2008). Characterization of the promoter region of the human *PARG* gene and its response to PU.1 during differentiation of HL-60 cells, *Genes to Cells* 13.(12): 1229–1247.

Uchiumi, F., Watanabe, T. & Tanuma, S. (2010a). Characterization of various promoter regions of the human DNA helicase-encoding genes and identification of duplicated *ets* (GGAA) motifs as an essential transcription regulatory element, *Experimental Cell Research* 316.(9): 1523–1534.

Uchiumi, F., Enokida, K., Shiraishi, T., Masumi, A. & Tanuma, S. (2010b). Characterization of the promoter region of the human *IGHMBP2* (*Sμbp-2*) gene and its response to TPA in HL-60 cells, *Gene* 436.(1-2): 8–17.

Uchiumi, F., Higami, Y. & Tanuma, S. (2010c). Regulations of telomerase activity and *WRN* gene expression, *in* Gagnon, A.N. (ed.), *Telomerase: Composition, Functions and Clinical Implications*, Nova Science Publishers, Inc., Hauppauge, NY, pp. 95–103.

Uchiumi, F., Watanabe, T., Hasegawa, S., Hoshi, T., Higami, Y. & Tanuma, S. (2011a). The effect of resveratrol on the werner syndrome RecQ helicase gene and telomerase activity, *Current Aging Science* 4.(1): 1–7.

Uchiumi, F., Miyazaki, S. & Tanuma, S. (2011b). The possible functions of duplicated ets (GGAA) motifs located near transcription start sites of various human genes, *Cellular and Molecular Life Sciences* 68.(12): 2039-2051.

van der Horst, A. & Burgering, B.M. (2007). Stressing the role of FoxO proteins in lifespan and disease, *Nature Reviews. Molecular Cell Biology* 8.(6): 440–450.

Vijg, J. (2007). Genome instability and accelerated aging, *in* Vijg, J. (ed.), *Aging of the Genome*, Oxford University Press, Oxford, pp. 151–180.

Zhou, B., Ikejima, T., Watanabe, T., Iwakoshi, K., Idei, Y., Tanuma, S. & Uchiumi, F. (2009). The effect of 2-deoxy-D-glucose on Werner syndrome RecQ helicase gene, *FEBS Letters* 583.(8): 1331–1336.

Zoncu, R., Efeyan A., & Sabatini, D.M. (2011). mTOR: from growth signal integration to cancer, diabetes and aging, *Nature Reviews. Molecular Cell Biology* 12.(1): 21–35.

30

Roles of DNA Repair Proteins in Telomere Maintenance

Masaru Ueno
Hiroshima University
Japan

1. Introduction

Most eukaryots have specialized protein-DNA complexs, called telomeres at the ends of natural linear chromosomes. Telomeric DNA consists of a tandemly repeated G-rich sequence. The lengths of telomeric DNAs in *S. pombe, S. cerevisiae,* and human are ~300 nucleotids, ~350 nucleotides, and ~10 kb, respectively. The ends of the telomeric DNA have 3′ single-stranded overhangs. The protein components of telomeres consists of double-stranded telomere-binding proteins, such as human TRF1 and TRF2, S. pombe Taz1, and single-stranded telomere-binding proteins, such as *S. cerevisiae* Cdc13, *S. pombe* Pot1, and human POT1. DNA double-strand breaks (DSBs) must be repaired to maintain genomic integrity. In contrast, natural chromosome ends should not be recognized as DSBs. The telomere is capped to protect from DNA repair activity. If this capping function is lost, this uncapped telomere is recognized as DNA damage and becomes substrate for DNA repair proteins. The first step in homologous recombination (HR) repair is processing of DNA ends by 5′ to 3′ degradation to create 3′ single-stranded overhangs. The proteins involved in this steps include *S. cerevisiae* Mre11-Rad50-Xrs2 complex (MRX), Sae2, Sgs1, and Dna2. Recent works revealed that proteins involved in the processing of DNA DSB ends are also involved in the processing of capped or uncapped telomere. These facts raised new question of how these proteins are regulated at telomere ends. This chapter will focus on the roles of proteins involved in the processing of DBS ends at capped (functional) and uncapped (dysfunctional) telomere in *S. pombe, S. cerevisiae* and human. This chapter will also focus on the functional interactions between telomere-binding proteins and proteins involved in the processing of DBS ends. Resent works revealed that double-stranded and single-stranded telomere-binding proteins play critical roles to control proteins involved in DNA repair at chromosome ends.

2. Roles of proteins involved in DNA end-processing in telomere maintenance

DNA DSBs are repaired by HR or non-homologous end-joining (NHEJ) [1]. *S. cerevisiae* MRX is involved in both HR and NHEJ [2]. MRX is suggested to be involved in the processng of DSB ends in HR repair. Recently, several other proteins involved the processing have been discovered. Some of the these proteins are also involved in the processing of telomere ends. In this section, the roles of these proteins in telomere maintenance will be discussed.

2.1 Roles of proteins involved in DNA end-processing at DSB ends

Role of *S. cerevisiae* MRX in HR is well studied both in vivo and in vitro (Mimitou and Symington 2009) (Mimitou and Symington 2008) (Zhu et al. 2008) (Gravel et al. 2008) (Cejka et al. 2010) (Niu et al. 2010). MRX cooperates with Sae2 to initiate 5′ resection at DNA DSB end. Although both MRX and Sae2 have nuclease activities, it remains unclear the contribution of these nucleases to DSB resection. The resultant 3′ single-stranded ovehangs are further resected by two redundant pathways. One is dependent on Sgs1 helicase, a conserved RecQ family member, and the Dna2. Dna2 has both helicase and nuclease domains, but nuclease activity is enough for DSB resection (Zhu et al. 2008). The other is dependent on Exo1 5′-3′ exonuclease. *S. cerevisiae* Yku70-Yku80 heterodimer (Ku) binds to DSB ends and recruits downstream NHEJ factors (Critchlow and Jackson 1998). Ku inhibits 5′ resection by MRX (Mimitou and Symington 2010) (Shim et al. 2010). Similar model is proposed in *S. pombe*(Tomita et al. 2003). *S. pombe* Mre11-Rad50-Nbs1 (S. cerevisiae Xrs2 homologue) complex (MRN) is also suggested to be involved in 5′ resection at DNA DSB end. *S. pombe* Ku also inhibits 5′ resection by MRN. In the absence of MRN, Exo1 can resect DSB ends. Contribution of *S. pombe* RecQ helicase Rqh1 and Dna2 in the resection of DSB ends remains unclear. It has been shown that human BLM, a RecQ helicase family, and DNA2 interact to resect DNA end and helicase activity of BLM and nuclease activity of DNA2 are required for this reaction (Nimonkar et al. 2011). The functional conservation of these proteins from yeast to human suggests that the functions of these proteins in *S. pombe* are also conserved.

2.2 Roles of proteins involved in DNA end-processing in telomere maintenance in *S. pombe* and in *S. cerevisiae*

Telomere ends should not be recognized as DSB ends, because telomere ends should no be repaired by HR or NHEJ. However, proteins involved in HR or NHEJ are also involved in telomere maintenance (Longhese et al. 2010). The chromosome end replicated by lagging-strand synthesis has 3′ single-stranded overhangs. In contrast, the chromosome end replicated by leading-strand synthesis is blunt-end. However, most eukaryotes have 3′ single-stranded overhangs at both ends, suggesting that the chromosome end replicated by leading-strand synthesis is resected (Wellinger et al. 1996; Makarov, Hirose, and Langmore 1997). *S. cerevisiae* MRX is suggested to be involved in this resection (Diede and Gottschling 2001). However, MRX independent resection has been suggested, which may be produced at lagging-strand telomere after DNA replication without any nuclease activity (Larrivee, LeBel, and Wellinger 2004). MRX mainly binds to the leading-strand telomere, further suggesting that MRX is involved in this resection at leading-strand telomere (Faure et al. 2010). An inducible short telomere assay revealed that artificial telomere ends is resected by the same DNA repair factors (Bonetti et al. 2009) (Longhese et al. 2010) (Iglesias and Lingner 2009) (Fig. 1). MRX and Sae2 act in the same resection pathway. Concomitant inactivation of Sae2 and Sgs1 abolishes end resection, suggesting that they have redundant function for the resection. Dna2 acts redundantly with Exo1, but not with Sgs1, suggesting that Dna2 supports Sgs1 activity. The lack of Sgs1, Dna2 or Exo1 by itself does not affect the resection, suggesting that Exo1 and Sgs1-Dna2 may less important for the resection than MRX and Sae2. These results were obtained by using artificial telomere, which initially produces blunt-end telomere by nuclease. However, leading-strand synthesis in wild-type cells also produces blunt-end telomere. Consistently, Sae2 and Sgs1 also play redundant functions in natural telomere end-processing (Bonetti et al. 2009), suggesting that an inducible short telomere assay mimic wild-type telomere end. In wild-type *S. cerevisiae* cells, 3′ single-stranded overhangs increase in S phase at telomeres (Wellinger, Wolf, and Zakian 1993) (Dionne and Wellinger 1996). In contrast, 3′ single-stranded overhangs can be detected at telomeres throughout the cell cycle in the absence of *S. cerevisiae* Ku, suggesting that Ku inhibits resection at telomere (Gravel et al. 1998) (Polotnianka, Li, and Lustig 1998). This function of Ku is conserved in *S. pombe* Ku (Kibe et al. 2003). However, proteins involved in the resection of telomere ends are not well studied in *S. pombe*. In *S. pombe*, Dna2 is involved in the resection of telomere ends (Tomita et al. 2004).

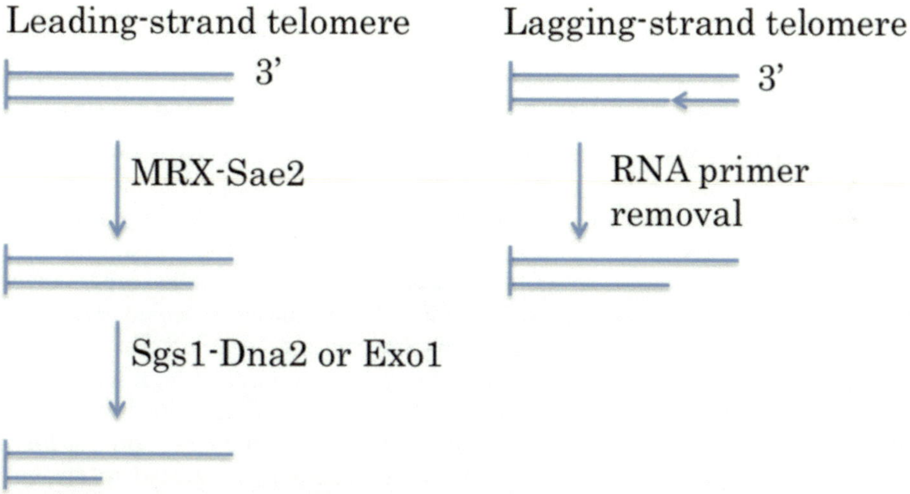

Fig. 1. Model for DNA end-processing at *S. cerevisiae* telomere. DNA replication will create blunt-end at leading-strand telomere and 3′ single-stranded overhangs at lagging-strand telomere after removal of the last RNA primer. Similar to the case at DSB ends, MRX and Sae2 play a major role to produce 3′ single-stranded overhangs at telomeres. Sgs1-Dna2 and Exo1 can provide compensatory activities to produce 3′ single-stranded overhangs.

2.3 Proteins involved in DNA end-processing in *S. pombe taz1Δ* cells

S. pombe Taz1 binds telomeric double-stranded DNA (Cooper, Watanabe, and Nurse 1998). Deletion of *taz1* causes massive telomere elongation. Asynchronous wild-type *S. pombe* cells have small amount of 3′ single-stranded overhangs (Kibe et al. 2003). In contrast, *taz1* disruptant has very long 3′ single-stranded overhangs (Tomita et al. 2003). In this mutant background, roles of MRN, Ku, Dna2, and Exo1 are studied (Fig. 2). MRN and Dna2 are responsible for the production of 3′ single-stranded overhangs (Tomita et al. 2004). But, 3′ single-stranded overhangs are produced by concomitant deletion of Ku and MRN, suggesting that unknown nuclease can produce the overhangs in the absence of both MRN and Ku in *taz1* disruptant. Exo1 is not involved in this activity. Telomere ends in *taz1* disruptant is partially unprotected. Indeed, RPA foci and Rad22^{Rad52} foci are produced at telomere in *taz1* disruptant (Carneiro et al. 2010). Therefore, proteins involved in the resection in *taz1* disruptant may not be same as that in wild-type cells. However, Dna2 is involved in the resection in both wild-type and *taz1Δ* background, suggesting that some of the proteins involved in the resection in *taz1* disruptant are also involved in the resection in wild-type cells.

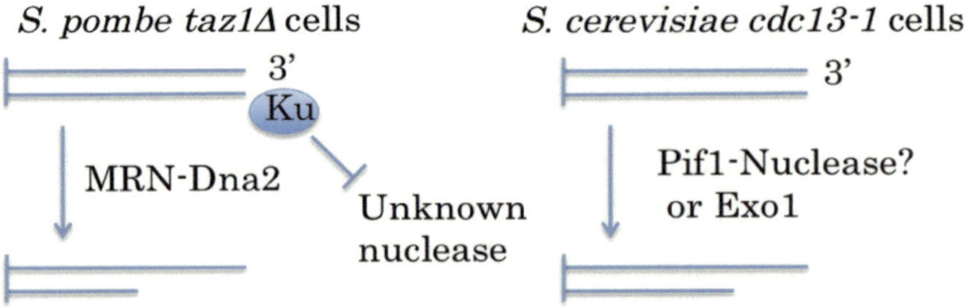

Fig. 2. Model for DNA end-processing at dysfunctional telomere. 3′ single-stranded overhangs are produced by MRN and Dna2 in *S. pombe taz1Δ* cells (Left). Ku inhibits unknown nuclease, but not nuclease activity depending on MRN-Dna2. 3′ single-stranded overhangs are produced by Pif1 or Exo1 in *S. cerevisiae cdc13-1* cells (Right). Unknown nuclease is suggested to function together with Pif1 helicase.

2.4 Proteins involved in DNA end-processing in *S. cerevisiae cdc13-1* cells

S. cerevisiae Cdc13 binds telomeric single-stranded DNA (Garvik, Carson, and Hartwell 1995). *cdc13-1* temperature sensitive mutant is used to study proteins that are involved in the resection at uncapped telomeres (Lydall 2009). These studies revealed that the single-stranded DNA at telomeres in *cdc13-1* mutants resembles a DSB end. However, there are some differences between these ends (Fig. 2). In *cdc13-1* mutants at high temperature, Pif1 helicase and Exo1 are redundantly involved in the resection of uncapped telomere (Dewar and Lydall 2010). It remains unclear how Pif1 contribute to the resection. As Pif1 has no nuclease activity, involvement of the unknown nuclease is suggested to cleave single-stranded DNA unwound by Pif1 helicase. Sgs1 also contributes to resection of telomeres in *cdc13-1* mutants (Ngo and Lydall 2010). However, unlike *pif1 exo1* double mutant, resection of telomeres in *cdc13-1* mutant background occurs in *sgs1 exo1* double mutant, demonstrating that Pif1 and Exo1 play major roles in the resection of uncapped telomere at high temperature.

3. Roles of RecQ helicase in telomere maintenance

RecQ helicase is conserved from *E. coli.* to human and play a critical role in genome stability (Bernstein, Gangloff, and Rothstein 2010). Werner Syndrome (WS) is a premature aging syndrome resulting from loss of function of one of the human RecQ helicase WRN. The roles of *S. cerevisiae* RecQ helicase Sgs1 in homologous recombination are well studied. RecQ helicase is also involved in telomere maintenance especially at dysfunctional telomere. In this section, roles of RecQ helicase in telomere maintenance will be discussed. Functional interaction between RecQ helicase and POT1 in *S. pombe* and in human will be also discussed.

3.1 Roles of RecQ helicase in DNA repair

S. cerevisiae RecQ helicase Sgs1 is involved in several steps in HR (Ashton and Hickson 2010). As discussed above, Sgs1 is involved in the resection of DSB ends. Genetic and in vitro studies also suggest that Sgs1 inhibits unscheduled recombinogenic events, but promotes the resolution of recombination intermediates. Strains deleted for *SGS1* display hyperrecombination phenotype, but are defective in DNA damage-induced heteroallilic recombination (Watt et al. 1996) (Onoda et al. 2001). *S. cerevisiae* Sgs1 and Top3 migrate and disentangle a double Holliday junction (dHJ) to produce non-crossover recombination products in vitro (Cejka et al. 2010). This activity is also detected in human RecQ helicase BLM and human topoisomerase IIIa (Wu and Hickson 2003). Mutant of *S. pombe* RecQ helicase *rqh1* is sensitive to DNA damage and has high frequency of recombination under normal growth conditions and following DNA damage, suggesting that Rqh1 is also involved in HR repair both positively and negatively (Murray et al. 1997) (Stewart et al. 1997) (Doe et al. 2000) (Caspari, Murray, and Carr 2002).

3.2 Roles of RecQ helicase in telomere maintenance in *S. cerevisiae*

As mutation of *S. cerevisiae SGS1* does not affect telomere length, Sgs1 has no apparent role in telomere maintenance in the presence of telomerase activity (Watt et al. 1996). However, the double mutant between telomerase RNA component *TLC1* and *SGS1* shorten telomeres at an increased rate per population doubling and Sgs1 affects telomere-telomere recombination in the absence of telomerase, demonstrating that Sgs1 plays roles at telomere in the absence of telomerase activity (Johnson et al. 2001) (Cohen and Sinclair 2001) (Huang et al. 2001). X-shaped structures are accumulated at telomeres in senescing *tlc1 sgs1* double mutants and these structures are suggested to be the recombination intermediates related to hemicatenanes. This result suggests that Sgs1 is required for the efficient resolution of telomere recombination intermediates in the absence of telomerase (Lee et al. 2007; Chavez, Tsou, and Johnson 2009).

3.3 Roles of RecQ helicase in telomere maintenance in mammals

Human RecQ helicase WRN binds to telomere in S phase in primary human IMR90 fibroblasts and is required for efficient replication of the G-rich telomeric DNA strand, suggesting that WRN is required for replication of telomeric DNA in telomerase-negative primary human fibroblasts (Crabbe et al. 2004). In Werner syndrome (WS) cells, replication-associated telomere loss results in the chromosome fusions, causing genomic instability (Crabbe et al. 2007). The life span of normal human skin fibroblasts derived from WS patients can be extended by expression of the catalytic subunit human telomerase reverse transcriptase (hTERT) (Wyllie et al. 2000; Ouellette et al. 2000). These facts demonstrate that dysfunctional telomere is a major determinant of the premature aging syndrome and WRN plays important role at dysfunctional telomere and telomerase activity can suppress the defect in WRN deficient cells. Consistently, Wrn-deficient mouse, which has telomerase activity, has no disease phenotype, but telomerase-Wrn double null mouse elicits a Werner-like premature aging syndrome (Chang et al. 2004). Telomere sister chromatid exchange (T-SEC) increases in cells from telomerase-Wrn double null mouse, suggesting that WRN are required to repress inappropriate telomere recombination (Laud et al. 2005) (Multani and Chang 2007). Human WRN and other RecQ helicase BLM co-localizes with telomere in human cancer cells that lack telomerase, ALT cells (Johnson et al. 2001; Opresko et al. 2004; Lillard-Wetherell et al. 2004). As telomeres in ALT cells are maintained by HR, human WRN and BLM are suggested to be involved in the recombination at telomere in ALT cells. Possible roles of WRN in telomere maintenance will be discussed in the next section.

3.4 Functional interaction between RecQ helicase and POT1 in *S. pombe* and in human

Pot1 is conserved from *S. pombe* to human and binds to single-stranded telomeric DNA sequence specifically (Baumann and Cech 2001). Deletion of *S. pombe pot1* causes rapid telomere loss and chromosome circularization and this circularization is mediated by single strand annealing (SSA) (Wang and Baumann 2008). In *S. cerevisiae*, Rad52, Rad1/Rad10 nuclease, RPA, Srs2 helicase, and Sgs1 are involved in SSA (Fishman-Lobell and Haber 1992) (Ivanov and Haber 1995) (Ivanov et al. 1996) (Paques and Haber 1997), (Sugawara, Ira, and Haber 2000; Umezu et al. 1998) (Zhu et al. 2008). Consistently, the double mutants between *S. pombe* homologue of these proteins and *pot1* are synthetically lethal (Wang and Baumann 2008). *S. pombe* telomerase disruptant can survive either by maintaining telomere by HR or chromosome circularization(Nakamura, Cooper, and Cech 1998). In contrast, *pot1* disruptant survives only by chromosome circularization (Baumann and Cech 2001). One possible explanation is that Pot1 is required for prevention of rapid telomere loss, which would lead chromosome circularization dominantly. Recently our group has reported that the double mutant between *rqh1-hd* (helicase dead point mutant) and *pot1* is not synthetically lethal (Takahashi et al. 2011). The chromosome ends of the *pot1 rqh1-hd* double mutant are maintained by HR. There are several possible explanations for this. First, helicase dead Rqh1 may bind to the chromosome ends in *pot1* disruptant to inhibit rapid telomere loss, allowing cells to maintain chromosome ends by HR. Second, helicase activity of the Rqh1 may be involved in the rapid telomere loss in the *pot1* disruptant, because *S. cerevisiae* RecQ helicase is involved in the processing of telomere ends. This will also allow cells to maintain chromosome ends by HR. Third, helicase activity of the Rqh1 may be required for the suppression of recombination at telomere. This will also allow cells to maintain chromosome ends by HR. The exact role of the helicase dead Rqh1 in pot1 disruptant remains unclear. Interestingly, *pot1 rqh1-hd* double mutant is sensitive to anti-microtubule drug thiabendazole (TBZ) (Takahashi et al. 2011). The *pot1 rqh1-hd* double mutant has recombination intermediates even in the M phase at the chromosome ends. This physical link between the sister chromatids in M phase will inhibit chromosome segregation, especially in the presence of TBZ, which would lender cells sensitive to TBZ. Interestingly, concomitant

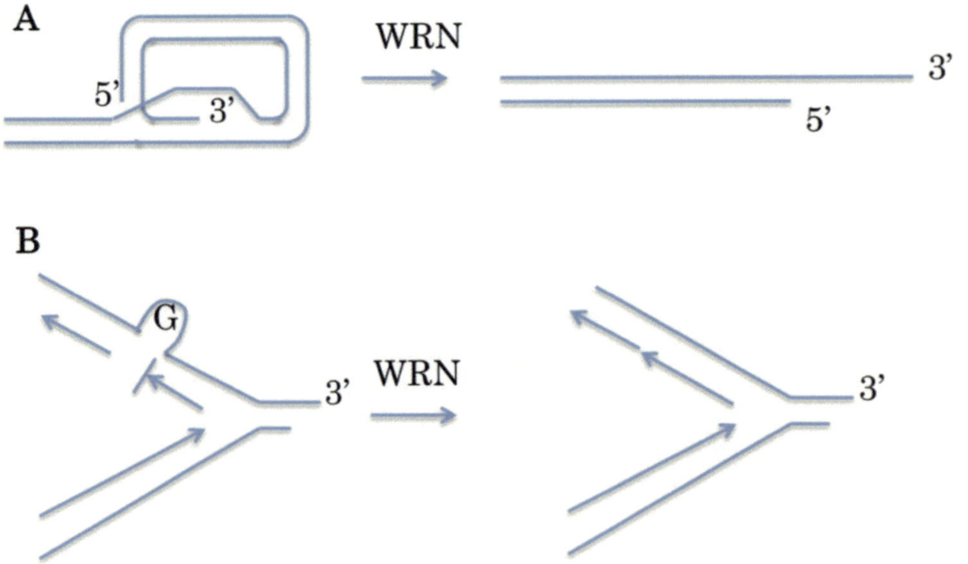

Fig. 3. WRN activities on a telomeric D-loop structure (A) and on a lagging strand telomere (B) during S phase. **A**. The model shows that WRN helicase releases the invading strand during S phase. **B**. WRN resolves G-quartet (G) formed on the lagging telomeric DNA.

inhibition of WRN and POT1 also lender human cells sensitive to anti-microtubule drug vinblastine, implying the functional conservation between human POT1 and WRN and *S. pombe* Pot1 and Rqh1(Takahashi et al. 2011). The other double knockdown experiments of WRN and POT1 in human cells show that human POT1 is required for efficient telomere C-rich strand replication in the absence of WRN (Arnoult et al. 2009). The functional interaction between human POT1 and RecQ helicase WRN is also suggested by in vitro experiment. Purified human POT1 binds to WRN and POT1 binding on telomeric DNA regulates the unwinding activity of WRN (Opresko et al. 2005; Sowd, Lei, and Opresko 2008; Opresko, Sowd, and Wang 2009). Based on these and other data, several possible roles of WRN at telomere are suggested (Rossi, Ghosh, and Bohr 2010) (Fig. 3). Telomere is capped by telomere binding proteins called shelterin and the chromosome end is protected through strand invasion of the duplex telomeric repeat by the 3′ single-stranded overhangs, which is called t-loop (Palm and de Lange 2008). As WRN acts to release the 3′ invading tail from a telomeric D loop in vitro, WRN may be involved in the regulation of the t-loop (Opresko et al. 2004). Single-stranded overhangs can fold into G-quadruplex DNA, which may inhibit DNA polymerase and telomerase at telomere (Zaug, Podell, and Cech 2005). Therefore, WRN may disrupt telomeric G-quadruplex with POT1 to facilitate DNA replication and/or telomere elongation at telomeres.

4. Roles of RPA in telomere maintenance

Replication protein A (RPA) is a heterotrimeric single-stranded non-specific DNA-binding protein consisting of a large (70 kDa), middle (32 kDa) and small (14 kDa) subunit. RPA is conserved from yeast to human and is essential for DNA replication, repair, and recombination (Binz, Sheehan, and Wold 2004). The large subunits of RPA in human, *S, cerevisiae* and *S. pombe* are named as RPA70, Rfa1 and Rad11, respectively. RPA is involved in HR repair by binding the single-stranded DNA generated by DNA end-processing at DSB ends. Single-stranded DNA is also produced at telomere. But RPA is suggested to be excluded from single-stranded telomere overhangs because it will lead to DNA damage checkpoint activation and cell cycle arrest. However, genetic evidences suggest the role of RPA in telomere maintenance. In this section, possible roles of RPA in telomere maintenance will be discussed. The functional relationship between RPA, RecQ helicase, and Taz1 will be also discussed.

4.1 Roles of RPA in DNA repair

Mutations in *S, cerevisiare rfa1* lender cells to sensitive to DNA damage and affect recombination efficiency, suggesting the involvement of RPA in recombination and repair processes (Smith and Rothstein 1995; Firmenich, Elias-Arnanz, and Berg 1995; Umezu et al. 1998). *S. pombe rad11* mutants are also sensitive to DNA damage and *rad11-D223Y* mutant is epitatic to *rad50* mutant, suggesting that RPA is involved in the HR repair (Parker et al. 1997; Ono et al. 2003). The roles of RPA in HR repair is well studied by in vitro system using *S. pombe* proteins (Kurokawa et al. 2008; Murayama et al. 2008). These in vitro and other genetic studies suggest that RPA binds to the single-stranded DNA generated by processing at DSB end. Then Rad22 (the *S. pombe* Rad52 homolog) helps Rad51 to displace RPA from single-stranded DNA. RPA bound to the single-stranded DNA recruits DNA damage checkpoint proteins to the DSB site to activate DNA damage checkpoint (Zou and Elledge 2003).

4.2 Roles of RPA in telomere maintenance

Telomere ends have single-strand overhangs, which may serve substrates for RPA. However, it is believeaved that RPA is excluded from telomere to suppress DNA damage checkpoint activation at telomere. Indeed, binding of human and mouse POT1 to telomeric ssDNA inhibits the localization of RPA to telomeres (Barrientos et al. 2008) (Gong and de Lange 2010). However, there are several genetic evidences suggesting that RPA is involved in telomere maintenance. Mutation of *S. cerevisiae RFA1* gene, *rfa1-D228Y* in *Yku70* mutant background causes telomere shortening, demonstration that RPA is required for telomere length regulation at dysfunctional telomere (Smith, Zou, and Rothstein 2000). Moreover, certain mutant alleles of *RFA2* gene, encoding the middle subunit of RPA, in wild-type background causes telomere shortening, demonstration that RPA is required for telomere length regulation (Mallory et al. 2003). In addition, *S. cerevisiae* RPA binds to telomere especially in S phase and cells expressing truncated Rfa2 show impaired binding of the Est1, a component of telomerase (Schramke et al. 2004). Based on these data, they proposed that RPA activates telomerase by loading Est1 onto telomeres during S phase. *S. pombe rad11-D223Y* mutant, which corresponds to the *S.cerevisiae rfa1-D228Y* mutant, has short telomere in wild-type background. Moreover, *S. pombe* RPA binds to telomere especially in S phase (Ono et al. 2003; Moser et al. 2009). A genome-wide screen for *S. pombe* deletion mutants shows that deletion of *ssb3*, the small subunit of RPA, affects telomere length(Liu et al. 2010). These facts suggest that RPA plays important role in telomere maintenance in both *S. cerevisiae* and *S. pombe*. Human RPA is also enriched at telomere during S phase, possibly due to exposure of single-stranded DNA during telomere replication (Verdun and Karlseder 2006). The aspartic acid at position 223 in *S. pombe* Rad11 is important for telomere length regulation, which corresponds to the position 227 in human RPA70 (Ono et al. 2003). Similarly, expression of RPA70-D227Y mutant protein in human fibrosarcoma HT1080 cells causes telomere shortening, suggesting that human RPA also plays role in telomere length regulation (Kobayashi et al. 2010). Possible role of RPA at telomere is the regulation of the processing of telomere ends by controlling accessibility of DNA repair proteins and/or Pot1 to single-stranded overhang (Fig. 4).

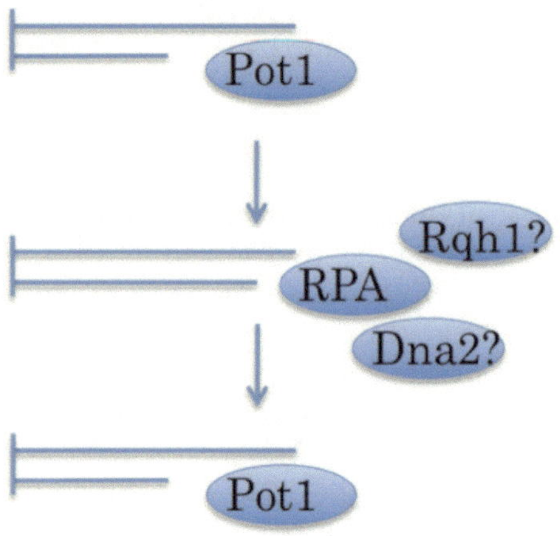

Fig. 4. The model shows that *S. pombe* RPA regulates the localizations and/or activities of proteins involved in the telomere maintenance. RPA may regulate Dna2 and/or Rqh1 during S phase.

4.3 Functional interaction between *S. pombe* Taz1, RPA and RecQ helicase

S. pombe taz1 rad11-D223Y double mutant lose telomere very rapidly, demonstrating that Taz1 and RPA collaborate to maintain telomere (Kibe et al. 2007). This rapid telomere loss can be suppressed by overexpression of Pot1. One possible explanation for this data is that Taz1 and RPA are required for the function of Pot1 at telomere and overexpression of Pot1 can rescue this defect. The rapid telomere loss of *taz1 rad11-D223Y* double mutant can be also suppressed by deletion of *rqh1*. Sgs1 is involved in the processing of telomere ends in *S. cerevisiae*. Similarly, *S. pombe* Rqh1 may be involved in the rapid telomere loss, possible by degradation of C-rich strand in *taz1 rad11-D223Y* double mutant (Fig. 5). The other functional relationship between Taz1 and Rqh1 is reported by Cooper group. *taz1* disruptant is sensitive to low temperature (Miller and Cooper 2003). Telomere entanglement is suggested to be a reason for this cold sensitivity. They found that unsumoylated Rqh1 mutant can suppress this cold sensitivity (Rog et al. 2009). Trt1 is a catalitic subunit of telomerase in *S. pombe*. *trt1* single mutant loses telomeric DNA gradually (Nakamura, Cooper, and Cech 1998). In contrast, *taz1 trt1* double mutant lose telomere very rapidly (Miller, Rog, and Cooper 2006). The replication fork stalling at the telomeres and resultant DSB is suggested to be a season for the rapid telomere loss in *taz1 trt1* double mutant. Unsumoylated Rqh1 mutant can also suppress this rapid telomere loss. Based on these data, they propose that sumoylated Rqh1 promotes telomere breakage and entanglement in *taz1* disruptant. This data demonstrate that the activity of Rqh1 at telomere is regulated to protect telomere. However, it remains unclear how Rqh1 and other DNA repair proteins are regulated at telomere. The functional interactions between human TRF1/TRF2 (*S. pombe*

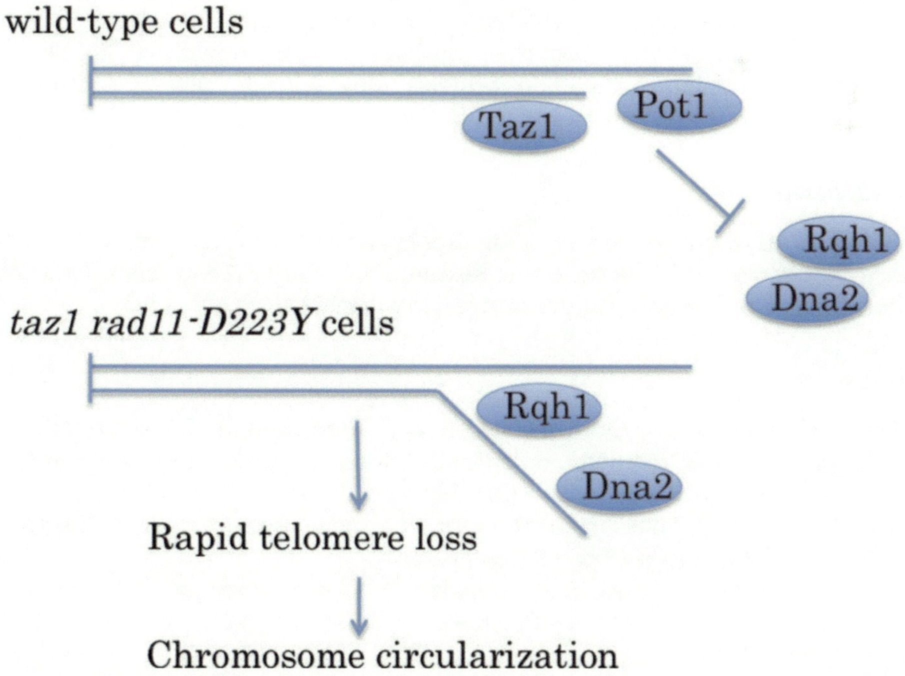

Fig. 5. The model shows that *S. pombe* Taz1 and RPA are required for prevent rapid telomere loss. In *taz1 rad11-D223Y* double mutant, Pot1 can not function properly and Rqh1 and possibly Dna2 resects telomere ends, which causes rapid telomere loss.

Taz1 ortholog) and human RecQ homolog WRN and BLM in telomere maintenance are also suggested (Opresko 2008). TRF2 interacts with WRN and stimulates helicase activity of WRN in vitro (Opresko et al. 2002; Machwe, Xiao, and Orren 2004). Expression of a TRF2 lacking the amino terminal basic domain induces the telomeric circle formations and rapid telomere deletions (Wang, Smogorzewska, and de Lange 2004). These events are dependent on WRN (Li et al. 2008). TRF2 also protects the displacement of Holliday junctions with telomeric arm by WRN in vitro (Nora, Buncher, and Opresko 2010). These facts suggest that the regulation of WRN activity by TRF2 is required to protect telomere.

5. Conclusion

This chapter focused on the roles of proteins involved in the processing of DBS ends at functional and dysfunctional telomere in *S. pombe, S. cerevisiae* and human. We found that MRN, Dna2, and possibly RecQ helicase Rqh1 are involved in the processing at telomere ends in *S. pombe*. Lydall group and other group found that Exo1, RecQ helicase Sgs1, Dna2, and Pif1 are involved in the processing at telomere ends in *S. cerevisiae*. Interestingly, most of these proteins were also involved in the processing of DNA double-strand break ends. These facts raise a new question of how these proteins are regulated at telomere ends. This chapter also focused on the functional interactions between telomere capping proteins and proteins involved in the processing of DBS ends mainly in *S. pombe*. We found that Taz1 and RPA collaborate to inhibit DNA end-processing, possibly by RecQ helicase, to prevent telomere loss. We also found that single-stranded telomere-binding protein Pot1 and RecQ helicase Rqh1 collaborate to inhibit homologous recombination at telomere. Cooper group found that RecQ helicase Rqh1 makes *taz1* disruptant sensitive to cold temperature by creating telomere entanglement. From these analyses, we learned that both double-stranded and single-stranded telomere binding proteins play critical roles to control proteins involved in DNA repair at chromosome ends.

6. Acknowledgment

I wish to thank all of my collaborators for support on my research. Part of this work was supported by Grants-in-Aid for Scientific Research on Priority Areas from the Ministry of Education, Science, Sports and Culture of Japan to Masaru Ueno.

7. References

Arnoult, N., C. Saintome, I. Ourliac-Garnier, J. F. Riou, and A. Londono-Vallejo. 2009. Human POT1 is required for efficient telomere C-rich strand replication in the absence of WRN. *Genes Dev.* 23 (24):2915-24.

Ashton, T. M., and I. D. Hickson. 2010. Yeast as a model system to study RecQ helicase function. *DNA Repair (Amst)* 9 (3):303-14.

Barrientos, K. S., M. F. Kendellen, B. D. Freibaum, B. N. Armbruster, K. T. Etheridge, and C. M. Counter. 2008. Distinct functions of POT1 at telomeres. *Mol. Cell. Biol.* 28 (17):5251-64.

Baumann, P., and T. R. Cech. 2001. Pot1, the putative telomere end-binding protein in fission yeast and humans. *Science* 292 (5519):1171-5.

Bernstein, K. A., S. Gangloff, and R. Rothstein. 2010. The RecQ DNA helicases in DNA repair. *Annu Rev Genet* 44:393-417.

Binz, S. K., A. M. Sheehan, and M. S. Wold. 2004. Replication protein A phosphorylation and the cellular response to DNA damage. *DNA Repair (Amst)* 3 (8-9):1015-24.

Bonetti, D., M. Martina, M. Clerici, G. Lucchini, and M. P. Longhese. 2009. Multiple pathways regulate 3' overhang generation at *S. cerevisiae* telomeres. *Mol. Cell* 35 (1):70-81.

Carneiro, T., L. Khair, C. C. Reis, V. Borges, B. A. Moser, T. M. Nakamura, and M. G. Ferreira. 2010. Telomeres avoid end detection by severing the checkpoint signal transduction pathway. *Nature* 467 (7312):228-32.

Caspari, T., J. M. Murray, and A. M. Carr. 2002. Cdc2-cyclin B kinase activity links Crb2 and Rqh1-topoisomerase III. *Genes Dev.* 16 (10):1195-208.

Cejka, P., E. Cannavo, P. Polaczek, T. Masuda-Sasa, S. Pokharel, J. L. Campbell, and S. C. Kowalczykowski. 2010. DNA end resection by Dna2-Sgs1-RPA and its stimulation by Top3-Rmi1 and Mre11-Rad50-Xrs2. *Nature* 467 (7311):112-6.

Chang, S., A. S. Multani, N. G. Cabrera, M. L. Naylor, P. Laud, D. Lombard, S. Pathak, L. Guarente, and R. A. DePinho. 2004. Essential role of limiting telomeres in the pathogenesis of Werner syndrome. *Nat Genet* 36 (8):877-82.

Chavez, A., A. M. Tsou, and F. B. Johnson. 2009. Telomeres do the (un)twist: helicase actions at chromosome termini. *Biochim Biophys Acta* 1792 (4):329-40.

Cohen, H., and D. A. Sinclair. 2001. Recombination-mediated lengthening of terminal telomeric repeats requires the Sgs1 DNA helicase. *Proc Natl Acad Sci U S A* 98 (6):3174-9.

Cooper, J. P., Y. Watanabe, and P. Nurse. 1998. Fission yeast Taz1 protein is required for meiotic telomere clustering and recombination. *Nature* 392 (6678):828-31.

Crabbe, L., A. Jauch, C. M. Naeger, H. Holtgreve-Grez, and J. Karlseder. 2007. Telomere dysfunction as a cause of genomic instability in Werner syndrome. *Proc. Natl. Acad. Sci. U. S. A.* 104 (7):2205-10.

Crabbe, L., R. E. Verdun, C. I. Haggblom, and J. Karlseder. 2004. Defective telomere lagging strand synthesis in cells lacking WRN helicase activity. *Science* 306 (5703):1951-3.

Critchlow, S. E., and S. P. Jackson. 1998. DNA end-joining: from yeast to man. *Trends Biochem Sci* 23 (10):394-8.

Dewar, J. M., and D. Lydall. 2010. Pif1- and Exo1-dependent nucleases coordinate checkpoint activation following telomere uncapping. *EMBO J* 29 (23):4020-34.

Diede, S. J., and D. E. Gottschling. 2001. Exonuclease activity is required for sequence addition and Cdc13p loading at a de novo telomere. *Curr Biol* 11 (17):1336-40.

Dionne, I., and R. J. Wellinger. 1996. Cell cycle-regulated generation of single-stranded G-rich DNA in the absence of telomerase. *Proc. Natl. Acad. Sci. U. S. A.* 93 (24):13902-7.

Doe, C. L., J. Dixon, F. Osman, and M. C. Whitby. 2000. Partial suppression of the fission yeast *rqh1-* phenotype by expression of a bacterial Holliday junction resolvase. *EMBO J.* 19 (11):2751-62.

Faure, V., S. Coulon, J. Hardy, and V. Geli. 2010. Cdc13 and telomerase bind through different mechanisms at the lagging- and leading-strand telomeres. *Mol Cell* 38 (6):842-52.

Firmenich, A. A., M. Elias-Arnanz, and P. Berg. 1995. A novel allele of Saccharomyces cerevisiae RFA1 that is deficient in recombination and repair and suppressible by RAD52. *Mol Cell Biol* 15 (3):1620-31.

Fishman-Lobell, J., and J. E. Haber. 1992. Removal of nonhomologous DNA ends in double-strand break recombination: the role of the yeast ultraviolet repair gene RAD1. *Science* 258 (5081):480-4.

Garvik, B., M. Carson, and L. Hartwell. 1995. Single-stranded DNA arising at telomeres in cdc13 mutants may constitute a specific signal for the RAD9 checkpoint. *Mol. Cell. Biol.* 15 (11):6128-38.

Gong, Y., and T. de Lange. 2010. A Shld1-controlled POT1a provides support for repression of ATR signaling at telomeres through RPA exclusion. *Mol Cell* 40 (3):377-87.

Gravel, S., J. R. Chapman, C. Magill, and S. P. Jackson. 2008. DNA helicases Sgs1 and BLM promote DNA double-strand break resection. *Genes Dev.* 22 (20):2767-72.

Gravel, S., M. Larrivee, P. Labrecque, and R. J. Wellinger. 1998. Yeast Ku as a regulator of chromosomal DNA end structure. *Science* 280 (5364):741-4.

Huang, P., F. E. Pryde, D. Lester, R. L. Maddison, R. H. Borts, I. D. Hickson, and E. J. Louis. 2001. SGS1 is required for telomere elongation in the absence of telomerase. *Curr Biol* 11 (2):125-9.

Iglesias, N., and J. Lingner. 2009. Related mechanisms for end processing at telomeres and DNA double-strand breaks. *Mol Cell* 35 (2):137-8.

Ivanov, E. L., and J. E. Haber. 1995. RAD1 and RAD10, but not other excision repair genes, are required for double-strand break-induced recombination in Saccharomyces cerevisiae. *Mol Cell Biol* 15 (4):2245-51.

Ivanov, E. L., N. Sugawara, J. Fishman-Lobell, and J. E. Haber. 1996. Genetic requirements for the single-strand annealing pathway of double-strand break repair in Saccharomyces cerevisiae. *Genetics* 142 (3):693-704.

Johnson, F. B., R. A. Marciniak, M. McVey, S. A. Stewart, W. C. Hahn, and L. Guarente. 2001. The Saccharomyces cerevisiae WRN homolog Sgs1p participates in telomere maintenance in cells lacking telomerase. *EMBO J* 20 (4):905-13.

Kibe, T., Y. Ono, K. Sato, and M. Ueno. 2007. Fission yeast Taz1 and RPA are synergistically required to prevent rapid telomere loss. *Mol. Biol. Cell.* 18 (6):2378-87.

Kibe, T., K. Tomita, A. Matsuura, D. Izawa, T. Kodaira, T. Ushimaru, M. Uritani, and M. Ueno. 2003. Fission yeast Rhp51 is required for the maintenance of telomere structure in the absence of the Ku heterodimer. *Nucleic Acids Res.* 31 (17):5054-63.

Kobayashi, Y., K. Sato, T. Kibe, H. Seimiya, A. Nakamura, M. Yukawa, E. Tsuchiya, and M. Ueno. 2010. Expression of mutant RPA in human cancer cells causes telomere shortening. *Biosci Biotechnol Biochem* 74 (2):382-5.

Kurokawa, Y., Y. Murayama, N. Haruta-Takahashi, I. Urabe, and H. Iwasaki. 2008. Reconstitution of DNA strand exchange mediated by Rhp51 recombinase and two mediators. *PLoS Biol* 6 (4):e88.

Larrivee, M., C. LeBel, and R. J. Wellinger. 2004. The generation of proper constitutive G-tails on yeast telomeres is dependent on the MRX complex. *Genes Dev.* 18 (12):1391-6.

Laud, P. R., A. S. Multani, S. M. Bailey, L. Wu, J. Ma, C. Kingsley, M. Lebel, S. Pathak, R. A. DePinho, and S. Chang. 2005. Elevated telomere-telomere recombination in WRN-deficient, telomere dysfunctional cells promotes escape from senescence and engagement of the ALT pathway. *Genes Dev.* 19 (21):2560-70.

Lee, J. Y., M. Kozak, J. D. Martin, E. Pennock, and F. B. Johnson. 2007. Evidence that a RecQ helicase slows senescence by resolving recombining telomeres. *PLoS Biol* 5 (6):e160.

Li, B., S. P. Jog, S. Reddy, and L. Comai. 2008. WRN controls formation of extrachromosomal telomeric circles and is required for TRF2DeltaB-mediated telomere shortening. *Mol Cell Biol* 28 (6):1892-904.

Lillard-Wetherell, K., A. Machwe, G. T. Langland, K. A. Combs, G. K. Behbehani, S. A. Schonberg, J. German, J. J. Turchi, D. K. Orren, and J. Groden. 2004. Association and regulation of the BLM helicase by the telomere proteins TRF1 and TRF2. *Hum Mol Genet* 13 (17):1919-32.

Liu, N. N., T. X. Han, L. L. Du, and J. Q. Zhou. 2010. A genome-wide screen for Schizosaccharomyces pombe deletion mutants that affect telomere length. *Cell Res* 20 (8):963-5.

Longhese, M. P., D. Bonetti, N. Manfrini, and M. Clerici. 2010. Mechanisms and regulation of DNA end resection. *EMBO J* 29 (17):2864-74.

Lydall, D. 2009. Taming the tiger by the tail: modulation of DNA damage responses by telomeres. *EMBO. J.* 28 (15):2174-2187.

Machwe, A., L. Xiao, and D. K. Orren. 2004. TRF2 recruits the Werner syndrome (WRN) exonuclease for processing of telomeric DNA. *Oncogene* 23 (1):149-56.

Makarov, V. L., Y. Hirose, and J. P. Langmore. 1997. Long G tails at both ends of human chromosomes suggest a C strand degradation mechanism for telomere shortening. *Cell* 88 (5):657-66.

Mallory, J. C., V. I. Bashkirov, K. M. Trujillo, J. A. Solinger, M. Dominska, P. Sung, W. D. Heyer, and T. D. Petes. 2003. Amino acid changes in Xrs2p, Dun1p, and Rfa2p that remove the preferred targets of the ATM family of protein kinases do not affect DNA repair or telomere length in Saccharomyces cerevisiae. *DNA Repair (Amst)* 2 (9):1041-64.

Miller, K. M., and J. P. Cooper. 2003. The telomere protein Taz1 is required to prevent and repair genomic DNA breaks. *Mol. Cell* 11 (2):303-13.

Miller, K. M., O. Rog, and J. P. Cooper. 2006. Semi-conservative DNA replication through telomeres requires Taz1. *Nature* 440 (7085):824-8.

Mimitou, E. P., and L. S. Symington. 2008. Sae2, Exo1 and Sgs1 collaborate in DNA double-strand break processing. *Nature* 455 (7214):770-4.

Mimitou, E. P., and L. S. Symington. 2009. Nucleases and helicases take center stage in homologous recombination. *Trends Biochem Sci* 34 (5):264-72.

Mimitou, E. P., and L. S. Symington. 2010. Ku prevents Exo1 and Sgs1-dependent resection of DNA ends in the absence of a functional MRX complex or Sae2. *EMBO J* 29 (19):3358-69.

Moser, B. A., L. Subramanian, Y. T. Chang, C. Noguchi, E. Noguchi, and T. M. Nakamura. 2009. Differential arrival of leading and lagging strand DNA polymerases at fission yeast telomeres. *EMBO. J.* 28 (7):810-20.

Multani, A. S., and S. Chang. 2007. WRN at telomeres: implications for aging and cancer. *J. Cell. Sci.* 120 (Pt 5):713-21.

Murayama, Y., Y. Kurokawa, K. Mayanagi, and H. Iwasaki. 2008. Formation and branch migration of Holliday junctions mediated by eukaryotic recombinases. *Nature* 451 (7181):1018-21.

Murray, J. M., H. D. Lindsay, C. A. Munday, and A. M. Carr. 1997. Role of *Schizosaccharomyces pombe* RecQ homolog, recombination, and checkpoint genes in UV damage tolerance. *Mol. Cell. Biol.* 17 (12):6868-75.

Nakamura, T. M., J. P. Cooper, and T. R. Cech. 1998. Two modes of survival of fission yeast without telomerase. *Science* 282 (5388):493-6.

Ngo, H. P., and D. Lydall. 2010. Survival and growth of yeast without telomere capping by Cdc13 in the absence of Sgs1, Exo1, and Rad9. *PLoS Genet* 6 (8):e1001072.

Nimonkar, A. V., J. Genschel, E. Kinoshita, P. Polaczek, J. L. Campbell, C. Wyman, P. Modrich, and S. C. Kowalczykowski. 2011. BLM-DNA2-RPA-MRN and EXO1-BLM-RPA-MRN constitute two DNA end resection machineries for human DNA break repair. *Genes Dev* 25 (4):350-62.

Niu, H., W. H. Chung, Z. Zhu, Y. Kwon, W. Zhao, P. Chi, R. Prakash, C. Seong, D. Liu, L. Lu, G. Ira, and P. Sung. 2010. Mechanism of the ATP-dependent DNA end-resection machinery from Saccharomyces cerevisiae. *Nature* 467 (7311):108-11.

Nora, G. J., N. A. Buncher, and P. L. Opresko. 2010. Telomeric protein TRF2 protects Holliday junctions with telomeric arms from displacement by the Werner syndrome helicase. *Nucleic Acids Res* 38 (12):3984-98.

Ono, Y., K. Tomita, A. Matsuura, T. Nakagawa, H. Masukata, M. Uritani, T. Ushimaru, and M. Ueno. 2003. A novel allele of fission yeast *rad11* that causes defects in DNA repair and telomere length regulation. *Nucleic Acids Res.* 31 (24):7141-9.

Onoda, F., M. Seki, A. Miyajima, and T. Enomoto. 2001. Involvement of SGS1 in DNA damage-induced heteroallelic recombination that requires RAD52 in Saccharomyces cerevisiae. *Mol Gen Genet* 264 (5):702-8.

Opresko, P. L. 2008. Telomere ResQue and preservation--roles for the Werner syndrome protein and other RecQ helicases. *Mech. Ageing Dev.* 129 (1-2):79-90.

Opresko, P. L., P. A. Mason, E. R. Podell, M. Lei, I. D. Hickson, T. R. Cech, and V. A. Bohr. 2005. POT1 stimulates RecQ helicases WRN and BLM to unwind telomeric DNA substrates. *J. Biol. Chem.* 280 (37):32069-80.

Opresko, P. L., M. Otterlei, J. Graakjaer, P. Bruheim, L. Dawut, S. Kolvraa, A. May, M. M. Seidman, and V. A. Bohr. 2004. The Werner syndrome helicase and exonuclease cooperate to resolve telomeric D loops in a manner regulated by TRF1 and TRF2. *Mol Cell* 14 (6):763-74.

Opresko, P. L., G. Sowd, and H. Wang. 2009. The Werner syndrome helicase/exonuclease processes mobile D-loops through branch migration and degradation. *PLoS One* 4 (3):e4825.

Opresko, P. L., C. von Kobbe, J. P. Laine, J. Harrigan, I. D. Hickson, and V. A. Bohr. 2002. Telomere-binding protein TRF2 binds to and stimulates the Werner and Bloom syndrome helicases. *J. Biol. Chem.* 277 (43):41110-9.

Ouellette, M. M., L. D. McDaniel, W. E. Wright, J. W. Shay, and R. A. Schultz. 2000. The establishment of telomerase-immortalized cell lines representing human chromosome instability syndromes. *Hum Mol Genet* 9 (3):403-11.

Palm, W., and T. de Lange. 2008. How shelterin protects mammalian telomeres. *Annu. Rev. Genet.* 42:301-34.

Paques, F., and J. E. Haber. 1997. Two pathways for removal of nonhomologous DNA ends during double-strand break repair in Saccharomyces cerevisiae. *Mol Cell Biol* 17 (11):6765-71.

Parker, A. E., R. K. Clyne, A. M. Carr, and T. J. Kelly. 1997. The *Schizosaccharomyces pombe rad11*+ gene encodes the large subunit of replication protein A. *Mol. Cell. Biol.* 17 (5):2381-90.

Polotnianka, R. M., J. Li, and A. J. Lustig. 1998. The yeast Ku heterodimer is essential for protection of the telomere against nucleolytic and recombinational activities. *Curr Biol* 8 (14):831-4.

Rog, O., K. M. Miller, M. G. Ferreira, and J. P. Cooper. 2009. Sumoylation of RecQ helicase controls the fate of dysfunctional telomeres. *Mol. Cell* 33 (5):559-69.

Rossi, M. L., A. K. Ghosh, and V. A. Bohr. 2010. Roles of Werner syndrome protein in protection of genome integrity. *DNA Repair (Amst)* 9 (3):331-44.

Schramke, V., P. Luciano, V. Brevet, S. Guillot, Y. Corda, M. P. Longhese, E. Gilson, and V. Geli. 2004. RPA regulates telomerase action by providing Est1p access to chromosome ends. *Nat. Genet.* 36 (1):46-54.

Shim, E. Y., W. H. Chung, M. L. Nicolette, Y. Zhang, M. Davis, Z. Zhu, T. T. Paull, G. Ira, and S. E. Lee. 2010. Saccharomyces cerevisiae Mre11/Rad50/Xrs2 and Ku proteins regulate association of Exo1 and Dna2 with DNA breaks. *EMBO J* 29 (19):3370-80.

Smith, J., and R. Rothstein. 1995. A mutation in the gene encoding the *Saccharomyces cerevisiae* single-stranded DNA-binding protein Rfa1 stimulates a RAD52-independent pathway for direct-repeat recombination. *Mol. Cell. Biol.* 15 (3):1632-41.

Smith, J., H. Zou, and R. Rothstein. 2000. Characterization of genetic interactions with *RFA1*: the role of RPA in DNA replication and telomere maintenance. *Biochimie* 82 (1):71-8.

Sowd, G., M. Lei, and P. L. Opresko. 2008. Mechanism and substrate specificity of telomeric protein POT1 stimulation of the Werner syndrome helicase. *Nucleic Acids Res* 36 (13):4242-56.

Stewart, E., C. R. Chapman, F. Al-Khodairy, A. M. Carr, and T. Enoch. 1997. *rqh1*+, a fission yeast gene related to the Bloom's and Werner's syndrome genes, is required for reversible S phase arrest. *EMBO J.* 16 (10):2682-92.

Sugawara, N., G. Ira, and J. E. Haber. 2000. DNA length dependence of the single-strand annealing pathway and the role of Saccharomyces cerevisiae RAD59 in double-strand break repair. *Mol Cell Biol* 20 (14):5300-9.

Takahashi, K., R. Imano, T. Kibe, H. Seimiya, Y. Muramatsu, N. Kawabata, G. Tanaka, Y. Matsumoto, T. Hiromoto, Y. Koizumi, N. Nakazawa, M. Yanagida, M. Yukawa, E. Tsuchiya, and M. Ueno. 2011. Fission yeast Pot1 and RecQ helicase are required for efficient chromosome segregation. *Mol Cell Biol* 31 (3):495-506.

Tomita, K., T. Kibe, H. Y. Kang, Y. S. Seo, M. Uritani, T. Ushimaru, and M. Ueno. 2004. Fission yeast Dna2 is required for generation of the telomeric single-strand overhang. *Mol Cell Biol* 24 (21):9557-67.

Tomita, K., A. Matsuura, T. Caspari, A. M. Carr, Y. Akamatsu, H. Iwasaki, K. Mizuno, K. Ohta, M. Uritani, T. Ushimaru, K. Yoshinaga, and M. Ueno. 2003. Competition between the Rad50 complex and the Ku heterodimer reveals a role for Exo1 in processing double-strand breaks but not telomeres. *Mol Cell Biol* 23 (15):5186-97.

Umezu, K., N. Sugawara, C. Chen, J. E. Haber, and R. D. Kolodner. 1998. Genetic analysis of yeast RPA1 reveals its multiple functions in DNA metabolism. *Genetics* 148 (3):989-1005.

Verdun, R. E., and J. Karlseder. 2006. The DNA damage machinery and homologous recombination pathway act consecutively to protect human telomeres. *Cell* 127 (4):709-20.

Wang, R. C., A. Smogorzewska, and T. de Lange. 2004. Homologous recombination generates T-loop-sized deletions at human telomeres. *Cell* 119 (3):355-68.

Wang, X., and P. Baumann. 2008. Chromosome fusions following telomere loss are mediated by single-strand annealing. *Mol. Cell* 31 (4):463-73.

Watt, P. M., I. D. Hickson, R. H. Borts, and E. J. Louis. 1996. SGS1, a homologue of the Bloom's and Werner's syndrome genes, is required for maintenance of genome stability in Saccharomyces cerevisiae. *Genetics* 144 (3):935-45.

Wellinger, R. J., K. Ethier, P. Labrecque, and V. A. Zakian. 1996. Evidence for a new step in telomere maintenance. *Cell* 85 (3):423-33.

Wellinger, R. J., A. J. Wolf, and V. A. Zakian. 1993. *Saccharomyces* telomeres acquire single-strand TG_{1-3} tails late in S phase. *Cell* 72 (1):51-60.

Wu, L., and I. D. Hickson. 2003. The Bloom's syndrome helicase suppresses crossing over during homologous recombination. *Nature* 426 (6968):870-4.

Wyllie, F. S., C. J. Jones, J. W. Skinner, M. F. Haughton, C. Wallis, D. Wynford-Thomas, R. G. Faragher, and D. Kipling. 2000. Telomerase prevents the accelerated cell ageing of Werner syndrome fibroblasts. *Nat Genet* 24 (1):16-7.

Zaug, A. J., E. R. Podell, and T. R. Cech. 2005. Human POT1 disrupts telomeric G-quadruplexes allowing telomerase extension in vitro. *Proc Natl Acad Sci U S A* 102 (31):10864-9.

Zhu, Z., W. H. Chung, E. Y. Shim, S. E. Lee, and G. Ira. 2008. Sgs1 helicase and two nucleases Dna2 and Exo1 resect DNA double-strand break ends. *Cell* 134 (6):981-94.

Zou, L., and S. J. Elledge. 2003. Sensing DNA damage through ATRIP recognition of RPA-ssDNA complexes. *Science* 300 (5625):1542-8.

Part 6

Measuring DNA Repair Capacity

31

DNA Repair Measured by the Comet Assay

Amaya Azqueta[1], Sergey Shaposhnikov[2] and Andrew R. Collins[2]
[1]*University of Navarra*
[2]*University of Oslo*
[1]*Spain*
[2]*Norway*

1. Introduction

The stability of the genome is of crucial importance, and yet the DNA molecule is prone to spontaneous loss of bases, and damage from exogenous and endogenous sources - with potentially mutagenic consequences. Damage can take the form of small alterations to bases (alkylation or oxidation); breaks in the sugar-phosphate backbone involving one or both strands (single or double strand breaks - SSBs or DSBs); bulky adducts combined with bases; and covalent bonds between adjacent bases (intra-strand cross-links), across the double helix (inter-strand cross-links), or between DNA and protein. These lesions can disrupt replication, or cause incorporation of the wrong base.

Cells possess repair enzymes that correct almost all the damage before it can result in permanent change to the genome. Different pathways deal with the various kinds of damage. Repair of SSBs is in most cells a rapid process, consisting of little more than ligation. DSBs are more complicated (and potentially more serious) since the continuity of the double helix is disrupted. Homologous recombination ensures restoration of the correct DNA sequence by using the DNA of the sister chromatid or homologous chromosome as a template, while non-homologous end-rejoining is less precise and can entail loss of sequence. Base excision repair (BER) is concerned with small base alterations and starts with removal of the damaged base by a more or less specific glycosylase, leaving a base-less sugar or AP-site (apurinic/apyrimidinic site). An AP endonuclease or lyase cleaves the DNA at this site, and - after trimming of the broken ends of DNA - the one-nucleotide gap is filled by DNA polymerase β. Ligation is the final stage. Nucleotide excision repair (NER) is a more complex affair, involving recognition of a bulky adduct or helix distortion (such as is caused by the dimerisation of adjacent pyrimidines by UV(C) radiation), endonucleolytic incision on each side of the lesion, and removal of an oligonucleotide containing the damage. This is then filled in by DNA polymerase δ, κ or ε and the new patch of nucleotides is ligated into the DNA, completing the repair. NER enzymes are also involved in repair of inter-strand cross-links, removing the linking molecule from one strand, leaving it attached to the other strand as a mono-adduct to be removed in a second NER reaction (according to the simplest, and possibly simplistic, model).

Individual DNA repair capacity is regarded as a biomarker of susceptibility to mutation and cancer. A person with high repair rate is assumed to be at lower risk than one with low repair rate. DNA repair is partially determined genetically, and polymorphisms in repair genes will affect overall repair activity. However, this variation cannot account for the wide range of individual repair rates as measured in human populations. The intrinsic repair rate is likely to be affected by environmental conditions such as the presence of DNA-damaging agents that induce repair activity, and there is accumulating evidence that nutritional and lifestyle factors - for instance, micronutrients - can also modulate DNA repair.

Levels of mRNA corresponding to DNA repair pathways are frequently assessed by DNA microarray techniques, or by RT-PCR for selected genes. However, gene expression does not necessarily correlate with enzyme activity, and there is no substitute for measurement of repair capacity, i.e. phenotype. This is where the comet assay can be most usefully applied.

The comet assay, with modifications, can measure various kinds of damage, and the corresponding repair pathways. The basic comet assay detects strand breaks (see section 2.1. "The comet assay"), and so is readily applied to SSB repair by monitoring the rejoining of breaks. With a modification to detect particular classes of damage by incorporating a digestion with lesion-specific endonuclease, repair of oxidised and alkylated bases, as well as dimerised pyrimidines, can be followed. There are other specialised modifications of the assay to study cross-link repair. In addition to these assays based on following the removal of damage, there is a method for measuring NER in cells in culture by blocking repair synthesis and accumulating incision events as DNA breaks. Another approach to measuring BER or NER involves an '*in vitro*' assay in which a cell extract is incubated with a DNA substrate containing specific lesions, and again the occurrence of breaks is monitored.

A quite distinct application of the comet assay is to the study of repair rates in different genes, taking advantage of the ability to identify - by the use of specific hybridisation probes - particular regions of the genome.

Here we will describe the different methods, and give examples of their application to cell culture, animal and human studies, where appropriate, without providing an exhaustive review of the literature.

2. Methods

2.1 The comet assay

The comet assay (single cell gel electrophoresis) is a simple, sensitive, economical method for measuring DNA SBs. Cells are embedded in agarose on a microscope slide, lysed, and electrophoresed. Broken DNA is drawn towards the anode, forming a 'comet tail'; it is stained with a DNA-binding dye and observed with fluorescence microscopy (Figure 1a). The assay depends on the fact that DNA in the mammalian nucleus is organised as a series of DNA loops, attached to the nuclear framework, or matrix, at intervals. The DNA is (negatively) supercoiled, by virtue of its arrangement as nucleosomes, and each supercoiled loop should be regarded as a structural unit. Lysis of cells with detergent and high salt (removing membranes, soluble cell components and most histones), leaves the DNA still attached to the matrix, and known as a nucleoid; the supercoiling is still present, and when this supercoiling is relaxed by a DNA SB, only the loop containing the break is affected. The assay can be carried out at 'neutral' pH (around 10 - not high enough to denature DNA [Ostling & Johanson, 1984] or at high pH above pH 13 [Singh et al., 1988]). Both neutral and alkaline versions detect SSBs, since a single SB is sufficient to relax supercoiling. The assay does not depend on alkaline denaturation to reveal SSBs (unlike other assays such as neutral/alkaline elution, and alkaline unwinding), but the apparent analogy has led to much confusion, and it is often stated that the neutral assay only detects DSBs. The neutral and alkaline comet assays do, however, differ in one important respect; at a high pH, AP-sites are converted to breaks.

The more breaks are present, the more loops are relaxed, and the more intense is the fluorescence of the comet tail relative to the nucleoid core when the nucleoids are stained with an appropriate DNA-binding dye (Figure 2). Comets (normally 30 to 100 per gel) are scored, most commonly, by computer-based image analysis, with '% tail DNA' as the preferred parameter, although an alternative 'visual scoring' technique is still widely used (Collins, 2004). For statistical analysis, the unit of analysis is the mean or median % tail DNA from the comets representing one independent sample of cells. % Tail DNA can be converted to 'real' units such as breaks per 10^9 Da by use of a calibration curve, based on γ- or X-irradiation of cells, since the breakage rate per Gy is known.

The comet assay can be applied to virtually any eukaryotic cell type that can be obtained as a single cell or nuclear suspension. Cell cultures and white blood cells are widely used, but also methods have been developed for disaggregating many kinds of tissue without causing damage to the cells' DNA. Sperm, with highly compacted DNA, can be subjected to comet analysis after treating with protease or dithiothreitol. The most commonly adopted strategy with plant cells is to release the nuclei by simply chopping the plant tissue with a sharp blade. The presence of chloroplasts in leaf tissue can lead to release of free radicals and oxidative damage to DNA unless the isolation is carried out under safelight conditions.

The basic comet assay is limited in its usefulness because only strand breaks (and alkali-labile sites) are detected. An additional step - digestion of the nucleoid DNA, after lysis, with a lesion-specific enzyme - converts various other kinds of DNA damage to DNA breaks (Figure 1b). Thus formamidopyrimidine DNA glycosylase (FPG) recognises oxidised purines, principally 8-oxoguanine (8-oxoG), but also ring-opened purines or formamidopyrimidines (and in addition some alkylated bases). Endonuclease III (EndoIII) converts oxidised pyrimidines to breaks, while 3-methyladenine DNA glycosylase II (AlkA) acts on alkylated bases (principally 3-methyladenine). UV-induced cyclobutane pyrimidine dimers are detected by the UV endonuclease, T4 endonucleaseV (T4endoV).

2.2 Measuring DNA repair with the "challenge assay"

The simplest assay for DNA repair is the so-called 'challenge assay' (Au et al., 2010), whereby cells are treated with a damaging agent and the removal of the damage is monitored over time to study the kinetics of repair. Different assays can be used to assess the level of damage remaining at different time points; the comet assay is one of them. It is commonly used to monitor rejoining of SBs by cells, but by incorporating the digestion of DNA (nucleoids) with a lesion-specific endonuclease the removal of different DNA lesions can also be assessed. With this aim FPG is used to convert oxidised purines into SBs, Alk A to convert the alkylated bases and T4endoV to convert the cyclobutane pyrimidine dimers induced by UV. Using all the possibilities, this assay allows us to measure SSB rejoining, BER (removal of oxidised and alkylated bases) and NER (removal of UV-induced cyclobutane dimers).

Different agents are used to induce the desired type of lesion in the DNA depending on the repair pathway to be studied. SSBs are easily induced by a brief treatment with H_2O_2 or by irradiation with X- or γ-rays. Oxidized purines, mainly 8-oxoG, are induced by treating the cells with the photosensitiser Ro 19-8022 plus visible light. Methyl methanesulfonate (MMS) can be used to produce alkylated bases and UV(C) radiation induces cyclobutane dimers.

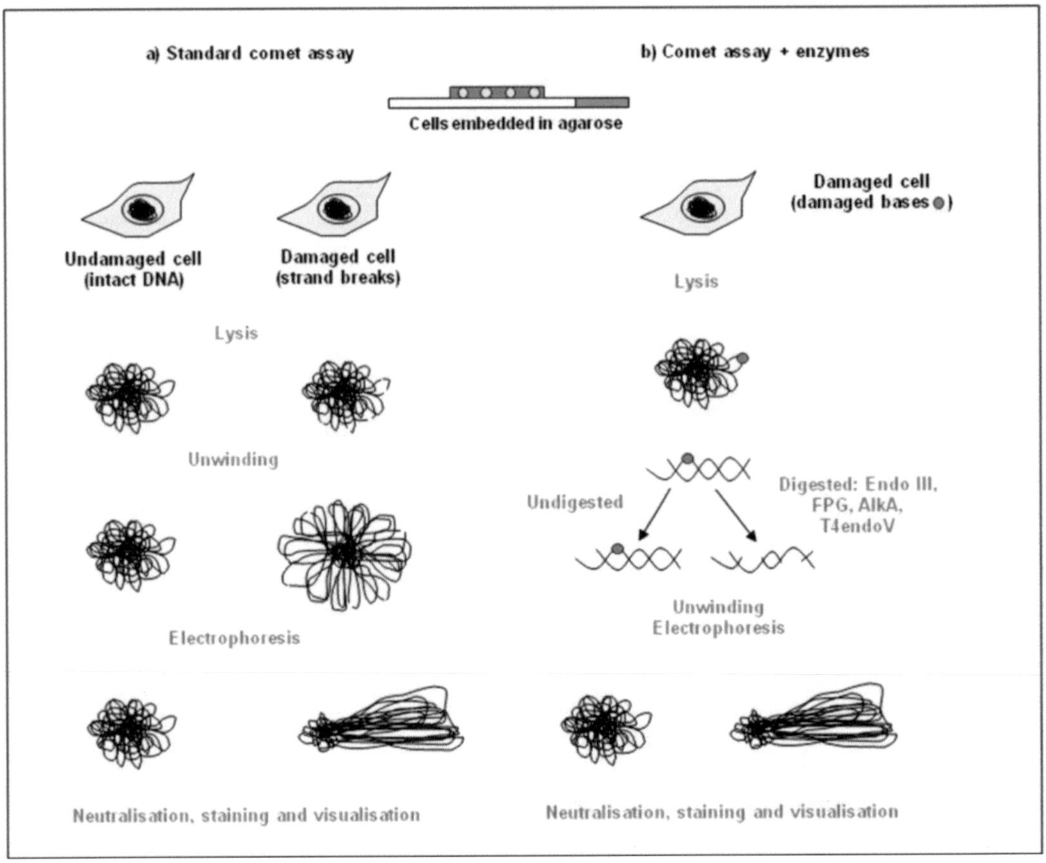

Fig. 1. Scheme of the standard comet assay (a), and the modified assay including digestion with lesion-specific enzymes (b).

The conditions of the treatment can vary depending on the cell type, and it is recommended first to establish optimal conditions; a high level of induced lesions, but not enough to saturate the assay or the capacity of the cells to repair the damage without entering apoptosis.

After the treatment cells are incubated in the appropriate cell culture medium and conditions (normally in an incubator at 37°C with 5% of CO_2) for different times. Just after the treatment (time 0) an aliquot of the cells is taken to check the level of induced damage. Further aliquots are taken at different times of incubation, including times soon after the start of incubation in order to estimate the initial rate of repair accurately.

In the case of adherent cells it is necessary to set up as many cell cultures as there are time-points (in multi-well plates or petri dishes) because at each time-point cells should be trypsinized. If cells are growing in suspension, an aliquot can be removed from the whole cell culture at each time-point. Setting the right times is a very important issue, influenced by the cell type and the repair pathway to be studied and so a prior investigation should be done on this topic also.

To avoid continuing repair of DNA damage while processing the cells after sampling at the different time-points, cells should be kept on ice during their manipulation. This is particularly important when very short intervals of time are tested.

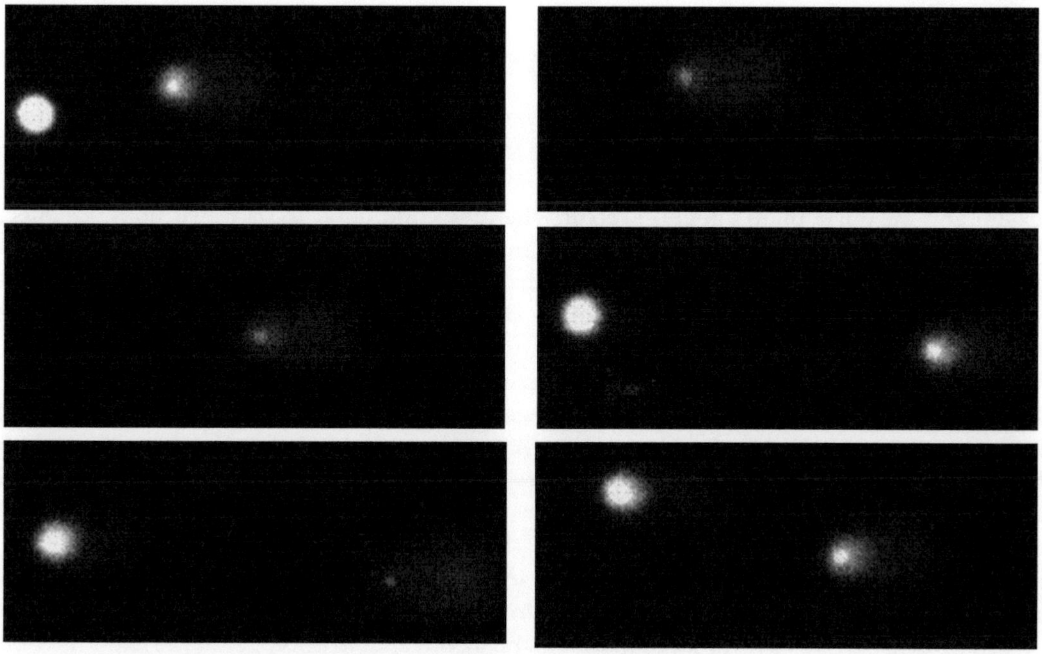

Fig. 2. Comet images with different levels of DNA damage.

The comet assay is done as described above; either the basic version (to assess SSB rejoining) or with an enzyme digestion (to assess BER or NER). The lysis step of the comet assay can last between 1 h and 24 h (or even longer) so gel-embedded cells/nucleoids can be kept in the lysis solution until all of the samples have been processed. Then samples from all time-points can be run in the same experiment, which as well as being practically convenient, avoids experimental variability.

To be able to compare different kinetics of repair, the half time of damage removal ($t_{1/2}$) should be calculated. To obtain an accurate estimation of this parameter the choice of the different time points is crucial. Generally the repair of SSBs is rapid, with a $t_{1/2}$ of 10 minutes or so while the repair of oxidized and alkylated bases and UV-induced cyclobutane dimers takes a few hours (Lorenzo et al., 2009). Another useful parameter is the initial repair rate, but this is difficult to estimate accurately if repair is rapid.

As in all of the assays, proper controls should be included to interpret the results correctly. A non-damaged cell culture should be included at all time points (including time 0) to check for any variation in or problem with experimental conditions.

2.2.1 Applications of the challenge assay

The challenge assay is used in cell culture experiments to check the influence of different compounds on the cellular repair rate. It is also used in animal studies and in human biomonitoring, normally studying lymphocytes.

The residual damage should always be measured at several time points after the incubation, so that the kinetics of the repair can be quantified and compared between different cell types or experimental conditions. Ideally, residual damage should be measured at shorter intervals immediately after treatment, since the initial rate of removal of damage is considered the defining step of the process. Another option, as explained before, is to calculate the $t_{1/2}$ for lesion removal. Measuring residual damage at a unique late point when most of the damage has been repaired, as is often reported, gives limited and ambiguous information.

For a valid comparison of different cell types or lymphocyte samples, the level of induced damage to be removed should ideally be the same in all cells/samples in the study, a state that in many cases is not easily achieved. It is a good assay to use with cell lines for examining the effect of an agent on repair when the compound to be tested does not affect the level of induced DNA damage. But sometimes cell cultures can be protected from DNA damage by the compound being studied; thus, for example, when an antioxidant micronutrient is tested for an effect on repair, it will obviously decrease the level of induced oxidative damage.

Compared with cell lines, animals and humans have more variability that can affect the level of damage achieved with the challenge compound. In biomonitoring, one subject group can have a higher antioxidant status that protects them against the damaging agent. This problem may well arise and is very difficult to solve. One possibility is to arrange for different doses of damage to each group to ensure the same initial level of lesions but this is in general impracticable.

Another disadvantage of this assay is that it involves a lot of cell culturing, specially when adherent cells are used and trypsinization is needed at all time points; the scheduled times to carry out the assay of residual damage can be inconvenient, and overall the experiment is complicated to perform. This is especially the case in biomonitoring studies, since the large number of samples to be tested precludes such complicated procedures - and there is inevitably day-to-day variation in culture conditions and results. On the other hand its endpoint is the removal of lesions and restoration of normal DNA structure, i.e. overall repair, whereas other methods tend to look only at one step in the repair process.

2.2.2 The challenge assay in cell culture studies

The "challenge assay" is the most suitable comet assay-based approach to measure DNA repair in cell culture and it has been used with different purposes. In 2003, Blasiak et al. demonstrated the temperature-dependence of the DNA repair process with the aim of using hyperthermia in the modulation of cancer therapy. They treated human peripheral lymphocytes and two variants of a human myelogenous leukemia cell line (K562 and its doxorubicin-resistant variant) with doxorubicin and studied the removal of the damage at 37°C and 41°C. They found an increase in the repair rate of the cells incubated at 41°C compared with 37°C. Tsai-Hsiu et al. (2003) studied the effect of S-adenosylhomocysteine (SAH), an inhibitor of most methyltransferases, on the repair rate of a mouse endothelial cell line and a human intestinal cell line. Cells were treated with H_2O_2 before incubating them with different concentrations of SAH or homocysteine as control and the removal of the damage was monitored. They showed that SAH decreased the DNA repair rate in a dose-dependent manner.

Ramos et al. (2008) studied the chemoprotective effects of the flavonoids quercitin and rutin, and the phytochemical ursolic acid, on the DNA damage induced by tert-butyl hydroperoxide (t-BHP) in a human hepatoma cell line. They checked the removal of the DNA damage induced by t-BHP after incubating the cells with different concentrations of quercitin, rutin or ursolic acid for 24h. There was an increase in the DNA repair rate of cells incubated with quercitin and ursolic acid, when the remaining lesions were measured 2 h after the treatment. The same group showed an enhancement in the repair rate when the human colon carcinoma cell line Caco-2 was preincubated with Salvia extracts or luteonil-7-glucoside before H_2O_2 treatment; but there was no effect when the compounds were just present during the repair time (Ramos et al., 2010a).

The repair of both SBs and oxidized bases (induced by treatment with H_2O_2 or with a photosensitiser plus visible light, respectively) were assessed in the human cervical cancer cell line HeLa and in Caco-2 cells incubated with different concentrations of the carotenoid β-cryptoxanthin (Lorenzo et al., 2009). This carotenoid induced a faster removal of both kinds of lesions in both cell lines at very low concentrations. The effect of β-cryptoxanthin on the removal of the 8-oxoG in Caco-2 cells is shown in Figure 3a.

Rejoining of X-ray-induced SBs by mouse leukocytes was studied by Gudkov et al. (2009) The natural ribonucleosides guanosine and inosine were present during the repair period, and SBs were measured after irradiation. Both ribonucleosides increased the repair rate. Moreover, in the presence of the repair inhibitor nicotinamide (prior to the irradiation and during the repair process), repair was slower and ribonucleosides did not induce any effect.

2.2.3 The challenge assay in animal studies

Although this approach is not ideal for application in *in vivo* animal studies, the lack of a good alternative makes it very common. Gover et al. (2001) studied the repair of DNA lesions induced by different concentrations of the fungicide mercuric chloride in leucocytes of rats. The comet assay was performed in whole blood at different times after an oral administration of a single dose. The level of the DNA damage decreased from 48 h and reached the control level at 2 weeks after the treatment. Very similar studies have been done to check the effects of the insecticide JS-118 (Zhang et al., 2010) and of copper sulfate (Saleha Banu et al., 2004) in mice.

This approach has also been applied to DNA repair in organs. Cells from the liver, kidney and bone marrow of mice were used to check the effect of the intraperitoneal administration of (MMS), a known genotoxic compound, and acetaminophen, an analgesic drug (Oshida et al., 2008). The level of DNA damage found at 4 h was less than at 24 h in all the organs and with both compounds. According to the authors this decrease can be due to detoxification, repair of the lesions induced by the treatment, or cell turnover.

The effect of intraperitoneal administration of the phytochemical feluric acid on repair of the DNA damage induced in lymphocytes by whole body γ-irradiation of mice was studied by Maurya et al. (2005). The disappearance of the induced SBs was faster in animals which received feluric acid compared to controls.

In these studies the challenging agent is given to the animals and repair occurs in physiological conditions (inside the animal). The assay has also been applied in animal studies where the challenge occurs *ex vivo*. Miranda et al. (2008) studied the protective effect of intragastric administration of aqueous extracts form Yerba mate tea in mice over a period of 60 days. After this period cells were isolated from liver, kidney and bladder and embedded in agarose before treating them with H_2O_2. There was an enhancement of DNA repair in liver cells.

2.2.4 The challenge assay in human studies

As explained before, the challenge assay presents many inconveniences when used in humans, but there are several studies that use this approach to measure the DNA repair capacity of individuals.

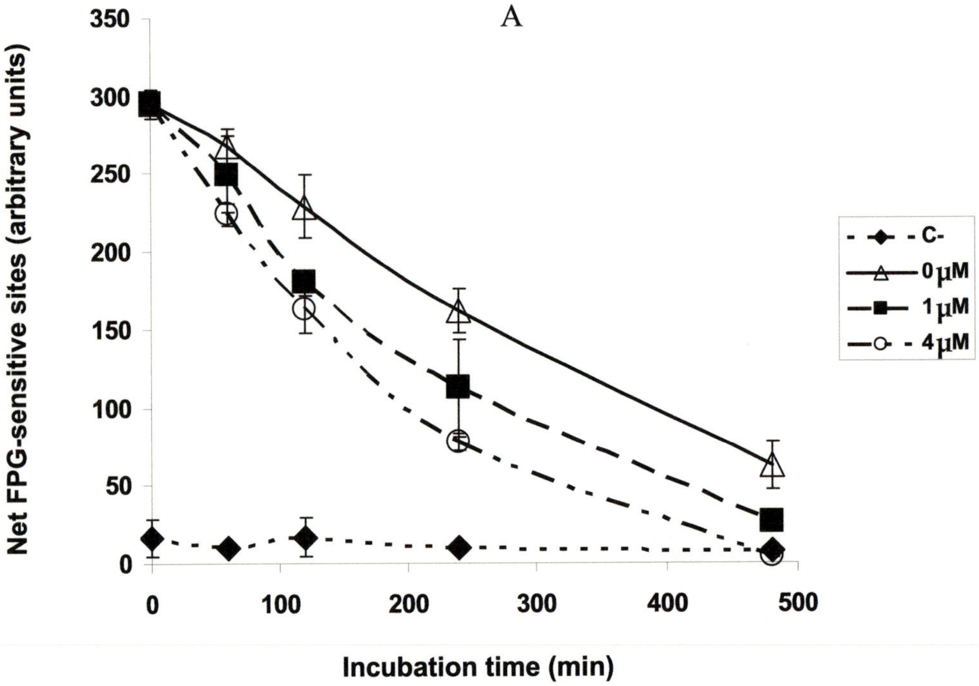

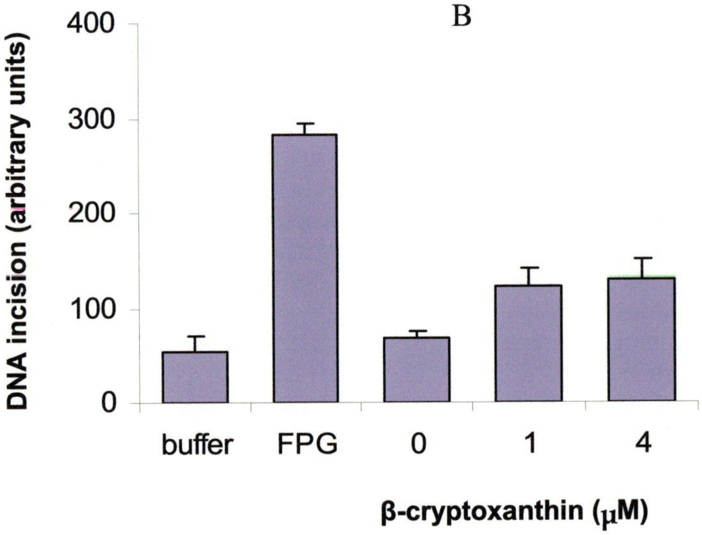

Fig. 3. Effect of β-cryptoxanthin on BER in Caco-2 cells: "challenge assay" (a) and *in vitro* repair assay (b). From Lorenzo Y, Azqueta A, Luna L, Bonilla F, Dominguez G, Collins AR (2009) The carotenoid β-cryptoxanthin stimulates the repair of DNA oxidation damage in addition to acting as an antioxidant in human cells. Carcinogenesis 30 (2):308-314, by permission of Oxford University Press.

In a case-control study the DNA repair capacity of lymphocytes from 44 healthy donors and 38 patients with squamous cell carcinoma of head and neck (before treatment) was measured (Palyvoda et al., 2003). Repair of γ-ray induced lesions showed a high variability between individuals ($t_{1/2}$ from about 10 min to more than 1 h). Lymphocytes from patients showed lower repair rates and a higher amount of non-repaired damage after the incubation period.

This approach has also been used to monitor DNA repair in relation to occupation, environment or lifestyle. The repair rates of stimulated lymphocytes from 10 nuclear power plant workers chronically exposed to low doses of ionizing radiation and 10 controls were assessed (Touil et al., 2002). The interindividual variation in the rates of repair of γ-irradiation-induced DNA damage was high but there were no significant differences between groups. In a similar study, the repair rate of lymphocytes from 104 asbestos-exposed workers and 101 control workers was studied (Zhao et al., 2006). Lymphocytes from asbestos-exposed workers showed slower repair of H_2O_2 induced damage.

The challenge assay has also been applied in nutritional studies to check the influence of phytochemicals or whole foods on DNA repair. To study the effect of lutein, lycopene and β-carotene, 8 healthy volunteers were given supplements daily during 1 week in a cross over study with a wash-out period of 3 weeks (Torbergsen & Collins, 2000). Lutein did not have any effect on the DNA repair rate, but lycopene and β-carotene apparently accelerated the rejoining of the SBs. However, an increase in the level of SBs in non-irradiated cells during approximately the first 4 h of the incubation period was seen. This could be due to the oxidative stress that lymphocytes suffer from sudden exposure to atmospheric oxygen. This transient increase was less pronounced in lymphocytes taken after lycopene or β-carotene supplementation so the apparent acceleration of repair could be explained by an antioxidant protection exerted by the presence of carotenoids. In another study (Astley et al., 2004) healthy volunteers followed a dietary intervention with a mixed carotene capsule, a daily portion of cooked minced carrots, a portion of mandarin oranges, a vitamin C tablet or a matched placebo (about 10 volunteers per group). Only the lymphocytes from individuals taking mixed carotene capsules showed an improvement in rate of repair of H_2O_2 induced DNA damage.

As explained above, crucial information is lost when just one time of recovery is used in the challenge assay, and - especially if starting levels of damage are not the same - it can be misleading to compare repair rates on the basis of residual damage.

2.3 Measuring NER by inhibiting DNA synthesis

Many years ago, inhibitors of the DNA polymerase species that participate in NER were employed to block repair synthesis after UV(C) irradiation of cells in culture: the earlier steps of repair continue, leading to an accumulation of DNA breaks which normally occur as very transient repair intermediates. Aphidicolin, or cytosine arabinoside in combination with hydroxyurea, are equally effective as inhibitors. As methods for measuring DNA breaks, alkaline unwinding and alkaline elution were used. The principle was then combined with the comet assay, and used as early as 1992 (Gedik et al., 1992), detecting the accumulation of breaks in HeLa cells irradiated with 0.5 Jm^{-2} of UV(C) and incubated for just 5 min.

This approach was adapted by Speit et al. (2004) as a way of enhancing the detection of damage done to DNA by a range of different agents (benzo[a]pyrene diolepoxide [BPDE], bischloroethylnitrosourea, and MMS). It is particularly useful in the detection of 'bulky adducts', which are repaired by NER, but are not recognised by T4endoV, and so are not amenable to the enzyme-modified comet assay. (The bacterial enzyme complex, uvrABC, detects bulky DNA adducts as well as UV-induced pyrimidine dimers. Many efforts have been made to incorporate this enzyme complex to the comet assay but, until now, it seems to detect only a small fraction of the available lesions [Dusinska & Collins, 1996]).

This inhibitor-based incision assay can be used as a simple and sensitive method to measure repair capacity, reflected in the rate of accumulation of breaks. Incision is generally considered to be the rate-limiting step of NER. Before the introduction of the comet assay, the accumulation of incision events was used to investigate the molecular defects in the disease xeroderma pigmentosum (Squires et al., 1982) and to characterise DNA repair-defective mutant cell lines (Stefanini et al., 1991).

2.3.1 Applications of the inhibitor assay for NER

This assay has not been widely used but it has considerable potential, particularly in human studies. Actually it seems that in the case of freshly isolated lymphocytes, the DNA breaks present as NER intermediates persist long enough to be detected with the comet assay without using aphidicolin or cytosine arabinoside (Collins et al., 1995; Green et al., 1994). Repair synthesis is unable to proceed due to the lack of enough DNA precursors (dNTPs). If deoxyribonucleosides are added to the medium, breaks are no longer detected. However, it seems wise to include aphidicolin or cytosine arabinoside to ensure that DNA resynthesis is completely blocked and so to be sure of detecting all the breaks.

Cipollini *et al.* (2006) treated lymphocytes with 1.5 Jm^{-2} of UV(C) and observed breaks accumulating to a maximum at about 60 min with then a decrease. This decline can be due to eventual completion of repair even with the low concentrations of precursors, or to a synthesis of DNA precursors induced as a response to the DNA damage. Experimental variation and inter-individual differences in kinetics were seen in 4 subjects. This could be explained by individual differences in the precursor pool size rather than differences in the repair capacity. The characterisation of several UV-sensitive rodent mutant cell lines included the measurement of their ability to carry out incision after irradiation with 0.1 Jm^{-2} of UV(C) (Collins et al., 1997).

The assay has been used to look for effects of *in vivo* exposure to different genotoxic agents by looking for an enhanced level of breaks when lymphocytes are incubated with DNA sythesis inhibitors. Crebelli et al. (2002) found a higher level of breaks (with cytosine arabinoside) in aluminium workers compared with controls; while Speit et al. (2003) did not detect such a difference between smokers and non-smokers.

The best use of the assay in human biomonitoring is probably as an *ex vivo* assay, i.e. treating the subjects' lymphocytes with UV(C) (or some other agent whose damage is repaired by NER) and incubating them with inhibitor *in vitro*. The Kirsch-Volders group recently carried out a pilot study with 22 subjects, treating peripheral blood mononucleated cells with BPDE for 2 h with and without preincubation with aphidicolin (Vande Loock *et al.*, 2010). They quantified repair capacity as the amount of SBs induced by BPDE with aphidicolin, minus the SBs induced by aphidicolin (a very small amount) and by BPDE alone – reckoning that this equates to the incision activity of the NER enzymes. (UV(C) is a cleaner agent to use, since it does not directly induce significant levels of SBs; all the SBs detected are NER intermediates.)

As a biomonitoring assay for human studies, the inhibitor assay for NER is still in the development phase. A comparison of results from this assay and from a UV challenge assay and an *in vitro* NER assay would be very informative.

2.4 Measuring BER and NER with an *in vitro* assay

2.4.1 Practical details

The comet assay has been modified to measure the excision repair activity in an extract of cells (or a nuclear extract). In this *in vitro* approach a substrate, in the form of agarose-embedded nucleoids derived by lysis of cells containing a specific lesion, is incubated with the extract whose excision repair activity is to be measured by the comet assay (Collins et al., 2001; Gaivão et al., 2009; Langie et al., 2006) (Figure 4). The nature of the DNA lesion in the substrate defines the repair pathway that is measured. Substrate containing 8-oxoG is used to measure the BER activity of 8-oxoG DNA glycosylase (OGG) in the extracts tested (Collins et al., 2001); if substrate contains bulky adducts or cyclobutane pyrimidine dimers NER is measured (Gaivão et al., 2009; Langie et al., 2006). More recently an assay for cross-link repair has been developed (Herrera et al., 2009). In all cases the enzymes contained in the extract will carry out the initial steps of repair by recognizing the lesion and introducing a break at or near its site. The rate of accumulation of breaks, assessed by alkaline electrophoresis, is a measure of the repair capacity of the cells.

The substrate nucleoids should contain a high level of specific base damage so that the enzymes in the extract have an excess of lesions to work on. This level should be more than enough to saturate the comet assay but the background level of breaks as well as other unwanted lesions should be very low. To reach this equilibrium is not always an easy task and as a result it is not always possible to produce substrate with the desired lesion.

Furthermore breaks do not continue to increase indefinitely but reach a saturation. This means that the longer the incubation, the less difference will be detected in activity between different extracts - so the time of incubation is crucial.

The description of the assay is divided into 5 steps: preparation of cells for the substrate, preparation of cells for the extract, preparation of the substrate nucleoids, preparation of the extract and incubation of the substrate with the extract.

Preparation of cells for the substrate for BER and NER: A substrate to measure BER is prepared by treating the cells with the photosensitiser Ro 19-8022 plus visible light to induce oxidized purines, mainly 8-oxoG. For NER, cells are irradiated with UV(C) to induce cyclobutane pyrimidine dimers (they can also be treated with BPDE or oxaliplatin to produce bulky adducts or cross-links respectively but we do not have experience with such treatments). Non-treated cells should be used to prepare a control substrate. The cell type used for substrate is not important.

After treatment cells are slowly frozen in aliquots and kept at -80°C (for months or even years).

Preparation of cells for the extract: Extract is normally prepared from lymphocytes or cultured cells (recently animal tissue has been successfully used [Langie et al., 2011] in this assay but this will not be covered in this article). In the order of 5-10 million cells are needed to perform about 6 determinations of repair activity.

Cells are washed, spun, suspended at 10^7 per 100 µl in extraction buffer and aliquots flash-frozen in liquid nitrogen before storage (for at least months) at -80°C. In fact there are three alternative methods to prepare cells for making extract: (1) direct preparation in extraction buffer, as above; (2) preparation of a dry pellet of the cells, snap-frozen and kept at 80°C (the rest of the extraction being done on the day of the assay); (3) cells frozen slowly in freezing medium to maintain viability, with complete extraction procedure carried out on day of experiment. Each method gives comparable results but experience shows that with method (2) the presence of residual supernatant when the pellet is thawed presents problems.

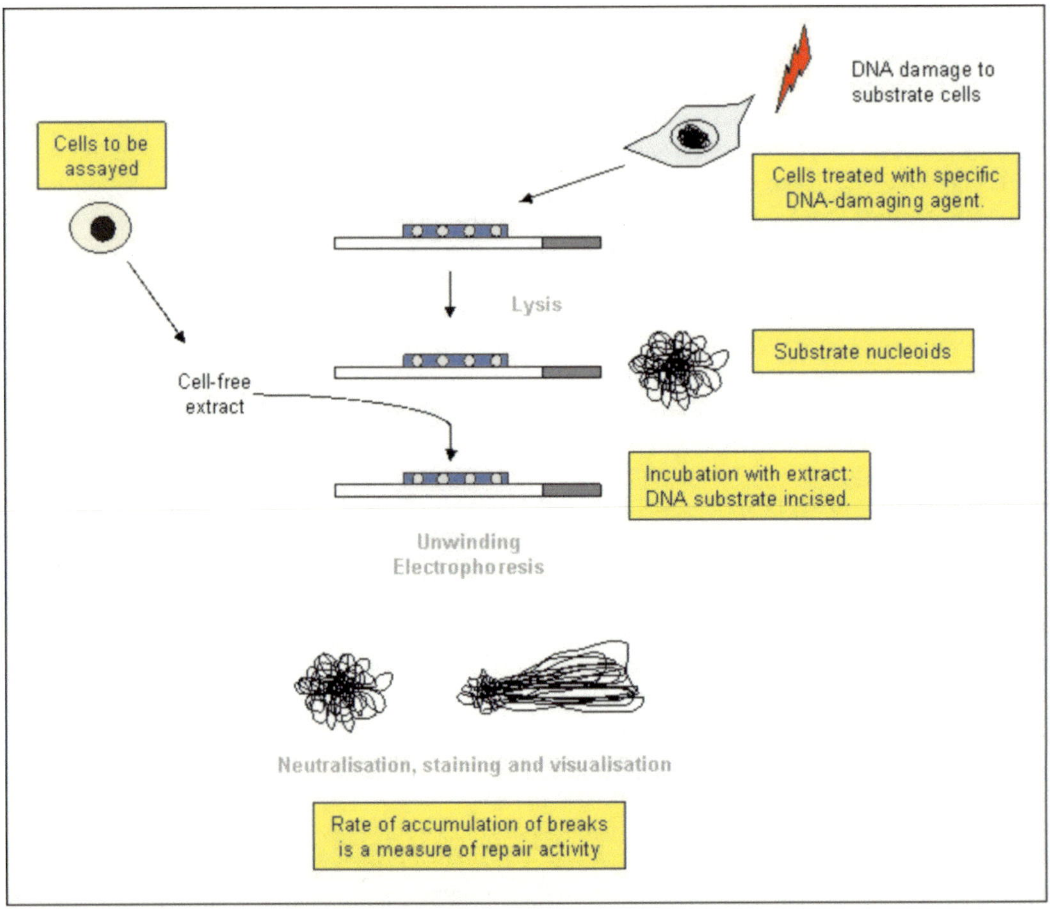

Fig. 4. Scheme of the *in vitro* repair assay

Preparation of the substrate nucleoids: Cells are thawed and embedded in agarose on a microscope slide as explained before (see section 2.1. "The comet assay"). Then slides are placed in the lysis solution for at least one hour to produce nucleoids. Control cells, without any induced damage, should always be included to check for unspecific nuclease activity in the extracts.

Preparation of the extracts: On the day of the experiment, after preparing substrate gels, an aliquot of the cells frozen for preparing the extract is thawed and kept on ice. Triton X-100 is added (final concentration 0.2%) to destabilize the membranes and complete lysis. After centrifugation at high speed to remove nuclei and cell debris, the supernatant is then diluted 4-fold in reaction buffer. All the procedures should be done on ice to avoid loss of activity.

Incubation of the substrate with the extracts: Substrate gels should be washed with the reaction buffer before the incubation with the extracts. Extracts are incubated with the substrate gels for between 10 and 30 min at 37°C in a humidified atmosphere. The optimal time should be established in each laboratory. If the 2 gels per slide format is used about 45 μl of extract is added on the top of the gel and a cover slip (or a Parafilm square) is placed on top. After that the standard comet assay protocol is followed.

Substrate nucleoids should be also treated with a buffer control (extraction buffer + Triton + reaction buffer) and with enzymes to test the level of DNA damage contained in the nucleoids. FPG is used for BER substrates and T4endoV for NER. Therefore the standard experiment should include substrate for BER or NER and substrate without damage, incubated with extracts, the buffer control and FPG or T4endoV.

To express the results the values of the activity of the extracts and controls obtained from the substrate without damage, representing the non-specific activity, should be subtracted from the values obtained from the BER or NER substrate.

It is crucial that the number of cells to prepare the extract is the same in all the samples. Counting is always time consuming and not accurate; it is useful to measure the protein concentrations in the extract residues left after an experiment, and to express repair activity relative to the protein concentration, thus allowing for variation in cell numbers. However, this correction is valid only over a narrow range, since repair activity deviates from linearity at high concentrations. Therefore, care must be taken to work with similar and appropriate protein concentrations or cell densities in all extracts.

2.4.2 Applications of the *in vitro* DNA repair assay

The *in vitro* DNA repair assay has been used in some cell culture and animal studies but it is mostly used in human biomonitoring. It is a very useful tool in this type of study since it can be used on extracts prepared from lymphocyte samples and stored frozen until a batch of extracts are ready to be measured at the same time.

This approach does not measure the whole process, but only the initial step of repair.

2.4.3 Cell culture studies with the *in vitro* assay

Very few examples of the *in vitro* repair assay applied to cell culture studies can be found in the literature. Ramos et al. (2010a) evaluated the incision activity of extract from Caco-2 cells treated for 24 h with water extracts of *Salvia* species, rosmarinic acid and luteonil-7-glucoside on nucleoid substrate containing 8-oxoG. All extracts from treated cells showed an increase. It was significant in the case of one of the *Salvia* species and with luteonil-7-glucoside. In the same way, Ramos and colleagues showed an increase in the BER activity of extract from Caco-2 cells incubated with ursolic acid (a triterpenoid) while the incubation with luteolin (a flavonoid) had no effect (Ramos et al., 2010b). The effect of β-cryptoxanthin in BER was also assessed in extracts from HeLa and Caco-2 cells incubated for 2 h with different concentrations of β-cryptoxanthin, on HeLa nucleoids. A significant increase in BER was shown by extracts of cells treated with β-cryptoxanthin, even at very low concentration (Lorenzo et al., 2009). They also incubated β-cryptoxanthin with nucleoids to check whether β-cryptoxanthin present in the extract could directly induce breaks in the nucleoids, but did not find any effect. The increase in the incision activity of Caco-2 cells incubated with β-cryptoxanthin is shown in Figure 3b.

The effect of STI571, the most used drug in the treatment of chronic myeloid leukemia, on NER was assessed using the *in vitro* DNA repair assay (Sliwinski et al., 2008). STI571 inhibits the activity of the BCR/ABL oncogenic kinase, and so 3 different cell lines were used: human myeloid leukemic cells expressing BCR/ABL, human lymphoid leukemia cells also expressing BCR/ABL, and human lymphoid leukemic cells which do not express BCR/ABL. Extracts were prepared after treating the cells with STI571 for 2 h, and incubated with UV-treated nucleoid DNA. The NER activity of extract from BCR/ABL cells showed a drastic and highly significant decrease after treatment with the drug - in contrast with the control cells, not expressing BCR/ABL, in which the drug did not induce any change in NER activity.

2.4.4 Animal studies with the *in vitro* assay

The *in vitro* repair assay has been mostly used on humans; applications in animal studies are extremely limited. Obtaining sufficient lymphocytes from rodents to prepare extract is not easy.

Recently Langie et al. (2011) have optimised the assay to measure the BER in extracts from rodent tissues. Various attempts have been made before, but they were hampered by the high non-specific nuclease activity present in the extracts. Langie et al. successfully measured the incision activity of extracts from liver and brain from C57/BL mice. Optimisation of the protein concentration in the tissue extract as well as the use of aphidicolin were the key steps to get rid of the non-specific activity. The assay was validated by using tissues from BER deficient OGG1 knockout mice where a low activity was found, significantly lower than with wild-type mice. In the same paper the assay was used to determine the effect of aging on the incision activity of extracts from mouse brain and the effect of diet on the incision activity of extracts from mouse liver. The BER activity of brain decreases with age, and in liver it is induced under dietary restriction.

2.4.5 Human studies

The *in vitro* repair assay has been widely used to measure BER and NER activities in human lymphocytes. The BER capacity of lymphocytes from 86 workers in a plastics factory, exposed to styrene, and 52 controls was studied (Vodicka et al., 2004a). The incision activity on HeLa nucleoids containing 8-oxoG was higher in styrene-exposed workers. The same group carried out a similar study to determine the effect of the occupational exposure to different xenobiotics from a tire plant on the DNA repair capacity of the workers (Vodicka et al., 2004b). No differences in repair activity were reported in lymphocytes of 15 workers with a high risk of exposure, 11 with a low risk and 12 employed in checking and quality control. In the same way the BER repair capacity was determined in 61 exposed workers from an asbestos cement plant and 21 controls (Dusinska et al., 2004). Females exposed to asbestos showed a decrease in their BER capacity compared with non-exposed ones but there were no differences between exposed and non-exposed males.

This approach has also been widely used in nutritional intervention studies. BER activity was measured in lymphocytes from 6 subjects before and after the intake of coenzyme Q_{10} during 1 week (Tomasetti et al., 2001). A significantly higher OGG1 activity was seen after the supplementation. Very recently a nutritional intervention study has been published, where not only BER but also NER in UV-treated nucleoids was measured (Brevik et al., 2011). A randomized parallel study with 3 groups (a high phytochemical group with a high intake of a variety of antioxidant-rich plant products, a kiwifruit group supplemented with three kiwifruits per day and a control group without supplementation) and 8 weeks of intervention was carried out. BER activity was measured in lymphocytes from 23, 25, and 21 subjects from each group respectively, while NER was measured in lymphocytes from 13, 11 and 12 subjects from each group. BER showed an increase in both supplemented groups, being significant in the high phytochemical group, while NER showed significant decreases in both these groups. The control group did not show any changes.

It is important to include in *in vitro* repair experiments an incubation of extract with an undamaged substrate, to check for possible non-specific nuclease activities in the extract. It is not always clear in publications whether this has been done.

2.5 Following DNA repair at the level of the gene (FISH-comet assay)

The special feature of the comet assay is the ability to study DNA damage in individual cells. By combining fluorescent *in situ* hybridization (FISH) and applying labelled probes to particular DNA sequences, an even finer level of resolution can be achieved. Fig 5 illustrates general principles of the comet assay combined with FISH.

Depending on the target sequence, different probes are applied to comets. The most widely used FISH probes are centromere, telomere and ribosomal DNA repeats, short interspersed repetitive elements (SINEs) and long interspersed repetitive elements (LINEs). Those repetitive probes produce strong signals and are often commercially available. Other popular commercially available non-gene-specific probes are chromosome arm- or band-specific painting probes (DNA from microdissected chromosomes) and whole-chromosome painting probes (DNA from flow-sorted chromosomes).

Probes for specific DNA sequences can consist of PCR products, cDNAs or genomic DNA cloned in cosmids, P1 artificial chromosomes, bacterial artificial chromosomes (BACs) or yeast artificial chromosomes. Large unique probes that are not commercially available can be prepared for FISH using standard molecular biology techniques. Another useful design of probe is the 'padlock probe'—a linear oligonucleotide designed so that the two end segments, connected by a linker region, are complementary—in opposite orientations—to adjacent target sequences (Larsson et al., 2004). On hybridization, the two juxtaposed probe ends can be joined by a DNA ligase, circularizing the padlock probe and leaving it physically catenated to the target sequence. The reaction requires a perfect match between the probe ends and the target sequence and therefore, it is stable and extremely specific. The crucial feature of these probes when applied to comets is that the reaction steps are performed at 37^{0}C so that there is no tendency for the agarose to melt or become unstable.

When analysing FISH-comets results, visualization and scoring depend entirely on direct observation. In most cases it is not possible to score the signals automatically because of the complexity of the preparations (for instance, the occurrence of signals in the same cell in different optical planes). Figure 5 illustrates different appearances of the signals: a linear array or separate spots.

An important question related to FISH signal visualization, is how many signals to expect. Based on our hypothesis that DNA organisation in comets reflects the DNA loop organization in living cells, it is reasonable to expect that the number of signals detected in comets will be related to the number of signals observed on chromosome spread preparations. Our results with chromosome 16 probes confirmed this hypothesis: twice as many signals were observed in the alkaline version of the assay relative to the number seen under neutral conditions (Shaposhnikov et al., 2008). This can be explained by DNA denaturation in alkaline comets since each strand of DNA will act as a target for the FISH probe. Furthermore, the average numbers of signals seen per cell corresponded closely with the numbers expected according to the gene copy number in a random interphase cell population.

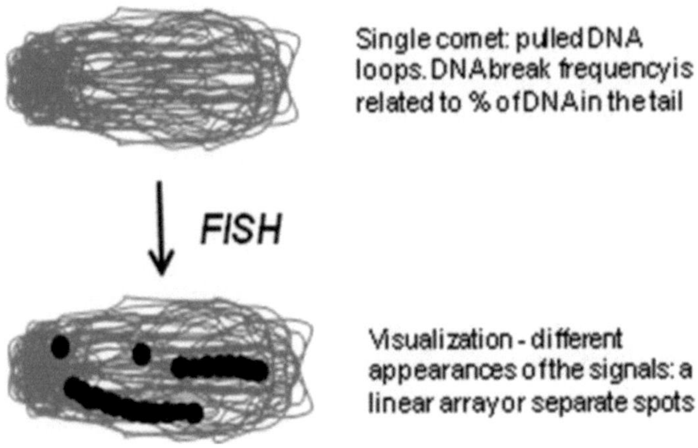

Fig. 5. General principles of the FISH-comet assay

Santos et al. (1997) published the first successful results of combining FISH with the (neutral) comet assay. Their aim was to investigate how centromeric and telomeric DNA behaves under electrophoresis. Probes to all centromeres, all telomeres, as well as chromosome-specific centromere and telomere DNA, and 3 segments of the gene *MGMT* (coding for the repair enzyme O6-methylguanine DNA methyltransferase) were used. Telomere probes were seen mostly over the comet head, consistent with their attachment to the nuclear membrane. The signals from the much larger centromere DNA (1000 kb in size) appeared as long strings of dots, extending well into the comet tail. *MGMT* gave signals that were found in the head as well as the tail, the 3 segments generally forming a linear array.

2.5.1 Gene-specific DNA repair

The FISH-comet assay can be used to monitor gene-specific DNA repair by following the 'retreat' of the gene-specific signals from tail to head during the incubation period. Thus it is possible to compare the kinetics of overall genomic and gene-specific repair.

McKenna et al. (2003) examined the repair of γ-ray-induced SBs in human cells. Using a probe for the *TP53* gene, they found that the number of signals increased immediately after irradiation (most being in the comet tails), and decreased over the first 15 min at which point most were in comet heads. By 60 min, the normal, lower number of signals was restored, while in contrast the % tail DNA (representing total DNA) was still elevated. Thus *TP53* repair was faster than total genomic repair.

We studied the repair of the *DHFR* gene (coding for dihydrofolate reductase), *MGMT*, and the *TP53* gene using a different approach (Horvathova et al., 2004). Probes were designed for each end of the gene and detected using antibodies giving different coloured signals so that the gene had red and green ends after hybridization. After H_2O_2-treatment, Chinese hamster ovary (CHO) cells gave comets with about 50% of the DNA in the tail. Almost all *DHFR* probe signals were in comet heads, whereas we had expected them to have a similar distribution to total DNA. The probable explanation is that a 'matrix associated region' or MAR is present in this gene, and this prevents the DNA from escaping from the head. For the *MGMT* gene, CHO cells were treated either with H_2O_2 or with Ro 19-8022 and light to create 8-oxoG residues (FPG-sensitive sites). In contrast to the *DHFR* result, signals appeared over tail DNA - though they were predominantly green dots, while almost all red dots were located over the head. Thus one end of the gene appeared to be attached to the matrix. Green signals were restored to the head region of the comets with similar kinetics to the total DNA, indicating similar time courses for total DNA repair and repair of *MGMT*. H_2O_2-treated human lymphocytes, hybridized with *TP53* probes, gave signals of both colours in the tail; after 20 min incubation, virtually all *TP53* signals were in the head, while the % of total DNA in the tail had decreased by only about one-third. Thus, the region of DNA containing *TP53* was apparently repaired significantly faster than genomic DNA overall. Kumaravel et al. (2005) also reported preferential repair of *TP53*, after ionising radiation or H_2O_2 treatment.

We recently used padlock probes and rolling circle amplification (RCA) to investigate the repair of two DNA repair genes, 8-oxoguanine-DNA glycosylase-1 (*OGG1*) and xeroderma pigmentosum group D (*XPD*), and the housekeeping gene for hypoxanthine-guanine phosphoribosyltransferase (*HPRT*) (Henriksson et al., 2011). The repair rates of these genes after H_2O_2 damage were compared with the repair rates of *Alu* repeats and of total genomic DNA. The signals were mainly detected in comet tails. The *HPRT* gene showed rapid repair compared to total DNA, and after approximately 10 min the *HPRT* gene signals were almost completely absent, whereas the mean % tail DNA, indicating total DNA damage, decreased from 67 to 43% over 2 h (consistent with the slow repair of SBs by lymphocytes, as described by Torbergsen and Collins, 2000). *HPRT* and *XPD* were repaired more rapidly and *OGG1* more slowly than *Alu* repeats.

3. Conclusion

The comet assay has proved to be remarkably versatile. Far from being just another way of measuring DNA breaks, it can give quantitative information about base damage if lesion-specific endonucleases are included in the protocol, and by extension it can be used to monitor the cellular repair of such damage (the challenge assay). The NER pathway for helix distortions and bulky adducts can be blocked at the repair synthesis stage by DNA polymerase inhibitors, and this leads to an accumulation of SBs - readily measured with the comet assay. A more biochemical approach to DNA repair is exemplified by the *in vitro* repair assay, in which a cell extract is incubated with a specifically damaged DNA substrate - again leading to an accumulation of DNA breaks - repair intermediates, for which the comet assay is ideally suited as a detector. These different approaches have found application in cell culture studies (e.g. investigating inhibitors and enhancers of repair, and repair mutant phenotypes), in animal experiments, and in human biomonitoring (particularly in relation to occupational exposure, and nutrition). Finally, DNA repair has been examined at the level of specific genome regions, using fluorescent *in situ* hybridisation with probes recognising different genes; it is clear that the rate of repair varies greatly between genes - as it does between people.

4. References

Astley, S., Elliott, R.M., Archer, D.B., & Southon, S. (2004). Evidence that dietary supplementation with carotenoids and carotenoid-rich foods modulates the DNA damage: repair balance in human lymphocytes. *British Journal of Nutrition*, Vol. 91, No. 1, (January 2004), pp. (63-72), 0007-1145

Au, W.W., Giri, A.A., & Ruchirawat, M. (2010). Challenge assay: A functional biomarker for exposure-induced DNA repair deficiency and for risk of cancer. *International Journal of Hygiene and Environmental Health*, Vol. 213, No. 1, (January 2010), pp. (32-39), 1438-4639

Blasiak, J., Widera, K., & Pertyński, T. (2003). Hyperthermia can differentially modulate the repair of doxorubicin-damaged DNA in normal and cancer cells. *Acta Biochimica Polonica*, Vol. 50, No. 1, (month and year of the edition), pp. (191-195), 0001-527X

Brevik, A., Karlsen, A., Azqueta, A., Estaban, A.T., Blomhoff, R., & Collins, A.R. (2011). Both base excision repair and nucleotide excision repair in humans are influenced by nutritional factors. *Cell Biochemistry and Function*, Vol. 29, No. 1, (January 2011), pp. (36-42), 0263-6484

Cipollini, M., He, J., Rossi, P., Baronti, F., Micheli, A., Rossi, A.M., & Barale, R. (2006). Can individual repair kinetics of UVC-induced DNA damage in human lymphocytes be assessed through the comet assay? *Mutation Research*, Vol. 601, No. 1-2, (October 2006), pp. (150-161), 0027-5107

Collins, A.R. (2004). The comet assay for DNA damage and repair: principles, applications, and limitations. *Molecular Biotechnology*, Vol. 26, No. 3, (March 2004), pp. (249-261), 1073-6085

Collins, A.R., Dusinska, M., Horvathova, E., Munro, E., Savio, M., & Stetina, R. (2001). Inter-individual differences in DNA base excision repair activity measured *in vitro* with the comet assay. *Mutagenesis*, Vol. 16, No. 4, (July 2001), pp. (297-301), 0267-8357

Collins, A.R., Ma, A., & Duthie, S.J. (1995). The kinetics of repair of oxidative DNA damage (strand breaks and oxidised pyrimidines) in human cells. *Mutation Research*, Vol. 336, No. 1, (January 1995), pp. (69-77), 0027-5107

Collins, A.R., Mitchell, D.L., Zunino, A., de Wit, J., & Busch, D. (1997). UV-sensitive rodent mutant cell lines of complementation groups 6 and 8 differ phenotypically from their human counterparts. *Environmental and Molecular Mutagenesis*, Vol. 29, No. 2, (1997), pp. (152-160), 0893-6692

Crebelli, R., Carta, P., Andreoli, C., Aru, G., Dobrowolny, G., Rossi, S., & Zijno, A. (2002). Biomonitoring of primary aluminium industry workers: detection of micronuclei and repairable DNA lesions by alkaline SCGE. *Mutation Research*, Vol. 516, No. 1-2, (April 2002), pp. (63–70), 0027-5107

Dusinska, M., & Collins, A.R. (1996). Detection of oxidised purines and UV-induced photoproducts in DNA of single cells, by inclusion of lesion-specific enzymes in the comet assay. *Alternatives to Laboratory Animals*, Vol. 24, (1996), pp. (405-411), 0261-1929.

Dusinska, M., Collins, A.R., Kazimirova, A., Barancokova, M., Harrington, V., Volkovova, K., Staruchova, M., Horska, A., Wsolova, L., & Kocan, A. (2004). Genotoxic effects of asbestos in humans, *Mutation Research*, Vol. 553, No. 1-2, (September 2004), pp. (91-102), 0027-5107

Gaivão, I., Piasek, A., Brevik, A., Shaposhnikov, S., & Collins, A.R. (2009). Comet assay-based methods for measuring DNA repair *in vitro*; estimates of inter- and intra-individual variation. *Cell Biology and Toxicology*, Vol. 25, No. 1, (February 2009), pp. (45-52), 0742-2091

Gedik, C.M., Ewen, S.W., & Collins, A.R. (1992). Single-cell gel electrophoresis applied to the analysis of UV-C damage and its repair in human cells. *International Journal of Radiation Biology*, Vol. 62, No. 3, (September 1992), pp. (313-320), 0955-3002

Green, M.H.L., Waugh, A.P.W., Lowe, J.E., Harcourt, S.A., Cole, J., & Arlett, C.F. (1994). Effect of deoxyribonucleosides on the hypersensitivity of human peripheral blood lymphocytes to UV-B and UV-C irradiation. *Mutation Research*, Vol. 315, No. 1, (July 1994), pp. (25-32), 0027-5107

Grover, P., Banus, B.S., Devi, K.D., & Begum, S. (2001). *In vivo* genotoxic effects of mercuric chloride in rat peripheral blood leucocytes using comet assay. *Toxicology*, Vol. 167, No. 3, (October 2001), pp. (191–197), 0300-483X

Gudkov, S.V., Gudkova, O.Y., Chernikov, A.V., & Bruskov, V.I. (2009). Protection of mice against X-ray injuries by the post-irradiation administration of guanosine and inosine. *International Journal of Radiation Biology*, Vol. 85, No. 2, (February 2009), pp. (116-125), 0955-3002

Henriksson, S., Shaposhnikov, S., Nilsson, M., & Collins, A.R. (2011). Study of gene-specific DNA repair in the comet assay with padlock probes and rolling circle amplification. *Toxicology Letters*, Vol. 202, No. 2, (April 2011), pp. (142-147), 0378-4274

Herrera, M., Dominguez, G., Garcia, J.M., Peña, C., Jimenez, C., Silva, J., Garcia, V., Gomez, I., Diaz, R., Martin, P., & Bonilla, F. (2009). Differences in repair of DNA cross-links between lymphocytes and epithelial tumor cells from colon cancer patients measured *in vitro* with the comet assay. *Clinical Cancer Research*, Vol. 15, No. 17, (September 2009), pp. (5466-5472), 1078-0432

Horvathova, E., Dusinska, M., Shaposhnikov, S., & Collins, A.R. (2004). DNA damage and repair measured in different genomic regions using the comet assay with fluorescent *in situ* hybridization. *Mutagenesis*, Vol. 19, No. 4, (July 2004), pp. (269-276), 0267-8357

Kumaravel, T.S., & Bristow, R.G. (2005). Detection of genetic instability at HER-2/neu and p53 loci in breast cancer cells using comet-FISH. *Breast Cancer Research and Treatment*, Vol. 91, No. 1, (May 2005), pp. (89-93), 0167-6806

Langie, S.A., Cameron, K.M., Waldron, K.J., Fletcher, K.P., von Zglinicki, T., & Mathers, J.C. (2011). Measuring DNA repair incision activity of mouse tissue extracts towards singlet oxygen-induced DNA damage: a comet-based *in vitro* repair assay. *Mutagenesis*, Vol. 26, No. 3, (May 2011), pp. (461-471), 0267-8357

Langie, S.A., Knaapen, A.M., Brauers, K.J.J., van Berlo, D., van Schooten, F.J., & Godschalk, R.W.L. (2006). Development and validation of a modified comet assay to phenotypically assess nucleotide excision repair. *Mutagenesis*, Vol. 21, No. 2, (March 2006), pp. (153-158), 0267-8357

Larsson, C., Koch, J., Nygren, A., Janssen, G., Raap, A. K., Landegren, U., & Nilsson, M. (2004). *In situ* genotyping individual DNA molecules by target-primed rolling-circle amplification of padlock probes. *Nature Methods*, Vol. 1, No. 3, (December 2004), pp. (227-232), 1548-7091

Lorenzo, Y., Azqueta, A., Luna, L., Bonilla, F., Dominguez, G., & Collins, A.R. (2009). The carotenoid β-cryptoxanthin stimulates the repair of DNA oxidation damage in addition to acting as an antioxidant in human cells. *Carcinogenesis*, Vol. 30, No. 2, (February 2009), pp. (308-314), 0143-3334

Maurya, D.K., Salvi, V.P., & Nair, C.K. (2005). Radiation protection of DNA by ferulic acid under *in vitro* and *in vivo* conditions. *Molecular and Cellular Biochemistry,* Vol. 280, No. 1-2, (December 2005), pp. (209-217), 0300-8177

McKenna, D.J., Rajab, N.F., McKeown, S.R., McKerr, G., & McKelvey-Martin, V.J. (2003). Use of the comet-FISH assay to demonstrate repair of the *TP53* gene region in two human bladder carcinoma cell lines. *Radiation Research,* Vol. 159, No. 1, (January 2003), pp. (49-56), 0033-7587

Miranda, D.D., Arçari, D.P., Pedrazzoli, J.Jr., Carvalho, O., Cerutti, S.M., Bastos, D.H., & Ribeiro, M.L. (2008). Protective effects of mate tea (*Ilex paraguariensis*) on H_2O_2-induced DNA damage and DNA repair in mice. *Mutagenesis,* Vol. 23, No. 4, (July 2008), pp. (261-265), 0267-8357

Oshida, K., Iwanaga, E., Miyamoto-Kuramitsu, K., & Miyamoto, Y. (2008). An *in vivo* comet assay of multiple organs (liver, kidney and bone marrow) in mice treated with methyl methanesulfonate and acetaminophen accompanied by hematology and/or blood chemistry. *The Journal of Toxicological Sciences,* Vol. 33, No. 5, (December 2008), pp. (515-524), 0388-1350

Ostling, O., & Johanson, K.J., (1984). Microelectrophoretic study of radiation-induced DNA damages in individual mammalian cells. *Biochemical and Biophysical Research Communications,* Vol. 123, No. 1, (August 1984), pp. (291-298), 0006-291X

Palyvoda, O., Polanska, J., Wygoda, A., & Rzeszowska-Wolny, J. (2003). DNA damage and repair in lymphocytes of normal individuals and cancer patients: studies by the comet assay and micronucleus tests. *Acta Biochimica Polonica,* Vol. 50, No. 1, (2003), pp. (181-190), 0001-527X

Ramos, A.A., Azqueta, A., Pereira-Wilson, C., & Collins A.R. (1010a). Polyphenolic compounds from Salvia species protect cellular DNA from oxidation and stimulate DNA repair in cultured human cells. *Journal of Agricultural and Food Chemistry,* Vol. 58, No. 12, (June 2010), pp. (7465-7471), 0021-8561

Ramos, A.A., Lima, C.F., Pereira, M.L., Fernandes-Ferreira, M., & Pereira-Wilson, C. (2008). Antigenotoxic effects of quercetin, rutin and ursolic acid on HepG2 cells: evaluation by the comet assay. *Toxicology Letters,* Vol. 177, No. 1, (February 2008), pp. (66–73), 0378-4274

Ramos, A.A., Pereira-Wilson, C., & Collins, A.R. (2010b). Protective effects of ursolic acid and luteolin against oxidative DNA damage include enhancement of DNA repair in Caco-2 cells. *Mutation Research,* Vol. 692, No. 1-2, (October 1010), pp. (6-11), 0027-5107

Saleha Banu, B., Ishaq, M., Danadevi, K., Padmavathi, P., & Ahuja, Y.R. (2004). DNA damage in leukocytes of mice treated with copper sulfate. *Food and Chemical Toxicology,* Vol. 42, No. 12, (December 2004), pp. (1931-1936), 0278-6915

Santos, S.J., Singh, N.P. & Natarajan, A.T. (1997). Fluorescence in situ hybridization with comets. *Experimental Cell Research,* Vol. 232, No. 2, (May 1997), pp. (407-411), 0014-4827

Shaposhnikov, S.A., Salenko, V.B., Brunborg, G., Nygren, J., & Collins, A.R. (2008). Single-cell gel electrophoresis (the comet assay): loops or fragments?. *Electrophoresis,* Vol. 29, No. 14, (July 2008), pp. (3005-3012), 0173-0835

Singh, N.P., McCoy, M.T., Tice, R.R., & Schneider, E.L. (1988). A simple technique for quantitation of low levels of DNA damage in individual cells. *Experimental Cell Research*, Vol. 175, No. 1, (March 1988), pp. (184-191), 0014-4827

Sliwinski, T., Czechowska, A., Szemraj, J., Morawiec, Z., Skorski, T., & Blasiak, J. (2008). STI571 reduces NER activity in BCR/ABL-expressing cells. *Mutation Research*, Vol. 654, No. 2, (July 2008), pp. (162-167), 0027-5107

Speit, G., Schütz, P., & Hoffmann, H. (2004). Enhancement of genotoxic effects in the comet assay with human blood samples by aphidicolin. *Toxicology Letters*, Vol. 153, No. 3, (November 2004), pp. (303-310), 0378-4274

Speit, G., Witton-Davies, T., Heepchantree, W., Trenz, K., & Hoffmann, H. (2003). Investigations on the effect of cigarette smoking in the comet assay. *Mutation Research*, Vol. 542, No. 1-2, (December 2003), pp. (33–42), 0027-5107

Squires, S., Johnson, R.T., & Collins, A.R. (1982). Initial rates of DNA incision in UV-irradiated human cells; differences between normal, xeroderma pigmentosum and tumour cells. *Mutation Research*, Vol. 95, No. 2-3, (August 1982), pp. (389-404), 0027-5107

Stefanini, M., Collins, A.R., Riboni, R., Klaude, M., Botta, E., Mitchell, D.L., & Nuzzo, F. (1991). Novel Chinese hamster ultraviolet-sensitive mutants for excision repair form complementation groups 9 and 10. *Cancer Research*, Vol. 51, No. 15, (August 1991), pp. (3965-3971), 008-5472

Tomasetti, M., Alleva, R., Borghi, B., & Collins, A.R. (2001). *In vivo* supplementation with coenzyme Q_{10} enhances the recovery of human lymphocytes from oxidative DNA damage. *The FASEB Journal*, Vol. 15, No. 8, (June 2001), pp. (1425-1427), 0892-6638

Torbergsen, A.C., & Collins, A.R. (2000). Recovery of human lymphocytes from oxidative DNA damage; the apparent enhancement of DNA repair by carotenoids is probably simply an antioxidant effect. *European Journal of Nutrition*, Vol 39, No. 2, (April 2000), pp. (80-85), 1436-6207

Touil, N., Aka, P.V., Buchet, J.P., Thierens, H., & Kirsch-Volders, M. (2002). Assessment of genotoxic effects related to chronic low level exposure to ionizing radiation using biomarkers for DNA damage and repair. *Mutagenesis*, Vol. 17, No. 3, (May 2002), pp. (223-232), 0267-8357

Tsai-Hsiu, Y., Nae-Cherng, Y., & Miao-Lin, H. (2003). S-adenosylhomocysteine enhances hydrogen peroxide-induced DNA damage by inhibition of DNA repair in two cell lines. *Nutrition and Cancer*, Vol. 47, No. 1, (2003), pp. (70-75), 0163-5581

Vande Loock, K., Decordier, I., Ciardelli, R., Haumont, D., & Kirsch-Volders, M. (2010). An aphidicolin-block nucleotide excision repair assay measuring DNA incision and repair capacity. *Mutagenesis*, Vol. 25, No. 1, (January 2010), pp. (25-32), 0267-8357

Vodicka, P., Kumar, R., Stetina, R., Musak, L., Soucek, P., Haufroid, V., Sasiadek, M., Vodickova, L., Naccarati, A., Sedikova, J., Sanyal, S., Kuricova, M., Brsiak, V., Norppa, H., Buchanova, J., & Hemminki, K. (2004b). Markers of individual susceptibility and DNA repair rate in workers exposed to xenobiotics in a tire plant. *Environmental and Molecular Mutagenesis*, Vol. 44, No. 4, (2004), pp. (283-292), 0893-6692

Vodicka, P., Tuimala, J., Stetina, R., Kumar, R., Manini, P., Naccarati, A., Maestri, L., Vodickova, L., Kuricova, M., Jarventaus, H., Majvaldova, Z., Hirvonen, A., Imbriani, M., Mutti, A., Migliore, L., Norppa, H., & Hemminki, K. (2004a).

Cytogenetic markers, DNA single-strand breaks, urinary metabolites, and DNA repair rates in styrene-exposed lamination workers. *Environmental Health Perspectives,* Vol. 112, No. 8, (June 2004), pp. (867-871), 0091-6765

Zhang, T., Hu, J., Zhang, Y., Zhao, Q., & Ning, J. Leucocytes DNA damage in mice exposed to JS-118 by the comet assay. *Human & Experimental Toxicology*. DOI:10.1177/ 0960327110388960

Zhao, X.H., Jia, G., Liu, Y.Q., Liu, S.W., Yan, L., Jin, Y., & Liu, N. (2006). Association between polymorphisms of DNA repair gene XRCC1 and DNA damage in asbestos-exposed workers. *Biomedical and Environmental Sciences*, Vol. 19, No. 3, (June 2006), pp. (232-238), 0895-3988